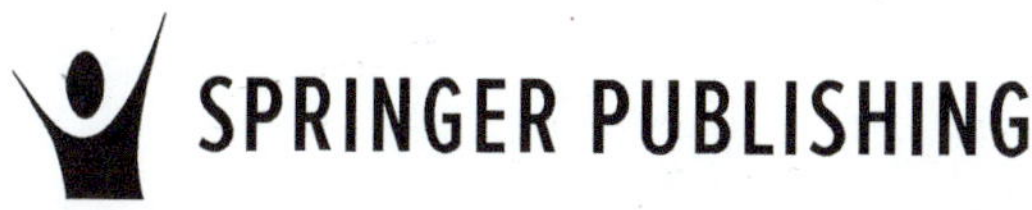

GET THE MOST FROM YOUR BOOK

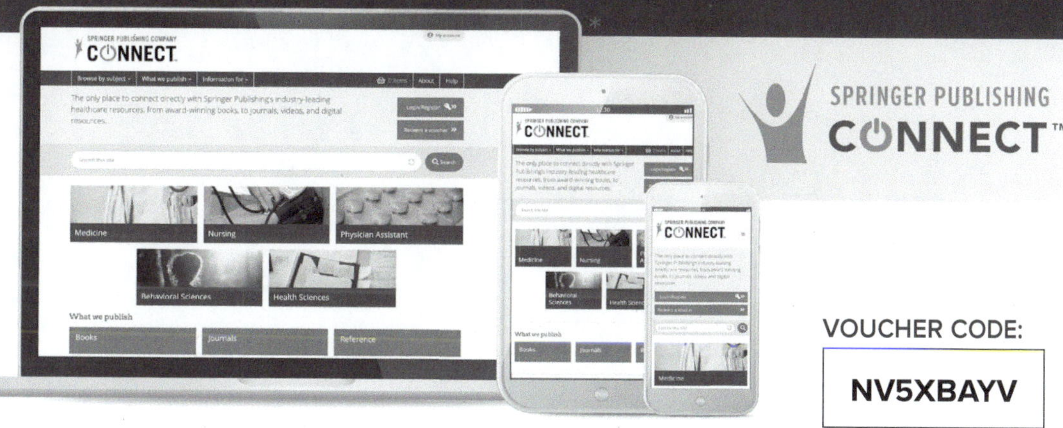

VOUCHER CODE:

NV5XBAYV

Online Access

Your print purchase of *Fetal and Neonatal Pharmacology for the Advanced Practice Nurse*, includes **online access via Springer Publishing Connect**™ to increase accessibility, portability, and searchability.

Insert the code at http://connect.springerpub.com/content/book/978-0-8261-5884-0 today!

Having trouble? Contact our customer service department at cs@springerpub.com

Instructor Resource Access for Adopters

Let us do some of the heavy lifting to create an engaging classroom experience with a variety of instructor resources included in most textbooks SUCH AS:

INSTRUCTOR MANUAL

POWERPOINTS

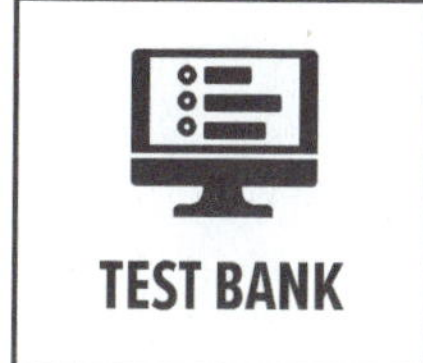

TEST BANK

Visit **https://connect.springerpub.com/** and look for the **"Show Supplementary"** button on your **book homepage** to see what is available to instructors! First time using Springer Publishing Connect?

Email **textbook@springerpub.com** to create an account and start unlocking valuable resources.

Fetal and Neonatal Pharmacology for the Advanced Practice Nurse

Amy J. Jnah, DNP, APRN, NNP-BC, is a veteran of the U.S. Navy Nurse Corps, an alumna of the Marquette University College of Nursing (BSN), East Carolina University College of Nursing (MSN), and University of Alabama at Birmingham (DNP). Dr. Jnah is currently an associate professor and director of the neonatal nurse practitioner program at the East Carolina University College of Nursing. She also serves as an assistant professor (adjunct) at the University of North Carolina at Chapel Hill School of Medicine. Her clinical interests include hyperbilirubinemia, neonatal resuscitation, the transition to extrauterine life, and issues that affect late-preterm infants. Dr. Jnah is a master trainer for the American Academy of Pediatrics Helping Babies Breathe program and an instructor-mentor for the Neonatal Resuscitation Program. Her academic interests include mentoring, role modeling, and the integration of multisensory teaching innovations within distance education. Dr. Jnah has received numerous awards and honors, which include the Reserve Officer Training Corps academic scholarship (1994–1998), distinguished graduate of the East Carolina University neonatal nurse practitioner program (2007–2008), and East Carolina University Scholar-Teacher of the Year (2017–2018). She is an active member of the National Association of Neonatal Nurses, the National Association of Neonatal Nurse Practitioners, and the Academy of Neonatal Nursing, as well as the Carolinas Association of Neonatal Nurse Practitioners.

Christopher McPherson, PharmD, BCPPS, graduated from the University of North Carolina School of Pharmacy and completed a fellowship in Neonatal Pharmacotherapy at The Women's Hospital of Greensboro. He is currently a clinical pharmacist in the neonatal intensive care unit at St. Louis Children's Hospital and an associate professor at the Department of Pediatrics at Washington University School of Medicine.

Fetal and Neonatal Pharmacology for the Advanced Practice Nurse

Amy J. Jnah, DNP, APRN, NNP-BC
Christopher McPherson, PharmD, BCPPS

Editors

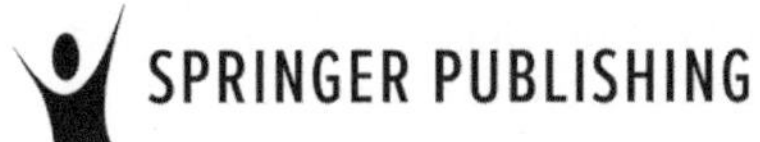

Springer Publishing Company, LLC
11 West 42nd Street, New York, NY 10036
www.springerpub.com
connect.springerpub.com/

Acquisitions Editor: Joseph Morita
Senior Content Development Editor: Lucia Gunzel
Compositor: Amnet

ISBN: 978-0-8261-5883-3
ebook ISBN: 978-0-8261-5884-0
DOI: 10.1891/9780826158840

SUPPLEMENTS:

Test Bank ISBN: 978-0-8261-5885-7

23 24 25 26 27 / 5 4 3 2 1

Medicine is an ever-changing science. Research and clinical experience are continually expanding our knowledge, in particular our understanding of proper treatment and drug therapy. The authors, editors, and publisher have made every effort to ensure that all information in this book is in accordance with the state of knowledge at the time of production of the book. Nevertheless, the authors, editors, and publisher are not responsible for any errors or omissions or for any consequence from application of the information in this book and make no warranty, expressed or implied, with respect to the content of this publication. Every reader should examine carefully the package inserts accompanying each drug and should carefully check whether the dosage schedules therein or the contraindications stated by the manufacturer differ from the statements made in this book. Such examination is particularly important with drugs that are either rarely used or have been newly released on the market.

Library of Congress Cataloging-in-Publication Data
Names: Jnah, Amy J., author, editor. | McPherson, Christopher, author, editor.
Title: Fetal and neonatal pharmacology for the advanced practice nurse / Amy J. Jnah, Christopher McPherson.
Description: First edition. | New York, NY : Springer Publishing Company, LLC, [2024] | Includes bibliographical references and index.
Identifiers: LCCN 2022049416 (print) | LCCN 2022049417 (ebook) | ISBN 9780826158833 (paperback) | ISBN 9780826158840 (ebook) | ISBN 9780826158857 (Test Bank)
Subjects: MESH: Infant, Newborn, Diseases--drug therapy | Fetal Diseases--drug therapy | Pharmaceutical Preparations | Pharmacological Phenomena | Nurses Instruction
Classification: LCC RG627 (print) | LCC RG627 (ebook) | NLM WS 421 | DDC 618.3/206--dc23/eng/20230124
LC record available at https://lccn.loc.gov/2022049416
LC ebook record available at https://lccn.loc.gov/2022049417

Amy J. Jnah: 0000-0002-3798-6470

Publisher's Note: **New and used products purchased from third-party sellers are not guaranteed for quality, authenticity, or access to any included digital components.**

Printed in the United States of America by Gasch printing.

Contents

Contributors

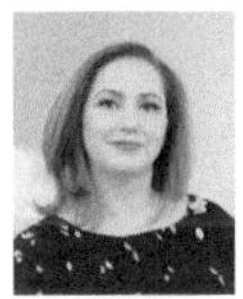

Jodi Amador, DNP, APRN, NNP-BC
Atrium Health, Charlotte, North Carolina; Rady Children's Hospital, San Diego, California; Adjunct Faculty, University of South Alabama, Mobile, Alabama; Catawba Valley Medical Center, Hickory, North Carolina

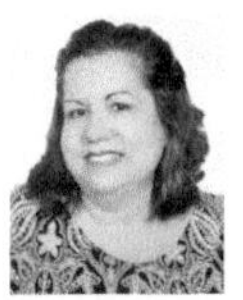

Valarie A. Artigas, DNP, APRN, NNP-BC
Assistant Clinical Professor, University of Connecticut, Neonatal Nurse Practitioner Program, Storrs, Connecticut

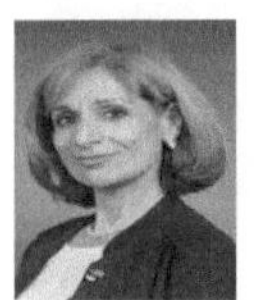

Mehran Nesari Asdigha, PharmD
Clinical Pharmacy Specialist, Neonatal Intensive Care, UMass Memorial Health Care, Worcester, Massachusetts; Adjunct Assistant Clinical Professor, Bouve College of Health Sciences, Northeastern University, Boston, Massachusetts; Adjunct Assistant Professor, Massachusetts College of Pharmacy, Boston, Massachusetts; Medical Advisory Board Member, Mother's Milk Bank of New England, Newton, Massachusetts

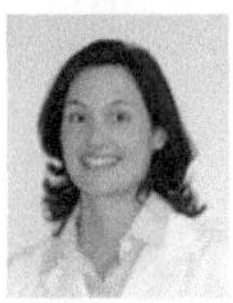

Teresa Baker, MD
Professor, Department of Obstetrics and Gynecology, InfantRisk Center of Excellence, Texas Tech University Health Sciences Center, Amarillo, Texas

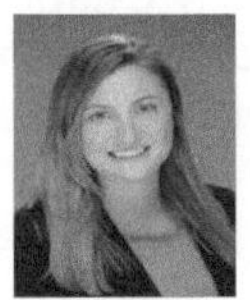

Jennifer Barnes, PharmD, BCPPS
Clinical Pharmacy Specialist, Neonatal-Perinatal Medicine, Atrium Health Levine Children's Hospital, Charlotte, North Carolina

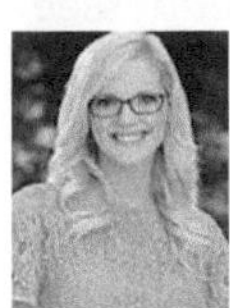

Kelley Baumgartel, PhD, RN
Assistant Professor, College of Nursing, University of South Florida, Tampa, Florida

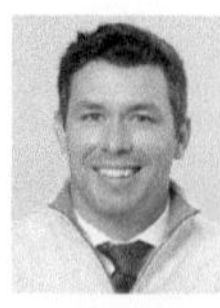

Alexander Berwick, DO, FAAP
Neonatologist, Children's Hospital at Erlanger, Chattanooga, Tennessee

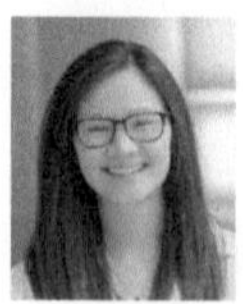

Deborah S. Bondi, PharmD, FCCP, BCPS, BCPPS
Pediatric Clinical Coordinator and NICU Clinical Pharmacy Specialist, Department of Pharmacy, University of Chicago Medicine, Comer Children's Hospital, Chicago, Illinois

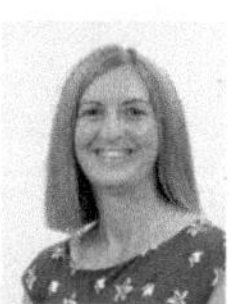

Amy L. Brown, PharmD, BCPS, BCPPS
Pediatric Clinical Pharmacist—Neonatology, UNC Medical Center Department of Pharmacy; Assistant Professor of Clinical Education, UNC Eshelman School of Pharmacy, Chapel Hill, North Carolina

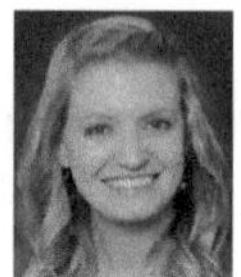

Meredith Chanas, PharmD, MSCR, BCPPS
Clinical Pharmacy Specialist—Pediatrics, Vidant Medical Center, Greenville, North Carolina

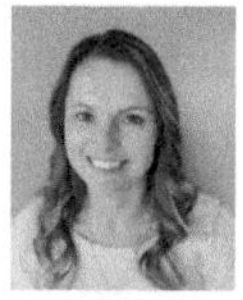

Lisa Clevenger, MSN, APRN, NNP-BC
Neonatal Intensive Care Unit, Atrium Health Levine Children's Hospital, Charlotte, North Carolina; Adjunct Assistant Professor, East Carolina University, Greenville, North Carolina

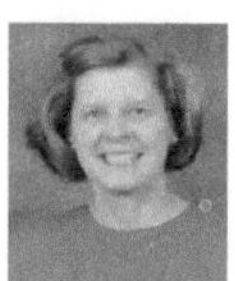

Robin Webb Corbett, PhD, RNC, FNP-C
Associate Professor, Chair—Advanced Nursing Practice and Education, East Carolina College of Nursing, Greenville, North Carolina

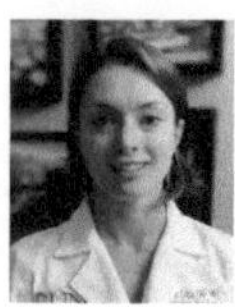

Sarah Croop, DNP, APRN, NNP-BC
Neonatal Nurse Practitioner, UNC Health, Newborn Critical Care Center, Chapel Hill, North Carolina; Adjunct Assistant Professor, Department of Pediatrics, Division of Neonatal-Perinatal Medicine, University of North Carolina at Chapel Hill, Chapel Hill, North Carolina

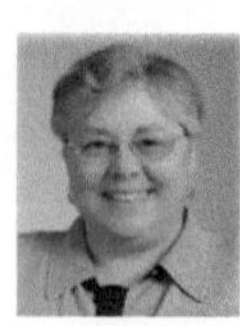

Karen D'Apolito, PhD, NNP-BC, FAAN
Professor Emeritus, School of Nursing, Vanderbilt University, Nashville, Tennessee

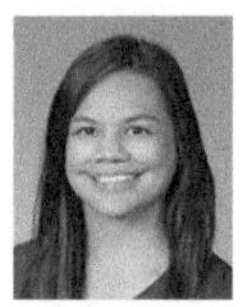

Erica Davenport, DO
Neonatologist, WellSpan Neonatology, York, Pennsylvania

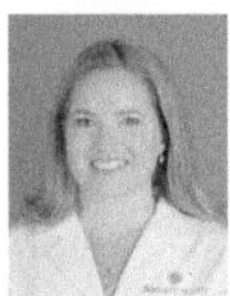

Patricia L. Dias, MD
Neonatologist, Neonatal-Perinatal Medicine, Atrium Health Levine Children's Hospital, Charlotte, North Carolina

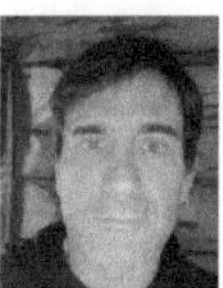

William Diehl-Jones, PhD, RN, MSc, BScN
Associate Professor, Faculty of Health Disciplines, Athabasca University, Athabasca, Alberta, Canada

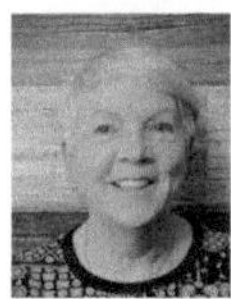

Debbie Fraser, MN, NNP, CNeoN(C), FCAN
St. Boniface Hospital, Winnipeg, Manitoba, Canada; Athabasca University, Athabasca, Alberta, Canada

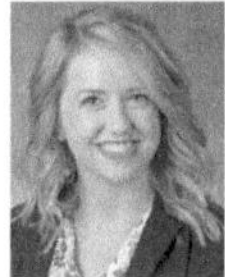

Allison Jones Guider, PharmD, BCPPS
Field Medical Director, Rare Neurology, Pfizer, Inc., Knoxville, Tennessee

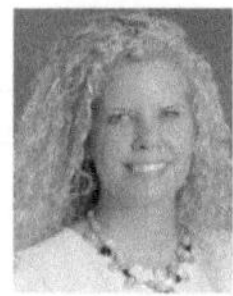

Tiffany Gwartney, DNP, APRN, NNP-BC
Associate Professor, School of Nursing, University of Connecticut, Storrs, Connecticut; Neonatal Nurse Practitioner, Neonatal Intensive Care, Nemours Children's Health System, Orlando, Florida; Neonatal Nurse Practitioner, Neonatal Intensive Care, Johns Hopkins All Children's Hospital, St. Petersburg, Florida

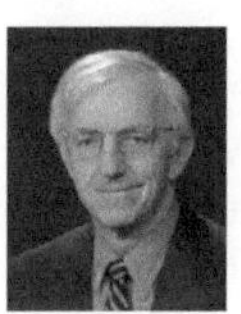

Thomas W. Hale, PhD
Professor, Department of Pediatrics, InfantRisk Center, Texas Tech University Health Sciences Center, Amarillo, Texas

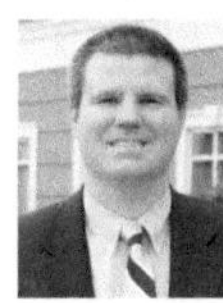

John Brock Harris, PharmD, BCPS, BCPPS, FCCP
Assistant Dean of Assessment and Accreditation, Associate Professor of Pharmacy, Wingate University School of Pharmacy, Wingate, North Carolina

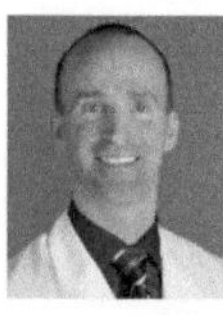

Andrew Heling, MD
Neonatologist, Assistant Professor, Pediatrics Department, Atrium Health, Charlotte, North Carolina

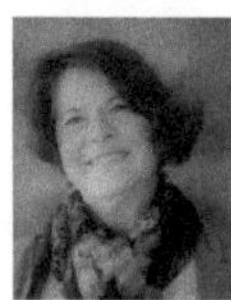

Carolyn J. Herrington, PhD, RN, NNP-BC
Adjunct Faculty, Wayne State University, College of Nursing, Detroit, Michigan

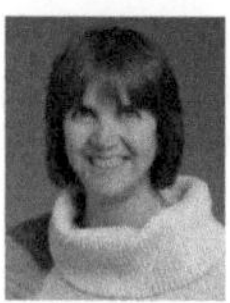

Jacqui Hoffman, DNP, ARNP, NNP-BC
Assistant Professor, Neonatal Nurse Practitioner, Doctor of Nursing Practice Program, Department of Women, Children and Family Nursing, Rush University College of Nursing, Chicago, Illinois

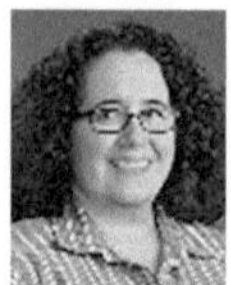

Amy P. Holmes, PharmD, BCPPS, FPPA
Neonatal Intensive Care Unit Staff Pharmacist, Department of Pharmacy, Atrium Health Wake Forest Baptist, Winston-Salem, North Carolina

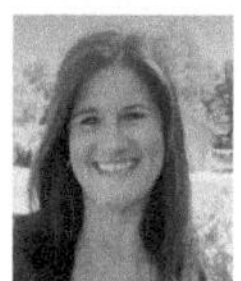

Mary Hurley, DNP, APRN, NNP-BC
Neonatal Nurse Practitioner, Department of Pediatrics, University of Chicago Medicine, Comer Children's Hospital, Chicago, Illinois

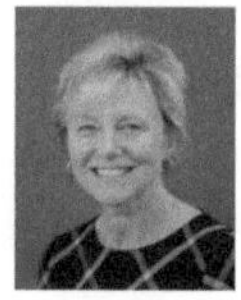

Jane Ierardi, MD, MBA, FAAP, CPE
Neonatologist, Neonatal Intensive Care Unit, Nemours Children's Health System, Orlando, Florida; Chief Partnership Office for Florida and Interim Chief, Division of Neonatology, Nemours Children's Health System, Orlando, Florida; Associate Professor of Pediatrics, College of Medicine, University of Central Florida, Orlando, Florida; Associate Professor of Pediatrics, Sidney Kimmel School of Medicine, Thomas Jefferson University, Philadelphia, Pennsylvania

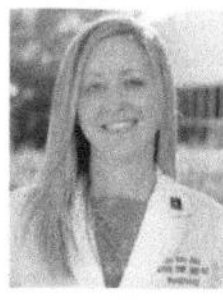

Amy J. Jnah, DNP, APRN, NNP-BC
Associate Professor, East Carolina University, Greenville, North Carolina; Neonatal Nurse Practitioner, UNC Health, Newborn Critical Care Center, Chapel Hill, North Carolina

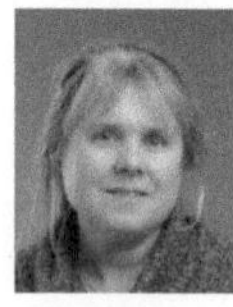

Denise Kirsten, DNP, APRN, NNP-BC
Assistant Professor, Department of Women, Children and Family Nursing, Rush University College of Nursing, Chicago, Illinois

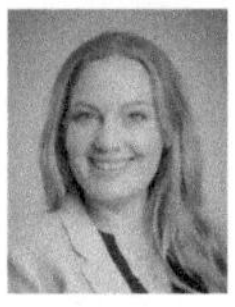

Kaytlin Krutsch, PharmD, MBA
Assistant Professor, Department of Obstetrics and Gynecology, InfantRisk Center of Excellence, Texas Tech University Health Sciences Center, Amarillo, Texas

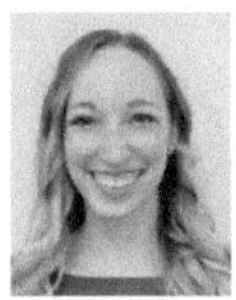

Macrina Liguori, MD, FAAP
Fellow, Neonatology, UNC Health, Newborn Critical Care Center, Chapel Hill, North Carolina

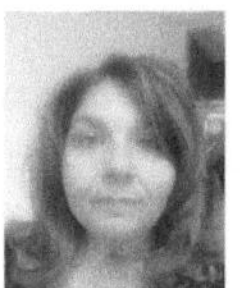

Mirjana Lulic-Botica, PharmD, BCPS
Neonatal Clinical Pharmacy Specialist, Hutzel Women's Hospital, Detroit Medical Center, Detroit, Michigan; Assistant Professor, Wayne State University, College of Nursing, Detroit, Michigan; Adjunct Assistant Professor, Wayne State University, College of Pharmacy, Detroit, Michigan

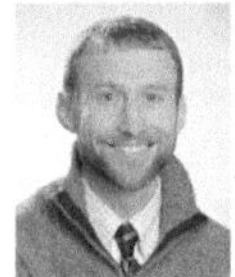

Christopher McPherson, PharmD, BCPPS
Clinical Pharmacy Specialist, Neonatal Intensive Care Unit, St. Louis Children's Hospital, St. Louis, Missouri; Associate Professor, Department of Pediatrics, Washington University School of Medicine, St. Louis, Missouri

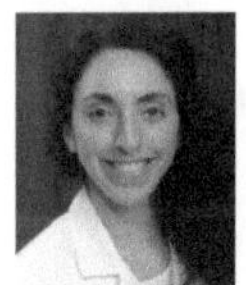

Stephanie Merlino Barr, MS, RDN, LD
Neonatal Dietitian, Department of Pediatrics, MetroHealth Medical Center, Cleveland, Ohio

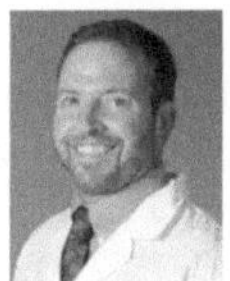

Ryan Moore, MD
Division Chief, Neonatal Intensive Care Unit, East Carolina University/James and Connie Maynard Children's Hospital, Greenville, North Carolina

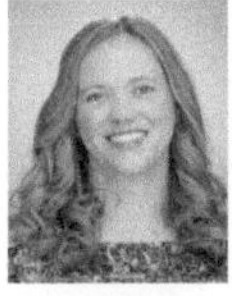

Colleen Moss, DNP, APRN, NNP-BC
Assistant Professor and Director, Neonatal Nurse Practitioner Specialty, Vanderbilt University School of Nursing, Nashville, Tennessee; Neonatal Nurse Practitioner, Monroe Carell Jr. Children's Hospital at Vanderbilt, Nashville, Tennessee

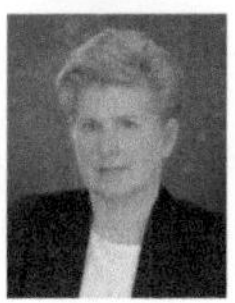

Leanne Nantais-Smith, PhD, RN, NNP-BC
Associate Clinical Professor, Wayne State University, College of Nursing, Detroit, Michigan

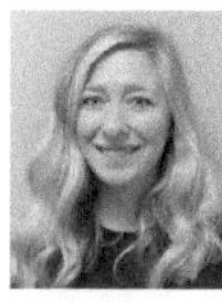

Keliana O'Mara, PharmD, BCPPS
Staff Pharmacist, Neonatal Intensive Care Unit, WakeMed Health and Hospitals, Raleigh, North Carolina

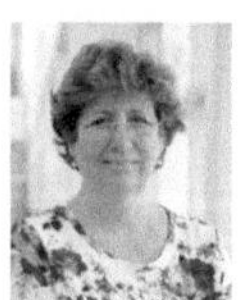

Stephanie M. Prescott, PhD, MSN, APRN, NNP-BC
Assistant Professor, University of South Florida College of Nursing, Tampa, Florida; Neonatal Nurse Practitioner, Fairfax Neonatal Associates PC, Fairfax, Virginia

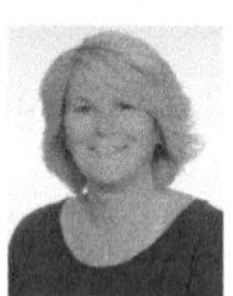

Tracy Rickard, MSN, APRN, NNP-BC
Clinical Instructor, Neonatal Nurse Practitioner Program, East Carolina University College of Nursing, Greenville, North Carolina; Neonatal Nurse Practitioner Coordinator, Neonatal Nurse Practitioner, Fairfax Neonatal Associates PC, Fairfax, Virginia

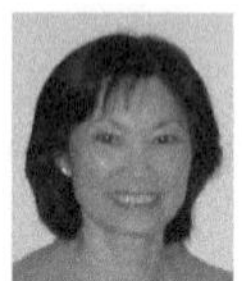

Elizabeth Sharpe, DNP, APRN, NNP-BC, VA-BC, FAANP, FAAN
Associate Professor Clinical Nursing, Neonatal Nurse Practitioner Specialty Track Director, The Ohio State University, Columbus, Ohio

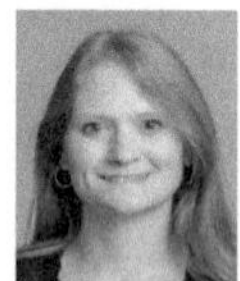

Carrie Smith, MS, RD, CSP, LD
Registered Dietitian, Cincinnati Children's Hospital Medical Center, Cincinnati, Ohio

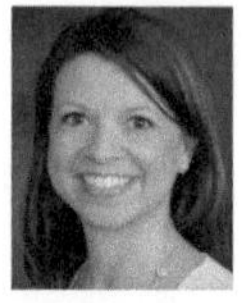

April Smithwick, MSN, APRN, NNP-BC
Neonatal Nurse Practitioner, UNC Health, Newborn Critical Care Center, Chapel Hill, North Carolina

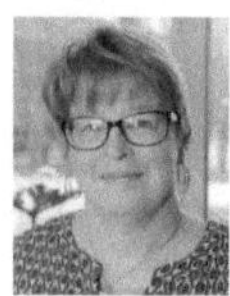

Renee Oakley Spain, MAEd, DNP, CNM
Clinical Assistant Professor, Department of Advanced Nursing Practice and Education, College of Nursing, East Carolina University, Greenville, North Carolina

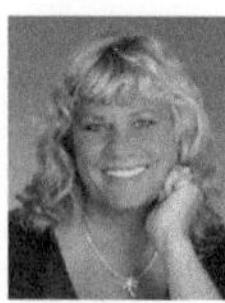

Diane L. Spatz, PhD, RN-BC, FAAN
Professor of Perinatal Nursing and the Helen M. Shearer Professor of Nutrition, Family and Community Health Department, University of Pennsylvania School of Nursing, Philadelphia, Pennsylvania; Nurse Scientist—Lactation, Center for Pediatric Nursing Research & Evidence-Based Practice, Children's Hospital of Philadelphia, Philadelphia, Pennsylvania

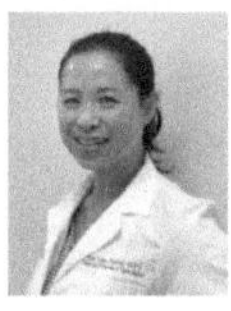

Van Tran, PharmD, BCPS, BCPPS, MBA
Clinical Pharmacy Specialist, Department of Pharmacy, L.J. Murphy's Inova Children's Hospital, Falls Church, Virginia

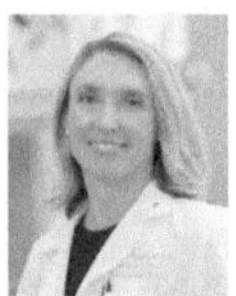

Andrea N. Trembath, MD, MPH, FAAP
Professor of Pediatrics, Neonatologist, University of North Carolina at Chapel Hill, Chapel Hill, North Carolina

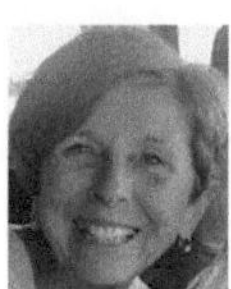

Mary Whalen, DNP, APRN, NNP-BC
Associate Professor, University of Connecticut, Storrs, Connecticut; Clinical Instructor, Department of Pediatrics, University of Massachusetts Medical School, Worcester, Massachusetts; Neonatal Nurse Practitioner, UMass Memorial Health Care, Worcester, Massachusetts

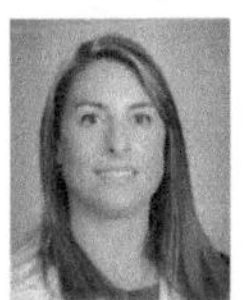

Amy Williford, MSN, APRN, NNP-BC
Assistant Professor, College of Nursing, East Carolina University Greenville, North Carolina; Neonatal Nurse Practitioner, Vidant Medical Center, Greenville, North Carolina

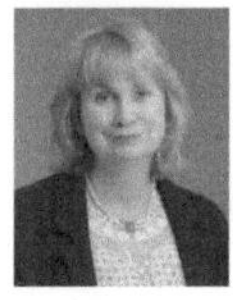

Karen Wright, PhD, APRN, NNP-BC
Assistant Professor and Director, Department of Women, Children and Family Nursing, Rush University College of Nursing, Chicago, Illinois

Foreword

APRNs are an influential and growing force in healthcare around the globe. APRNs include certified nurse midwives, certified registered nurse anesthetists, certified clinical nurse specialists, and certified nurse practitioners, such as pediatric nurse practitioners (PNPs) and neonatal nurse practitioners (NNPs). PNPs and NNPs play a significant role in caring for neonates and infants requiring intensive care due to critical or severe conditions until they reach a certain age. In any case, APRNs cannot provide optimal care by working in silos; they must collaborate with intra- and interprofessional colleagues to achieve the best possible patient and population health outcomes.

APRNs play a crucial role in leading interprofessional teams, overseeing patient care, and generating synergy to promote efficient, safe, and high-quality patient care. This book is a rare find for APRNs, especially PNPs and NNPs, and provides excellent APRN collaboration instances in everyday clinical and academic settings. The chapters are written by interprofessional healthcare providers, such as NNPs and PharmDs, and provide information and practice guidelines from a collaborative perspective. Each chapter contains artwork and concept maps of key content, offering readers the means to turn the written content into easy-to-understand, practical cues. This will appeal to visual and tactile learners, encouraging students to engage with the material and demonstrate cognitively active learning behaviors.

The book includes 10 parts and 31 chapters. The 10 parts are: Part I, Basic Principles of Fetal and Neonatal Pharmacology; Part II, Common Central Nervous System Problems; Part III, Common Respiratory Problems; Part IV, Common Cardiovascular Problems; Part V, Common Gastrointestinal Problems; Part VI, Common Hematopoietic and Endocrine Problems; Part VII, Common Infectious Disease Problems; Part VIII, Common Ocular Problems; Part IX, Special Circumstances; and Part X, Appendix.

The key features of each chapter include

- **Mind Maps,** which provide visual and tactile learners with tools to engage and demonstrate active learning;
- **clear, concise descriptions** of the fetal and neonatal pharmacology principles that include answers to essential questions for students transitioning to advanced practice roles;
- **Learning Objectives and Discussion Prompts** to guide learning activities for faculty and students;
- **a medication reference** which presents a table with about 100 of the most common medications prescribed in the NICU for quick reference in the academic and clinical arenas; and
- **advanced knowledge for APRNs** that explores the genesis, evolution, and current knowledge surrounding pharmacologic therapies to treat common problems afflicting preterm and critically ill neonates.

The setup of the book mimics real-world situations and offers graduate APRN students in neonatal and pediatric courses insight into the core pharmacologic concepts in a logical, systematic fashion. The text introduces the core concepts and discusses perinatal and intrapartum pharmacologic therapies and their implication on fetuses and neonates. The book also explores important topics such as postnatal concepts, including human milk, maternal drug addiction, and pharmacologic medications commonly used in the newborn nursery. This book covers the core curricular content that meets the accreditation requirements for MSN and DNP programs offering the 3P courses (physical assessment, physiology/pathophysiology, and pharmacology) to neonatal and pediatric nurse practitioner students, clinical nurse specialist students, and midwifery students. It is an excellent resource and hands-on guide for graduate APRN students.

The editors of the book, Dr. Amy J. Jnah, the director of the neonatal nurse practitioner concentration at the East Carolina University College of Nursing, and Dr. Christopher McPherson, a PharmD and clinical pharmacist at the Department of Pediatrics at Washington University School of Medicine in St. Louis, purposefully designed and organized the book following the principles and guidelines of interprofessional collaboration. They partnered together, simulating the interprofessional unity found in pediatric intensive care units and NICUs in real-world situations, to avoid perpetuating a model in which APRNs practice in silos.

As indicated in the convergent care theory (Wei, 2022), achieving the best optimal health outcomes requires all stakeholders' combined efforts. The four domains of the convergent care theory are all-inclusive organizational care, effective interprofessional collaborative care, person-centered precision patient care, and patients' and clinicians' self-care. The underlying foundation for effective collaboration of all stakeholders is a caring culture that promotes human connection among healthcare team members. Effective partnerships among healthcare professionals can be nurtured and fostered through seven processes: developing shared goals and values, building trusting and caring relationships, sharing resources, increasing an ownership mentality through involvement, providing constructive feedback by using effective communication skills, applying the strengths-based practice appreciating one another's contributions, and taking responsibility and accountability. Facilitating interprofessional collaboration is one of the essentials of doctoral education for advanced nursing practice and the underpinning principle of *Fetal and Neonatal Pharmacology for the Advanced Practice Nurse.*

This book provides an excellent example of the integration of theory into practice and doctoral education. This theory-based approach to doctoral education meets the new American Association of Colleges of Nursing Essentials, which endorse integrating theories into nursing education and practice both at the entry and doctoral levels. The purpose of healthcare clinicians' convergent and collaborative care is to promote interprofessional care and unity, not competition or division. Learning to collaborate is a "must-have" not a "good-to-have" practice principle in healthcare. This book is highly recommended for all clinicians and APRN students, especially pediatric and neonatal graduate students.

Holly Wei, PhD, RN, CPN, NEA-BC, FAAN
Professor
Assistant Dean for the PhD Program
University of Louisville School of Nursing
Louisville, Kentucky

REFERENCE

Wei, H. (2022). The development of an evidence-informed convergent care theory: Working together to achieve optimal health outcomes. *International Journal of Nursing Science*, *9*(1), 11–25. https://www.sciencedirect.com/science/article/pii/S2352013221001216

Preface

Dear neonatal nurse practitioner students,

You are more than likely a neonatal nurse and quite possibly a neonatal nurse practitioner (NNP) student. Therefore, I probably do not need to tell you that there is no better career in healthcare than neonatal nursing. We are trusted and respected professionals, yet we approach each shift with the mind-set that trust is earned, not given. We genuinely partner with families of critically ill infants and, in doing so, help parents and guardians through some of their darkest days. We accept challenges as opportunities, not inconveniences. We care deeply—about our babies, their family members, and our colleagues.

You might agree that the NICU is, more often than not, an unrelenting environment. The unexpected *is* expected and silence is unnerving at best. As a result, we are always prepared to respond to an emergency at a moment's notice. For every plan "A," there also is a plan "B" and "C" (because triplets *are* a thing, you know). Every code team has a backup. Every nurse has another to lean on, ask questions of, or assist in their time of need. The same is true for the NNPs, neonatologists, dietitians, and pharmacists. The NICU is its own unique melting pot of expertise, and *every expert is valued*. You see, I believe that we do our best work in teams, not in silos. Retired Admiral William H. McRaven said, "For the boat to make it to its destination, everyone must paddle… to truly get from your starting point to your destination takes friends, colleagues, the good will of strangers, and a strong coxswain to guide them. If you want to change the world, find someone to help you paddle" (The University of Texas at Austin, 2014).

Fortunately, the NICU is a team-based environment (Admiral McRaven would surely be proud of this). It is also a mecca for NNP students, medical students, residents, fellows, and allied health interns. Experts (nurses, neonatologists, NNPs, pharmacists, dietitians) can be found in hallways, corridors, patient rooms, and staff workrooms. Help is never far away and that is reassuring for students. The same should hold true in the academic setting. You should never learn in a silo. Faculty engagements (e.g., routine, live teaching lectures) are crucial, as they stir intellectual curiosity and facilitate learning. When you have the opportunity to get to know your faculty (and they get to know you), trusting relationships form, your self-efficacy and self-confidence increase, and your role transition from bedside nurse to novice NNP begins.

Readers, we (the authors and editors) want to help support your role transition. In doing so, we are counting on you to demonstrate accountability to your learning outcomes. Resist complacency; no clinician is entitled to defer swaths of knowledge to preceptors or colleagues. Rather, constantly question the state of the science, both in the classroom and in the clinical setting. Seek answers to your questions, and clarify your understanding with a trusted faculty member or preceptor. Do not stop there! Also consider the principle of self-directed mastery through repetition. As the daughter of a Montessori teacher (thanks, Mom!) and parent to two Montessori-educated young adults, I know that self-directed learning and repetitious practice works—with children and adults. This encourages mastery and enhances your ability to retrieve (remember) information in high-stress situations (e.g., during an exam, advanced neonatal resuscitation, or while standing in front of a perceivably intimidating expert during patient rounds).

You will notice that the chapters in this book were deliberately written by teams of experts. Therefore, the content reflects a synergy of perspective from nurses, physicians, pharmacists, and dietitians. No chapter reflects a siloed perspective, just as no clinician in a NICU practices in a silo.

I am forever grateful to my colleagues who authored the chapters and who provided behind-the-scenes support (Dr. Marc Collin, thank you for your help!). Collectively, we succeeded in filling the largest chasm in NNP education, as this book is the *first* fetal/neonatal pharmacology textbook published specifically for graduate-level NNP students. This was no small undertaking. But then again, *good things come to those who work hard and never give up.*

Students, *thank you* for choosing neonatal nursing as your profession and *thank you* for embracing the challenges embedded within graduate studies. Your hard work will pay great dividends and faster than you think. I hope to meet you, either in my online classroom or at a professional conference in the near future!

All my best,

Amy J. Jnah

P.S. For those of you who would benefit from a short "primer" before diving into the content contained within this book, please read on.

CORE TERMS AND DEFINITIONS

Before progressing to the major chapters in this textbook, it may help to refresh your understanding of the core pharmacologic terms listed herein. Be assured that all contributors made a concerted effort to clarify unique or complex terms through the use of parentheticals. In reviewing this material, you may not have to pause, interrupt your thought process, and seek clarification from other sources. However, should you stumble upon an unfamiliar term, I encourage you to engage in the process of "word anatomy." Break the term apart into its prefix, root or combining form, and suffix. Then, define each word part and put those definitions together. This tends to yield a long-lasting understanding of the term. In fact, repetitious use of this method leads to efficient decoding, saving you time in the long run.

Example: **Intravenous**
Intra / ven / ous
Intra (prefix)—defined as *within*
ven/o (combining form)—defined as *vein*
ous (suffix)—defined as *pertaining to*

Pharmacology is defined as the scientific study of drugs, their sources, biochemical actions, and uses. *Pharmaco-* refers to chemicals that exert an effect on the body and *-ology* refers to the study of something, which in this case is drugs. Pharmacology is divided into several subdisciplines.

Pharmacy, the first and probably most well-known subdiscipline of pharmacology, focuses on the preparation and dispensing of drugs. Given that there are thousands of drugs used to treat individuals of all ages, most hospitals assign pharmacists to a specific population of focus. This gives pharmacists margin to maintain awareness of the most common drugs used to treat that subpopulation, as well as participate in research, quality improvement, or other scholarly projects. Most U.S. NICUs are staffed with at least one pediatric pharmacist for this very reason. Pediatric pharmacists are an integral part of the NICU cross-disciplinary team.

Pharmacokinetics, the second subdivision of pharmacology, focuses on the movement of a drug throughout the body. *Pharmaco-* is defined as the study of drugs. *Kinetics* is defined as effects of forces on the motions of material bodies or with changes in a physical or chemical system. Therefore, *pharmacokinetics* refers to the study of the movement of a drug throughout the body. This is divided into four phases (absorption, distribution, metabolism, and excretion).

Pharmacodynamics, the third subdivision of pharmacology, involves the analysis of the mechanism of action of a drug and associated physiologic effect(s). For example, some drugs inhibit enzymes, whereas others interact with receptors as agonists or antagonists. These concepts are investigated in more detail in Chapter 3, "Pharmacokinetics and Pharmacodynamics."

The final two subdisciplines of pharmacology are **toxicology** and **pharmacognosy**. Recall that the prefix *toxic-* means poisonous. Therefore, *toxicology* involves the study of harmful, adverse effects that a drug imposes on the body. Last, *pharmacognosy* focuses on the botanical study of naturally occurring drugs.

DRUG NOMENCLATURE

Drug nomenclature tends to be one of the most confusing aspects of pharmacology coursework. Every drug is given multiple additional names, so many that it is nearly impossible for clinicians to recall each one. These names are divided into three major categories: (a) chemical name, (b) generic name, and (c) trade names (Table 1). The chemical name, assigned by the International Union of Pure and Applied Chemistry (IUPAC), describes the molecular structure of the drug. The generic name (also known as the *nonproprietary* or *official* name), is an adopted name assigned by the U.S. Pharmacopeia (USP). The trade name is also referred to as the *proprietary* name, *brand* name, or *registered* name. It is typically a three-syllable name that is selected, registered, and copyrighted by the drug manufacturer.

Clearly, this is a complicated web of nomenclature! However, only the **generic name** (issued by the USP) is used in clinical practice. This is also true as it relates to test questions on standardized board examinations.

Now, off you go! I wish you the very best as you (and your peers) embark on this fascinating and high-yield study of fetal and neonatal pharmacology!

TABLE 1 Drug Nomenclature Exemplars

	EXAMPLE 1: AMPICILLIN	EXAMPLE 2: LIDOCAINE
Chemical name	(2S,5R,6R)-6-([(2R)-2-amino-2-phenylacetyl]amino) -3,3-dimethyl-7-oxo-4-thia-1-azabicyclo [3.2.0]heptane-2-carboxylic acid	2-diethylamino-2,6-acetoxylidide
Generic name	Ampicillin (USP)	Lidocaine hydrochloride (USP)
Trade name[a]	Ampi® Binotal® Cillin® Omnipen® Principen®	Dalcaine® Lidoject® Nervocaine® Octocaine® Xylocaine®

[a]List of trade names associated with ampicillin and lidocaine is not all inclusive.
USP, U.S. Pharmacopeia.

REFERENCE

The University of Texas at Austin. (2014). *Adm. McRaven urges graduates to find courage to change the world.* https://news.utexas.edu/2014/05/16/mcraven-urges-graduates-to-find-courage-to-change-the-world/

Acknowledgments

We would like to thank several individuals who made this book possible:

To my husband, Lieutenant Colonel Eric Jnah, and our children, Mya and Ryan:
Your uncompromising support for my professional endeavors over the past two decades and sustained patience throughout the duration of this project have been a source of inspiration, motivation, and reassurance. Thank you for keeping the house stocked with caffeine. Eric, thank you for graciously sacrificing numerous hours of family time for this project. Mya, thank you for being a source of encouragement and hope, and creating artwork for this book! Ryan, thank you for consistently demonstrating curiosity and determination (and your sense of humor)!

—AJ

To my wife, Cindy, my NICU pharmacy colleagues, Brandy and Caren, and the Women's Hospital of Greensboro and SLCH NP teams:
Cindy, you motivate me to be a better person and inspire me both personally and professionally. Brandy and Caren, you are the real pharmacists in our NICU and keep the unit running while I edit textbooks. Strong women run the world. The senior nurse practitioners in Greensboro and St. Louis literally raised me, encouraging my growth as a pharmacist and a human. The midcareer and junior NPs in St. Louis continue to inspire me as we work and learn together. Strong NPs run the NICU.

—CCM

To our contributing-author teams, East Carolina University NNP/NCNS student artists, authors in the Class of 2022 and Class of 2023, and East Carolina University NNP alumni who graciously donated intellectual material from their tenure in the program:
Thank you for faithfully supporting NNP education and the greater nursing profession! Special thanks to Roxane Warren of Photography, Eh! for our cover image.

—AJ & CCM

Instructor Resources

A set of instructor resources designed to supplement this text is located at http://connect.springerpub.com/content/book/978-0-8261-5884-0. Qualifying instructors may request access by emailing textbook@springerpub.com.

Instructor Resources Include:

- Test Bank
- Mapping to AACN Essentials: Core Competencies for Professional Nursing Education

PART I

Basic Principles of Fetal and Neonatal Pharmacology

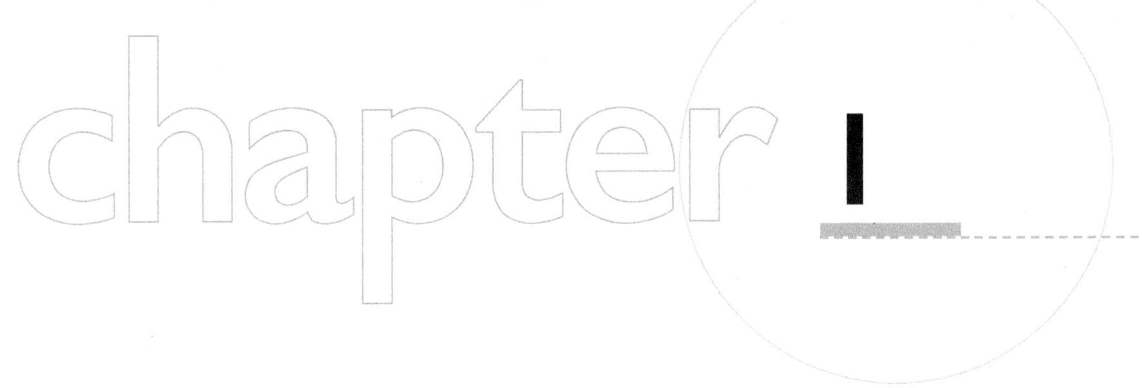

Pediatric Drug Regulation in the United States

Amy J. Jnah and April Smithwick

LEARNING OBJECTIVES

After completing this chapter, the reader should be able to:

- Review the evolution of federal drug regulation and oversight.
- Understand the purpose for the Pediatric Pharmacology Research Unit Network (1994), Pediatric Labeling Rule (1994), U.S. Food and Drug Administration (FDA) Modernization Act (1997), and Pediatric Rule (1998) as they pertain to early efforts to stimulate neonatal and pediatric drug research.
- Investigate the relationship between the Best Pharmaceuticals for Children Act (2002) and Pediatric Research Equity Act (2003).
- Identify the prevalence and implications associated with off-label prescribing in neonatal intensive care.
- Investigate current pediatric drug labeling rules and regulations.

INTRODUCTION

Pediatric drug regulation has drastically changed over the past 25 years. In fact, it is now considered unethical to design a drug trial that excludes neonates (birth–28 days of life), infants (29 days–1 year of life), and fragile pediatric patients. This is, in part, due to changes in federal legislation that require new medicines to be studied in neonates, infants, and children. Formerly, the fragility of this population was used as a basis for excluding neonates and infants from studies. Now, regulatory changes deem the exclusion of neonates and infants to be unethical. This has led to an increase in neonatal-specific labeling information; 40% of drugs prescribed to extremely low-birth-weight (ELBW) infants have U.S. Food and Drug Administration (FDA) infant labeling (Stark et al., 2022). However, numerous drugs that are commonly prescribed in NICUs remain devoid of neonatal-specific information. Healthcare providers are left with an incomplete understanding of the efficacy and safety of these drugs. Clearly, there is much work to be done.

This chapter offers readers a unique view through the looking glass, specific to the evolution of regulatory oversight and pediatric drug research. We begin with a review of several noteworthy tragedies involving untoward fetal and neonatal drug exposures. Next, we review key pieces of legislation that influenced pediatric drug research. Last, we review the current prescribing landscape in NICUs and identify strategies to increase the number of drug studies conducted in neonates and infants in the coming years.

TRIAL AND ERROR: THE EVOLUTION OF REGULATORY OVERSIGHT

Consider the number of medication exposures neonates and infants in NICUs are subject to during the birth hospitalization. Infants larger than 1 kg at birth receive an average of two unique medications (interquartile range [IQR] 0–3), whereas infants born at an ELBW less than 1 kg are exposed to an average of nine medications (IQR 5–14; Stark et al., 2022). Most ELBW infants receive one or more drug doses per day, most unlabeled for use in ELBW infants. As a result, more than 70% of ELBWs experience at least one drug–drug interaction (Costa et al., 2021). In fact, furosemide, fentanyl, and fluconazole, the seventh, eighth, and 15th most commonly prescribed drugs in the NICU, respectively, are *not* labeled for use in the ELBW population (Costa et al., 2021; Stark et al., 2022).

Neonatal clinicians are well aware that high-level drug safety and efficacy studies are critical to advance the state of the science and inform regulatory bodies as well as bedside prescribers. Historically, randomized controlled trials (RCTs) are the gold standard for generating drug safety and efficacy data; however, recruitment can delay data collection and, in some situations, yield smaller participant numbers than what can be generated by using electronic medical record warehouse data. Whether future data are obtained primarily from RCTs, real-world data, and/or off-label use registries remains to be seen. Regardless, federal oversight is necessary to ensure that research is designed and conducted ethically, and conclusions are data driven. This section of the chapter offers a review of accidents and lessons learned that hastened the enactment of drug legislation, which benefitted the pediatric population (Table 1.1).

TABLE 1.1 Milestones in the Evolution of Pediatric Drug Regulation

1906	Original "Food and Drug Act" is passed by Congress and signed by President Theodore Roosevelt. This law prevented the "manufacture, sale or transportation of adulterated or misbranded or poisonous or deleterious food, drugs, medications... ."
1937	Diethylene glycol (contained in Elixir Sulfanilamide) kills 107 children and adults. This prompted officials to reexamine the Food and Drug Act for vulnerable loopholes.
1938	Federal Food, Drug, and Cosmetic Act is passed by Congress. This modified the original Food and Drug Act and extended the FDA's regulatory authority. Now, drug safety had to be established prior to marketing and distribution.
1951	Durham-Humphrey Amendment is passed by Congress. This amendment established that habit-forming or potentially harmful drugs could only be dispensed by a pharmacist with a prescription and were to be labeled "Caution: Federal Law prohibits dispensing without prescription."
1962	Thalidomide, a drug prescribed in Western Europe to treat nausea, is the cause for fetal toxicity and major congenital malformations. This same year, the National Institute for Children's Health and Development was founded.
1970	First FDA-regulated package insert is included with oral contraceptive packaging. This regulation required that patients receive a printed summary of risks and benefits at the time a medication is dispensed by a pharmacy.
1977	The American Academy of Pediatrics Committee on Drugs issues guidelines for ethical conduct in pediatric studies.
1979	The FDA requires pediatric clinical trials prior to including pediatric information in the "Indications and Usage" and "Dosage and Administration" sections of a label. In addition, "pregnancy categories" (A, B, C, D, X) were established.
1983	The Orphan Drug Act is passed. This Act permitted the FDA to offer financial incentives to drug manufacturers in order to stimulate drug research and development for the treatment of rare diseases.

(continued)

TABLE 1.1 Milestones in the Evolution of Pediatric Drug Regulation (*continued*)

1994	The PPRU Network is formed. Data from clinical trials was compiled into the PPRU Clinical Data Repository and made accessible to the pharmaceutical industry, regulatory agencies, healthcare providers, and general public.
1997	The Food and Drug Modernization Act is enacted, giving the FDA authority to encourage the inclusion of pediatric patients in drug trials.
1998	The "Pediatric Rule" is enacted. This rule required manufacturers of selected new and existing drugs to include pediatric assessments if 50,000 or more pediatric patients were expected to use the drug or if the drug was expected to offer a meaningful therapeutic benefit.
2002	Washington DC Federal Court rules the Pediatric Rule invalid, stating that the rule exceeded the regulatory authority conferred to the FDA at the time. The BPCA is passed. Now, pediatric-specific drug safety reviews were mandated as was drug labeling for pediatric use. Information on pediatric use is to be extrapolated from adult pharmacokinetic data and based on data from pediatric-specific studies (if the disease and drug response was similar in children and adults). In addition, the FDA offices of Pediatric Therapeutics and Pediatric Advisory Committee were established.
2003	PREA is passed. This Act gave the FDA authority to require drug or biologic agent-specific research in pediatric patients to ensure safety and efficacy. This applied to products submitted to the FDA for approval by way of the New Drug Application.
2012	The FDA Safety and Innovation Act (Title V) **permanently** reauthorized the BPCA and PREA. Now, pharmaceutical companies were required to provide a rationale if neonates were to be excluded from a drug trial. This Act is renewed every 5 years.

BPCA, Best Pharmaceuticals for Children Act; FDA, U.S. Food and Drug Administration; PPRU, Pediatric Pharmacology Research Units; PREA, Pediatric Research Equity Act.

Federal Food, Drug, and Cosmetic Act (1938)

The original Food and Drug Act was enacted in 1906 and already becoming obsolete in the 1930s. Ongoing discussions to update the law continued, but arguments among politicians consistently stalled congressional action. In the meantime, drugs were incepted and prescribed, many in the absence of relevant efficacy and safety data.

Consider, for example, the devastating effects of Elixir Sulfanilamide. In 1932, German chemist Gerhard Domagk, who worked for Bayer Pharmaceuticals, discovered the antibiotic Prontosil. This drug was famously prescribed to Franklin Delano Roosevelt's son to treat a bacterial infection of the throat. The antibiotic cured the infection and was celebrated as a lifesaving medication.

Meanwhile, other scientists began investigating the composition of Prontosil, a patented drug. In doing so, they discovered that 50% of each drug molecule was biologically active and capable of killing bacteria. This portion of the drug was sulfanilamide. Pharmaceutical companies quickly realized that the patent on sulfanilamide was expired and sought to capitalize on the drug. However, a significant problem challenged this pursuit: sulfanilamide was hydrophobic.

Harold Watkins, a chemist employed by the Massengill Company, resolved this conundrum by combining diethylene glycol with sulfanilamide. This combination effectively dissolved sulfanilamide, and with the addition of artificial flavoring made it palatable and appealing for use in children and adults. The solution was labeled "Elixir Sulfanilamide," produced by the gallons, and initially prescribed to over 100 individuals. Use of the term *elixir* inferred that the antibiotic was made from ethanol; however, it was made from diethylene glycol, also known as *antifreeze*, a deadly poison. The medicine had been unintentionally "mislabeled." Within 1 week of exposure to the drug, patients developed abdominal pain, nausea, and vomiting, which led to more advanced and ominous complications, including renal failure, cardiac arrythmias, stupor, convulsions, coma, and death (Ballentine, 1981). In an act of desperation, one mother wrote the following note to President Roosevelt:

> The first time I ever had the occasion to call in a doctor for [Joan] and she was given Elixir of Sulfanilamide. All that is left to us is the caring for her little grave. Even the memory of her is mixed with sorrow for we can see her little body tossing to and fro and hear that little voice screaming with pain and it seems as though it would drive me insane. ... It is my plea that you

> will take steps to prevent such sales of drugs that will take little lives and leave such suffering behind and such a bleak outlook on the future as I have tonight. (as cited in Ballentine, 1981, p. 4)

The FDA, American Medical Association, media, and other agencies worked tirelessly to recapture all distributed Elixir Sulfanilamide. Then, FDA Commissioner Walter Campbell publicly released the following statement in response to the deaths:

> It is unfortunate that under the terms of our present inadequate Federal law, the Food and Drug Administration is obliged to proceed against this product on a technical and trivial charge of misbranding ... the distribution of highly potent drugs should be controlled by an adequate Food and Drug law. (as cited in Ballentine, 1981, pp. 4–5)

Dr. Campbell went on to remind legislators of prior drug-induced injuries, including blindness and death from dinitrophenol exposure, hepatic injury from cinchophen exposure, and poisonings from thyroid and radium formulations (Ballentine, 1981). He emphasized the dangers associated with releasing untested, unregulated drugs and implored Congress to act quickly. Lawmakers and scientists had not heeded lessons learned through the use of trial and error.

Dr. Campbell's efforts hastened the enactment of the **Federal Food, Drug, and Cosmetic Act of 1938 (FFDCA)**. This new law required manufacturers to prove their compounds were safe, with no false labels or claims. In addition, factories had to undergo quality inspections. Violations would be taken to federal court, and criminals would be prosecuted.

Although a step toward better federal oversight, the FFDCA did not regulate or discourage off-label drug use and did not prioritize drug safety and efficacy research in the pediatric population. As a result, trial and error persisted. One particularly noteworthy error involved the administration of vitamin K in newborns, which began in the early 1940s as a means to reduce the incidence of hemorrhagic disease (Robertson, 2003). In the absence of standardized dosing recommendations, small (1 mg) and large (10 mg) doses of water-soluble synthetic vitamin K were prescribed to newborns, including those born premature. Over the following decade, numerous preterm neonates developed severe unconjugated hyperbilirubinemia (>18 mcg/dL) and concerns were raised that the water-soluble vitamin K analogue (Synkavit) was to blame. Bound and Telfer (1956) published outcomes of a small study that compared the effect of small- and large-dose vitamin K on plasma bilirubin levels and concluded that the larger dose (10 mg) of vitamin K was positively associated with severe hyperbilirubinemia, death, and autopsy-confirmed kernicterus. In response, the American Academy of Pediatrics (AAP; 1961) recommended one standardized dose of natural vitamin K for prophylactic use. Had drug studies been available in the 1940s and regulatory mandates in place, error (neurologic injury) could have been avoided.

Antibiotic prophylaxis for newborns at risk for early-onset sepsis offers a second example of the downstream risks of off-label prescribing. Throughout the 1950s, physicians customarily prescribed antibiotics, some new to the market, to empirically treat premature and term infants at risk for sepsis. In 1953, a new sulfonamide, sulfisoxazole, was introduced to pediatricians and quickly gained favor because fewer doses were required compared to traditional antibiotics on the market (Robertson, 2003). Sulfisoxazole was administered subcutaneously in combination with penicillin over a period of 5 days. By 1955, concerns were raised about a possible connection between sulfisoxazole exposure and kernicterus. One particularly noteworthy report was published by William Silverman and colleagues. He performed a single-center controlled trial of sulfisoxazole/penicillin compared with penicillin/oxytetracycline prophylaxis and concluded that sulfisoxazole exposure was associated with a 51% mortality risk (compared to 13% mortality in the control group, $p < .001$) and substantial risk for kernicterus (16 of 35 deaths in the sulfisoxazole group, $p < .001$; Silverman et al., 1956). The study went on to issue the following warning: "the likelihood of a causal association between sulfisoxazole administration and kernicterus is sufficiently strong to justify a warning that until further evidence is available, sulfisoxazole treatment of premature infants in the first 5 days of life should be discontinued" (Silverman et al., 1956, p. 746). In 1959, scientists discovered that sulfisoxazole displaced bilirubin from albumin, which increased unconjugated bilirubin concentrations and the risk for bilirubin-induced neurologic dysfunction and kernicterus. Yet another avoidable error illuminated the need for prospective pediatric drug trials monitored by federal agencies.

Chloramphenicol was also in use at the time that sulfisoxazole was being dispensed. Some pediatricians preferred to pair chloramphenicol with penicillin and administer this prophylactic regimen over the first 5 days of life in neonates at risk for sepsis. Like sulfisoxazole, several years passed before clinicians recognized that a subset of newborns, and in particular low-birth-weight newborns, exposed to chloramphenicol manifested with hypotension and shock, which progressed to cardiovascular collapse and death. Several reports were published between 1959 through 1961 that described the gradual and fatal onset of "gray baby syndrome" after 72 to 96 hours of chloramphenicol exposure. Newborns would develop a worsening feeding intolerance complicated by abdominal distension and emesis, as well as hypotonia, hypothermia, and a conspicuous "gray" skin tone (Meissner & Smith, 1979). Formal investigations of chloramphenicol use in newborns ensued and each study linked the drug to an increased risk of cardiovascular collapse and death. By 1960, chloramphenicol use ceased. Here again, tragedy was the impetus for prioritizing research into the efficacy and safety of drugs in the pediatric population.

Kefauver–Harris Drug Amendment (1962)

Next, in 1962, thalidomide was marketed in Europe and other nearby countries as a therapeutic agent for pregnancy-induced nausea. Obstetric providers took a liking to this medication and numerous women and fetuses were exposed to the drug. The manufacturer (William S. Merrill Company) sought to expand the reach of this drug in the United States and applied for FDA approval in 1962. Per the requirements set forth in the FFDCA, Dr. Frances Oldham Kelsey, a senior FDA official, was assigned to review the application for thalidomide, and in doing so noticed the absence of scientifically reliable data. Dr. Kelsey adamantly denied the request for FDA approval. Sadly, unbeknownst to FDA officials, the Merrill Company had already distributed thalidomide to 1,200 U.S. physicians ahead of FDA approval. Before the FDA could reclaim all dispensed doses (similar to efforts required to retrieve Elixir Sulfanilamide), 17 fetuses were exposed to thalidomide and developed major congenital malformations (Geraghty, 2001). Dr. Kelsey is credited with preventing the authorized distribution of a teratogen and was awarded the President's Award for Distinguished Federal Civilian Service for her role in protecting scores of pregnant women and fetuses from thalidomide exposure.

As a consequence of these lessons learned, Congress passed amendments to the FFDCA. The intent was to provide the FDA with broader regulatory oversight. One particularly noteworthy amendment was the **Kefauver–Harris Drug Amendment** (1962), an amendment initially aimed to curb drug costs that was expanded after the thalidomide tragedy and passed by a unanimous vote. This legislation mandated the following (FDA, 2012):

- No drug can be marketed in the United States without FDA approval.
- Pharmaceutical manufacturers are required to provide the FDA with evidence of drug efficacy, based on data from well-powered clinical studies, conducted by qualified experts.
- FDA review of a new drug application is extended to 180 days.
- After approval, all reports of major side effects are to be reported to the FDA.
- All drugs approved between 1938 and 1962 are subject to a focused safety review.
- The FDA is responsible for establishing drug manufacturing regulations and coordinating routine inspections of manufacturing facilities, drug advertising, and marketing of generic drugs to ensure fair pricing for consumers.

It is interesting to note that although the intent of the 1962 Kefauver–Harris amendment was to safeguard vulnerable populations, it unintentionally gave manufacturers margin to exclude infants and children from drug research. They voiced the following perspective: *Is it ethically just to subject neonates, infants, and children to drugs without any prior understanding of the pharmacokinetics and pharmacodynamics of the drug in this vulnerable population?* Manufacturers and scientists found themselves in a catch-22; the need to collect scientific study data to establish drug efficacy and safety conflicted with the ethics of human experimentation. As a result, many refused the call for research; pediatricians became notably concerned. Dr. Harry Shirkey, a pediatrician and pediatric pharmacologist, published a powerful editorial in which he argued that excluding infants and children from drug trials would relegate them to a status of "therapeutic orphan" (Shirkey, 1968). He argued that off-label prescribing would persist to the detriment of the pediatric population, as would the use of the dead-end phrase, "not recommended for use in children" on drug labels.

Clearly, regulations implemented through 1962 primarily benefitted adults. Insufficient pediatric dosing information increased the risk for toxicity or subtherapeutic dosing that could otherwise be averted with efficacy data from clinical trials. Further, insufficient pediatric safety data increased the risk for adverse effects; the consensus among pediatric clinicians was that adverse effects observed in adults may not be inclusive of adverse effects in children. In response, the FDA (Labeling and Prescription Drug Advertising, 1979) published a requirement that manufacturers clarify whether safety and efficacy were established in the pediatric population; this was to be printed on each drug label. However, the clarification was to be based on an analysis of data from clinical trials that included pediatric patients. Given the preexisting resistance from manufacturers and lack of research due to ethical and economic concerns, little progress was made.

Pediatric Labeling Rule (1994)

Pediatric drug research was relatively static over the following 15 years. By 1994, only 2,000 studies had been published and 80% of FDA-approved drug labels were devoid of pediatric information (Burkhart & van den Anker, 2021; Friedman Ross, 2018). This prompted two noteworthy changes. First, the National Institutes of Health (NIH) formed the Pediatric Pharmacology Research Unit Network in 1994 to strategize ways to spur pediatric drug research. Second, the FDA instituted the **Pediatric Labeling Rule** in 1994. The Labeling Rule required manufacturers to examine existing data and determine whether the drug was indicated for use in the pediatric population and whether pediatric use information should be added to the label (Zajicek, 2009). Although this prompted a purposeful look at the state of the science at the time, a paucity of data was available, and manufacturers were not required to conduct safety and efficacy studies to fill the gap.

Food and Drug Administration Modernization Act (1997)

By 1997, pediatric labeling information was available on only 430 drug and biologic labels. This meant 76% of all drug labels were devoid of pediatric labeling information (FDA, 1998; Rakhmanina & van den Anker, 2006). Clearly, drug manufacturers were not amenable to voluntary pediatric drug research. In response, Congress passed the **FDA Modernization Act** of 1997. This legislation included the Better Pharmaceuticals for Children Act, a subsidiary piece of legislation that incentivized pediatric research. Now, pharmaceutical companies that conducted pediatric drug safety and efficacy research were offered marketing exclusivity (FDA approval of generic versions of the drug were deferred for an additional 6 months) or patent protection. However, like the Pediatric Rule, it did not require manufacturers to conduct pediatric research as a requisite for obtaining FDA approval for use in adults. As a result, many declined.

Pediatric Rule (1998)

To make matters worse, the incentives tied to the Modernization Act did not apply to antibiotics, biologics, and off-patent products. This further deterred manufacturers from pursuing costly research in the pediatric population (FDA, 1998). Manufacturers were outspoken about the economic burden linked to pediatric research and the fact that the current incentives did not offset research costs associated with drugs projected to yield a low profit margin. Therefore, the FDA implemented a stricter regulatory mandate, the **Pediatric Rule**, in 1998. This rule gave the FDA authority to mandate that manufacturers conduct pediatric efficacy and safety studies for certain new active ingredients, indications, dosages and regimens, or administration routes (FDA, 1998). Certain drugs (e.g., those with orphan designation) were waived of this requirement. Pediatricians applauded the FDA's initiative.

Best Pharmaceuticals for Children Act (2002)

However, as of the turn of the 21st century, 75% of drugs prescribed to children remained unlabeled for pediatric use. Then, in December 2000, the Association of American Physicians and Surgeons, Competitive Enterprise Institute, and Consumer Alert filed a federal lawsuit against the FDA. These agencies claimed that the FDA did not hold the necessary authority to enforce mandated drug trials. The AAP responded with an amicus brief in support of the Pediatric Rule. Ultimately, the presiding judge, Henry H. Kennedy, Jr. of the U.S. District Court for the District of Columbia, opined that the FDA could not require drug manufacturers to pursue drug trials for indications not listed by the manufacturer in the FDA application. For example, if the manufacturer submitted an application for a drug intended for use in adults, the FDA could not mandate pediatric trials to determine safety and efficacy for use in infants and children. Next, Judge Kennedy compared the terms of the Pediatric Rule to new legislation, the **Best Pharmaceuticals for Children Act (BPCA)** of 2002. This new legislation was introduced in 2001 by Senator Christopher Dodd of Connecticut on behalf of the Senate Health, Education, Labor, and Pensions Committee chaired by Senator Edward Kennedy and passed the Senate by unanimous consent. The bill maintained the exclusivity incentive, defined pediatric age groups to include neonates, encouraged voluntary research of NIH-approved off-patent drugs for use in pediatric patients, and gave priority review status to pediatric supplemental applications (Avant et al., 2018; Thaul, 2012). This necessary research was funded by a $200 million annual NIH fund. Given that the BPCA was passed by Congress and called for voluntary participation, Judge Kennedy ruled that the FDA must also accept the voluntary approach as customary. The Pediatric Rule was struck down on October 17, 2002.

Pediatric Research Equity Act (2003)

Congress responded in 2003 with passage of the **Pediatric Research Equity Act (PREA)**. Many of the requirements listed within the former Pediatric Rule were adopted into PREA. Two noteworthy changes implemented with the 2012 reauthorization involved the requirement for drug manufacturers to submit an "initial pediatric study plan (iPSP)," followed by a "pediatric assessment," with each application for new active ingredients, new indications, dosages and regimens, or administration routes. The purpose of the iPSP was to facilitate early identification of gaps in knowledge and begin to formulate pediatric studies early into the drug development process. Congress defined the term *pediatric assessment* in FFDCA 505B(a)(2)(A), as follows:

> The assessments referred to in paragraph (1) shall contain data, gathered using appropriate formulations for each age group for which the assessment is required, that are adequate—(i) to assess the safety and effectiveness of the drug or the biological product for the claimed indications in all relevant pediatric subpopulations; and (ii) to support dosing and administration for each pediatric subpopulation for which the drug or the biological product is safe and effective. ... If the course of the disease and the effects of the drug are sufficiently similar in adults and pediatric patients, the Secretary may conclude that pediatric effectiveness can be extrapolated from adequate and well-controlled studies in adults, usually supplemented with other information obtained in pediatric patients, such as pharmacokinetic studies. (ii) Extrapolation between age groups. A study may not be needed in each pediatric age group if data from one age group can be extrapolated to another age group. (iii) Information on extrapolation. A brief documentation of the scientific data supporting the conclusion under clauses (i) and (ii) shall be included in any pertinent reviews for the application under section 355 of this title or section 262 of title 42.

Under PREA, the FDA's authority was limited to drugs under review for use in adults. In those circumstances, the FDA would review the sponsor's iPSP and pediatric assessment, and notify drug manufacturers at either the end-of-phase-1 (safety evaluation in a small group of human subjects) or end-of-phase-2 (efficacy and safety evaluation in a larger group of human subjects) clinical trial meeting (between the FDA representative and drug manufacturer) if data from pediatric studies would be required with the final submission for FDA approval, or if the review of drug-specific pediatric data would be deferred until after FDA approval was rendered.

In comparison, BPCA permitted the FDA to proactively contact pharmaceutical companies and provide a "written request" for new research on an already approved moiety specific to the pediatric population (Figure 1.1). The caveat was the voluntary nature of participation; manufacturers could agree to conduct research in exchange for pediatric exclusivity and federal funding support or they could provide a rationale for not including pediatric studies. Of the studies that qualified for exclusivity, 87% yielded sufficient data for the addition of pediatric labeling information (U.S. Government Accountability Office [USGAO], 2007).

FIGURE 1.1 Best Pharmaceuticals for Children Act incentive program.

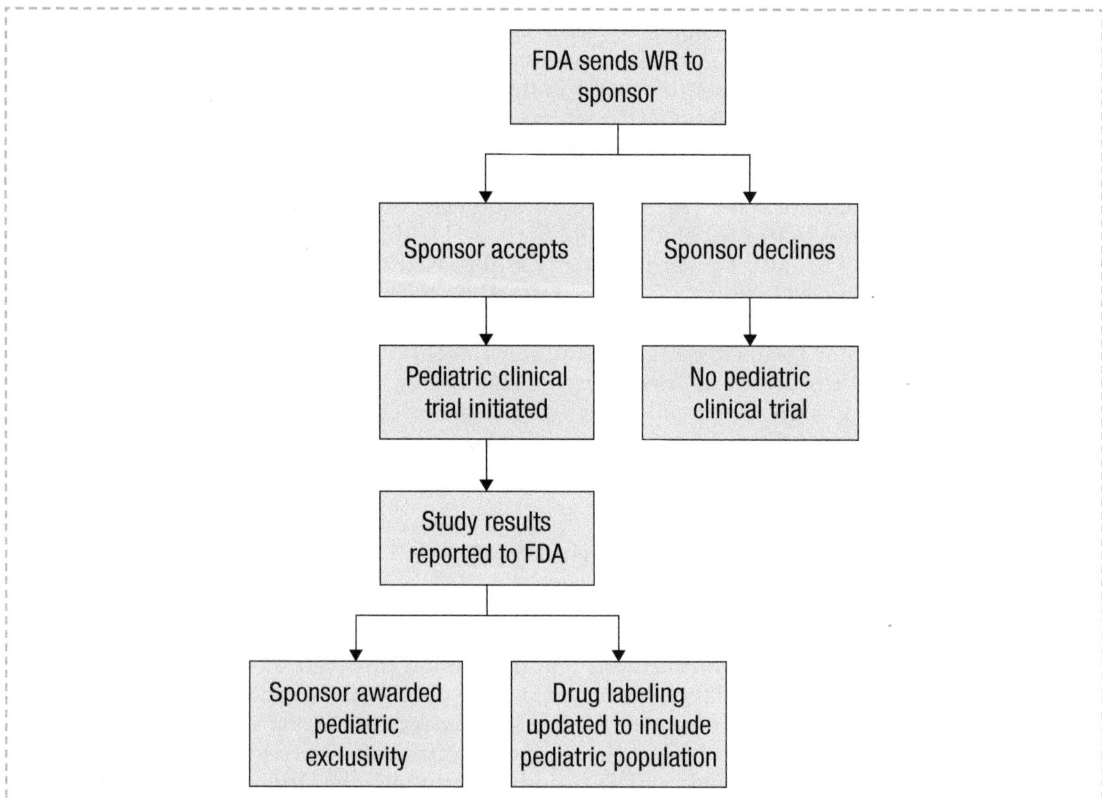

Note: The BPCA grants the FDA permission to directly contact manufacturers (sponsors) who hold the rights to a particular drug and provide a formal written request for a pediatric drug trial involving the active moiety (molecule or ion responsible for eliciting a physiologic or pharmacologic action) of interest. As of August 2021, the FDA had issued 517 WRs for pediatric studies.
FDA, Food and Drug Administration; WR, written request.
Source: From U.S. Food and Drug Administration (n.d.). *Approved active moieties to which FDA has issued a written request for pediatric studies under Section 505A of the Federal Food, Drug, and Cosmetic Act.* U.S. Department of Health and Human Services. https://www.fda.gov/drugs/development-resources/written-requests-issued

Food and Drug Administration Safety and Innovation Act (2012) and Food and Drug Administration Reauthorization Act (2017)

PREA was reauthorized as part of the **FDA Safety and Innovation Act** (2012) and **FDA Reauthorization Act** (2017). Of note, Section 505(d)(2) of the FDA Reauthorization Act required that guidance on the inclusion of neonates in drug and biologic product studies was to be issued within 2 years (FDA, 2017). This draft guidance was published in August 2019; final guidance has yet to be issued.

OFF-PATENT MEDICATION USE

From 2003 through 2009, an increasing number of drugs and biologic agents were labeled for pediatric use, but few included neonatal/infant-specific information. These data supported the renewal of the BPCA and continued efforts toward the inclusion of neonates and infants in drug studies. As part of the renewal, Congress reauthorized the $200 million appropriation for NIH-approved pediatric drug studies; research funding required the submission of a research proposal, review by an expert panel that scored the submission, site visits, and the negotiation of a funding contract

FIGURE 1.2 Drugs unlabeled for use in infants (1994–2021).

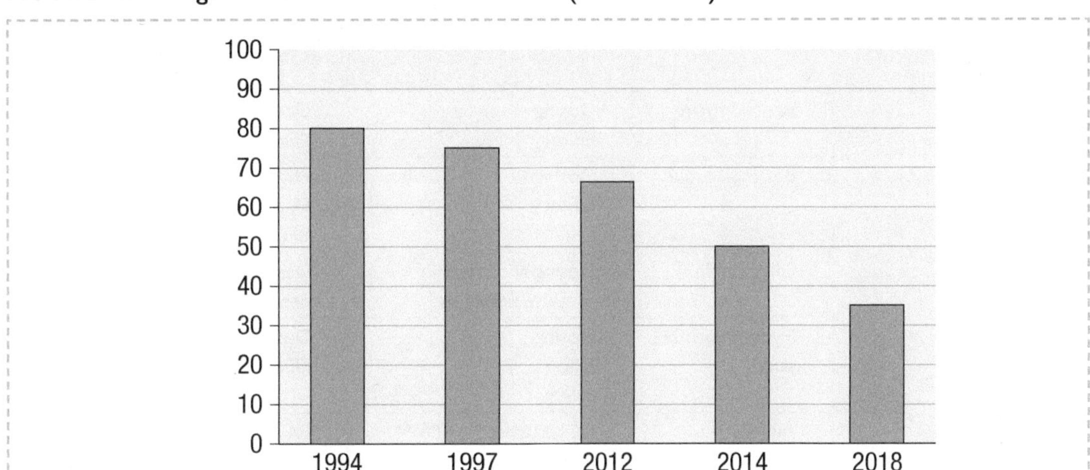

Sources: Ali, A. A., Charoo, N. A., & Abdallah, D. B. (2014). Pediatric drug development: Formulation considerations. *Drug Development and Industrial Pharmacy, 40*(10), 1283–1299. https://doi.org/10.3109/03639045.2013.850713; Burkhart, G. J., & van den Anker, J. N. (2021). Neonatal and pediatric dose selection: Quo vadis? *Journal of Clinical Pharmacology, 61*(S1 Suppl.), S7–S8. https://doi.org/10.1002/jcph.1888; Friedman Ross, L. (2018). 50 years ago in *The Journal of Pediatrics. The Journal of Pediatrics, 192*, 59. https://doi.org/10.1016/j.jpeds.2017.07.017; Laughon, M. M., Avant, D., Tripathi, N., Hornik, C. P., Cohen-Wolkowiez, M., Clark, R. H., Smith, P. B., & Rodriguez, W. (2014). Drug labeling and exposure in neonates. *JAMA Pediatrics, 168*(2), 130–136. https://doi.org/10.1001/jamapediatrics.2013.4208.

(Zajicek, 2009). This NIH appropriation was a noteworthy stimulus for pediatric drug research. By 2012, 67% of drugs remained devoid of pediatric labeling information, and in particular devoid of information specific to infants (Figure 1.2; Ali et al., 2014). Given the success of the appropriation, the NIH went on to publish a priority list of needs to encourage drug trials that included neonates (Table 1.2). One noteworthy outcome of that call for research, issued in 2014, were data accrued from a multicenter trial of antibiotic safety and efficacy in premature infants with intra-abdominal infections (Smith et al., 2021). We direct readers to Chapter 24, "Necrotizing Enterocolitis," for additional details specific to that study.

National Institutes of Health Priority List (2020–2021)

The current NIH priority list (2020–2021) includes some of the same priorities from the 2014 list as well as new therapeutic areas or drugs of interest (Table 1.3). Although this list is relatively new, some research that aligns with the priority list has been underway for several years. For example, the Duke Clinical Research Institute used published, prospective RCT data along with novel retrospective data from the Pediatrix Medical Group and the National Institute of Child Health and Human Development (NICHD) cofunded Prematurity and Respiratory Outcomes Program to evaluate the safety and efficacy of caffeine citrate in premature infants, a drug previously labeled for use in pediatric patients (Smith et al., 2018). In March 2020, as a result of this study, pediatric drug labeling for caffeine citrate was expanded to include dosing information for preterm neonates. We refer readers to Chapter 10, "Apnea of Prematurity," for an expanded discussion of caffeine therapy.

EXPANDED PEDIATRIC DRUG LABELING: WHERE ARE WE NOW?

Between 2007 and 2016, data from 292 pediatric studies were presented to the FDA for the purpose of new drug approvals and labeling changes. Of those studies, only 7.9% (n = 23) were inclusive of neonates, infants, and children younger than 2 years of age (Avant et al., 2018). Given this information, it should be of little surprise that by 2014, merely 35% of all drugs prescribed to neonates/infants were FDA approved, and of the 100 most commonly prescribed drugs in the NICU, only two (famotidine, linezolid) were properly labeled for use in neonates (Hsieh et al., 2014).

TABLE 1.2 National Institutes of Health Neonatal-Specific Priority List (2014)

THERAPEUTIC AREA	DRUG OF INTEREST	KNOWLEDGE OR LABELING GAP(S)	TYPE OF BPCA STUDY OR SCIENTIFIC NEED(S)
BPD	Azithromycin	Dosing Efficacy	Dosing Efficacy
	Betamethasone	Dosing Efficacy	PK Efficacy (ureaplasma infection) BPD prevention
	Furosemide	Dosing and safety in preterm neonates	Dosing and safety in preterm neonates
	Hydrochlorothiazide	Dosing Efficacy Safety	Dosing Efficacy
Infection	Ampicillin	PK and safety in VLBW neonates	PK Safety
	Fluconazole	PK and safety in VLBW neonates	PK Safety
	Metronidazole	PK and efficacy with abdominal infections	PK
Necrotizing enterocolitis	Meropenem	PK Safety	Not specified
NAS	Methadone	PK Safety	Treatment of NAS in opioid-exposed neonates
Pain	Morphine	Pain	Optimization of dosing and biomarkers of pain
Seizures	Not specified	Safety	Safety secondary to exposure for maternal seizure disorder

BPCA, Best Pharmaceuticals for Children Act; BPD, bronchopulmonary dysplasia; NAS, neonatal abstinence syndrome; PK, pharmacokinetics; VLBW, very low birth weight.
Source: National Institutes of Health. (2014). *Best Pharmaceuticals for Children Act (BPCA) priority list of needs in pediatric therapeutics.* U.S. Department of Health and Human Services. https://www.nichd.nih.gov/sites/default/files/inline-files/Priority_List_07082014.pdf

As of April 2023, 1,050 FDA-approved drugs included new or revised pediatric labeling information, a significant increase in pediatric labeling activity from 1997 (FDA, 2023). While promising, many of these pediatric labeling changes are not inclusive of term or preterm neonates, suggesting that pediatric drug research does not include a sample population which extends to the cusp of viability. In fact, the most common requests for pediatric drug studies (autism spectrum disorders, attention deficit hyperactivity disorder [ADHD]-induced insomnia, tinea capitis, Kawasaki disease, and delayed puberty) submitted to the FDA between 2007 and 2016 did not inform neonatal prescribing practices at all (Avant et al., 2018). Presently, 40% of medications prescribed to preterm infants weighing less than 1 kg at birth are FDA approved, leaving a majority (94%) of preterm infants exposed to at least one medication that is not labeled for use in preterm neonates (Table 1.4; Stark et al., 2022).

In order to continue to increase the number of drugs labeled for use in neonates and infants, scientists must overcome challenges associated with executing pharmacokinetic studies in neonates and infants. Commonly reported logistical challenges include study-related expenses; processes involving institutional review board and regulatory agency reviews and approvals; patient recruitment; obtaining parental informed consent; patient retention; and the allocation of time necessary to collect, analyze, and report data (Raju, 2019; Stark et al., 2022; Woolfall et al., 2013). Other population-specific challenges include the immature physiologic function observed in preterm and term neonates, increased morbidity and mortality risks compared to older children and adults, the need to minimize painful procedures, and difficulty obtaining blood samples for analysis.

TABLE 1.3 National Institutes of Health Neonatal-Specific Priority List (2020–2021)

THERAPEUTIC AREA	DRUG OF INTEREST	KNOWLEDGE OR LABELING GAP(S)	TYPE OF BPCA STUDY OR SCIENTIFIC NEED(S)
Apnea of prematurity	Caffeine	Dosing Safety	Dosing and long-term safety in preterm neonates
BPD	Azithromycin	Dosing Efficacy	Dosing Efficacy
	Betamethasone	Dosing Efficacy	PK Efficacy (ureaplasma infection) BPD prevention
	Furosemide	Dosing and safety in preterm neonates	Dosing and safety in preterm neonates
	Hydrochlorothiazide	Dosing Efficacy Safety	Dosing Efficacy
Necrotizing enterocolitis	Meropenem	PK Safety	Not specified
NAS	Methadone	PK Safety	Treatment of NAS in opioid-exposed neonates
Pain	Morphine	Pain	Optimization of dosing and biomarkers of pain
	Hydromorphone Ketamine	Dosing	Optimization of dosing and biomarkers of pain
Seizures	Levetiracetam	Dosing Safety	Safety secondary to exposure for maternal seizure disorder Platform trial design for dosing and safety evaluations
Medication exposure in breast milk	Azithromycin Clindamycin Escitalopram Labetalol Metformin Nifedipine Ondansetron Oxycodone Sertraline Tranexamic acid	Dosing Safety	Opportunistic PK sampling of medications in mother–infant dyads to determine relative concentrations in breast milk

BPCA, Best Pharmaceuticals for Children Act; BPD, bronchopulmonary dysplasia; NAS, neonatal abstinence syndrome; PK, pharmacokinetics.
Source: National Institutes of Health. (2020). *Best Pharmaceuticals for Children Act (BPCA) priority list of needs in pediatric therapeutics.* U.S. Department of Health and Human Services. https://www.nichd.nih.gov/sites/default/files/inline-files/2020PriorityListFeb20.pdf

CONCLUSIONS

Fortunately, legislation has been enacted over the years that prioritizes justice, or fair access to clinical trials. This is true for neonates, infants, children, and adults. As a result of the legislation discussed in this chapter and the efforts of myriad organizations, including the International Neonatal Consortium, which was incepted in 2015, nearly 14,000 pediatric drug studies have been published to date (Burkhart & van den Anker, 2021). Additional neonatal-specific drug efficacy and safety studies are needed to reduce the incidence of off-label prescribing and drug–drug interactions in the NICU. As the state of the science grows and pediatric labeling expands to include neonatal-specific information, sponsors might be able to use this information to develop novel drugs for use in preterm neonates. After all, 27 years has elapsed since the first novel drug

TABLE 1.4 Top 25 Drugs Prescribed in the NICU (2014–2018)

2014	2018
1. Ampicillin	1. Ampicillin[a,b]
2. Gentamicin	2. Gentamicin[a]
3. Caffeine citrate	3. Caffeine citrate[a,b]
4. Vancomycin	4. Poractant alfa[a]
5. Beractant	5. Morphine[b]
6. Furosemide	6. Vancomycin
7. Fentanyl	7. Furosemide[a]
8. Dopamine	8. Fentanyl
9. Midazolam	9. Midazolam[a]
10. Calfactant	10. Acetaminophen[a,b]
11. Metoclopramide	11. Dopamine
12. Ranitidine	12. Calfactant[a]
13. Poractant alfa	13. Beractant[a]
14. Morphine	14. Phenobarbital
15. Cefotaxime	15. Fluconazole[b]
16. Acetaminophen	16. Erythromycin[a,b]
17. Indomethacin	17. Hydrocortisone
18. Phenobarbital	18. Indomethacin[a]
19. Albuterol	19. Lorazepam[b]
20. Epoetin alfa	20. Cefotaxime[a]
21. Lorazepam	21. Albuterol[b]
22. Hydrocortisone	22. Ranitidine[c]
23. Tobramycin	23. Acyclovir[b]
24. Erythromycin	24. Dexamethasone[b]
25. Dobutamine	25. Epoetin alfa

[a]FDA approved for use in infants.
[b]To date, this drug has been studied in response to a written request (WR) under the Best Pharmaceuticals for Children Act (BPCA) and/or Pediatric Research Equity Act (PREA).
[c]Black-box warning, withdrawn from use.
Sources: Best Pharmaceuticals Act for Children. (2022). *Clinical studies publications.* https://www.nichd.nih.gov/research/supported/bpca/publications; Hsieh, E. M., Hornik, C. P., Clark, R. H., Laughon, M. M., Benjamin, D. K., Smith, P. B. (2014). Medication use in the neonatal intensive care unit. *American Journal of Perinatology, 31*(9), 811–822. https://doi.org/10.1055/s-0033-1361933; Stark, A., Smith, P. B., Hornik, C. P., Zimmerman, K. O., Hornik, C. D., Pradeep, S., Clark, R. H., Benjamin, D. K., Jr., Laughon, M., & Greenberg, R. G. (2022). Medication use in the neonatal intensive care unit and changes from 2010 to 2018. *Journal of Pediatrics, 240*, 66–71.e4. https://doi.org/10.1016/j.jpeds.2021.08.075

(surfactant) was developed for use in the NICU! Of equal importance, focused study and expanded labeling improves the quality and safety of pharmacotherapy required to optimize the outcomes of vulnerable, sick neonates.

ACKNOWLEDGMENT

The authors thank Edress Darcy, PharmD, FPPAG, for her critical review, feedback, and support during the development of this chapter.

LEARNING TOOLS AND RESOURCES

Advice From the Authors

Amy J. Jnah, DNP, APRN, NNP-BC

We learn valuable lessons from history. Fortunately, we have abundant access to historical facts. Take pause to understand how we arrived at this current state of knowledge specific to drugs and drug research. It will make you a more conscientious clinician, teacher, and scholar.

April Smithwick, MSN, APRN, NNP-BC

It is important that neonatal advanced practice nursing students learn about the evolution of drug regulation and implications for babies born during the time when drugs were far less regulated. We must continue to pursue research inquiries which provide clinicians with appropriate safety and efficacy data on drugs prescribed in neonatal intensive care, as is the case in pediatric and adult medicine.

Discussion Prompts

1. Analyze the NIH priority lists for neonatal drug research. Identify at least one published study linked to each priority list and discuss the implications of that research on APRN prescribing practices and neonatal outcomes.
2. Identify factors that may prolong the recruitment of neonates/families to a drug trial. How can APRNs help overcome these types of obstacles?
3. Discuss the impact of off-patent prescribing in the NICU and implications for APRN practice and prescriptive authority.

Mind Map

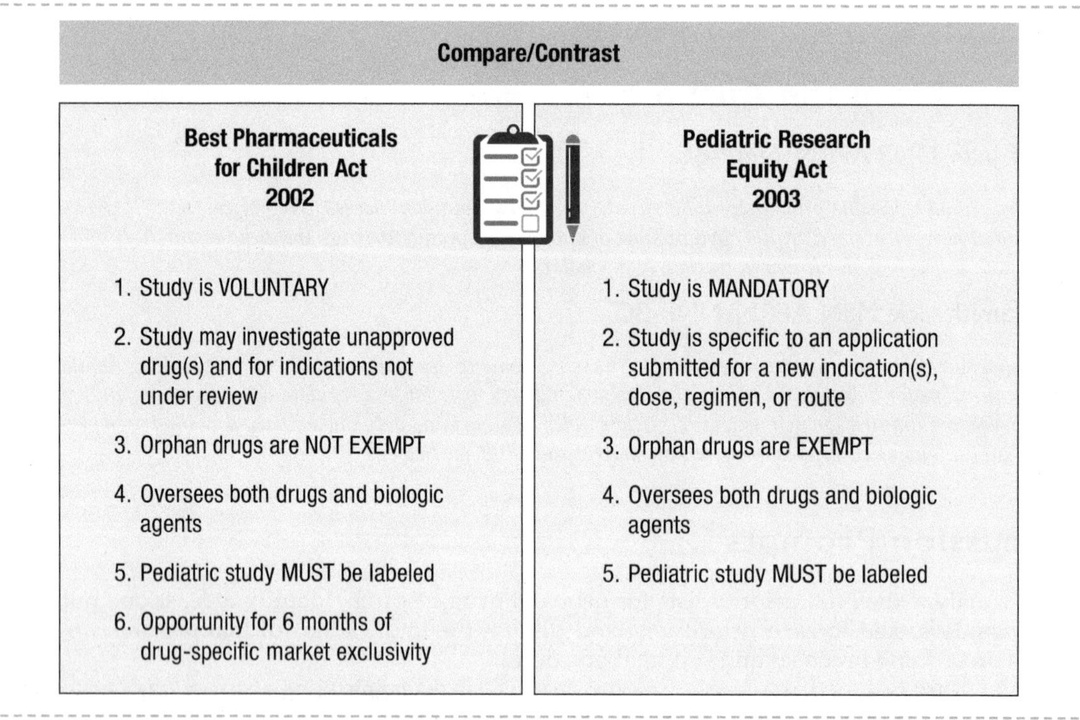

Design credit: Amy J. Jnah, created with Biorender.com.

REFERENCES

References for this chapter are online and available at https://connect.springerpub.com/content/book/978-0-8261-5884-0/part/partI/toc-part/ch1.

chapter 2

Prescriptive Authority

Colleen Moss

LEARNING OBJECTIVES

After completing this chapter, the reader should be able to:

- Compare the legal parameters associated with practice and prescriptive authority for APRNs.
- Differentiate the standards of care for prescribing and administering pharmacologic therapies.
- Evaluate the APRN collaborative practice agreement (CPA) and associated practice implications for APRNs.
- Examine the concept of primum non nocere as it relates to prescriptive authority.

INTRODUCTION

The act of prescribing medications was exclusive to the medical profession until the late 1960s, when a steady increase in demand for inpatient and outpatient physician services was observed. Neonatal, pediatric, and adult acute and primary care settings steadily accepted an increasing patient load, leaving physicians outnumbered and overworked. Within NICUs, this disproportionate increase in patient census (and acuity) illuminated the need for more clinicians with an advanced scope of practice and prescriptive authority.

In response, neonatologists invited select neonatal nurses to expand their scope of practice beyond basic bedside care (Slovis & Comerci, 1974). Neonatal nurses enrolled in 12-week intensive academic training programs (e.g., Georgetown University School of Medicine, Department of Pediatrics, Certificate Neonatal Nurse Practitioner Program). Upon successful completion of the designated certificate program, which at the time was not regionally accredited or linked with a graduate nursing degree, nurses were eligible for licensure as a neonatal nurse practitioner (NNP). The role of the NNP was intended to offset the work of neonatologists in NICUs by managing neonates in collaboration with the attending neonatologist, performing invasive technical procedures, writing medical orders, and prescribing medications.

It is prudent to emphasize that NNPs were not the first APRNs to prescribe medications. Rather, thanks to the work of two pediatricians, Dr. Loretta Ford and Dr. Henry Silver (Berg, 2020), the APRN role was created in the 1960s, and APRN-driven prescribing began in 1969 in Idaho. Thereafter, a ripple effect was observed as boards of nursing in all U.S. states drafted and enacted rules and regulations governing APRN practice and prescriptive authority. This paved the way for graduates of certificate NNP programs to obtain licensure and prescriptive authority without encountering barriers.

Although the aforementioned efforts advanced the nursing profession, the regulations and statutes that composed each state's Nurse Practice Act (NPA) were unique to that state. The creation of a single, unifying body of rules and regulations was not considered; barriers to APRN practice emerged as a result. Some APRNs could independently/autonomously write prescriptions without a physician cosignature and practice to the full extent of their training and scope of practice, whereas APRNs in other states remained restricted by a collaborative practice agreement (CPA) that mandated physician supervision and cosignatures, as well as restricted prescriptive authority. This holds true today. APRNs must apply for and maintain individual state licenses to practice across state lines. Faculty who teach in online graduate programs are also required to hold a costly APRN license and maintain a record of state-required continuing education in certain states (e.g., Washington) despite never intending to clinically practice in that state.

Inconsistencies with APRN scope-of-practice and prescriptive authority rules are also observed across 12 (of 195) countries in the world that permit nurses to prescribe medications. The United States, New Zealand, and Australia require nurse prescribers to hold a minimum of a master's degree (Fong et al., 2017; Wilkinson, 2015). In stark contrast, the United Kingdom requires a minimum of 3 years of work experience and completion of the Nursing and Midwifery Council Independent Nurse Prescribing course for a nurse to apply for prescriptive privileges (Mitchell & Pearce, 2021; Ross et al., 2014). No graduate degree, national certification, or APRN license is required in the United Kingdom. These inconsistencies are confusing and unintentionally diminish the authoritative role of the APRN—in particular, in countries that grant prescriptive authority to non-APRNs.

Within the United States, the turn of the century marked the genesis of a shift toward regulatory uniformity. More than 40 nursing organizations came together, motivated by a sense of commitment to the APRN role, determination, and desire to help APRNs across the country practice without barriers. Their efforts led to the creation of the APRN Consensus Model (National Council of State Boards of Nursing [NCSBN], 2008), and later the APRN Compact (NCSBN, 2021b). Both are novel regulatory models that offer standardized regulatory criteria for graduate APRN education, accreditation, certification, and licensure. These models established full practice and prescriptive authority as the only authority commensurate with APRN practice. Key legislative efforts focused on advancing APRN prescriptive authority are summarized in Table 2.1.

This chapter, a first-of-its-kind for NNP students, offers readers a comprehensive discussion of APRN scope of practice and prescriptive authority; the three levels of regulatory structure of practice and prescriptive authority in the United States; the two primary regulatory models that seek to help APRNs practice to the full extent of their education and training; and relevant barriers to independent practice and prescriptive authority. These topics are tightly interwoven; therefore, conceptual overlap is observed throughout the chapter. Readers should be aware that the concept of APRN practice and prescriptive authority is contentious; several medical organizations are working tirelessly to keep primary care and some inpatient APRN subspecialties restricted to physician oversight. Fortunately for NNPs, neonatologists support the APRN role and recognize it as critical to providing high-quality care (Committee on Fetus and Newborn, 2003; Keels et al., 2019; Wallman & Committee on Fetus and Newborn, 2009). Competition is pushed to the side in exchange for collaboration and shared decision-making, as the life-threatening illnesses that plague neonates demand conversation and consensus building among all stakeholders, including the family, before treatments are prescribed. Novice neonatal APRNs who are exploring these concepts for the first time are encouraged to pause and recognize the tremendous responsibility associated with practice and prescriptive authority. By doing so, we all can develop a deeper appreciation for the efforts of lobbyists and others who are advocating for the benefit of the APRN profession and the collaborative culture found in NICUs in the United States.

APRN PRACTICE AUTHORITY

A question that often surfaces during legislative meetings, conferences, and committee meetings is: *Should APRNs be permitted to practice without direct physician oversight?* Many APRNs advocate for this level of full (independent) practice authority. Quality data supporting the APRN as a competent and knowledgeable prescriber are widely available in the literature (Hamric et al., 1998; Mahoney, 1992; Rosenaur et al., 1984). Of all indemnity claims filed between 2012 and 2016, 1% were linked to neonatal APRN-related diagnostic or prescriptive errors (Flynn & Pierce, 2017).

TABLE 2.1 Key Legislation for Advancing APRN Prescriptive Authority

YEAR	ORGANIZATION/ PUBLICATION	POLICY
2000	DEA	APRNs are assigned DEA registration numbers.
2001	*Crossing the Quality Chasm* (Institute of Medicine, 2010)	APRNs provide care that is: • Safe • Effective • Patient centered • Timely • Effective • Equitable
2008	*Campaign for Consensus* (NCSBN, 2008)	This is an initiative used to encourage states to implement a consensus model for the standardization of regulatory requirements, such as licensure, accreditation, certification, and education for APRNs.
2010	*The Future of Nursing* (Institute of Medicine [renamed National Academy of Medicine])	This advocates for the removal of practice barriers and FPA for APRNs.
2012	NGA, 2012	Literature indicates that NPs provide safe and effective care. NGA calls for states to reduce barriers to APRN practice and reimbursement.
2014	Federal Trade Commission	APRNs are safe and effective as independent providers of many healthcare services within the scope of their training, licensure, certification, and current practice.
2020	NCSBN APRN Compact	APRNs with a minimum of 2,080 clinical practice hours can hold a multistate license with a privilege to practice in other states that recognize the Compact (not active at this time; will implement when seven states enact this legislation).

DEA, Drug Enforcement Administration; FPA, full practice authority; NCSBN, National Council of State Boards of Nursing; NGA, National Governors Association; NP, nurse practitioner.

Despite this, some medical organizations lobby against full practice authority for APRNs, whereas others remain firmly in support of the role.

The American Academy of Pediatrics (AAP) was one of the first medical organizations to support the role of the APRN. In fact, the AAP went so far as to endorse the role of NNPs by stating that NNPs possess requisite advanced knowledge and demonstrate psychomotor skill commensurate with that of a physician (Harper et al., 1982). This endorsement helped universities develop and fund weeks-long training programs for the advanced practice role. Graduates were awarded a certificate of completion and could go on to apply for APRN licensure and prescriptive authority. Later, in the 1990s, the AAP's endorsement helped NNP faculty garner the necessary support and momentum to develop formal graduate-level curricula. Weeks-long certificate training programs were retired, and the master's degree in nursing (with NNP concentration) was adopted as the minimum education necessary for licensure and prescriptive authority as an NNP in all U.S. states. The NNP concentration, as opposed to a family nurse practitioner (NP) or pediatric NP concentration, allowed a graduate to sit for the NNP national certification exam and, upon successful completion, attain licensure and prescriptive authority as an NNP within the United States. The AAP has consistently renewed its endorsement of the APRN role over the years (Committee on Fetus and Newborn, 2003; Keels et al., 2019; Wallman & Committee on Fetus and Newborn, 2009).

Next, in 2010, the Institute of Medicine (IOM) published a powerful position statement titled "The Future of Nursing," which advocated for full practice authority for all APRNs. The IOM wrote that APRNs should continue to *partner* with physicians and other healthcare professionals to redesign healthcare in the United States. This concept of partnership versus supervisorship would allow APRNs to practice to the full extent of their education and training. Following the

IOM's report, the National Governors Association (NGA) issued a report highlighting their finding that APRN scope of practice, to include rules and licensure requirements, varied significantly among states. The NGA recommended that states reduce barriers to APRN practice and reimbursement (NGA, 2012). This was followed by a statement from the Federal Trade Commission (FTC) that endorsed APRNs as "safe and effective as independent providers of many health care services within the scope of their training, licensure, certification, and current practice" (FTC, 2014, p. 38).

In response, the American Medical Association (AMA) published a scathing statement in opposition of full practice authority: "Patients deserve care led by physicians—the most highly educated, trained and skilled health care professionals. Through research, advocacy and education, the AMA vigorously defends the practice of medicine against scope of practice expansions that threaten patient safety" (American Medical Association, 2021). Similar to the aforementioned sentiment, the AMA recently opposed an expanded scope of practice for pharmacists and pharmacy interns. This position statement was issued in response to the U.S. Department of Health and Human Services' (HHS) "Third Amendment to Declaration Under the Public Readiness and Emergency Preparedness Act for Medical Countermeasures Against COVID–19." The amendment declared that pharmacists and technicians may administer vaccines to children and provide parents with a vaccination record, outside the purview of a physician (e.g., at a local pharmacy). In the absence of quality evidence, the AMA contended that this expanded scope of practice for pharmacists and technicians threatened patient safety.

Scope of Practice

But what does the term *scope of practice* mean for a regulated profession like nursing? Broadly speaking, the scope of practice describes profession-specific procedures, actions, and activities (services) that clinicians are permitted to perform. These services are unique to each healthcare discipline. Further, the scope (breadth) of permissions expands with graduate-level training and advanced certifications. The scope of practice for a neonatal nurse is narrow compared with the scope of practice for an NNP, who can perform invasive procedures and prescribe medications.

Policy makers define the scope of practice for each discipline commensurate with (a) competencies defined by the population-specific certifying body, (b) policy statements and standards published by related professional organizations, and (c) the NPA enacted by the respective state board of nursing (National Association of Neonatal Nurse Practitioners [NANNP], 2014).

The National Certification Corporation (NCC) is the population-specific certifying body for NNPs. The NCC lists the following as core competencies for NNPs:

- Demonstrate the knowledge inherent in the role and scope of NNP practice.
- Apply knowledge of basic sciences to the provision of neonatal healthcare.
- Obtain and interpret a comprehensive perinatal history and a systematic assessment of all body systems.
- Obtain clinical laboratory information and interpret the resultant data.
- Institute diagnostic procedures and techniques and interpret the resultant data.
- Apply critical thinking to diagnose reasoning and clinical decision-making with the caregiver and family.
- Evaluate the benefits and risks of diagnostic and therapeutic intervention.
- Use adult learning principles when teaching about the care, growth, and development of high-risk infants up to 2 years of age.
- Formulate diagnosis and plan of care in collaboration with physicians, other healthcare professionals, and family.
- Initiate appropriate therapeutic and educational interventions, including consultations and referral.
- Evaluate and document responses to interventions and modify the plan of care as indicated.
- Maintain current knowledge regarding advances in neonatal healthcare.
- Apply knowledge of basic research principles to practice.
- Integrate legal and ethical principles into neonatal healthcare.

Complementary to the NCC's competencies is the scope of practice position statement issued by the NANNP (2014). According to the NANNP, "the scope of the neonatal APRN is expected to evolve through experience, education (formal and informal), evidence-based practice, developing technology, and changes in the healthcare delivery system. The neonatal APRN's practice may be extended through continued advanced practice experience congruent with the accepted scope of practice (National Organization of Nurse Practitioner Faculties, 2013). There are finite limits, however, to the expansion of scope of practice without completing additional formal education. An APRN licensed in one role and population cannot practice in another APRN role or population without additional formal education, certification, and board of nursing recognition in the second role and/or population. APRNs are expected to seek and document appropriate education and competencies when expanding their scope of practice" (NANNP, 2013, pp. 6–7). This position statement helped solidify the role of the NNP as the APRN best suited to work in the NICU, as NNP education is the only formal, accredited, population-specific graduate education pathway that trains neonatal nurses to care for acutely ill preterm and term neonates from birth through 2 years of age (NANNP, 2022). Further, this educational pathway prepares graduates to extend their practice outside the NICU and into chronic care and primary care environments, offering families a unique opportunity for exceptional continuity of care.

Unlike the NCC competencies and the NANNP policy statement, and as alluded to earlier in this chapter, the language used in NPAs differs among states. Each board of nursing considers guidance put forth by national organizations and the safety of citizens, and creates regulations and statutes that compose the NPA. In its entirety, this legislation frames the APRN's scope of practice (NCSBN, 2012; Russell, 2012). Generally speaking, most NPAs in the United States include the following services as core components of APRN scope of practice:

- Evaluate neonates and infants.
- Diagnose neonates and infants.
- Order and interpret diagnostic tests.
- Initiate and manage medical treatment regimens.
- Prescribe pharmacotherapies.

The laws and rules that govern the aforementioned services are regularly reviewed and readopted, or, in some circumstances, amended. For example, until recently, NNPs in Ohio could not prescribe schedule II controlled substances. As of 2017, NNPs in Ohio can prescribe schedule II to IV controlled substances. Therefore, APRNs must remain "in the know."

Figure 2.1 shows the North Carolina Board of Nursing's (NCBON) scope of practice (rule 21NCAC36.0802). The NCBON requires APRNs to attain population-specific graduate-level education at the master's or doctoral level and pass a population-specific national board certification examination. In addition, all APRNs must identify a supervising and collaborating physician; the name and contact information for that physician are required before a license is issued and must be reviewed and confirmed when the license is due for renewal.

Similarly, the Ohio Board of Nursing (OBON) Nurse Practice Act, Ohio Revised Code (ORC) Chapter 4723, defines the scope of practice for the certified nurse practitioner (CNP) as shown in Figure 2.2. As with the NCBON, APRNs seeking to practice in Ohio must attain population-specific graduate-level education at the master's or doctoral level and pass a population-specific national board certification examination. In addition, the OBON also requires APRNs to identify a collaborating physician. Unlike North Carolina rules and regulations, applicants must provide proof of completion of 45 contact hours of advanced population-specific pharmacology training commensurate with rules published in ORC 4723.482.

Next, consider APRN scope of practice as defined by the Washington State Legislature WAC 246-840-300 (Figure 2.3). Like the NCBON and the OBON, the Washington Department of Health (WaDOH) requires applicants to provide proof of graduate-level, population-specific nursing education and national certification. Prescriptive authority is conferred with proof of completion of one course in advanced pharmacology. Unlike the NCBON and the OBON, the state of Washington does not require APRN applicants to establish or maintain a collaborative agreement with a supervising physician. Therefore, newly certified NNPs can apply for and obtain state licensure before employment is secured, which can expedite the credentialing process.

FIGURE 2.1 The North Carolina Board of Nursing scope of practice (Rule 21NCAC36.0802).

21 NCAC 36 .0802 SCOPE OF PRACTICE

The nurse practitioner's scope of practice is defined by academic educational preparation and national certification and maintained competence. A nurse practitioner shall be held accountable by both Boards for a broad range of personal health services for which the nurse practitioner is educationally prepared and for which competency has been maintained, with physician supervision and collaboration as described in Rule .0810 of this Section. These services include:

(1) promotion and maintenance of health;
(2) prevention of illness and disability;
(3) diagnosing, treating, and managing acute and chronic illnesses;
(4) guidance and counseling for both individuals and families;
(5) prescribing, administering, and dispensing therapeutic measures, tests, procedures, and drugs;
(6) planning for situations beyond the nurse practitioner's scope of practice and expertise by consulting with and referring to other health care providers as appropriate; and
(7) evaluating health outcomes.

History Note: *Authority G.S. 90-18(c)(14); 90-18.2; 90-171.23(b)(14);*
Recodified from 21 NCAC 36 .0227(b) Eff. August 1, 2004;
Amended Eff. August 1, 2004;
Readopted Eff. January 1, 2019;
Amended Eff. June 1, 2021.

Source: From http://reports.oah.state.nc.us/ncac/title%2021%20-%20occupational%20licensing%20boards%20and%20commissions/chapter%2036%20-%20nursing/21%20ncac%2036%20.0802.html.

Consider that certain state boards of nursing do not retain statutory authority to regulate APRN practice. For example, APRN prescribing practices in Georgia are regulated by the Georgia Composite Medical Board (https://medicalboard.georgia.gov/professionals/list-nurse-protocols-reviewed-board-prescribing-privileges). In other states, such as in North Carolina, APRN practice is dually regulated by the NCBON and the North Carolina Medical Board. NNPs who practice in New York are licensed by the New York Board of Nursing. However, neonatology is not a recognized patient population. Therefore, NNPs are licensed as pediatric NPs, and population-specific national certification is not required.

LEVELS OF PRACTICE AUTHORITY AND THE COLLABORATIVE PRACTICE AGREEMENT

Determining which states reduce or restrict APRN practice may seem daunting. Fortunately, the American Academy of Nurse Practitioners (AANP) created a user-friendly, color-coded U.S. map that clearly presents the levels of practice authority, per state, and that is frequently updated to maintain accuracy (Figure 2.4; AANP, 2022). States that reduce (medium gray) or restrict (dark gray) APRN scope of practice require APRNs to maintain a CPA with a supervising physician (Table 2.2). This section of the chapter begins with a review of the CPA, followed by a discussion of the three levels of practice authority.

COLLABORATIVE PRACTICE AGREEMENT

By definition, a CPA is a written legal document that delineates the terms of a supervisory relationship between the APRN and a physician (Table 2.3; Ritter et al., 2018). The CPA outlines tasks that an APRN is permitted to perform, as well as the type and amount of physician supervision and involvement required (Fauteux et al., 2017). Currently, 44% (n = 21) of all U.S. states require

FIGURE 2.2 The Ohio Board of Nursing Nurse Practice Act, Ohio Revised Code Chapter 4723, definition of scope of practice for the certified nurse practitioner.

CNP Scope of Practice, Section 4723.43(C), ORC

- CNP practice requires a written SCA with a qualified collaborating physician or podiatrist. Section 4723.431, ORC.
- CNPs may provide preventive and primary care services, provide services for acute illnesses, and evaluate and promote patient wellness, consistent with the CNP's advanced formal education, training, and clinical experience, in their population focus, national certification, and in accordance with rules adopted by the Board.
- A CNP may, in collaboration with one or more physicians, prescribe drugs and therapeutic devices. When collaborating with a podiatrist, the CNP's scope of practice is limited to the procedures that the podiatrist has authority to perform under Section 4731.51, ORC.

CNP, certified nurse practitioner; ORC, Ohio Revised Code; SCA, standard care arrangement.
Source: From Ohio Revised Code, Section 4723.43. Available at: https://codes.ohio.gov/ohio-revised-code/section-4723.43. Accessed on November 30, 2023.

FIGURE 2.3 APRN scope of practice as defined by the Washington State Legislature, WAC 246-840-300.

WAC 246-840-300 ARNP scope of practice. The scope of practice of a licensed ARNP is as provided in RCW 18.79.250 and this section.

(1) The ARNP is prepared and qualified to assume primary responsibility and accountability for the care of patients.

(2) ARNP practice is grounded in nursing process and incorporates the use of independent judgment. Practice includes collaborative interaction with other health care professionals in the assessment and management of wellness and health conditions.

(3) The ARNP functions within his or her scope of practice following the standards of care defined by the applicable certifying body as defined in WAC 246-840-302. An ARNP may choose to limit the area of practice within the commission approved certifying body's practice.

(4) An ARNP shall obtain instruction, supervision, and consultation as necessary before implementing new or unfamiliar techniques or practices.

(5) Performing within the scope of the ARNP's knowledge, experience and practice, the licensed ARNP may perform the following:

(a) Examine patients and establish diagnoses by patient history, physical examination, and other methods of assessment;

(b) Admit, manage, and discharge patients to and from health care facilities;

(c) Order, collect, perform, and interpret diagnostic tests;

(d) Manage health care by identifying, developing, implementing, and evaluating a plan of care and treatment for patients;

(e) Prescribe therapies and medical equipment;

(f) Prescribe medications when granted prescriptive authority under this chapter;

(g) Refer patients to other health care practitioners, services, or facilities; and

(h) Perform procedures or provide care services that are within the ARNP's scope of practice according to the commission approved certifying body as defined in WAC 246-840-302.

[Statutory Authority: RCW 18.79.050, 18.79.110, and 18.79.160. WSR 16-08-042, § 246-840-300, filed 3/30/16, effective 4/30/16. Statutory Authority: RCW 18.79.010, [18.79.]050, [18.79.]110, and [18.79.]210. WSR 09-01-060, § 246-840-300, filed 12/11/08, effective 1/11/09. Statutory Authority: RCW 18.79.110 and 18.79.050. WSR 00-21-119, § 246-840-300, filed 10/18/00, effective 11/18/00. Statutory Authority: Chapter 18.79 RCW. WSR 97-13-100, § 246-840-300, filed 6/18/97, effective 7/19/97.]

APRNs to maintain a CPA in order to obtain licensure and associated practice and prescriptive authority (Latner, 2016; Ritter et al., 2020). Should an APRN practice at more than one institution, a CPA is required for each place of employment.

FIGURE 2.4 Nurse practitioner practice authority in the United States (2021).

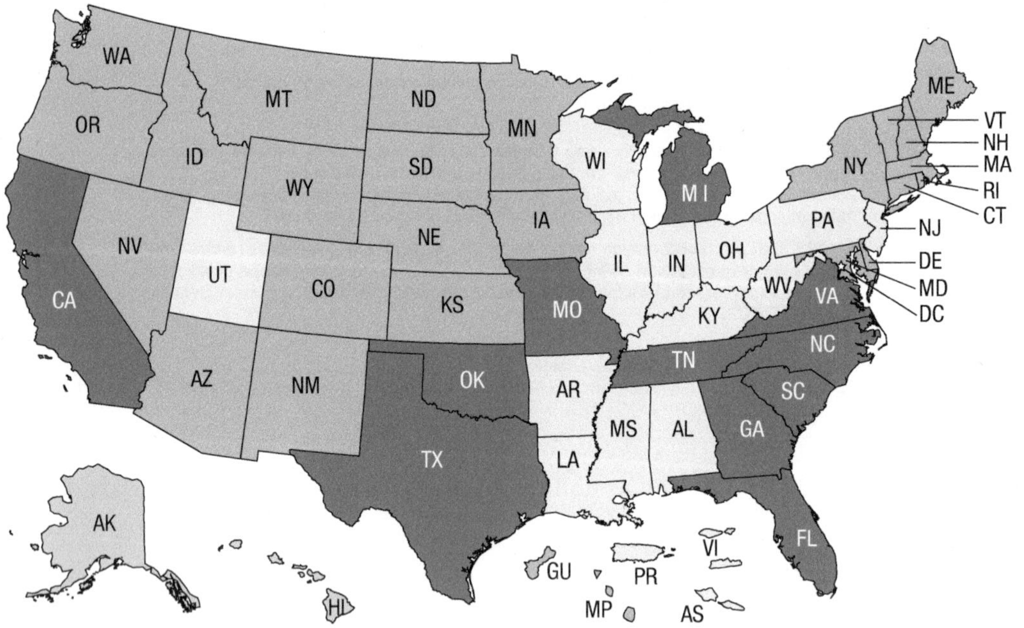

Note: Medium gray represents states with full practice authority, light gray indicates states with reduced practice authority, and dark gray indicates states with restricted practice authority.
Source: From the American Academy of Nurse Practitioners (2022). *State practice environment.* https://www.aanp.org/advocacy/state/state-practice-environment

TABLE 2.2 Levels of Practice Authority

	WASHINGTON	OHIO	NORTH CAROLINA
LEVEL OF PRACTICE AUTHORITY	FULL	REDUCED	RESTRICTED
Autonomous practice	NPs in Washington are fully authorized by state law to see patients, provide diagnoses, and prescribe.	Physicians and NPs must enter into a collaborative agreement for one or more elements of NP practice.	Physicians and NPs must enter into a collaborative agreement for one or more elements of NP practice.
PCPs	Full: State statute and/or administrative code recognize NPs as PCPs.	Full: State statute and/or administrative code recognize NP as PCPs.	No law: State statute and/or administrative code do not define whether NPs can be PCPs.
Independently prescribe schedule II drugs	Reduced: NPs may prescribe certain drugs after a specified number of hours of experience and pharmacotherapeutics education.	Restricted: NPs are not authorized to prescribe schedule II controlled substances in convenience care clinics.	Reduced: Depending on their education and certification, NPs may prescribe limited amounts of legend drugs and controlled substances.
Order PT	Full: NPs may make referrals for PT.	Full: NPs may make referrals for PT.	Full: NPs may make referrals for PT.
Sign death certificates	Full: NPs can sign death certificates.	Restricted: Only a licensed physician can sign death certificates.	Full: NPs can sign death certificates.
Medical staff membership	Full: NPs may join medical staff.	Reduced: The facility's bylaws determine the composition of medical staff.	Full: NPs may join medical staff.

NP, nurse practitioner; PCP, primary care provider; PT, physical therapy.

TABLE 2.3 Common Categories in a Collaborative Practice Agreement

CATEGORY	DESCRIPTION OF CUSTOMARY INFORMATION INCLUDED IN CATEGORY
Demographic information	APRN's name, license, and certification information Primary supervising physician name and practice site
Setting	Unit/clinic where APRN will be practicing
Patient population	Patient population to be served by the APRN, including name of hospital unit/clinic and address
Scope of practice and clinical responsibilities	Employer-specific expectations regarding APRNs' required education and training, requirement to practice commensurate with the acceptable standard of care, maintain awareness of boundaries of competency, and consult other members of healthcare team when boundaries are reached
Phyisician supervision	Physician is ultimately responsible for the provision of high-quality care and must maintain oversight of the APRN
Physician consultation	Delineates acceptable forms of communication (e.g., in-person, telephonic, email) between APRN and supervising physician
Prescriptive authority	Specifies the need for the APRN to maintain DEA licensure and delineates the category of drugs that the APRN can prescribe, per state board of nursing rules
Documentation	Specifies whether the APRN and the supervising physician must maintain evidentiary proof of a signed CPA and interval for renewals
Education plan	Specifies the interval in which the APRN and the supervising physician must meet to review clinical care and quality improvement, as well as documentation required to establish proof of such meetings

CPA, collaborative practice agreement; DEA, Drug Enforcement Administration.

Restricted Practice Authority

Currently, 22% ($n = 11$) of all states (e.g., North Carolina, Tennessee) restrict APRN practice. APRN practice is typically jointly regulated by the state board of nursing and medical board. These states require "career-long supervision, delegation, or team-management by another health provider in order for the NP to provide patient care" (AANP, 2022). Two regulatory restrictions are (a) physician cosignatures for prescriptions written by an APRN and (b) a regulated CPA with a physician (AANP, 2021b). Prescriptive authority is restricted; the Drug Enforcement Administration (DEA) license offers limited prescriptive permissions.

The majority of NNPs practice in the southeastern portion of the United States, where restricted practice is most prevalent. Of all southeastern states, Tennessee imposes the most practice restrictions on APRNs (Myers & Alliman, 2018). APRN applicants must obtain licensure as an RN, provide proof of attainment of a graduate degree in nursing with the appropriate population-specific focus, as well as national certification. Physicians maintain control and responsibility for all prescriptive services provided by an APRN (Tennessee Board of Nursing, 2021). Further, a "certificate of fitness" from the state board of nursing must be obtained prior to obtaining authority to prescribe limited controlled substances. The certificate of fitness is issued with proof of an active and unrestricted nursing license, completion of a master's or doctoral degree in nursing, population-specific national certification, and completion of 45 hours of advanced pharmacology instruction (Tennessee Board of Nursing, 2021). In order to renew the certificate of fitness each year, APRNs must log a minimum of 2 contact hours of continuing education specific to controlled substance prescribing practices, regardless of the APRN's specialty area.

Of note, Florida formerly imposed similarly significant APRN practice restrictions. However, Florida Statute 464.0123, passed in 2020, now permits certain APRNs who practice in a primary care environment to break free from the CPA requirement and establish an autonomous practice. Those who seek this level of independent practice must provide evidence of an unencumbered license, 3,000 physician-supervised practice hours within a 5-year period, and successful completion of graduate-level credits focused on differential diagnosis (three credits) and pharmacology (three credits). At present, NNPs who practice within the inpatient acute care setting in the state of Florida remain subject to practice restrictions.

Restricted practice authority restricts the ability of APRNs to engage in at least one aspect of full APRN practice. State law requires the APRN to maintain a career-long CPA with a qualifying physician and physician supervision or collaboration in order for the APRN to provide patient care.

Reduced Practice Authority

States with limited scope of practice (e.g., Ohio) reduce the ability of APRNs to engage in at least one element of NP practice (e.g., prescribing a specific class of controlled substances, performing a specific invasive procedure). Currently, 26% (n = 13) of these states require one or both of the following: (a) physician cosignatures for prescriptions written by an APRN or (b) a regulated CPA with a physician (AANP, 2021b). In addition, the board of medicine retains partial authority over APRN practice.

Some states have successfully passed statutes that permit APRNs to "transition to independent practice" by logging a specified number of physician-supervised clinical hours. For example, APRNs in Illinois can log 4,000 hours of supervised clinical experience and apply for full practice authority (Chapman et al., 2019). Until 2020, Colorado required APRNs to develop an "Articulated Plan for Safe Prescribing" that "includes a quality assurance plan and mechanism for ongoing consultation with a physician or NP mentor"; however, this is currently optional (Chapman et al., 2019, p. 39).

Reduced practice authority reduces the ability of APRNs to engage in at least one aspect of full APRN practice. State law requires the APRN to maintain a career-long CPA with a qualifying physician or limits the setting of one or more elements of APRN practice.

Full Practice Authority

Full practice authority is the gold standard level of authority for APRNs. In these states (e.g., Washington), APRN practice is regulated by the state board of nursing or the Department of Health, not the state medical board. APRNs can practice to the full extent of their license, population-specific certification, and education. As of November 22, 26 states award APRNs full practice authority (AANP, 2022).

NPs employed in states with full practice authority have greater potential to identify creative approaches for solving healthcare problems (Bosse et al., 2017). For example, Oregon grants full scope of practice to the state's APRNs. NPs in Oregon have had independent practice since the 1970s and were granted prescriptive authority in 1979. In 2013, Oregon passed a payment parity law requiring that APRNs be "paid 100% of what physicians are paid for providing the same services in primary care and mental health" (Chapman et al., 2019, p. 38).

Full practice authority permits APRNs to independently evaluate patients, order diagnostic tests, diagnose, manage treatment plans, and prescribe medications and controlled substances. This authority is under the exclusive purview of the state board of nursing. This is the "gold standard" model recommended by the National Academy of Medicine (formerly IOM) and the NCSBN.

CONSENSUS MODEL FOR APRN REGULATION

Clearly, there are varied levels of APRN practice and prescriptive authority observed across the United States. At present, no APRN can practice across state lines without applying for and maintaining a license in each respective state. This is costly and time-consuming and can be confusing because each state's NPA is unique. Practice and prescriptive authority differ, and continuing education requirements often differ, as do fees and the interval for license renewal. To decrease variation, more than 40 nursing organizations convened with the goal of drafting a regulatory model that would standardize APRN education, certification, and licensure requirements across the United States. After months and years of tireless work, the *Consensus Model for Advanced Practice Registered Nurse Regulation: Licensure, Accreditation, Certification, and Education* (LACE; APRN Consensus Work Group & National Council of State Boards of Nursing APRN Advisory Committee, 2008) was presented to boards of nursing across the United States. To protect patient safety and promote a consistent scope of practice across states, the document aligned graduate program accreditation and education as well as APRN certification and licensure requirements to protect patient safety and promote a consistent scope of practice across states (Hudspeth and Klein, 2019; Kleinpell et al., 2012). Consequently, barriers to nursing practice and nursing care would be permanently retired. Participating state boards of nursing were required the following:

- Limit APRN licensure to graduates of accredited graduate programs who successfully complete a national certification exam, both of which must include curricula specific to the APRN core, role, and population-specific competencies for APRN licensure.
- License APRNs within one of four populations: certified registered nurse anesthetist (CRNA), certified nurse midwife (CNM), clinical nurse specialist (CNS), or CNP when the applicant's education and certification are congruent.
- Remain solely responsible for APRN licensure, eliminating the reach of state medical boards.
- Eliminate temporary APRN licensure.
- License APRNs as independent practitioners (full practice authority).
- Adopt the APRN Compact to allow for interstate recognition of advanced practice registered nursing.

According to policy expert Suzanne Staebler, DNP, APRN, NNP-BC, "[t]his document united APRNs. The goal of the Consensus Model was for full implementation, including legislative pieces, by 2015. Although it was a lofty goal, it gave APRNs a roadmap and common language across specialties to make progress with legislation" (personal communication).

No specific timeline for implementation of all requirements was imposed and, as a result, state boards of nursing were given ample time to incrementally revise their NPA. Over the years, experts have tracked the implementation of the consensus model. At present, all 50 state boards of nursing have *endorsed* the consensus model, making it the guiding document for regulatory purposes. However, not all states have *implemented* the consensus model in its entirety. An interactive map with up-to-date information is available (https://www.ncsbn.org/5397.htm).

APRN Compact

As mentioned in the prior section, states that implement the consensus model should enact laws that permit APRNs to practice within other participating states. Promoting this form of interstate practice for APRNs increases access to care for patients, particularly those living in rural and underserved areas (Chesney & Duderstadt, 2017). Benefits associated with this Compact include

- professional portability with the uninterrupted ability to provide services across state lines (e.g., secondary to a military relocation),
- increased access to healthcare clinicians during crisis or calm,
- increased access to higher education through elimination of barriers to faculty licensing requirements,
- cost containment, and
- retention of state-specific NPAs and associated regulatory autonomy.

Under the current terms of the APRN Compact, APRNs who have accrued a minimum of 2,080 practice hours may be granted a multistate, Compact license (NCSBN, 2021b). At present, North Dakota and Delaware have enacted the APRN Compact; however, 10 states must enact the Compact for it to be considered active in participating states. Ongoing lobbying will be necessary to activate and expand the APRN Compact across all states that adopted the APRN consensus model, as no deadline exists.

The AMA and other organizations, including the American Society of Anesthesiologists and the American Academy of Family Physicians (AAFP), oppose the APRN consensus model and APRN Compact and have spoken out against both pieces of legislation for decades. The basis for their vehement opposition is the elimination of physician oversight as a requisite requirement for APRN practice (Chesney & Duderstadt, 2017). A 2012 report from the AAFP warned against creating a two-class system of healthcare: one that is led by physicians and another led by "less qualified health professionals" (Goertz, 2012, p. 572). In 2013, the AMA launched an unrelenting campaign in favor of restricted APRN scope of practice, at both the state and the national level. Medical professionals argued that APRNs should remain part of a physician-led multidisciplinary team to ensure quality and safety of patient care (AMA, 2013). Members of the AMA are leading efforts to restrict the scope of practice with the belief that the expansion of NP's scope of practice is a threat to patient safety (O'Reilly, 2020).

These efforts certainly altered the perceptions of members of the public and elected officials. Multiple studies demonstrate that APRNs provide equivalent or better care compared with physicians on quality metrics, including physical exams, education/counseling, and medication use (Kapu et al., 2014; Kurtzman & Barnow, 2017). More data are needed to raise eyebrows and convince lobbyists that expanded APRN practice and prescriptive authority benefits communities across the United States.

Further, altered perceptions prompted institutions to develop barriers embedded within credentialing and privileging, which limited APRN scope of practice despite prerequisite education and experience, certifications, and licensure (The Joint Commission, n.d.). These efforts were intended to ensure public safety. However, restricting APRN practice does not necessarily protect the public, particularly in times of crisis. Recall that patient demand for healthcare increased with the onset of the coronavirus disease 2019 (COVID-19) global pandemic. Clinician attrition, secondary to retirements, deaths, and voluntary resignations, left institutions devastatingly short-handed. In response, emergency regulatory legislation and policy changes were enacted to increase the pool of frontline clinicians. In some states, new-graduate APRNs were permitted to enter the workforce immediately after graduation and prior to successfully passing their population-specific national certification examination. The same was true for new graduate RNs. Some states also removed barriers to practice and permitted retirees or those with inactive licenses to return to the workforce. As a result, RNs and APRNs were thrust into a noticeable and value-added role, one that caught the attention of the general public and elected officials.

Now, APRNs are positioned to educate the public about this crucial role during both crisis and calm (Stucky et al., 2021). Empowering nurses at all levels to support healthcare reform is essential to advancing full practice authority within the United States. Realigning organizational credentialing and privileging with state-regulated APRN scope of practice will reduce both practice and prescriptive barriers (Gigli et al., 2018).

APRN PRESCRIPTIVE AUTHORITY

> "Prescriptive authority is not about what your employer requires—it is about what NNPs should do as professionals to safeguard our practice." —Suzanne Staebler, DNP, APRN, NNP-BC

As presented throughout this chapter, prescriptive authority is a key component of APRN scope of practice (NCSBN, 2021a). By definition, prescriptive authority confers permission to prescribe legend (prescriptive) and controlled medications, devices, healthcare services, durable medical and other equipment, and supplies to provide timely, cost-effective, and quality healthcare (AANP, 2020). APRNs are required to maintain state-level prescriptive authority, which is often tied to the APRN license. In addition, some APRNs must maintain a DEA certificate in order to prescribe controlled substances. The extent to which an APRN can prescribe drugs depends on the state NPA and associated statutes. Over time, as more states adopt the consensus model, prescribing practices will become less restricted.

State-Issued Prescriptive Authority

In order to attain prescriptive authority, APRNs customarily must provide the state board of nursing with proof of a current and unrestricted APRN license, CPA (in limited and restrictive states), and in some cases a copy of the DEA certificate (for controlled substances). Prescriptive authority is issued as an adjunct to the APRN license and is renewed with the APRN license. The interval for license renewal varies by state.

Drug Enforcement Administration Certificate for Prescribing Controlled Substances

The DEA regulates prescriptive authority specific to scheduled controlled substances (Table 2.4). APRNs who write prescriptions for controlled substances must have an active DEA certificate, which can be requested upon employment. Prescribers are granted any combination of the following authorities: to prescribe, procure, dispense, or administer controlled substances, which varies by state (Table 2.5). In addition, APRNs are permitted to participate in research and instructional activities specific to the controlled substances approved by the DEA and state statutes.

All DEA numbers begin with the letter *M*, followed by the first initial of the NP's last name and a unique seven-digit number. The registration period for the DEA certificate is 3 years; as of 2020, application and renewal fees cost $888 (DEA, 2020). Some employers reimburse DEA-related expenses, whereas NNPs employed by federal (e.g., military hospital, Veterans Health Administration) or state-operated healthcare facilities may qualify for a fee exemption.

Principles of Ethical Prescribing

APRNs are responsible for maintaining ethical prescribing practices (Table 2.6). However, many neonatal APRNs, nurses, and other neonatal clinicians find themselves morally distressed due to the uncertainties tied to pharmaceutical decisions. After all, most drugs are prescribed off-label in the NICU. In these situations, the desire to know as much as possible about the drug prior to writing the prescription is hindered by a lack of available or sufficient data.

In order to minimize moral distress, APRNs are encouraged to exemplify ethical prescribing practices. First, APRNs should ensure that the drug serves a specific, validated need. Next, shared decision-making that includes the APRN, neonatologist, pediatric pharmacist, and family should be pursued. In addition, proper resources (e.g., Lexicomp, NeoFax) should be consulted when making decisions about dosage, interval, and route. These efforts underpin the ethical principles of beneficence and nonmaleficence, or primum non nocere.

TABLE 2.4 Drug Enforcement Administration Schedule Categories for NICU Patients

SCHEDULE CATEGORY	DESCRIPTION	EXAMPLES
Schedule I	High abuse potential No acceptable medical use in the NICU	Heroin, marijuana
Schedule II/IIN	Schedule II drugs: narcotics Schedule IIN drugs: non-narcotics High abuse potential (both categories) Increased risk for physical dependence (both categories)	Schedule II: morphine, hydromorphone, methadone Schedule IIN: amphetamine, methamphetamine
Schedule III/IIIN	High abuse potential but less than schedule I or II	Schedule III: tylenol with codeine, buprenorphine Schedule IIIN: ketamine
Schedule IV	Drugs with an abuse potential less than those listed in schedule III	Phenobarbital, chloral hydrate
Schedule V	Drugs with an abuse potential less than schedule IV contain limited quantities of certain narcotic and stimulation drugs for antidiarrheal and analgesic purposes	Lomotil, gabapentin

TABLE 2.5 Controlled Substance Authority for Neonatal Nurse Practitioners Per State[a]

STATE	SCHEDULE CATEGORY OF CONTROLLED SUBSTANCES
Alabama	2, 2N, 3, 3N, 4, 5 Prescribe, administer Special permit required for 2/2N
Alaska, Connecticut, Maine, Maryland	2, 2N, 3, 3N, 4, 5 Prescribe, procure, dispense, administer
Arizona	2, 2N, 3, 3N, 4, 5 Prescribe, order, procure, administer
Arkansas	3, 3N, 4, 5 Prescribe, order, administer Hydrocodone products only with a CPA; may be extended to C2 and C2N drugs if in accordance with Arkansas Act 593
California	2, 2N, 3, 3N, 4, 5 Prescribe, dispense, administer Note: Schedule 2 requires continuing education.
Colorado	2, 2N, 3, 3N, 4, 5 Prescribe, procure May dispense and administer samples
Delaware, Idaho, Indiana, Iowa, Minnesota, Mississippi, Montana, Nevada, New Hampshire, New York, North Dakota, Oregon, Rhode Island, South Dakota, Tennessee, Utah, Vermont, Virginia, Washington, Wisconsin, Wyoming, Commonwealth of the Northern Mariana Islands	2, 2N, 3, 3N, 4, 5 Prescribe, procure, dispense, administer
District of Columbia, Guam, Kentucky, New Jersey	2, 2N, 3, 3N, 4, 5 Prescribe only
Florida	2, 2N, 3, 3N, 4, 5 Prescribe, dispense, administer only in accordance with state law
Georgia	3, 3N, 4, 5 Prescribe, dispense, administer
Hawaii, Ohio	2. 2N, 3, 3N, 4, 5 Prescribe, administer
Illinois	2N, 3, 3N, 4, 5: prescribe, dispense, administer Schedule 2: only prescribe 30-day supply
Kansas	2, 2N, 3, 3N, 4, 5 Prescribe, administer, dispense
Louisiana	3, 3N, 4, 5: prescribe 2, 2N: prescribe and dispense for attention deficit disorder only
Massachusetts	2, 2N, 3, 3N, 4, 5 Prescribe, procure, administer
Michigan	2, 2N, 3, 3N, 4, 5 Prescribe Schedule 2 prescribing requires physician authorization letter, renewed annually.[b]

(continued)

TABLE 2.5 Controlled Substance Authority for Neonatal Nurse Practitioners Per State[a] (*continued*)

STATE	SCHEDULE CATEGORY OF CONTROLLED SUBSTANCES
Missouri	3, 3N, 4, 5: administer, dispense, prescribe Schedules 2 and 3: 5-day supply only Schedule 2: only for hydrocodone products CS Rx license and BNDD and professional license needed (CPA)
Nebraska	2, 2N, 3, 3N, 4, 5 Prescribe only
New Mexico	2, 2N, 3, 3N, 4, 5 Prescribe, procure, dispense
North Carolina	2, 2N, 3, 3N, 4, 5 Prescribe, dispense, procure Schedule 2–3N: limited to 30-day supply
Oklahoma	3, 3N, 4, 5 Except CRNAs administer only 2, 2N, 3, 3N, 4, 5
Pennsylvania	2, 2N: 30-day supply 3, 3N, 4, 5: 90-day supply, prescribe only
Puerto Rico	No authority
Texas	3, 3N, 4, 5: prescribe, administer Schedule 2, 2N: limited to prescribing, ordering for hospital/hospice only
Virgin Islands	4, 5 Prescribe, dispense only
West Virginia	2, 2N: prescribe only 3, 3N, 4, 5: prescribe, administer, dispense

[a]Information current as of December 16, 2021. [b]https://www.law.cornell.edu/regulations/michigan/Mich-Admin-Code-R-338-2411.
BNDD, Bureau of Narcotics and Dangerous Drugs; CPA, collaborative practice agreement; CRNA, certified registered nurse anesthetist; CS, controlled substance; Rx, prescription.
Source: From Drug Enforcement Administration (2021). https://www.deadiversion.usdoj.gov/drugreg/practioners/mlp_by_state.pdf.

TABLE 2.6 Customary Duties of a Prescribing Neonatal Nurse Practitioner

LEGAL AND ETHICAL RESPONSIBILITIES
Link the diagnosis to the prescribed medication to establish a medical need for therapy
Discuss the mechanism of action and dosing parameters with NICU pharmacist and other healthcare team members to determine the therapeutic objective of drug therapy
Identify and discuss the benefits and risks of therapy with the healthcare team and family
Use an electronic medical record to prescribe the medication to reduce the risk for error
Discuss the order with the administering nurse and clarify questions, as needed
Follow up with the nurse after the medication is administered to assess patient response
Provide appropriate follow-up and teaching with the family, in particular if a medication is to be continued after discharge

Source: Courtesy of Amy J. Jnah.

Duties of the Licensed APRN Prescriber

Licensed APRNs are obligated to act with beneficence and nonmaleficence, best summarized by the Hippocratic adage *primum non nocere,* or *do no harm.* This precept serves as an important reminder that the pharmacologic decisions APRNs make have the potential to harm vulnerable and preverbal infants. The duties of an APRN prescriber include the following:

- Monitor for safety alerts or recalls linked to drugs commonly prescribed in the NICU.
- Use a shared decision-making model with all prescriptive decisions.
- Link a diagnosis (at least one) to the need for the drug.
- Discuss the mechanism of action, benefits and risks, dosage, route, and length of therapy with the interdisciplinary team, which includes the family (life-threatening emergencies may warrant a modified approach).
- Cross-check dosage decisions with appropriate resources (Lexicomp, NeoFax).
- Communicate the medication order to the administering nurse.
- Clarify questions that the nurse (or the family, if present) may have about the medication.
- Follow up with the bedside nurse after the medication is administered, and over the course of therapy, to assess patient response.

Duties of the Student APRN Prescriber

NNP students are not permitted to prescribe, dispense, or administer drugs, as student learners do not hold the appropriate licensure, permissions, or scope of practice. However, NNP students should be encouraged to discuss drug therapies during medical rounds and privately with preceptors. This helps establish or refine the student's knowledge base and, in doing so, facilitates the role transition from an RN to an APRN. Over time, NNP students learn to integrate scientific knowledge into clinical know-how. Recommended learning behaviors for NNP students include the following:

- Identify a medical diagnosis (at least one) with the indication for pharmacotherapy.
- Discuss the mechanism of action and dosing parameters with the NNP preceptor, neonatologist, or pediatric pharmacist.
- Determine whether the drug will be prescribed on- or off-label.
- Identify the benefits and adverse effects of therapy.
- Communicate the medication order directly with the administering nurse and clarify questions that the nurse (or family, if present) may have about the medication.
- Follow up with the bedside nurse after the medication is administered, and over the course of therapy, to assess patient response.
- Debrief with the preceptor at the end of each clinical shift to identify strengths and weaknesses, so that the student can develop an appropriate study plan in-between shifts.

Providers, both students and licensed APRNs, are clearly obligated to consider myriad factors when prescribing medications; this process may seem daunting for novice clinicians. In these situations, use of a prescriptive decision-making flowchart can help. The OBON recently published an APRN prescribing tool (Figure 2.5). Upon closer inspection, readers will ascertain that this tool can be used in any practice setting, including the NICU. The initial questions—*Is prescribing the drug: (a) within the scope of practice? (b) consistent with the CPA? (c) within the authority of the collaborator? (d) not excluded by the Formulary? (e) in accordance with Ohio and federal law? (f) within a valid patient–prescriber relationship? and (g) if to a family member, does it comply with Ohio Administrative Code?*—force APRNs to pause and consider legal and ethical implications. Then, if conditions are met and the drug is not a controlled substance, the APRN can execute the prescription. However, if the drug of choice is a controlled substance, the flowchart assists the APRN in determining whether the drug may be prescribed (or whether a neonatologist must write the prescription). Student learners are encouraged to create a similar flowchart that aligns with state statutes and DEA permissions.

FIGURE 2.5 APRN prescribing process in Ohio.

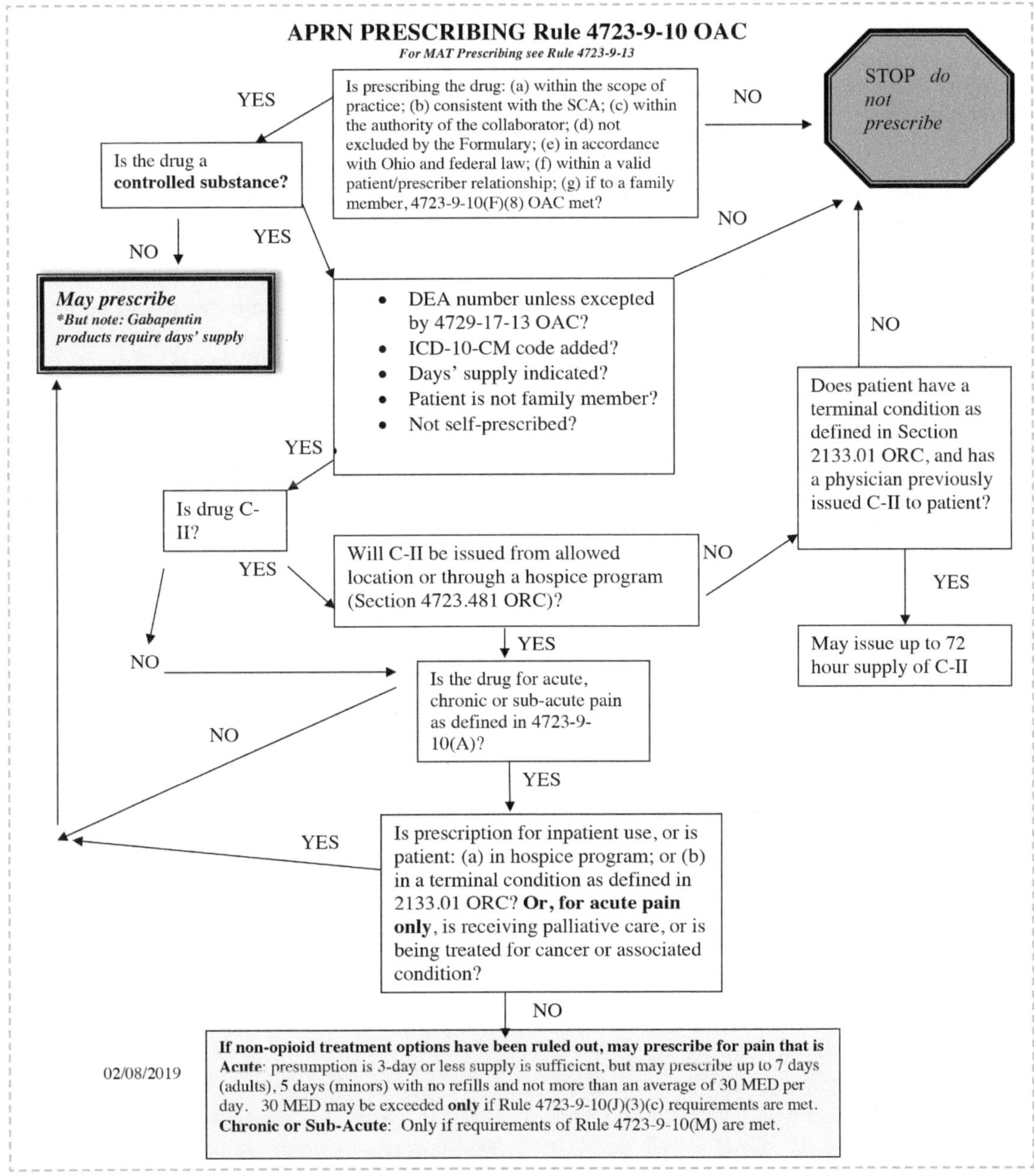

OAC, Ohio Administrative Code; ORC, Ohio Revised Code; SCA, standard care arrangement (also known as *collaborative practice agreement*).
Source: Reprinted with permission from the Ohio Board of Nursing.

CONCLUSIONS

NNPs are highly skilled APRNs who play an integral part in the delivery of acute care services to one of the most vulnerable populations in the healthcare system. Currently, NNPs provide evidence-based, high-quality, safe care in practice environments, including level I to level IV NICUs, critical care transport, and pediatric clinics (Williams, 2019). Given the complexity of the role and the variety of practice environments available to NNPs, it is crucial that we maintain awareness of DEA-regulated and state-specific scope of practice and prescriptive regulations. Practicing outside one's scope threatens the health of our tiniest patients and the work of tireless lobbyists fighting for full practice authority.

It is also important to recognize that many NNPs find themselves in a unique position relative to practice and prescriptive authority, compared with our primary care counterparts. After all, most (but not all) NNPs practice in the inpatient acute care setting. The NICU environment demands the use of a shared decision-making model. For NNPs, this involves career-long consultations with neonatologists, pediatric pharmacists, radiologists, and other pediatric subspecialists, before, during, and after patient rounds. NNPs should not consider this collaborative model commensurate with reduced or restricted practice authority. Rather, this culture of collaboration builds trust among clinicians and embeds valuable checks and balances that optimize quality and safety. Collaboration should not infringe on the APRN's scope of practice or prescriptive authority. Licensing rules and regulations, however, do directly affect the APRN's ability to practice to the full extent of their education, training, and skill, and for this that reason they should be revised accordingly.

In closing, readers interested in supporting efforts to optimize APRN scope of practice and prescriptive authority are encouraged to join their state nurses' association. State-level nursing associations monitor policy and report the status and implications of proposed legislative changes to their membership. Some states employ lobbyists whose main role is to be the representative voice of nurses at the state capital. State nursing associations also educate members on the legislative process and how to best influence policy. These organizations work in harmony with one another to ensure that nurses' collective voices are heard and respected by legislators.

LEARNING TOOLS AND RESOURCES

Advice From the Author

Colleen Moss, DNP, APRN, NNP-BC

The transition from expert nurse to novice nurse practitioner is stressful and challenging. It is humbling to consider the amount of information you learn each day! Your decision to return to school offers you significant opportunities for professional growth and development. Embrace the change; find a mentor who is willing to encourage and challenge you. It's amazing what words of encouragement can accomplish! Practice and prescriptive authority can be complicated, but commit to understanding the rules and regulations of your state. Be an advocate for your patients and your profession.

Discussion Prompts

1. Compare and contrast full, reduced, and restrictive practice authority for APRNs.
2. Discuss the internal and external barriers to achieving full practice authority in all 50 states.
3. Consider the statement: "NNPs need to be involved and active in the advocacy and policy arena for full practice authority." If you live in a state that does not grant full practice authority, how can you engage in advocacy for full practice authority at the local and state levels? If your state grants full practice authority, how can you be a champion for other APRNs?

REFERENCES

References for this chapter are online and available at https://connect.springerpub.com/content/book/978-0-8261-5884-0/part/partI/toc-part/ch2.

chapter 3

Pharmacokinetics and Pharmacodynamics

Amy J. Jnah and Amy P. Holmes

LEARNING OBJECTIVES

After completing this chapter, the reader should be able to:

- Define and explore principles specific to pharmacokinetics (PK) and pharmacodynamics (PD).
- Apply the basic concepts of drug absorption, distribution, metabolism, and excretion to neonatal medicine (gestational age, postnatal age, disease state).
- Describe first-order, zero-order, and one-compartment pharmacokinetics.
- Analyze the concept of adaptive pharmacology as a mechanism used to evaluate the efficacy of various pharmacotherapies prescribed in NICUs.

INTRODUCTION

Two phases of drug–host interactions occur when a clinician, most often a neonatal RN, administers a prescribed, properly dispensed, and verified medication. These phases include the pharmacokinetic (PK) phase and pharmacodynamic (PD) phase. For readers new to these terms, or any complex medical term, a bit of "word anatomy" can help illuminate its meaning. We apply this strategy by breaking the terms *pharmacokinetics* and *pharmacodynamics* into "anatomic" parts. *Pharmaco-* is defined as "relating to drugs" (Box 3.1). The term *kinetic* refers to movement. Therefore, the *pharmacokinetic phase* describes the events that occur from the time the drug is administered, moves into the plasma, and a serum drug concentration is achieved. Next, the term *dynamic* implies change. Therefore, the *pharmacodynamic phase* describes the biophysiological effects that manifest once the drug reaches the target tissues.

An understanding of PK and PD specific to the neonatal population is essential to ensure that dosing regimens for term and preterm infants are safe and effective. Factors, such as genetics, gestational age, weight, and comorbid conditions, must be considered, as these factors often complicate dosing decisions. This chapter describes these core pharmacologic principles and explores how prematurity or critical illness implicate therapeutic regimens.

PHARMACOKINETICS

When clinicians consider drug kinetics, they consider what the body does with the drug, or the processes that occur between when the dose is administered and a drug concentration is achieved. This begins with the absorption and distribution of a drug. Next, a drug may be metabolized. Finally, all drugs are eliminated from the body through the renal or biliary systems (Figure 3.1).

BOX 3.1 Important Terms

Drug: A therapeutic agent (other than food) used in the prevention, diagnosis, alleviation, treatment, or curing of a disease process.

Xenobiotic: A chemical or drug considered pharmacologically (endocrinologically) active but NOT endogenously produced (within the body). Therefore, xenobiotics are foreign to the human body.

Pharmaco-: A combining form that means *relating to drugs*.

Kinetics: A branch of biochemistry focused on measuring and studying rates of chemical or biochemical reactions.

Dynamics: A branch of biochemistry focused on measuring and studying the effect of chemicals on the body.

Therapeutics: The act of preventing and treating disease.

An understanding of PK allows clinicians to answer common questions, including, "What dose should be ordered to achieve the desired effect?" "What route should be used to administer this medication?" "What drug administration interval should be ordered?" and "What unique patient-specific factors could affect the action of this drug at its desired site?" Understanding the PK profile of drugs informs the likelihood of intended effects versus untoward side effects (and toxicity), which helps clinicians determine a drug of choice and concentration (or amount) necessary to exert the desired effect.

For a drug to exert a positive or negative effect, the medication must first enter the body (i.e., intravenous, oral, dermal, rectal, or submucosal route) and then enter the bloodstream. Once in the bloodstream, the drug is distributed and ultimately reaches the site (target tissue or receptor) in the body where it may produce the desired effect. After the drug-receptor interaction, the medication returns to the bloodstream. It is taken to the liver and other organs, where it is metabolized into more easily eliminated substances in the urine or feces.

Drug Absorption

Absorption refers to the movement of a drug across one or more biomembranes, from the site of administration and into the systemic circulation. *Bioavailability* refers to the fraction of the absorbed dose that enters the bloodstream and is available to target tissues/receptor sites.

$$Bioavailability\ (F) = \frac{Concentration\ following\ oral\ dose}{Concentration\ following\ intravenous\ (IV)\ dose}$$

Drugs administered intravenously are considered immediately and wholly (100%) bioavailable; the total dose of the drug directly enters the systemic circulation (without being absorbed through membranes). Intravenously administered drugs are 100% bioavailable because they are *not* subject to hepatic metabolism before reaching the systemic circulation. In comparison, drugs administered extravascularly (e.g., oral, intramuscular, rectal, and percutaneous drugs) must cross multiple membranes through passive aqueous or lipid diffusion or carrier-mediated facilitated transport before reaching the liver and then the systemic circulation. The process of crossing these biomembranes, in addition to location-specific rate-limiting factors, reduces drug bioavailability (Table 3.1). Furthermore, the onset of the drug's effect is contingent upon the absorption rate, which can vary based on blood flow.

Biomembranes consist of fatty acids, and these fatty acids create a lipophilic barrier, which limits the absorption of some drugs. Therefore, the lipid solubility of a drug is the most crucial factor to consider when analyzing drug absorption, distribution, and the ability of the drug to cross the blood–brain barrier. **Lipophilicity** refers to a drug's affinity, or attraction, to body fat. Lipophilic drugs (e.g., fentanyl, morphine, phenobarbital) are highly lipid soluble and can readily

FIGURE 3.1 Absorption, distribution, metabolism, excretion.

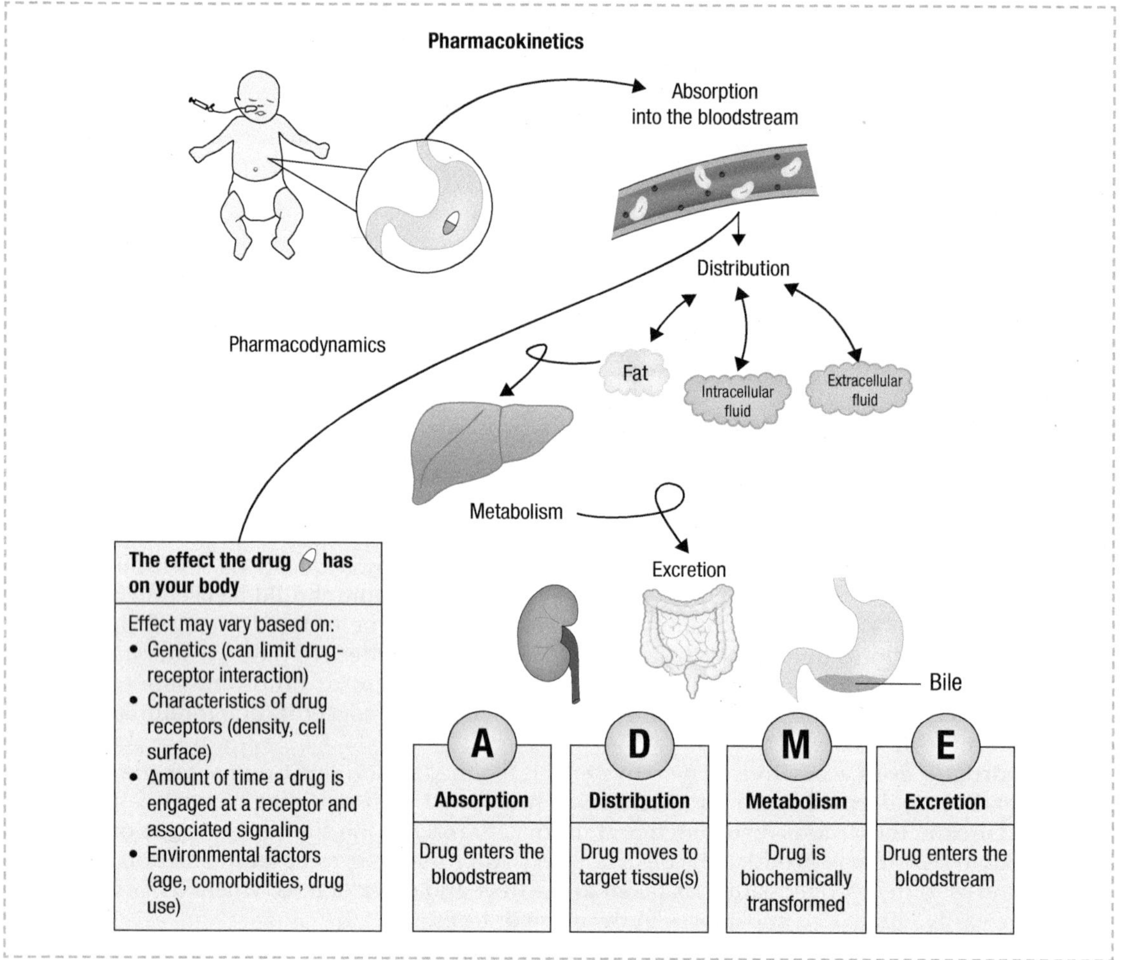

Source: Design credit: Rebecca Judy, MSN, APRN, NNP, East Carolina University College of Nursing, Neonatal Nurse Practitioner Program.

TABLE 3.1 Factors That Affect Drug Absorption and Bioavailability in Neonates

ORAL	TOPICAL	INTRAMUSCULAR	RECTAL/ MUCOSAL	INHALATIONAL
• Gastric pH is elevated • Irregular/delayed gastric emptying time • Reduced intestinal motility and circulation • Immature biliary function (reduced bile acid synthesis)	• Thin stratum corneum • Large surface area: body weight (ratio)	• Decreased muscle mass • Reduced muscular perfusion • Decreased contractility (of muscles)	• Erratic rate of absorption • Risk of injury • Risk of premature evacuation of medication (e.g., suppository)	• Drug volatility • Size of droplets or particles that are administered • Clinician technique • Lung volume

cross biomembranes. As a consequence, a higher volume of distribution occurs. These and other lipophilic drugs cross membranes by one of three kinetic mechanisms: (a) passive aqueous diffusion, (b) passive lipid diffusion, or (c) carrier-mediated transport.

Passive aqueous diffusion refers to the diffusion of a drug through the aqueous phase, using a concentration gradient, from the side of a membrane with a high concentration to the other side with a lower concentration. An example of aqueous diffusion involves the movement of a hydrophilic drug from the capillary bed to the extravascular space. *Hydrophilicity* refers to a drug's affinity, or attraction, to water. Water-soluble (hydrophilic/lipophobic) drugs stay within water compartments and demonstrate a low volume of distribution and poor absorption by surrounding tissues. Examples of water-soluble drugs include aminoglycosides and penicillin. These drugs are readily excreted from the body.

Passive lipid diffusion describes the movement of a drug from a high to a low concentration. The rate at which these lipophilic drugs cross a membrane depends on the concentration gradient, lipid solubility, available surface area, molecular size, and polarity (ionized versus unionized state).

Carrier-mediated transport involves binding a drug to a carrier or transporter for transport across a membrane. Unlike passive transport, carrier-mediated transport can occur up or down a concentration gradient. Facilitated carrier-mediated transport describes movement down a concentration gradient. Active carrier-mediated transport requires adenosine triphosphate (ATP) because activity occurs up (or against) a concentration gradient.

Each of the aforementioned extravascular routes of medication administration is associated with individual rate-limiting factors that affect drug bioavailability. Orally (PO) administered medications are absorbed primarily in the small intestine (Reinus & Simon, 2014). Therefore, gastric pH, brush border enzyme function, and surface area will affect the bioavailability of PO drugs. The newborn gastrointestinal tract is relatively neutral at birth because amniotic fluid is relatively neutral. It is widely accepted that there is a gradual reduction in gastric pH to an average of 1 to 3 over the first 2 weeks of postnatal life (Sage et al., 2014). This initial state of achlorhydria alters oral drug absorption. Basic drugs (unionized) are readily absorbed, whereas acidic drugs (ionized) are poorly absorbed (Reiter, 2002). These factors offer a valid rationale for delaying the administration of PO medications until full enteral feedings are attained and tolerated.

Newborns, in particular preterm newborns, exhibit limited gastrointestinal absorptive capacity due to two factors: decreased brush border enzymes and gastrointestinal surface area. The reduced complement of brush border enzyme concentrations limits functionality, which reduces absorptive capacity. Second, decreased gastrointestinal surface (compared to adults) offers less physical space for drug absorption.

A formerly uncontested and widely accepted rate-limiting factor specific to neonates was gastric motility; for years, experts believed that preterm infants and newborns exhibited delayed gastric transit time compared to children and adults. The belief was that this stalled the absorption of drugs, attainment of a therapeutic drug concentration, and desired clinical effect. However, in 2015, a novel meta-analysis challenged this theory; the results yielded no significant difference in gastric emptying time among preterm neonates, infants, children, and adults (Bonner et al., 2015). Additional studies are indicated to generalize these findings, but, at present, motility is not widely accepted as a primary limiting factor to gastrointestinal drug absorption.

In conclusion, the introduction of enteral feedings helps lower the gastric pH and increases the absorption of some drugs but decreases absorption of others, including acid-labile drugs (e.g., penicillin G, nafcillin). As such, most PO medication regimens are initiated after an infant has an established tolerance for enteral nutrition (Tetelbaum et al., 2005).

Medications administered per rectum (PR) are typically absorbed more slowly than those administered PO. This is attributed to an absence of villi, microvilli, and reduced surface area (the average rectal surface area is 18 cm^2 in infants compared to 230 cm^2 in older children; Hua, 2019). Once introduced into the rectum, the drug is solubilized in rectal fluid and absorbed across a layer of goblet cells (mucus layer) and epithelium. The rate at which the drug is absorbed depends on a few factors, including (a) the formulation (e.g., enema versus suppository), (b) state (lipophilic versus lipophobic), and (c) physiochemical properties (e.g., solubility, size) of the drug. Drug bioavailability is also subject to the position at which the drug is inserted into the rectum and the retention time.

Let's apply these principles to the administration of an acetaminophen rectal suppository (Figure 3.2). If the suppository is inserted further up the rectum, at the region of the superior rectal vein, it will be absorbed and subject to the first-pass effect (covered in more detail later in this

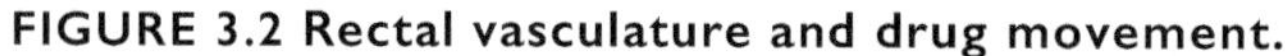

FIGURE 3.2 Rectal vasculature and drug movement.

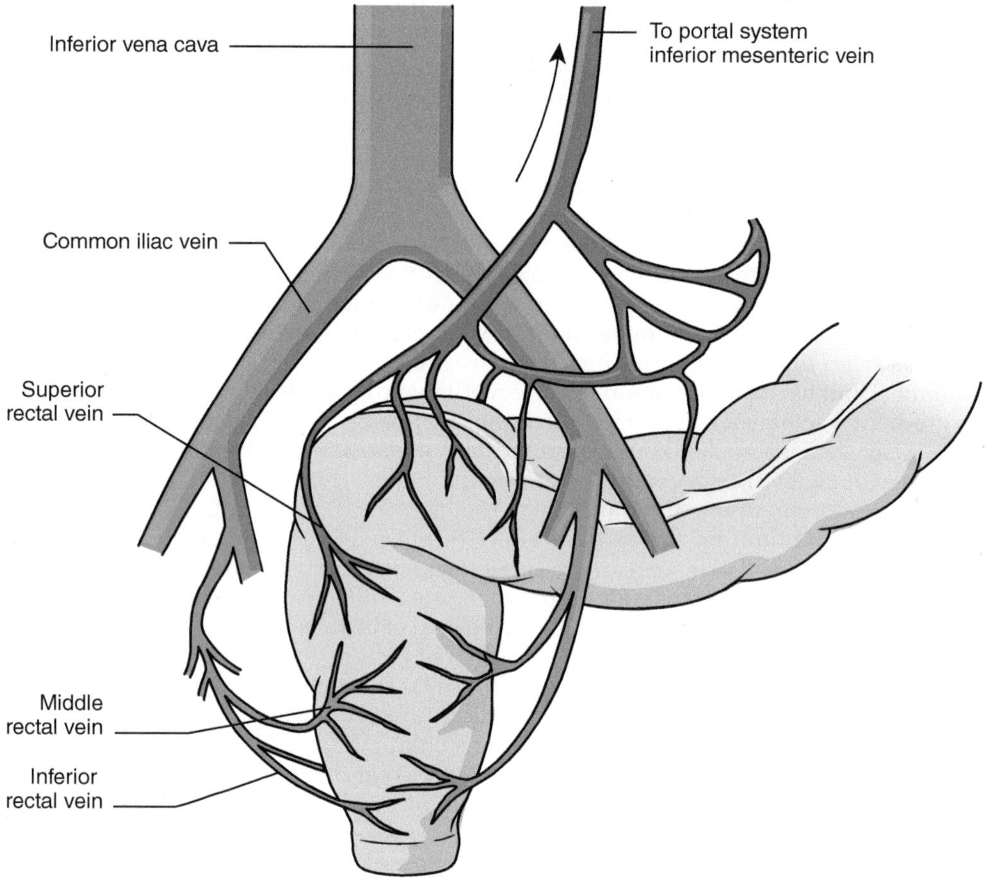

chapter). The drug will travel through the superior rectal vein to the inferior mesenteric vein and portal system (hepatic first-pass effect) before reaching the systemic circulation. On the other hand, a suppository administered at a lower position, at the region of the middle and inferior veins, will be subject to direct transport to the inferior vena cava and systemic circulation, yielding increased bioavailability (Reiter, 2002). Among infants (both preterm and term), rectal drug administration is associated with irregular absorption, an increased risk for trauma to the epithelial membrane, and infection (Jannin et al., 2014). For these reasons, PR medications (e.g., acetaminophen suppositories) may be avoided in NICUs when more reliable routes exist (e.g., intravenous acetaminophen).

Intramuscularly (IM) administered medications are subject to decreased absorption (and bioavailability) secondary to factors including (a) body water content, (b) reduced muscle volume, (c) decreased blood flow to the muscle tissue, and (d) weakened contractile potential compared to children and adults. The absorption rate may be further limited among infants with reduced or absent muscle movement, secondary to prematurity or the use of paralytics (Lim & Pettit, 2019; Yaffe & Aranda, 2011).

Contrary to the aforementioned medication administration routes, percutaneous administration is associated with an increased risk for abundant, rapid absorption. This, of course, increases the risk for unintended drug toxicity. Several factors explain this risk. First, total body surface area (per kg) is increased in infancy compared to childhood and adulthood. Second, hydration at the epidermal layer is increased, which encourages absorption. Third, perfusion to the cutaneous skin layer is increased, which facilitates rapid drug movement into the systemic circulation. Among preterm infants, the thin and immature stratum corneum may permit increased (and potentially toxic) drug absorption.

Drug Distribution

Once a drug is absorbed, it travels throughout the body in fluids (blood, extracellular, lymphatic, or cerebrospinal fluid) and diffuses into target organ tissue(s). Depending on the properties of the drug, it may require binding to plasma proteins or dissolution into body fat to reach the target site. To produce the desired effect, enough drug (concentration) must reach the desired site of action.

Unfortunately, the precise amount of drug that reaches the target site and leads to the desired effect is impossible to measure. However, clinicians can measure the plasma drug concentration and consider this measurement in the context of other factors that affect drug distribution. This plasma drug concentration is regarded as a proportion of the total amount of the drug in the body (before it is metabolized) and referred to as the *volume of distribution* (V_d). The following formula calculates the volume of distribution:

$$V_d\,(\text{L}/\text{kg}) = \text{dose}\,(\text{mg}/\text{kg}) \div \text{plasma drug concentration}\,(\text{mg}/\text{L}).$$

Drugs primarily contained within the intravascular space have a low V_d, whereas drugs that readily diffuse to the tissues have a high V_d. Written differently, a low V_d is associated with an increased amount of drug in the plasma and decreased amount of drug within target tissue(s), excluding the vasculature. A high V_d is associated with a reduced amount of drug in the plasma and increased drug within the target tissue(s).

Among premature and term infants, certain factors affect the V_d. These factors include (a) drug hydrophilicity, (b) drug lipophilicity, (c) drug–protein and tissue binding, and (d) body composition (Table 3.2). As stated earlier in this chapter, *hydrophilicity* refers to a drug's affinity for water. *Lipophilicity* refers to a drug's affinity for body fat. The total body water is estimated at 86% among extremely preterm infants and 78% among term infants (Lindower, 2017). Among newborns classified as appropriate for gestational age (AGA), total body fat is customarily between 10% and 20%. Infants subject to intrauterine growth restriction (IUGR) and who are small for gestational age (SGA) manifest with less than 10% body fat (Schmelzle et al., 2007). Based on these data, neonatal clinicians should recognize that lipophilic drugs do not distribute as readily (decreased V_d) in infants compared to children and adults.

Let's apply these factors to a typical clinical situation: weight-based dosing of aminoglycoside antibiotics. These antibiotics are hydrophilic and diffuse freely in water (high V_d; tobramycin > gentamicin). Generally speaking, the V_d of infants is nearly *twice* that of children and adults. Given that preterm newborns have an increased proportion of extracellular and total body water compared to term newborns, aminoglycoside dosing is highest for the extremely preterm neonate and lowest for the term neonate (Figure 3.3).

Neonates also have a decreased drug–protein binding affinity relative to children and adults. Recall that only unbound drugs can diffuse across membranes and exert a biological effect. Factors that contribute to the observed decrease in plasma protein binding in neonates include reduced albumin and alpha-fetoprotein concentrations, abnormal free fatty acid-to-albumin ratios, acidosis, and neonatal hyperbilirubinemia. Reduced albumin and alpha-fetoprotein concentrations, as

TABLE 3.2 Factors That Commonly Affect Drug Distribution in Neonates

BODY COMPOSITION	PLASMA PROTEIN BINDING	BLOOD–BRAIN BARRIER
• Increased total body water and ECF volume (water-soluble drugs) • Preemies have lowest percentage of body fat (lipid-soluble drugs)	• Reduced in term newborns, even more in preemies • Reduce plasma proteins (especially albumin) for first 10 months of life • Potential for higher levels of free drug in plasma	• Functionally incomplete in neonates (especially preemies) • Penetration favored with lipid-soluble drugs • Some drugs penetrate BBB easier (i.e., meningitis abx, opioids, sedatives)

Note: Drug distribution significantly influences the pharmacodynamics (efficacy) of a drug. Distribution is influenced by drug-related factors (i.e., molecular size and weight, acid dissociation constant), availability of drug transporters and plasma proteins, systemic pH, and tissue perfusion. abx, antibiotics; BBB, blood–brain barrier; ECF, extracellular fluid.

FIGURE 3.3 Clinical application—Volume of distribution of gentamicin in neonates.

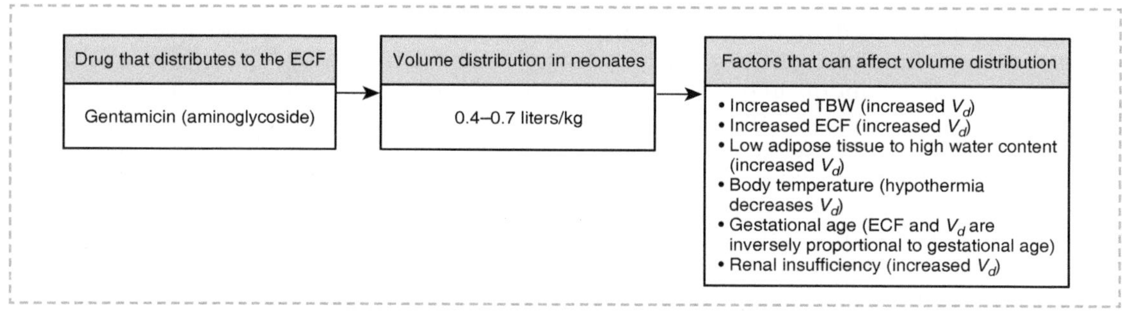

ECF, extracellular fluid; TBW, total body water.

well as fatty acid dissociation from albumin molecules, permit an increase in unbound drug molecules within the systemic circulation, which can exacerbate drug toxicity. Acidosis also favors the dissociation of drug molecules from plasma proteins, which increases the amount of unbound drug molecules in the systemic circulation. Finally, unconjugated bilirubin molecules may compete with drug molecules for albumin, increasing the risk for the accumulation of unbound drug or bilirubin in the bloodstream and associated hyperbilirubinemia or drug toxicity. Drugs known to dissociate bilirubin from albumin (e.g., ceftriaxone) should be used with caution in newborns due to the potential risk for drug-induced kernicterus (Table 3.3; Meyers et al., 2020).

The term *half-life* refers to the amount of time it takes for the concentration of a drug to reduce by half in the body (Table 3.4). As a rule of thumb, *a newly prescribed drug generally takes four to five half-lives to reach a steady-state concentration*. Conversely, it takes approximately five half-lives for near-complete drug elimination to occur. Steady-state concentration is reached when equilibrium is achieved between dose and interval, and the peak and trough serum concentrations do not vary significantly between doses (Figure 3.4). Drugs with a long half-life will take a long time to reach a steady-state; however, using a loading dose can decrease the amount of time it takes to reach a therapeutic concentration (e.g., caffeine, phenobarbital).

Drug Metabolism

Drug metabolism involves the biotransformation of medications by organs within the body. The primary organ for drug metabolism is the liver, but it may also include the gastrointestinal mucosa, skin, kidneys, blood cells, or lungs (van den Anker et al., 2018). This transformation may be necessary to convert an inactive substance into an active substance, such as the case when the prodrug fosphenytoin is converted to phenytoin. Metabolism is most often the process by which the body breaks down medication for elimination. This process may create both biologically active and inactive metabolites. Numerous factors affect drug metabolism and are summarized in Table 3.5.

Drugs administered by the gastrointestinal route are subject to first-pass metabolism (Figure 3.5). This phenomenon occurs when medication absorbed via the gastrointestinal mucosa is carried in the bloodstream through the liver before reaching the target organ. The metabolism that occurs during this "first pass" through the liver accounts for some loss of bioavailability of enterally administered medications. Morphine is a medication subject to first-pass metabolism, resulting in a reduction of bioavailability (e.g., in adults, morphine 10 mg IV is considered equivalent to 30 mg PO due to this first-pass effect). Because these metabolic processes are not developed or are underdeveloped, first-pass metabolism generally occurs less in the neonatal period.

DRUG METABOLISM: PHASES I AND II

Drug metabolism by the liver is divided into Phase I and Phase II. Phase I metabolism refers to biotransformation performed by CYP450 hepatic enzymes and includes oxidation, reduction, hydrolysis, and demethylation (Martin et al., 2020). This process makes molecules more water soluble for urinary excretion. Phase II metabolism matures more slowly than Phase I and includes synthetic conjugation reactions such as glucuronidation, sulfation, glutathione conjugation, and acetylation

TABLE 3.3 Drugs to Use With Caution in Neonates and Infants Through Age 2

DRUG NAME	RISK/RATIONALE	EXPERT RECOMMENDATION
Benzocaine	Methemoglobinemia	Avoid use in infants who are teething or with pharyngitis
Chloramphenicol	Gray baby syndrome	Avoid in neonates unless serum drug monitoring is utilized
Dopamine agonists (e.g., metoclopramide)	Acute dystonia; IV use associated with increased risk for respiratory depression, extravasation, and death	Avoid in infants Use with caution in children
Gentamicin ophthalmic ointment	Severe ocular reaction	Avoid in neonates
Hexachlorophene	Neurotoxicity	Avoid in neonates
Indinavir	Hyperbilirubinemia Nephrolithiasis	Avoid in neonates Avoid in children
Lamotrigine	Serious skin rash	Caution in children; titration needed
Lidocaine 2% viscous	Arrhythmia, CNS depression, death, seizures	Avoid among teething infants
Loperamide	Ileus, lethargy	Avoid in infants with acute infectious diarrhea
Macrolide antibiotics (e.g., azithromycin, erythromycin IV and PO)	Hypertrophic pyloric stenosis	Avoid in neonates EXCEPT if treating *Bordetella pertussis* (azithromycin indicated) or *Chlamydia trachomatis* pneumonia (azithromycin and erythromycin indicated); caution indicated if using for ureaplasma (azithromycin indicated)
Meperidine	Respiratory depression	Avoid in neonates Use with caution in children
Midazolam	Severe IVH, PVL, or death	Avoid in VLBW infants
Naloxone	Seizure	Avoid in neonates for use in postnatal resuscitation
Olanzapine	Hyperlipidemia, hyperglycemia, metabolic syndrome	Use caution with long-term use >2 years in children
Opium tincture	Respiratory depression	Avoid in neonates Use with caution in children
Paregoric	CNS depression, gasping syndrome, hypoglycemia, seizures	Avoid in children
Propofol	Propofol-related infusion syndrome	Avoid doses >4 mg/kg/hr administered for >48 hours
Sodium phosphate solution, rectal (enema)	Acute kidney injury, arrythmia, electrolyte disturbance, death	Avoid in infants
Tetracyclines (e.g., demeclocycline, tetracycline)	Stunted skeletal development and bone growth in preterm neonates (tetracycline use), enamel hypoplasia (tetracycline use), tooth discoloration (demeclocycline and tetracycline)	Use with caution in neonates Use with caution in children <8 years
Valproic acid and derivatives	Fatal hepatotoxicity, pancreatitis	Avoid in infants Use with caution in children <6 years

Note: Data listed in this table were extrapolated from the KIDS List and are associated with high quality of evidence and moderate/strong recommendations by the research team. Low-quality evidence and weak recommendations were excluded.

CNS, central nervous system; IV, intravenous; IVH, intraventricular hemorrhage; PO, by mouth; PVL, periventricular leukomalacia; VLBW, very low birth weight.

Source: From Meyers, R., Thackray, J., Matson, K., McPherson, C., Lubsch, L., Hellinga, R., & Hoff, D. (2020). Key potentially inappropriate drugs in pediatrics: The KIDS list. *The Journal of Pediatric Pharmacology and Therapeutics, 25*(3), 175–191. https://doi.org/10.5863/1551-6776

TABLE 3.4 Drug Half-Life

DECREASE IN SERUM DRUG CONCENTRATION	HALF-LIFE
50% of the peak level	1
25% of the peak level	2
12.5% of the peak level	3
6.25% of the peak level	4 (~94% of the drug is eliminated from the body)
3.125% of the peak level	5 (~97% of the drug is eliminated from the body)

Note: One (1) half-life = the amount of time required for the concentration of a drug to decrease by 50%. This time frame will remain consistent as long as the processes modulating drug metabolism and excretion remain unchanged. **It takes approximately four half-lives for a drug to reach a "steady state."**

Source: From Ito, S. (2011). Pharmacokinetics 101. *Paediatrics & Child Health, 16*(9), 535–536. https://doi.org/10.1093/pch/16.9.535

FIGURE 3.4 Steady state.

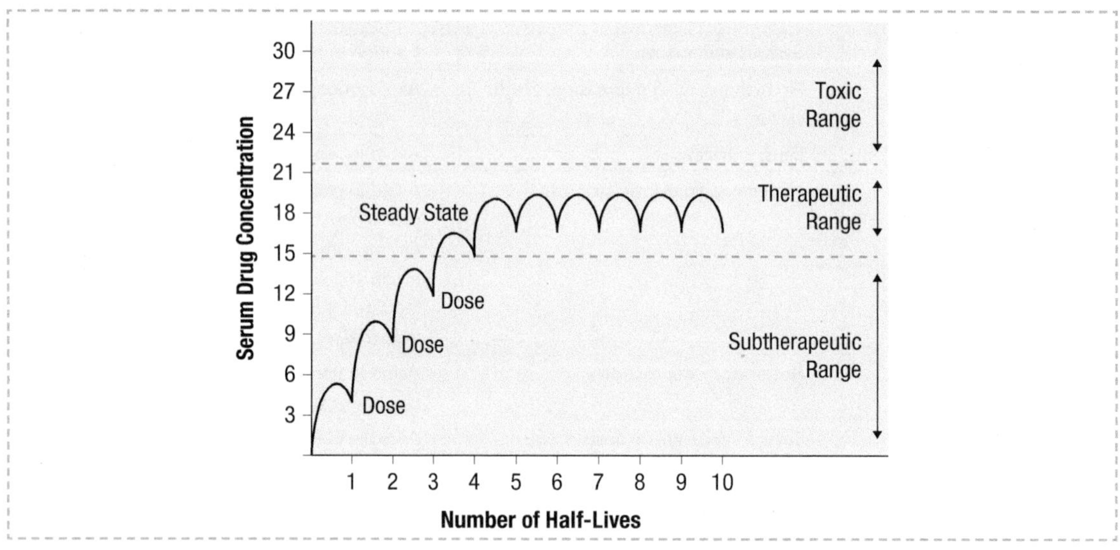

Source: Design credit: Amy Jnah via BioRender.

TABLE 3.5 Summary of Common Factors That Affect Drug Metabolism Across the Life Span

	FETUS	NEONATE	ADULT
Skin	Immature epidermis	Immaturity inversely proportional to GA at birth	Fully keratinized Mature innate defenses
Body composition	Increased TBW Decreased adipose tissue	Increased TBW (decreasing) Decreased adipose tissue (increasing)	Mature (unless disease develops)
Renal function	Low RBF	Low RBF Low GFR Immature tubular function	Mature capacity (unless disease develops)
Hepatic blood flow	Reduced	Closure of ductus venosus alters hepatic BF	All BF from GI tract passes through liver first
Hepatic enzymes	Absent or reduced early in development	Gradual accumulation/ maturation	Mature function (unless disease present)
GI enzymes	Absent/partially present	Present but immature Low absorptive capacity	Mature function
Stomach acid/pH	No acid Neutral pH	Some acid (increases) Neutral pH (decreases)	High acid Low pH

BF, blood flow; GA, gestational age; GI, gastrointestinal; GFR, glomerular filtration rate; RBF, renal blood flow; TBW, total body weight.

FIGURE 3.5 First-pass metabolism.

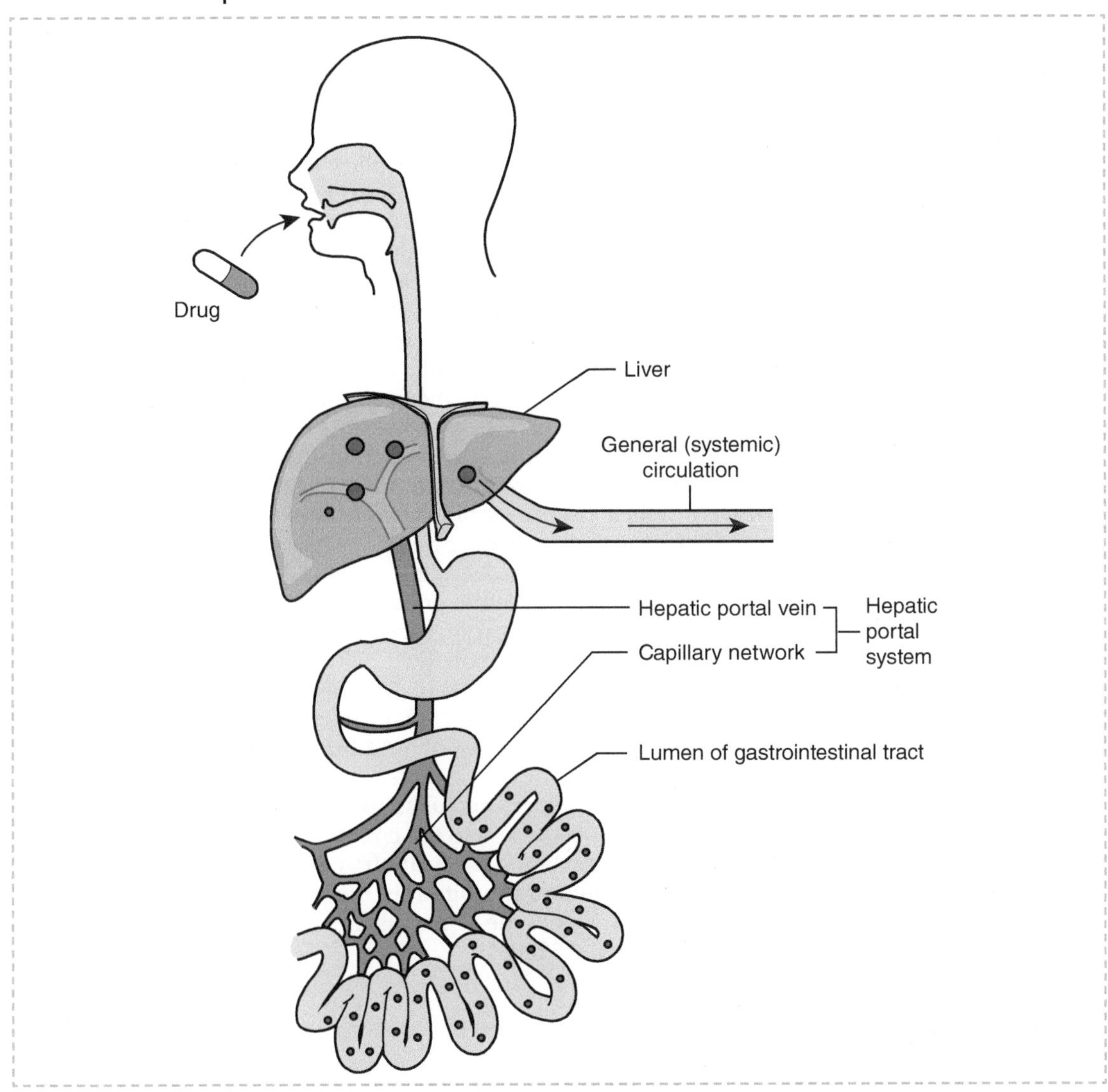

(Martin et al., 2020). These reactions create a more water-soluble moiety that can easily be cleared through renal elimination. The uridine 5′-diphospho-glucuronosyltransferase (UGT) enzyme group performs glucuronidation for approximately one-third of Phase II reactions in adults, but the level of UGT enzymes in children is reduced, affecting drug clearance (Lim & Pettit, 2019). Medications that are metabolized by the UGT enzyme system include acetaminophen, chloramphenicol, and morphine. Chloramphenicol, a broad-spectrum antibiotic previously used to treat sepsis and meningitis in neonates, is a notorious example of toxicity related to immature metabolism. Due to the low activity of UGT2B7, chloramphenicol accumulates in neonates and leads to a significant adverse event known as gray baby syndrome (Table 3.3).

Cytochrome P450 Enzymes

The most well-known enzyme collection is the cytochrome P450 (CYP450) system. The CYP450 system is composed of over 50 isoenzymes (e.g., CYP3A4, CYP1A2), found predominantly in the hepatic system, which are responsible for the biotransformation of most medications during Phase I drug metabolism. CYP450 expression varies across fetal and postnatal life. Some enzymes are abundant during fetal development, whereas others are not expressed until after birth. This observed variance, particularly among the CYP enzymes responsible for the bulk of drug biotransformation, can alter the disposition of drugs in neonates. Clinicians may observe a failed response to therapy, signs of drug toxicity, or unique drug–drug reactions that threaten physiologic homeostasis. We explore this concept of CYP450 maturation, given its significance to prescribing practices within the neonatal population. The enzymes we focus on include CYP3A4, CYP3A7, CYP2E1, and CYP1A2 (Figure 3.6).

CYP3A4 is found within the hepatic system and is the primary enzyme responsible for the biotransformation of at least 50% of drugs prescribed to neonates (Lim & Pettit, 2019). Drugs that require CYP3A4 include fentanyl, midazolam, and sildenafil. CYP3A4 is also responsible for the biotransformation of endogenously produced substances, for example, cortisol. The ontogeny of CYP3A4 is noteworthy in that levels are *very low* across fetal development. Enzyme expression slowly increases beginning after birth; therefore, the low circulating CYP3A4 in the neonatal period and most of infancy reduces drug clearance. Levels slowly increase over the first year of life and reach 50% of adult function by 1 year (de Wildt et al., 1999; Lacroix et al., 1997). Neonatal clinicians must understand that although CYP3A4 levels increase postnatally, certain drugs (e.g., dexamethasone, phenobarbital) can upregulate CYP3A4 expression (Vital Durand et al., 1986). This will increase drug biotransformation and clearance, lowering serum drug levels to potentially subtherapeutic levels. Other drugs can inhibit the expression of CYP3A4 (e.g., erythromycin, not commonly prescribed in the NICU), which decreases biotransformation and risks toxicity. It is essential to pause and consider these factors before dosing decisions are made.

Unlike CYP3A4, CYP3A7 is the most abundant isoenzyme present during fetal development and immediately after birth. CYP3A7 is a fetoprotective enzyme; this enzyme can catalyze the breakdown of substances, such as retinoic acid, and protect the fetus from what otherwise could be toxic exposure to maternal drug therapy with retinoic acid. CYP3A7 levels peak during the third trimester and then decline to adult levels shortly after birth. Concurrently, CYP3A4 enzymes increase and assume the primary role of catalyzing the biotransformation of substrates and drugs. Of note, CYP3A7 can metabolize the same substrates as CYP3A4 but less efficiently, making this postnatal shift in enzyme levels quite protective for the neonate.

CYP2E1 expression begins in the second trimester and substantively increases after birth (Johnsrud et al., 2003). The extent to which CYP2E1 is present in the circulation is contingent upon gene expression and advancing postnatal age, not gestational age at birth. As with other CYP enzymes, CYP2E1 expression can be affected (upregulated or inhibited) in the presence of xenobiotics. Specific to neonates, adequate expression of this enzyme is necessary for the biotransformation of acetaminophen to its toxic metabolite (Bolt et al., 2003).

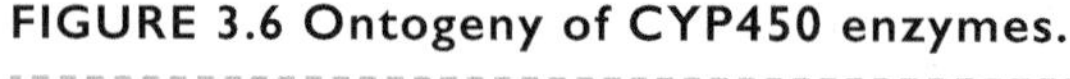

FIGURE 3.6 Ontogeny of CYP450 enzymes.

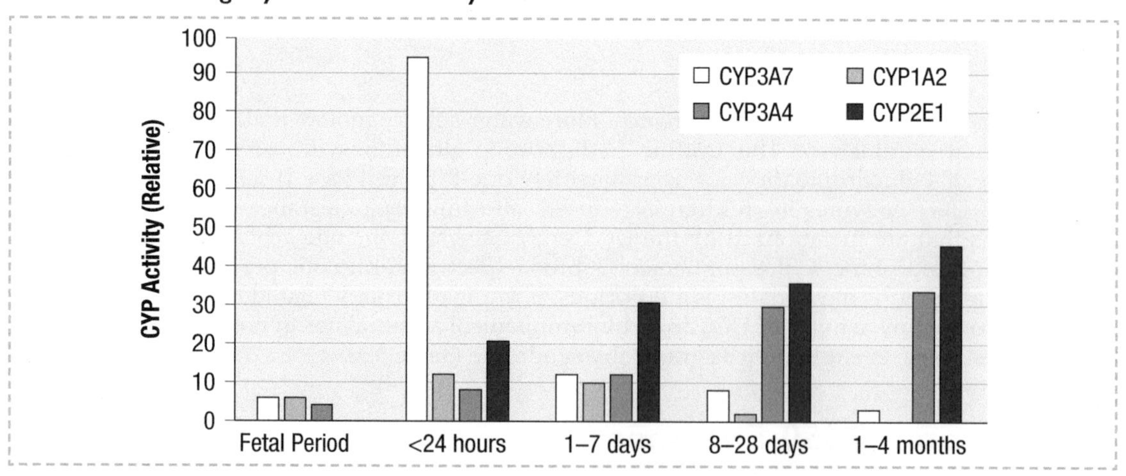

Note: This graph offers a visual depiction of changes in CYP450 enzyme levels over time, from fetal development to 4 months postnatal age. The relative activity reflected in the graphic is estimated (based on original data from Crestell, 1998) and only intended for conceptual learning purposes.

Source: From Blake, M. J., Castro, L., Leeder, S., & Kearns, G. L. (2005). Ontogeny of drug metabolizing enzymes in the neonate. *Seminars in Fetal and Neonatal Medicine, 10*(2), 123–138. https://doi.org/10.1016/j.siny.2004.11.001

CYP1A2 is expressed within the hepatic system and nearly entirely (90%) responsible for the biotransformation and clearance of caffeine (Kalow & Tang, 1993). Very little CYP1A2 is noted in the fetal liver and the immediate postnatal period. In fact, adequate enzyme expression is not observed until 4 months postnatal age (Sonnier & Cresteil, 1998). Similar to CYP3A4, certain drugs can either exacerbate or inhibit the expression of CYP1A2. Phenobarbital and omeprazole are known to upregulate CYP1A2 expression, whereas erythromycin and a diet that includes human milk inhibit enzyme expression. Recall that erythromycin similarly inhibits the expression of CYP3A4. A human milk diet is associated with prolonged caffeine clearance, leading scientists to conclude that dietary choices also influence enzyme activity (Blake et al., 2004).

Given the essential function of the CYP450 system and maturational changes in individual enzyme levels across fetal development and postnatal life, let's apply this information to a common clinical situation. Neonates at risk for bronchopulmonary dysplasia or who manifest with apnea of prematurity are often treated with caffeine. CYP1A2 and CYP2E1 hepatically metabolize caffeine (Aranda & Beharry, 2020). Recall that both CYP1A2 and CYP2E1 enzymes are deficient for the first several months of life. As a result, biotransformation is decreased, and neonates excrete 85% of the caffeine they receive unchanged in the urine.

In contrast, adults excrete 2% unchanged caffeine in the urine. The reason for this is the deficient state of CYP enzymes in neonates compared to adults. This explains why the half-life for caffeine is prolonged in neonates (20–99 hours) compared with adults (5 hours; Taketomo, 2023).

Drug Elimination

Drug elimination (or excretion) removes drugs and any metabolites from the body by organs, primarily the kidneys and, to a lesser extent, the gastrointestinal tract. The majority of drugs administered to neonates are eliminated by **first-order kinetics**. In these circumstances, a constant proportion (or fraction) of drug molecules are eliminated per unit of time. Therefore, since the proportion or fraction of the eliminated drug is constant, increasing the dose will result in a proportional increase in elimination.

In contrast, when the elimination rate is constant per unit of time, the rule of **zero-order kinetics** applies (Figure 3.7). In these situations, any excess drug molecules will exhaust the capacity of hepatic enzymes and/or drug transporters while a constant amount of drug is eliminated per unit of time. Drugs, including caffeine and furosemide, exhibit zero-order kinetics when administered at therapeutic doses. Interestingly, phenytoin exhibits first-order kinetics when administered at low doses and switches to zero-order kinetics when administered at high doses; therefore, close monitoring of serum concentrations is indicated when the dosage is increased to the upper limit of the dosing range.

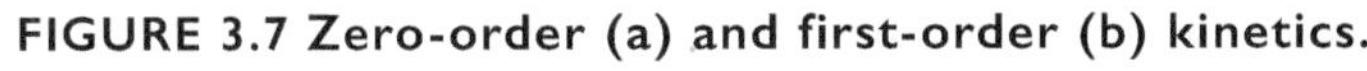

FIGURE 3.7 Zero-order (a) and first-order (b) kinetics.

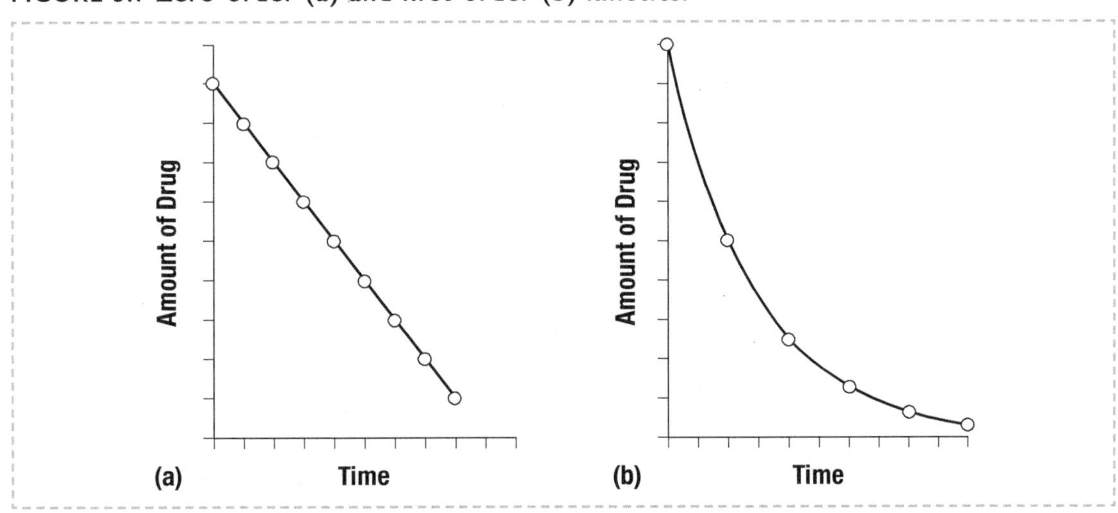

Source: From Raffa, R. B. (2010). Drug disposition and response. In J. Boullata & V. Armenti (Eds.), *Handbook of drug-nutrient interactions* (pp. 27–43). Humana Press. https://doi.org/10.1007/978-1-60327-362-6_2

The kidneys remove drug molecules and drug by-products by glomerular filtration or tubular secretion, both of which are immature at birth (Lim & Pettit, 2019). Nephrons become functional as early as 8 weeks of gestation, and formation of the kidney is considered complete at 36 weeks' gestational age (Jnah & Trembath, 2019). However, term infants have a glomerular filtration rate (GFR) 50% lower than adult levels, and preterm infants may display as little as 1% of adult GFR, given that preterm birth interrupts nephrogenesis (Guignard, 2017; Muhari-Stark & Burckart, 2018). GFR reaches adult levels in term infants by 6 to 12 months of age and 2 years of age among infants born preterm (Guignard, 2017). Drugs that are eliminated by glomerular filtration include aminoglycosides and vancomycin. Tubular secretion, which plays a less significant role in drug excretion, reaches adult capacity by 1 year of age (Lim & Pettit, 2019). Examples of medications eliminated by tubular secretion are furosemide, morphine, and penicillin.

Blood enters the glomerulus by way of the afferent arteriole. Structurally, the glomerulus consists of a network of capillaries, which accept the inflow of blood from the afferent arteriole and distribute that blood across the glomerular membrane. Blood is selectively filtered across the glomerular capillary wall, basement membrane, and Bowman capsule; the remaining filtrated plasma enters the Bowman capsule. The rate at which blood is filtered is contingent upon several factors: (a) blood flow into the glomerulus; (b) differences between osmotic pressure within the capillary bed and hydrostatic pressure within the glomerulus; and (c) available surface area for filtration, glomerular capillary permeability in particular, at the basement membrane. Disease states (e.g., asphyxia, acute hemorrhage, hypertension, hypotension/shock, left-to-right patent ductus arteriosus), prematurity, and drugs may pathologically alter any factors mentioned previously and increase or decrease GFR. Angiotensin-converting-enzyme (ACE) inhibitors (e.g., captopril, enalapril) and nonselective cyclooxygenase inhibitors (e.g., ibuprofen) are known to decrease the GFR. On the contrary, methylxanthines (e.g., caffeine) increase osmotic pressure at the capillary membrane, GFR, and urinary output (Gillot et al., 1990). Given that GFR cannot be directly measured, neonatal clinicians consider creatinine clearance as a surrogate. Under normal circumstances, creatinine is excreted at the same rate at which it is produced. Therefore, a normal creatinine level suggests normal glomerular filtration.

Clinicians must consider factors unique to preterm infants when analyzing creatinine as an index of renal function. First, fetal creatinine levels reach equilibrium with maternal values during pregnancy, and, as a result, creatinine levels in newborns reflect maternal levels immediately after birth (Guignard & Drukker, 1999). Among preterm infants weighing less than 1.5 kg at birth, creatinine levels continue to increase over the first few days of life. This transient increase is attributed to increased reabsorption in the renal tubule secondary to temporarily "leaky capillaries." Tubular function normalizes over the following month of postnatal life, and creatinine levels recede toward normal neonatal values (Guignard & Drukker, 1999). Second, creatinine clearance is a less reliable marker of GFR in the setting of renal failure. Recall that creatinine is typically distributed in body water and, to a small degree, in the gut. However, creatinine accumulates in the setting of renal failure, given the decrease in GFR. In this circumstance, creatinine deposition within the gut may increase as a compensatory mechanism to reduce serum concentrations, masking its presence with routine renal function testing. In these situations, creatinine levels overestimate GFR (Guignard, 2017).

ADAPTIVE PHARMACOLOGY

Given that gestational age at birth and many disease states affect the PK and PD of drug therapies, neonatal APRNs must be prepared to observe the efficacy and kinetics of prescribed drugs. The process by which clinicians establish therapeutic goals, select a therapeutic agent, determine a dosing regimen, observe the infant's clinical and biochemical response to therapy, and adjust pharmacotherapies can be referred to as *adaptive pharmacology* (Figure 3.8). Based on the infant's clinical presentation and outcome of the diagnostic reasoning process, clinicians will establish a therapeutic goal. A drug is selected based on the therapeutic goal, infant's gestational age, risk factors, and disease process. When logistically feasible, the neonatal APRN, pharmacist, neonatologist, family, and allied health clinicians (i.e., neonatal dietician, respiratory therapist, clinical nurse) will collectively discuss the drug of choice, risks, benefits, and alternatives. In the absence

FIGURE 3.8 Principles of adaptive pharmacology.

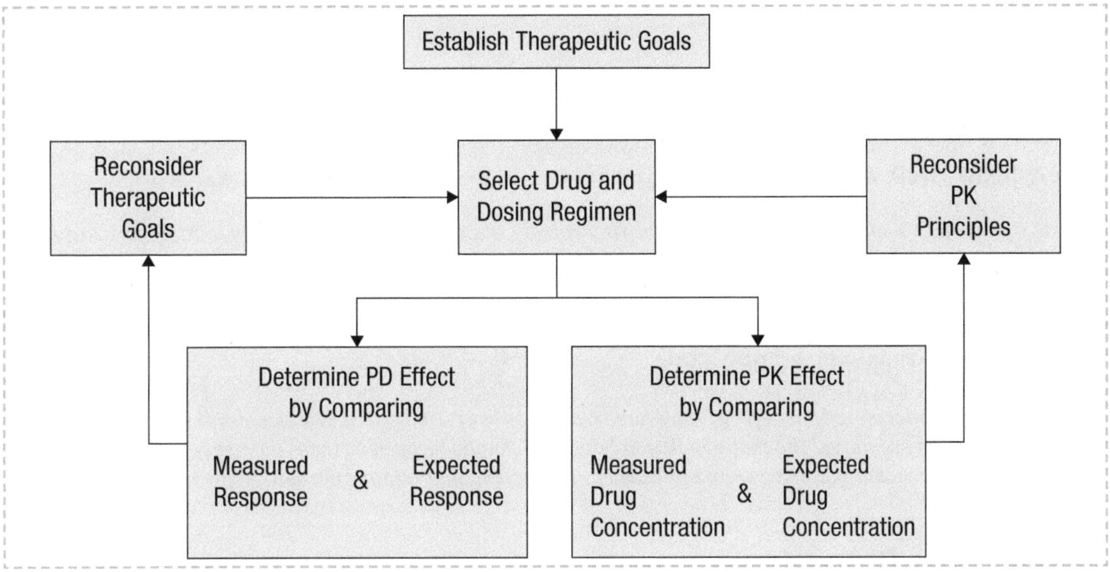

PD, pharmacodynamic; PK, pharmacokinetic.
Source: Design credit: Amy Jnah via BioRender.

of a robust pharmacy team, tertiary references or local drug monographs that consider emerging PK and dynamics should be consulted. Once the therapeutic agent is administered, drug efficacy is appraised based on the infant's observable response to the therapy (i.e., vital sign monitoring and physical, radiographic, or biochemical examination). In neonatal intensive care, serum drug concentrations inform the kinetics of a prescribed drug. This limited PK profile reduces iatrogenic blood loss.

CORE PRINCIPLES OF PHARMACODYNAMICS

Pharmacodynamics refers to the relationship between a pharmacologic agent and a physiologic or biochemical effect. Simply stated, clinicians consider "what the body does with the drug." A drug's effect on the human body will vary based on several factors. Genetic factors may limit drug-receptor interactions. The density and cellular surface of drug receptors can affect the efficacy of a drug. Further, the length of time a drug is engaged at a receptor may affect associated signaling and alter drug efficacy. In addition, environmental factors, including age, the presence of comorbidities, and even exposure to secondhand smoke, can alter the PD of a drug.

The therapeutic range is a window framed by the minimum serum concentration at which a medication is known to exert an effect and the range at which toxic effects are observed. Toxic effects of medications, which occur when excessive amounts of a substance are present, should not be confused with adverse drug effects, which can present at any point on the therapeutic spectrum.

CONCLUSIONS

PK, what the body does to drugs, differ in neonates due to their different body composition and organ immaturity. Likewise, PD, what the drug does to the body, differs for similar reasons. Understanding these principles will lay a foundation for optimal medication use in the neonatal population.

LEARNING TOOLS AND RESOURCES

Advice From the Authors

Amy J. Jnah, DNP, APRN, NNP-BC

Be sure you achieve a solid understanding of the concepts discussed in this chapter before moving forward in this textbook. Then, cycle back to this chapter as you read about disease processes and pharmacotherapeutics. This cycling of curricular concepts will help you establish easily retrievable memories! And last, DRAW! Take the time to draw out complex concepts. This activity will pay great dividends!

Amy P. Holmes, PharmD, BCPPS, FPPA

Sometimes these concepts are just "facts" you have read until you see them in practice. I call them "light bulb" moments when you see in real life that which you have read about. Be open to those moments and revisit the material to reinforce what you have seen and learned. It will help you retain information for the future.

Discussion Prompts

1. Based on what you have learned about caffeine metabolism, are there scenarios when twice-daily dosing may become necessary? If so, what might affect metabolism in a way that would require this dosing change?
2. Based on what you have learned about half-lives, how long of a washout period would you need before starting a corticosteroid (e.g., dexamethasone for ventilation weaning protocol) after a course of indomethacin for patent ductus arteriosus closure if the half-life of indomethacin is ~ 30 hours?
3. What are some potential pitfalls of using a pediatric or adult dosing guide to estimate dosing for the neonatal population based on some of the differences you have learned in PK/PD of neonates (e.g., think about morphine, which is subject to a sizeable first-pass effect in older children and adults, or gentamicin, which is hydrophilic and excreted through renal elimination)?

Mind Map

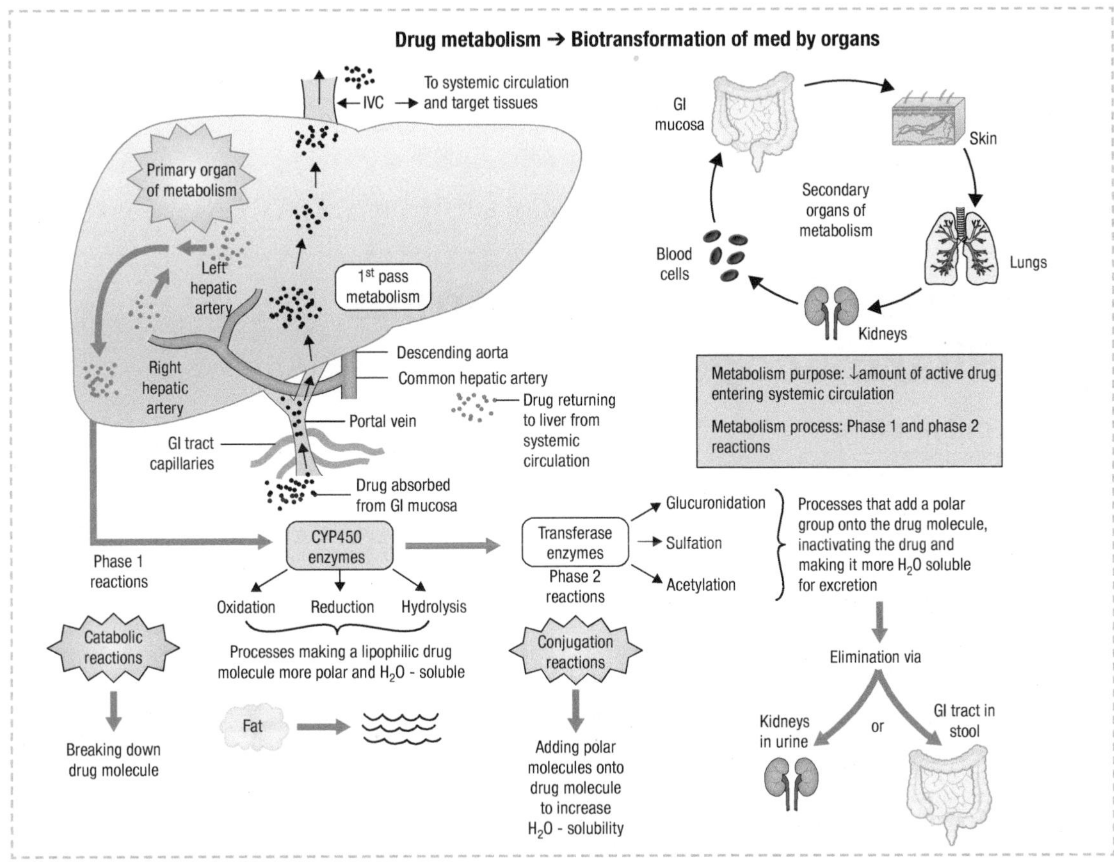

Note: This mind map reflects the design team's interpretation of a portion of one or more concepts addressed in this chapter. Readers should regard the mind maps woven throughout this textbook as examples of multisensory study tools that can be developed to encourage conceptual understanding. Readers are encouraged to develop their own unique mind maps in consultation with academic faculty or clinical preceptors. Design credit: Joanna Reynolds, MSN, APRN, NNP, RNC-NIC, RNC-LRN, RNC-mNN, East Carolina University Neonatal Nurse Practitioner Program.

REFERENCES

References for this chapter are online and available at https://connect.springerpub.com/content/book/978-0-8261-5884-0/part/partI/toc-part/ch3.

chapter 4

Neonatal Pharmacogenomics and Pharmacogenetics

William Diehl-Jones

LEARNING OBJECTIVES

After completing this chapter, the reader should be able to:

- Define *pharmacogenetics* (*PGe*) and *pharmacogenomics* (*PGx*).
- Describe causes of interindividual and interpopulation variability in neonatal drug response.
- Discuss the basic mechanisms of transcription and translation.
- Define the following: *phenotype, haplotype, single nucleotide polymorphisms, tandem number variable repeats, polymerase chain reaction,* and *restriction fragment length polymorphism.*
- Describe polymorphism types and their impact on pharmacokinetics and pharmacodynamics.
- Analyze current methods of PGe and PGx testing.
- List clinically significant PGe variants involved in differential drug responses in neonates.
- Discuss the potential of model-based tools for integrating genetic data with neonatal prescribing.

INTRODUCTION

Drug therapy is a mainstay in the treatment of most diseases; however, there is a wide variation in drug response among individuals. In fact, among the adult population, only 25% to 80% of individuals respond beneficially to a given drug therapy (Twycross et al., 2015). Furthermore, some individuals respond adversely to drug therapy. Most of these variations are secondary to pharmacokinetic processes, including absorption, distribution, protein binding, and elimination, although pharmacodynamic processes such as drug-receptor binding also account for variability in drug response.

In the neonatal population, a further complication exists; according to a comprehensive 2013 review (Hsieh et al., 2014), of the 10 most commonly used drugs in NICUs, which include anti-infectives, surfactant, caffeine, furosemide, dopamine, fentanyl, and midazolam, only one—surfactant—was developed specifically for neonatal use. Although a necessary tenet of neonatal care, according to a one-decade-old estimate, up to 90% of medications prescribed for neonates are either unauthorized, unapproved, or off-label (Tayman et al., 2011). What may be surprising is that this estimate has changed little in more recent times (Costa et al., 2018). One other drug not on this list—nitric oxide—was initially targeted for neonatal use, but with respect to most pharmacotherapeutic applications neonates have the dubious distinction of being "therapeutic orphans" (Lewis & Leeder, 2018).

Although physicians and nurse practitioners in the NICU have become adept at prescribing these drugs for neonates, in comparison with other mainstay therapies, such as ventilation, infection control, and surgery, it must be admitted that neonatal pharmacotherapeutics lag behind (Lewis & Leeder, 2018). An existential problem has been the wide interindividual variability in drug response in the neonatal population (Tayman et al., 2011). This at times has made the determination of safe and effective drug doses challenging, although there have been advances in our understanding of the factors that cause such variability (van den Anker et al., 2018). Aside from the aforementioned problem of necessary off-label and unauthorized drug use, we can attribute the essential challenges of neonatal pharmacotherapeutics to three factors: (a) infant health, (b) developmentally related changes in pharmacokinetics (PK) and pharmacodynamics (PD), and (c) genetic heterogeneity that can affect drug PK and PD.

This chapter focuses on the influence of genetics on PK processes (absorption, distribution, metabolism, and elimination) and PD (a drug's effects on the body, often mediated via drug–receptor interactions). The two terms often interchangeably used to describe these fields are *pharmacogenetics* (*PGe*) and *pharmacogenomics* (*PGx*). As will become evident, there are subtle differences between these terms, but the unifying concept underpinning both these fields is that variations in a gene may affect either PK or PD, and in turn affect drug efficacy and/or toxicity.

PK and PD in the context of the neonate were reviewed in Chapter 3, "Pharmacokinetics and Pharmacodynamics." However, given the importance of developmental processes on both PK and PD, we begin this chapter with another, albeit briefer, overview of developmental variations in PK and PD that can influence drug response in neonates. This is followed by a more fulsome definition of PGe and PGx. This chapter is written with the nonspecialist in mind, such that the reader who does not have a background in genetics will find the concepts easy to comprehend. Thus, I summarize some of the foundational principles and concepts underlying genetic variations in drug responses, and from there review some of the current methodologies used in PGe and PGx research. We then consider the current state of PGe and PGx related to neonates and identify genes of specific interest to the neonatal prescriber. Finally, we consider the current and future state of neonatal PGx and discuss the feasibility of routine genomic sequencing in the NICU and the potential of using combined physiologic and genetic models as a means of individualized pharmacotherapy for neonates.

DEVELOPMENTAL VARIATIONS IN PHARMACOKINETICS AND PHARMACODYNAMICS

It is well understood that neonates are unlike adults with respect to drug prescribing. Simply scaling down drug dosing used for adults is unreliable, owing to developmental variations in both PK and PD processes. Ruggiero et al. (2019) presented an excellent review of neonatal pharmacology, and rather than recapitulate the contents of their paper we summarize some of the key points, which we will subsequently relate to PGe and PGx. The neonatal period is generally considered to include the first 28 days of life in term infants and up to 44 weeks of age in preterm infants (Ruggiero et al., 2019). There is a wide variation in the anatomic and physiologic maturity of many organ systems. As a consequence, genetic variations notwithstanding, these physiologic differences can have significant impacts on both PK and PD processes. This of course further complicates the impact of inborn genetic differences, and any PGx analysis must be based on an understanding of the developmental trajectories of maturing organ systems before genomic differences can be addressed. In the proceeding sections, the developmental variables affecting PK and PD are summarized.

As depicted in Figure 4.1, PK processes are impacted by a variety of factors in the neonate. Of all the PK processes, enteral absorption is most dependent on the maturity of the gastrointestinal (GI) tract of neonates (Neal-Kleuver et al., 2019). Drug absorption may be either delayed or accelerated, depending on factors such as GI pH and motility. There have been many studies on neonatal GI pH, dating from the early 1950s to the present era (Barbero et al., 1952; Palla et al., 2018; Ruggiero et al., 2019). Although there is poor consensus among studies on average GI pH in preterm (<37 weeks'

FIGURE 4.1 Developmental variability in neonatal pharmacokinetics.

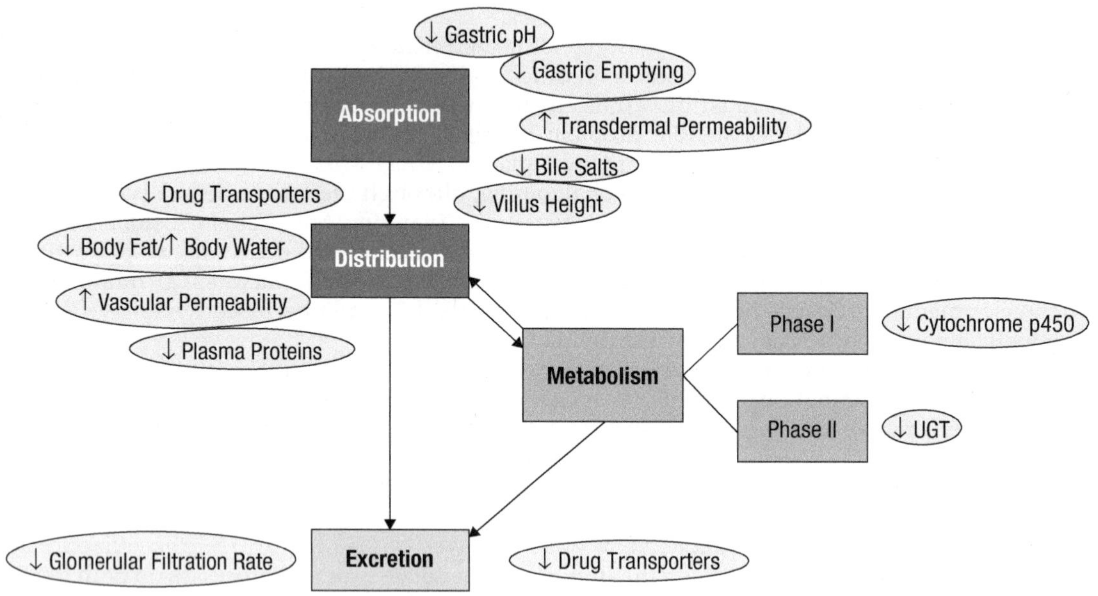

UGT, uridine glucuronyl transferases.

gestational age) and term (>37 weeks' gestational age) infants, on average, gastric pH is less acidic in preterm infants than in full-term infants, which in turn is less acidic than in adults. Gastric pH can affect the ionization state of a drug; for example, indomethacin, which is sometimes used to treat a patent ductus arteriosus (PDA), is a weak acid. Such drugs become less ionized in a more neutral pH and therefore may be better absorbed. If drug dosage is based on an adult model, a simple scaling back of dosage based on body mass could result in a higher-than-anticipated plasma level. Delayed GI emptying, lower bile salt production, and decreased villus height also affect drug absorption, although this can depend on drug pKa (acid–base dissociation constant). For example, lower stomach acidity facilitates the uptake of drugs that are weak acids, whereas the reverse is true of basic drugs. In contrast, transdermally administered drugs are typically better absorbed in preterm neonates owing to low keratinization and a thin hypodermal layer (Ruggiero et al., 2019). One drawback is that topical agents, such as povidone-iodine, can cause iodine toxicity (Mancini, 2004).

Drug distribution is also altered in neonates, depending on drug ionization state, molecular weight, and lipid solubility. Preterm infants in particular have a greater percentage of total body water, thus allowing for a greater volume of distribution of lipophobic drugs (Modi, 2003). The implication of this physiologic property is that some drugs need to be administered at higher weight-based doses to reach therapeutic levels (Smits et al., 2013). Drug transporters, such as P-glycoprotein, which we return to when discussing PGe variability in neonates, also show a marked ontogenic functionality in the intestine and lungs (van den Anker et al., 2018). Finally, in neonates, there is a relative lack of abundance of plasma proteins, such as albumin and alpha 1-acidic glycoproteins, offset to some extent by fetal albumin, persisting for up to 2 years of age. Coupled with the decreased drug-binding affinity, this results in an increased proportion of several free drugs in neonates compared with adults (Ruggiero et al., 2019).

Drug metabolism is an area in which both physiologic and genetic differences intersect. Most, although not all, acts of drug biotransformation occur in the liver, and both phase I and phase II enzymes are highly developmentally regulated. We will not consider the role(s) of phase II enzymes, such as glucuronosyltransferases (UGT), in this context and will focus on phase I enzymes. The cytochrome p450 (CYP450) family is functionally the most significant group of enzymes active during phase I and predominantly (although not exclusively) found in the liver. There are currently over 50 members of the CYP450 family, and alternative splicing (as discussed later) can extend the number of variants even further (Annalora et al., 2017). In this review, we focus on a few clinically significant CYP450 enzymes: CYP1A2, CYP2C9, and CYP2C19.

At birth, cumulative CYP450 enzyme activity is anywhere from 50% to 70% that of adults, although the function of individual enzymes is highly variable. CYP1A2 is one of the enzymes involved in demethylation of caffeine. CYP1A2 levels are barely measurable at birth and show slight increases by 3 months of age (Ruggiero et al., 2019). For this reason, efficacious doses of caffeine for apnea are approximately 10 mg/kg/d (Erenberg et al., 2000). CYP2C9 is also at extremely low levels at birth and this impacts dosing of the antiseizure drug phenytoin. At birth, the recommended dose for term infants is 5 mg/kg/d, contrasted with 8 to 10 mg/kg/d by 6 months of age (Suzuki et al., 1994). Finally, CYP2C19 is worthy of note in that it metabolizes a class of drugs frequently used in the NICU, namely proton pump inhibitors (PPIs). CYP2C19 is also coded by a gene that has several genetic variants, as discussed later. According to Duan et al. (2019), CYP2C19 expression reaches 15% or less of adult levels during the prenatal period and increases linearly after birth within the first 5 postnatal months. Thus, care must be taken in dosing PPIs such as pantoprazole. The pharmacology of PPIs is made even more interesting by the fact that another PPI, esomeprazole, is an inhibitor of CYP2C19. Furthermore, as we discuss later in this chapter, there are several well-known genetic variants of CYP2C19.

Finally, both metabolism and renal function in neonates have an overall effect of increasing the half-life of many drugs. Decreased renal blood flow and glomerular filtration rate, as well as the relatively low expression and activity of organic anion transporters (OATs), organic cation transporters (OCTs), and ABC transporters such as P-glycoprotein, all contribute to relatively low elimination rates of many drugs. These include nonsteroidal anti-inflammatory drugs and beta-lactam antibiotics, which have increased drug half-lives in neonates compared with adults (Ruggiero et al., 2019). We also take a closer look at P-glycoproteins and their genetic variants.

In comparison with developmentally related changes in PK, PD in the neonate is still poorly understood, with few exceptions. According to Kearns et al. (2003), "little information exists about the effect of human ontogeny on interactions between drugs and receptors and the consequence of these interactions" (p. 1162). Most differences in drug response in neonates are due to PK variations. There are, however, age-related differences in the relationship between the plasma level and pharmacologic effect. This is seen in warfarin, cyclosporine, midazolam, and valproate, implying a developmental trajectory in the expression of receptors or targets for these drugs (van den Anker et al., 2018). In most studies of neonatal and infant PD, investigators have relied on biomarkers of disease or response to assess developmental change; for example, endpoints such as blood pressure, CYP expression for PPIs, and PET imaging and functional MRI have been used as indirect measures of PD (Kearns & Artman, 2015). Certainly, this field requires further investigation.

An appreciation of some of the PK and PD variations in neonates underpins the main thesis of this chapter, which is the role of genetic variation in neonatal drug response. We begin with a description of and comparison between PGe and PGx.

PHARMACOGENETICS VERSUS PHARMACOGENOMICS

For several decades, it has been understood that genetic components also affect drug metabolism and response. This initially led to the melding of the disciplines of pharmacology and genetics into PGe, which began as the study of the role of single genes in the context of drug response. The earliest study to explicitly link a gene to an altered drug response involved a surgical patient who died after injection of succinylcholine, due to the genetic lack of "pseudocholinesterase" (Kalow, 1956). Since then, the field of PGe has evolved considerably and has been extended to the study of genetic differences across populations (Kalow, 2006).

We have also come to appreciate that the controls of most drug responses are in fact multifactorial: multiple genes and/or gene families and their protein products regulate drug responses. Moreover, some drugs themselves elicit changes in gene expression. Enter the field of PGx, in which the expression of multiple genes or gene patterns involved in drug responses is studied. In comparison with PGe, PGx involves population-wide analysis of genes regulating drug efficacy and toxicity (Pirmohamed, 2001). A key distinction between PGe and PGx is that, although these terms are often used interchangeably and these fields use some of the same methodologies, PGx has the broader scope. PGx studies were able to mature concomitantly with the development of novel technologies that gave researchers the ability to observe the expression of multiple genes simultaneously and to use more advanced computational tools. At its core, however, PGx aims to correlate specific genetic variants with associated drug responses; such variants occur primarily in the form of single nucleotide polymorphisms, but also include copy number variants (multiple copies of the same gene), deletions, and duplications (Corsello et al., 2013). In our context, PGx can be applied to fetal, maternal, neonatal, and even placental drug responses; in this review, we focus primarily on neonatal PGx.

PRINCIPLES AND CONCEPTS

Before discussing some of the mechanisms underlying genetic causes of variations in drug disposition, a brief review of the central paradigm of molecular biology and relevant terminology may be helpful. We begin with what is called the *central dogma of cell biology:* namely, that DNA carries the genetic code or blueprint for proteins, which in turn help regulate cellular activity. The basic unit of DNA is a *nucleotide*, which is a molecule consisting of a five-carbon sugar (ribose) with an attached phosphate molecule, and one of four different *nitrogenous bases* (adenine, cytosine, guanine, thymine), as depicted in Figure 4.2.

Nitrogenous bases form complementary pairs via hydrogen bonding: Cytosine (C) binds to guanine (G), and adenine (A) binds to thymine (T). Adjacent nucleotides form polynucleotide sequences, which ultimately comprise the alpha double helix that is DNA. Although DNA is understood to form the basis for chromosomes, it is important to remember that DNA is usually tightly packed by associating with *histone proteins*. When DNA is either replicated or the genetic code is being read, it is unwound and "unzippered" into *sense* and *antisense* strands (Figure 4.3).

The actual genetic code is carried by the sequence of nucleotides in DNA, which include adenine (A), cytosine (C), thymine (T), guanine (G), and uracil (U). Each sequence of three nucleotides (e.g., ATG) on the sense strand corresponds to a complementary sequence in messenger RNA (mRNA). For example, ATG corresponds to UAC on mRNA, and ultimately this codes for the amino acid tyrosine, whereas GGC codes for glycine and GUG for valine (Figure 4.4).

FIGURE 4.2 Basic structure of DNA.

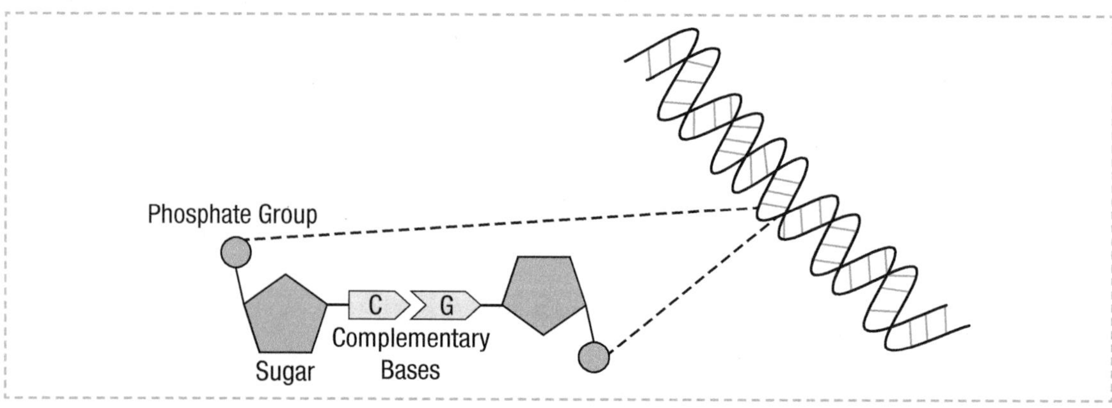

FIGURE 4.3 Sense and antisense strands of DNA.

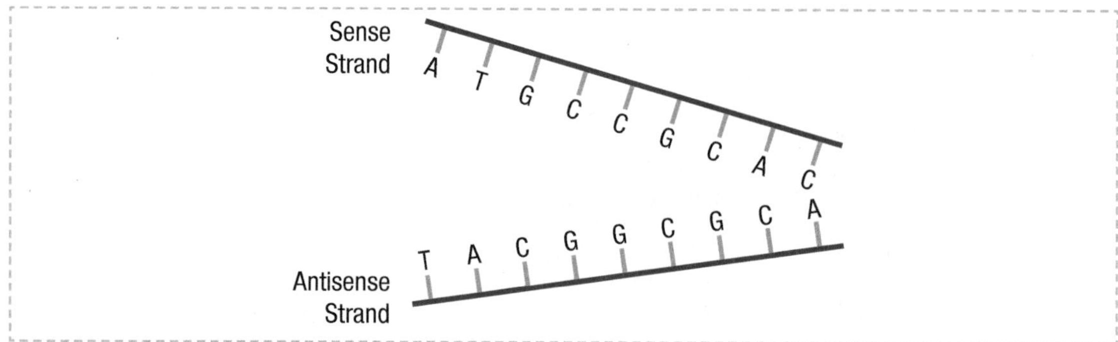

Source: From Wright, K., & Diehl-Jones, W. L. (2019). An introduction to clinical genetics. *Neonatal Network, 38*(5), 266–273. https://dx.doi.org/10.1891/0730-0832.38.5.266.

This leads us to a brief review of the structure of a gene. Although there are varying degrees of complexity, the nucleotide sequence of a gene codes for what we call the *promoter sequence*, to which an enzyme known as *RNA polymerase* binds, a process that is usually facilitated by another protein called a *transcription factor*. Upstream of the promoter is the coding sequence, which ultimately determines the specific *mRNA transcript*, discussed in the text that follows. Finally, another nucleotide sequence known as the *terminator* ceases transcription or reading of the coding sequence (Figure 4.5).

The above model represents the simplest case. In fact, most nucleotide sequences are not part of any gene; nucleotides, which are part of the structure of a gene, are organized into *introns* and *exons*. The actual coding sequence of DNA consists of exons, which can essentially be mixed and matched by splicing out the introns and combining different exons, a process known as *alternative splicing* (Figure 4.6).

In this way, a single gene may actually code for several different types of proteins, and alternative splicing can be considered a mechanism used to adapt to physiologic demands. An example discussed later in the chapter is alternative splicing of CYP450 genes, whose protein products are a key enzyme involved in drug metabolism.

The nucleobase sequence of the gene is used to eventually produce small amino acid sequences called *peptides* and longer sequences called *proteins*. This is a multistep process, beginning with the production of single-stranded mRNA within the nucleus, a process referred to as *transcription*. After mRNA leaves the nucleus, the genetic message is "read" or translated by ribosomes, during which individual amino acids are carried by *transfer RNA* (tRNA; Figure 4.7).

FIGURE 4.4 The genetic code.

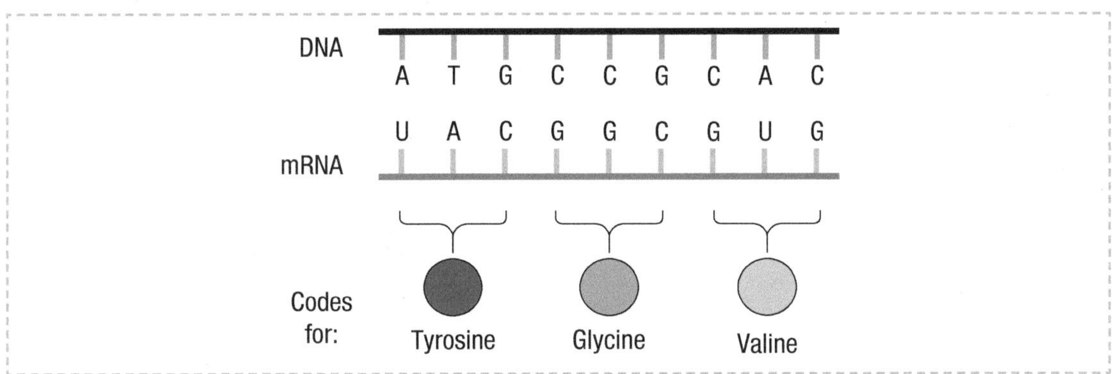

mRNA, messenger RNA.

Source: From Wright, K., & Diehl-Jones, W. L. (2019). An introduction to clinical genetics. *Neonatal Network, 38*(5), 266–273. https://dx.doi.org/10.1891/0730-0832.38.5.266.

FIGURE 4.5 Gene structure.

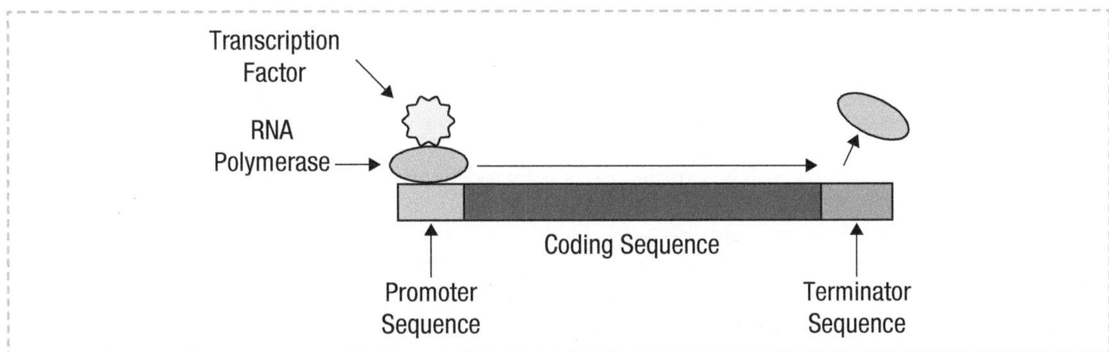

Source: From Wright, K., & Diehl-Jones, W. L. (2019). An introduction to clinical genetics. *Neonatal Network, 38*(5), 266–273. https://dx.doi.org/10.1891/0730-0832.38.5.266.

FIGURE 4.6 Alternative splicing.

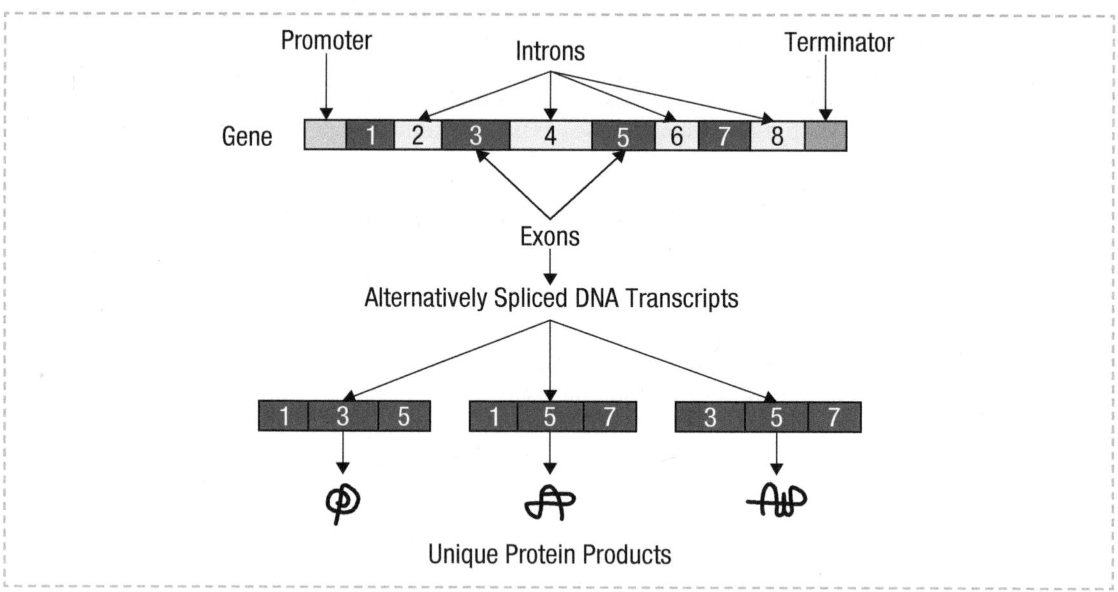

FIGURE 4.7 Messenger RNA and transfer RNA.

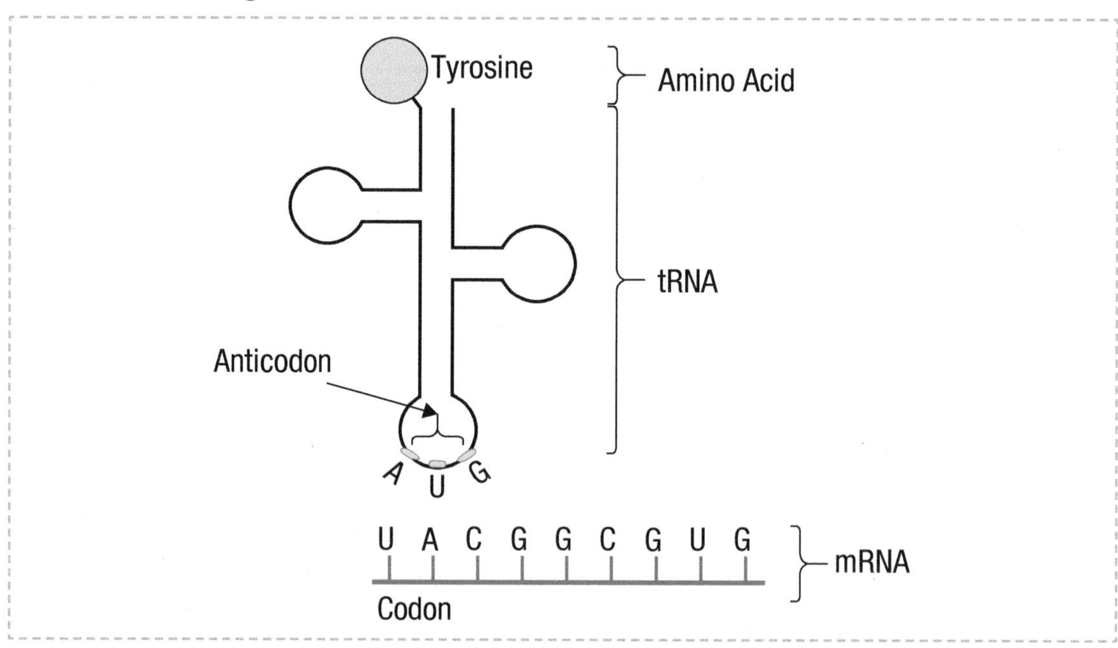

mRNA, messenger RNA; tRNA, transfer RNA.

Source: From Wright, K., & Diehl-Jones, W. L. (2019). An introduction to clinical genetics. *Neonatal Network, 38*(5), 266–273. https://dx.doi.org/10.1891/0730-0832.38.5.266.

The triplet of UAC on the mRNA molecule is referred to as a *codon*. The corresponding nucleobases on the specific, paired tRNA molecule are referred to as an *anticodon*, and a tRNA with this anticodon carries a specific amino acid, in this case tyrosine. The pairing of mRNA codons with tRNA anticodons occurs in the cytoplasm at specific sites on ribosomes. As the codon on an mRNA transcript matches with its corresponding tRNA, the mRNA moves through the ribosome, making available the next codon of triplet bases. During this process, called *translation*, amino acids become covalently linked into a growing polypeptide chain. We can put this together and depict the processes of transcription (formation of mRNA from template DNA) and translation (the building of polypeptides and proteins from mRNA) in Figure 4.8.

Specific genes are located at discrete locations along chromosomes. Different versions of genes are called *alleles*, and humans normally have two copies (one on each *homologous chromosome*) of a given gene. Alleles include coding sequences that are considered typical, or *wild type*, whereas variations of the nucleotide sequence generate different alleles of that gene. Recall that the term *genotype* refers to a set of two alleles a person carries, whereas the *phenotype* refers to the actual expression of the gene. It is useful at this point to introduce another term, namely *haplotype*, which refers to a set of alleles at neighboring positions on the same homologous chromosome, or even within the same gene (Figure 4.9).

Haplotypes are typically found within a relatively short distance of one another and thus are unlikely to be transferred between homologous chromosomes during recombination events. We return later to the importance of haplotypes as we discuss sources of genetic variation that can affect PK and PD processes in neonates.

FIGURE 4.8 Transcription and translation.

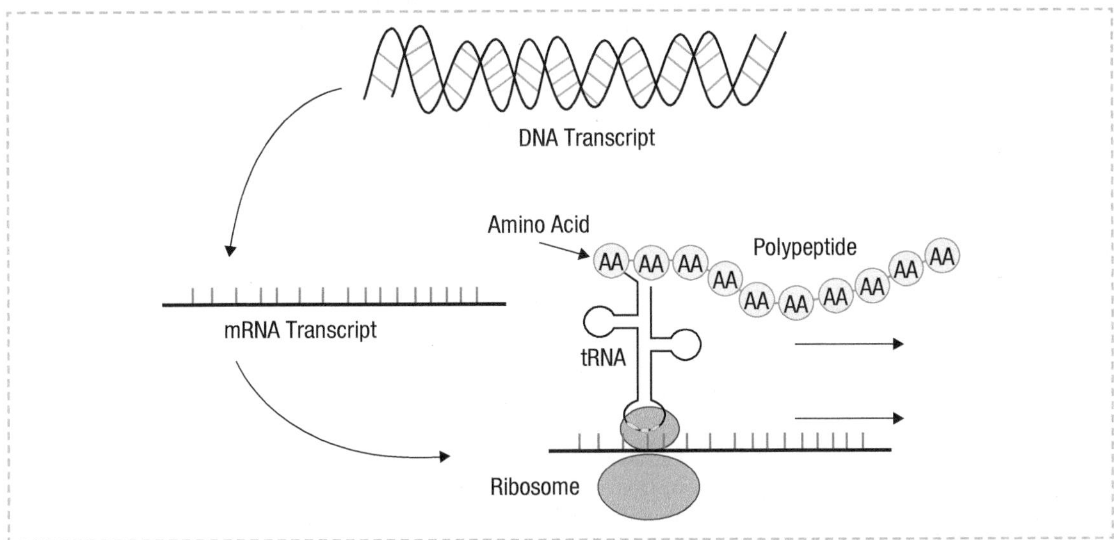

mRNA, messenger RNA; tRNA, transfer RNA.
Source: From Wright, K., & Diehl-Jones, W. L. (2019). An introduction to clinical genetics. *Neonatal Network, 38*(5), 266–273. https://dx.doi.org/10.1891/0730-0832.38.5.266.

FIGURE 4.9 Homologous chromosomes and haplotypes.

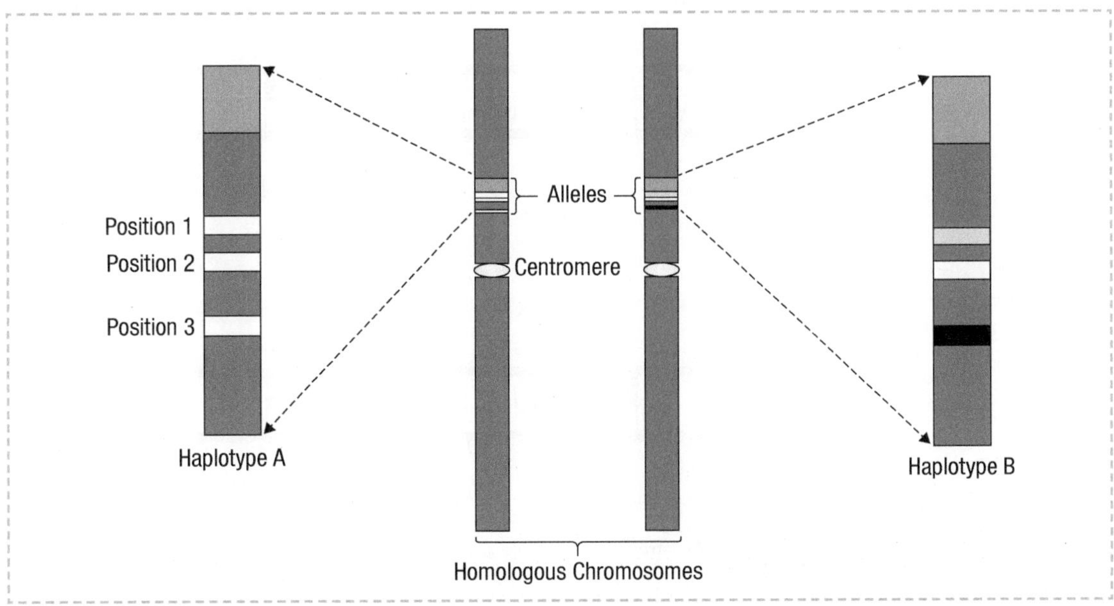

GENE POLYMORPHISMS AFFECTING DRUG DISPOSITION

Based on the preceding brief review, we may now discuss some of the main sources of genetic variation that account for differences in PK and PD processes. A *polymorphism* is a variation in DNA sequence that is present in more than 1% of the population; if the variation is present in less than 1% of the population, it is considered a mutation of that allele (Karki et al., 2015). There are several different polymorphisms that impact PK and/or PD, including *SNPs*, *variable number tandem repeats*, *gene deletions*, and *copy number variants*.

We begin with the single nucleotide polymorphism, or *SNP* (pronounced *snip*), which is by far the most common type of polymorphism (Figure 4.10). In this case, a single nucleotide has been substituted in the sense strand and matched in the antisense strand of DNA. Such substitutions are very common: In the human genome, it is estimated that there is 1 SNP in every 100 to 300 nucleotides, or at least 30 million SNPs in the human genome (Robert & Pelletier, 2018).

It is useful to understand some of the nomenclature used to refer to clinically significant SNPs. For example, in the SNP nomenclature, an SNP which we will refer to later is identified as follows:

- VKORC1 1173 C>T

The first few letters or numbers identify the specific gene (in this case, VKORC1). The numbers after the gene name indicate the position of the nucleotide in the gene, or position 1173. The first letter, *C* or cytosine, refers to the original nucleotide in the wild-type gene, and the second letter, *T* or thymine, represents the changed or variant nucleotide in the SNP.

The *reference SNP* or *rs* nomenclature consists of a number assigned by the SNP database (dbSNP), a central repository for all SNPs thus far identified.

The *Star nomenclature* also refers to SNPs but conveys different information. For example, let's consider two different alleles of one of the CYP450 family of enzymes (abbreviated as *CYP*) also involved in drug metabolism:

- CYP2C19*1
- CYP2C19*2

In the preceding example, the allele of interest is cytochrome P4502C19. The **1* always designates the normal, or wild-type gene. The *2 indicates the SNP form of the allele, and in this case the allele codes for a protein that has no enzyme activity. It is important to understand that the *2 does not always indicate the gene product is inactive; depending on the gene, the SNP may have decreased or even increased activity. Thus, this system simply designates the wild-type allele and the SNP.

FIGURE 4.10 Single nucleotide polymorphism.

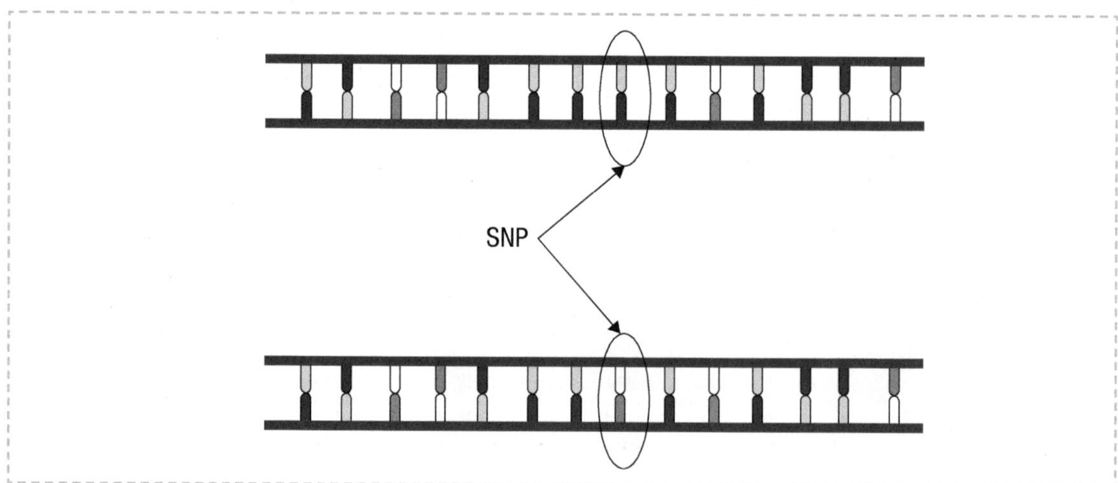

SNP, single nucleotide polymorphism.

Source: From Wright, K., & Diehl-Jones, W. L. (2019). An introduction to clinical genetics. *Neonatal Network, 38*(5), 266–273. https://dx.doi.org/10.1891/0730-0832.38.5.266.

Genotype nomenclature refers to two alleles (one on each homologous chromosome) inherited for a specific gene. For example, a person may carry two copies of the *1 allele (both wild type), two copies of the *2 allele, or one of each of the CYP2C19 alleles, in which case the genotypes (and corresponding phenotypes) would be the following:

- CYP2C19*1/*1 (normal enzyme activity)
- CYP2C19*2/*2 (no enzyme activity)
- CYP2C19*1/*2 (reduced enzyme activity)

The CYPC19 *1/*2 highlights the inheritance of the two alleles, one on each of the homologous chromosomes. In such instances of heterozygosity with no dominant or recessive allele, it is common that the phenotype expressed will be an intermediate of the two alleles. Other SNPs with similar or differing activity levels exist and are designated by specific number codes.

SNPs can occur outside the protein-coding regions of genes and have no effect on the protein itself, or may alter the expression level of the gene. When an SNP is present in the coding region of a gene, it again may or may not alter protein synthesis. Consistent with this concept, SNPs occurring within genes can be classified as *synonymous polymorphisms*, *nonsynonymous polymorphisms*, or may induce a premature stop codon.

As an example of a synonymous polymorphism, we can consider the gene ABCB1, whose protein product is P-glycoprotein, a transmembrane drug transporter that is part of the multidrug resistance (MDR) gene family, which enables the efflux and/or secretion of several drugs, including morphine (Lam et al., 2015). The expression of the ABCB1 MDR protein is relatively low in neonates, thus explaining the enhanced opioid sensitivity in this population. The allele ABCB1 345 C>T (rs1045642) has a nucleotide change wherein cytosine at position 345 has been transposed into thymine, changing the codon from ATC to ATT. This does not cause an amino acid change; many amino acids have more than one nucleotide coding sequence. In this case, both ATC and ATT code for the amino acid isoleucine (Lam et al., 2015).

Another enzyme involved in drug metabolism is thiopurine methyltransferase (TPMT), which codes for the enzyme thiopurine methyltransferase. The gene product of TPMT metabolizes thiopurine drugs, such as azathioprine, an immune inhibitor, and is actually expressed at higher levels in term infants than in adults (McLeod et al., 1995). In this case, there are SNPs that demonstrate a nonsynonymous haplotype named TPMT*3A (Wang & Weinshilboum, 2006), which has two SNPs:

- TPMT 615 G>A
- TPMT 847 A>G

In this instance, both SNPs consist of nucleotide substitutions that do result in different codons for different amino acids: changing from alanine to threonine and tyrosine to cysteine. The end result is a TMPT enzyme with less activity and more azathioprine toxicity due to the metabolites produced (Dean, 2012).

Finally, SNPs can generate a premature stop codon within the coding sequence. An example involves another CYP450 enzyme called *CYP2C19*, and an SNP-linked allele, *CYP2C19*3*. The wild-type gene product is involved in the metabolism of many drugs, including PPIs (Deshpande et al., 2016), which are often used in neonatal practice (Safe et al., 2016). In the wild-type allele, the TGG (which represent the nucleotide sequence thymine, guanine, guanine) codon codes for the amino acid tryptophan. In the CYP2C19*3 allele, the nucleotide guanine is replaced by adenine to yield TAG, which is a stop codon. This results in a truncated protein that does not metabolize PPIs, resulting in increased drug toxicity.

SNPs are continually added to the dbSNP, and we discuss other SNPs that affect either PK or PD in neonatal pharmacology in a later section of this chapter.

In contrast to single nucleotide substitutions, other gene variations may involve two or more nucleotide changes. For example, variable number tandem repeats involve dinucleotide sequences that may be repeated several times. For example, an important enzyme in phase II metabolism is UDP-glucuronyl transferase 1A1, which glucuronidates metabolites in the liver and increases their water solubility. UDP-glucuronyl transferase is of primary importance to neonates in that it is the only enzyme that metabolizes bilirubin (Sumida et al., 2013). The gene UGT1A1 codes for this enzyme, and the wild-type includes 6 "T-A" dinucleotide repeats:

- UGT1A1: ...GTATATATATATAGTAA...

In contrast, the UGT1A1 *28 has an extra dinucleotide *T′*:

- UGT1A1 *28: ...GTATATATATATATAGTAA...

The result is a decrease in UGT1A1 transcription and glucuronidation levels, which results in a hyperbilirubinemia disorder known as *Gilbert syndrome* (Gil & Sąsiadek, 2012) and *Crigler–Najjar syndrome* (Maruo et al., 2016), and which may contribute to hyperbilirubinemia and kernicterus in some infants (Watchko, 2021). In terms of its relevance to PGe, this allele increases the toxicity of irinotecan, an anticancer drug, and atazanavir, an antiviral used in the treatment of HIV-1 (Barbarino et al., 2014), neither of which is yet approved for use in neonates less than 3 months of age.

The aforementioned genes and alleles primarily impact PK mechanisms, and all but one of these are related to metabolism. In addition, the vast majority of PGe and PGx studies have focused on the nuclear genome. More recently, another source of genetic variation in drug responses has been identified: the mitochondrial genome. Human *mitochondrial DNA* (mtDNA) is circular, approximately 16,569 base pairs in length, and codes for only 37 genes (Jones et al., 2021). mtDNA is also unique in that it is generally believed to be inherited exclusively from the maternal germline and has a high rate of replication errors and poor repair capacity compared with nuclear DNA. Thus, it has a 10- to 17-fold higher mutation rate compared with genomic DNA, making mtDNA a rich source of SNPs (Wallace & Chalkia, 2013). mtDNA variants have been associated with altered responses in adults to drugs, ranging from antimicrobials and antivirals to anticancer agents (Jones et al., 2021). As of this writing, however, there are no published accounts of mtDNA variants and variations in either neonatal and/or pediatric drug responses, although further research in this area may add yet another component to PGx modeling.

Another frontier in PGx research may be *microRNAs*, or *miRNAs*. These are 18- to 22-nucleotide molecules that are involved in post translation modulation of the expression of multiple protein-encoding genes (Zhang & Dolan, 2010). Within the last decade, evidence has been accumulating on a role of miRNAs that impact both PK and PD, and it is speculated that variations in the levels of circulating miRNAs contribute to interindividual variability in drug response (Latini et al., 2019). Given that miRNAs are stable and easily identifiable, they are believed to be potential biomarkers of individual response to drugs. As with mtDNA, miRNAs await further validation before they can fully enter the arsenal of PGx tools.

METHODOLOGIES

PGe studies have traditionally relied on the identification of a single gene variant responsible for abnormal or adverse drug responses. In some of the earliest PGe studies, enzymes responsible for such drug responses were purified and gene sequenced. This time-intensive approach has been significantly improved upon with the advent of increasingly sophisticated techniques. It is beyond the scope of this chapter to review these methodologies in depth, although it may be useful to highlight some of the more common and/or promising techniques. For example, we previously discussed the role(s) of SNPs in PK variations. One of the earliest and more common SNP detection techniques used *restriction fragment length polymorphism* (*RFLP*). Essentially, purified DNA is collected from individuals who may have different drug responses and subjected to digestion with *restriction enzymes* that cut DNA at specific sites dictated by specific nucleotide sequences. This would result in DNA fragments of varying size, which could be *electrophoretically* separated (an electric field is used to separate molecules based on size and charge), and DNA sequences with SNPs could then be detected on the basis of differences in DNA fragments (Figure 4.11). Later advances in this technique used the *polymerase chain reaction* (*PCR*) to amplify the amount of DNA in samples.

This "global" search strategy for SNPs was very laborious and expensive and did not permit identification of sequence differences among RFLPs unless DNA sequencing was performed (Kwok & Chen, 2003). Two methodologic advances that made advanced SNP analysis possible and allowed broader PGx studies were the sequencing of the human genome and *microarray analysis*. Currently, SNP microarrays may be used to detect thousands of SNPs. The basic principles are demonstrated in Figure 4.12.

In this type of analysis, plates or glass chips are printed with known oligonucleotide probes for specific SNPs derived from SNP databases such as the dbSNP previously discussed. DNA from a test subject is amplified and labeled with a fluorescent molecule. If there are nucleotide sequences that are complementary to any of the "designer nucleotides" immobilized on the

FIGURE 4.11 Identification of single nucleotide polymorphisms by restriction fragment length polymorphism analysis.

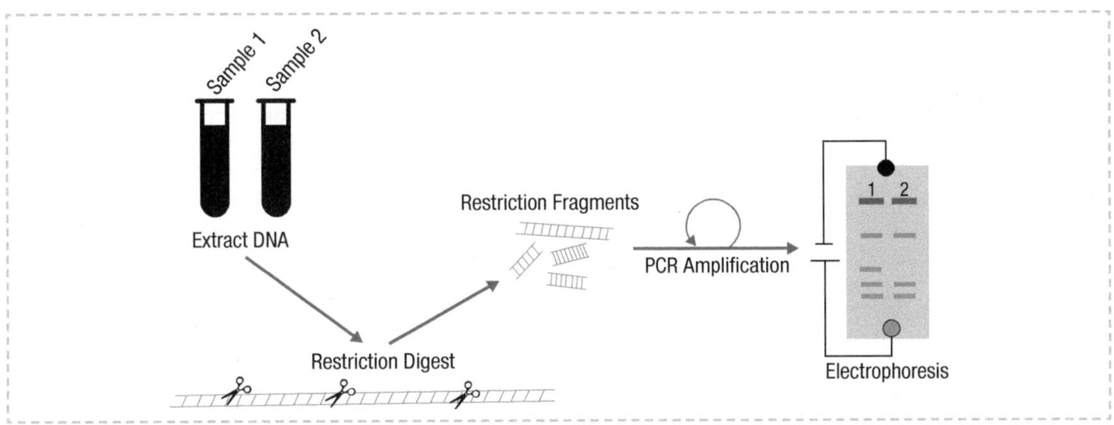

PCR, polymerase chain reaction.

FIGURE 4.12 Microarray single nucleotide polymorphism analysis.

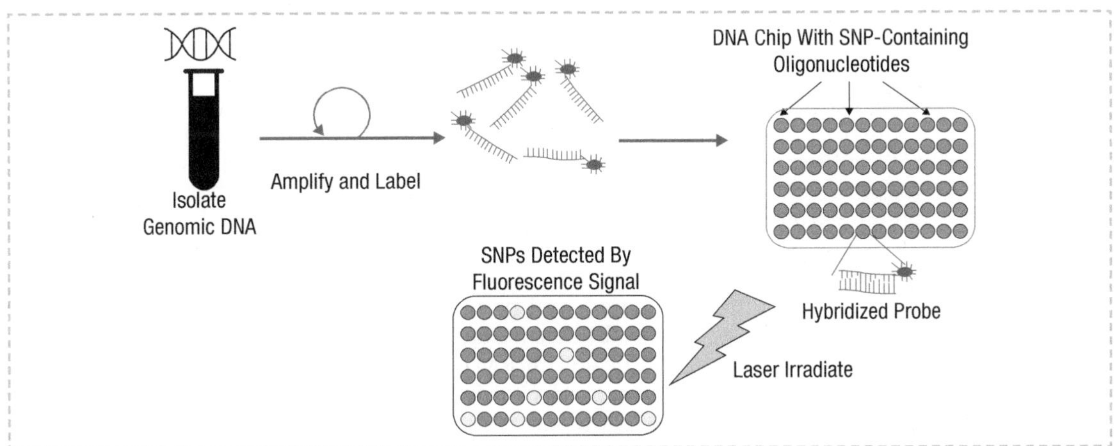

SNP, single nucleotide polymorphism.

microarray chip, they can bind or hybridize to the plate, whereas noncomplementary nucleotide sequences are washed away. Hybridization can then be detected by irradiating the microarray chip with laser light and the fluorescence signal detected (Mishra et al., 2017).

Other "high throughput" analytical techniques have now made it possible to conduct PGx studies at the population level. Today we have at our disposal techniques such as genotyping by *real-time PCR* (Bothos et al., 2021), as well as the so-called big data and deep analytics approaches to identify drugs associated with genes carrying relevant SNPs (Bachtiar et al., 2019). The latter is able to evaluate SNPs based on two properties: (a) whether the allele frequency of the SNP in one population is significantly different from the frequency in another population, and (b) whether the SNP is predicted to be potentially functional, affecting either gene/protein expression or activity. SNPs that fulfill either the first criteria alone (*population-differentiated* SNP [pdSNP]) or both criteria (*potentially functional, population-differentiated* SNPs [pf-pdSNPs]) can be mapped to their corresponding genes. Genes containing pf-pdSNPs can then be mapped to specific drug pathways using open-source drug–gene databases.

As might be evident, such PGx analytical techniques are complex and require multidisciplinary approaches and complex data handling. However, due to the complexity of PK and PD variability, coupled with physiologic variability, such methods are becoming validated as tools necessary to translate PGx into clinically actionable information. Moreover, *next-generation sequencing* platforms now allow the rapid, relatively inexpensive sequencing of DNA or RNA to study genetic variations associated with diseases and differential drug responses (Cousin et al., 2017).

PHARMACOGENOMICS AND NEONATAL PHARMACOLOGY

This brings us back to the application of PGx in the NICU. As much as PGx has advanced our knowledge of the genetic components underlying variability to drug response, an inescapable fact is that genetics comprises but one factor determining how premature or ill infants respond to drug therapy (Lewis & Leeder, 2018). As indicated earlier in this chapter, all aspects of PK have developmental trajectories in the neonatal population, from variations in enteral drug absorption to age-specific drug metabolism and excretion. Also, the type of feeds, neonatal health, and drug therapies themselves have the potential to increase or decrease drug efficacy, or to cause adverse drug reactions (Lewis & Leeder, 2018). Environmental factors can also generate unexpected drug responses in neonates: Exposure to xenobiotics, such as benzo(a)pyrenes, which are present in cigarette smoke, can cause differential splicing of the CYP450 gene (Annalora et al., 2017).

Another hurdle to implementing PGx research into the NICU *is genotype–phenotype discordance*; in other words, a specific genotype may not be functionally expressed to yield the expected phenotype. Usually, this is the result of immature systems in the neonate (Lewis & Leeder, 2018). Let us consider two members of the CYP450 family. Neonates with the wild-type CYP2D6 *1/*1 alleles biotransform tramadol as early as 37 weeks' postmenstrual age, whereas infants with variant alleles clearly expressed this activity at lower levels (Allegaert et al., 2008). In contrast, a discordance is evident in CYP2C19 (which, recall, was highlighted previously in this chapter); infants who have the variant alleles and who are poor metabolizers of oral pantoprazole cannot be distinguished from infants who carry the wild-type CYP2C19 alleles until 45 weeks' postmenstrual age (Ward et al., 2010).

Amid such background variables, a few inroads have been made with respect to applying PGx research into practice in the NICU. As mentioned previously, metabolism of tramadol by neonates is dependent on which CYP2D6 alleles they possess. In another example of applied PGx, indomethacin, a drug sometimes used to treat PDA (Evans et al., 2021), is metabolized by CYP2C9. In a study of infants treated with indomethacin, individuals were assigned to either the "responder" or the "nonresponder" group. It is interesting to note that two CYP2C9 SNPs (rs2153628 and rs1799853) were associated with increased odds of response to the drug (Smith et al., 2017).

Pain is routinely assessed in NICU, and opiates are frequently the drug of choice (Hall & Anand, 2014). Failure to adequately treat neonatal pain is often in conflict with the risk of overdose, and these are complicated by PK variabilities (Anand & Hickey, 1987). Three genes in particular appear to be associated with opioid efficacy: OPRM1, which codes for the opioid mu receptor; ABCB1, an MDR gene previously discussed; and COMT, the gene for catechol-o-methyltransferase (an inactivator of catecholamine neurotransmitters, including dopamine, epinephrine, and norepinephrine). Research by Matic et al. (2014) suggests that combined *OPRM1* 118A>G and *COMT* 472G>A genotypes serve as predictors of the need for rescue morphine in mechanically ventilated infants.

In a study of antenatal corticosteroids (ACS), Borowski et al. (2015) studied candidate genes associated with steroid metabolism and respiratory function. The authors were able to show that neonates with allelic SNPs of the genes CRHBP, CRH, and SCNN1B were at greater risk of continuous positive airway pressure (CPAP)/ventilator use (CPV or cardiopulmonary ventilation), and SNPs in CRH and CRHR1 conferred a decreased likelihood of CPV. Considering the concerns about growth and brain development associated with ACS, such genotypic data may be helpful in determining risk/benefit in specific members of the patient population (Lewis & Leeder, 2018).

Although our focus has been on neonatal PGx, it is clear that maternal and placental PK processes also affect drug disposition in neonates; this has been starkly highlighted by the deleterious impact of maternal CYP2D6 and CYP3A4 variants of codeine metabolism (Gasche et al., 2004; Koren et al., 2006). Mothers with specific CYP2D6 variants ultra rapidly metabolize codeine, one of the metabolites of which is morphine, which is transferred in breast milk. This has led to neonatal morbidity and mortality, and clinicians in the NICU are now well aware of this PGe interaction.

Genetic variations in other fetal/placental metabolic pathways have also been characterized, including enzymes that metabolize nicotine and other xenobiotics (Bieche et al., 2007; Hakkola et al., 1998). Some of the other key maternal and fetal/placental enzymes with variants that have been linked to neonatal effects, as well as neonatal enzyme variants, are summarized in Table 4.1.

TABLE 4.1 Pharmacokinetic Enzymes Associated With Variable Neonatal Drug Responses

MATERNAL ENZYME	FETAL-PLACENTAL ENZYMES	NEONATAL ENZYMES
CYP2D6, CYP3A4 • Codeine metabolism	CYP1A1, CYP2E1 • Upregulated by placenta by nicotine	CYP2D6 • Opioid metabolism
CY2D6, CYP2C19 • Antidepressant metabolism	CYP3A7 • Primary cytochrome P459 gene in fetal liver	SLC6A4 serotonin transporter promoter • Adverse effects of SSRIs
ALDH1B, ALDH2, CYP2E1 • Alcohol metabolizing enzymes		NAT1, GSTM1 • Phase II enzymes affecting

ALDH, aldehyde dehydrogenase; GSTM1, glutathione S-transferase mu 1; NAT1, novel APOBEC1 target 1; SLC, solute carrier; SSRIs, selective serotonin uptake inhibitors.

Source: Adapted from Blumenfeld, Y. J., Reynolds-May, M., Altman, R., & El-Sayed, Y. (2010). Maternal–fetal and neonatal pharmacogenomics: A review of current literature. *Journal of Perinatology, 30*(9), 571–579. https://doi.org/10.1038/jp.2009.183.

NEONATAL PHARMACOGENOMICS: PAST, PRESENT, FUTURE

One of the great hopes underpinning both PGe- and PGx-based research is that it will translate into a more personalized approach to pharmacotherapy. Rather than the current one-size-fits-all prescribing, a more tailored, or patient-centered, means of prescribing could be informed by genetic testing, thus reducing treatment failure or harm to the patient (Lewis & Leeder, 2018). Another hope is that, especially with respect to the neonatal population, PGe and PGx research will also yield insights into fetal and neonatal developmental processes (Blumenfeld et al., 2010).

In this chapter, we have discussed some of the past and present practices around the discovery and application of genetic studies as they relate to neonatal pharmacology. Recent advances in high-throughput screening of genes inspire hope that we will graduate to increasingly individualized drug therapy (Corsello et al., 2013). In addition to the extant PGx screening tools, other "-omics" technologies are opening up the possibilities for comprehensive neonatal screening. For example, *proteomics*, *transcriptomics*, and *metabolomics* allow global assessment of hundreds of thousands of expressed proteins, transcripts, and metabolites, respectively (Corsello et al., 2013; Ernst et al., 2021; Huang et al., 2020; Ling & Sylvester, 2011). Genomic prescribing tools have also been developed for "bedside PGx" (Danahey et al., 2017). Whole genome sequencing in support of such tools is now a possibility, and there is increasing support for genetic sequencing of neonates (Johnston et al., 2018). In as much as these technologies have tremendous potential for PGx research and eventual clinical translation, there are some significant caveats.

In an ideal world, PGx research is a potential pathway toward personalized medicine, increased drug efficacy, and harm reduction. Before embracing all these promising technologies, particularly universal sequencing of neonates in support of PGx, perhaps the most serious concern should be an ethical one. Johnston et al. (2018) provide an insightful analysis of the ethics of newborn screening, as well as the challenges of interpreting complex data, and potential benefits versus risks. Genomic sequencing does raise the specter of both long-term monitoring and also of discriminatory use by employers and other entities. A key point made by these authors is that any such screening must hold the well-being of both infants and family in mind first. Holm et al. (2018) suggest that there is a tremendous opportunity for lifelong impact by sequencing the neonatal genome and have initiated the "BabySeq" project to examine medical, behavioral, and economic impacts of integrated genomic sequencing of healthy and sick newborns.

More targeted sequencing approaches have also been suggested. For example, *whole exome sequencing* (*WES*) is a tool for sequencing all the protein-coding regions of the genome (known as the *exome*). Adhikari et al. (2020) suggest a role of exome sequencing in screening newborns for inborn errors of metabolism; Meng et al. (2017) suggest that exome sequencing may be a powerful diagnostic tool in the NICU. Cousin et al. (2017) reported their PGx results as secondary findings in pediatric patients during clinical WES. It is notable that 91% of their patients had at least one variant allele, with potential immediate pharmacotherapeutic implications for 20% of this cohort.

In the preceding sections of this chapter, we have already highlighted some of the other challenges to applying PGx research to neonatal medicine. Genotype–phenotype discordance is particularly challenging in neonatal medicine due in large part to varying levels of maturity and underdeveloped body systems. Physiologic variations also complicate the application of PGx in the neonatal population, which brings us to the need for more comprehensive models. Toward this end, Kamisoglu et al. (2017) assert the need for statistical and model-based methods that can integrate transcriptomic, proteomic, and metabolomic information to better understand the dynamic nature of both disease state and pharmacotherapy. Any such model also needs to integrate all the factors we have discussed herein: gene expression, developmental variation, physiologic and environmental factors, all of which impact PK and PD in neonates (Figure 4.13).

Ultimately, we should consider whether the goal of using PGx to inform a new era of neonatal pharmacotherapy is even feasible, or are there simply too many variables to make it practicable? Lewis and Leeder (2018) make the point that, "even if instant-return comprehensive PGx results were available to all NICUs starting today, clinical care would not necessarily change" (p. 1233). At the same time, these same authors espouse a sense of "realistic optimism" regarding the current state of PGx. In summary, the full potential of PGx to inform neonatal medicine will likely be realized only with the development and application of model-based dosing tools based on multidisciplinary collaboration.

CONCLUSIONS

A central notion developed in this review is that PGe explores the role(s) of single genes in altered drug responses, whereas PGx aims to capture the role(s) of multiple genes and gene families in drug responses. Variations in the nucleotide sequences account for many of the differences we see in drug responses, and the most common source of gene variants is SNPs. Most of the SNPs identified so far code for enzymes that affect pharmacodynamic processes, and one of the best studied of these enzymes is the CYP450. Several CYP450 variants have been identified to affect neonatal drug metabolism. How and whether we are able to integrate PGx data into clinical neonatal practice will depend on an integrated approach that combines this information with physiologic and genetic models. Finally, clinicians and researchers need to be aware of the ethical implications of PGx screens.

FIGURE 4.13 Integrative modeling of genetic, developmental, environmental, and physiologic factors impacting pharmacokinetics and pharmacodynamics.

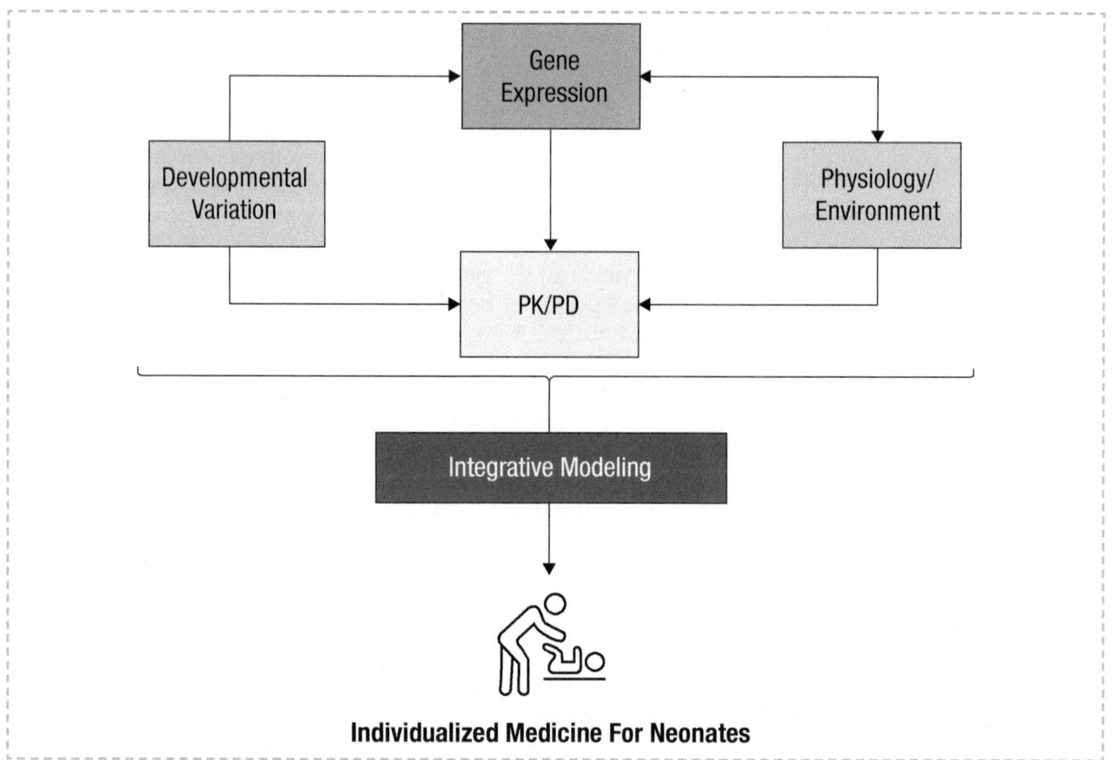

PD, pharmacodynamics; PK, pharmacokinetics.

LEARNING TOOLS AND RESOURCES

Advice From the Author

William Diehl-Jones, PhD, RN, MSc, BScN

Most of us forget the minutiae of courses or content we once learned as undergraduates unless they become part of our everyday professional lives. I think this is especially true with topics such as genetics and cell biology. With that in mind, I have tried to reintroduce some of the foundational concepts and terms from these disciplines so that some of the subsequent discussion in this chapter becomes easier to follow. You will find many words italicized as a means of highlighting some of this terminology. You will also note that I have reiterated some concepts in PK and PD, although these were most excellently reviewed in Chapter 3, "Pharmacokinetics and Pharmacodynamics." This was intentional; so much of pharmacogenetics relates to specific elements of PK and PD, and the aim was to provide context and to allow the current chapter to be read (and understood) as a stand-alone piece.

Once you get past the terminology and nomenclature, I trust that you will gain an appreciation of the potential of pharmacogenetics and pharmacogenomics to advance clinical practice toward more personalized prescribing for neonates. At the same time, it is my hope that you will also consider the multitude of developmental, physiological, and ethical factors that must guide this aspiration. After reading this chapter, it may be helpful to test and consolidate your learning by reviewing some of the discussion questions below.

(Dedicated to my daughter, Chloe Denise Diehl-Jones. Etiam in morte, superest amor.)

Discussion Prompts

1. How can genome sequencing inform PGx studies?
2. How do developmental considerations among neonates impact PGx?
3. How have PGx and PGe informed current neonatal prescribing?
4. If you were to design a PGx study, what techniques would you use? What drug pathways or gene targets would you choose?
5. Is it possible for PGx to inform personalized medicine for neonates? What are some of the benefits? What are some of the barriers?

Mind Map

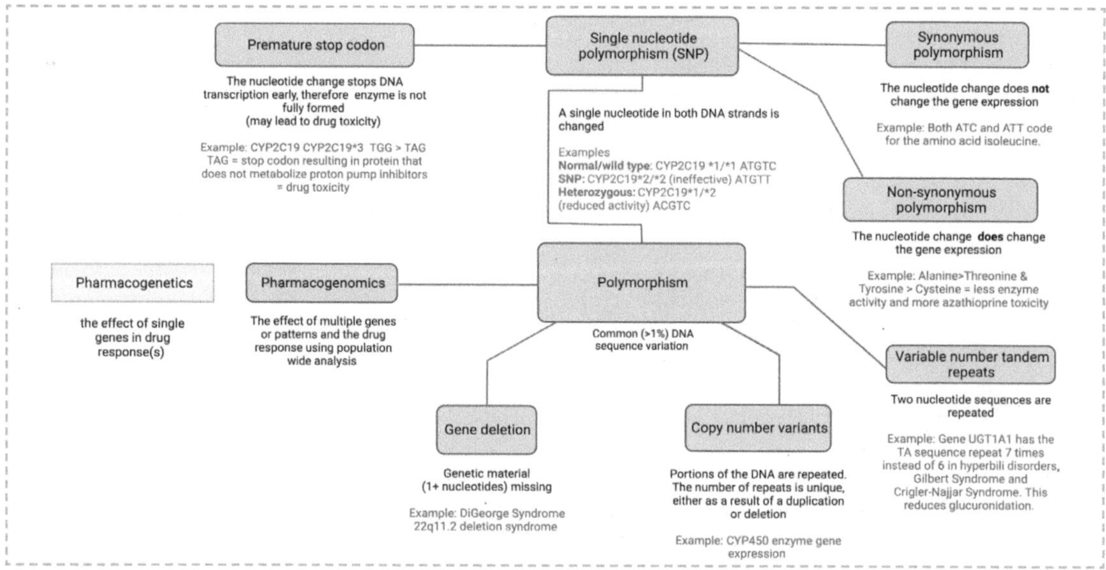

Note: This mind map reflects the design team's interpretation of a portion of one or more concepts addressed in this chapter. Readers should regard the mind maps woven throughout this textbook as examples of multisensory study tools that can be developed to encourage conceptual understanding. Readers are encouraged to develop their own unique mind maps in consultation with academic faculty or clinical preceptors.
SNP, single nucleotide polymorphism.
Design credit: Alison McFarland, BSN, RNC-NIC, and Kelly Kubsien, MSN, RNC-NIC, C-ELBW, East Carolina University Neonatal Nurse Practitioner Program and Neonatal Clinical Nurse Specialist Program.

REFERENCES

References for this chapter are online and available at https://connect.springerpub.com/content/book/978-0-8261-5884-0/part/partI/toc-part/ch4.

chapter 5

Perinatal Pharmacology

Robin Webb Corbett, John Brock Harris, Renee Oakley Spain, and Amy J. Jnah

LEARNING OBJECTIVES

After completing this chapter, the reader should be able to:

- Review common physiologic changes that occur during pregnancy and that implicate maternal/fetal pharmacokinetics.
- Investigate the relationship between the maternal circulation during pregnancy and pharmacokinetics.
- Analyze pharmacokinetic principles that apply to placental transfer of drugs.
- Apply maternal/fetal pharmacokinetics to the principles of absorption, distribution, metabolism, and elimination of maternally ingested drugs.
- Explore common diseases that affect the pregnant female, customary pharmacologic treatment regimens, and implications for the fetus/newborn.
- Explore common medications prescribed during the intrapartum period and implications for the fetus/newborn.

INTRODUCTION

Seventy percent of pregnant women ingest at least one licit prescription drug. In comparison, 90% of pregnant women ingest at least one licit over-the-counter (OTC) *or* prescription drug, beginning in the first trimester of pregnancy, the most vulnerable developmental period for the fetus (Thorpe et al., 2013). Of all commonly ingested OTC drugs during pregnancy, 63% have been studied in pregnant women, and the quality of the available data is deemed *limited to fair*. Merely 2% of commonly ingested OTC drugs have been studied in a manner that yielded *good to excellent* data (Thorpe et al., 2013). Clearly, numerous drugs that pregnant women ingest have not been adequately studied.

Maternally ingested drugs can reach the placenta, a semiprotective portal for drugs and nutrients. Drug molecules enter through the maternal spiral arteries, conduits to the intervillous space that increase in number across gestation. Next, drug molecules reach the syncytiotrophoblast layer and are subject to one of two fates: (a) metabolism by cytochrome P450 (CYP450) enzymes located at the chorion and excretion, or (b) transport into the fetal circulation by way of influx transporters. The relative risk for fetal toxicity is inversely proportional to gestational age, but risk extends across gestation, even if to a lesser degree as the fetus approaches term.

This chapter begins with a review of rather interesting theories of placental function. Readers will come to understand that medical advances progressed at a very slow pace across the first 20 centuries of the Common Era. Seminal discoveries made during the Renaissance and other time frames transitioned focus from mystical views of the placenta toward scientific inquiries focused upon better understanding of placental anatomy and function. After this intriguing historic context is presented, we move to a discussion of the current state of the science specific to placental anatomy. This is followed by a necessary review of maternal physiologic adaptations to pregnancy. Common maternal diseases, both chronic and pregnancy induced, are presented in order to illuminate causal relationships among these diseases, physiologic adaptations, dosages, maternal and hepatic drug metabolism, placental drug metabolism, and drug transport to the fetus. Last, we offer readers a discussion of common drugs prescribed during labor, as well as fetal and postnatal implications. Learning tools and resources provided at the end of this chapter are offered to stimulate additional scholarly conversation both in the classroom and clinical setting, as well as to encourage active learning habits for those preparing for clinical rotations or a board certification examination.

THE PLACENTA: SEMINAL AND OTHER NOTEWORTHY DISCOVERIES

The role of the placenta in human reproduction was a topic of wild conjecture dating back to BCE times (De Witt, 1959). Most individuals who lived prior to the first century CE believed the placenta possessed a spiritual essence capable of imposing good or evil on humans. This animistic view of the placenta largely persisted through the 14th century. For example, Arapesh of New Guinea hung placentas in trees to avoid animal attacks. Mannus of New Guinea believed the placenta was an evil structure (Mead, 1939). Certain African tribes expressed deep respect for the placenta. Other cultures considered the placenta was a symbol of good fortune (Kofoid, 1937). Egyptians believed careful handling and preservation of the placenta was essential, as it contained a portion of the newborn's soul. In fact, royal placentas were accounted for by an office of the "Opener of the King's Placenta" and ceremoniously "opened" at the end of each pharaoh's reign.

Acceptance of this mystical view waxed and waned over the years. The first known challenger was the physician Diogenes of Apollonia of Ionia, present-day Turkey. Circa 480 BCE, he correctly theorized that the placenta was an organ system capable of nourishing a developing fetus (De Witt, 1959). Next, Aristotle (384–322 BCE) incorrectly theorized there was a direct connection between the maternal circulation and fetal circulation via the placenta (Blits, 1999; Bloch, 1904). Galen of Pergamum, physician–philosopher (ca. 200 CE), thoughtfully considered prior theories and incorrectly theorized maternal blood permitted the formation of an embryo, female "semen" formed the allantois, and male semen formed the chorion. He went on to explain that females carried a developing fetus because their bodies were "colder" than males' bodies, making that environment ideal for a developing fetus. While an interesting historic conversation piece, this theory is clearly littered with flaws.

The Renaissance and Reformation periods catalyzed additional scientific inquiry, mainly because artists were enthralled with the mystery of human anatomy. Leonardo da Vinci (1452–1519) was a prominent anatomist whose drawings helped advance the understanding of placental and human anatomy. His anatomic drawings and other theories helped J. C. Arantius (1530–1589) propose the maternal and fetal circulations were separate, noncommunicating entities and the placenta served as a filtration system for the developing fetus (Huisman & Wladimiroff, 1993). This school of thought was later advanced by Walter Neeham (1631–1691), who proposed fetal nutritional intake occurred by way of the placenta and umbilical veins (De Witt, 1959). In addition, A. Spigelius (1578–1625) proposed that waste products were removed from the fetus through two umbilical arteries and deposited into the placenta for maternal uptake and clearance (Bloch, 1904).

These findings helped establish the general consensus that the fetus could not survive without intake from the maternal circulation. Therefore, scientists who lived during the Enlightenment Period focused on reconciling how these two separate circulations communicated with one another. This began with William Hunter (1718–1783) and John Hunter (1728–1792), who correctly identified the decidua as a product of the mucosal lining of the uterus and chorion as the outermost layer of the placenta connected to the embryo by way of the allantois. These brothers also correctly described the yolk sac as an early conduit for fetal nutritional intake. Around this same time, British apothecary Sir William Watson (1717–1787), whose research involved deliberate and unethical inoculation of children with smallpox, discovered that fetuses of mothers who acquired smallpox demonstrated acquired immunity after birth (Needham, 1934). The 18th century ended with the consensus that certain immunoglobulins and toxins crossed the placenta from mother to fetus. However, additional research was needed to examine the effect of fetal exposures to other substances, including drugs. In order to do so, a more granular understanding of the chorion was necessary.

Noteworthy discoveries made during the 19th century included the identification and labeling of layers of cells found within the chorion. Dr. A. A. W. Hubrecht, at the Anatomical Congress at Wurzburg, Germany, in 1888 termed these cells *trophoblast*. Serendipitously, *tropho* refers to nourishment and *blast* refers to bud (i.e., early embryo). Next, the cells were noted to present in a layered arrangement. The outermost layer of the chorion, which does, in fact, communicate with the maternal blood, was labeled the *syncytiotrophoblast*. The middle layer of the chorion was labeled the *cytotrophoblast* layer, and the innermost layer labeled the *extraembryonic mesoderm*. Therefore, in order for substances to reach the fetal circulation, molecules had to penetrate each of these layers of cells.

Numerous advances are documented across the 20th and 21st centuries, many of which focused on where the placenta attaches to the uterus. The physician–scientist who pioneered these and other investigations, Dr. William B. Robertson, studied the placental bed of hypertensive women to understand proximate causes for reduced fetal blood flow (Brosens, 2017). Dr. Robertson discovered that maternal spiral arteries located within the decidual layer of the placenta were full of fat-filled macrophages and appeared similar to atherosclerotic vessels. Around this time, ultrasonography use increased, tissue sampling methods were simplified, and histochemical and electron microscopic procedures refined to better investigate pathologic and pathogenic mechanisms impacting the placental bed. This shifted scientific inquiry toward the pursuit of a better understanding of placental maturation and function across pregnancy, in particular in the face of disease.

One additional initiative worthy of mention is the National Institutes of Health (NIH)-funded **Human Placenta Project (HPP)**. The HPP was initiated in 2014 to further investigate and understand placental anatomy and function (Guttmacher et al., 2014). Its primary research objectives are summarized here:

- Improve current methods and develop new technologies for real-time assessment of placental development across pregnancy.
- Apply these technologies to understand and monitor, in real time, placental development and function in normal and abnormal pregnancies.
- Develop and evaluate noninvasive markers for the prediction of adverse pregnancy outcomes.
- Understand the contributions of placental development to long-term health and disease.
- Develop interventions to prevent abnormal placental development and hence improve pregnancy outcomes.

To date, outcomes data from over 370 HPP-supported investigations have been published in the literature. These and other scientific advances are critical to reduce the impact of maternal disease and pregnancy-induced diseases on the developing fetus and, ideally, reduce the incidence of preterm birth.

MEDICATION USE DURING PREGNANCY AND TERATOGENIC RISK

Consider the following question: "Can maternally ingested drugs cross the placenta and affect the fetus?" Much to our dismay, this fundamentally important question went relatively unanswered until thalidomide was introduced as a therapy for pregnancy-induced hyperemesis and nausea. The use of thalidomide began in the 1950s in Australia, Europe, and Japan. As a result of unregulated distribution, over 10,000 fetuses were exposed to thalidomide and developed major birth defects, including limb defects (phocomelia), congenital heart defects, and ear and eye abnormalities (Miller & Strömland, 1999). After years of information sharing among physician–scientists, thalidomide was identified as the proximate cause for these catastrophic birth defects and removed from formularies for this indication.

Although thalidomide, a teratogen, is no longer accessible to pregnant women, other teratogens (e.g., alcohol) are consumed to this day because they do not require a prescription. For example, maternal alcohol consumption is associated with an increased risk for fetal alcohol syndrome (FAS). Thanks to decades of research, we know that socioeconomic status, race, siblings with FAS, and other factors increase the risk for FAS. This guides prenatal education initiatives. Research also elucidated clinical manifestations of FAS, including facial abnormalities (e.g., thin philtrum), poor growth, and neurocognitive delays. These data help clinicians identify, diagnose, and initiate early-intervention therapies to optimize long-term outcomes.

Research and data sharing also led to the inception of the U.S. Food and Drug Administration (FDA) pregnancy risk categories (PRC) in 1979. Pharmaceutical companies were mandated to include the risk categories on drug information sheets to help clinicians make informed prescribing decisions. Then, on December 4, 2014, the FDA announced plans to retire the PRC in exchange for the *Pregnancy and Lactation Labeling Rule (PLLR)*, a more expansive repository of drug-specific information organized into three categories. Subsection 8.1 ("Pregnancy Considerations") would provide clinicians and pregnant women with a risk summary, clinical considerations, data (as available), and clarification if there is a pregnancy exposure registry for the drug. Subsection 8.2 ("Breastfeeding Considerations") would clarify the risks, clinical considerations, and data (as applicable) specific to drug use during lactation. Subsection 8.3 ("Reproductive Considerations") would provide recommendations for pregnancy testing before, during, or after drug exposure, as well as data specific to drug-associated fertility risks (FDA, n.d.). The PLLR was implemented on June 30, 2015, and all information for new prescription drugs follows this labeling system. Older medications and products are being transitioned to the PLLR, which takes time. Therefore, PRC-specific data are still present on some drug labels (Harris et al., 2021).

Although the PLLR is a helpful tool for obstetric prescribers, adequate pharmacokinetic, pharmacodynamic, and fetal safety data are lacking for more than 90% of commonly prescribed drugs (University of Washington, 2021). Therefore, a complementary resource that clinicians refer to when making prescribing decisions is the Teratogen Information System (TERIS). This is an online, subscription-based database overseen by an advisory panel composed of expert scientists that provides up-to-date teratology risks, pregnancy and neonatal outcomes data, and neurodevelopmental outcomes. Data reported in the TERIS are qualified as *limited to fair, fair to good, good to excellent,* or *excellent*, and used to generate a teratogenic risk assignment (*none, minimal, moderate, high*).

Last, readers are alerted to the **B**irth **D**efects **S**tudy **T**o **E**valuate **P**regnancy Exposure**S** (BD-STEPS) database (Centers for Disease Control and Prevention [CDC], n.d.). This is yet another repository of valuable data reported between 1997 through 2011. To date, scientists refer to this database to investigate and illuminate causal relationships between fetal exposures to drugs and resultant birth defects (e.g., antiherpetic medications and gastroschisis, smoking and choanal atresia; CDC, n.d.). Others, including the TERIS advisory panel and individual clinicians, use the database to better understand the interplay between maternally ingested drugs and fetal outcomes.

PHYSIOLOGY REVIEW: THE INTERVILLOUS SPACE

For drugs to reach the fetus and potentially exert a therapeutic or toxic effect, drug molecules must migrate through two layers of trophoblast cells found within the intervillous space. We present a focused review of placental development in order to orient readers to this important locus. A conceptual understanding of the anatomy and function of the intervillous space is essential before studying the remainder of this chapter.

Within just a few days after conception, the conceptus differentiates into a blastocyst. The blastocyst is regarded as a simplistic ball consisting of two layers of highly capable cells. The inner layer of cells differentiates into the embryo. The exterior layer of cells, composed of trophoblasts, gives rise to the chorion, placenta, amniotic sac, and yolk sac. Trophoblasts consist of two lineages of highly specialized cells: cytotrophoblasts and syncytiotrophoblasts. Cytotrophoblasts form extensions off the blastocyst and penetrate into the endometrium. Some cytotrophoblasts differentiate into anchoring cells to hold the placenta to the endometrial wall, whereas others continue the migratory process toward endometrial blood vessels. These cells penetrate the blood vessels, form blood-filled sinuses, and migrate toward the maternal spiral arteries to invoke a process of vascular remodeling. This establishes a connection between the spiral arteries and future intervillous space and lowers vascular resistance, which permits future maternal/fetal gas and nutrient exchange. Other cytotrophoblasts, which become syncytialized (syncytiotrophoblasts), secrete hormones, including human chorionic gonadotropin (hCG) and endothelial growth factor (EGF). The hCG primes the uterine endometrium for implantation, whereas EGF stimulates the continued production of trophoblasts across pregnancy. The aforementioned sinuses (also referred to as *pools*) nourish these newly formed trophoblasts (Nantais-Smith et al., 2019).

By approximately week 3 of development, trophoblastic proliferation, migration, differentiation, and organization yield "leaf-like" projections, which surround the developing embryo and amniotic cavity. These leaf-like projections are chorionic villi, which comprise a significant portion of the aggregate intervillous space. As this space expands commensurate with embryologic and fetal growth, maternal blood rich with oxygen, nutrients, and immunoglobulins (and potentially drug molecules) enters the intervillous space by way of spiral arteries. Clinically significant blood flow through the spiral arteries is observed at 13 weeks of gestation, and as the number of spiral arteries and blood flow increases over time, the effective surface area for drug transfer increases, whereas diffusion distance decreases (Bertholdt et al., 2019; Roberts et al., 2017; Tashev et al., 2021). Blood thereby enters the intervillous space and saturates the outermost layer of each chorionic villi (syncytiotrophoblast layer). If not ushered away by efflux transporters or metabolized by cytochrome (CYP450) enzymes, drug molecules will become subject to fetal uptake by tiny extensions of the umbilical vein, suspended within the innermost portion of each individual villi.

MATERNAL ADAPTATIONS TO PREGNANCY

Pregnant females are subject to numerous physiologic changes during pregnancy that affect nearly all body systems. Most of these changes begin during the first trimester of fetal development, are primarily hormonally driven, and are necessary to sustain a pregnancy to term. Maladaptation to pregnancy, which can be exacerbated by the presence of disease or acquisition of disease during pregnancy, can alter uteroplacental blood flow and implicate fetal health.

Hematologic and Cardiovascular Adaptations

A constellation of dynamic hematologic and cardiovascular adaptations is observed during early pregnancy. A 20% to 30% increase in mean corpuscular volume (MCV) 45% to 55% increase in plasma volume, and 35% to 48% increase in whole blood volume is observed across pregnancy, likely in response to erythropoietin upregulation (Aguree & Gernand, 2019; Chandra et al., 2012; Sanghavi & Rutherford, 2014). This occurs in the setting of a static red blood cell count and incremental increase in total body water (TBW) by approximately 6 to 8 liters. Albeit a necessary adaptation, this yields a state of hemodilution and physiologic anemia of pregnancy.

The aforementioned hematologic adaptations elicit changes in the mother's heart rate (HR), preload, stroke volume (SV), and cardiac output (CO). HR increases by approximately 17%, or by 10 to 15 beats per minute (Odendaal et al., 2018). Preload increases, which yields an increase in SV. Given that the product of SV and HR is CO, it is no surprise that CO increases by 30% to 50% over the first trimester of pregnancy (Hunter & Robson, 1992). This is necessary to perfuse the uterus and placenta. In fact, by 40 weeks of gestation, 30% of maternal CO is routed to the placenta (Tetro et al., 2018).

The maternal vasculature relaxes in response to these physiologic changes; this is primarily observed through the second trimester. Systemic vascular resistance (SVR), pulmonary vascular resistance (PVR), and blood pressure (BP) decrease by 21% to 34%; the physiologic nadir is observed at midgestation (22–24 weeks; Poppas et al., 1997). Albeit a necessary adaptation, this yields a transient state of hypotension. Thereafter, all indices steadily increase and return to the pre-pregnant baseline by term gestation.

Renal Adaptations

The aforementioned increase in TBW elicits an increase in renal blood flow (50%–75%) and glomerular filtration (50%; Hussein & Lafayette, 2014). The renal system responds with a state of hyperfiltration and upregulation of the renin–angiotensin–aldosterone system (RAAS). Hyperfiltration yields a consequential decrease in baseline serum creatinine, blood urea nitrogen, and uric acid levels. Upregulation of the RAAS elicits increased sodium and water reabsorption at the distal collecting duct. The net effect is the retention of approximately 5 to 8 liters of *added* water volume during pregnancy and a state of physiologic (or dilutional) hyponatremia (Widen & Gallagher, 2014).

The increase in TBW and glomerular filtration impacts the pharmacokinetics of maternally ingested drugs. Higher dosages or more frequent administrations may be required to elicit a therapeutic effect. Increased filtration at Bowman capsule may decrease drug half-life and increase clearance.

Respiratory Adaptations

It is well documented that increased upper respiratory secretions, vascularity, and diaphragmatic elevation (up to 4 cm above baseline) develop with pregnancy (Popa et al., 2021; Taylor, 1961). Increased circulating estrogen and progesterone precipitate an increase in respiratory secretions and a compensatory 20% to 50% increase in minute ventilation (MV) and oxygen consumption (Hegewald & Crapo, 2011; McAuliffe et al., 2002; Schaeffer et al., 2021). Of note, progesterone levels increase from approximately 25 ng/mL in early pregnancy to 150 ng/mL by term (Popa et al., 2021). Clinically, otherwise healthy pregnant women report dyspnea and air hunger. Biochemically, a primary respiratory alkalosis is observed, with metabolic compensation through increased renal excretion of bicarbonate. These maternal adaptations are advantageous to the fetus, as they encourage the elimination of carbon dioxide from the fetal circulation. Manifestations associated with asthma, the most common respiratory disease treated during pregnancy, are presented later in this chapter.

The passive diffusion of carbon dioxide from the fetal to maternal circulation is explained by the Bohr and Haldane effects. Due to its perceived complexity, as reported by numerous APRN students over the years, we digress to offer a timely refresher. Given that ions move from the mother to the fetus, and fetus to the mother, the terms *double Bohr* and *double Haldane* are used. We describe these effects in a cause-and-effect format for conceptual purposes. Readers are encouraged to review the interactions that align with each individual effect (Bohr/Haldane). In addition, review of the oxyhemoglobin dissociation curve may be necessary. Increased $PaCO_2$ levels at the placental interface drive the pH into the acidic range and decrease the affinity of oxygen for maternal hemoglobin. As a result, oxygen is readily released for optimal fetal uptake. As fetal oxygen levels increase, carbon dioxide is offloaded and discarded to the placenta by way of the fetal umbilical artery. Concurrently, as oxygen uptake in the fetus is optimized and maternal oxygen levels decrease, the maternal blood takes on an affinity for $PaCO_{2.}$ Therefore, the carbon dioxide being discarded by the fetus is easily taken up by maternal hemoglobin for efficient removal (by way of increased MV, as previously described; Nantais-Smith et al., 2019).

Gastrointestinal Adaptations

The increase in progesterone synthesis, as previously mentioned, also implicates gastrointestinal function. Smooth muscle relaxation is observed, which reduces motility, delays gastric emptying, and may elicit nausea (Parry et al., 1970). One particularly undesirable adaptation is vomiting, which is observed in a majority (70%–80%) of pregnant women and typically resolves by the end of the first trimester (Lee & Saha, 2011). If severe, dehydration, electrolyte imbalances, and poor maternal nutritional intake are observed, which can affect the pharmacokinetics and pharmacodynamics of maternally ingested drugs. Gallbladder function may also decrease, which risks the formation of painful gallstones. This type of obstruction can decrease the absorption of enterally ingested medications and reduce drug efficacy.

Hepatic Adaptations

Albumin, A1A glycoprotein, and glucocorticoid binding protein are three prominent plasma proteins that bind to and distribute drugs. However, albumin and A1A glycoprotein concentrations decrease across pregnancy (Seong et al., 2010; Solano & Arck, 2020). This may increase the fraction of unbound drug available for transfer to the fetus. Alternatively, glucocorticoid binding protein levels increase during pregnancy. This protects the fetus from excess unbound corticosteroid transfer, in particular, when corticosteroids are administered during threatened preterm labor.

TABLE 5.1 Commonly Prescribed Maternal Medications That Require Major Cytochrome P450 Enzymes for Phase I Drug Metabolism

THERAPEUTIC CATEGORY	DRUGS METABOLIZED BY CYP3A4	DRUGS METABOLIZED BY CYP2D6
Acne, topical	Dapsone	N/A
Adrenergic blocker	N/A	Debrisoquine
Analgesic	Lidocaine	N/A
Antianxiety agent	Buspirone	N/A
Antiarrhythmic agent	N/A	Flecainide, mexiletine, propafenone
Antiemetic agent	N/A	Promethazine
Antifungal agent	Itraconazole	N/A
Antihistamine	Chlorpheniramine, loratadine	N/A
Antilipemic agent	Simvastatin	N/A
Antimuscarinic agent	N/A	Tolterodine
Antipsychotic agent	N/A	Haloperidol, risperidone, thioridazine
Antiretroviral agent	Efavirenz,[a] indinavir,[a] nelfinavir[a]	N/A
Antitussive	N/A	Dextromethorphan
Benzodiazepine	Alprazolam, midazolam	N/A
Beta-adrenergic blocker	N/A	Metoprolol, propranolol
Calcium channel blocker	Amlodipine, felodipine, isradipine, nicardipine, nifedipine	N/A
Hypnotic	Zolpidem	N/A
Immunosuppressant	Cyclosporine, tacrolimus	N/A
Macrolide antibiotic	Erythromycin[a]	N/A
Opioid analgesic	Alfentanil, fentanyl, methadone, oxycodone	Codeine, hydrocodone
SNRI	N/A	Venlafaxine
SSRI	Citalopram	Fluoxetine, fluvoxamine, paroxetine
Tricyclic antidepressant	N/A	Amitriptyline, clomipramine, doxepin, imipramine, nortriptyline

Note: List is not inclusive of all drugs metabolized by CYP3A4 or CYP2D6.
[a] These drugs may *inhibit* CYP3A4 activity.
N/A, not applicable (no drug available); SNRI, serotonin and norepinephrine reuptake inhibitor; SSRI, selective serotonin reuptake inhibitor.
Sources: From Ke, A. B., Rostami-Hodjegan, A., Zhao, P., & Unadkat, J. D. (2014). Pharmacometrics in pregnancy: An unmet need. *Annual Review of Pharmacology and Toxicology, 54*(1), 53–69. https://doi.org/10.1146/annurev-pharmtox-011613-140009; Mattison, D., & Halbert, L.-A. (Eds.). (2021). *Clinical pharmacology during pregnancy* (2nd ed.). Academic Press/Elsevier; Taketomo, C.K. (Ed.). (2023). *Pediatric & neonatal dosage handbook: An extensive resource for clinicians treating pediatric and neonatal patients* (29th ed.). Lexicomp/Wolters Kluwer. Ward, R. M., & Varner, M. W. (2019). Principles of pharmacokinetics in the pregnant woman and fetus. *Clinics in Perinatology, 46*(2), 383–398. https://doi.org/10.1016/j.clp.2019.02.014

In addition, consider that most drugs are ingested in an active form and are subject to hepatic Phase I and Phase II metabolism. Phase I reactions convert drugs to metabolites by way of oxidation, hydrolysis, or reduction. CYP450 enzymes are necessary for Phase I metabolism of numerous drugs (Table 5.1). Two particular CYP enzymes that metabolize the majority (90%) of drugs prescribed to pregnant women are CYP3A4 and CYP2D6. CYP3A4 enzyme levels remain consistent with pre-pregnant levels until the third trimester, when levels increase by more than 100% (Ke et al., 2014). CYP2D6 enzyme levels are more than 120% of pre-pregnant levels during the first trimester, exceed 130% of pre-pregnant levels during the second trimester, and are greater than 140% of pre-pregnant levels during the third trimester (Ke et al., 2014). Phase II reactions conjugate drug metabolites with substances, including sulfates, glucuronic acid, or other amino acids (Mattison & Halbert, 2021; Ward & Varner, 2019).

BASIC PRINCIPLES OF MATERNAL–FETAL DRUG TRANSPORT

Although a relatively prescription drug-free pregnancy is desirable, the reality is that nine out of 10 women consume an average of more than two prescription drugs daily throughout pregnancy (Mitchell et al., 2011). Most medications prescribed during the antepartum period are orally ingested and subject to first-pass hepatic metabolism. These drugs are thereby biotransformed by CYP enzymes, namely, CYP3A4 and CYP2D6. Remaining unbound, active drug molecules may enter one of the 180 to 320 maternal spiral arteries and intervillous space by one of four well-known mechanisms:

- passive diffusion,
- facilitated diffusion,
- active transport, or
- pinocytosis.

Passive diffusion is concentration dependent; drug molecules (e.g., oxygen, fat-soluble vitamins, opioids, barbiturates, anesthetics) some nutrients move across lipid membranes from higher to lower concentration compartments, until concentrations equalize between the maternal and fetal circulations. *Facilitated diffusion* requires specialized protein transporters found in lipid membranes; drug molecules (e.g., cephalosporins, glucocorticoids) bind with protein transporters and then move across lipid membranes from a higher to lower concentration gradient, until concentrations equalize between the maternal and fetal circulations. *Active transport* is energy dependent; nutrients (e.g., glucose) and drug molecules (e.g., amino acids, iron, potassium, water-soluble vitamins, calcium, phosphate) bind with a transport molecule (e.g., adenosine triphoshate [ATP]) for transport against a concentration gradient and into the fetal circulation (Nantais-Smith et al., 2019). *Pinocytosis* involves the formation of a vesicle around larger molecules (e.g., immunoglobulin G [IgG]) for transport into the fetal circulation.

Barriers to Placental Drug Transfer

It is important to recognize that some maternally administered drugs (e.g., insulin, heparin) and substances (e.g., immunoglobulin M [IgM], thyroid-stimulating hormone) cannot cross the placenta by any of the aforementioned mechanisms. This may be due to differences between the maternal blood pH and the drug's hydrogen ion concentration (pKa), lipophilicity, or molecular weight. In contrast, other drugs can successfully cross the placenta. Syncytiotrophoblast cells detect these drug molecules and attempt to reduce the risk for toxic fetal exposure by synthesizing select CYP enzymes and efflux transporters, which reduce the proportion of unbound drug molecules available for uptake by the branches of the umbilical vein located in each villus (Mason & Weiner, 2011).

MATERNAL pH AND DRUG pKa

By definition, pKa is the dissociation constant of a drug; that is, a numeric value that informs the strength of the drug as an acid or a base in a specific solution. Recall that only unionized drug molecules can cross lipid membranes. The degree of ionization of any drug is determined by the pH of the medium and the pKa of the drug. Therefore, the pKa helps clinicians understand the pH necessary for 50% of the drug (acid or base) to exist in an unionized form, able to cross a lipid membrane such as the placenta, and the other 50% of the drug to exist in an ionized form unable to cross a lipid membrane (Griffiths & Campbell, 2015). This state of equilibrium is represented as:

Unionized drug molecules (50%) : ionized drug molecules (50%)

Crosses placenta *Does not cross placenta*

Generally speaking, no drug exists at equilibrium. Rather, drugs are either weakly acidic or weakly basic. Given that the pH of extracellular fluid is approximately 7.4 under normal physiologic conditions, drugs with a pKa of 7.4 or greater are considered weakly basic, unionized, lipophilic, and capable of crossing the placenta. Drugs with a pKa lower than 7.4 are weakly acidic, ionized, more hydrophilic, and less capable of crossing the placenta. Circumstances that alter body pH (e.g., hyperventilation-induced alkalosis) may alter the ionized proportion of a drug available for transport across the placenta and increase the risk for fetal toxicity.

Practical Application for Neonatal Clinicians

Local anesthetics, like bupivacaine and lidocaine, are often used in maternal epidural anesthesia during labor and delivery. Bupivacaine and lidocaine are weak bases and cross the placenta readily via passive diffusion at physiologic pH. However, as fetal pH decreases, these agents become *ionized* and hence are trapped in the fetus (Gaylard et al., 1990). In addition, as the concentration of unionized drug drops in the acidic fetus, unionized drug transfer from maternal to fetal circulation appears to also *increase* in an effort to equilibrate the concentration of unionized drug (Johnson et al., 1996). After delivery, the impacted neonate risks cardiovascular (bradycardia, dysrhythmia, collapse) and neurologic toxicity (apnea, hypotonia, seizures) from the local anesthetic, additive to any risk acquired from in utero acidemia (Dontukurthy & Tobias, 2021). The risk of toxicity is likely augmented further in preterm neonates by low levels of blood esterases necessary for drug metabolism. Readers should note that these outcomes are limited due to local (versus systemic) administration.

LIPID SOLUBILITY

As discussed in the prior section, obstetric clinicians must consider the lipophilicity of a drug that a pregnant woman ingests. Highly lipid-soluble drugs (e.g., antihypertensive drugs, barbiturates) can readily cross the placenta. One noteworthy exception to this principle involves the transfer of fentanyl (or analogues). Although fentanyl is highly lipid-soluble, drug molecules become bound (trapped) within the lipid membrane, which reduces fetal exposure (Krishna et al., 1997; Mason & Weiner, 2011).

MOLECULAR WEIGHT

Clinicians must consider the molecular weight of drugs, as this implicates the ability of the drug to cross the placenta by any of the aforementioned mechanisms. Drugs with a molecular weight of less than 500 daltons (e.g., antiretroviral nucleoside reverse transcriptase inhibitors [NRTIs]) readily cross the placenta, whereas drugs with a molecular weight greater than 1,000 daltons (e.g., protease inhibitor) do not cross in significant amounts (Mason & Weiner, 2011; Pacifici & Nottoli, 1995).

Practical Application for Neonatal Clinicians

Consider, for example, maternal therapy for HIV infection. NRTIs are low molecular weight drugs that readily cross the placenta. NRTI uptake by the fetus offers protection from perinatal HIV infection. NRTIs are commonly paired with a protease inhibitor as combination therapy. This synergistic therapy helps control the maternal viral load, and, in doing so, reduces the risk for perinatal transmission by as much as 98% (Gulati & Gerk, 2009). But unlike NRTIs, protease inhibitors are high molecular weight drugs that cannot cross the placenta in sufficient amounts to directly suppress fetal viral load; therefore, monotherapy is not beneficial to the fetus.

PLACENTAL CYTOCHROME P450 ENZYMES, INFLUX TRANSPORTERS, AND EFFLUX TRANSPORTERS

Once drug molecules are detected in the intervillous space, syncytiotrophoblast cells secrete CYP enzymes and activate influx and efflux transporters. Similar to the principles of hepatic drug biotransformation, CYP enzymes in the placenta metabolize unbound drug molecules to reduce the proportion of free/unbound drug available to the fetal circulation (Mason & Weiner, 2011; Nanovskaya et al., 2011). Influx transporters courier drugs into the fetal circulation, whereas efflux transporters remove active drug molecules that absorb into the syncytiotrophoblast layer. In addition, efflux transporters can remove drug molecules or metabolites from the fetal circulation.

Practical Application for Neonatal Clinicians

Methadone ingestion during pregnancy is tightly linked to the development of fetal dependence on methadone. With birth comes the abrupt cessation of methadone intake. Consequently, the newborn manifests with neonatal abstinence syndrome (NAS). Methadone is orally ingested and subject to hepatic first-pass metabolism by CYP3A4 enzymes. However, when methadone is consumed in large amounts, excess unbound drug reaches the placenta.

Two protective mechanisms are present at the placenta to minimize fetal methadone exposure. First, efflux transporters are present in the syncytiotrophoblast layer and can courier drug molecules away from the fetal circulation. Second, CYP19/aromatase (a surrogate for CYP3A4) is synthesized by syncytiotrophoblast cells and can metabolize methadone molecules (Mason & Weiner, 2011). CYP19/aromatase levels are produced in small quantities during early fetal development and incrementally increase across gestational development, whereas efflux transporters are abundant in early gestation and decrease as the fetus approaches term (Nanovskaya et al., 2011). These factors reduce but cannot eliminate the passage of unbound methadone from the mother to the fetus. Therefore, long-term intrauterine methadone exposure is tightly correlated with fetal methadone dependence. The abrupt cessation of methadone uptake that occurs at birth is the catalyst for the onset of neonatal withdrawal.

Fetal Drug Absorption

Medications are delivered to the fetus via the bloodstream. Although possible, other routes, including oral and transcutaneous absorption, have few data regarding their use. Transcutaneous absorption is hindered by a lipid membrane. Hydrophilic medications and compounds do not diffuse through the membrane inhibiting absorption (Ward & Varner, 2019).

Fetal Drug Distribution

Distribution of medications in the fetus is directly related to the fat and water composition of the body. In early gestation (16 weeks), the fetus is approximately 94% water and 0.5% fat. By term gestation, body composition has shifted to 75% water and 15% fat (Ward & Varner, 2019). This shift in body composition may partially explain differences in the incidence of NAS between preterm and term neonates. Preterm neonates consistently have a lower incidence and severity of NAS compared to term neonates with similar exposures (Dysart et al., 2007). Although this may reflect a difference in symptomology/scoring, preterm neonates also experience lower exposure to lipophilic opioids (both duration and concentration) due to a lower total body fat composition (as compared to water).

Fetal Drug Metabolism

Most fetal metabolic enzyme activity varies over the course of pregnancy and after birth. Enzyme function has been grouped into three categories: enzymes with greatest function early in gestation that tapers over time (CYP3A7), enzymes with fairly consistent function from early in gestation to adulthood (CYP3A5, CYP2C19), and enzymes with little function early in gestation that increase over time (remaining CYP enzymes including 1A2, 2C9, 2D6, 2E1, and 3A4; Hines, 2013). Phase II enzyme activity (sulfate and glycine conjugation) is well developed throughout gestation, compensating for low activity of glucuronyl transferases (UGTs; Ring et al., 1999). For example, antenatally administered corticosteroid primarily undergo sulfate conjugation in the fetus, whereas UGT1A1 conjugation and CYP3A4 oxidation predominate in the maternal host. However, the ontogeny of specific UGT enzymes remains an area of active study, as the conjugation of morphine by UGT2B7 to potent and neuroexcitatory metabolites has been documented in fetal animal models.

Fetal Drug Excretion

Fetal drug excretion occurs predominantly through the placenta. Metabolites (and waste products such as urea and creatinine) are transferred by diffusion across the placenta, carried by the umbilical arteries into the maternal blood, and further metabolized or eliminated by the maternal liver, kidneys, and/or gastrointestinal system. The fetal kidneys account for the minority of drug excretion for water-soluble drugs; however, this pathway increases during gestation. For example, many antibiotics (most notably, penicillin) concentrate in the fetal urine and are excreted in significant amounts late in gestation. As a result, amniotic fluid concentrations of these agents often exceed concentrations in maternal or fetal plasma (Bray et al., 1966).

COMMON DISEASES THAT REQUIRE PHARMACOTHERAPIES DURING PREGNANCY

Pregnancies complicated by preexisting or acquired diseases often require the implementation or continuation of pharmacotherapies. Prior to the 1990s, in the absence of adequate data and in the setting of historic crises (e.g., thalidomide crisis), obstetric providers were hesitant to expose a fetus to maternally ingested medications. In the minds of healthcare providers, the risk for structural malformations and long-term neurocognitive impairment were high. Fortunately, during this time period, obstetricians increasingly relied on ultrasonography to monitor fetal development and promptly identify structural or pathologic problems. These data prompted scientific inquiries in the form of drug-therapy studies, as clinicians desired to elucidate causal relationships between maternal physiologic adaptations during pregnancy, maternal disease, pharmacotherapies, and fetal anatomic and physiologic outcomes.

Asthma

Asthma complicates approximately 3% to 12% of pregnancies, with about 63% of those affected using medications to manage the illness (Murphy, 2015). Likely the result of progesterone changes during pregnancy, affected women often manifest with dyspnea *plus* wheezing or coughing.

Currently, the American College of Obstetricians and Gynecologists (ACOG) and Global Initiative for Asthma (GINA) endorse the prospective use of asthma-specific pharmacotherapies, individualized to the patient because they enhance pregnancy outcomes by reducing the risk for comorbid gestational diabetes, acute exacerbations (some precipitated by psychologic stress associated with pregnancy), asthma-related hospitalizations, and preterm birth (Table 5.2; ACOG, 2008; Kim et al., 2015; Namazy & Schatz, 2017). Neonatal clinicians may notice that monotherapy or combination therapy (inhaled corticosteroids with long-acting beta-2-agonists) was prescribed throughout pregnancy. Commonly prescribed medications include inhaled corticosteroids (e.g., budesonide, fluticasone) and short-acting beta-2-agonists (e.g., albuterol), long-acting beta-2-agonists (e.g., formoterol, salmeterol), muscarinic antagonists (e.g., tiotropium), and leukotriene receptor antagonists (e.g., zileuton, montelukast).

Given concerns specific to teratogenic risks, a summary of key systematic reviews and meta-analyses, which helped inform the position statements listed previously, is provided for readers seeking additional context. Murphy and Gibson (2011) reported that unmanaged maternal asthma is associated with an increased risk for preeclampsia and preterm birth, low birth weight (<2,500 grams), and small-for-gestational-age birth weight (<10th percentile). In contrast, active management of asthma throughout pregnancy reduced the risk for the aforementioned outcomes to nonsignificant levels (Murphy & Gibson, 2011). In 2013, Murphy and colleagues explored additional risk factors, including congenital malformations, stillbirth, neonatal death, perinatal death, neonatal respiratory distress syndrome (RDS), transient tachypnea of the newborn (TTNB), and neonatal sepsis. Asthma management did not increase the risk for stillbirth, neonatal death, perinatal death, RDS, or neonatal sepsis. Increased risk for congenital malformations (cleft lip/cleft palate) was exclusively associated with oral corticosteroid use during early pregnancy, a therapy that is used only when absolutely necessary in the United States (Murphy et al., 2013). Last, the relative risk for TTNB may increase among offspring of asthmatic mothers; however, data were limited to two studies and women with acute exacerbations were subject to cesarean section, a causative factor for TTNB. In addition, Eltonsy and colleagues (2015) investigated the risk for congenital malformations with combination therapy, defined as concurrent use of inhaled corticosteroids and long-acting beta-2-agonists. The authors concluded that combination therapy posed no additional risk when compared to monotherapy (with inhaled corticosteroids alone).

TABLE 5.2 Common Asthma Therapies and Safety Considerations

DRUG CATEGORY	DRUG NAME	TERIS CONSIDERATIONS*	PREGNANCY CONSIDERATIONS (SUBSECTION 8.1)	LACTATION CONSIDERATIONS (SUBSECTION 8.2; HALE, 2021)	REPRODUCTIVE CONSIDERATIONS (SUBSECTION 8.3)
Inhaled corticosteroid	Budesonide		No teratogenic warning	Compatible with breastfeeding; RID 0.3%	Discontinuation is not recommended prior to conception.
	Fluticasone		No teratogenic warning	Probably compatible with breast-feeding; RID unknown	
Short-acting Beta-2-agonist	Albuterol		No teratogenic risk; preferred over long-acting beta-2-agonists	Compatible with breastfeeding; RID unknown	
Long-acting Beta-2-agonist	Formoterol		No teratogenic warning	Probably compatible with breast-feeding; RID unknown	
	Salmeterol		No teratogenic warning	Probably compatible with breast-feeding; RID unknown	
Muscarinic antagonist	Tiotropium		No teratogen-specific outcomes data is available; use is probably accept-able; monthly monitoring of maternal symptoms is recommended	Probably compatible with breast-feeding; RID unknown	
Leukotriene receptor antagonists	Zileuton		No teratogenic warning	Probably compatible with breast-feeding; RID unknown	
	Montelukast		**Pediatric black-box warning** *(consider with teen pregnancy)* No teratogenic warning	Possibly hazardous; RID 0.68%	

Note: Breastfeeding is considered safe when the relative infant dose (RID) is less than 10%. Drugs provided in this table are representative examples and not inclusive of all drugs that may be prescribed by an obstetrician or certified midwife. *The Organization of Teratology Information Specialists continues to collect data specific to infant outcomes after exposure to the therapies listed in this table. Parents may independently enroll exposed infants by visiting https://mothertobaby.org

RID, relative infant dose; TERIS, Teratogen Information System.

Sources: From Global Initiative for Asthma. (2020). *Global strategy for asthma management and prevention*. https://ginasthma.org/wp-content/uploads/2020/04/GINA-2020-full-report_-final-_wms.pdf; Hale, T. W. (2021). *Hale's medications & mothers' milk 2021: A manual of lactational pharmacology* (19th ed.). Springer Publishing; Taketomo, C. K. (Ed.). (2023). *Pediatric & neonatal dosage handbook: An extensive resource for clinicians treating pediatric and neonatal patients* (29th ed.). Lexicomp/Wolters Kluwer.

Diabetes

Diabetes mellitus (DM) may exist prior to conception or present as a gestationally acquired disease process. Approximately 6% to 9% of pregnancies are complicated by diabetes, and of these cases, 90% are associated with gestational diabetes mellitus (GDM; Bishop et al., 2019). ACOG-derived and endorsed prenatal screening modalities that begin between 24 and 28 weeks of gestation have been used by obstetric clinicians for decades to promptly identify women at risk for or with definitive GDM (ACOG, 2018b). Infants at risk for exposure to unmanaged GDM include extremely low-birth-weight infants and infants of mothers who do not seek prenatal care.

GDM increases the risk for preeclampsia, cesarean or operative vaginal birth, and latent diabetes among women of childbearing age (ACOG, 2018b; Cheng et al., 2009). Women with preexisting (and uncontrolled) type 1 or 2 DM also incur increased risk for preeclampsia as well as diabetic ketoacidosis, retinopathy, and neuropathy. Fetuses subject to a persistently elevated glucose load are often large for gestational age (>90th percentile) at birth and develop macrosomia. Other noteworthy risks to the fetus include birth trauma with injury to the brachial plexus, in particular with an operative vaginal birth secondary to shoulder dystocia, respiratory distress, polycythemia, hypoglycemia, hyperbilirubinemia, and congenital heart disease (e.g., hypertrophic cardiomyopathy; Jnah & Trembath, 2019).

The ACOG and Society for Maternal-Fetal Medicine (SMFM) recommend that women with DM refractory to diet and exercise regimens receive pharmacotherapies with close monitoring; this strategy optimizes fetal and maternal outcomes (ACOG, 2018b; SMFM Publications Committee, 2018). Currently, the ACOG (2018b) and American Diabetes Association recommend insulin as a first-line therapy, whereas the SMFM Publications Committee (2018) recommends metformin. An alternative medication commonly prescribed to affected women is glyburide, a second-generation sulfonylurea (Table 5.3; ACOG, 2018b). Insulin does not cross the placenta, whereas both

TABLE 5.3 Common Diabetic Therapies and Food and Drug Association–Regulated Considerations

DRUG CATEGORY	DRUG NAME	FDA PREGNANCY CONSIDERATIONS (SUBSECTION 8.1)	FDA LACTATION CONSIDERATIONS (SUBSECTION 8.2; HALE, 2021)	FDA REPRODUCTIVE CONSIDERATIONS (SUBSECTION 8.3)
Insulin aspart	NovoLog	No teratogenic warning; does not cross the placenta; dose requirements often increase across pregnancy	Probably compatible with breastfeeding; RID unknown	Adequate contraception is recommended until euglycemia is achieved.
Insulin lispro	Humalog			
Insulin humulin	NPH			
Long-acting insulin glargine	Lantus			
Long-acting insulin detemir	Levemir			
Biguanide analog	Metformin	No teratogenic warning; crosses the placenta; no long-term safety data is available	Compatible with breastfeeding; RID unknown	
Second-generation sulfonylurea	Glyburide	No teratogenic warning; crosses the placenta; no long-term safety data is available; contraindicated as a first-line therapy for DM	Probably compatible with breastfeeding; RID unknown	

Note: Breastfeeding is considered safe when the RID is less than 10%. Drugs provided in this table are representative examples and not inclusive of all drugs that may be prescribed by an obstetrician or certified midwife. The Organization of Teratology Information Specialists continues to collect data specific to infant outcomes after exposure to the therapies listed in this table. Parents may independently enroll exposed infants by visiting https://mothertobaby.org

DM, diabetes mellitus; FDA, U.S. Food and Drug Administration; NPH, neutral protamine hagedorn; RID, relative infant dose.

Sources: From the American College of Obstetricians and Gynecologists. (2018b). ACOG practice bulletin no. 190: Gestational diabetes mellitus. *Obstetrics & Gynecology, 131*(2), e49–e64. https://doi.org/10.1097/aog.0000000000002501; Hale, T. W. (2021). *Hale's medications & mothers' milk 2021: A manual of lactational pharmacology* (19th ed.). Springer Publishing. https://doi.org/10.1891/9780826189264; Taketomo, C. K. (Ed.). (2023). *Pediatric & neonatal dosage handbook: An extensive resource for clinicians treating pediatric and neonatal patients* (29th ed.). Lexicomp/Wolters Kluwer; Society of Maternal-Fetal Medicine Publications Committee. (2018). SMFM statement: Pharmacological treatment of gestational diabetes. *American Journal of Obstetrics and Gynecology, 218*(5), B2–B4. https://doi.org/10.1016/j.ajog.2018.01.041

metformin and glyburide cross into the fetal circulation by passive diffusion. Fetal metformin drug concentrations often equilibrate to maternal levels. Studies have consistently shown that fetal glyburide levels are at least 70% lower than maternal levels (Caritis & Hebert, 2013; Schwartz et al., 2015). Neonatal clinicians should note that compared to insulin and metformin, maternal glyburide therapy is associated with a significant risk for prolonged postnatal hypoglycemia. Pregnant women may be advised to discontinue glyburide 14 days prior to delivery or the anticipated due date, to mitigate postnatal hypoglycemia.

Hypertensive Disorders

Hypertensive disorders that affect pregnant women include chronic hypertension, gestational hypertension, preeclampsia/eclampsia, and preeclampsia/eclampsia superimposed on chronic hypertension. The incidence of hypertensive disorders in pregnancy ranges between 2% and 25%; preeclampsia accounts for 2% to 8% of cases (Garovic et al., 2020; Topel et al., 2018). Perinatal risks include birth weight less than 2,500 grams, preterm birth, and a prolonged birth hospitalization often requiring neonatal intensive care. From a neurodevelopmental standpoint, studies have reported an association between gestational hypertension or preeclampsia and language delay in exposed infants and children between the ages of 2 and 15 years (Palatnik et al., 2021; Whitehouse et al., 2012). Prompt identification and treatment of the affected mother is essential to optimize neonatal outcomes.

Currently, the ACOG (2019a) recommends labetalol as a first-line therapy for chronic and gestational hypertension; contraindications include asthma, cardiomyopathy, heart block, and bradycardia (Table 5.4; ACOG, 2019a, 2020b; Battarbee et al., 2020). An alternative first-line therapy, when labetalol is contraindicated, is nifedipine. Other common treatment regimens include methyldopa and hydrochlorothiazide. The treatment of acute hypertension differs in that intravenous hydralazine, labetalol, or oral nifedipine are commonly prescribed first-line agents. Daily low-dose aspirin may be prescribed as prophylaxis for preeclampsia (ACOG, 2020b; Grab et al., 2000). Magnesium sulfate may be administered intravenously for eclampsia prophylaxis. Angiotensin-converting enzyme (ACE) inhibitors are specifically contraindicated during pregnancy due to a potential association with congenital anomalies (e.g., esophageal atresia, congenital heart defects); however, it remains unclear whether the proximate cause for these malformations is exposure to antihypertensive medications or the hypertensive state (Battarbee et al., 2020).

Neonatal clinicians should be aware that labetalol use is associated with neonatal respiratory depression, bradycardia, and hypoglycemia (Taketomo, 2023). Maternal hydrochlorothiazide use is associated with an increased risk for hyperbilirubinemia and thrombocytopenia (Taketomo, 2023). Extended magnesium sulfate exposure is associated with sedation and decreased gastrointestinal motility; neonatal clinicians should be prepared to provide appropriate resuscitative support at delivery and may consider a delayed or slow enteral feeding advance while monitoring serum calcium and magnesium levels until values normalize.

Psychiatric Disorders: Anxiety and Major Depressive Disorder

Two common psychiatric disorders treated during pregnancy are anxiety and depression. Anxiety disorders (AD) affect between 8% and 39% of pregnant women, with approximately 20% of affected pregnant women manifesting with one of eight ADs (Table 5.5).

Major depressive disorder (MDD) is a mood disorder characterized by symptoms of generalized anxiety and depression (e.g., fatigue, irritability, low energy; Martin-Key et al., 2021). The American Psychiatric Association (APA; 2013) considers perinatal depression, which begins during pregnancy or within the first postpartum month, an MDD. The prevalence of perinatal MDD ranges between 10% and 25% in high- and low-income countries, respectively (APA, 2013; Hasin et al., 2018; Woody et al., 2017). Of all pregnant women affected by MDD in the United States, 4% to 10% require antidepressant therapy to stabilize their mental health, with 6.3% of cases involving the use of selective serotonin reuptake inhibitors (SSRIs; Brajcich et al., 2021; Xing et al., 2020).

TABLE 5.4 Common Hypertensive Therapies and Food and Drug Administration-Regulated Considerations

DRUG CATEGORY	DRUG NAME	FDA PREGNANCY CONSIDERATIONS (SUBSECTION 8.1)	FDA LACTATION CONSIDERATIONS (SUBSECTION 8.2; HALE, 2021)	FDA REPRODUCTIVE CONSIDERATIONS (SUBSECTION 8.3)
Beta-adrenergic antagonist	Labetalol	No teratogenic warning; crosses the placenta; maternal use associated with IUGR	Probably compatible; RID 0.2%–0.6%	Preferred agent for the treatment of chronic hypertension; discontinuation is not indicated prior to conception
Calcium-channel blocker	Nifedipine	No teratogenic warning; crosses the placenta; maternal use associated with increased risk for perinatal asphyxia, prematurity, IUGR, and cesarean delivery	Probably compatible; RID 2.3%–3.4%	
Alpha-2 adrenergic agonist	Methyldopa	No teratogenic warning; crosses the placenta	Probably compatible; RID 0.1%–0.4%	Discontinuation is not indicated prior to conception unless contraindications exist
Vasodilator	Hydralazine	No teratogenic warning; crosses the placenta	Probably compatible; RID 1.2%	
Thiazide diuretic	Hydrochlorothiazide	No teratogenic warning; crosses the placenta	Probably compatible; RID 1.68%	Not applicable; therapy initiated after conception
NSAID	Aspirin (low dose, preeclampsia prophylaxis)[a]	No teratogenic warning; crosses the placenta	Probably compatible; RID 2.5%–10.8%	
Anticonvulsant	Magnesium sulfate[b]	No teratogenic warning; crosses the placenta	Compatible; RID 0.2%	

Note: Breastfeeding is considered safe when the RID is less than 10%. Drugs provided in this table are representative examples and not inclusive of all drugs that may be prescribed by an obstetrician or certified midwife. The Organization of Teratology Information Specialists continues to collect data specific to infant outcomes after exposure to the therapies listed in this table. Parents may independently enroll exposed infants by visiting https://mothertobaby.org.

[a] Low-dose aspirin is used for preeclampsia prophylaxis.

[b] Intravenous magnesium sulfate therapy is utilized for eclampsia prophylaxis.

FDA, U.S. Food and Drug Administration; IUGR, intrauterine growth restriction; NSAID, nonsteroidal anti-inflammatory drug; RID, relative infant dose.

Sources: From the American College of Obstetricians and Gynecologists. (2019a). ACOG practice bulletin no. 203: Chronic hypertension in pregnancy. *Obstetrics & Gynecology, 133*(1), e26–e50. https://doi.org/10.1097/AOG.0000000000003020; American College of Obstetricians and Gynecologists. (2020b). ACOG practice bulletin, number 222: Gestational hypertension and preeclampsia. *Obstetrics & Gynecology, 135*(6), e237–e260. https://doi.org/10.1097/AOG.0000000000003891; Hale, T. W. (2021). *Hale's medications & mothers' milk 2021: A manual of lactational pharmacology* (19th ed.). Springer Publishing. https://doi.org/10.1891/9780826189264; Taketomo, C. K. (Ed.). (2023). *Pediatric & neonatal dosage handbook: An extensive resource for clinicians treating pediatric and neonatal patients* (29th ed.). Lexicomp/Wolters Kluwer.

TABLE 5.5 Common Perinatal Anxiety Disorders

OBSESSIVE-COMPULSIVE AND RELATED DISORDERS	TRAUMA- AND STRESSOR-RELATED DISORDERS	ANXIETY DISORDERS
Obsessive-compulsive disorder	Acute stress disorder Posttraumatic stress disorder	Agoraphobia Generalized anxiety disorder Panic disorder Social phobia Specific phobia

Note: Categories align with the *Diagnostic and Statistical Manual of Mental Disorders* (5th ed.; *DSM-5*; APA, 2013).

TABLE 5.6 Congenital Malformations Associated With Fetal Exposure to Mood Stabilizers

DRUG NAME	ASSOCIATED FETAL MALFORMATIONS
Valproic acid	Cleft palate Congenital heart defects Hypospadias Neural tube defects
Carbamazepine	Congenital diaphragmatic hernia Facial dysmorphism Hypospadias Myelomeningocele
Lithium	Diabetes insipidus Ebstein anomaly Goiter Hypotonia

Sources: From Bromley, R. L., Mawer, G. E., Briggs, M., Cheyne, C., Clayton-Smith, J., García-Fiñana, M., Kneen, R., Lucas, S. B., Shallcross, R., & Baker, G. A. (2013). The prevalence of neurodevelopmental disorders in children prenatally exposed to antiepileptic drugs. *Journal of Neurology, Neurosurgery, and Psychiatry, 84*(6), 637–643. https://doi.org/10.1136/jnnp-2012-304270; Christensen, J., Grønborg, T. K., Sørensen, M. J., Schendel, D., Parner, E. T., Pedersen, L. H., & Vestergaard, M. (2013). Prenatal valproate exposure and risk of autism spectrum disorders and childhood autism. *Journal of the American Medical Association, 309*(16), 1696–1703. https://doi.org/10.1001/jama.2013.2270; Cohen, L. S., Friedman, J. M., Jefferson, J. W., Johnson, E. M., & Weiner, M. L. (1994). A reevaluation of risk of in utero exposure to lithium. *Journal of the American Medical Association, 271*(2), 146–150. https://doi.org/10.1001/jama.1994.03510260078033; Moretti, M. E. (2009). Psychotropic drugs in lactation—Motherisk update 2008. *Canadian Journal of Clinical Pharmacology, 16*(1), e49–e57. https://jptcp.com/index.php/jptcp/article/view/292/240; Pearlstein, T. (2013). Use of psychotropic medication during pregnancy and the postpartum period. *Women's Health, 9*(6), 605–615. https://doi.org/10.2217/whe.13.54

ADs and MDD are associated with an increased risk for preeclampsia or eclampsia as well as cesarean and operative vaginal delivery. Rejnö and colleagues (2019) reported a significant correlation between anxiety *or* depression and preeclampsia or eclampsia (adjusted odds ratio [aOR] = 1.17; 95% CI, 1.12, 1.22) as well as cesarean delivery (aOR = 1.62; 95% CI, 1.57, 1.68). Other studies have reported similar correlations between anxiety or depression and hypertensive disorders (Kurki et al., 2000, Miyasaka et al., 2018). The significance in these findings for neonatal clinicians relates to the aggregate comorbid risks imposed on fetuses when anxiety or depression and a hypertensive disorder (or any combination of these diseases) complicate a pregnancy. Fetal/neonatal risks include preterm birth, cesarean delivery, respiratory complications (e.g., RDS, TTNB), hyperbilirubinemia, and hypoglycemia. Some of these postnatal disease states require neonatal intensive care.

Psychotropic medications are frequently prescribed to pregnant women with ADs and MDD; antidepressants are prescribed more often than antianxiety medications (Hanley & Oberlander, 2014). Mood stabilizers, including valproic acid, carbamazepine, and lithium, are not prescribed during pregnancy due to a significant risk for congenital anomalies (Table 5.6). In some cases, antipsychotic drugs (e.g., risperidone, haloperidol) may be prescribed; these drugs are associated with maternal obesity and GDM, as well as birth weight in the 90th percentile or greater, as well as neonatal hypoglycemia (Newham et al., 2008).

ANTIDEPRESSANTS

Antidepressant medications include SSRIs (e.g., citalopram), serotonin and norepinephrine reuptake inhibitors (SNRI; e.g., duloxetine), dopamine reuptake inhibitors (DRI; e.g., bupropion), serotonin modulators (SM; e.g., trazodone), and tricyclic antidepressants (TCA; e.g., amitriptyline).

Despite adequate and well-powered data supporting the relative safety of antidepressant use during pregnancy, fears persist among some clinicians and pregnant women. Longstanding concerns relate to SSRI exposure and the development of fetal anomalies and postnatal complications, including congenital heart defects, persistent pulmonary hypertension of the newborn, preterm birth, birth weight less than 2,500 grams, and childhood autism. More recent studies, which properly controlled for risk factors and behaviors prevalent among women with psychiatric disorders, reported no significant associations (Chisolm & Payne, 2016; Huybrechts et al., 2014, 2015; Jarde et al., 2016; Kobayashi et al., 2016; Wang et al., 2015).

Although no teratogenic risks are linked to fetal antidepressant exposure, there are reports of transitional postnatal side effects of which neonatal clinicians should remain cognizant, specific to SSRI/SSNI exposure. Poor neonatal adaptation syndrome (PNAS) is a complication that affects 33% of neonates exposed to SSRI/SSNIs with or without adjunct dopamine-reuptake inhibitor or antipsychotic drug use during the third trimester of pregnancy (Hendson et al., 2021; Webster, 1973). PNAS, first reported in 1973, is a consequence of serotonin toxicity. Commonly reported manifestations include irritability, hypertonia, tremors, reduced sleep intervals, seizures, respiratory distress, and feeding intolerance (Brajcich et al., 2021). Postnatal management is limited to supportive care, as this condition is transient and self-limiting. Families benefit by receiving consistent emotional support and encouragement, and instruction when performing daily care and providing consoling techniques, including skin-to-skin care and lactation support.

ANTIANXIETY DRUGS

Drugs used to treat anxiety in pregnant women include benzodiazepines (e.g., lorazepam) and anticonvulsants (e.g., gabapentin). Of note, the following anticonvulsants are associated with teratogenic risks when consumed during the first trimester of pregnancy: carbamazepine, hydantoin, phenobarbital, and valproate; these drugs were marketed prior to 1976 and used to control maternal seizure activity.

Single-drug therapy for anxiety is limited to benzodiazepines and is associated with a low risk for facial deformities, namely cleft lip and palate (Iqbal et al., 2002; Lin et al., 2004). Combination therapy (SSRI/SSNI plus benzodiazepine) is associated with an increased risk for congenital heart defects (Oberlander et al., 2009). Alternatively, gabapentin is considered a safer alternative to benzodiazepine therapy. To date, no reports linking gabapentin use and congenital malformations have been published. However, some reports suggest that fetal exposure to gabapentin may increase the risk for preterm birth and birth weight less than 2,500 grams. As mentioned earlier in this section of the chapter, additional research is needed to control for confounders and to determine whether gabapentin exposure versus behaviors associated with anxiety are to blame for these potential adverse effects. Presently, clinicians are challenged to weigh the risks of fetal drug exposure against the risks of untreated anxiety disorder. Table 5.7 offers a summary of drug therapies used in pregnant women with AD and MDD.

DRUGS IN LABOR AND THE EFFECT ON THE FETUS AND NEWBORN

Neonates may be exposed to various pharmacologic agents in the immediate peripartum period. Drugs may be administered to the laboring mother for the fetoprotective effect or to treat maternal conditions. Tocolytics delay delivery, magnesium sulfate and antenatal corticosteroids protect the neonate's brain and lungs, induction agents facilitate a safe delivery, and analgesics/anesthetics provide maternal comfort. All these agents have unique pharmacologic properties in this setting and expose the neonate to both benefits and risks. Knowledge of these properties aids the neonatal medical team in providing optimal care.

TABLE 5.7 Common Psychiatric Drug Therapies and U.S. Food and Drug Administration-Regulated Considerations

PRIMARY DIAGNOSIS	DRUG CATEGORY	DRUG NAME	FDA PREGNANCY CONSIDERATIONS (SUBSECTION 8.1)	FDA LACTATION CONSIDERATIONS (SUBSECTION 8.2; HALE, 2021 RECOMMENDATIONS)	FDA REPRODUCTIVE CONSIDERATIONS (SUBSECTION 8.3)
MDD	SSRI	Citalopram	No teratogenic warning; crosses the placenta	Probably compatible; RID 3.56%–5.37%	Discontinuation is not indicated prior to conception; single therapy is preferred; preferred SSRI for first-time treatment of MDD.
	SNRI	Duloxetine	No teratogenic warning; crosses the placenta	Probably compatible; RID 0.12%–1.12%	Discontinuation is not indicated prior to conception; not recommended as first-line treatment.
	DRI	Bupropion	No teratogenic warning; crosses the placenta	Probably compatible; RID 0.11%–1.99%	Discontinuation is not indicated prior to conception; associated with less risk for sexual dysfunction compared to other antidepressants.
	SM	Trazodone	No teratogenic warning; crosses the placenta	Probably compatible; RID 2.8%	Discontinuation is not indicated prior to conception; **not** recommended as first-line treatment for new-onset MDD during pregnancy.
	TCA	Amitriptyline	No teratogenic warning; crosses the placenta	Probably compatible; RID 1.08%–2.8%	
AD	Benzodiazepine	Lorazepam	**Teratogenic warning;** crosses the placenta	Probably compatible; RID 2.6%–2.9%	Adequate contraception is recommended until alternative therapy is established.
	Anticonvulsant	Gabapentin	No teratogenic warning; crosses the placenta	Probably compatible; RID 6.6%	Folic acid supplementation is recommended prior to conception.

Note: Breastfeeding is considered safe when the RID is less than 10%. Drugs provided in this table are representative examples and not inclusive of all drugs that may be prescribed by an obstetrician or certified midwife.

AD, anxiety disorder; DRI, dopamine reuptake inhibitors; MDD, major depressive disorder; RID, relative infant dose; SM, serotonin modulators; SNRI, serotonin and norepinephrine reuptake inhibitors; SSRI, selective serotonin reuptake inhibitors; TCA, tricyclic antidepressants.

Sources: From Hale, T.W. (2021). Hale's medications & mothers' milk 2021: A manual of lactational pharmacology (19th ed.). Springer Publishing. https://doi.org/10.1891/9780826189264; Taketomo, C. K. (Ed.). (2023). Pediatric & neonatal dosage handbook: An extensive resource for clinicians treating pediatric and neonatal patients (29th ed.). Lexicomp/Wolters Kluwer.

Threatened Preterm Labor and Fetal Neuroprotection

MAGNESIUM SULFATE

Magnesium sulfate readily crosses the placenta within an hour of maternal administration (Ting et al., 2018). Due to its rapid placenta transit, magnesium sulfate has been studied as a fetal neuroprotective agent. Proposed neuroprotective mechanisms of action based on animal models include inhibition of excitatory neurotransmitter receptors, tempering of proinflammatory cytokines, and reduction of intracellular calcium influx (Beloosesky et al., 2016; Mami, Ballesteros, Fritz, et al., 2006; Mami, Ballesteros, Mishra, et al., 2006; Tam Tam et al., 2011). Antenatal magnesium sulfate produces a decreased risk for cerebral palsy (Doyle, 2012; Doyle et al., 2009; Shepherd et al., 2017) and the combined outcome of cerebral palsy and death in preterm neonates (Crowther et al., 2017). Antenatal magnesium sulfate also reduces the risk of cerebellar hemorrhage in preterm neonates less than 33 weeks' gestation (Gano et al., 2016). Data assessing cerebral palsy risk reduction with antenatal use of magnesium sulfate in term neonates are lacking (Nguyen et al., 2013).

Magnesium sulfate dosing for fetal neuroprotection is a 4-gram loading dose followed by a continuous infusion of 1 gram per hour for up to 24 hours (Crowther et al., 2003; Marret et al., 2007). Loading doses of up to 6 grams may be used when treating preeclampsia or eclampsia (ACOG, 2020a). Maternal characteristics may impact fetal magnesium exposures. Obstetric patients receiving magnesium sulfate with higher body weight or renal dysfunction eliminate magnesium at a lower rate, possibly contributing to increased fetal exposure (da Costa et al., 2020). Fetal and neonatal adverse events may have a dose-dependent and/or time-dependent exposure relationship (Greenberg et al., 2013). The ratio of umbilical vein serum magnesium concentration to maternal serum concentration at birth is 0.94 ± 0.15 (Brookfield et al., 2016). Consequently, serum magnesium concentrations at birth are higher in neonates exposed to magnesium in utero compared to neonates who are not exposed (McGuinness et al., 1980; Pritchard, 1980). Given that magnesium is renally excreted, the steady improvement in renal function that occurs during the newborn period helps normalize serum magnesium concentrations.

Magnesium sulfate may increase the risk of clinically significant adverse effects in preterm and term neonates. The relationship between magnesium sulfate and gastrointestinal morbidity in preterm neonates remains an area of active investigation. Retrospective studies have produced mixed results (Kim et al., 2021; Rattray et al., 2014; Sung et al., 2022), although randomized controlled trials have not detected increased risk (Shepherd et al., 2019). Diligent monitoring is warranted. Prolonged fetal hypermagnesemia may lead to toxicity resulting in osteopenia. An obstetric patient was treated with magnesium sulfate for tocolysis from 22 weeks' to 30 weeks' gestation when triplets were born. The two surviving siblings experienced fractures and osteopenia due to demineralization of bone (Wedig et al., 2006). Observational cohort studies of late preterm and term neonates, published over 50 years ago, reported conflicting evidence specific to hyporeflexia and respiratory depression after antenatal magnesium sulfate administration (Lipsitz & English, 1967; Stone & Pritchard, 1970). More recent investigations have associated maternal magnesium sulfate administration for preeclampsia or eclampsia at greater than 36 weeks' gestation with increased risk of NICU admissions requiring both fluid and nutritional support (Greenberg et al., 2013). A contemporary study demonstrated decreasing Apgar scores with increasing antenatal magnesium dose. The study also demonstrated increased hypotonia, asphyxia, intubation, and NICU admission with higher doses (Das et al., 2015).

CORTICOSTEROIDS

Intramuscular antenatal corticosteroids reduce the risk of adverse neonatal outcomes, including perinatal and neonatal death and RDS (McGoldrick et al., 2020). Antenatal corticosteroids mature alveoli, increase pulmonary surfactant synthesis, and improve lung compliance. Peak efficacy is experienced between 2 and 7 days after course completion (ACOG, 2017). Corticosteroid use for fetal lung maturation is an off-label indication. However, antenatal corticosteroids are indicated for obstetric patients at risk for delivery within 7 days and any of the following:

- 23 0/7 to 23 6/7 weeks' gestation based on the family's decision regarding resuscitation,
- 24 0/7 to 33 6/7 weeks' gestation, or
- 34 0/7 to 36 6/7 weeks' gestation with no previous course of corticosteroid administration.

A repeat course may be administered if at least 14 days have passed since the completion of the first series and the fetus is under 34 0/7 weeks' gestation and at risk for delivery in the next 7 days (ACOG, 2016, 2017, 2020a).

The two recommended corticosteroids for fetal lung maturation are betamethasone and dexamethasone. Both corticosteroids cross the placenta in their active forms with similar activity and are partially metabolized via placental 11β-HSD2, inactivating a percentage of the parent corticosteroid (Murphy et al., 2007). The two compounds are stereoisomers varying by a single methyl group's spatial orientation. Although structurally similar, betamethasone has a higher volume of distribution and a longer half-life (Fanaroff & Hack, 1999). Fetal and neonatal outcomes are consistent for both regimens (Brownfoot et al., 2013). Limited long-term outcome data are available comparing the two regimens. The betamethasone dosing regimen is 12 mg intramuscularly every 24 hours for two doses. The dexamethasone dosing regimen is 6 mg intramuscularly every 12 hours for four doses. A first dose should be administered even if course completion is not anticipated prior to delivery. Any exposure to betamethasone or dexamethasone, even in a limited capacity, is beneficial to the fetus (ACOG, 2016). Decreasing the dosing interval (e.g., every 24 hours to every 12 hours) in order to complete an antenatal corticosteroid regimen does not improve fetal and neonatal outcomes (ACOG, 2016).

TOCOLYTICS

Terbutaline. Terbutaline relaxes uterine smooth muscle by agonizing beta-2 cells, causing tocolysis. Short-term terbutaline (≤72 hours) is used off-label for tocolysis preventing preterm labor. Terbutaline carries the following black-box warning:

> Terbutaline sulfate has not been approved and should not be used for prolonged tocolysis (beyond 48 to 72 hours). In particular, terbutaline sulfate should not be used for maintenance tocolysis in the outpatient or home setting. Serious adverse reactions, including death, have been reported after administration of terbutaline sulfate to pregnant women. In the mother, these adverse reactions include increased heart rate, transient hyperglycemia, hypokalemia, cardiac arrhythmias, pulmonary edema and myocardial ischemia. Increased fetal heart rate and neonatal hypoglycemia may occur as a result of maternal administration. (Bedford Laboratories, 2011)

Enteral terbutaline administration is not approved or recommended for tocolysis. The subcutaneous dosing regimen is 0.25 mg every 20 minutes to every 3 hours with dose-holding parameters for maternal HRs over 120 beats per minute (ACOG, 2016). The intravenous infusion regimen is initiated at 2.5 or 5 mcg per minute, titrated every 20 to 30 minutes by 2.5 or 5 mcg per minute to a maximum of 25 mcg per minute. Note that intravenous dosing is in micrograms and the subcutaneous dosing is in milligrams. Once tocolysis has occurred, wean terbutaline to the lowest effective dose to reduce adverse event risk (ACOG, 2016; Hearne & Nagey, 2000; Travis & McCullough, 1993). Terbutaline has a shorter half-life and higher clearance in pregnant patients compared to 3 to 6 months' postpartum (Lyrenas et al., 1986). Terbutaline should be used with caution in patients also receiving magnesium sulfate due to the increased risk of maternal complications (ACOG, 2016). Terbutaline crosses the placenta, reaching therapeutic concentrations in the fetus, although the medication is relatively hydrophilic (Bergman et al., 1984), leading to the possible fetal/neonatal adverse events of tachycardia and hypoglycemia (ACOG, 2016).

Nifedipine. Nifedipine is a calcium channel blocker that inhibits the influx of calcium into smooth muscles, ultimately relaxing the muscle. Nifedipine has two enteral formulations, immediate-release and extended-release. Immediate-release formulations have been used off-label as a tocolytic agent for up to 48 hours. The dosing strategy begins with a loading dose of 20 to 30 mg followed by a maintenance dose of 10 to 20 mg every 3 to 8 hours, with a maximum daily dose of 180 mg. Most dosing intervals are every 6 to 8 hours (ACOG, 2016). Nifedipine is highly protein bound. Recall that a bound drug is less likely to cross the placenta and impact the fetus. Once the maternal nifedipine serum concentration has reached steady state, fetal umbilical cord blood nifedipine serum concentrations approximate 77% of the maternal concentration (Silberschmidt, 2008). One underpowered, randomized placebo-controlled trial of nifedipine for tocolysis compared neonatal outcomes between the groups. No differences were seen between groups for necrotizing enterocolitis (NEC), sepsis, intracranial hemorrhage, or periventricular leukomalacia (Nijman et al., 2016). Secondary outcomes in another small, underpowered study comparing neonatal outcomes for patients whose mothers were randomized to receive nifedipine or terbutaline for tocolysis did not conclude a statistically significant difference among NEC, sepsis, intracranial hemorrhage, or jaundice in the groups (Padovani et al., 2015). Transient, acute neonatal complications requiring careful monitoring may include tachycardia/arrhythmia and hypotension. Like terbutaline, nifedipine should be used with caution when coadministered with magnesium sulfate due to the increased risk of maternal adverse events (ACOG, 2016).

Drugs Used to Induce or Augment Labor

OXYTOCIN

Oxytocin is indicated for induction or augmentation of labor, promoting vaginal delivery, as well as postpartum hemorrhage control. Oxytocin stimulates oxytocin receptors, promoting the production of localized prostaglandins and release of intracellular calcium, ultimately inducing uterine contractions. Oxytocin receptors begin to appear around the start of the second trimester and increase in concentration until term gestation (Page et al., 2017). As receptor concentrations increase, less oxytocin is needed to stimulate uterine contractions. Multiple oxytocin dosing regimens have been studied. Oxytocin, a continuous infusion, is titrated and weaned based on uterine contraction patterns and fetal heart rates (FHRs). Initial infusion rates range from 0.5 to 6 milliunits per minute and are titrated by 1 to 6 milliunits per minute based on specific protocol (Alhafez & Berghella, 2020; Simpson, 2020). Some protocols have been referred to as high- or low-dose regimens. A pharmacokinetic study concluded that increased infusion rates merely increase the serum concentration of oxytocin without reflecting progressing labor or uterine activity (Perry et al., 1996). Institutions should have set oxytocin protocols in order to reduce possible medication errors. The onset and duration of action is 1 minute and 60 minutes, respectively (Taketomo, 2023). Peak serum concentrations are achieved approximately 40 minutes after administration (Seitchik et al., 1984). Maternal clearance is unchanged with pregnancy (Zeeman et al., 1997). A serious maternal adverse effect is tachysystole, or excessive uterine contractions, defined as five contractions over 10 minutes within a 30-minute window (Simpson, 2020). The use of oxytocin to promote uterine contractions may impact the FHR. Oxytocin may require weaning or stopping if the FHR remains abnormal. Neonates born to primiparous mothers receiving oxytocin have increased odds of cord blood pH less than 7.20 (OR = 2.84, 95% CI = 1.27–6.34; Hidalgo-Lopezosa et al., 2016).

DINOPROSTONE

Dinoprostone is a prostaglandin, E_2 specifically, which relaxes cervical smooth muscles allowing for dilation of the cervix. Dinoprostone is administered locally to the cervix as a gel, insert, or suppository. The onset of action is approximately 10 minutes postadministration. Product selection does impact the duration of action. The vaginal insert provides dinoprostone at 0.3 mg per hour for 12 hours, whereas the vaginal suppository's duration is 2 to 3 hours (Forest Pharmaceuticals, 2006; Pfizer, 2017). Like oxytocin, FHR should be monitored and tachysystole may occur, which may require removing the dinoprostone suppository or insert. Fetal adverse events are related to the effects of maternal contractions versus systemic drug exposure (Simpson, 2020).

Drugs in Early Labor

Additional medications may be used as adjunctive therapies during labor that are not directly related to tocolysis or induction or augmentation of labor. These medications may treat or prevent accompanying comorbidities like nausea or vomiting, anxiety, or pain. Information for two medications is provided in Table 5.8 (ACOG, 2018a; Serreau et al., 2005).

NEURAXIAL ANESTHESIA

Neuraxial anesthesia is a broad term encompassing spinal and epidural anesthesia. Epidural anesthesia is administered via catheter into the fatty epidural space near nerve roots, and spinal anesthesia is administered into the subarachnoid space and enters the cerebrospinal fluid. Local anesthetics, such as bupivacaine and ropivacaine, are used in epidural anesthesia. Although epidural anesthesia

TABLE 5.8 Peripartum Treatments for Nausea/Vomiting

MEDICATION	INDICATION	COMMENTS	FETAL AND NEONATAL CONSIDERATIONS
Promethazine	• PINV • Opioid adjunctive medication	• Adjunct therapy when first-line nausea and vomiting agents are ineffective • Reduces the opioid dose required for maternal pain management	• Crosses the placenta • Possible inhibition of neonatal platelet aggregation up to 2 weeks after delivery
Hydroxyzine	• Peripartum anxiety • PINV • Opioid adjunctive medication	• Contraindicated in early pregnancy for PINV • Reduces the opioid dose required for maternal pain management	• Crosses the placenta • Possible neonatal withdrawal with prolonged in utero exposure

PINV, pregnancy-induced nausea and vomiting.

is a localized administration, some systemic absorption may occur, resulting in maternal, fetal, or neonatal cardiovascular and neurologic adverse events. Both bupivacaine and ropivacaine cross the placenta readily via passive diffusion. Both are also highly protein bound, limiting the available free drug to cross the placenta (Fresenius Kabi, 2018; Hospira, 2011). It is important to note that only the 0.25% and 0.5% bupivacaine is indicated for obstetric use (Hospira, 2011).

Drugs in Active Labor

Labor is an event that causes significant pain in the person giving birth. Some pregnant individuals choose to labor without pain-relieving medications, but many use pharmacologic assistance to support the labor experience. Births that occur at home are considered completely natural, with no availability of medications for pain relief. Births occurring in a birthing center may have the availability of nitrous oxide (NO). Additional pharmacologic options for pain relief are found within a hospital setting. The ACOG (2019b) states that analgesia should be allowed for any laboring person who makes the request and has no medical contraindications. There are a number of options for pain relief, including analgesia, such as opioids, which reduce the pain sensation yet allow muscle movement; anesthesia that blocks pain sensation and may prevent motor function; and NO, which is an inhalation analgesic. Each of these is discussed in this section.

OPIOIDS

Opioids have been used to minimize labor pain, but they rarely block it completely. Tolerance after repetitive administration further limits efficacy; therefore, these medications are generally not given until active labor. Opioids used during labor have a range of pharmacokinetic properties that should be carefully considered when determining the optimal dosing interval for the mother and potential impacts on the neonate. Recall that opioids cross the placenta via passive diffusion, and fetal exposure is relatively robust despite protective placenta mechanisms. The most common adverse effect in the neonate is respiratory depression, highlighting the vital role of postnatal respiratory support after recent/repetitive exposure. Commonly prescribed opioids and core pharmacokinetic principles are listed in Box 5.1.

GENERAL ANESTHESIA

General anesthetics are indicated when neuraxial anesthesia is insufficient during a complicated cesarean section. These agents generally have a rapid onset and short duration of action, but also rapidly cross the placenta and impact the fetus. Neonatal respiratory depression is common and often necessitates the presence of a skilled resuscitation team. However, neonatal impact is dramatically mediated by neonatal pharmacokinetics. For example, fetal concentrations of the mild inhalational anesthetic nitrous oxide are 80% of the maternal concentration; however, the neonatal

BOX 5.1 Commonly Prescribed Opioids and Core Pharmacokinetic Principles

Butorphanol (Stadol)
Typical dose: 1–2 mg IV or IM
PK data: Onset within minutes IV, ≤ 15 minutes IM
Duration: 3–4 hours

Nalbuphine (Nubain)
Typical dose: 10 mg IV, 10 mg IM
PK data: Onset: 2–3 min IV, 10–15 min IM
Duration: 3–6 hours

Remifentanil (Ultiva)
Typical dose: 0.05–1 mcg/kg/min
PK data: Onset: 1–3 minutes
Duration: 3–10 minutes

Fentanyl (Sublimaze)
Typical dose: 25–50 mcg IV, PCA: Loading dose 50–100 mcg IV; patient bolus 10–25 mcg IV; lockout 5–12 minutes
PK data: Onset: 1–3 min IV
Duration: 30–60 minutes IV

IM, intramuscular; IV, intravenous; PK, pharmacokinetic; PCA, patient-controlled analgesia.
Source: Lexicomp. (n.d.). Lexi-Drugs online. UpToDate. Retrieved 2023, from https://online.lexi.com

half-life is ~3 minutes, resulting in limited neonatal impact (Rosen, 2002). In contrast, propofol elimination is slow and highly variable in early neonatal life. When used for maternal anesthesia, propofol easily crosses the placenta and commonly suppresses Apgar scores in the newborn.

CONCLUSIONS

Greater than 90% of pregnant women ingest at least one licit OTC or prescription drug during pregnancy, with most pregnant women taking two drugs daily. Therefore, neonatal clinicians must carefully review the maternal history and consider the known effects of fetal exposures to maternally ingested drugs (licit and illicit). The PRC was initiated in 1979, followed by the PLLR of 2014, and supplemented by the TERIS. Each of these systems provides obstetric and neonatal clinicians with all known pregnancy, lactation, and reproductive-related implications of maternally ingested medications. That being said, gaps exist, and much work remains to be done for this information to be complete. For example, research focused on maternal and placental physiology, per week of gestation, is needed to better understand the safety and efficacy profile of drugs that are accessed, metabolized, and excreted by the fetus. Postnatally, long-term population-based studies are needed that investigate the effect of maternally ingested drugs on the transition to extrauterine life, the immediate newborn period, and across the life span. We are optimistic that with each upcoming edition of this textbook, new data will be available to share with readers!

LEARNING TOOLS AND RESOURCES

Advice From the Authors

Robin Webb Corbett, PhD, RNC, FNP-C

Obstetrics is providing care to two patients; the mother–infant dyad. You always have to clarify whether the medication to be taken is needed and safe for both of these patients. To do otherwise, may result in lifelong complications for one or both patients.

John Brock Harris, PharmD, BCPS, BCPPS, FCCP

When evaluating medication use in patients, the risks and benefits must be compared. The evaluation of medication use in obstetric patients is vital considering the risks and benefits are impacting both mom and fetus. Both mom and fetus have built-in physiologic protection mechanisms mitigating medication risk. Data and information are consistently being added to the body of literature that continues to recalibrate pharmacotherapeutic approaches to obstetric care.

Renee Oakley Spain, MAEd, DNP, CNM

Don't be afraid to say, "I don't know but I will find out." Read to stay up to date and take care of yourself.

Amy J. Jnah, DNP, APRN, NNP-BC

Collaborative information sharing between obstetric and neonatal clinicians should be intentional and timely. Please proactively seek dialogue with your obstetric team. Prioritize completing a thorough review and analysis of the maternal history and engage the family in conversation, as this yields additional valuable information. Your understanding of placental physiology, pathophysiology, and the effect of maternally ingested drugs on the fetus, in combination with knowledge of the maternal medical and pregnancy history, is critical to identifying at-risk neonates and optimizing outcomes.

Discussion Prompts

1. Diagram placental development, formation of the maternal spiral arteries, and blood flow from the maternal spiral arteries to the intervillous space. Why is maternal blood flow regarded as the primary rate-limiting factor for fetal nutrient uptake and growth? How does maturation of the chorionic villi affect the transfer of nutrients and drug molecules from the mother's circulation to the fetal circulation?
2. Discuss the risks associated with DM and pregnancy. Which congenital anomalies are associated with DM and when during fetal development are they likely to present? How might these anomalies affect the transition to extrauterine life?
3. Maternal ultrasonography can detect major fetal anomalies as early as 16 weeks of gestation. Discuss the effect of major anomalies (e.g., congenital heart defect, myelomeningocele, hydrops fetalis) diagnosed during early gestation and the role of the neonatal APRN during the intrapartum and immediate postnatal period.

Mind Map

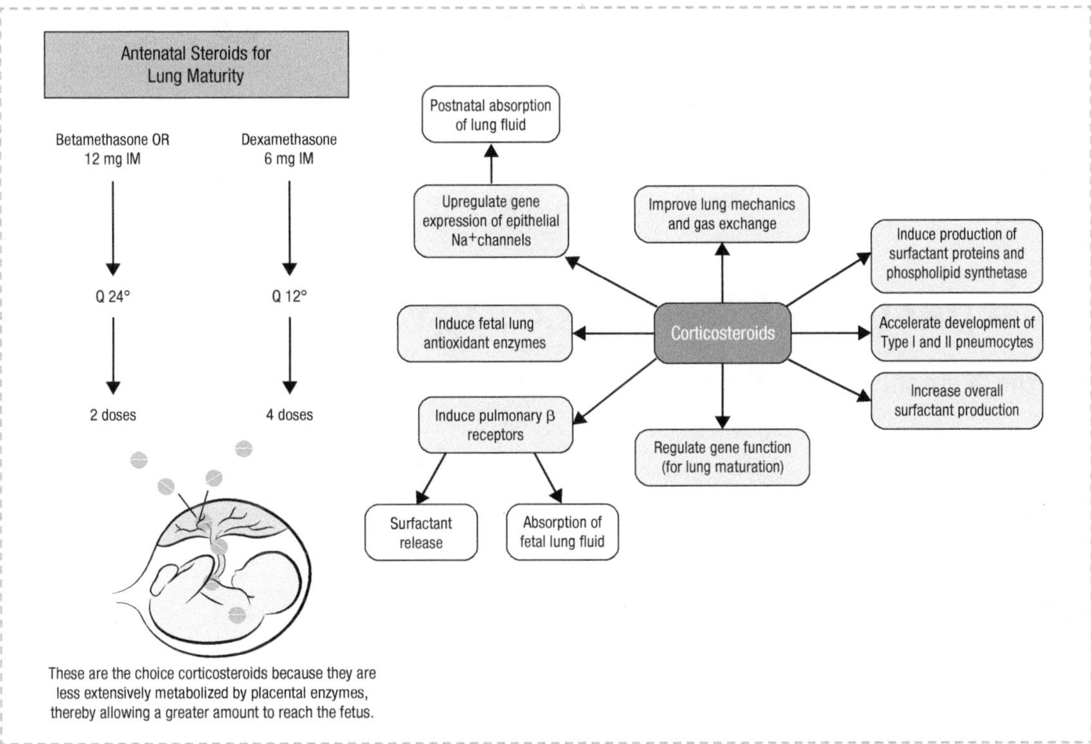

Note: This mind map reflects the design team's interpretation of a portion of one or more concepts addressed in this chapter. Readers should regard the mind maps woven throughout this textbook as examples of multisensory study tools that can be developed to encourage conceptual understanding. Readers are encouraged to develop their own unique mind maps in consultation with academic faculty or clinical preceptors. Design credit: Sarah Byler, MSN, APRN, NNP, and Kristen Landis, BSN, RNC-NIC, East Carolina University Neonatal Nurse Practitioner Program.

REFERENCES

References for this chapter are online and available at https://connect.springerpub.com/content/book/978-0-8261-5884-0/part/partI/toc-part/ch5.

chapter 6

Postpartum Pharmacology

Kaytlin Krutsch, Teresa Baker, and Thomas W. Hale

LEARNING OBJECTIVES

After completing this chapter, the reader should be able to:

- Explain the importance of breastfeeding from the standpoint of maternal and infant gain.
- Assess which medications are transmitted through breast milk to infants.
- Evaluate which infant situations pose the highest risk.
- Determine appropriate risk mitigation strategies to limit infant exposure to drugs when appropriate.
- Recall available evidence-based resources for selecting the safest medications.

INTRODUCTION

The benefits of breastfeeding are numerous and well documented for infants and their mothers. Breastfed infants have a lower risk of sudden infant death syndrome (SIDS), respiratory tract infections, otitis media, gastroenteritis, and necrotizing enterocolitis, among other morbidities (Bowatte et al., 2015; N. Christensen et al., 2020; Frank et al., 2019; Hauck et al., 2011; Holman et al., 2006; Ip et al., 2007). Lactation affords the mother protective benefits against hypertension, type 2 diabetes, some cancers, and heart disease long after the cessation of breastfeeding (Bajaj et al., 2017; Li et al., 2014; Collaborative Group on Hormonal Factors in Breast Cancer, 2002; Li et al., 2014; Nguyen et al., 2017; Zhang et al., 2015).

Historically, clinicians opted to discontinue breastfeeding while breastfeeding patients consumed almost any medication. However, there are few cases known to have caused infant harm (Anderson et al., 2016). The breast is incredibly efficient not only in producing the nutritional components of milk but also in excluding substances that may be of harm. Simultaneously, maternal health is an essential influencer for infant health. Maternal medication use is one of the most common reasons patients are advised to stop breastfeeding in the first year (Kirkland, 2001). In reality, very few medications are known to be incompatible with breastfeeding (Berlin & van den Anker, 2013; Centers for Disease Control and Prevention [CDC], 2022; Sachs & Committee on Drugs, 2013). In most cases, a practical solution can be found to safely keep patients breastfeeding despite medication use. This chapter describes how medications penetrate breast milk; how to evaluate the infant's risk from breast milk residues; and how to support breastfeeding mothers in safe, informed decision-making.

Disclaimer: We seek to be inclusive of all people in our material. We recognize that not all people who give birth and lactate identify as female, and some identify as neither male nor female. Our readers should be aware that the information included in this chapter is intended for all persons, including those who breastfeed, chest feed, or feed with donated expressed human milk.

PHYSIOLOGY REVIEW: BREAST MILK PRODUCTION AND REGULATION

The compositions of colostrum, transitional milk, and mature milk all differ due to changes in the production and transfer of milk components. Prior to pregnancy, secretory epithelial cells in the mammary gland, also called *lactocytes*, function similarly to other semipermeable membranes in the body. Lobular alveoli clusters, lined with lactocytes, extend into a ductal system ending at the nipple (Figure 6.1). During early pregnancy, hormonal changes induce mammogenesis, increasing the number and size of lactocytes and duct systems to prepare for the unique function of producing milk. Lactocytes extract the necessary building blocks of milk from the maternal blood supply and transform them into a highly regulated milk secretion.

Lactogenesis starts in late pregnancy and persists through the first few weeks postpartum. Upon suckling, oxytocin is released and initiates alveolar smooth muscle contraction, thus ejecting milk. During the colostral phase, white blood cells, antibodies, and other cellular components from maternal circulation may pass freely into the colostrum via paracellular passive diffusion. These components are thought to provide vital support to the infant for gastrointestinal (GI) growth, seeding the developing infant gut and microbiome while suppressing hazardous bacterial growth (Martín et al., 2003). During the initial phase, exogenous substances, such as maternal medications, are likely to transfer through this permeable membrane into the milk even if they are large molecules. When progesterone levels abruptly drop after delivery, mammary epithelial cells finalize their differentiation into lactocytes and migrate closer together to form tight apical junctions (Figure 6.2; Neville et al., 2002). Then, full milk production (also called *lactation*) is completely established. Subsequently, tight junctions inhibit paracellular diffusion, preventing large molecules present in maternal serum from entering the milk. By 2 weeks' postpartum, tight junctions have been fully developed between lactocytes, producing mature milk. This process is maintained until involution.

Regulation of Milk Supply

Frequent and complete emptying of the ducts is needed for high-volume milk production. Anything that interferes with emptying the breast, such as blocked ducts or a poor infant latch, may lead to a sharp decrease in milk supply. Most cases of inadequate milk supply are due to incomplete removal

FIGURE 6.1 Physiology of the breast.

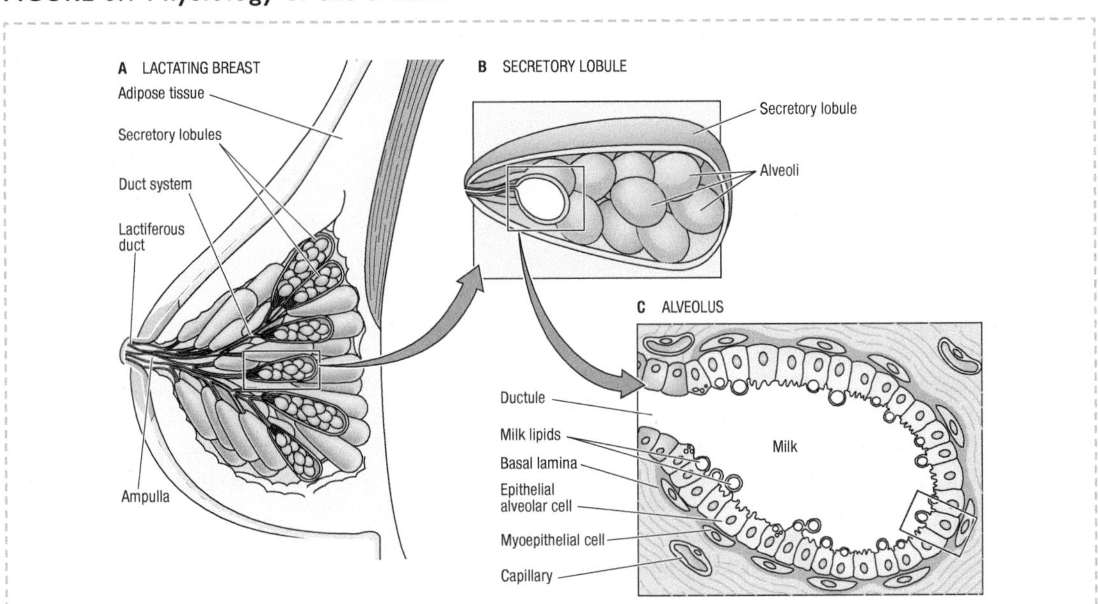

Source: From Mesiano, S., & Jones, E. (2017). Fertilization, pregnancy, and lactation. In W. Boron & E. Boulpaep (Eds.), *Medical physiology* (pp. 1129–1150, Fig. 56.11). Elsevier.

of milk from the breast. In some cases, this may be reversible without medications, but some patients may require a galactagogue (e.g., metoclopramide) to maintain adequate milk production.

Milk supply primarily depends on maternal prolactin levels remaining greater than the pre pregnancy baseline (>50 ng/mL). Prolactin is a hormone produced and stored by lactotrophs in the anterior pituitary gland during pregnancy and throughout lactation. It promotes alveolar survival, maintenance of tight junctions, production of protein and lactose synthesis, and more. Prolactin levels rise steadily throughout pregnancy, peaking at levels of 400 ng/mL. Even with these high levels, milk production is apparently inhibited by progesterone until delivery (Cox et al., 1999). Then, prolactin levels decline, and by day 3 or 4 suckling and milk removal are required to sustain milk production. Upon infant feeding, pulses of prolactin are released; without these frequent pulses, milk production will wane. Readers should also note that, although prolactin is required for milk synthesis, the volume of milk secreted is not necessarily directly related to plasma prolactin concentration (Figure 6.3).

Certain neurotransmitters inhibit prolactin synthesis and secretion. The most common inhibitory neurotransmitter is dopamine, also known as *prolactin-inhibiting hormone (PIH)*. Figure 6.4 describes the mechanism of action of dopamine specific to prolactin inhibition. Clinicians should

FIGURE 6.2 Pathways for drug secretion into the milk throughout stages of lactation.

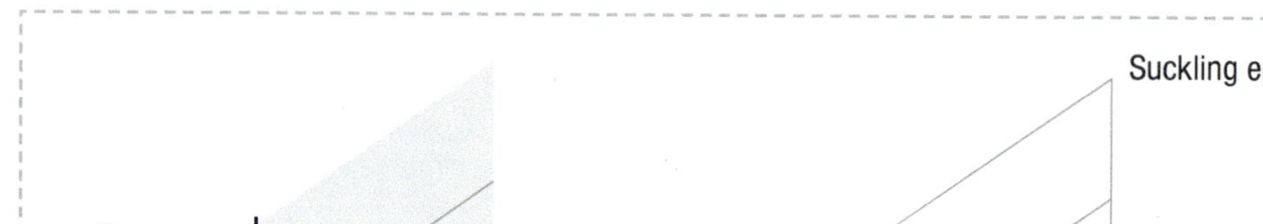

Source: From Medina Poeliniz, C., Engstrom, J. L., Hoban, R., Patel, A. L., & Meier, P. (2020). Measures of secretory activation for research and practice: An integrative review. *Breastfeeding Medicine, 15*(4), 191–212. https://doi.org/10.1089/bfm.2019.0247.

FIGURE 6.3 Hormonal changes in the peripartum period.

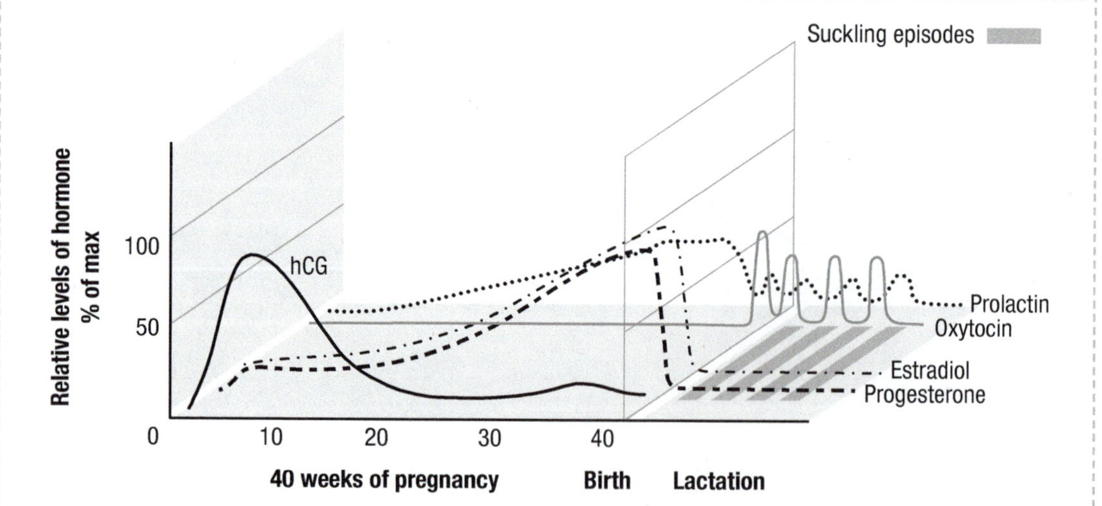

hCG, human chorionic gonadotropin.
Source: From Grattan, D. R., & Ladyman, S. R. (2020). Neurophysiological and cognitive changes in pregnancy. In E. A. P. Steegers, M. J. Cipolla, & E. C. Miller (Eds.), *Handbook of clinical neurology* (pp. 25–55). Elsevier.

recognize that dopamine agonists may inhibit lactation, whereas dopamine antagonists may stimulate lactation. These drugs are discussed in the sections titled "Lactation Inhibitors" and "Galactagogues," respectively.

DRUG TRANSFER INTO BREAST MILK

To some degree, all substances ingested (e.g., foods, preservatives, environmental substances, medications) are transferred to the breast milk. The concentrations of these substances in the milk are usually low and deemed clinically irrelevant. With ultra sensitive analytical procedures available today, medication concentrations can be detected down to picograms per milliliter. Thus, it is almost always possible to quantify some level of drug in the milk. These levels are attributed to the living nature of the lactocyte barrier. At 6 months postpartum, alveolar lactocytes age and begin to shed, reducing the production of milk. Thus, the resultant minimal transfer of drug may not be clinically relevant to the infant's health.

Ideally, the degree of transfer and the subsequent effects of a drug on the infant would be studied and known before use by a breastfeeding patient. However, only about 400 currently available drugs have been evaluated to establish their concentrations in breast milk (U.S. Department of Health and Human Services et al., 2017). Even fewer have follow-up data for infant outcomes. For all other drugs, methods of estimating transfer and risk are necessary.

FIGURE 6.4 Regulation of lactation.

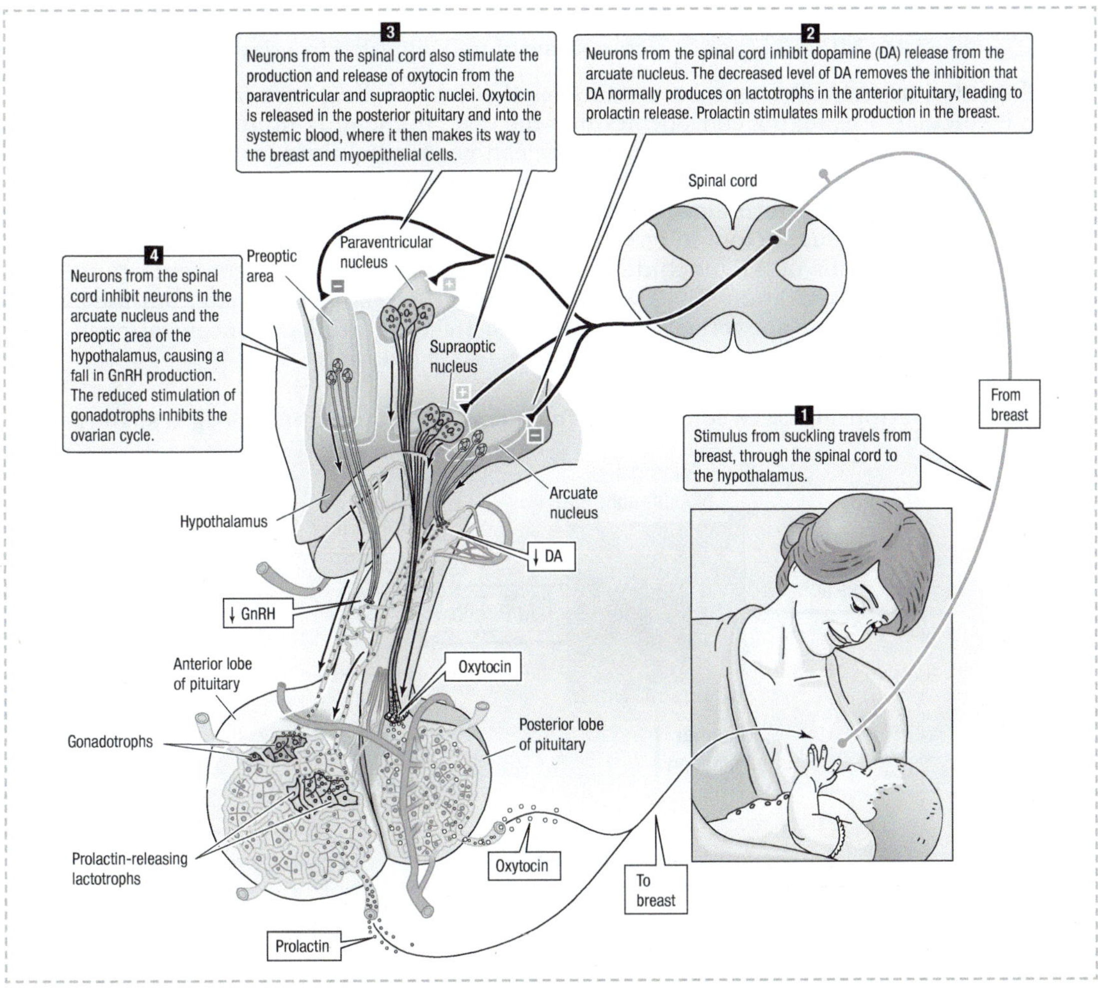

DA, dopamine; GnRH, gonadotropin-releasing hormone.
Source: From Mesiano, S., & Jones, E. (2017). Fertilization, pregnancy, and lactation. In W. Boron & E. Boulpaep (Eds.), *Medical physiology* (pp. 1129–1150, Fig. 56.12). Elsevier.

Ultimately, the risk to the infant is determined by considering drug toxicity and the dose transferred to the infant, either by passive diffusion (transcellular or paracellular) or by active transport from maternal plasma (Ilett & Kristensen, 2005). Most medications transfer into the milk by way of a passive transcellular diffusion gradient. However, few drugs transfer via active transport, which raises legitimate concerns for unstudied drugs.

The amount of drug that transfers into the milk is directly related to the level of drug in the maternal plasma. Milk to plasma ratios are commonly reported in breastfeeding literature; however, without significant context, they are clinically irrelevant. Fortunately, multiple pharmacokinetic scenarios prohibit drug transfer into maternal plasma, which in turn prohibits drug transfer into the milk. Drugs that are not systemically absorbed by the patient do not have the opportunity to enter the breast milk. For example, many inhaled medications, nasal sprays, or topical preparations never leave the application site. Some oral medications, like loperamide or budesonide, cannot leave a healthy GI tract. Other drugs have such limited durability in serum that they do not persist long enough to enter the milk in clinically relevant amounts, like many anesthetics. In short, if a drug is not present in maternal plasma, it will not be normally found in milk.

Scientists quantify the infant's exposure using two methods: (a) the absolute infant dose (AID) and (b) the relative infant dose (RID; Begg et al., 2002). The relationship between these metrics is described in Figure 6.5. None are perfect indicators of infant risk. A comparison of the pros and cons of each metric is described in Table 6.1.

Absolute Infant Dose

$$\text{AID} = (C_{max} \text{ or } C_{ave}) \times (\text{volume of milk ingested in a day}).$$

The absolute (theoretical) infant dose estimates the dose of drug an infant is exposed to per day. It is calculated using the concentration of the drug in the milk multiplied by the volume (total fluid) of milk ingested by the infant. The estimated total fluid (milk) intake used with this calculation is 150 mL/kg/d. Clearly, this is an average and may not represent the milk intake of preterm infants, term newborns, or toddlers. When pediatric doses of a medication exist, AID can be a valuable tool to use to compare with the infant's exposure, to determine relative toxicity. Pitfalls of AID include the lack of standardization of concentration to use. Using maximum concentration (C_{max}) will always result in an overestimate, but the average concentration (C_{ave}) may not reflect an infant breastfeeding at peak concentrations. AID is also sometimes referred to as the *theoretical infant dose (TID)*.

FIGURE 6.5 Relationship between metrics for quantifying lactational drug transfer.

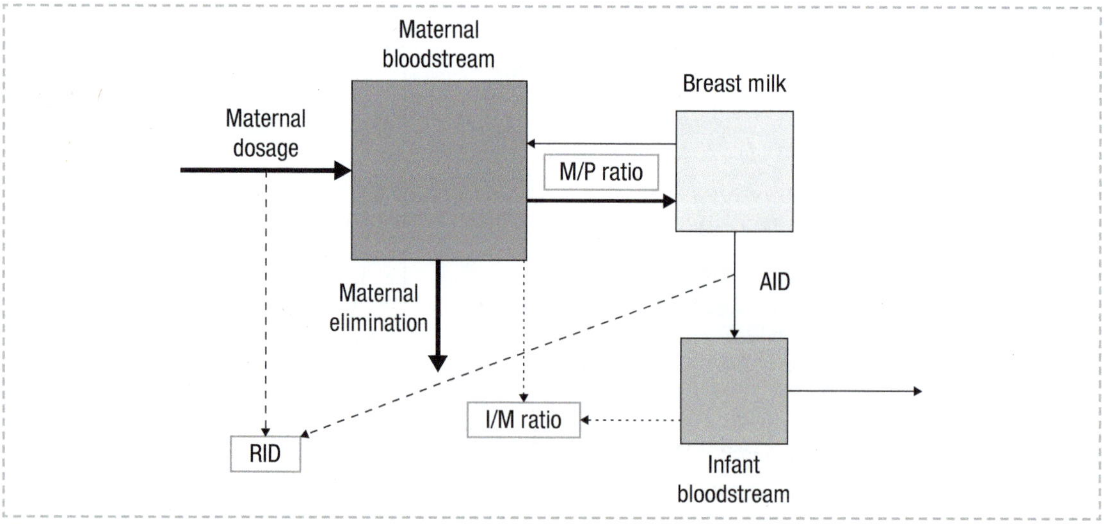

Note: M/P ratio, I/M ratio, and RID indicate the various metrics describing the extent of drug passage.
AID, absolute infant dose; I/M, infant to maternal plasma concentration ratio; M/P, milk to maternal plasma concentration ratio; RID, relative infant dosage.
Source: From Anderson, P. O. (2018). Drugs in lactation. *Pharmaceutical Research, 35*(3), 45. https://doi.org/10.1007/s11095-017-2287-z.

TABLE 6.1 Summary of Parameters

	M/P	AID	RID
Quantifies drug transfer	Yes	Yes	Yes
Estimates infant exposure	No	Yes	Yes
Adjusts for an infant-sized dose	No	No	Yes
Considers maternal dose	No	No	Yes
Considers infant absorption	No	No	No
Considers relative toxicity	No	No	No
Conventional safety standard	No	No	<10%

AID, absolute infant dose; M/P, milk to plasma ratio; RID, relative infant dose.
Sources: From Bennett, P. (1988). *Drugs and human lactation* (1st ed.). Elsevier; Bennett, P. N., & Jensen, A. A. (1996). *Drugs and human lactation: A comprehensive guide to the content and consequences of drugs, micronutrients, radiopharmaceuticals, and environmental and occupational chemicals in human milk* (2nd ed.). Elsevier.

Relative Infant Dose

RID (%) = absolute infant dose (milk; mg/kg/d) / maternal dose (mg/kg/d) × 100.

RID is a practical tool for assessing drug safety in breastfeeding. It is more than simply the percentage of a maternal dose that is excreted in the milk. RID standardizes the maternal dose to a referential weight-adjusted infant-sized dose. For example, if a 70-kg patient takes a 1,000-mg dose of medication and their infant consumes a milk volume containing 5.7 mg of the drug, the infant consumes 0.57% of the maternal dose. Using this example, the RID is 8%.

Unfortunately, RID does not include all factors needed for a risk–benefit evaluation, particularly the infant's tolerance or the influence of the maternal dose. Doses exceeding those studied to attain RID may result in disproportionately increased risk.

STANDARDS OF COMPATIBILITY

An RID benchmark for safety was arbitrarily set at less than 10% in the late 1980s/early 1990s (Bennett, 1988; Bennett & Jensen, 1996). At the same time, RIDs greater than 25% were considered risky and to be avoided. Although there were no data to support these cutoffs, they have been commonly used for decades without significant detriment. Since then, a lower safety benchmark of 5% (again, arbitrary) has been suggested for psychotropic drugs (Larsen et al., 2015). In practice, each case is different. Proper evaluation of risk and benefit for breastfeeding mothers and their infants requires consideration of several factors.

MATERNAL DOSE

Some degree of standardization has been achieved in developing the parameters mentioned earlier to assess medication transfer into the milk. However, they each come with limitations. A significant limitation is the lack of consideration for the maternal dose. Many doses commonly used in practice fall far below doses reported in lactation studies. Ultimately, the level of transfer of all medications into the milk is dependent on the dose. Assuming all else is constant, if a patient takes a 500-mg dose of a drug with a 15% RID, and another patient takes double the dose, that patient's infant will receive double the drug via milk. Figure 6.6 illustrates this example.

Active Transport of Medications

The transcellular movement of a drug (or any substance) against an electrical, pressure, or concentration gradient, and across a cell membrane with the help of a specialized carrier protein and the expenditure of energy, is called active transport. Active transport is capable of moving drugs into or out of the breast milk. While this transport pathway poses a legitimate risk to infant safety, very few drugs are known to be actively transported into and out of the breast milk.

FIGURE 6.6 Influence of maternal dose on infant exposure.

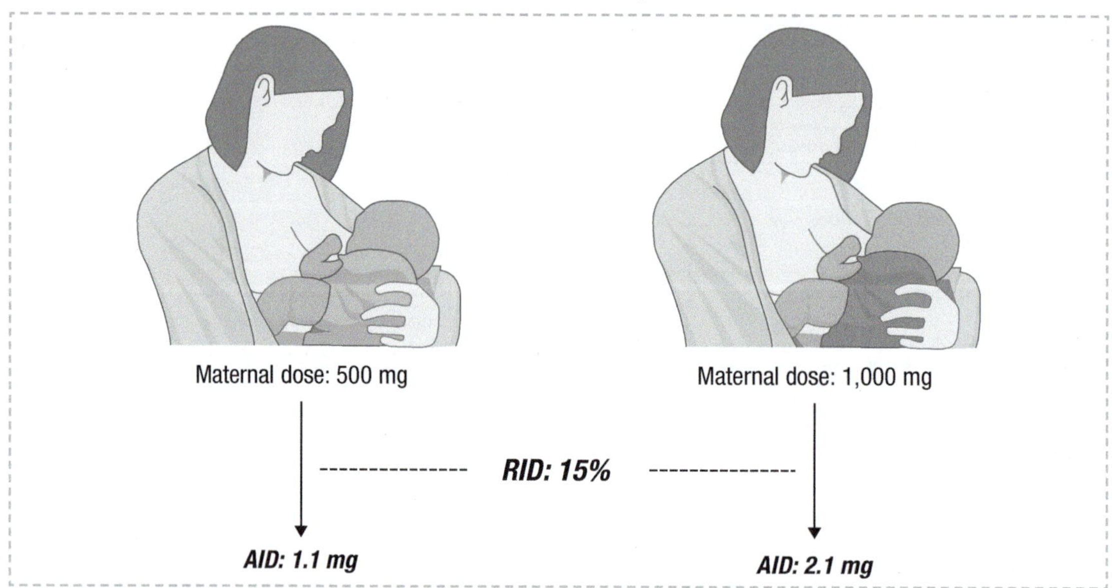

Note: Visualization of relative infant dose versus absolute infant dose. Note that in this example, maternal and infant weights are equivalent, and only the dosage of the drug changes.
AID, absolute infant dose; RID, relative infant dose.

When milk to plasma ratios contradict expectations based on the physiochemical properties of a drug, active transport may be a primary suspect. Some drugs may be actively transported out of the breast milk compartment as a protective mechanism in the same manner as used by the blood–brain barrier. For example, when evaluating the pharmacokinetic parameters of metformin, estimated transfer into the milk should be significant (Hale et al., 2002). However, studies evaluating its actual concentration in milk are five fold lower than expected. The lower observed drug levels may be due to an active efflux transporter pumping metformin out of the milk and back into the maternal plasma. To the contrary, active transport of iodide, by the sodium iodide symporter (solute carrier transporter [SLC] family), is extensive. Iodine is transported so extensively that levels in milk may evoke neonatal hypothyroidism (Delange et al., 1988). Other drugs are actively transported by the breast cancer resistance protein (ABC family). These include cimetidine, nitrofurantoin, acyclovir, and ranitidine. Although these are concentrated in milk, they usually do not attain clinically relevant levels in infants.

Given that drugs are often designed to mimic endogenous substances and likewise fit onto transporters found naturally throughout the body, it is not surprising that transport proteins on lactocytes are capable of actively transporting certain drugs into and out of the milk. Unfortunately, active transporters on human lactocytes are relatively undefined. Once an accurate mapping of these transporters is achieved, it may be more feasible to predict which drugs are actively transported into the milk (Nauwelaerts et al., 2021). At present, we know of only about five drugs that are actively transported into human milk (Table 6.2).

Passive Diffusion of Medications

Paracellular passive diffusion of substances occurs when solutes move from a highly concentrated region to a region of lower concentration. In the lactocyte, this occurs when a nonionized, unbound drug moves from maternal plasma into the breast milk across the mammary epithelial cells. Because passive diffusion happens without energy expenditure, the physiochemical properties of medications can be used somewhat to estimate their degree of transfer. It is easier for drugs with low molecular weight, low protein binding, and high pKa to pass through the lactocytes. Therefore, these drugs find equilibrium between maternal plasma and milk at higher drug-in-milk concentrations. Several drug attributes affect passive diffusion across lactocytes and are discussed next.

TABLE 6.2 Medications With Active Transport Into the Milk

DRUG	REFERENCES	M/P	RID (%)	CLINICAL EFFECT
Radioactive iodine	Delange et al., 1988; Postellon & Aronow, 1982	23	n/a	HAZARDOUS; limit to <150 mcg daily. There are also reports of neonatal hypothyroidism.
Nitrofurantoin	Gerk et al., 2001	6	6.8	Not clinically significant in older infants. This drug can displace bilirubin from albumin binding sites—use caution in premature infants and infants with hyperbilirubinemia or G6PD deficiency.
Acyclovir	Lau et al., 1987	4	<1.5	Therapy in neonates is common and produces few toxicities. Calculated intake by infant would be less than 0.87 mg/kg/d. Comparable neonatal doses are 60 mg/kg/d. Avoid application directly to nipples.
Ranitidine	Kearns et al., 1985	7–24	2.5–9.1	Therapy in neonates is common and produces few toxicities. Estimated infant ingestion is 0.4 mg/kg/d. Comparable pediatric doses are 2–10 mg/kg/d.
Cimetidine	Oo et al., 1995	5	9.8–32.6	Therapy in neonates is common and produces few toxicities. Estimated infant ingestion is 5.6 mg/kg/d. Comparable pediatric doses are 20–40 mg/kg/d.

G6PD, glucose-6-phosphate dehydrogenase; M/P, milk to plasma ratio; n/a, not available; RID, relative infant dose.

MOLECULAR WEIGHT AND PROTEIN BINDING

The primary drug attribute that affects passive diffusion across lactocytes is the size of the molecule. Small drugs, like lithium (less than 200 daltons), pass readily through cell membranes and into the milk. Drugs larger than 500 to 800 daltons have difficulty entering milk without a transporter. Many drugs today are quite large, such as monoclonal antibodies (~150,000+ daltons), botulinum toxin (150,000 daltons), enoxaparin (8,000 daltons), and insulin (6,000 daltons). Their size alone prevents entry into the milk in clinically relevant amounts. Although adverse effect profiles may seem concerning for these examples, they are all considered compatible with breastfeeding.

Protein binding works similarly. Most drugs in plasma travel bound to plasma proteins, namely albumin. Albumin weighs 65,000 daltons. Therefore, a drug–protein (albumin) complex will be far too large to diffuse out of the plasma and into the lactocyte. For example, warfarin (308 daltons) is 99% protein-bound in the plasma, making it a large drug–protein complex that has yet to be detected in milk samples with maternal use up to 12 mg daily (McKenna et al., 1983; Orme et al., 1977). Based on current data, drugs that exhibit protein binding exceeding 85% exhibit low transfer into the milk (G. D. Anderson, 2006). Only the free (unbound) drug passively diffuses out of plasma.

VOLUME OF DISTRIBUTION

Recall from Chapter 4, "Neonatal Pharmacogenomics and Pharmacogenetics," that the theoretical amount of water in which a given dose would have to be dissolved to produce an experimentally measured maximum plasma concentration is called the *volume of distribution (Vd)*. Practically speaking, a drug with a high Vd yields a lower plasma concentration than the same dose of a drug with a low Vd. Taking this one step further, drugs with a Vd that exceeds the estimated plasma volume (3.5 L or 0.05 L/kg) reside outside the plasma and in select tissues (e.g., adipose tissue, skeletal muscle, bone). Recall the previous discussion which established that the concentration of a drug in milk is almost entirely determined by the concentration of free (unbound) drug in the breastfeeding mother's *plasma*. Therefore, after the absorption phase, drugs with a high Vd, such as digoxin (Vd: 6 L/kg) and marijuana (Vd: 10 L/kg), primarily concentrate in the peripheral tissues and do not transfer in clinically relevant amounts into the milk.

LIPID SOLUBILITY

Cell membranes are predominantly composed of lipid bilayers; thus, drugs must exhibit some lipophilicity (fat solubility) to transfer across most membranes. Lipophilic drugs (which exhibit an affinity for fats) passively dissolve through basilar and apical cell membranes and into the milk. Milk fat also can concentrate lipid-soluble drugs, increasing the total drug quantity in milk. The clinical relevance of this phenomenon is limited by the estimated fat content in human milk relative to total milk consumed by the infant. Milk has a high lipid content, ranging from 2.3% in foremilk to as much as 8% in hindmilk. Lipid content is highly variable, fluctuating among individual people, time of day, and type of milk expression (e.g., hand expression vs. electric pump).

Furthermore, lipid-soluble medications frequently cross the blood–brain barrier, producing high levels in the central nervous system (CNS). If a drug is active in the CNS, it may also produce higher levels in the breast milk. Unfortunately, these drugs often exhibit neurologic adverse effects, such as sedation, using the same rationale. A classic example of this phenomenon is the antidepressant mirtazapine. A drug's lipophilicity is measured in a laboratory setting by its octanol-to-water partition coefficient (cLogP). Mirtazapine's cLogP is 2.8, meaning it is almost three times more soluble in lipids than in water. Similarly, its concentration in fatty hindmilk is 2.3 times higher than in foremilk (Kristensen et al., 2007). Although this is often a theoretical concern, it does not always mean the proportional difference in drug levels is clinically significant. For example, duloxetine has a cLogP greater than 4 and concentrations do rise in hindmilk, but RID is less than 1% for both hindmilk and foremilk.

EVALUATING DRUG RISK TO THE INFANT

The assessment of the safety of drugs in breast milk depends on five major factors: toxicity, maternal dose, amount of medication present in the breast milk available for infant absorption, oral bioavailability, and the ability of the infant to clear the medication. Even though numerous studies review the levels of drugs in breast milk and their bioavailability, each infant's ability to tolerate many medications is still highly variable and requires close evaluation by the attending clinician.

Toxicity

Some drugs are inherently more toxic than others. Even in miniscule doses, cancer chemotherapy drugs, radioisotopes, and antimetabolites may be hazardous to an infant. Other drugs are toxic only at high doses, such as opioid pain relievers. Still other drugs may not be overly toxic at therapeutic levels via breast milk when comparing alternative options in a risk–benefit analysis. Basic knowledge of the drug at hand is required to make an appropriate risk–benefit determination.

Infant Absorption of Drugs in Milk

Simply because a drug is present in an infant's milk does not mean it will reach the infant's systemic circulation. GI systems designed to break down compounds to ready them for utilization are often protective, destroying the activity of drugs. Although it has not been extensively studied, it is commonly assumed that infant oral bioavailability is similar to that of an adult soon after birth (Alcorn & McNamara, 2003). However, because of underdeveloped digestive systems in prematurity, absorption may be altered in this population. Slower intestinal absorption in these infants is often advantageous in this respect, as it keeps plasma concentrations of drugs low (Besunder et al., 1988). Additionally, an infant's liver is comparatively larger than in an adult.

Oral Bioavailability

The proportion of a dose that reaches the systemic circulation after oral administration is referred to as *oral bioavailability*. The movement of solutes (nutrients in food, liquids, and drugs) from the GI tract to portal circulation of the gut uses the same principles of transfer discussed previously. The portal circulation initially delivers all drugs to the liver, which sequesters and metabolizes many of them before reaching peripheral blood circulation. This "first-pass" effect may exponentially reduce the amount of drug available to the body. Examples of drugs that have protective low oral bioavailability include morphine. Choosing medications with low oral bioavailability ultimately leads to reduced drug exposure in the infant. Table 6.3 lists medications with poor oral bioavailability in adults.

Many drugs are specially formulated to circumvent pharmacokinetic challenges with oral absorption. For example, women with gastric reflux may take a proton pump inhibitor, such as omeprazole, which cannot withstand acidic environments. For that reason, omeprazole is contained within acid-resistant granules designed to dissolve in the basic environment of the intestines. Upon release from the granules, the drug is absorbed into systemic circulation. Other drugs are injected subcutaneously (e.g., insulin, enoxaparin) or even intravenously (IV). These drugs exhibit their intended effect in the patient, and whatever amount of drug is then present in the patient's breast milk would be rendered inert and/or not be absorbed by the infant's GI tract.

Even if a drug is sequestered in the infant's GI tract, some medications present in breast milk can exert negative effects on the infant (e.g., antibiotics). These drugs may irritate the mucosa, disturb the gut flora, or serve as an osmotic laxative. The most common symptoms are diarrhea and constipation, although others are possible. Because local GI adverse effects do not appear during clinical trials with protectively formulated mechanisms (e.g., nonoral routes, enteric coating), these may not be mentioned in drug labels or be easily predicted. Clinically speaking, signs of feeding intolerance could result from drug-induced iatrogenic disturbances of the breast milk and should be considered in differential diagnoses in infants who present with a mild feeding intolerance.

Clearance of Drugs Transferred Through Milk

Placental drug transfer, especially when drugs are ingested over a prolonged period of time, can yield clinically significant drug levels in the neonate. If a patient continues taking a drug while lactating, and the drug is readily transferred into their breast milk, it is possible for serum levels in the breastfed neonate to rise over the first few weeks of life, even to a dangerous level. Infants must clear and eliminate drugs after birth; however, these pathways are immature. As hepatic and renal function improves, this risk resolves. A typical example of this phenomenon is seen with lithium, which is discussed at length in Chapter 2, "Prescriptive Authority."

Other factors that affect drug clearance include postnatal age, hepatic and renal function, and volume of milk ingested. These factors are discussed in this section.

POSTNATAL AGE

Infant age is a suggestive predictor of risk from exposure to maternal medications that pass into the milk. Approximately 63% of adverse reactions reported in the literature (in case reports) are from neonates (0–28 days of life; P. O. Anderson et al., 2016). An additional 15% of adverse reactions

TABLE 6.3 Medications With Low Oral Bioavailability

DRUG	ORAL BIOAVAILABILITY (%)
Acyclovir	20
Atorvastatin	14
Benzoyl peroxide	5
Budesonide	37
Cefdinir	15–25
Ceftriaxone	0
Chlorothiazide	13
Gentamycin	5
Linaclotide	0
Morphine	24
Vancomycin	0

Note: Percentages reflect adult values.
Source: From Hale, T. W. (2020). *Hale's medications & mothers' milk 2021*. Springer Publishing Company.

occur in the second month of life. These trends are likely attributable to several factors, including existing infant drug load upon delivery, higher milk consumption, and metabolic capacity. A comparison of these events over time is described in Figure 6.7.

HEPATIC FUNCTION

Recall from Chapter 4, "Neonatal Pharmacogenomics and Pharmacogenetics," that many drugs are hepatically metabolized, in large part through the action of cytochrome P450 (CYP) enzymes. Preterm and critically ill term neonates are uniquely vulnerable over the first few months of life. Hepatic function is immature and often incapable of compensating for minor drug exposures; drugs are not metabolized as expected. In general, neonates born ≤30 weeks' gestational age possess 28% of adult total CYP protein mass (Alcorn & McNamara, 2002). Infants aged 1 to 3 months exhibit about 20% to 50% of their adult enzymatic activity, which finally peaks at age 12 months (Grijalva & Vakili, 2013; Piñeiro-Carrero & Piñeiro, 2004).

Because hepatic biotransformation pathways are immature in infants, drugs that are purely metabolized in the liver have prolonged drug elimination and extended plasma half-lives. Careful scrutiny of the ontogeny of the specific enzymes at hand is required to evaluate specific drugs for neonates. As metabolic capacity improves, the risk of a negative drug effect is reduced. By 4 months of life, most term infants can metabolize and handle drugs efficiently.

RENAL FUNCTION

Nephrogenesis begins as early as week 8 of gestation, glomerular filtration commences during week 9, and urine production is observed by week 10 (Jnah & Trembath, 2019). Nephrogenesis is considered 80% complete by 36 weeks of gestation; completion by term gestation is typical. Infants born at term have the total number of nephrons they will have in their lifetime. Premature infants undergo postnatal nephrogenesis, due to glomerular hypertrophy and tubular elongation, for up to 40 days postnatally (Dyson & Kent, 2019). Regardless, kidney function develops quickly over the first 2 weeks of life.

By 2 months' postpartum, term infants exhibit almost 80% of their adult renal function (Atiyeh et al., 1996). By that time, they are more capable of metabolizing drugs following exposure via breast milk. Many drugs that are considered nephrotoxic, arousing caution in the neonatal

FIGURE 6.7 Infant events over time.

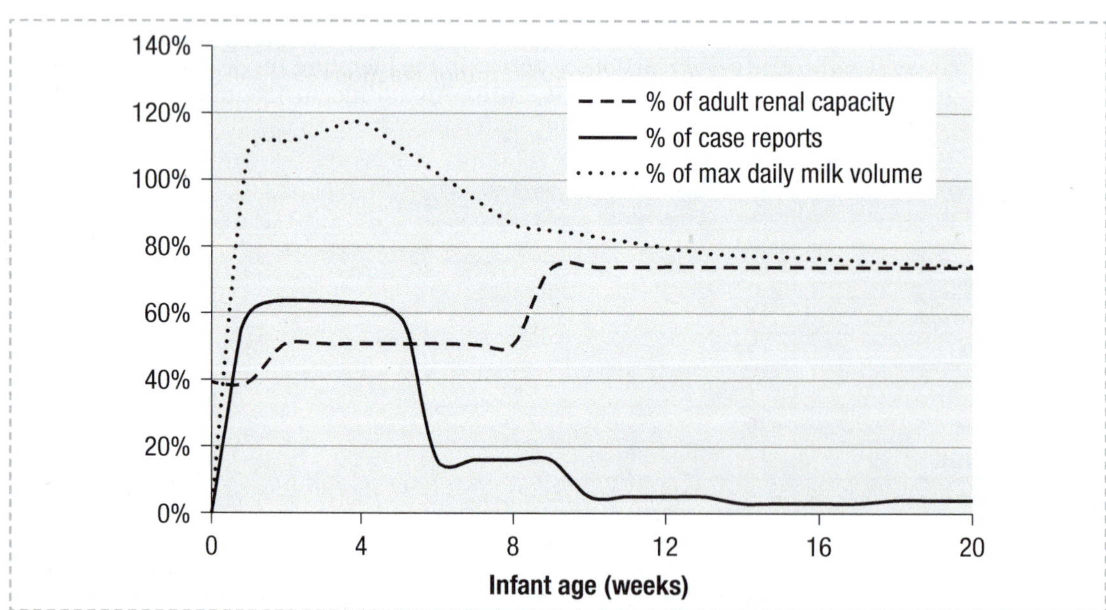

Note: Comparison of case reports, infant renal function, and milk volume over time. As renal function matures and milk volume decreases, case reports decrease sharply.

population, are also poorly orally bioavailable, limiting their risk of acute kidney injury through breast milk (Hanna et al., 2016). For example, vancomycin, aminoglycosides, amphotericin B, and acyclovir are all less than 20% orally bioavailable.

VOLUME OF MILK CONSUMPTION

As previously discussed, when progesterone inhibition of lactation is removed after delivery of the placenta, lactocytes finalize their maturation and colostrum can be expressed. The lactocyte barrier grows tighter during the same early postpartum period when milk volume expands. The transition of low volume with leaky junctions to high volume with tight junctions somewhat balances the risk of toxicity of drugs in the colostrum and transitional milk.

Many breastfeeding mothers who do not pump are unaware of the amount of milk they feed to their infants. Further, the volume of mature milk ingested is highly variable to each mother–infant dyad. Vital factors for prediction are the extent to which an infant is breastfed and postnatal age. The standard reference used to estimate the amount of milk ingested by an exclusively breastfed infant is 150 mL/kg/d. However, this is an estimated average and does not accurately represent average consumption for neonates during the immediate postnatal period. Neonates feeding during the colostral period, infants supplemented with formula or donor milk, or infants of those with milk supply difficulties may ingest far less milk. Mother–term infant dyads who are exclusively breastfeeding typically benefit from assistance from trained lactation consultants, who can help establish an effective latch and milk transfer. Once lactation is established, the actual volume of intake is likely higher over the first months of life and then decreases over time (P. O. Anderson & Valdes, 2015). The peak in volume of milk consumed aligns with the trend of reports of infant adverse events, suggesting that the events may be related. Thus, the congruence of low metabolic capacity and high milk volumes corresponds with infant risk.

CONTEXTUALIZING INFANT RISK

The risk of infant harm due to maternal medication ingestion is widely overestimated (P. O. Anderson et al., 2003, 2016; Soussan et al., 2014; Verstegen et al., 2020). Over 17 years, U.S. poison centers received 2,300 calls related to infant adverse effects attributed to breast milk-associated medication exposures (Beauchamp et al., 2019). Major reactions (e.g., respiratory depression, arrest) were confirmed in only eight instances and attributed to only two drug classes: opioids, benzodiazepines, or a combination of both. More than 53 million infants were breastfed during this time, yielding an incidence of one severe reaction per more than six million breastfed infants (CDC, 2020). Less severe cases (e.g., drowsiness, agitation, diarrhea) involving moderate reactions were limited to 43 infants, and 170 infants displayed minor reactions (Beauchamp et al., 2019).

Other studies have reviewed trends in case reports of infant harm thought to be attributed to maternal medication exposure through breast milk over decades. One hundred cases were evaluated using the Naranjo algorithm to assess a causal relationship between a clinical event and a potential drug cause. Of these reports, none could be definitively attributed to milk exposures, and less than half (47%) of events were found to be a "probable" adverse event (P. O. Anderson et al., 2003).

Another analysis suggested two identifiable factors that predict infant risk: infant age and drug class (P. O. Anderson et al., 2016). However, evaluating case reports alone without an understanding of medication usage inevitably leads to major shortcomings. Medications that are commonly used are also the most likely to be represented in case reports. Breastfeeding is the most prevalent in the early postpartum days; at the same time, there are higher numbers of case reports. Without a method to standardize case reports per exposure, conclusions from these counts must be limited.

MATERNAL DRUGS COMMONLY ASSOCIATED WITH ADVERSE EFFECTS IN INFANTS

When evaluating maternal medication safety, it is prudent to consider the likelihood and possible severity of adverse effects specific to the maternal drug chosen (Table 6.4). Case reports of infants with adverse effects are most frequently due to opioids, antidepressants, anticonvulsants, and the simultaneous use of multiple drug classes (Figure 6.8; P. O. Anderson et al., 2016).

TABLE 6.4 Common Medications That May Impact Lactation

DRUGS THAT INCREASE MILK SUPPLY	DRUGS THAT REDUCE MILK SUPPLY
• Metoclopramide: major • Domperidone: major	• Bromocriptine: major • Cabergoline: major • Aripiprazole: minor/moderate • Combination estrogen contraceptives: none/minor (>12 weeks' postpartum), moderate/major (<12 weeks' postpartum) • High estrogen doses: moderate/major • Pseudoephedrine: moderate • Epinephrine: major • Ropinirole: possible

Note: "Major" indicates a substantial increase/decrease in milk supply. "Moderate" indicates a noticeable increase/decrease. "Minor" indicates a slight increase/decrease.

FIGURE 6.8 Rates of adverse effects of most common drug classes.

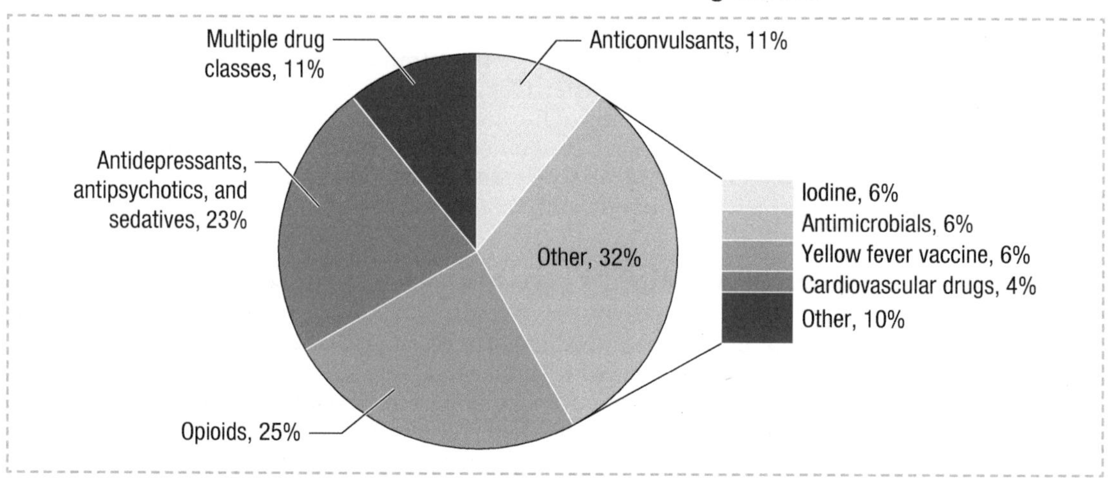

Note: Drugs capable of crossing the blood–brain barrier have the most reported adverse effects.
Source: From Anderson, P. O., Manoguerra, A. S., & Valdés, V. (2016). A review of adverse reactions in infants from medications in breastmilk. *Clinical Pediatrics, 55*(3), 236–244. https://doi.org/10.1177/0009922815594586.

The following section describes the transfer of many medications and medication classes into human milk. It does not provide a comprehensive list of all conceivable pharmaceuticals; rather, it is a sampling of some of the most prevalent and intriguing ones. Kinetics can be used to approximate the amounts in milk, but nothing is superior to clinical research in breastfeeding individuals. Significant progress has been made in breastfeeding pharmacovigilance over the past 30 years. The data from these studies are summarized in part by drug category. Drugs with RID of less than 10% are generally regarded as safe to use while breastfeeding. A discussion of notable exceptions and illustrative examples follows.

Labor and delivery, neonatal, and postpartum clinicians are encouraged to maintain strong lines of communication with lactating patients, so that breastfeeding or pumping begins within the first hour after birth and any issues can be quickly identified. Mothers of hospitalized neonates and infants may need intermittent lactation support, which can preserve and even increase milk supply. Given the strong evidence that supports the use of human milk as the primary source of enteral nutrition for neonates and infants, efforts to support a lactating patient reap great rewards for both the patient and the infant.

Galactagogues

Recall that inhibiting dopamine encourages the release of prolactin from the pituitary gland. Therefore, drugs that antagonize dopamine, like metoclopramide and domperidone, are commonly used to stimulate milk production. They may be effective choices for lactating patients who have failed to increase milk production after counseling and who historically have had elevated prolactin levels, but whose levels are now low. If milk supply is low while prolactin levels are high, dopamine antagonists will not be effective. However, it is difficult to predict who will respond well to these drugs. It must be noted that dopamine antagonists also come with significant maternal risk.

METOCLOPRAMIDE

Upward of 50% to 85% of patients with a low milk supply may respond to metoclopramide (Grzeskowiak & Amir, 2014). In successful scenarios, it can increase milk production by as much as 100% (Betzold, 2004). A standard oral dose is 10 mg three times per day. Drug response appears to be dose-related, and maximum effects are seen at doses up to 135 mg/d (Betzold, 2004). Milk production typically responds quickly, with the patient noticing significant volume increases within 24 to 48 hours. The amount of metoclopramide in milk rarely exceeds 0.16 mcg/mL, even at the highest maternal doses, resulting in a theoretical exposure of 0.024 mg/kg/d (Kauppila et al., 1981). In comparison, metoclopramide is prescribed directly to infants at a dose of 0.8 mg/kg/d (Custer et al., 2009). Although this infant dose presents significant safety concerns in neonates, metoclopramide residues in breast milk are minute in comparison and have not resulted in reports of infant harm.

Metoclopramide easily crosses the blood–brain barrier. Drug-induced depression is a common adverse complaint in breastfeeding patients. Other side effects include extrapyramidal symptoms, gastric cramping, and tardive dyskinesia. If a patient discontinues the drug without weaning slowly, a rebound drop in milk production may occur.

DOMPERIDONE

Domperidone is used successfully worldwide to increase milk production, but it is not approved in the United States (Brouwers et al., 1980; da Silva et al., 2001; Hofmeyr & van Iddekinge, 1983). Unlike metoclopramide, domperidone does not cross the blood–brain barrier. Unfortunately, domperidone is associated with arrhythmias. Although this side effect is rare and more common in older adults, this drug should not be used in patients with existing rhythm disorders such as prolonged QT syndrome. Levels of domperidone in milk are extraordinarily low (around 1.2 mcg/L), and oral bioavailability is less than 20%, further reducing infant exposure (Brouwers et al., 1980).

The lowest effective dose of domperidone should be used for the shortest duration necessary. Slow titration is essential when discontinuing this drug. Maximum effects of domperidone are seen at doses totaling 30 mg/d. Even standard doses sometimes result in severe withdrawal symptoms after tapering of the dose. These symptoms include severe anxiety and psychosis, even with slow tapering (Doyle & Grossman, 2018; Papastergiou et al., 2013).

HERBAL GALACTAGOGUES

A variety of herbal and complementary therapies, such as fenugreek, milk thistle, and fennel, have a long history of use in increasing milk flow. Even though many of these plants contain biologically active compounds, their effectiveness in increasing milk production is questionable. The existing literature in this field is scant and contradictory.

Lactation Inhibitors

Many medications can interfere with hormonal homeostasis and reduce milk supply. A list of drugs that affect lactation can be found in Table 6.5. Here again, through the establishment of open lines of communication and reciprocal trust, labor and delivery, neonatal, and postpartum clinicians can identify behaviors that threaten optimal milk supply. Often, breastfeeding patients do not realize that some over-the-counter medications can decrease milk supply. Ongoing and cyclical education, which begins in the antepartum arena and extends into the postpartum arena, is critical.

TABLE 6.5 Nonopioid Analgesics

DRUG CLASS	GENERIC DRUG	REFERENCES	RID (%)	LACTATION RISK
Other	Acetaminophen	Berlin et al., 1980; Bitzen et al., 1981; Craig et al., 2011; Kulo et al., 2012; Notarianni et al., 1987; Serinken et al., 2011	6–9	Very low
NSAID	Aspirin	Datta et al., 2017	0	Low
	Celecoxib	Gardiner, Doogue, et al., 2006; Hale et al., 2004; Knoppert et al., 2003	<0.7	Low
	Ibuprofen	Rigourd et al., 2014; Townsend et al., 1984; Walter & Dilger, 1997; Weibert et al., 1982	<0.7	Very low
	Indomethacin	Eeg-Olofsson et al., 1978; Lebedevs et al., 1991	1	Low
	Ketorolac	Cohen et al., 2011; Wischnik et al., 1989	<0.2	Low
	Naproxen	American Academy of Pediatrics Committee on Drugs, 2001; Brogden et al., 1975; Ito, Blajchman, et al., 1993; Jamali & Stevens, 1983	3	Low (short term), moderate (chronic)

NSAID, nonsteroidal anti-inflammatory drug; RID, relative infant dose.

BROMOCRIPTINE AND CABERGOLINE

Dopamine agonists are effective at suppressing lactation. The risks may outweigh the benefits. Bromocriptine was used historically but is no longer recommended due to reports of cardiac dysrhythmias, stroke, intracranial bleeding, cerebral edema, convulsions, and myocardial infarction (Dutt et al., 1998; Iffy et al., 1998; Pop et al., 1998). Cabergoline, a similar drug, is typically well tolerated and may be a safer off-label alternative. However, sufficient data on safety and efficacy are not available (Ferrari et al., 1995; Webster et al., 1992). Therefore, nonpharmacologic methods are generally preferred.

ANTIHISTAMINES

It is commonly thought that antihistamines may reduce milk volume. Mammary glands have no parasympathetic innervation. Their sympathetic nerves are associated only with arteries, not with alveoli (Rezaei et al., 2016). Rather, alveolar functions are primarily controlled by hormonal mediations. First-generation antihistamines (like diphenhydramine) have antimuscarinic and anticholinergic properties, both components of the parasympathetic nervous system. The lack of these nerve receptors in the breast means that antihistamines cannot affect milk supply directly. However, antihistamines may indirectly impact hormonal regulation. It is thought that anticholinergic drugs may decrease oxytocin, growth hormone, and prolactin, but there are very few data to support these claims (Daniel et al., 1997; Masala et al., 1982; Messinis et al., 1985; Svennersten et al., 1992).

Although their effect on milk volume is questionable, first-generation antihistamines (e.g., diphenhydramine, chlorpheniramine) may pose a threat of sedation, although minimal, to young infants. Second-generation antihistamines (e.g., loratadine, cetirizine) are preferred in lactating patients.

PSEUDOEPHEDRINE

Pseudoephedrine has long been known to reduce milk volume. Because it is a sympathomimetic vasoconstrictor, blood supply is reduced to the breast, reducing liquid diffusion. It may also reduce prolactin by 10% to 15%, enough to potentially halt late-stage lactation when prolactin levels wane. In one trial, a single 60-mg oral dose of pseudoephedrine reduced milk supply by 24% over the following 24 hours (Aljazaf et al., 2003).

Pain Control: Nonopioid Analgesics

Used briefly and in low doses, nonopioid analgesics likely pose little risk to a breastfed infant. Known milk concentrations are all low, and toxicity is minuscule.

A common concern is the risk of Reye syndrome with maternal aspirin use (acetylsalicylic acid). However, acetylsalicylic acid is sequestered and transformed into salicylic acid immediately by the liver. There is currently no known association between salicylic acid and Reye syndrome. As only salicylic acid is found in milk, low-dose maternal aspirin use (<325 mg/d) is not expected to cause infant harm (Datta et al., 2017).

Pain Control: Opioid Analgesics

To some extent, all opioids transfer into human milk. They all pose a potential risk of sedation and apnea in the infant. To ensure the safety of breastfeeding patients, maternal doses should always be considered. Dose stability is vital to mitigate the risk of respiratory depression in the infant. For acute pain control, the lowest dose to adequately control pain is recommended. Chronic use of opioids is expected to induce tolerance of opioids in both the patient and the infant. However, both maternal dose and infant milk consumption must remain stable to balance the risks of overdose or withdrawal. If this is achievable, higher doses of opioids may be reasonable.

Over the past 40 years, clinicians have had extensive experience with morphine, hydrocodone, methadone, and codeine in lactating patients. Morphine appears to be safe when taken sparingly in low to moderate dosages (10–30 mg oral dose, 5–15 mg intramuscularly [IM], or 2.5–5 mg IV every 4 hours, as needed; Hale, 2021). It is an excellent choice for those with severe pain due to its poor oral bioavailability in the breastfeeding patient, potentially limiting infant exposure. Millions of breastfeeding patients have undoubtedly used codeine in the last half-century, with few problems reported. Codeine and tramadol are thought to have pharmacogenetic variation in metabolism, suggesting inconsistent safety and efficacy. Codeine has been linked to one infant death, prompting warnings against its usage in breastfeeding patients; however, recent evaluations have demonstrated the implausibility of this case report. Although tramadol has the same warnings, there is even less evidence suggesting it causes deleterious events in breastfed infants. For decades, hydrocodone has been the predominant opioid administered postnatally in the United States, with excellent results. Maximum recommended maternal doses are reported in Table 6.6. These are based on doses seen in current literature. For more information about the effect of opioids on the fetus and neonate, please see Chapter 9, "Neonatal Abstinence Syndrome."

TABLE 6.6 Opioids

GENERIC DRUG	REFERENCES	RID (%)	ORAL BIOAVAILABILITY (%)	MME	LACTATION RISK	MAXIMUM DOSE RECOMMENDED WITH FULL BREASTFEEDING
Tramadol	Ilett et al., 2008	3	60	0.1	Low	[b]
Codeine	Koren et al., 2006; Lam, Matlow, et al., 2012; Meny et al., 1993	0.6–8	53	0.15	Moderate	[b]
Hydrocodone	Anderson et al., 2007, 2011	3	25	1	Low	40 mg/d[a]
Oxycodone	Lam, Kelly, et al., 2012; Seaton et al., 2007	1–5	60–87	1.5	Low	30 mg/d[a]
Morphine	Feilberg et al., 1989; Robieux et al., 1990; Wittels et al., 1990	9–35	26	1	Low	80 mg/d[a] (oral)

[a]Maximum recommended maternal dose per day in opioid-naïve breastfed patients.
[b]Please refer to chapter text; not recommended per Food and Drug Association position statement.
MME, morphine milligram equivalent; RID, relative infant dose.

Central Nervous System Medications

It has always been debated whether psychoactive drugs should be used in the early postpartum period. Concerns about an infant's exposure to medications that enter the CNS during a critical period of neural development typically make it difficult to justify their usage in the breastfeeding population. Given that detrimental consequences can be subtle or manifest over a lengthy period, these suspicions are paramount. Long-term research of second-generation antipsychotics (e.g., olanzapine, risperidone) have found that exposure during lactation has limited to no negative effects on neurobehavioral development (Field, 2008; Weissman et al., 2004). Furthermore, recent information suggests that untreated depression, mania, or psychosis significantly interferes with optimal parenting and results in neurobehavioral delay in infants (C. M. Lee & Gotlib, 1991; Sinclair & Murray, 1998; Zekoski et al., 1987).

ANTIDEPRESSANTS

The most commonly used psychotropic drugs in lactating patients are selective serotonin reuptake inhibitors (SSRIs; Table 6.7). They have low RIDs, and uptake by the infant further reduces exposure. Many of these drugs are undetectable in infant plasma (Berle et al., 2004; Weissman et al.,

TABLE 6.7 Antidepressants

DRUG CATEGORY	GENERIC DRUG	REFERENCES	RID (%)	LACTATION RISK
SSRI	Sertraline	Altshuler et al., 1995; C. N. Epperson et al., 1997; N. Epperson et al., 2001; Kristensen et al., 1998; Mammen et al., 1997; Stowe et al., 1997	0.5–2	Low
SSRI	Paroxetine	Begg et al., 1999; Hendrick et al., 2001; Misri et al., 2000; R. Ohman et al., 1999; Spigset et al., 1996; Stowe, 2000; Weissman et al., 2004	1–3	Low
SSRI	Citalopram	Briggs et al., 2015; Heikkinen et al., 2002; Jensen et al., 1997; A. Lee, Woo, et al., 2004; Rampono et al., 2000; Schmidt et al., 2000; Spigset et al., 1997	3–5	Low
SSRI	Escitalopram	Bellantuono et al., 2013; Castberg & Spigset, 2006; Rampono et al., 2006	5–8	Low
SSRI	Fluoxetine	Brent & Wisner, 1998; Burch & Wells, 1992; Hale et al., 2001; Isenberg, 1990; Kristensen et al., 1999; Lester et al., 1993; Mohan & Moore, 2000; Taddio et al., 1996	2–15	Low
SNRI	Duloxetine	Boyce et al., 2011; Briggs et al., 2009; Lobo et al., 2008	0.1–1	Low
SNRI	Venlafaxine	Ilett et al., 2002; Newport et al., 2009	7–8	Low
DNRI	Bupropion	Baab et al., 2002; Briggs et al., 1993; Chaudron & Schoenecker, 2004; Davis et al., 2009; Haas et al., 2004	<0.2–2	Low
TCA	Amitriptyline	Breyer-Pfaff et al., 1995; Brixen-Rasmussen et al., 1982; Misri & Sivertz, 1991	1–3	Low
TCA	Doxepin	Frey et al., 1999; Kemp et al., 1985; Matheson et al., 1985	0.3–3	High
Other	Trazodone	Verbeeck et al., 1986	3	Low
Other	Vortioxetine	Marshall et al., 2021	1–2	Low

DNRI, dopamine–epinephrine reuptake inhibitor; RID, relative infant dose; SNRI, serotonin–norepinephrine reuptake inhibitor; SSRI, selective serotonin reuptake inhibitor; TCA, tricyclic antidepressant.

2004). Newer serotonin–norepinephrine reuptake inhibitors (SNRIs), such as duloxetine and vortioxetine, are also both excellent options with low transfer to milk. Doxepin has fallen out of favor in lieu of newer drugs, as multiple cases of severe infant CNS depression have been reported due to breast milk exposures (Frey et al., 1999; Kemp et al., 1985; Matheson et al., 1985).

Serotonin Discontinuation Syndrome

Of infants exposed to serotonin-modulating drugs during pregnancy, 30% exhibit serotonin discontinuation syndrome (SDS), also known as *poor neonatal adaptation syndrome* (*PNAS*; not to be confused with neonatal abstinence syndrome [NAS] from opioid withdrawal). Neonatal serotonin withdrawal manifests similarly to serotonin toxicity: poor adaptation, irritability, jitteriness, tachypnea, hypertonicity, diarrhea, and temperature instability. It should not be confused with opiate withdrawal, although it appears similar. Although toxicity should resolve shortly after birth, SDS does not present until 48 hours after delivery and persists for 4 days. Although there is no standard treatment for SDS, supportive treatment may include breastfeeding and clonidine (Burdine & Luedtke, 2021). Breastfeeding is encouraged in these situations as it may mitigate symptoms of withdrawal. In the case of concurrent opioid and SSRI use, withdrawal symptoms are traditionally more severe and breastfeeding significantly improves symptoms (Bakhireva et al., 2021).

SDS is more common in neonates exposed to SSRIs with short half-lives, like paroxetine (t½: 21 hours), sertraline, and venlafaxine (t½: 10 hours); it occurs at a rate of approximately 30%. Fluoxetine, with a half-life of 240 hours, is much less likely to cause SDS. However, the risk of SDS is probably inversely proportional to the amount of infant exposure, as long half-lives typically increase maternal and infant serum drug levels (Chambers et al., 1996; Holland & Brown, 2017; Levinson-Castiel et al., 2006; Spencer, 1993; Stiskal et al., 2001). Regardless, all of these choices still present a low risk to the infant due to lactational exposure.

ANXIOLYTICS

Although benzodiazepine use has been suspected with a significant proportion of adverse infant events (Soussan et al., 2014), they are still commonly prescribed to breastfeeding patients. A small, prospective study identified significant sedation in 2 of 124 mother–infant pairs taking a range of benzodiazepines (Lam, Kelly, et al., 2012). The dose or breastfeeding intensity did not seem to influence sedation.

Lorazepam is the preferred benzodiazepine for intermittent use in breastfeeding patients (RID 3%). It has a short half-life, limited maternal sedation, no active metabolites, limited infant exposure, and minimal accumulation. Long-term use of diazepam should be avoided due to its long half-life and reported RID of up to 9.1% (including its even longer acting desmethyldiazepam metabolite). Any benzodiazepine in combination with other sedating medications, such as opioids, may contribute to poorer outcomes.

Buspirone is an attractive anxiolytic choice due to its lack of sedation and dependence. Data are sparse but promising on the limited extent of its transfer into the breast milk. It is presently used more often as prescribing trends diverge from benzodiazepines. There is only one report of infant adverse effects (seizure-like activity and cyanosis), but it was attributed to concomitant fluoxetine use (Brent & Wisner, 1998).

ANTIPSYCHOTIC AND ANTIMANIC DRUGS

If at all possible, psychotropic polypharmacy should be avoided, as well as any concurrent drugs that increase infant exposure (Table 6.8). Some typical antipsychotics, such as chlorpromazine, have been linked to neonatal apnea and SIDS and should never be used by breastfeeding patients (Boutroy, 1994; Pollard & Rylance, 1994). However, starting at approximately 4 months of age, the risk of SIDS declines rapidly. If the breastfeeding patient requires these drugs past this time frame, the risks should be reevaluated. Second-generation atypical antipsychotics olanzapine and quetiapine demonstrate low RIDs, are reasonably safe, and are definitely preferred. Symptoms of concern in the infant include sedation, apnea, irritability, and extrapyramidal symptoms. Most second-generation atypical antipsychotics can produce hyperprolactinemia in patients, even galactorrhea in male patients. Aripiprazole is the exception; instead, it suppresses prolactin levels. This may reduce milk supply, particularly early after delivery (Lozano et al., 2014).

TABLE 6.8 Antipsychotics

DRUG CATEGORY	GENERIC DRUG	REFERENCES	RID (%)	LACTATION RISK
Antipsychotic (first generation)	Haloperidol	Ohkubo et al., 1992; Stewart et al., 1980; Whalley et al., 1981; Yoshida et al., 1998	0.2–12	Low
Antipsychotic (second generation)	Olanzapine	Ambresin et al., 2004; Brunner et al., 2013; Croke et al., 2002; Gardiner et al., 2003; Gilad et al., 2011	0.3–2	Low
	Risperidone	Hill et al., 2000; Ilett et al., 2004	3–9	Low
	Quetiapine	A. Lee, Giesbrecht, et al., 2004; Misri et al., 2006; Rampono et al., 2007	<0.1	Low
	Aripiprazole	Nordeng et al., 2014; Schlotterbeck et al., 2007; Watanabe et al., 2011	1–6	Low
Mood stabilizer	Lithium	Moretti et al., 2003; Sykes et al., 1976; Tunnessen & Hertz, 1972	0.9–7	Moderate

RID, relative infant dose.

Due to a paucity of breast milk data, newer atypical drugs, such as lurasidone and brexpiprazole, are not yet preferred. Cariprazine, another second-generation antipsychotic, has an active metabolite (DDCAR; didesmethyl-cariprazine) whose half-life may be up to 3 weeks in adults. DDCAR is detectible in adults for over 8 weeks after a single 1-mg dose of cariprazine. It has been implicated in at least one anecdotal case of reversible infant tardive dyskinesia in an infant who was exposed during both pregnancy and lactation. Cariprazine should be avoided during pregnancy and lactation until more is known.

Lithium

Lithium may require dose elevations throughout pregnancy, and caution must be taken in the peripartum period to prevent maternal and infant toxicity as lithium requirements quickly return to normal. Relatively high levels in milk are the result of its low molecular weight and low protein binding. Some toxicity has been reported in infants (Llewellyn et al., 1998; Sykes et al., 1976; Tunnessen & Hertz, 1972). Although plasma levels of lithium in breast fed infants are moderate, approximately 30% to 40% of the maternal level (Frees, 1970; Sykes et al., 1976), the situation can dramatically worsen if the infant becomes dehydrated. There are many recommendations for testing regimens for lithium-breastfed infants. The most practical of these is to measure serum lithium, thyroid, and renal function 10 days after delivery to allow transplacental lithium to clear (Bolton, 1990). Further monitoring is required only if serum lithium is equal to or greater than 0.3 mEq/L, or signs of toxicity are present. These signs include elevated thyroid-stimulating hormone, cyanosis, lethargy, or EKG T-wave inversion.

Antiepileptics

Even with the high RIDs found with antiepileptic medications, only 49% of infants have detectable serum levels of the drugs (Birnbaum et al., 2020). Antiepileptic drug use in a breastfeeding patient is associated with impaired neonatal social and fine motor development regardless of breastfeeding status, presumably due to altered in utero development. Continuous breastfeeding is somewhat protective against these adverse effects. In a Norwegian study examining antiepileptic effects (primarily of lamotrigine, carbamazepine, and valproate) during pregnancy and lactation, breastfed infants scored higher for autistic traits, communication, and gross motor skills early in life. No harmful effects were observed due to breastfeeding in this study (Veiby et al., 2013). These results support mother's taking standard doses of up to two or three antiepileptics to continue breastfeeding. Preferably, this would apply to the few medications that have been well studied in breast milk and have a history of clinical use, as listed in Table 6.9.

TABLE 6.9 Antiepileptics

GENERIC DRUG	REFERENCES	RID (%)	LACTATION RISK
Valproate	Meador et al., 2014; Nau et al., 1981; Philbert et al., 1985; Piontek et al., 2000; Stahl et al., 1997; Tsuru et al., 1988; von Unruh et al., 1984; Wisner & Perel, 1998	1–6	High
Carbamazepine	Froescher et al., 1984; Kaneko et al., 1979; Merlob et al., 1992; Niebyl et al., 1979; Pynnonen et al., 1977; Shimoyama et al., 2000; Wisner & Perel, 1998	4–6	Low
Lamotrigine	Liporace et al., 2004; I. Öhman et al., 2000; Page-Sharp et al., 2006; Tomson et al., 1997	9–18	Low
Levetiracetam	Johannessen et al., 2005; Krämer et al., 2002	3–8	Low
Oxcarbazepine	Bulau et al., 1988; Lutz et al., 2007	1.7	Low
Topiramate	I. Öhman et al., 2002	3–23	Low

Note: Valproate use is associated with a possible risk of neurodevelopmental delay in exposed infants. High-dose carbamazepine (>850 mg) is associated with infant apnea.
RID, relative infant dose.

Migraines: Prevention and Treatment

Migraines are notoriously difficult to treat. Until recently, medications used to treat and prevent migraines were repurposed from treatments for other disorders. Anticonvulsants, antidepressants, antihypertensives, and monoclonal antibodies are most commonly used and are discussed elsewhere in the chapter. Botulinum toxin can also be used to prevent migraines. Although it has not been studied in milk, it is not detectible in maternal serum post administration, making its presence in milk unlikely (Bodkin et al., 2005; de Oliveira Monteiro, 2006; Kuczkowski, 2007). Dietary supplements have also been used to prevent migraines, with limited success. Doses of riboflavin exceeding 400 mg daily (Food and Drug Administration [FDA] tolerable upper intake level: 1.6 mg daily) have anecdotally caused milk to turn yellow and thus should probably be avoided.

Triptans are now the mainstay of migraine treatment, and many have been studied during breastfeeding (Amundsen et al., 2021). Sumatriptan has the most data, with an RID ranging from 0.2% to 3.5%. The pharmaceutical manufacturer of eletriptan submitted data from eight breastfeeding patients in their application for drug approval with a reported RID of 0.6%. Naratriptan so far exhibits the highest transfer at 5.0% RID. Due to these low RIDs, as-needed use in the breastfeeding patient, and poor bioavailability, these drugs are good choices for lactating patients and require no interruption of breastfeeding.

Calcitonin gene-related peptide (CGRP) receptor antagonists have recently become available for treatment and prevention of migraines. More recent formulations of this drug category are orally available. Rimegepant is currently the only oral example of this drug class that has been studied in breastfeeding. Levels in milk of breastfeeding patients were exceedingly low, with an RID of <0.5% (Baker et al., 2021). Many CGRP antagonists, like erenumab, are monoclonal antibodies. See the section titled "Monoclonal Antibodies" for a discussion of these agents.

Analgesics and opioids are among the drugs used as migraine treatments and are discussed elsewhere in the chapter. Products containing ergot alkaloids, or combinations with butalbital (e.g., Fioricet, Fiorinal), while unstudied, may cause infant sedation and are not preferred.

Antimicrobials

Antibiotics and antifungals are probably the most common medications used in lactating patients. For short durations (less than 3 weeks in a healthy term infant), maternal antimicrobial use should be minimally disruptive. In a prospective cohort of breastfeeding patients who took antibiotics, 19.3% reported minor adverse effects in their infant (Ito, Koren, et al., 1993). Two-thirds of these were attributed to diarrhea. After an infection requiring antibiotics, a separate study found that 7% stopped breastfeeding (Ito, Koren, et al., 1993). It is not understood whether this is more attributable to the infection or the medication. Chronic use of antibiotics requires further consideration. Research is currently being conducted to determine the impact of maternal antibiotics on the developing infant microbiome. For premature neonates, maternal antibiotic use can present a challenging scenario. The benefit of breast milk in this population is undisputed; partially supplementing breast milk with donor milk may be necessary to reduce the risk of infant GI effects.

Most antibiotics are considered safe for short durations, typically less than 2 weeks. In certain cases (e.g., Lyme disease) the recommended duration or potency of therapy requires further consideration of breastfeeding risks versus benefits (Table 6.10). Acyclovir, fluconazole, metronidazole, and erythromycin are further discussed in the following text because they are common causes of questions.

ACYCLOVIR

Acyclovir is thought to be actively transported into the milk, but concentrations in milk are reportedly low (Lau et al., 1987). Acyclovir therapy in neonates is common and produces few toxicities. Calculated intake by an infant would be less than 0.87 mg/kg/d via milk; comparable neonatal doses are 60 mg/kg/d. Topical therapy on herpetic lesions elsewhere than the nipple is probably safe. Patients with lesions on or close to the nipple should not breastfeed on that side.

FLUCONAZOLE

The RID of fluconazole is estimated to be as high as 21%. Although this greatly exceeds the conventional safety benchmark, this drug is used extensively in infant populations. The AID from milk is far lower than the direct doses used clinically.

TABLE 6.10 Antibiotics

DRUG CLASS	GENERIC DRUG	REFERENCES	RID (%)	LACTATION RISK
Beta-lactam	Amoxicillin	Kafetzis et al., 1981	1	Low
	Cephalexin	Ilett et al., 2006; Kafetzis et al., 1981; Matsuda, 1984	<1.5	Low
	Cefotaxime	Kafetzis et al., 1980; Matsuda, 1984	<0.3	Low
Sulfonamide	Sulfamethoxazole	Durant & Miller, 1973; Hale, 2021	2–3	Low
Fluroquinolone	Ciprofloxacin	Cover & Mueller, 1990; Gardner et al., 1992; Giamarellou et al., 1989; Harmon et al., 1992	0.5–6	Low
	Levofloxacin	Cahill et al., 2005	11–17	Low
Tetracycline	Doxycycline	Briggs et al., 2015; Jha et al., 1989; Koren, 2007	4–13	Low
Macrolide	Azithromycin	Kelsey et al., 1994	6	Low
Other	Clindamycin	Mann, 1980; Smith et al., 1975; Stéen & Rane, 1982	1–2	Low
	Metronidazole	Erickson et al., 1981; Heisterberg & Branebjerg, 1983; Passmore et al., 1988	13	Low
	Linezolid	Lim et al., 2017; Rowe et al., 2014	1–16	Low
	Vancomycin	Briggs et al., 2015; Reyes et al., 1989	7	Low
	Nitrofurantoin	Gerk et al., 2001; Varsano et al., 1973	7	Avoid during hyperbilirubinemia
Antifungal	Nystatin	Hale, 2021; Nystatin, 2006	0	Very low
	Fluconazole	Force, 1995	16–21	Low
Antiviral	Acyclovir	Lau et al., 1987	<1.5	Low

RID, relative infant dose.

METRONIDAZOLE

Although metronidazole has a significant RID, it is fairly benign and no adverse effects have been documented in neonates. Some infants might be disinclined to eat because it may give milk a metallic taste. To avoid the peak plasma concentration, large oral dosages (such as the single 2-gram dose for treatment of vaginal trichomoniasis) should be followed by a temporary break in breastfeeding for 12 hours.

ERYTHROMYCIN

Extensive data now suggest that the use of erythromycin in the early postnatal period increases the risk of hypertrophic pyloric stenosis (Sørensen et al., 2003). When a macrolide is indicated, azithromycin or clarithromycin is preferred.

Antidiabetics

Diabetes in its various forms is common during the postnatal period. Although insulin and metformin have been studied in milk and in breastfed infants, very little research has been conducted in other drug classes (Table 6.11). Monitoring neonatal blood glucose in the infants of patients with diabetes is highly recommended regardless of drug choice.

Maternal diabetes is known to cause perinatal and postnatal complications, including neonatal hypoglycemia. In utero, infants are inundated with both maternal insulin and hyperglycemia. After birth, however, the neonate may experience prolonged hypoglycemia. Initial treatments for hypoglycemia in breastfed late-preterm and term neonates include glucose gel and formula (see Chapter 24, "Necrotizing Enterocolitis" Harris et al., 2013; Wight & Academy of Breastfeeding Medicine, 2021).

INSULIN

Insulin is endogenously produced and is a normal component of human milk. It may have local activity in the GI tract that has not been elucidated, but its oral absorption is negligible, preventing adverse infant effects. Although there are many formulations of insulin, none have proven harmful to breastfeeding. Different formulations are the result of minor adjustments to the amino acid sequence of regular human insulin (Mane et al., 2012). These adjustments cause wide differences in the absorption of the drug from the subcutaneous maternal depot to the maternal systemic circulation (e.g., insulin lispro acts within 15 minutes and is cleared within 2–4 hours; insulin glargine does not have a peak and lasts 24 hours). However, all insulins are peptides that exhibit limited oral bioavailability.

TABLE 6.11 Pharmacokinetic Estimates of Transfer of Antidiabetic Drugs

CLASS	SUFFIX	ORAL BIOAVAILABILITY	MOLECULAR WEIGHT	PROTEIN BINDING	VOLUME OF DISTRIBUTION	HALF-LIFE	HYPOGLYCEMIC RISK
DPP-4 inhibitors	-gliptin	High	300–500	Variable	Moderate/high	Long	Low
GLP-1R agonists	-tide	Low	High	Variable	Low	Variable	Low
SGLT2 inhibitors	-gliflozin	High	400–500	High	Moderate	Moderate	Low
TZD	-glitazone	High	300–400	High	Low	Short/ moderate	Low

DPP-4, dipeptidyl peptidase-4; GLP-1R, glucagon-like peptide-1 receptor; SGLT2, sodium–glucose cotransporter 2; TZD, thiazolidinedione.
Sources: From Harris, D. L., Weston, P. J., Signal, M., Chase, J. G., & Harding, J. E. (2013). Dextrose gel for neonatal hypoglycaemia (the Sugar Babies Study): A randomised, double-blind, placebo-controlled trial. *The Lancet, 382*(9910), 2077–2083. https://doi.org/10.1016/S0140-6736(13)61645-1; Wight, N. E. & Academy of Breastfeeding Medicine. (2021). ABM clinical protocol #1: Guidelines for glucose monitoring and treatment of hypoglycemia in term and late preterm neonates, revised 2021. *Breastfeeding Medicine, 16*(5), 353–365. https://doi.org/10.1089/bfm.2021.29178.new.

METFORMIN

Metformin is the first-line choice of therapy for most patients with type 2 diabetes. Although it was expected to significantly transfer into the milk, clinical studies demonstrated that RIDs are less than 0.5% (Briggs et al., 2005; Gardiner, 2003; Hale et al., 2002). As discussed previously, this suggests a protective mechanism in which the drug is removed from the milk via a transporter. Adverse effects were not documented in a prospective study of infants consuming milk during metformin use (Glueck et al., 2006).

SULFONYLUREAS

Glyburide and glipizide have been studied in eight breastfeeding patients with promising results (Feig et al., 2005). Neither drug was detectible in breast milk. All breastfed infants from these studies had no changes in blood glucose levels. In breastfeeding patients for whom sulfonylureas are being considered, these drugs are preferred choices from this class of medications because they have minimal safety data suggesting toxicity in the infant.

OTHERS

Few other drugs have been studied for safety during breastfeeding. Many of these drugs may be compatible with breastfeeding because they are unlikely to result in infant hypoglycemia after delivery. However, pharmacokinetic estimations do suggest differences in drug transfer among medications in the same therapeutic class. For example, canagliflozin is less orally bioavailable than the rest of the sodium–glucose cotransporter 2 (SGLT2) inhibitors and is 99% protein-bound, making it the best choice for this class. SGLT2 inhibitors theoretically pose some risk to developing kidneys, so this class is still not an ideal option.

Antihypertensives

Most antihypertensives have been proven safe for breastfeeding patients. However, postpartum preeclampsia is sometimes treated with doses that reflect a five fold increase versus studied doses. Although each drug at a standard dose may have been studied and deemed "safe," combinations of high doses, particularly in fragile infants, warrant caution.

BETA-BLOCKERS

Caution is warranted for atenolol, acebutolol, and nadolol. Data seem to indicate that atenolol secretion into the breast milk is highly variable but may be as high as 10 times greater than for propranolol. This may explain case reports of cyanosis and bradycardia in breastfed infants. Acebutolol has an active metabolite, diacetolol, that together can reach a concerning RID. Nadolol has an extended half-life and larger RID of 7%, making it a less attractive choice than other options.

Metoprolol, propranolol, and labetalol all have long histories of use in breastfeeding patients. Labetalol's RID may be dose-related. Current data include breast milk from patients taking up to 1,200 mg/d. However, this resulted in a subclinical RID of 0.58%. Hypotension and hypoglycemia should be watched for in newborns exposed to high maternal doses.

CALCIUM CHANNEL BLOCKERS

Calcium channel blockers are considered safe for use in breastfeeding. Many of these drugs have been studied in breast milk. Nifedipine is the preferred choice in breastfeeding due to its low RID (<3.5%), long history of postpartum usage, and lack of adverse reports in infants. However, many other choices are reasonable; for example, nimodipine has an RID of <0.01% and a low oral bioavailability of 13% (Tonks, 1995).

ANGIOTENSIN-CONVERTING ENZYME INHIBITORS AND ANGIOTENSIN RECEPTOR BLOCKERS

Captopril, benazepril, and enalapril are the preferred angiotensin-converting enzyme (ACE) inhibitors for breastfeeding. They have all been quantified and their RIDs are less than 0.2%. Other ACE inhibitors (including lisinopril) and angiotensin-receptor blockers (ARBs) are expected to transfer similarly but have no data.

ACE inhibitors are avoided in pregnancy due to known fetotoxic effects, likely due to impaired renal morphogenesis. Recall that nephrogenesis is complete by approximately 36 weeks of gestation; this process is interrupted with preterm birth. As premature infants are still undergoing significant kidney nephrogenesis after birth, there is some concern about the potential renal effects of ACE inhibitor exposure through breast milk and possible drug accumulation. After these nephrons are in place, the risk of ACE and ARB residues in milk harming a premature infant is greatly reduced. This is most easily identified by urine production.

DIURETICS

Diuretics are often a topic of interest for breastfeeding patients. Hydrochlorothiazide (HCTZ) transfers into the milk with an RID of 1.6%, but absolute infant exposures are still low and the drug has been undetectable in infant plasma. Some authors suggest that HCTZ can produce thrombocytopenia in nursing infants, although this is unsubstantiated. Thiazide diuretics could potentially reduce milk production by depleting maternal blood volume, although it is seldom observed. Although furosemide has not been quantified in milk, pediatric use is common. It is unlikely that the amount transferred into human milk would produce any effects in a nursing infant, although its maternal use could suppress lactation.

Anticoagulants and Antiplatelet

Patients requiring antithrombotic therapy would likely disproportionately benefit from the cardioprotective mechanisms apparent to lactation (Countouris et al., 2020). To confer this benefit, safe anticoagulant choices can be made to encourage continued breastfeeding. Warfarin has been used for decades without harm to the infant; very little is secreted into human milk. In multiple studies totaling 15 people, the maximum concentration in milk was found to be less than 0.08 µmol/L, and no warfarin was detected in the infants' plasma (McKenna et al., 1983; Orme et al., 1977). Heparins and low-molecular-weight heparins, such as enoxaparin, are too large to enter the milk compartment. In one study of 12 people using 20 to 40 mg of enoxaparin daily, no change in anti-factor Xa level was noted in any of the 12 breastfed infants (Guillonneau et al., 1996).

Some newer direct oral anticoagulants (DOACs) pose challenges to this population. The pharmacokinetic estimates paired with severity of possible adverse effects make them a poor choice for breastfeeding parents until more research is available. Most factor Xa inhibitors and the direct thrombin inhibitor dabigatran have not been studied. In multiple studies totaling six people taking rivaroxaban, the maximum RID was as high as 4% (Muysson et al., 2020; Zhao et al., 2020). Of four parents taking apixaban, the maximum RID ranged from 12.8% to a highly concerning 21%, suggestive of active transport (Datta et al., 2021; Zhao et al., 2020). Rivaroxaban and other suitable alternatives to therapy like warfarin and enoxaparin are preferred while breastfeeding.

Low-dose aspirin, as previously discussed, is a reasonable choice for antiplatelet action in a lactating patient, with low infant risk. Unfortunately, the more efficacious clopidogrel has not been studied, but the severity of possible infant risk warrants caution. It is 98% protein-bound, but the active metabolite has a long half-life of 11 days and irreversibly inhibits platelet aggregation. The manufacturer reports some post marketing use of clopidogrel in a lactating patient without infant adverse effects.

Immunosuppressants

SYSTEMIC CORTICOSTEROIDS

Endogenous steroid production likely overshadows the minimal amounts secreted into the breast milk (Katz & Duncan, 1975; McKenzie et al., 1975; Öst et al., 1985). Even large IV doses, such as those used in organ transplants, redistribute out of the plasma compartment quickly, limiting clinically relevant transfer into the milk. In these extreme cases, interrupting breastfeeding for a maximum of 12 hours should sufficiently mitigate infant risk (Cooper et al., 2015; Hale & Ilett, 2002).

METHOTREXATE

Animal studies demonstrate that methotrexate is retained in tissues for extended time frames (Oliverio & Davidson, 1962). This is also evident in the long-term association of methotrexate with fetal malformations during pregnancy, even when administered 3 months prior to conception (Walden & Bagshawe, 1979). As a result, even though methotrexate has an especially low RID of 0.1%, interrupting breastfeeding by 24 to 48 hours after a single dose is prudent (Baker, Datta, Rewers-Felkins, & Hale, 2018; Johns et al., 1972). The safety of long-term treatment with methotrexate while breastfeeding is questionable.

T-CELL INHIBITORS

Post transplant populations have long advocated for their ability to breastfeed while understanding the need for medication treatment for their health. Azathioprine and tacrolimus are commonly used during pregnancy for these populations; therefore, they have been studied in lactation. Both have low RIDs and no case reports of infant harm with decades of use (Angelberger et al., 2011; Bramham et al., 2013; L. A. Christensen et al., 2008; Coulam et al., 1982; French et al., 2003; Gardiner & Begg, 2006; Gardiner, Gearry, et al., 2006; Grekas et al., 1984; Moretti et al., 2006; Sau et al., 2007; Zelinkova et al., 2009; Zheng et al., 2013). Cyclosporine has been studied with mixed results and is not considered a first-line option. Due to the potential for toxicity, use of well-studied drugs is necessary when possible. When patients take these medications, careful monitoring of the newborn, including laboratory measurements of drug levels, can help limit the risk of toxicity.

Monoclonal Antibodies

There are many monoclonal antibodies available today for many different conditions, ranging from neoplasms to migraines. These medications are similar in that they are close congeners of endogenous immunoglobulin G (IgG) antibodies, but each product has a specific target that varies broadly across this drug type. Targets range from exogenous pathogens, like venoms or viruses, to receptors to receptor substrates, all modulating systems up or down to various degrees. As a drug "class," monoclonal antibodies with different targets or mechanisms are not easily comparable.

Natural IgG antibodies are present in human milk, but in limited amounts due to their large molecular weight. These molecules typically exceed 150,000 daltons, and their RIDs are usually on the order of 1% to 2%. This should not be confused with neutralizing secretory immunoglobulin A (IgA) antibodies that are actively transported into human milk and stabilized by an additional protein (J-chain).

Even with low RIDs, these medications often cause concern during lactation due to their potency and long half-lives. Monoclonal antibodies might exhibit limited absorption via the IgG-transporting neonatal Fc receptor (FcRn) expressed in the intestinal cells of adults and fetuses to form an entero-mammary link (Fritzsche et al., 2012). This suggests that systemic absorption of these large molecules is possible by the infant (although it is not well supported by evidence). Certolizumab presents an interesting case of this phenomenon. To remove the risk of transport via the Fc receptor in pregnancy, this drug was designed without the Fc region of the antibody. This inhibits infant recycling of any orally bioavailable portion of the drug that persists in the breastfed infant's gut. RIDs for this drug are exceedingly low at less than 0.3%, making it an excellent option for breastfeeding patients (Clowse et al., 2017).

Even for drugs without this special design, the amount of drug available to the infant is likely very low. This can be demonstrated in a worst-case scenario using the highest drug concentration quantified in the monoclonal antibodies with the highest RID, natalizumab (Figure 6.9). Natalizumab has an extremely long half-life and requires 24 weeks to reach steady state. In one lactation study, the drug levels rose five fold over the first 12 weeks after injection, peaking at 2.83 mcg/L of milk (Fritzsche et al., 2012). If 5% infant absorption of IgG is assumed, only 0.085 mcg of natalizumab would be systemically available per day per kilogram in an infant. Using the most conservative adult parameters for Vd (0.034 L/kg) to estimate infant serum concentrations, in a single day an infant would need to consume more than 500 L/kg of milk to reach even 10% of the mean trough steady-state concentrations seen in the breastfeeding mother (23 mcg/mL).

FIGURE 6.9 Worst-case scenario of monoclonal antibody exposure through milk.

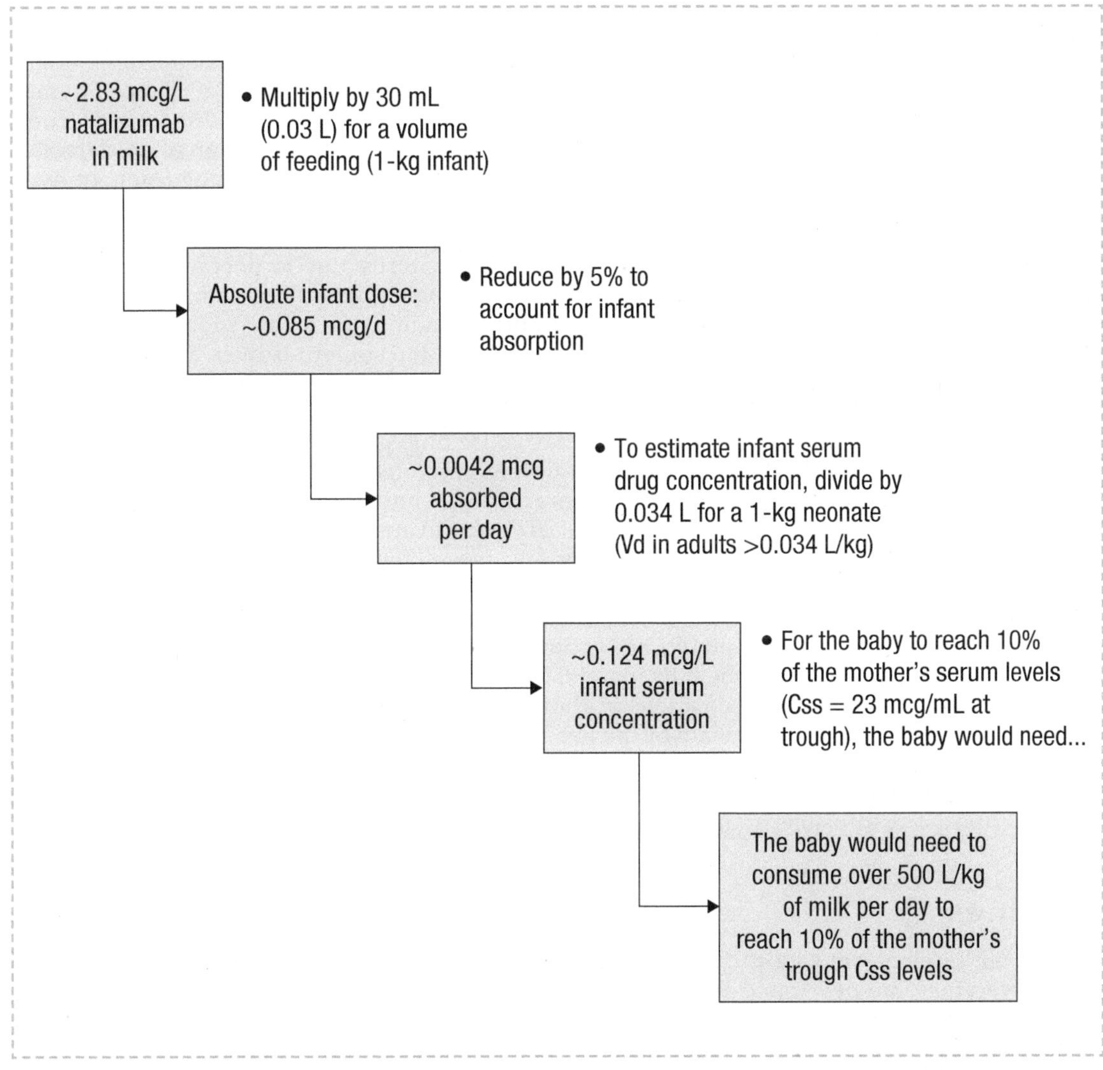

Css, steady-state drug concentration; Vd, volume of distribution.

Another theoretical risk is presented by monoclonal antibodies whose target resides in the infant's GI tract (e.g., vedolizumab binding α4β7 integrin expressed on the surface of mucosal endothelial cells). Although these drugs may lead to the potential for adverse effects without systemic absorption, they have not been recognized in clinical practice (LaHue et al., 2020). While knowledge in this area continues to evolve, the current evidence is starting to favor the use of these medications in breastfeeding patients.

Chemotherapy

Alkylating and antimetabolite drugs, including anthracyclines, topoisomerase inhibitors, and mitotic inhibitors, are all dangerous to use during breastfeeding. Even though the average dose in milk is minor, these drugs are extremely toxic and can cause substantial long-term damage. The risk to the infant is effectively eliminated after seven half-lives, when breastfeeding can be resumed. This withhold period can be as short as hours or as long as months depending on the drug. If a combination of chemotherapeutic drugs is employed, the agent with the longest half-life should determine the breastfeeding-withhold period.

Surgical Anesthetics

Current recommendations from the Academy of Breastfeeding Medicine and the American Society of Anesthesiologists suggest that lactating patients may safely resume breastfeeding as soon as they are awake, alert, and stable (American Society of Anesthesiologists, 2019; Reece-Stremtan et al., 2017). A new slogan, "sleep and keep," has been introduced to promote this concept (Kraus et al., 2020). Premature infants fall outside of these parameters, and interruption of breastfeeding is recommended for 6 to 12 hours after anesthesia to reduce risk of apnea, hypotension, or hypotonia. In more stable neonates, it is reasonable to dilute maternal milk with previously expressed milk, donor milk, or formula during this time.

Surgery may independently reduce milk volume temporarily due to operative volume loss, fluid and calorie restrictions, and stress. Inhalational anesthetics, neuromuscular blocking agents, and their reversal agents are all unlikely to impact breastfeeding or a breastfed infant due to their short duration and lack of oral bioavailability. By the time the surgery is over, and the patient is alert enough to breastfeed, these drugs pose little risk to the infant. This even applies for surgical use of opioids and benzodiazepines, except in cases of preexisting infant risk.

Propofol appears to have low transfer but may cause blue-green discoloration of milk (Bulut & Ovali, 2021; Nitsun et al., 2006). Dexmedetomidine is excreted only minimally even during infusion (Dodd et al., 2021). Data from ketamine are available only for IM injection with lower doses, but suggest minimal transfer (Wolfson et al., 2021). Local anesthetics used for nerve blockade, such as lidocaine or bupivacaine, can be used safely as well. However, large doses of tumescent lidocaine can be concerning (Dryden & Lo, 2000).

Postsurgical opioids pose the most risk to a breastfeeding infant. Pain interferes with successful breastfeeding, and pain control should be encouraged in breastfeeding parents. Because opioids transfer in small quantities into the milk, parents should be encouraged to continue breastfeeding with responsible use of these medications. Although they have an excellent safety record, breastfeeding parents should also be aware of the need to monitor the infant for rare cases of sedation and apnea.

These recommendations apply only to surgical situations. Long-term use of the same drugs, such as critical care infusions, requires additional consideration.

Vaccines

Almost all vaccines are safe to use while breastfeeding. Most present-day vaccines, including mRNA vaccines, are developed from nonliving or inactivated pathogens that pose no risk to a breastfed infant. Maternal antibodies elicited from vaccination transfer into the milk. They may neutralize pathogens in milk and on mucosal membranes, but they do not protect the infant from the pathogen later in life (CDC, 2019).

Live attenuated viral vaccines pose some risk as viruses can be detected in human milk and cause infection. Yellow fever vaccination has been associated with a few cases of encephalitis in neonates and is not generally recommended in breastfeeding patients with an infant younger than 9 months (CDC, 2010; Kuhn et al., 2011). However, in the case of endemic areas, the potential benefits of the vaccine outweigh the potential risks, and immunization should be considered.

Herbal Products

Seventy-five percent of women report believing "natural" products are safer than medications during breastfeeding, although they do not perceive them to be more effective. This misconception is dangerous, as herbal products can interact with one another as well as with prescription drugs. For example, a 2019 report demonstrated that fenugreek (an herbal galactagogue) interacted with the SSRI sertraline. This patient was admitted to a medical unit for diaphoresis, mydriasis, tachycardia, clonus, hyperreflexia, nausea, and anxiety and was diagnosed with serotonin syndrome (Doolabh et al., 2019).

Unfortunately, the U.S. FDA does not regulate herbal products. There can be considerable differences in potency and purity among various products or even among different lots of the same product. There are very few published data on the safety of these products in breastfeeding patients and almost none on combination herbal products. When deciding whether to take a supplement, both dangers and benefits should be considered. Herbal products should be evaluated for potential infant side effects with as much care as FDA-regulated medications.

Radioactive Isotopes

Radioactive drugs are used as tracers and as ablative chemotherapeutic agents. The radioisotope is usually coupled to a "carrier" compound that helps it find its target and facilitate elimination. In addition to a biological half-life that describes how quickly a drug is eliminated from the body, radioisotopes have a radioactive half-life that measures how quickly the drug decays into its more stable isotope.

Radioisotopes confront breastfeeding infants through ingestion of contaminated milk and direct exposure to radiation emitted from the mother's body. Radiation-contaminated milk must be withheld from infant consumption for a drug- and dose-dependent period. The risk of direct radiation must also be addressed through close contact restrictions. The Nuclear Regulatory Commission and the American Academy of Pediatrics issue guidelines for various radiopharmaceuticals to limit infants' effective dose to less than 1 mSv of radiation (1 mSv = 100 mrem) per procedure (U.S. Nuclear Regulatory Commission (NRC), 1997; Sachs & Committee on Drugs, 2013). The use of some radioactive isotopes may require discontinuing breastfeeding (iodine-131 [I-131]), whereas others may not require much interruption (technetium-99). Radioisotopes continue to degrade in stored milk samples, much like heat dissipates. In the right circumstances, it may be possible to reduce the risk of toxicity by storing milk for a period of time (e.g., some technetium-99 preparations). The impact of these medications on breastfeeding should be addressed carefully and in advance.

Radioactive Iodine

Radioactive iodine isotopes deserve special attention as iodine is one of the few products known to be actively transported into human milk. The effective dose of I-131 in human milk is approximately 28% of the dose (Robinson et al., 1994). Radioiodine concentrates in the thyroid glands and mammary tissue of the breastfeeding patient and their infant. Direct radiation exposure can occur from the close contact of breastfeeding. It is therapeutic in the breastfeeding patient, but their infant's thyroid can be suppressed. It also poses a risk of future thyroid carcinomas in the infant (Hale, 2021).

If the impacted milk is discarded or held for a suitable period, very low dosages of radioactive iodine tracers may be compatible with nursing. Even standard doses of I-131, I-125, and I-123 pose risks that exceed the benefits of breastfeeding (NRC, 1997). Contact restrictions should be referenced to ensure proper, temporary distancing of the patient from their infant.

Radiocontrast Agents

MRI and CT scanning sometimes requires techniques to improve contrast in a particular area of the body. Radiopaque substances can be formulated to travel to specific locations of interest to enhance these images. These substances are not radioactive; instead, they absorb or deflect x-ray radiation used in the imaging process. Because of the location-specific formulations, radiocontrast agents are designed to stay in their target compartment. Iodinated and gadolinium-based contrast agents both have RIDs of less than 1%. Infant oral absorption is also less than 1%, introducing minimal risk from the medication. The American College of Radiology has issued guidelines stating that these products are compatible with breastfeeding without restriction (ACR Committee on Drugs and Contrast Media, 2020). When indicated, these products are used for imaging in infants.

Tobacco

Environmental tobacco smoke is a known risk factor for increases in rates of infant allergies and SIDS. Nicotine and its active metabolite, cotinine, are both present in human milk. Studies have demonstrated a linear relationship between smoking rates in the breastfeeding parent, nicotine levels in the milk, and urine cotinine levels in the breastfed infant (Dahlström et al., 1990; Woodward et al., 1986). Urine cotinine levels in these infants can be up to five times higher than in newborns whose parents smoke but do not breastfeed (Becker et al., 1999). Secondhand smoke can also make an infant more susceptible to otitis media, respiratory tract infections, and asthma (*International Consultation on Environmental Tobacco Smoke (ETS) and Child Health Report*, 1999). Breastfeeding offsets some of this risk and is highly encouraged as a modifiable risk factor.

The current recommendations are for the parent to continue to breastfeed regardless of smoking habits but never to smoke in the presence of the infant (Yılmaz et al., 2009). Some smoking cessation aids can be used while breastfeeding. Bupropion and nicotine replacement therapy are both preferred to smoking. Varenicline has not been studied to date and is not first line.

Alcohol

Many patients resume alcohol consumption after delivery; it is common to hear of patients "pumping and dumping" milk after drinking alcohol. As with almost all medications, this is not necessary. A patient of average size will reduce milk alcohol level by 15 to 20 mg/dL/hr. This is equivalent to one "standard drink" in about 2 hours (Ho et al., 2001).

Ethanol inhibits oxytocin release; thus, it temporarily reduces milk delivery to the infant (Coiro et al., 1992). Occasional consumption of one to two alcoholic beverages with an appropriate waiting period before breastfeeding poses little risk to the infant. Any milk expressed during the waiting period should not be used for infant consumption.

Recreational Substances

In general, breastfeeding is contraindicated in those who use recreational substances. However, history of substance use can sometimes be managed in a way that is supportive of breastfeeding. Stable, engaged patients who have demonstrated a suitable commitment to abstinence (typically 90 days of sobriety) should be empowered to initiate breastfeeding.

CANNABIS/MARIJUANA

Emerging evidence suggests that exposure to delta-9-tetrahydrocannabinol (THC) in pregnancy or chronic use in adolescence may change the endocannabinoid system in the brain (Astley & Little, 1990; Volkow et al., 2014). As this system regulates mood, reward, and goal-directed behavior, cannabis in breast milk has created substantial perceptions of risk. However, at least with occasional use, the active ingredient in marijuana (THC) rapidly redistributes from the plasma to the adipose tissue, leaving milk levels low. In studies of 23.28 mg of smoked THC, the AID was estimated at 8 mcg daily, 2.5% of the weight-adjusted maternal dose (Baker, Datta, Rewers-Felkins, Thompson, et al., 2018). In addition, only 1% to 6% of this minuscule dose is absorbed orally. Although high milk to plasma ratios are commonly cited in the media, these do not correlate with the actual dose and are not clinically relevant. Chronic use has been unstudied, but it is possible that it could lead to accumulation in the breast milk. Determining who qualifies as a heavy or chronic cannabis user is challenging. Parents should be counseled to prevent smoke exposure to their infants.

COCAINE

The amount of cocaine contamination in breast milk varies greatly, with RID estimates ranging from 1% to 10% (Sarkar et al., 2005; Winecker et al., 2001). Cocaine is rapidly metabolized and redistributed out of the brain. Breast milk is likely to be cocaine-free after 24 hours, but infants may be drug screen-positive for much longer. Inactive metabolites of cocaine are excreted into the urine and breast for up to 7 days after the initial dose.

HALLUCINOGENS

Although there are no high-quality human studies on their transfer, hallucinogens are predicted to enter human milk. The signs and symptoms of hallucinogen intoxication have not been described in patients whose only exposure was through breast milk. Lysergic acid (LSD) and phencyclidine (PCP) are associated with altered consciousness levels in infants and young children

(Schwartz & Einhorn, 1986; Welch & Correa, 1980). Both have been detectable in human milk, but concentrations are unknown (Kaufman et al., 1983; Nicholas et al., 1982; Uyeno, 1970). With large maternal doses, more serious effects, such as seizures and coma, have been documented. Similar experiences are expected with other hallucinogens at high doses, such as dextromethorphan, 3,4-methylenedioxy-methamphetamine (MDMA), gamma hydroxybutyrate, and methamphetamines.

HEROIN

Heroin has many active metabolites, including 6-acetylmorphine and morphine, all of which may transfer into the breast milk. As with other opioid use disorders, chronic use results in tolerance, causing doses to climb in order to maintain the same effect. Lability in plasma levels can be dangerous, and dependent users are probably not appropriate candidates for breastfeeding.

Patients with opioid use disorder who are stable in treatment programs can successfully, and safely, breastfeed their infants (Table 6.12). Treatment with both buprenorphine and methadone has been extensively studied in breastfeeding. Transfer for both of these medications is low, as is oral bioavailability. The breastfed infants of patients on these medications demonstrate less severe NAS and require less direct pharmacologic intervention than formula-fed infants (Abdel-Latif et al., 2006; O'Connor et al., 2013; Welle-Strand et al., 2013). Some infants will undergo non life-threatening withdrawal symptoms with breastfeeding cessation.

STRATEGIES TO REDUCE INFANT RISK

A few basic techniques can help reduce the risks of drug exposure in infants:

- Use nondrug therapies whenever possible.
- Reduce infant exposure:
  - Supplement feedings: Diluting human milk with donor milk can be used as a strategy to reduce infant drug exposure. Donor milk is preferred as it is most similar in composition to the mother's own milk, but it may be available only for severe situations. Previously pumped frozen milk may also work for short-term situations, such as after surgery.
  - Medicated milk holiday ("pump and dump"): Sometimes it may be necessary to withhold freshly expressed human milk for a short period of time due to the presence of medications.
  - Time doses versus feedings: For drugs with a half-life of less than 4 hours, medication schedules can be managed to avoid feeding during peak medication levels. This can effectively reduce the AID to a more manageable level. However, for most medications, this method is not effective.

TABLE 6.12 Medications for Opioid Use Disorder

OPIOID	ORAL BIOAVAILABILITY (%)	RID (%)	MORPHINE MILLIGRAM EQUIVALENTS	MAXIMUM RECOMMENDED DOSE WITH FULL BREASTFEEDING
Buprenorphine	29	<1–3	10	22 mg/d[a]
Methadone	50	2–7	4–12[b]	180 mg/d[a]

[a]Maximum consistent maternal dose per day.
[b]Dose-dependent.
RID, relative infant dose.
Sources: From Abdel-Latif, M. E., Pinner, J., Clews, S., Cooke, F., Lui, K., & Oei, J. (2006). Effects of breast milk on the severity and outcome of neonatal abstinence syndrome among infants of drug-dependent mothers. *Pediatrics, 117*(6), e1163–e1169. https://doi.org/10.1542/peds.2005-1561; O'Connor, A. B., Collett, A., Alto, W. A., & O'Brien, L. M. (2013). Breastfeeding rates and the relationship between breastfeeding and neonatal abstinence syndrome in women maintained on buprenorphine during pregnancy. *Journal of Midwifery & Women's Health, 58*(4), 383–388. https://doi.org/10.1111/jmwh.12009; Welle-Strand, G. K., Skurtveit, S., Jansson, L. M., Bakstad, B., Bjarkø, L., & Ravndal, E. (2013). Breastfeeding reduces the need for withdrawal treatment in opioid-exposed infants. *Acta Paediatrica, 102*(11), 1060–1066. https://doi.org/10.1111/apa.12378.

- Choose breastfeeding-friendly medications:
  - Use medications with evidence on safety.
    - Choose medications that have been quantified for drug transfer. For example, captopril, benazepril, and enalapril are all known to have low transfer, whereas lisinopril has not been studied.
    - Choose medications commonly used in pediatric clinical practice.
    - When no other data exist, choose medications with a known history from clinical practice. For example, buspirone has not been studied for transfer but has been used widely in practice to avoid prescribing alternate anxiolytics like sedating benzodiazepines.
  - Use formulations that have local activity. For example, topical preparations are preferred to oral options when possible.
  - When no other data exist, use drugs with high molecular weights, high protein binding, high water solubility, and high Vd.

RESOURCES FOR EVALUATING INFORMATION

Drug references commonly used for pediatric or adult indications often do not include sufficient information for lactating patients. There have been significant improvements in the quality and quantity of breastfeeding data included in FDA-approved package inserts since the Pregnancy and Lactation Labeling Rule was implemented in 2014. Most medications on the market were approved prior to the changes. Older drug labels rarely cite any breastfeeding data, urging caution or incompatibility without evidence of harm. Even in situations in which independent post marketing research is available, the package inserts are not updated to reflect the results. Without regulation to include lactating patients in drug trials, pharmaceutical companies have no incentive to complete the research or take a proactive stance in their marketing materials. For these reasons, medication information provided by the pharmaceutical manufacturer is commonly the worst resource for lactation drug information.

Instead, lactation-specific drug references are the best repositories of drug-specific studies and clinical experience. Although PubMed is always an excellent resource for primary literature, including lactation studies, excellent lactation-specific references are available to summarize and contextualize this information.

LactMed

The National Library of Medicine maintain the Drugs and Lactation Database (LactMed) online, freely available to anyone (https://www.ncbi.nlm.nih.gov/books/NBK501922). It is updated monthly and is an excellent source of current data for each medication listed. Unfortunately, it is not all inclusive and does not have monographs for many common medications that have not been studied. Further, it does not provide personal information concerning doses and multiple drug use. When information is not available via research, LactMed will most often not provide conjecture.

Hale's Medications & Mothers' Milk

This book is produced in print every 2 years (Hale, 2020). It is also available in a mobile application and a digital portal format for institutional subscription. Electronic versions update monthly.

Drugs in Pregnancy and Lactation

This book (Briggs et al., 2015) is produced in print and electronically every 5 years. It is available through premium versions of the Lexicomp drug compendium.

InfantRisk Center

The InfantRisk Center has many resources for parents and providers regarding medication safety during pregnancy and lactation.

- InfantRisk.com has many articles on common topics for breastfeeding patients.
- The free InfantRisk Hotline has nurses available to answer breastfeeding medication questions for specific scenarios of parents or clinicians. They are available during regular business hours (Central Standard Time) at +1 (806) 352-2519.
- MommyMeds is a paid mobile application providing easy-to-digest information for parents.
- InfantRisk HCP is a paid mobile application for clinicians to use to quickly reference drug safety in pregnancy and lactation.

SHARED DECISION-MAKING

Most medications are compatible with breastfeeding. However, clinicians often fear adverse effects of maternal medications on a breastfeeding infant. Consequently, out of an excess of caution, they unnecessarily advise patients to either withhold medication treatments or discontinue breastfeeding, both of which impact maternal health (Davanzo et al., 2016; Sachs & Committee on Drugs, 2013). Unfortunately, breastfeeding patients often seek information from multiple medical providers (e.g., their provider, their infant's pediatrician, their pharmacist) and receive conflicting advice (McClatchey et al., 2018). Twice as many patients who were sick or had to take medicine did not breastfeed compared with their counterparts who did not take medication or experience illness (Odom et al., 2013). Taking extra time for shared decision-making with these patients can relieve maternal anxiety and improve breastfeeding behaviors.

CONCLUSIONS

In most cases, a practical solution can be found to safely allow patients to breastfeed despite medication use. Infant harm due to medicated human milk exposure is rare. The risk to the infant is due to the degree of drug toxicity, the dose of the drug, and the amount of drug absorbed. The infant's age and metabolic capacity also impact their ability to tolerate drug exposures. Some drugs have excellent information backed by research, whereas others must be estimated by physiochemical and pharmacokinetic parameters. Drug properties that make transfer more likely are active transport, low molecular weight, low protein binding, high lipophilicity, and low Vd. Drugs that are most concerning include radioactive iodine, chemotherapy and antimetabolites, drugs of abuse, and medications used for chronic sedation.

Some medication classes are safer than others, and there can be significant variability within the same class. Medications with an RID of less than 10% are generally considered compatible with breastfeeding. Lower thresholds may be necessary for more toxic drugs. Risk–benefit analyses should include not only the risk of the drug to the infant, but the benefits and risks of breastfeeding and maternal treatment or lack thereof. Multiple resources exist to facilitate these assessments.

LEARNING TOOLS AND RESOURCES

Advice From the Authors

Kaytlin Krutsch, PharmD, MBA

Neonatal care is challenging on its best day. The holistic balance of the maternal-infant dyad and the potential infant exposure to necessary maternal medications add another layer of complexity. Applying concepts of drug transfer is more than knowing the facts. It demands in-depth clinical consideration and integration of multiple fields; these patients' medical decisions influence each other's health. The wealth of knowledge is quickly growing in this field. Utilizing your understanding will require flexibility in accepting new data—research exists to improve clinical practice…but isn't successful until people implement it.

Teresa Baker, MD

As an obstetrics/gynecology physician, I can attest to the fact that clinical scenarios in today's mother–infant dyad are becoming more complex. Trying to help a mother–infant dyad to navigate breastfeeding with complex medical conditions can be very challenging. We hope that the growing body of literature and support services help all those involved in the care of breastfeeding mothers' infants to feel more confident in their decision-making and want to reiterate that support and guidance is always available.

Thomas W. Hale, PhD

Almost all breastfeeding mothers will use medications while feeding their infant. In addition, all drugs will penetrate the breast milk compartment to some degree. To determine the risk to the infant depends on multiple factors, but most important is the dose the drug in milk, and the innate hazard of the medication itself. Small levels of some drugs, such as penicillins, have little to no effect on the infant, but small levels of highly dangerous anticancer drugs may certainly be hazardous to an infant. Thus, to evaluate the risk to the infant requires some knowledge of pharmacology and perinatology.

Discussion Prompts

1. Describe the neuronal and hormonal regulation of lactation. Consider how changes in these pathways may alter milk secretion.
2. How would a drug with an RID of 18% compare with a drug with an RID of 1.3%? How does an increase in maternal dose affect RID? How does the increase affect the absolute infant dose?
3. Compare and contrast the roles of active and passive transport systems and their influence on drug concentration in milk.
4. Evaluate the influence of oral bioavailability, milk volume, and infant renal function on the potential for the development of adverse effects.
5. Differentiate the frequency and type of adverse effects seen among different drug classes, such as serotonin-modulating agents or antibiotics.
6. Summarize the effects of tobacco, alcohol, and recreational substances on milk production and their potential concentration in milk.
7. Outline strategies to limit drug exposure to infants while safely breastfeeding.

Mind Map

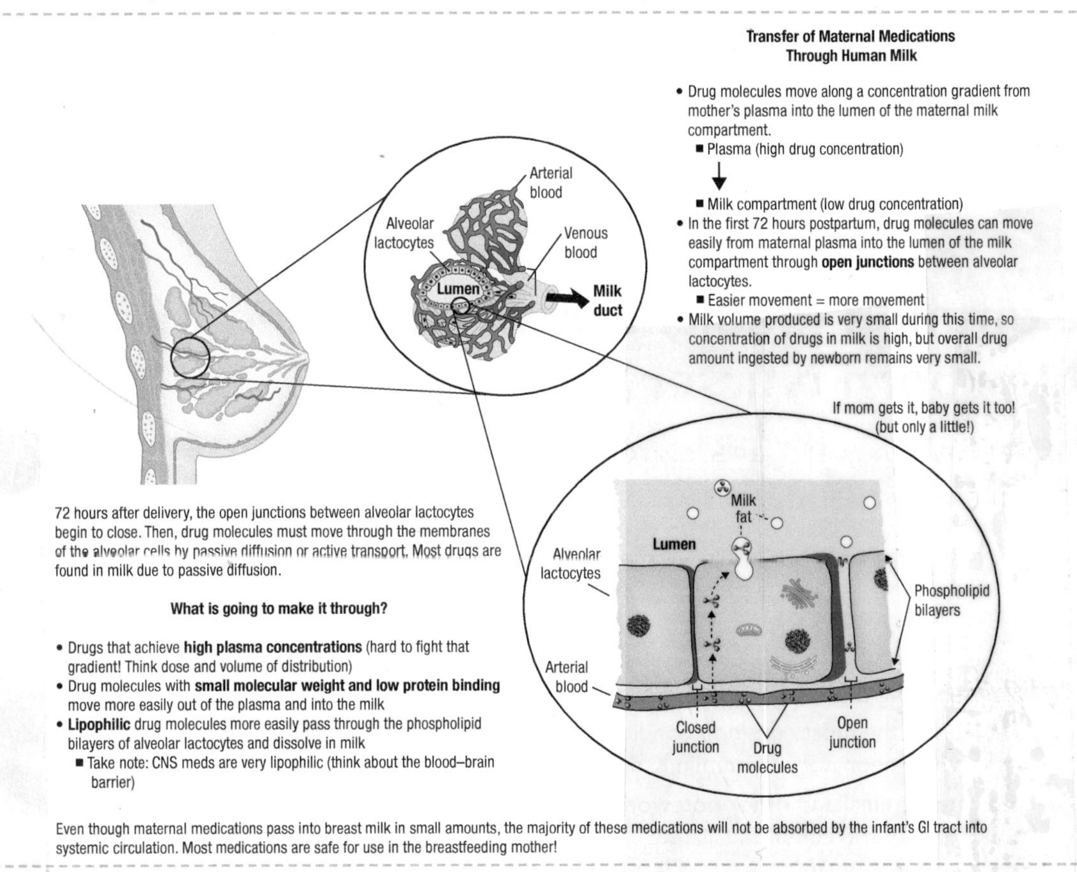

CNS, central nervous system; GI, gastrointestinal.
Design credit: Erin McDowell, MSN, RNC-NIC, and Kristen Landis, BSN, RNC-NIC, East Carolina University Neonatal Nurse Practitioner Program MSN students.

REFERENCES

References for this chapter are online and available at https://connect.springerpub.com/content/book/978-0-8261-5884-0/part/partI/toc-part/ch6.

chapter 7

Common Medications Prescribed in the Newborn Nursery

Tiffany Gwartney and Jane Ierardi

LEARNING OBJECTIVES

After completing this chapter, the reader should be able to:

- Enumerate the most common conditions frequently observed in the newborn nursery, including ophthalmia neonatorum, vitamin K deficiency, circumcision pain, hypoglycemia, and maternal HIV.
- Examine seminal and other noteworthy studies that shaped the state of the science specific to treatment of the conditions listed.
- Discuss pharmacotherapeutics available to the newborn infant in the newborn nursery.

INTRODUCTION

The goal of this chapter is to introduce a historical perspective of how and why pharmacotherapeutic interventions were developed and familiarize the reader with the pharmacokinetic principles, current dosing recommendations, and clinical monitoring pearls frequently used in the care of a late preterm and term newborn infant admitted to a well-baby nursery. We begin with a discussion of preventative and pharmacologic treatment strategies for ophthalmia neonatorum and vitamin K deficiency bleeding. Next, we present readers with core concepts specific to the pharmacologic treatment of hypoglycemia, an increasingly common problem with a potential link to childhood neurocognitive impairment. Last, we present the current state of the science specific to pharmacotherapeutics used with circumcision and perinatal HIV exposure.

PREVENTION OF OPHTHALMIA NEONATORUM AND VITAMIN K DEFICIENCY BLEEDING

Ophthalmia Neonatorum

Ophthalmia neonatorum, or newborn conjunctivitis, involves the infiltration of bacterial or viral pathogens, or chemical irritants, into the conjunctiva (Tesini, 2020). By definition, the disease state manifests within the first 30 days of life. The two most common bacteria associated with conjunctivitis are *Chlamydia trachomatis* and *Neisseria gonorrhoeae*. Chlamydia infection accounts for 2% to 40% of cases of conjunctivitis in the United States, whereas gonococcal infection is identified in fewer than 1% of all cases (Kimberlin et al., 2021; Jin, 2019). Viral infiltration is also rare; the incidence of herpetic conjunctivitis is estimated at less than 1% (Kimberlin et al., 2021).

PATHOGENESIS AND CLINICAL MANIFESTATIONS

The pathogenesis of ophthalmia neonatorum often begins with the vertical transmission of a pathogen (e.g., *C. trachomatis, N. gonorrhoeae,* herpes simplex virus [HSV]) from mother to fetus. This is followed by an incubation period and subsequent manifestation of the disease process. *C. trachomatis*-mediated conjunctivitis customarily manifests within 7 days (range: 5–12 days) of birth (Darville, 2005; Kimberlin et al., 2021). Common ocular manifestations include watery or mucopurulent discharge, lid edema and irritation (chemosis), and thickened conjunctiva (pseudomembranes; Hammerschlag, 2011; Zuppa et al., 2011). Spontaneous resolution of symptoms is common and long-term complications, namely blindness, are rare.

N. gonorrhoeae-mediated conjunctivitis customarily manifests within 2 to 5 days of delivery; however, a prolonged incubation with onset of disease 2 to 3 weeks after birth has been reported (Kimberlin et al., 2021; Zuppa et al., 2011). Manifestations can mimic chlamydia infection, complicating empiric treatment decisions in the absence of confirmatory testing. Common symptoms include abundant mucopurulent discharge, lid edema, and chemosis. Complications are far more serious compared to chlamydia conjunctivitis; the disease process progresses rapidly (within 24 hours), and, in the absence of treatment, can give rise to corneal scarring or ulcerations. Even more deleterious is perforation of the bulbus oculi, which contains the sclera, choroid, and retina (Woods, 2005).

Infants who develop viral conjunctivitis manifest with unique ocular findings. For example, herpes simplex-mediated conjunctivitis often involves the development of herpetic lesions on the eyelids, which present within 6 to 14 days after birth (Kimberlin et al., 2021; Zuppa et al., 2011). Adenovirus-mediated conjunctivitis usually presents 4 to 5 days into the viral process and involves the development of watery discharge, lid and conjunctival edema, pseudomembranes or true membranes, and pinpoint subconjunctival hemorrhages (Hoffman, 2020).

HISTORIC CONTEXT: SEMINAL AND OTHER NOTEWORTHY STUDIES

The evolution of understanding specific to the treatment of two diseases diagnosed in the newborn nursery setting, congenital gonorrhea and chylamydia infection, is well documented. We digress to offer a high-level review of the evolution of select events and studies, as trainees and novice clinicians benefit from establishing an awareness of these historic milestones.

Between the 1800s and early 1900s (the "preantibiotic era"), ophthalmia neonatorum, primarily caused by *N. gonorrhoeae,* was a common cause for ocular scarring and blindness in newborns (Castro Ochoa & Mendez, 2021). In fact, 10% of all newborns born in Germany manifested with this disease state, 3% went on to become blind, and 50% of school-age children enrolled in schools for the blind had been subject to untreated gonococcal ophthalmia neonatorum as newborns (Klauss & Fransen, 1994; Oriel, 1991).

On June 1, 1880, Dr. Carl Credé, a German obstetrician (who incidentally contributed to the development of modern-day isolettes), proposed the use of silver nitrate for prophylaxis of ophthalmia neonatorum (Dunn, 2000). An excerpt from the translated version of Credé's (1881) seminal publication "Prevention of Inflammatory Eye Disease in the Newborn" is provided:

> I am (...) publishing the following information concerning the prevention of inflammatory eye disease in the newborn (...) because the disease is almost invariably caused by infection during delivery and is therefore directly related to a diseased condition of the female genitals. Responsibility for prevention of the disease must lie solely with obstetricians and midwives. I shall confine my remarks exclusively to the practical question of prophylaxis.
>
> (...) Most obstetricians would probably share my view that the case of vaginal catarrh and infections that are so frequently encountered are attributable to gonorrheal infection and that the discharge remain infectious long after the specific symptoms of gonorrhea have disappeared; moreover, in some cases where there is virtually no further trace of discharge, the infection may still be considered to have occurred in the mother's vagina when an inflammatory eye condition develops in the first few days after birth.

Transmission of the infectious substance from another child with eye disease is inconceivable (...) inasmuch as every child who is suffering from inflammatory eye disease is moved with its mother to a ward that is entirely separate in all respects from the maternity ward. The possibility of mothers infecting their children, for example through fingers soiled by lochial discharge, is also remote because the child's cot is always placed beyond reach of the mother, who only comes into contact with the child when the nurse places it on her breast.

I am therefore convinced (...) that all affected children in (...) hospital (...) were infected solely by direct transmission of vaginal discharge to the eye during delivery. The infected eye usually begins to show symptoms of disease 2 or 3 days after birth, but also sooner or later—the sooner, the more serious the condition.

I initially focused on ensuring extensive and effective treatment and cleansing of the diseased vaginas of pregnant and delivering women. But the results were poor and unsatisfactory, although there were fewer cases of eye disease (...). I then began to disinfect the children's eyes themselves and from then on, the success recorded was surprisingly encouraging.

My experiments proceeded as follows: first, the vaginas of all pregnant and delivering women admitted to the hospital with gonorrhea or chronic vaginal catarrh were cleaned out with lukewarm water or a light solution (2:100) of carbolic or salicylic acid as frequently as possible—every half hour in the case of delivering women. The incidence of eye disease declined but the problem persisted (...).

In October 1879, I carried out my first test involving the introduction of prophylactic eye drops into the newborn babies immediately after birth, using a borax solution (1:60) because it seemed to be the mildest and least caustic substance. This was only done, however, in the case of children whose mothers were ill and whose vaginas had been cleansed during the whole delivery process in a manner described above. From December 1879, I replaced the borax by solutions of Argentum nitricum (1:40) [silver nitrate 2% solution], which were injected into the [middle of the] eyes [by way of a glass rod] shortly after birth. The eyes were carefully washed beforehand with a solution of salicylic acid (2:100). The children of sick mothers who were treated in this way remained healthy, while other children who had not been given preventive treatment (...) still fell ill, in two cases quite seriously.

From 1 June 1880, all eyes without exception were disinfected immediately after birth by means of a weaker solution of Argentum nitricum (1:50). (...) a glass stick was used to introduce a single drop of liquid into each eye, which was gently opened by an assistant, and which had been cleaned beforehand with ordinary water. Then the eyes were cooled for 24 h with a canvas cloth soaked in salicylic water (2:100). The numerous vaginal douches, on the other hand, were abandoned (...). All children treated in this way remained free from even mild attacks of inflammatory eye disease, although many mothers showed advanced symptoms of vaginal blenorrhea (...). Only one child (...) fell ill on the 6th day with a moderate inflammation of the conjunctiva of the left eye, without swelling of the eyelid, which healed within 3 days. It emerged that, quite by chance, owing to pressure of work, the prophylactic eye drops had not been administered to this child.

To date, no adverse effect on the treated eyes has been observed. Not infrequently the administration of the eye drops is followed by a slight hyperemia and in some cases by slight increased secretion from the conjunctiva in the first 24 hours. Then these symptoms disappear. They could perhaps be avoided if further tests indicate that a weaker solution of Argentum nitricum is sufficient.

As has been shown, the procedure is simple, (...) completely without risk and seemingly reliable in terms of its effect. (...) my set of observations is (...) still sufficiently extensive and striking to warrant further urgent application of the procedure. I wish to lay special emphasis on the finding that the desired effects are achieved through dis- infection of the eyes themselves rather than the vagina. It is to be hoped that the future will tell whether the eye procedure that I have been using is the best and most reliable one (...). For the time being, I have no reason to deviate from my own method.

Source: Credé, C. S. F. (1881). Die verhutung der augenentzundung der neugeborenen ("Prevention of inflammatory eye disease in the newborn"). *Bulletin World Health Organization, 79,* 265–266. https://apps.who.int/iris/handle/10665/74722

Over the next 2 years, Credé simplified his method. After birth, the umbilical cord was reduced, and the newborn was bathed. The eyes were cleansed with water and 2% silver nitrate solution was applied by way of a glass rod. All newborns subject to his treatment regimen were disinfected, and this thrust silver nitrate to the forefront. On January 31, 1883, Credé's method for providing prophylaxis against *N. gonorrhoeae*-mediated ophthalmia neonatorum was written into law in Austria. Due to the success of limiting the risk of blindness, many countries, including the United States, mandated its use in birthing centers and hospitals (Zar, 2005). This was despite the 50% to 90% incidence of severe and presumed painful chemical conjunctivitis from silver nitrate exposure.

By the mid to late 1900s, with a decrease in gonorrheal infections, *C. trachomatis* became the most common cause for blindness in the world (Moore et al., 2015). Like gonorrhea, chlamydia was identified as a vertically transmitted infection and associated with the development of pneumonia in infants. However, clinicians quickly realized that Credé's prophylactic regimen was ineffective against *C. trachomatis*. Even worse, the incidence of severe chemical conjunctivitis (secondary to silver nitrate exposure) had risen. Numerous countries, including the United States, abandoned silver nitrate protocols. Quickly, cases of *N. gonorrhoeae*-mediated conjunctivitis resurged. In Florida, for example, 55 new cases were reported between 1984 and 1989 (Schaller & Klauss, 2001). Experts voiced concerns and lobbied for the establishment of an enforceable prophylactic regimen for all newborns. This led to the introduction of several new drugs for this purpose.

In 1952, 0.5% erythromycin, a macrolide antibiotic, was trialed in newborns (Moore et al., 2015). Reports confirmed that erythromycin 0.5% was active against both *C. trachomatis* and *N. gonorrhoeae* and seemed to provide effective prophylaxis. However, many cautioned that widespread macrolide use could perpetuate the emergence of new drug-resistant strains. Other drugs used for prophylaxis included povidone-iodine 2.5% solution and tetracycline, both found to be effective treatments for neonatal conjunctivitis. Povidone-iodine 2.5% solution is very cost-effective ($0.10 per 5 mL) and likewise still used in many underserved countries. In comparison, the cost for erythromycin 0.5% ophthalmic ointment is $3 to $12 per tube. Povidone-iodine 2.5% solution is not currently commercially available in the United States and its effectiveness against gonorrhea remains unclear.

More recently, erythromycin-resistant strains of gonorrhea have emerged, leading many to question the cost-effectiveness of mandated universal eye prophylaxis that may or may not be effective against these newer strains. Many countries, including Canada, Denmark, Norway, Sweden, and the United Kingdom, continue to mandate screening during pregnancy and delivery but no longer mandate universal newborn prophylaxis (Kimberlin et al., 2021). However, experts in the United States attribute the overall decrease in the incidence of *N. gonorrhoeae* ophthalmia neonatorum (1980 to present) to existing standardized prenatal screening and treatment, as well as postnatal erythromycin 0.5% prophylaxis (Centers for Disease Control and Prevention [CDC], n.d.-b).

PRIMARY PREVENTION: PRENATAL SCREENING AND TREATMENT

Obstetric clinicians align their practice with current CDC screening guidance for the primary prevention of ophthalmia neonatorum. This involves routine first-trimester maternal surveillance for gonorrhea and chlamydia, often pursued during the first prenatal visit, as well as repeat screening of high-risk women in the third trimester. Maternal risk factors include inconsistent use of condoms during intercourse, multiple-partner sexual relationships, drug or alcohol abuse, or maintaining a residence within an endemic area (CDC, n.d.-b). Once a sexually transmitted infection is confirmed, repeat testing is indicated 3 months after treatment is completed (to establish a "test of cure"), and at the time of admission to the labor/delivery unit. Women who do not seek prenatal care and whose records cannot be obtained in a timely manner should be tested upon admission to the labor/delivery unit (CDC, n.d.-b).

SECONDARY PREVENTION: POSTNATAL PHARMACOLOGIC TREATMENT MODALITIES

Secondary prevention begins at birth and involves prophylactic (preventative) or targeted pharmacotherapies for ophthalmia neonatorum. We begin with a discussion of the use of erythromycin 0.5% ophthalmic ointment and then move to a discussion of postexposure antimicrobial therapies for infants born to a mother with confirmed and untreated chlamydial or gonococcal infection (CDC, n.d.-b).

Postnatal Prophylaxis

As discussed, erythromycin 0.5% ophthalmic ointment is the drug of choice in the United States for the prevention of infectious neonatal conjunctivitis (Dekker & Bertone, 2019). Erythromycin inhibits the proliferation of *C. trachomatis* and is active against most strains of *N. gonorrhoeae* and other gram-positive bacteria. The CDC, AAP, and American College of Obstetricians and Gynecologists (ACOG) currently recommend the universal use of erythromycin 0.5% ophthalmic ointment prophylaxis for all newborns, regardless of gestational age. A recent meta-analysis concluded with moderate certainty that preventative treatment reduces the risk for infectious conjunctivitis over the first month of postnatal life; the risk of disease outweighs the low risk of side effects or complications from the treatment (Bocchini, 2009; Kapoor et al., 2020).

Mechanism of Action/Pharmacokinetic Principles

Erythromycin inhibits protein synthesis by binding to the 50S ribosomal subunit of susceptible organisms. The drug is more permeable to cell membranes in alkaline environments (Tesini, 2020).

Dosing Recommendations

Using a single-dose tube, apply a ribbon of 0.5% erythromycin ointment, approximately 1 inch or 2.5 centimeters in length, along each lower conjunctival sac. Discard the tube after use. Do not flush the eye after application.

Treatment with oral erythromycin is reserved only for infants diagnosed with symptomatic disease. Prophylactic oral erythromycin for asymptomatic exposed infants is not recommended, due to the relatively low incidence of transmission of chlamydia and the relatively high incidence of the development of pyloric stenosis (Castro Ochoa & Mendez, 2021).

Clinical-Monitoring Pearls

Side effects in neonates are rare and limited to transient irritation with redness (Hammerschlag et al., 1989). However, drug efficacy in the treatment of *C. trachomatis* remains controversial due to the rise of resistant bacterial strains (Zar, 2005). Therefore, ongoing monitoring for signs of chlamydial pneumonia and conjunctivitis is indicated. Conjunctivitis may develop secondary to other common viruses, including HSV and adenovirus (Moore et al., 2015). Parents should be instructed to seek medical attention if inflammation or conjunctival discharge develops.

Postexposure Prophylaxis

Well-appearing infants born to women with a *confirmed* chlamydial infection do not routinely receive postexposure prophylaxis because the efficacy of antibiotic therapy has not been proven to date. On the contrary, the AAP Committee on Infectious Diseases (2021–2024) recommends that well-appearing infants born to women with *confirmed* gonococcal infection receive intravenous (IV) or intramuscular (IM) antibiotic prophylaxis (Kimberlin et al., 2021).

Mechanism of Action/Pharmacokinetic Principles

See Chapter 28, "Neonatal Sepsis and Meningitis," for a discussion of the mechanism of action and pharmacokinetic principles of cephalosporins and aminoglycosides.

Dosing Recommendations

Clinicians must choose one of three eligible treatments: a single dose of ceftriaxone, or a single dose of cefotaxime or gentamicin.

Single-dose ceftriaxone (25–50 mg/kg/dose IM or IV) may be given to well-appearing term infants. Alternative therapy is indicated for preterm infants, any infant at risk for severe hyperbilirubinemia, and infants receiving calcium-containing IV solutions. In these cases, therapy involves a single dose of cefotaxime (100 mg/kg/dose IV or IM), which is also a third-generation cephalosporin, or a single dose of gentamicin (2.5 mg/kg/dose IV or IM; Kimberlin et al., 2021). Importantly, gentamicin should not be used as treatment for neonates with confirmed or suspected gonococcal ocular disease due to inadequate penetration into the globe of the eye.

Clinical-Monitoring Pearls

Clinical monitoring involves ocular assessments performed at intervals and the provision of gentle saline flushes. This helps relieve irritation caused by the accumulation of mucopurulent drainage and prevents corneal abrasions. In addition, neonates should be carefully monitored for signs of systemic infection, which warrant a more comprehensive diagnostic evaluation, including blood and cerebrospinal fluid cultures for Gram-stain analysis.

Vitamin K Deficiency Bleeding

The term *vitamin K* does not represent one specific vitamin. Rather, this is a label given to a group of lipophilic (fat-soluble) compounds. Each compound consists of a 2-methyl-1,4-naphthoquinone (menadione) ring, but they differ from one another in that each has a unique isoprenoid side chain. The two naturally occurring forms of vitamin K are phylloquinone and phytonadione (vitamin K_1) and menaquinone (vitamin K_2). vitamin K_1 is naturally found in plants (e.g., green leafy vegetables, meat, eggs). vitamin K_2 is naturally found in dairy products (e.g., milk) and is synthesized in the colon through normal processes of fermentation (by *Bacteroides*).

PATHOGENESIS AND CLINICAL MANIFESTATIONS

Normally, vitamin K functions as a necessary cofactor to the enzyme γ-glutamyl carboxylase (GGCX). When activated, GGCX carboxylates specific glutamic acid residues, creating γ- carboxyglutamic acid (Gla). These Gla-containing proteins are capable of binding to calcium, a critical step in the activation of the vitamin K-dependent clotting factors (Table 7.1).

All components of the coagulation cascade are present in variable amounts by approximately 10 weeks of gestation. However, less than 10% of maternal vitamin K crosses the placenta and the fetal liver cannot store vitamin K for postnatal use. After birth, the infant has an insufficient amount of endogenous vitamin K and a relatively sterile gut devoid of adequate *Bacteroides* species necessary to stimulate endogenous synthesis of vitamin K. In addition, dietary intake of vitamin K after birth is insufficient; breast milk contains 1 to 4 mcg/L of vitamin K_1 and even less vitamin K_2 (Greer et al., 1988; Hiraike et al., 1988; Mandelbrot et al., 1988). Therefore, the pathogenesis of vitamin K deficiency bleeding (VKDB) in newborns involves failed activation of the vitamin K-dependent proteins.

Vitamin K-deficient bleeding in the newborn presents at three distinct time points (CDC, n.d.-c, n.d.-d). *Early vitamin K deficiency* usually occurs within the first 24 hours of life. The incidence is between 6% and 12% of infants who do not receive a vitamin K injection at birth. Common manifestations include a severe cephalohematoma, intracranial hemorrhage, or abnormal bleeding at puncture sites. It occurs primarily in infants who are exclusively breastfed and in mothers receiving vitamin K-inhibiting medications such as warfarin, carbamazepine, phenytoin, barbiturates, isoniazid, rifampin, and some cephalosporins (Autret-Leca & Jonville-Béra, 2001; Hand et al., 2022; Lippi & Franchini, 2011). *Classic vitamin K deficiency* typically occurs between 2 and 7 days of life. The incidence is between 0.25% and 1.5% of infants who do not receive a vitamin K injection at birth. It presents with easy bruising, gastrointestinal bleeding or bleeding from the umbilicus or puncture sites, and, rarely, intracranial hemorrhage. It is often idiopathic, but may be associated with a delay in feeding or insufficient intake of feeds (Autret-Leca & Jonville-Béra, 2001; Lippi & Franchini, 2011). *Late vitamin K deficiency* typically occurs between 1 week and 6 months of life, with severe abnormal bleeding and/or intracranial hemorrhage; the peak time frame of the onset of disease is between 2 and 8 weeks of life (Hand et al., 2022). The incidence is 1/15,000 to 1/20,000 among infants who are exclusively breastfed and do not receive a vitamin K injection at birth or are affected by cholestasis or malabsorption conditions. Mortality risk is estimated to be 20% (Autret-Leca & Jonville-Béra, 2001; Lippi & Franchini, 2011).

TABLE 7.1 Vitamin K-Dependent Clotting Factors

PROTEIN	FUNCTION
Factor II, VII, IX, X	Procoagulation
Protein C, S, Z	Anticoagulation

HISTORIC CONTEXT: SEMINAL AND OTHER NOTEWORTHY STUDIES

Hemorrhagic disease of the newborn was first identified by Wendell and Townsend in the late 19th century (Hand et al., 2022). Vitamin K was discovered in the 1930s by Danish biochemist Henrik Dam, who noticed that chickens would bleed easily if fed a low-fat or low-cholesterol diet (Lippi & Franchini, 2011). He discovered the responsible agent and referred to it as a *koagulation vitamin*. It soon became known as an *antihemorrhagic factor*. Approximately 1 decade later, Dam and Edward Doisy were awarded the Nobel Prize in Physiology for Medicine for their investigation of the chemical construct of vitamin K (Klebanoff et al., 1993). The controversy with neonatal vitamin K arose in the early 1990s when two retrospective British studies proposed an association between childhood leukemia and infants who received IM vitamin K_1 at birth (Golding et al., 1990, 1992). However, two subsequent large retrospective studies, one from the United States and one from Sweden, could not find any association (Lippi & Franchini, 2011). Subsequently, multiple studies confirmed the association to be erroneous. Roman and associates (2002) combined data from six cohorts (including subjects in the two studies published by Golding) and reported no significant association between vitamin K injection and childhood cancer (odds ratio [OR] = 1.09; 95% CI, 0.92–1.28). One year later, Fear and associates (2003), also British, published a single case-controlled study (N = 8,769) confirming no significant association between vitamin K and leukemia.

Despite a large amount of evidence to refute the initial two studies, concerns about the safety of administering IM vitamin K_1 in the newborn remain (Fear et al., 2003; Roman et al., 2002). In some European countries, parents who refuse the vitamin K injection are offered oral vitamin K_1. However, the efficacy of the oral form in preventing late vitamin K deficiency is low (McPherson, 2020). Since 2003, the AAP recommends routine IM vitamin K_1 for every newborn, and it is approved by the Food and Drug Administration (FDA; American Academy of Pediatrics Committee on Fetus and Newborn, 2003).

CURRENT PHARMACOLOGIC TREATMENT MODALITY

VKDB can be averted with the provision of IM vitamin K_1 within the first 6 hours after birth. Infants who do not receive vitamin K_1 may develop bleeding severe enough to warrant volume resuscitation with fresh frozen plasma (10–20 mL/kg), prothrombin complex concentrates, or recombinant Factor VIIa.

Phytonadione (Vitamin K_1)

Phytonadione is used for prophylaxis of hemorrhagic disease of the newborn. Parenteral vitamin K will lead to increased blood coagulation factors within 1 to 2 hours of administration. When treating for a hemorrhage or abnormal bleeding due to vitamin K deficiency, control is usually achieved within 3 to 6 hours of IV administration, yet a normal prothrombin level may not be reached until 12 to 14 hours.

Mechanism of Action

Vitamin K_1 promotes the activation of vitamin K-dependent clotting factors in the liver, including Factor II (active prothrombin), Factor VII (proconvertin), Factor IX, and Factor X.

Intramuscular Dosing Recommendations

Vitamin K_1 is supplied as a 2-mg/mL dispersion in a 0.5-mL ampule or syringe. **Note**: The ampule contains 0.9% benzyl alcohol as a preservative, which is considered insignificant (CDC, n.d.-c, n.d.-d; McPherson, 2020). The AAP-recommended dose for infants weighing more than 1,500 grams is 1 mg IM within 6 hours of birth (Hand et al., 2022). Larger or repeated doses may be required in infants whose mothers are taking anticonvulsants or oral anticoagulants (Hand et al., 2022; Prescriber's Digital Reference [PDR], n.d.). The AAP-recommended dose for infants weighing less than 1,500 grams is 0.3 to 0.5 mg/kg IM (Hand et al., 2022).

Oral Dosing (Not Licensed in the United States)

An alternative consideration, if parents refuse the IM dose, is oral vitamin K_1. Oral vitamin K is considered effective in preventing classic VKDB; however, the efficacy in preventing late-onset VKDB remains unclear (Hand et al., 2022). Oral vitamin K is absorbed by the jejunum and ileum, but requires the presence of bile salts and pancreatic enzymes. Ingestion of vitamin K simultaneously with fat will improve absorption. Once ingested, an increase in the concentration of blood coagulation factors occurs within 6 to 12 hours. The injection may be administered orally; however, this is costly (~$8 per dose for ampules, $45 per dose for syringes, $25–$50 per dose for tablets that must be crushed and suspended) and cumbersome. Although unlicensed in the United States, certain European countries offer 2 to 4 mg orally after the first enteral feeding, followed by 2 to 4 mg orally between 2 and 4 weeks of age and again between 6 and 8 weeks of age. Breastfed babies may receive 2 to 4 mg orally after the first feeding, followed by weekly doses of 2 mg orally while breastfeeding continues. A third regimen reported in the literature involves 2 mg orally after the first feeding followed by 2 mg orally in the first week of life, and 25-mcg oral doses each week for 13 consecutive weeks. Postdischarge parental compliance is critical to achieve a fraction of the efficacy that IM therapy offers; failure rates are high with all oral regimens. **Note:** Oral vitamin K_1 is contraindicated for preterm infants, infants receiving antibiotics, or infants with cholestasis or diarrhea.

Clinical-Monitoring Pearls

Side effects of vitamin K_1 use include associated pain and swelling at the injection site with IM administration. Although there is a black-box warning to avoid IM administration if a subcutaneous route is possible, this does not apply to newborns and the AAP recommends IM vitamin K_1 prophylaxis for all newborns. There have been reports of severe reactions with IV vitamin K_1 administration in adults, similar to anaphylaxis leading to shock, cardiac arrest, and even death. This is very rare and has not been reported in newborns.

SPECIAL CIRCUMSTANCES WARRANTING PHARMACOLOGIC TREATMENT

Postnatal Hypoglycemia and 40% Oral Glucose Gel

Hypoglycemia is considered the most commonly diagnosed metabolic disorder in newborns. Inadequate glycogen stores, increased glucose requirements, and hyperinsulinism account for the majority of cases. Preterm, late preterm, small for gestational age, and infants of diabetic mothers are considered high-risk populations. Researchers estimate that up to 50% of well-appearing newborns 36 weeks of gestation or older meet criteria for postnatal glucose monitoring, and, of those infants, 40% to 45% are likely to manifest with hypoglycemia.

HISTORIC CONTEXT: SEMINAL AND OTHER NOTEWORTHY STUDIES

Historically, oral glucose gel (OGG) has been used in the adult population since the 1970s, with some concern regarding its bioavailability and lack of absorption (Gunning & Garber, 1978). Prior to its introduction among the neonatal population in the 2000s, early feedings with breast milk, formula, and/or 5% dextrose in water were used as first-line interventions for transient neonatal hypoglycemia (TNH; Gibson et al., 2021; Gomella et al., 2020). Currently, 40% OGG is being used as a first-line intervention for TNH in the absence of the ability to place a peripheral IV line for a bolus or continuous dextrose infusion, such as in a well-baby or level I nursery (Gibson et al., 2021). Further, research outcomes support that use of 40% OGG as a cost-effective first-line intervention for TNH increases exclusive breastfeeding rates, reduces the mean number of heel lances required, and decreases admissions to the NICU (Gibson et al., 2021; Glasgow et al., 2018).

CURRENT PHARMACOLOGIC TREATMENT MODALITIES

A lack of consensus regarding appropriate screening intervals, blood glucose concentration (BGC) for newborns, and use of OGG as a first-line intervention for TNH in the immediate postnatal period is reflected in the literature. Current guidelines from the AAP and the Pediatric Endocrine Society (PES) recommend an ante cibum (AC) BGC of 45 mg/dL or more and 50 mg/dL or more, respectively, within the first 48 hours of life (Adamkin & Committee on Fetus and Newborn, 2011; Thornton et al., 2015). Although often asymptomatic, if left untreated TNH can lead to seizures, brain tissue injury, and subsequent developmental delay (Martin et al., 2014; Weston et al., 2016).

40% Oral Glucose Gel

The use of 40% OGG is intended as an adjunct to the provision of breast milk or formula. Combination therapy mitigates TNH and helps to prevent neurologic sequelae secondary to prolonged hypoglycemia or mother–infant separation secondary to NICU admission (Edwards et al., 2021).

Mechanism of Action

Glucose is a carbohydrate. In gel form, glucose is a solution that has been dissolved in water and can be rapidly absorbed into circulation via the highly vascularized buccal mucosa and lingual surface. If swallowed, absorption may also occur in the small intestine (Hegarty et al., 2016).

Dose and Administration

The recommended dosing for 40% OGG is 200 mg/kg (0.5 mL/kg; Hegarty et al., 2016). The maximum recommended doses of 40% OGG are six doses within 48 hours (Gomella et al., 2020). Harris and colleagues (2016) posit that fewer repeat doses of 40% OGG are required when used in tandem with breast milk versus formula feedings. In fact, 40% OGG is administered orally, onto the buccal mucosa and lingual surfaces, facilitating rapid systemic absorption (Weston et al., 2016).

Clinicians should be aware that it is important to dry the buccal mucosa with sterile gauze prior to administration. Next, massage a partial dose of 40% OGG into the buccal mucosa using a gloved finger, and repeat until the full dose is administered. Then, immediately following administration, the newborn should be fed.

Clinical-Monitoring Pearls

At-risk newborns should begin feeding within 1 hour of birth and BGC should be screened within 30 minutes of completion of the feeding (Gibson et al., 2021; Gomella et al., 2020). Skin-to-skin care with frequent breastfeeding over the first 12 hours of life minimizes newborn brown fat consumption, helps maintain euthermia, reduces stress, and encourages maternal breast milk synthesis (Adamkin, 2016; Chappe, 2020; Edwards et al., 2021). Use of 40% OGG as a first-line intervention for TNH remains controversial, making adherence to institutional guidelines highly recommended. Additional laboratory studies and a consultation with an endocrine specialist should be considered if hypoglycemia persists beyond 72 hours of life (Chappe, 2020; Gomella et al., 2020).

Last, clinicians must recognize that postnatal hypoglycemia may increase the risk for visual motor coordination disorders and reduced executive function psychometric test scores. A precise risk threshold has yet to be defined and conflicting data add to the difficulty in establishing neuroprotective standards of practice (Goode et al., 2016; McKinlay et al., 2017; Shah et al., 2019; Tin et al., 2012). The use of an evidence-based guideline for treatment of TNH that prioritizes an adequate provision of substrate for carbohydrate metabolism and appropriate fasting window in between feeding sessions, with consistent adherence by all healthcare providers, will result in the best patient outcomes.

Neonatal Circumcision

Circumcision remains an elective, cosmetic procedure offered to families of eligible male neonates prior to discharge. Depending on population and religious, cultural, and ethical beliefs, in the United States, the incidence of male circumcision remains between 42% to 80%, and is predominantly practiced among Caucasians (91%), followed by Black (76%) and Hispanic (44%) males (Rossi et al., 2021; Simpson et al., 2014).

HISTORIC CONTEXT: SEMINAL AND OTHER NOTEWORTHY STUDIES

Dating back centuries, male circumcision is one of the oldest surgical procedures in the world. Male circumcision is a surgical procedure described as removal of the skin on the penile shaft and inner foreskin, exposing the glans penis (Rossi et al., 2021). Although additional research is indicated, the purported health benefits of male circumcision are prevention of penile cancer, urinary tract infections, and decreased acquisition and transmission of sexually transmitted diseases, including HIV, human papilloma virus, syphilis, and HSV (AAP Task Force on Circumcision, 2012).

Although an abundance of supportive literature continues to be published regarding appropriate interventions for neonatal procedural pain, including male circumcision, a gap remains in terms of a gold standard for analgesic practice. Further, there is wide variability among professional organizations and providers regarding the application of evidence-based interventions for procedural pain in the neonatal population. The literature supports that painful stimuli during the newborn period can have long-term effects (Walker, 2019). A systematic review of studies published over the past 20 years revealed that a combination of non-pharmacologic and pharmacologic strategies provides best pain management during male circumcision (Rossi et al., 2021).

CURRENT PHARMACOLOGIC TREATMENT MODALITIES

The AAP Task Force on Circumcision (2012) and the literature support using a combination of pain-relieving strategies to achieve best outcomes. The foundation of pharmacotherapy is lidocaine or bupivacaine via dorsal penile nerve block (DPNB) or ring block (RB), with adjunctive interventions, including optimized nonpharmacologic comfort measures, EMLA cream, oral sucrose, and acetaminophen (Rossi et al., 2021; Stolik-Dollberg & Dollberg, 2005). In a retrospective study, Stolik-Dollberg and Dollberg (2005) showed that patients who received 0.5% bupivacaine versus 1% lidocaine required less acetaminophen postcircumcision; however, bupivacaine use is associated with increased risk for adverse cardiovascular effects.

Lidocaine 1%

Lidocaine 1% is administered into the tissue at the base of the penis either by way of a DPNB to the dorsal nerves or RB for analgesia prior to circumcision.

Mechanism of Action

Lidocaine is a local anesthetic that numbs tissue sensation by blocking sodium channels, preventing neurons from communicating the pain sensation to the brain (DrugBank Online, 2023b). When provided in the subcutaneous tissue for circumcision, the numbing effect lasts approximately 10 to 20 minutes (DrugBank Online, 2023b).

Dosing Recommendations

If providing a DPNB, 0.2 to 0.4 mL of 1% lidocaine hydrochloride (without epinephrine) or 0.5% bupivacaine can be injected using a tuberculin syringe and 27-gauge needle into the dorsal nerves at the junction of the pubic and pelvic skin (MacDonald et al., 2013). Repeat in the dorsolateral position, then wait 3 to 5 minutes for infiltration of the lidocaine to numb the ventral nerve at the base of the penis.

Clinical-Monitoring Pearls

Unintentional IV injection of bupivacaine increases the risk for side effects, including heart block, hypotension, bradycardia, and arrest, making its use for circumcision less preferable (Choi et al., 2003; Stolik-Dollberg & Dollberg, 2005).

EMLA Cream

EMLA cream is a topical anesthetic composed of a mixture of 2.5% lidocaine and 2.5% prilocaine (Gomella et al., 2020). Common indications for use include relief of procedural pain associated with the insertion of IV catheters, IM injections, venipuncture, or lumbar puncture (Gomella et al., 2020). EMLA tempers circumcision pain if applied 1 to 1.5 hours prior to the procedure. On the basis of available evidence, EMLA is generally used to provide topical anesthesia prior to instillation of subcutaneous lidocaine or bupivacaine.

Mechanism of Action

As a whole, local anesthetics block the transfer of sensory nerve impulses by altering the ability of ions to penetrate the cell membrane (Gomella et al., 2020).

Dosing Recommendations

In the patient population 0 to 3 months of age with weight of less than 5 kg, the maximum dosing is placement of 1 gram of EMLA cream, coating 10 cm^2 of intact skin, wrapped in an occlusive dressing for a maximum of 1 hour prior to the procedure (Gomella et al., 2020). For patients in the 3- to 12-month and greater-than-5-kg age and weight range, 20 cm^2 of intact skin is coated with 2 grams of EMLA cream and wrapped in an occlusive dressing for 4 hours prior to the procedure (Gomella et al., 2020).

Clinical-Monitoring Pearls

Clinicians should avoid massaging EMLA cream into the skin or applying repeat doses. Use of EMLA cream is contraindicated on mucous membranes, in eyes, in patients with methemoglobinemia, and among newborns less than 37 weeks' gestation or of low birth weight (AAP Task Force on Circumcision, 2012; Gomella et al., 2020). When used as a single analgesic intervention, EMLA topical cream is associated with higher pain scores, thereby making its use as an adjunctive pharmacotherapy most ideal (Sharara-Chami et al., 2017).

24% Oral Sucrose

A Cochrane review found that compared to water, oral sucrose provided via pacifier 2 minutes prior to the procedure was more effective in reducing the length of crying time associated with circumcision (Stevens et al., 2016). Although sucrose has been shown to provide behavioral comfort, it lacks an analgesic effect and is subsequently not recommended as a single intervention for reducing circumcision discomfort (Rossi et al., 2021).

Mechanism of Action

The mechanism of action for sucrose is not well understood, but potentially includes endogenous opioid system stimulation using taste receptors on the tongue (Thakkar et al., 2016).

Dosing Recommendations

A lack of consensus in the literature remains regarding an ideal volume of oral sucrose to provide prior to painful procedures. Sucrose should be placed directly on the tongue (one drop at a time) with a pacifier offered thereafter to infants who are able to suckle. Alternatively, a pacifier can be dipped in sucrose (approximately 0.2 mL) and offered to the infant. Maximal effect occurs after 2 minutes, with a duration of approximately 5 to 10 minutes (Lefrak et al., 2006, Thakkar et al., 2016). Repeat as needed.

Clinical-Monitoring Pearls

Clinicians should consider tandem administration with EMLA cream and injectable lidocaine to maximize analgesic effect throughout the invasive procedure. Additional sucrose may be provided 2 minutes into the procedure (Stevens et al., 2016). Appropriate use of a neonatal pain scale is indicated to appraise the efficacy of therapy and determine readiness for the invasive procedure.

Acetaminophen (Paracetamol)

Acetaminophen is an antipyretic and nonopioid analgesic commonly used to treat mild to moderate pain. Acetaminophen is a systemic analgesic and is recommended by the AAP for use with procedures such as circumcision; however, the three systematic reviews published between 2004 and 2019 concluded that a reduction in pain was not proven (AAP Task Force on Circumcision, 2012; Anand et al., 2005; Brady-Freyer et al., 2004; Ohlsson & Shah, 2020).

Mechanism of Action/Pharmacokinetic Principles

Acetaminophen exerts an analgesic effect during and after circumcision through some combination of inhibition of cyclooxygenase (COX) enzymes, and, more specifically, COX-2, to reduce prostaglandin synthesis, antagonism of central vanilloid and cannabinoid receptors, and stimulation of C-fibers in the spinal dorsal horn. These effects inhibit the transmission of pain impulses, making acetaminophen a desirable drug for mild to moderate pain relief (Marko & Dickerson, 2017). Acetaminophen is administered orally with circumcision procedures. The drug is primarily metabolized in the liver by way of sulfation and glucuronidation; premature infants less than 32 weeks' gestation, and/or infants with liver dysfunction, may require modified dosages. Acetaminophen is excreted in the urine with a half-life of 7 hours in neonates, which decreases to 4 hours in infants. The time to peak concentration with oral dosing is 10 to 60 minutes and the duration of action is approximately 4 to 6 hours (Pacifici & Allegaert, 2014). To achieve the maximum therapeutic effect, these data should be considered when timing the administration of acetaminophen prior to circumcision.

Dosing Recommendations

Oral dosing for prevention and treatment of circumcision pain includes a single 20- to 25-mg/kg loading dose, followed by a 12- to 15-mg/kg maintenance dose, every 6 hours (>37 weeks' gestational age), every 8 hours (32–36 6/7 weeks' gestational age), or every 12 hours (<32 weeks' gestational age; Marko & Dickerson, 2017). Rectal dosing of acetaminophen should be reserved for infants in whom enteral intake is contraindicated secondary to erratic absorption. As such, rectal dosing is not indicated for routine circumcision.

Clinical-Monitoring Pearls

Although uncommon, adverse effects include thrombocytopenia, leukopenia, and neutropenia (Marko & Dickerson, 2017). Appropriate use of a neonatal pain scale is indicated to appraise the efficacy of therapy and determine readiness for discontinuation. Clinical-monitoring pearls associated with extended use of acetaminophen are discussed in Chapter 11, "Analgesia and Sedation."

HIV

From 2014 to 2018, new diagnoses of HIV among children in the United States declined (CDC, n.d.-a). Of the 645 children younger than 13 years of age who received a diagnosis of HIV, 31% received the diagnosis within the first 6 months of life (CDC, n.d.-a). Although there is a lack of consensus regarding the number of HIV-infected individuals who give birth in the United States, experts estimate that 5,000 HIV-infected individuals give birth every year (Nesheim et al., 2019). The current goal in the United States is to decrease the incidence of perinatal HIV transmission to less than 1% (Neshiem et al., 2019). Among untreated HIV-positive women in the United States, perinatal transmission occurs in approximately 25% of infants (Kimberlin et al., 2021).

HISTORIC CONTEXT: SEMINAL AND OTHER NOTEWORTHY STUDIES

A landmark study in the 1990s discovered that in the absence of breastfeeding, perinatal transmission of HIV was decreased from 26% to 8% when zidovudine (ZDV) was administered during the ante-, intra-, and postpartum periods (Connor et al., 1994). Studies from the early 2000s worked to refine the practice of prophylactic antiretroviral therapy (ART) during the ante-, intra-, and postpartum periods, with a goal of adequate maternal viral suppression (Nesheim et al., 2019). The goals of ART for newborns are to suppress viral replication to a nondetectable level (if infected), preserve function of the immune system, and prevent clinical disease (Siberry, 2014).

CURRENT TREATMENT RECOMMENDATIONS (NATIONAL GUIDELINES)

The risk of perinatal transmission of HIV can be reduced to less than 2% if ART is initiated (Siberry, 2014) in accordance with the current recommendations by the U.S. Department of Health and Human Services Panel on Treatment of HIV Infection During Pregnancy and Prevention of Perinatal Transmission (DHHS Panel; 2023). However, there are a number of determinants of health, ethnic, and socioeconomic factors that influence barriers to successful adherence to the DHHS Panel's recommendations. These factors include the establishment of timely prenatal care and screenings, poor maternal ART adherence, and a lack of centralized electronic health records.

The DHHS Panel's recommendations were developed based on peer-reviewed evidence regarding the safety and efficacy of ART and are evaluated monthly (Panel, 2023). In accordance with the DHHS Panel's recommendations, if a maternal HIV RNA level of less than 1,000 copies per mL of serum near the time of delivery is not achieved using ART, a cesarean section delivery is strongly encouraged (Panel, 2023).

In the United States, breastfeeding is strongly discouraged among HIV-infected lactating parents (HIVLP). The most significant rationale for discouraging an HIVLP from breastfeeding is the known 5% residual transmission risk via breast milk, even among women who are compliant with ART therapy (Hale, 2019; Panel, 2023; Siberry, 2014). Additional rationales include access to safe and affordable alternative feeding options (e.g., donor breast milk, commercial formula), and a reported increase in risk for drug resistance to ART medications secondary to subtherapeutic exposure in breast milk (Panel, 2023). Safety data related to the transfer of ART medications in the breast milk are limited. The reported relative infant dose (RID) of zidovudine (0.01%–0.36%), lamivudine (0.49%–6.4%), and nevirapine (4.8%–17.84%) is low, yet all drugs are classified as "L5" (limited data—hazardous if maternal HIV infection) due to the risk for residual transmission (Hale, 2019). In the case of HIVLPs who live in the United States and choose to breastfeed despite evidence-based recommendations against it, clinicians should refer to the DHHS Panel's guidelines for counsel regarding risk–benefit ratio and management of the couplet for best patient outcomes (Panel, 2023). In contrast, breastfeeding is often necessary in resource-poor countries due to the lack of availability of commercial formulas; therefore, clinicians in these countries must exhaust all efforts to encourage postdischarge ART compliance for the mother–infant dyad.

Zidovudine (Retrovir)

ZDV is the backbone of neonatal ART. ZDV, a nucleoside reverse transcriptase inhibitor (NRTI), is a thymidine analogue that selectively inhibits HIV reverse transcriptase.

Mechanism of Action/Pharmacokinetic Principles

During reverse transcription, ZDV inhibits HIV replication by interrupting the viral DNA chain (DrugBank Online, 2023d). Readers are referred to Chapter 4, "Neonatal Pharmacogenetics and Pharmacogenomics," for additional discussion of the translation of RNA to DNA.

ZDV undergoes extensive first-pass hepatic glucuronidation; clearance is decreased among infants with impaired hepatic function. The immaturity of hepatic function accounts for higher oral bioavailability in more immature patients. However, incomplete enteral bioavailability accounts for differences in enteral and IV dosing. In addition, hepatic metabolism and renal elimination explain lower weight-based doses in premature neonates compared to term neonates and the requirement to increase the weight-based dose at specific postnatal ages as the baby matures. ZDV is excreted in the urine, with a half-life of 3 and 6 hours in full-term and premature neonates, respectively. The time to peak concentration with oral dosing is 30 to 90 minutes (ViiV Healthcare, 2021).

Dosing Recommendations

The initiation of ZDV for newborns at high risk for perinatal HIV transmission should begin as close to birth as possible, no later than 6 to 12 hours of life, and continue generally for 4 to 6 weeks (Table 7.2; Panel, 2023; Siberry, 2014). For drug and dosing recommendations, providers should refer to the most recent DHHS Panel's recommendations (https://clinicalinfo.hiv.gov/sites/default/files/guidelines/documents/perinatal-hiv/guidelines-perinatal.pdf and https://clinicalinfo.hiv.gov/en/guidelines/perinatal/management-infants-arv-hiv-exposure-infection). Consultation with a pediatric infectious disease specialist is recommended for antepartum counseling and planning and postpartum treatment and follow-up.

Clinical-Monitoring Pearls

Myelosuppression is the primary adverse effect of ART therapy; clinicians commonly obtain a baseline complete blood count and differential prior to starting therapy and monitor throughout therapy (complete details available in the DHHS Panel's guidelines). Other adverse effects that could manifest in infants up to 6 weeks of age include fatigue, weakness, respiratory distress, emesis, loss of appetite, diarrhea, dark-colored urine, acholic stools, or jaundice (Taketomo, 2023).

Given that therapy extends beyond discharge of the newborn, parents or guardians must be educated on the adverse effects associated with ZDV therapy and the importance of strict compliance with the dosing regimen. This teaching should occur prior to discharge and with each outpatient primary care appointment. Maintaining 100% patient (or parent) compliance with administering an oral medication regimen as prescribed is one of the most difficult aspects of outpatient medical management; poor compliance threatens the efficacy of therapy. Neonatal clinicians who practice in primary care settings should be aware that ZDV prophylaxis among HIV-exposed newborns

TABLE 7.2 Antiretroviral Therapy Management for Newborns

LEVEL OF TRANSMISSION RISK	RISK DESCRIPTION	MEDICATION	DOSING PER GESTATIONAL AGE AT BIRTH AND WEEKS OF AGE	
Low	• Maternal HIV+ • Adheres to antepartum ART • Subsequent viral suppression to <50 copies/mL	ZDV • Note: For newborns who are unable to tolerate PO ZDV, the IV dose is 75% of PO dose, given BID	≥35 weeks' GA at birth	• Birth to 4 weeks: 4 mg/kg/dose PO BID • Simplified weight-based dosing for newborn aged ≥35 weeks' gestation from birth to 4 weeks (volume based on ZDV 10 mg/mL oral syrup): ◦ 2 to <3 kg: 1 mL PO BID ◦ 3 to <4 kg: 1.5 mL PO BID ◦ 4 to <5 kg: 2 mL PO BID
			≥30 to <35 weeks' GA at birth	• Birth to 2 weeks: 2 mg/kg/dose PO BID • Age 2 to 6 weeks: 3 mg/kg/dose PO BID
			<30 weeks' GA at birth	• Birth to 4 weeks: 2 mg/kg/dose PO BID • Age 4 to 6 weeks: 3 mg/kg/dose PO BID
		3TC	Not recommended	
		NVP	Not recommended	
		RAL	Not recommended	
High	• Maternal acute/primary HIV+ • Nonadherence with or did not receive antepartum or intrapartum ART • Maternal receipt of only intrapartum ART • Adherence with ante/intrapartum ART without subsequent viral suppression to <50 copies/mL	ZDV	≥35 weeks' GA at birth	• Birth to 6 weeks: 4 mg/kg/dose PO BID; or • Simplified weight-based dosing for newborn aged ≥35 weeks' gestation from birth to 6 weeks (volume based on ZDV 10 mg/mlL oral syrup): ◦ 2 to <3 kg: 1 mL PO BID ◦ 3 to <4 kg: 1.5 mL PO BID ◦ 4 to <5 kg: 2 mL PO BID
			≥30 to <35 weeks' GA at birth	• Birth to 2 weeks: 2 mg/kg/dose PO BID • Age 2 to 6 weeks: 3 mg/kg/dose PO BID
			<30 weeks' GA at birth	• Birth to 4 weeks: 2 mg/kg/dose PO BID • Age 4 to 6 weeks: 3 mg/kg/dose PO BID

(*continued*)

TABLE 7.2 Antiretroviral Therapy Management for Newborns (*continued*)

LEVEL OF TRANSMISSION RISK	RISK DESCRIPTION	MEDICATION	DOSING PER GESTATIONAL AGE AT BIRTH AND WEEKS OF AGE		
High (*continued*)		3TC	≥32 weeks' GA at birth	• Birth to 4 weeks: 2 mg/kg/dose PO BID • >4 weeks: 4 mg/kg/dose PO BID	
		NVP	≥37 weeks' GA at birth	Birth to 4 weeks: 6 mg/kg/dose PO BID	
			≥34 to <37 weeks' GA at birth	Birth to 1 week: 4 mg/kg/dose PO BID	
				Age 1 to 4 weeks: 6 mg/kg/dose PO BID	
		RAL (10 mg/mL suspension)	≥37 weeks' GA at birth and weighing ≥2 kg	Birth to 1 week:	2 to <3 kg: 0.4 mL (4 mg) PO QD
					3 to <4 kg: 0.5 mL (5 mg) PO QD
					4 to <5 kg: 0.7 mL (7 mg) PO QD
				1 to 4 weeks:	2 to <3 kg: 0.8 mL (8 mg) PO BID
					3 to <4 kg: 1 mL (10 mg) PO BID
					4 to <5 kg: 1.5 mL (15 mg) PO BID
				4 to 6 weeks:	3 to <4 kg: 2.5 mL (25 mg) PO BID
					4 to <6 kg: 3 mL (30 mg) PO BID
					6 to <8 kg: 4 mL (40 mg) PO BID
Presumed HIV-exposed newborn	• Unconfirmed maternal HIV status with one positive HIV test at delivery or postpartum • Newborn with positive HIV antibody test	• Triple-drug ART (ZDV, 3TC, NVP [or RAL]) per recommendations for high risk of transmission • Discontinue ART if maternal HIV testing is reported as negative			
HIV-positive newborn	• Positive HIV NAT	• Triple-drug ART (ZDV, 3TC, NVP [or RAL]) per recommendations for high risk for transmission			

ART, antiretroviral therapy; BID, twice daily; GA, gestational age; IV, intravenous; NAT, nucleic acid test; NVP, nevirapine; PO, by mouth; QD, every day; RAL, raltegravir; 3TC, lamivudine; ZDV, zidovudine.

Sources: From Panel on Treatment of HIV During Pregnancy and Prevention of Perinatal Transmission. (2023, January 31). *Recommendations for the use of antiretroviral drugs during pregnancy and interventions to reduce perinatal HIV transmission in the United States. U.S. Department of Health and Human Services*. https://clinicalinfo.hiv.gov/en/guidelines/perinatal/management-infants-arv-hiv-exposure-infection?view=full; Siberry, G. (2014). Preventing and managing HIV infection in infants, children and adolescents in the United States. *Pediatrics in Review, 35*(7), 268–286. https://doi.org/10.1542/pir.35-7-268

may impact virologic assays. If the virologic assay is negative in a newborn receiving ART, testing should be repeated 2 to 6 weeks after prophylaxis is completed (Panel, 2023). In addition, some forms of ZDV contain high levels of metabolites of benzyl alcohol (sodium benzoate or benzoic acid); avoid and/or use caution with these formulations of ZDV (ViiV Healthcare, 2021).

Lamivudine

Mechanism of Action/Pharmacokinetic Principles

By way of HIV reverse transcriptase enzyme inhibition, lamivudine (3TC) is a synthetic nucleoside analogue that is incorporated into viral DNA, resulting in replication chain termination (DrugBank Online, 2023a). The drug is primarily metabolized in the liver and excreted by the renal system; clearance is reduced in infants with renal impairment (Taketomo, 2023). 3TC has a half-life of approximately 2 hours in children aged 4 months to 14 years; pharmacokinetic data specific to newborns are limited or unavailable (Taketomo, 2023).

Dosing Recommendations

The initiation of 3TC for newborns at high risk for perinatal HIV transmission should begin as close to birth as possible, no later than 6 to 12 hours of life, and continue generally for 4 to 6 weeks (Table 7.2; Panel, 2023; Siberry, 2014). For drug and dosing recommendations, providers should refer to the most recent DHHS Panel's recommendations (https://clinicalinfo.hiv.gov/sites/default/files/guidelines/documents/perinatal-hiv/guidelines-perinatal.pdf and https://clinicalinfo.hiv.gov/en/guidelines/perinatal/management-infants-arv-hiv-exposure-infection). Consultation with a pediatric infectious disease specialist is recommended for antepartum counseling and planning and postpartum treatment and follow-up.

Clinical-Monitoring Pearls

Breastfeeding is contraindicated among HIV-infected mothers living in the United States, as this greatly reduces the risk for residual transmission (5%) via breast milk (Hale, 2019; Siberry, 2014). Adverse effects of 3TC are similar to those of ZDV. Parental education about medication adherence is paramount (see previous clinical pearls for ZDV).

Nevirapine

Mechanism of Action/Pharmacokinetic Principles

In contrast to nucleoside analogues, such as ZDV and 3TC, nevirapine (NVP) is a non-nucleoside reverse transcriptase inhibitor that blocks HIV type 1 replication (DrugBank Online, 2023c). NVP is excreted in the urine, extensively metabolized in the liver, and is metabolized more quickly in children than in adults (Taketomo, 2023). NVP has a half-life of 30 to 44 hours in term infants and 59 hours in premature infants (Mirochnick et al., 2008).

Dosing Recommendations

The initiation of NVP for newborns at high risk for perinatal HIV transmission should begin as close to birth as possible, no later than 6 to 12 hours of life, and continue generally for 4 to 6 weeks (Table 7.2; Panel, 2023; Siberry, 2014). For drug and dosing recommendations, providers should refer to the most recent DHHS Panel's recommendations (https://clinicalinfo.hiv.gov/sites/default/files/guidelines/documents/perinatal-hiv/guidelines-perinatal.pdf and https://clinicalinfo.hiv.gov/en/guidelines/perinatal/management-infants-arv-hiv-exposure-infection). Consultation with a pediatric infectious disease specialist is recommended for antepartum counseling and planning and postpartum treatment and follow-up.

Clinical-Monitoring Pearls

Oral NVP therapy can be administered before, during, or after feedings. NVP exhibits synergy with other antiretrovirals; monotherapy may increase the risk for viral resistance (DrugBank Online, 2023c). Baseline alanine transaminase (ALT), aspartate aminotransferase (AST), and bilirubin levels should be obtained prior to the initiation of therapy and repeated at regular intervals (particularly during the first 6 weeks of treatment) or with a dosage escalation (Taketomo, 2023). The most common adverse reactions to NVP are rash and hyperbilirubinemia (DrugBank Online, 2023c).

Initiation and Cessation of Antiretroviral Therapy

As discussed earlier in this chapter, the initiation of ART for newborns at high risk for perinatal HIV transmission should begin as close to birth as possible, no later than 6 to 12 hours of life, and continue generally for 4 to 6 weeks (Table 7.2; Panel, 2023; Siberry, 2014). Maintaining nonjudgmental attitudes, developing trust, educating families, and identifying mutual treatment goals prior to initiating ART are critical components of medication adherence and viral suppression (Panel, 2023). Mobile phone technologies may assist in supporting adherence to ART medications.

CONCLUSIONS

Our understanding of pharmacotherapies commonly prescribed to well-appearing newborns has certainly evolved over the years. Early inquiries prompted decades of research and the development of policies and procedures that successfully prevent or treat the needs of newborns. Neonatal APRNs are encouraged to share these data with orientees and other junior staff, to expand awareness and clinical acumen. New data are on the horizon, thanks to the Best Pharmaceuticals for Children Act and Pediatric Drug Research Equity Act (Christensen, 2012). This legislation helps ensure that drug studies include neonates and infants, and in doing so addresses gaps in drug labeling and FDA approval.

LEARNING TOOLS AND RESOURCES

Advice From the Authors

Tiffany Gwartney, DNP, APRN, NNP-BC

As I look back through the content in this chapter and reflect on my career as a NICU nurse and a neonatal nurse practitioner (NNP) student, a few salient points come to mind. First, it is important to know the historical background and indication for each medication, in order to be well poised to educate families regarding these practices. Fueled by research in the 1980s that was later debunked, there is an emerging conglomerate of parents who are resistant not only to vaccinations, but also to many of the common medications used in the newborn nursery. Often, a bit of education is all that is necessary to garner parental approval for these medications. Knowing which medications are critical for positive patient outcomes is paramount. Second, it is important to open this dialogue with parents. Motivational interviewing techniques can assist in facilitating a dialogue regarding positive behavior change and is emerging as a tool to address parents who are hesitant, or completely against vaccinations, and so on. In short, a dialogue that is supported by motivational interviewing techniques may include the following points of conversation:

1. *Invite the parent to share information they already know about the topic.*
2. *Provide affirmation about their knowledge.*
3. *Ascertain permission to provide the parent with additional information.*
4. *Inquire about the integration of the additional information into the parents' previous constructs or habits.*

Third, some of the medications discussed in this chapter have been in practice for decades without much change in terms of how, when, where, and why they are used. Others, such as the medications for HIV, are ever changing as scientific discovery around the disease is continually evolving. Remember to flex your lifelong learner muscles and maintain your knowledge and understanding of these medications in particular.

Jane Ierardi, MD, MBA, FAAP, CPE

Generally speaking, the newborn nursery offers an incredible opportunity to refine skills related to recognizing clinical findings that are normal in order to be able to recognize clinical findings that are not. This in no way means that the newborn nursery is not full of challenges, but rather indicates that this patient population is unique compared to the neonatal intensive care population and requires a certain skill set to manage it properly.

Discussion Prompts

1. Discuss current information regarding the prevention of hemorrhagic disease of the newborn in preterm and term infants and develop a guide to counseling parents who refuse parenteral vitamin K.
2. Consider the following recommendation by the AAP (2022): "Pediatricians and other health care providers must be aware of the benefits of vitamin K administration as well as the risks of refusal and convey this information to the infant's caregivers." Discuss the essential information that must be presented to parents in order to ensure a complete discussion of risks of refusal and benefits of vitamin K administration.
3. Discuss the risks associated with poor adherence with ART and strategies that can be incorporated into discharge teaching to optimize the likelihood for parental compliance.

Mind Map

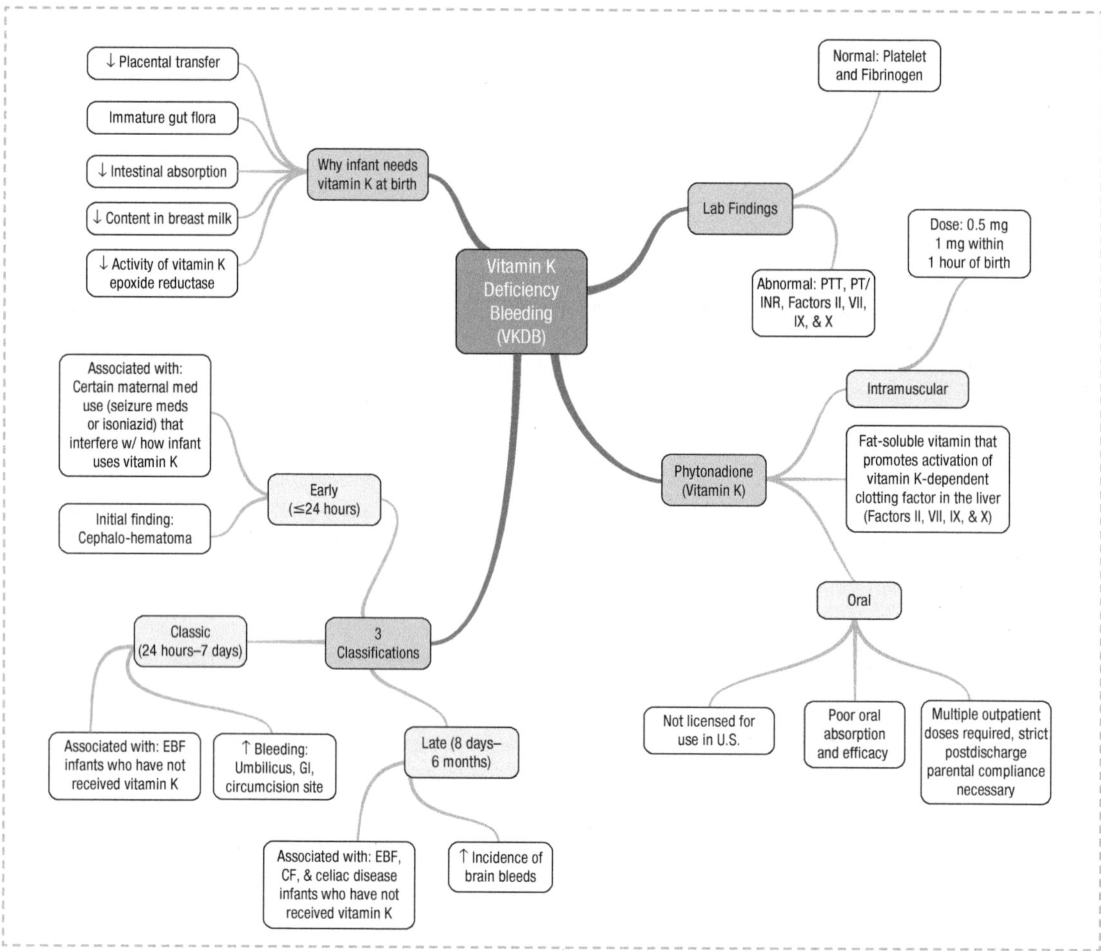

Note: This mind map reflects the design team's interpretation of a portion of one or more concepts addressed in this chapter. Readers should regard the mind maps woven throughout this textbook as examples of multisensory study tools that can be developed to encourage conceptual understanding. Readers are encouraged to develop their own unique mind maps in consultation with academic faculty or clinical preceptors.
CF, cystic fibrosis; EBF, exclusively breastfed; GI, gastrointestinal; INR, international normalized ratio; PT, prothrombin time; PTT, partial thromboplastin time.
Design credit: Briana Bitterman, BSN, RNC-NIC, and Rielee Welch, MSN, APRN, NNP, East Carolina University neonatal nurse practitioner program.

REFERENCES

References for this chapter are online and available at https://connect.springerpub.com/content/book/978-0-8261-5884-0/part/partI/toc-part/ch7.

chapter 8

Vaccines and Schedules

Amy P. Holmes

LEARNING OBJECTIVES

After completing this chapter, the reader should be able to:

- Explain the difference between active and passive immunity.
- Describe different types of vaccinations (e.g., live vs. inactivated, conjugated vs. polysaccharide).
- Discuss considerations related to vaccine spacing and timing.
- Discuss common adverse reactions related to vaccine use in neonates (and which are myths).

INTRODUCTION

Infectious diseases present a significant risk to mortality across the life span. The ability to prevent and treat infections has evolved throughout human history. Chinese literature dating back to the 11th century describes the use of insufflated smallpox scabs to immunize against the variola virus (Plotkin, 2005). Edward Jenner used the weaker cowpox virus to develop the first vaccination against smallpox. In fact, the word *vaccination* derives from the Latin word for cowpox, *vaccinia* (Riedel, 2005). Several decades after Jenner, Pasteur discovered that weakened or attenuated organisms stimulated immunity without causing infection (Plotkin, 2005). Vaccine technology has continued to develop over the centuries since Jenner's first vaccinations, with vaccines now available for prevention of 26 different human pathogens (Geoghegan et al., 2020). Development of a smallpox vaccine eventually led to complete eradication of the disease. Global eradication of other diseases is a realistic goal that some of you may see met in your lifetime. Figure 8.1 represents a chronological view of vaccine development.

Key progress in vaccinology included the development of methods to inactivate whole bacteria, the discovery of bacterial toxins and subsequent the development of antitoxin, and the recognition of substances in the serum of immune individuals (now called *antibodies*) that could neutralize toxins or bacterial replication (Plotkin & Plotkin, 2011). The so-called Golden Age in vaccine history was launched in the mid-20th century with the advent of virus growth in cell culture. Later in that same century came breakthroughs in the conjugation of bacterial polysaccharides to proteins, as well as genetic engineering. Vaccine development is still a very active area of research, and it is noteworthy that the coronavirus vaccines approved as recently as 2021 were the first to use mRNA vaccine technology in a licensed vaccine.

Vaccination hesitancy related to fear of adverse effects, autonomous decision-making, or religious beliefs has existed since the use of the first vaccine, limiting their full uptake (Conis, 2019). To eradicate vaccine-preventable diseases, legislation has been passed through the years to mandate the use of various vaccines, usually in conjunction with school attendance. In 1995, the Advisory

FIGURE 8.1 A timeline of vaccine development.

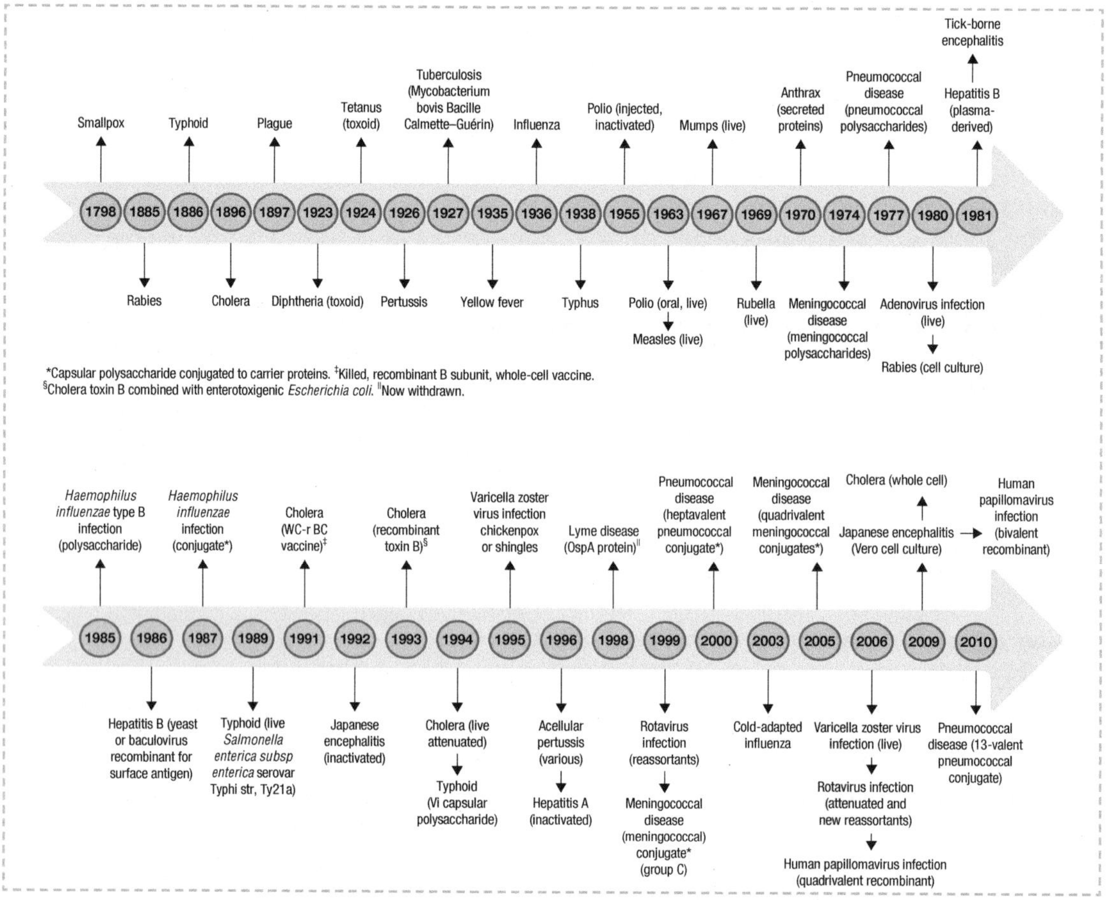

Tick-borne encephalitis

Smallpox | Typhoid | Plague | Tetanus (toxoid) | Tuberculosis (Mycobacterium bovis Bacille Calmette–Guérin) | Influenza | Polio (injected, inactivated) | Mumps (live) | Anthrax (secreted proteins) | Pneumococcal disease (pneumococcal polysaccharides) | Hepatitis B (plasma-derived)

1798 1885 1886 1896 1897 1923 1924 1926 1927 1935 1936 1938 1955 1963 1967 1969 1970 1974 1977 1980 1981

Rabies | Cholera | Diphtheria (toxoid) | Pertussis | Yellow fever | Typhus | Polio (oral, live) | Measles (live) | Rubella (live) | Meningococcal disease (meningococcal polysaccharides) | Adenovirus infection (live) | Rabies (cell culture)

*Capsular polysaccharide conjugated to carrier proteins. ‡Killed, recombinant B subunit, whole-cell vaccine.
§Cholera toxin B combined with enterotoxigenic *Escherichia coli*. ||Now withdrawn.

Haemophilus influenzae type B infection (polysaccharide) | *Haemophilus influenzae* infection (conjugate*) | Cholera (WC-r BC vaccine)‡ | Cholera (recombinant toxin B)§ | Varicella zoster virus infection chickenpox or shingles | Lyme disease (OspA protein)|| | Pneumococcal disease (heptavalent pneumococcal conjugate*) | Meningococcal disease (quadrivalent meningococcal conjugates*) | Cholera (whole cell) | Japanese encephalitis (Vero cell culture) | Human papillomavirus infection (bivalent recombinant)

1985 1986 1987 1989 1991 1992 1993 1994 1995 1996 1998 1999 2000 2003 2005 2006 2009 2010

Hepatitis B (yeast or baculovirus recombinant for surface antigen) | Typhoid (live *Salmonella enterica subsp enterica* serovar Typhi str, Ty21a) | Japanese encephalitis (inactivated) | Cholera (live attenuated) | Typhoid (Vi capsular polysaccharide) | Acellular pertussis (various) | Hepatitis A (inactivated) | Rotavirus infection (reassortants) | Meningococcal disease (meningococcal) conjugate* (group C) | Cold-adapted influenza | Varicella zoster virus infection (live) | Rotavirus infection (attenuated and new reassortants) | Human papillomavirus infection (quadrivalent recombinant) | Pneumococcal disease (13-valent pneumococcal conjugate)

Source: From Plotkin, S.A., & Plotkin, S. L. (2011). The development of vaccines: How the past led to the future. *Nature Reviews. Microbiology,* 9(12), 889–893. https://doi.org/10.1038/nrmicro2668.

Committee on Immunization Practices (ACIP), the American Academy of Pediatrics (AAP), and the American Academy of Family Physicians (AAFP) issued the first vaccine schedule (see The Development of the Immunization Schedule, 2021). This schedule is updated annually and guides vaccination practice nationally.

In this chapter, we explore basic immunology principles and vaccine pharmacology. We also take a look at the specific vaccines typically used in the NICU. Tables have been created for quick reference to organize vaccines by type as well as to help differentiate among some very similar sounding names. Questions at the end of the chapter have been formulated to prompt discussion and consideration of scenarios that you may face in clinical practice.

BASIC IMMUNOLOGY PRINCIPLES

The immune system allows us to differentiate between "self" and "nonself," or foreign, cells. This differentiation allows the immune system to attack invading organisms while preserving self. Once the immune system has been introduced to a foreign substance, it recognizes it more readily and can mount a more rapid and efficient response. Immunity may be cellular or humoral in nature (Sturgill, 2008). Cellular immunity is marked by activities of cells such as helper T lymphocytes, cytotoxic T lymphocytes, memory T-cell lymphocytes, suppressor T lymphocytes, and B lymphocytes. Antibody molecules confer humoral immunity.

Immunity developed in response to an active infection is considered *natural immunity*. Immunity developed in response to disease or vaccination is considered *active immunity*. When antibodies are passed from one person to the next, such as the placental transfer of antibodies from mother to fetus, passage of antibodies to infants through maternal milk, or the administration of medications such as palivizumab or intravenous immune globulin, it is considered *passive immunity*. Passive immunity is shorter lived than active immunity and has no memory. It is important to note that this passive immunity occurs later in pregnancy, peaking around 34 weeks of gestation (Healy et al., 2020). Transplacental transport of antibodies from mother to fetus can be influenced by conditions such as infections or malnutrition (Leuridan & Van Damme, 2007). In conjunction with the ability of the neonate's immune system to respond to a vaccine, determining the best time to initiate vaccination involves a delicate balance between waning of antibodies that have been passed from mother to child and susceptibility or risk of the specific pathogen.

A resurgence of pertussis, commonly known as *whooping cough*, in recent years has led to much study of the limits of maternal antibody protection of the newborn for this disease. Maternal antibodies to pertussis pass readily across the placenta and have half-lives of roughly 30 days: pertussis-specific immunoglobulin G (IgG) = 29.4 days (95% CI: 27.3–31.7); filamentous hemagglutinin = 29.8 days (95% CI: 27.7–32.2); pertactin = 31.2 days (95% CI: 28.9–33.7); and fimbrial proteins = 35.8 days (95% CI: 30.1–44.3; Healy et al., 2020). In order to optimize the amount of antibodies present at 34 weeks of gestation when placental transfer is at its peak, the ACIP and the Centers for Disease Control and Prevention (CDC) recommend a tetanus, diphtheria, and acellular pertussis (Tdap) booster during each pregnancy between 27 and 36 weeks of gestation, as well as to other caregivers who will have close contact with the infant (CDC, 2013). This practice of providing protection to the neonate by immunizing others is referred to as *cocooning*. The goal is to ensure a window of protection until vaccination begins at around 6 weeks of life.

Conversely to pertussis, for optimal vaccine response to the measles vaccine, immunization should occur when maternal antibodies can no longer interfere with vaccine response but before the infant is susceptible to disease (Leuridan & Van Damme, 2007). There are regional variations in the occurrence of this window of optimization. In the United States, it has been determined that the first dose of measles vaccine should be administered at age 12 to 15 months, whereas in developing countries age 9 months is the optimal time to vaccinate against measles based on waning of antibodies.

When the prevalence of immunity to a specific infectious disease reaches a certain point (this varies by disease), the number of active cases of the disease drops to nearly zero. This low incidence of cases prevents even those who do not have immunity from being affected by the disease. This is known as *herd immunity* (Figure 8.2).

GENERAL VACCINE PHARMACOLOGY

A *vaccine* is defined as "a biological product that can be used to safely induce an immune response that confers protection against infection and/or disease on subsequent exposure to a pathogen" (Pollard & Bijker, 2021, p. 83). Vaccines usually work by introducing some part of an organism to the immune system in order to stimulate a cellular and/or a humoral response. Various vaccine technologies exist and are described individually in the following text and illustrated in Figure 8.3.

Live Vaccines

Live attenuated vaccines include a form of the virus that is able to replicate but is weakened and unable to replicate rapidly enough to cause disease. Slow replication of the weakened virus allows for the development of subclinical disease and subsequent stimulation of both humoral and cell-mediated immune responses.

With the exception of the rotavirus vaccine, live vaccines are not indicated during the first year of life. Passive immunity, or the antibodies passed from mother to child through the placenta, can eliminate the live attenuated virus before the infant's immune system is able to mount an immune response. For this reason, any live attenuated vaccine administered prior to the first birthday will need to be repeated as part of the recommended vaccination series. Table 8.1 summarizes live virus vaccines that may be given in the NICU.

FIGURE 8.2 Herd immunity.

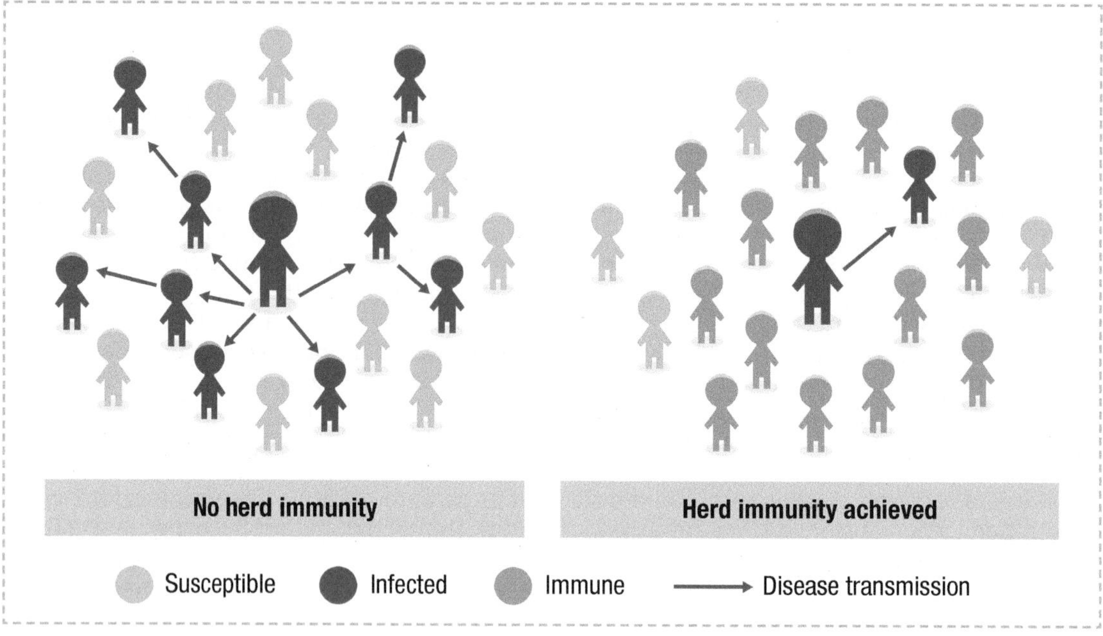

Source: From U.S. Government Accountability Office. *Science and tech spotlight: Herd immunity for COVID-19*. https://www.gao.gov/products/gao-20-646sp.

FIGURE 8.3 Types of vaccines.

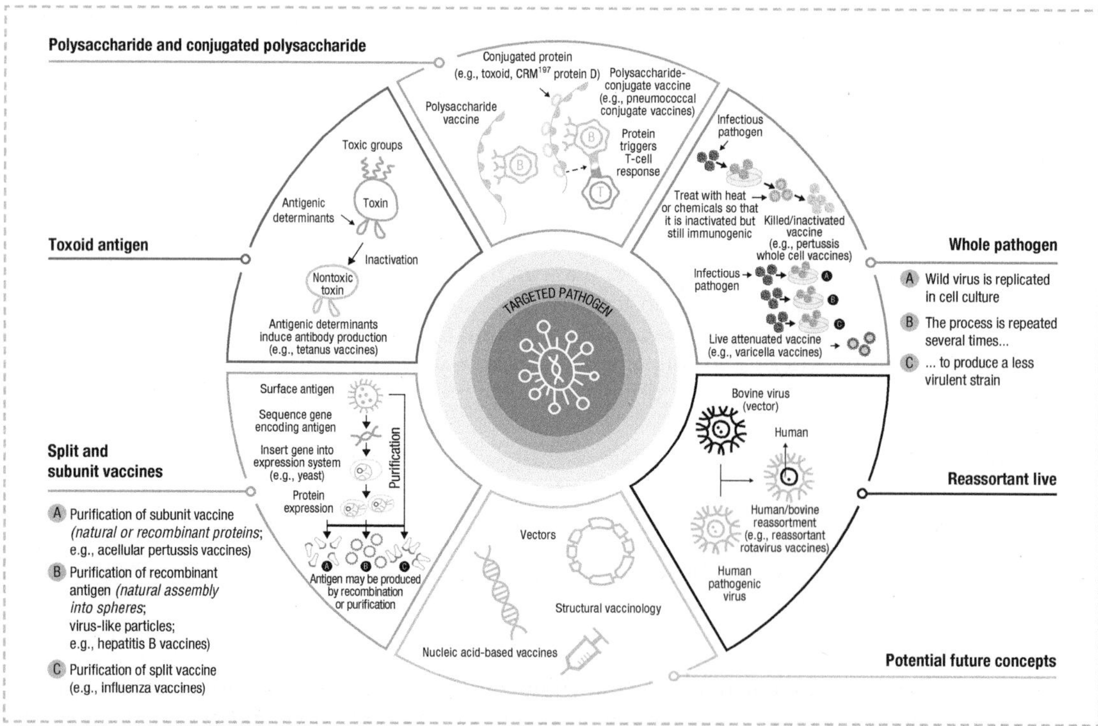

Source: From Vetter, V., Denizer, G., Friedland, L. R., Krishan, J., & Shapiro, M. (2018). Understanding modern-day vaccines: What you need to know. *Annals of Medicine, 50*(2), 110–120. https://doi.org/10.1080/07853890.2017.1407035.

TABLE 8.1 Live Virus Vaccines Given in the NICU

VACCINE (TRADE NAME)	COMPONENT	COMMENT OR CONSIDERATION
Rotarix®	One strain (type G1PA[8]) live attenuated human strain	Two-dose oral vaccine Dose = 1–1.5 mL (volume may be a consideration in some infants) Dose and buffered diluent must be mixed prior to administration; comes in oral syringe
RotaTeq®	Five reassortant strains developed from human and bovine strains	Three-dose oral vaccine Dose = 2 mL (volume may be a consideration in some infants)

Source: From GlaxoSmithKline Biologicals. (2019). *Rotarix: Highlights of prescribing information.* Author; Merck & Co., Inc. (2020b). *RotaTeq: Highlights of prescribing information.* Author.

Inactivated Vaccines

Inactivated (or "killed") vaccines include some piece of the virus or bacteria that cannot replicate. The immune reaction to inactivated vaccines is not as robust as the reaction to live vaccines and often requires more doses to gain the desired response. Inactivated vaccines can be further divided into polysaccharide, conjugate, and recombinant vaccines.

Several pathogenic bacteria, such as *Streptococcus pneumoniae* and *Haemophilus influenzae* type B, are protected by capsules (Vetter et al., 2018). These capsules are targets for antibodies; therefore, using the polysaccharides present in the capsule is the premise of polysaccharide vaccines. Unfortunately, these vaccines are poorly immunogenic and the protection they provide is short-lived. Polysaccharide vaccines are recognized by B cells and activate them directly without assistance of T cells, making them largely ineffective in children younger than 2 years. For this reason, polysaccharide vaccines are not used in the NICU, rather conjugate vaccines are used to immunize against *S. pneumoniae* and *H. influenzae* type B.

Conjugate vaccines were created to overcome the problem of B-cell-dependent immunogenicity of polysaccharide vaccination that is ineffective in children under 2 years of age. By conjugating a polysaccharide to a protein (frequently a toxoid), it transforms into a T-cell-dependent antigen and allows for the production of immune globulin and the development of immunologic memory (Snitkoff, 2008).

Recombinant DNA technology has been used to develop vaccines by using yeast or bacteria cells as hosts that replicate the desired antigen particles. The most successful example of recombinant technology is expression of hepatitis B surface antigen by *Saccharomyces cerevisiae* yeast for use in hepatitis B vaccine (Snitkoff, 2008). Table 8.2 summarizes inactivated vaccines commonly administered in the NICU.

Toxoids

Bacteria, such as *Clostridium tetani* and *Corynebacterium diphtheriae,* cause disease—tetanus, and diphtheria, respectively—through the toxins they produce. Toxoid vaccines were developed to provide protection from disease caused by these toxins. Toxoids are structurally similar to their toxin counterparts but are rendered inactive through chemical or thermal manipulation. Administration of the toxoid stimulates creation of neutralizing antibodies against the toxin (Snitkoff, 2008). Toxoids have good, although short-lived, immunogenicity; therefore, multiple doses over the span of a lifetime are necessary to confer and sustain immunity (Vetter et al., 2018). Toxoids administered in the NICU include tetanus toxoid and diphtheria toxoid and are usually given in combination with the acellular pertussis vaccine (DTaP).

Adjuvants

An *adjuvant* is any component whose addition enhances the activity of a vaccine. Through their ability to activate innate immune responses, adjuvants can improve the initial response to vaccines as well as improve memory response, especially in populations with typically low responses such as infants (Vetter et al., 2018). Adjuvants are defined by their activity and not by their physical or

TABLE 8.2 Inactivated Vaccines Given in the NICU

INACTIVATED VACCINE (TRADE NAME)	COMPONENT	COMMENT OR CONSIDERATION
Pneumococcal vaccine (Prevnar-13®)	13 serotypes of *Streptococcus pneumoniae*: 1, 2, 3, 4, 5, 6B, 7F, 8, 9N, 9V, 10A, 11A, 12F, 14, 15B, 17F, 18C, 19A, 19F, 20, 22F, 23F, and 33F	Uses a nontoxic variant of diphtheria toxoid as a carrier protein—does not immunize against diphtheria
Haemophilus *influenzae*, type B (Pedvax-HIB®)	*Haemophilus influenzae*, type B	Uses a meningococcal outer membrane carrier protein—does not immunize against meningococcus
Haemophilus *influenzae*, type B (ActHIB®)	*Haemophilus influenzae*, type B	Uses a tetanus toxoid carrier protein—does not immunize against tetanus
Polio	Polio virus	Is usually given in combination with DTaP
Pertussis (whooping cough)	Acellular pertussis	Is given as a component of DTaP
Influenza virus	Contains 3–4 strains of influenza A and B Changes annually	First-time immunization requires two doses 4 weeks apart
Meningococcus (Menveo®)	Covers serogroups A, C, W, and Y	Approved for use beginning at 2 months of age
Meningococcus (Menactra®)	Covers serogroups A, C, W, and Y	Approved for use beginning at 9 months of age
Hepatitis B (Engerix™-B; Recombivax HB®)	Recombinant hepatitis B	Dose volume the same for each vaccine (0.5 mL), although the amount of antigen per dose differs

DTaP, diphtheria, tetanus, acellular pertussis.
Sources: From Acosta, A. M., Moro, P. L., Hariri, S., & Tiwari, T. S. P. (2020). Diphtheria in Centers for Disease Control and Prevention. In J. Hamborsky, A. Kroger, & S. Wolfe (Eds.), *Epidemiology and prevention of vaccine-preventable diseases* (13th ed.). Public Health Foundation; Gierke, R., Wodi, A. P., & Kobayashi, M. (2021). Pneumococcal disease in Centers for Disease Control and Prevention. In J. Hamborsky, A. Kroger, & S. Wolfe (Eds.), *Epidemiology and prevention of vaccine-preventable diseases* (13th ed.). Public Health Foundation; Haber, P., & Schillie, S. (2021). Hepatitis B in Centers for Disease Control and Prevention. In J. Hamborsky, A. Kroger, & S. Wolfe (Eds.), *Epidemiology and prevention of vaccine-preventable diseases* (13th ed.). Public Health Foundation; Mbaeyi, S., Duffy, J., & McNamara, L. A. (2021). Meningococcal disease in Centers for Disease Control and Prevention. In J. Hamborsky, A. Kroger, & S. Wolfe (Eds.), *Epidemiology and prevention of vaccine-preventable diseases* (13th ed.). Public Health Foundation; Tiwari, T. S. P., Moro, P. L., & Acosta, A. M. (2020). Tetanus in Centers for Disease Control and Prevention. In J. Hamborsky, A. Kroger, & S. Wolfe (Eds.), *Epidemiology and prevention of vaccine-preventable diseases* (13th ed.). Public Health Foundation.

chemical composition. Broadly, adjuvants can be considered to work one of two ways: (a) as an immune potentiator acting directly on the immune cells to increase an immune response (e.g., liposomes, polymeric particles) or (b) as a "delivery system" working to promote the uptake of antigen into the immune cells (e.g., alum, emulsions; Brito et al., 2013). Alum-based adjuvants, including aluminum hydroxide, aluminum phosphate, and potassium aluminum sulfate, are the most widely used in currently available vaccines. Although the safety of these adjuvants is often challenged, they have been thoroughly studied and established to be not only effective, but also safe and well tolerated. The amount of aluminum salts delivered via vaccination is well within permissible safety limits. Table 8.3 lists vaccines commonly used in the NICU that contain adjuvants.

Vaccine Timing and Spacing

The ACIP sets forth the recommendations for the use of vaccines in the United States. The most up-to-date recommendations can be found on the CDC website (www.cdc.gov/vaccines). Timing for vaccine administration is based on multiple factors. First is the age-based risk of infectious disease, which creates the highest burden during the first 5 years of life (Pollard & Bijker, 2021). The organisms responsible for the most invasive diseases in childhood are targeted for the earliest vaccination. Second, initiation of vaccination with conjugate vaccines begins at 2 months of age to coincide with the development of T-cell-dependent immunogenicity and the ability to induce immune memory. Preterm infants who are medically stable should follow vaccination schedules based on postnatal age.

TABLE 8.3 Vaccines in the NICU That Contain Adjuvant(s)

VACCINE (TRADE NAME)	COMPONENT	ADJUVANT(S)
Daptacel®	DTaP	Aluminum phosphate 1.5 mg (0.33 mg aluminum)
Infanrix®	DTaP	Aluminum hydroxide (not more than 0.625 mg of aluminum/dose)
Pediarix®	DTaP/HepB/polio	Aluminum salts (not more than 0.85 mg aluminum/dose)
Pentacel®	DTaP/polio/Hib	Aluminum phosphate 1.5 mg (0.33 mg aluminum)
Vaxelis™	DTaP/polio/Hib/HepB	Aluminum salts (0.319 mg aluminum)
Engerix™-B	HepB	Aluminum hydroxide (0.25 mg aluminum)
RecombivaxHB®	HepB	Aluminum hydroxide (0.25 mg aluminum)
PedvaxHIB®	Haemophilus *influenzae*	Aluminum hydroxide (0.225 mg aluminum)
Prevnar®	Pneumococcus	Aluminum phosphate (0.125 mg aluminum)

DTaP, diphtheria, tetanus, acellular pertussis; HepB, hepatitis B; Hib, *Haemophilus influenzae* type B.
Sources: From Centers for Disease Control and Prevention. (2021b, December). *About diphtheria, tetanus, and pertussis vaccines.* https://www.cdc.gov/vaccines/vpd/dtap-tdap-td/hcp/about-vaccine.html; GlaxoSmithKline Biologicals. (2021). *Engerix-B: Highlights of prescribing information.* Author; Merck & Co., Inc. (2010). *Recombivax HB: Highlights of prescribing information.* Author; Merck & Co., Inc. (2020a). *PedvaxHIB: Highlights of prescribing information.* Author; Pfizer, Inc. (2017). *Prevnar 13: Highlights of prescribing information.* Author.

Considerations when developing a vaccination schedule also include initiation of vaccination before protection from maternal antibodies wanes. Vaccination schedules generally include several priming doses at initiation, with some vaccines requiring boosters in later years as immunity wanes. Recommendations for vaccine spacing take into consideration optimization of immune response as well as compliance (vaccine compliance is known to be better when doses are given close together). Caregivers may request alternative vaccine spacing to avoid giving multiple injections at once. Alternative schedules not only increase the risk for an important vaccine being omitted, but potentially create more stress for the infant. Ramsay and Lewis (1994) studied the stress response to one vaccination compared with two vaccinations administered concurrently and found no difference between the two groups in stress as represented by change in cortisol or by behavioral response.

VACCINES COMMONLY USED IN THE NICU

Hepatitis B

Hepatitis B virus is associated with both acute and chronic infections. As many as 90% of infants who contract hepatitis B will progress to chronic disease (Haber & Schillie, 2021). Chronic hepatitis B viral infection may lead to cirrhosis, liver failure, and hepatocellular carcinoma. In the early 1990s, the World Health Organization (WHO) targeted hepatitis B for worldwide eradication. A pillar of this initiative includes universal administration of the hepatitis B vaccine to all infants at birth to eliminate vertical transmission from mothers to their newborns. The hepatitis B vaccine is a three-dose series recombinant DNA vaccine. The CDC recommends that all infants 2 kg or greater receive the first dose of hepatitis B vaccine within the first 24 hours of life (Schillie et al., 2018). For infants less than 2 kg, the dose should be delayed until 1 month of age or prior to hospital discharge, whichever comes first, as long as the maternal hepatitis B status is negative (Table 8.4).

Streptococcus pneumoniae

At least 100 serotypes of the gram-positive bacteria *S. pneumoniae* are known to exist, although not all are pathogenic. Pneumococcal disease in children less than 2 years old primarily presents as bacteremia. It is also a significant cause of bacterial pneumonia in this age group.

TABLE 8.4 Recommendations for Administration of Birth Hepatitis B Vaccine

BIRTH WEIGHT	MATERNAL HEPATITIS B STATUS	IMMUNIZATION RECOMMENDATION
≥2 kg	Positive	Administer within 12 hours of delivery. Give concomitant HBIG 0.5 mL IM in the opposite thigh.
	Unknown	Administer vaccine within 12 hours of delivery. If the mother is determined to be positive, give HBIG within the first 7 days of life.
	Negative	Administer within 24 hours of birth.
<2 kg	Positive	Administer within 12 hours of delivery. Give concomitant HBIG 0.5 mL IM in the opposite thigh.
	Unknown	Administer within 12 hours of birth. Give concomitant HBIG 0.5 mL IM in the opposite thigh.
	Negative	Administer the first dose of vaccine at 1 month of life (if medically stable) or immediately prior to discharge, whichever is first.

HBIG, hepatitis B immune globulin; IM, intramuscular.
Source: From Schillie, S., Vellozzi, C., Reingold, A., Harris, A., Haber, P., Ward, J.W., & Nelson, N. P. (2018). Prevention of hepatitis B virus infection in the United States: Recommendations of the Advisory Committee on Immunization Practices. *Morbidity and Mortality Weekly Report. Recommendations and Reports*, *67*(No. RR-1), 1–31. https://doi.org/10.15585/mmwr.rr6701a1.

The first pneumococcal vaccine licensed for use in the United States was a 14-valent polysaccharide vaccine, followed several years later by a 23-valent polysaccharide vaccine that is still used in adults. The first conjugate pneumococcal vaccine contained seven serotypes; however, the current pneumococcal conjugate vaccine is a 13-valent vaccine (PCV13). The recommended vaccination schedule for PCV13 includes a three-dose primary series at 2, 4, and 6 months of age with one booster dose between 12 and 15 months of age.

Polio

Poliovirus was the cause of increasingly severe epidemics throughout the developed Northern Hemisphere in the early 20th century. Although 70% of polio infections in children were asymptomatic, paralytic polio was a devastating disease associated with often permanent paralysis and a mortality rate of 2% to 5% in children and 15% to 30% in adolescents (Estivariz et al., 2020). The initial polio vaccination was a live-virus vaccine that was administered orally. In areas of the world where polio is still active, the oral vaccine is still in use. The United States, where the last endemic or wild virus-associated case of polio was recorded several decades ago, uses an inactivated vaccine administered by injection. A total of four doses are required to complete the series, with the first dose beginning as early as 6 weeks of life and the fourth dose recommended between 4 and 6 years of age.

Diphtheria/Tetanus/Pertussis

Diphtheria is a disease caused by a toxin produced by *C. diphtheriae,* an aerobic, gram-positive bacteria (Acosta et al., 2020). Diphtheria vaccine is always accompanied by tetanus vaccine. Tetanus is an often-fatal disease caused by the toxin produced by *C. tetani,* a spore-forming, gram-positive anaerobic rod. Tetanus is contracted through contact with spores in contaminated soil or exposure to colonized animals such as horses, sheep, cattle, dogs, cats, rats, guinea pigs, or chickens. Tetanus cannot be spread by human-to-human contact.

Pertussis, also known as *whooping cough,* is the disease caused by the bacterium *Bordetella pertussis.* Early versions of the vaccine included inactivated whole-cell bacteria; however, concerns related to safety led to the development of a more purified, acellular version of the vaccine. The acellular vaccine is associated with less adverse effects, but has also proven to be less immunogenic, requiring multiple boosters later in life.

Several combinations of tetanus, diphtheria, and pertussis vaccines are available in the United States. The DTaP (diphtheria, tetanus, acellular pertussis) vaccines are approved for use in children less than 7 years old for primary immunization. The primary vaccination series consists of three doses given at 2, 4, and 6 months of age, with a booster at 15 to 18 months and another at 4 to 6 years of age. Diphtheria and tetanus (DT) vaccines are available without pertussis for use when pertussis vaccination is contraindicated. Contraindications to pertussis vaccination include a severe allergic reaction to any vaccine component or following a dose, or encephalopathy within 7 days after vaccination that is not attributable to another identifiable cause (Havers et al., 2020).

DTaP vaccines should not be confused with Tdap vaccines, which are used as a booster immunization in older children and adults. Notably, in order to protect newborns, it is recommended that parents and close contacts should receive the Tdap vaccine. Specifically, women are advised to get a Tdap vaccine during each pregnancy between 27 and 36 weeks to maximize the passage of antibodies to their newborn (CDC, 2013).

Haemophilus influenzae

Before effective vaccines were available, *H. influenzae* type B was the leading cause of invasive bacterial disease, including meningitis, in children under 5 years of age (Oliver et al., 2020). Since the vaccine has become available, there has been a 99% reduction in invasive disease caused by this organism. There are three *H. influenzae* conjugate vaccines available in the United States. Two use a tetanus carrier protein (ActHIB®, Hiberix®) and one uses a meningococcal outer membrane as the carrier protein (PedvaxHIB®). The primary series beginning at 2 months differs depending on which vaccine is used—three doses for ActHIB or Hiberix and two doses for PedvaxHIB. Regardless of which vaccine is used for the primary series, a booster dose is recommended between ages 15 and 18 months.

Neisseria meningitidis

Neisseria meningitidis, or meningococcus, is responsible for approximately half of the cases of meningitis in the United States (Mbaeyi et al., 2021). Meningococcal conjugate vaccines are currently only recommended for use in patients under 11 years of age with special circumstances. If infants have certain risk factors for meningococcal disease, including, but not limited to, complement deficiency and functional or anatomic asplenia, they should receive the meningococcal vaccine beginning as early as 2 months of age. Menveo® and Menactra® are quadrivalent meningococcal vaccines covering serogroups A, C, W, and Y (Mbaeyi et al., 2021). Menveo is approved for use beginning at 2 months of age and is a two- to four-dose series depending on age at initiation. Menactra is approved for use beginning at 9 months of age. It is a two-dose series that should be given 4 weeks or more after completion of the primary pneumococcal series.

Rotavirus

Young infants are especially prone to morbidity and mortality from rotavirus infection related to severe diarrhea, dehydration, electrolyte imbalance, and/or metabolic acidosis. There are two rotavirus vaccines currently available in the United States. Both are live attenuated vaccines administered orally. Rotarix® is a monovalent vaccine (RV1) containing the G1P[8] human rotavirus (GlaxoSmithKline Biologicals, 2019). It provides protection against G1 and non-G1 type (G3, G4, and G9) rotavirus through a two-dose series. RotaTeq® is a pentavalent vaccine (RV5) and contains G1, G2, G3, G4, and P1A strains derived from human and bovine sources (Merck & Co, Inc., 2020b). This three-dose series vaccine provides protection against rotavirus types G1, G2, G3, G4, and G9. Despite some difference in protection, the vaccines are interchangeable.

Timing of rotavirus vaccination involves some unique considerations. An earlier version of the vaccine was discontinued due to safety concerns related to high numbers of intussusception. Although these newer versions of the vaccine have not been linked to increased rates of intussusception, the ACIP recommends that the maximum age at which rotavirus vaccination can begin is 104 days of life. This is to ensure that vaccination is complete prior to the period of time when the risk of intussusception is highest.

In general, live virus vaccines are administered in inpatient settings immediately prior to discharge to prevent any possible transmission of vaccine virus to immune-compromised hosts within the facility. Many infants across the country miss the opportunity to be vaccinated against rotavirus because they remain admitted to an inpatient unit well past the maximum age for immunization. Several studies have established that despite postimmunization vaccine shedding, rotavirus vaccines can be safely administered in the NICU (Hofstetter et al., 2018, Monk et al., 2014, Thrall, 2015). The ACIP recommendations (Cortese, 2009) consider the risk from shedding to be greater than the benefit from inpatient vaccination; however, the most recent edition of the *Red Book: Report of the Committee on Infectious Diseases* states that there are limited studies on the transmission of vaccine virus in hospital settings: "Individual institutions may consider administering rotavirus vaccine at the recommended chronological age to otherwise eligible infants during hospitalization, including in the neonatal intensive care unit" (AAP, 2021, p. 647).

Influenza

Influenza is a seasonally occurring virus associated with respiratory illness ranging in severity from asymptomatic to severe. Historically, influenza pandemics recur a few times each century, with the most recent being the H1N1 pandemic of 2009 (Chung et al., 2020). The CDC recommends influenza vaccination for everyone beginning at 6 months of age during influenza season (Grohskopf et al., 2020). Some patients will still be in the NICU when they reach this age. Initial influenza vaccination requires two doses spaced 4 weeks apart for adequate immunogenicity (Chung et al., 2020). Multiple forms of the influenza vaccine are available, with annual changes to the three or four strains of influenza A and B predicted to be more active in the coming season (Vetter et al., 2018). For infants (6–35 months), any of the approved inactivated flu vaccines are acceptable for use. The dose varies from 0.25 mL to 0.5 mL in this population based on the individual product.

Combination Vaccines

Several combination vaccines are available on the market (e.g., Pentacel®, Pediarix®). Combination vaccines are beneficial in that they allow a reduced number of needlesticks for an equivalent number of vaccinations. It is helpful to be familiar with the products available in your practice to optimize compliance and reduce needlesticks. Table 8.5 contains combination vaccine products commonly used in the NICU. Use of combination vaccines may sometimes result in additional doses of a particular vaccine being administered (usually a fourth dose of hepatitis B). The ACIP considers this permissible in facilitating efforts to decrease overall needlestick burden or the number of shots to be administered (CDC, 2021a).

VACCINE ADVERSE EVENTS

Information on adverse reactions from vaccinations comes from clinical trials as well as from postmarketing surveillance, which depends on voluntary reporting. The most common adverse events reported with vaccines are mild and transient, including erythema or swelling at the injection site, fever, crying, and apnea (Omeñaca et al., 2018). With the exception of apnea, adverse effects are similar regardless of birth weight and whether or not there is a history of prematurity. Clinicians are encouraged to report any unusual or unanticipated adverse reaction from a vaccine to the Vaccine Adverse Event Reporting System (https://vaers.hhs.gov). Among other things, this program, comanaged by the CDC and the Food and Drug Administration (FDA), serves to recognize new or increasing trends in adverse events related to vaccine use. Voluntary reporting is necessary to detect rare or serious adverse effects (Vetter et al., 2018).

Myths and misconceptions regarding vaccination abound despite scientific evidence that disproves them. It may be helpful to stay apprised of what is circulating online and in your community to be prepared to thoroughly address questions from parents. Some common myths that have been debunked by substantial scientific data are included in Table 8.6 for reference. Advocating for timely vaccination is always in the best interest of the patient.

TABLE 8.5 Combination Vaccines Given in the NICU

COMBINATION VACCINE (TRADE NAME)	COMPONENTS	COMMENTS AND CONSIDERATIONS
Pediarix®	DTaP HepB Polio	
Pentacel®	DTaP Polio Hib	Packaged as two separate vials—one is used to reconstitute the other; vaccine omission has been linked to this packaging
Vaxelis™	DTaP Polio HepB Hib	Most recently approved Allows the fewest needlesticks
Infanrix®	DTaP	Combination products preferred but may be used if there are contraindications to other components of the combination vaccine or due to shortage or formulary issues
Daptacel®	DTaP	Combination products preferred but may be used if there are contraindications to other components of the combination vaccine or due to shortage or formulary issues

DTaP, diphtheria, tetanus, acellular pertussis; HepB, hepatitis B; Hib, *Haemophilus influenzae* type B.

TABLE 8.6 Key Concepts Addressing Common Vaccine Safety Concerns

COMMON VACCINE SAFETY MYTHS	KEY CONCEPTS
Too many vaccines too soon.	• The number of immunologic components in vaccines has declined over time. • The current 14 vaccines on the U.S. schedule contain 200 immunologic proteins in total; the smallpox vaccine contained 160.
Too many vaccines can "overwhelm" the immune system.	• Epidemiologic and biologic data show that cumulative increases in the number of vaccines have no effect on immune function.
MMR vaccine causes autism.	• Original study making this claim contained 12 children; the paper was subsequently retracted due to evidence of misrepresented data. • Multiple large-scale studies, including a study of half a million children, have shown no association between receipt of MMR and risk of autism.
HPV vaccine increases risk of AI disease.	• More than 270 million doses of HPV vaccine have been administered. • Repeated well-designed studies show no association between HPV and AI disease.
Influenza vaccine given in early pregnancy increases risk of miscarriage.	• A study of 2,762 women showed no association between influenza vaccine and spontaneous abortion.

AI, autoimmune; HPV, human papillomavirus; MMR, measles, mumps, rubella.
Source: From Geoghegan, S., O'Callaghan, K. P., & Offit, P. A. (2020). Vaccine safety: Myths and misinformation. *Frontiers in Microbiology, 11*(372), 1–7. https://doi.org/10.3389/fmicb.2020.00372.

Postimmunization Apnea

Apnea is an adverse reaction related to immunization that is specific to the neonatal population. Although this remains somewhat controversial, retrospective studies have demonstrated the rate of apnea following 2-month immunizations to be 8.4% in one study and up to 20% in others (Anderson et al., 2013). Risk factors for postimmunization apnea include preimmunization apnea, with a specific association in infants who experienced apnea within the 24-hour period prior to immunization. Other risk factors that have been associated with postimmunization apnea include weight less than 2,000 grams, postnatal age younger than 67 days, and more severe illness at birth

(Klein et al., 2008). Apnea has been documented to commence from 3 hours up to 20 hours post-vaccination, indicating that cardiorespiratory monitoring for a minimum of 24 hours following 2-month immunizations is a reasonable consideration in the NICU setting. There is mixed evidence on whether the risk of apnea persists with the 4-month vaccinations (Anderson et al., 2013).

Antipyretic Use With Vaccination

Antipyretics, such as acetaminophen and ibuprofen, have been routinely used for prophylaxis of immunization-related fever. In 2009, Prymula et al. found that although prophylactic administration of acetaminophen did reduce fever associated with vaccination, antibody response to several antigens was also impacted (Prymula et al., 2009). Several studies have followed to determine the reproducibility and clinical impact of these findings. Wysocki et al. compared five cohorts, namely groups 1 and 2, which received delayed or concomitant acetaminophen; groups 3 and 4, which received delayed or concomitant ibuprofen; and group 5, which received no prophylactic antipyretics (but could receive doses as needed for fever; Wysocki et al., 2017). Both timing and choice of antipyretic affected the outcomes. Acetaminophen coadministration affected the initial pneumococcal immunogenicity and ibuprofen affected the initial immune responses to tetanus toxoid and pertussis antigens. The difference in immunogenicity did not persist once the toddler doses were administered, with the majority of subjects achieving prespecified levels of antibody for each antigen.

Fever from vaccination is common and is generally both mild and self-limiting. With the clinical significance of these blunted antibody responses unknown, prophylactic antipyretics should be used with an abundance of caution, especially during infancy. Acetaminophen may be administered on an as-needed basis for postimmunization fever.

CONCLUSIONS

Vaccine-preventable infectious diseases have the potential to cause significant morbidity and mortality in the neonatal population. Adherence to the ACIP/CDC-recommended vaccination schedules can protect infants and mitigate risk. Understanding adverse effects related to vaccination can assist the provider in monitoring appropriately. Being aware of myths and misconceptions surrounding vaccination will prepare the provider for questions that parents may pose.

LEARNING TOOLS AND RESOURCES

Advice From the Author

Amy P. Holmes, PharmD, BCPPS, FPPA

Vaccination may seem like a low priority in the critical care setting but remember that your patients are more vulnerable to communicable disease than others. Take advantage of the opportunity to vaccinate medically stable infants according to the ACIP/CDC-recommended schedules when able.

Discussion Prompts

1. Steroids can be a contraindication to vaccine administration due to their immunosuppressive activity. The concern with live vaccines would be a potential breakthrough infection, whereas the concern for high-dose steroids is inadequate immune response to the vaccine. Discuss the benefits of vaccinating infants on time versus the potential risk of inadequate coverage.
2. Many neonates who are born prematurely require prolonged hospitalization to the point that they "age out" of rotavirus vaccination. Compare and contrast the risks and benefits of administering rotavirus vaccines during hospitalization versus only at discharge.
3. How can you advocate for timely vaccination by encouraging and/or educating family members who have incorrect perceptions of harm related to vaccines?

Mind Map

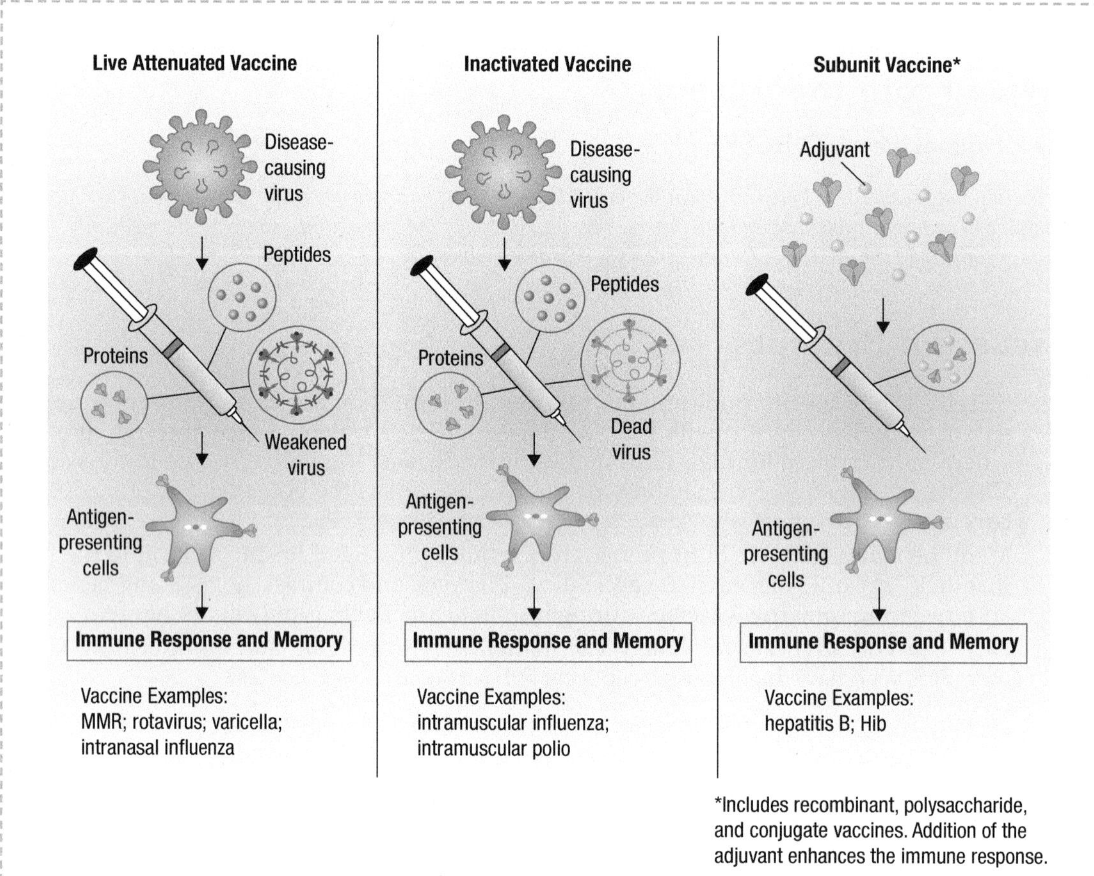

Hib, Haemophilus influenza, type B; MMR, measles, mumps, rubella.

Note: This mind map reflects the design team's interpretation of a portion of one or more concepts addressed in this chapter. Readers should regard the mind maps woven throughout this textbook as examples of multisensory study tools that can be developed to encourage conceptual understanding. Readers are encouraged to develop their own unique mind maps in consultation with academic faculty or clinical preceptors. Design credit: Jessica Mazzei, MSN, APRN, NNP, C-NPT, and Samantha Skeen, MSN, APRN, NNP-BC, East Carolina University Neonatal Nurse Practitioner Program.

REFERENCES

References for this chapter are online and available at https://connect.springerpub.com/content/book/978-0-8261-5884-0/part/partI/toc-part/ch8.

PART II

Common Central Nervous System Problems

chapter 9

Neonatal Abstinence Syndrome

Tiffany Gwartney, Karen D'Apolito, and John Brock Harris

LEARNING OBJECTIVES

After completing this chapter, the reader should be able to:

- Define *neonatal abstinence syndrome* (*NAS*) and identify the epidemiology of the disease process.
- Correlate the pathophysiology of NAS with the need for pharmacologic treatment.
- Appraise the historical evolution of pharmacologic management for NAS.
- Evaluate current nonpharmacologic and pharmacologic therapies for the treatment of NAS.

INTRODUCTION

Neonatal abstinence syndrome (NAS) involves the abrupt cessation of intrauterine opioid transfer from mother to fetus, which elicits central nervous system (CNS) hyperirritability, autonomic dysregulation, and gastrointestinal (GI) dysfunction. Although opioid exposure is the most significant etiology for NAS, and historically its primary cause, maternal ingestion of certain nonopioids (e.g., cocaine, benzodiazepines, tetracyclic antidepressants, selective serotonin reuptake inhibitors, nicotine) has also been associated with a milder and more transient degree of neonatal abstinence.

The incidence of NAS has steadily increased since the 1970s and continues to be a significant public health problem (Finnegan et al., 1975; Gomez-Pomar & Finnegan, 2018). Over the past 15 years, cases of NAS have increased 300%, from 1.5/1,000 to 7.3/1,000 live births in the United States (National Institute on Drug Abuse [NIDA], 2020). Maternal ingestion of opioids, either licit or illicit, is primarily responsible for the increase in cases of NAS. The two drugs most commonly associated with NAS, which are long-acting opioids, are methadone and buprenorphine. Heroin use in developed countries is also increasing. More specifically, NAS from heroin and misuse of opioid prescription drugs has increased fivefold over the past decade (NIDA, 2020).

Morbidity and mortality data related to intra- and extrauterine exposure to opioids are limited. Nonetheless, exposure to methadone during infancy has been shown to be associated with a lower IQ and attention deficit hyperactivity disorder (ADHD), among other behavioral disorders (Coyle et al., 2005). Among preterm infants, Zwicker and colleagues (2016) noted that morphine exposure was associated with a decrease in cerebellar volume ($p = .04$), poorer motor outcomes ($p < .001$), and poorer cognitive outcomes ($p = .006$) in early childhood.

This chapter has been purposefully developed to provide readers with an overview of the etiology and pathophysiology of NAS. We discuss the relevant assessment tools and their application in the clinical setting. Common signs of NAS are described to assist readers in using appropriate diagnostic skills in the clinical setting. Next, we discuss outcomes for NAS that garner significance for pharmacotherapies from a historical perspective. Finally, we examine current literature for innovative and evidence-based nonpharmacologic interventions, as well as review primary and adjunctive pharmacotherapies. Learning tools and resources are provided throughout the chapter as a method of providing quick reference for the seasoned clinician, as well as the novice clinician preparing for board examination.

REVIEW OF PATHOPHYSIOLOGY: NEONATAL ABSTINENCE SYNDROME

The cellular and molecular mechanisms of opioid withdrawal are not well understood in adults; therefore, even less is known about the mechanisms involved in neonatal opioid withdrawal. Experts have proposed that complex maternal–placental–fetal pharmacokinetics, in combination with immature neurologic development and impaired neurologic processing at birth, complicate the pathophysiology of neonatal withdrawal (Kocherlakota, 2014). We review major theories that seek to explain the current state of the science of neonatal opioid withdrawal in this section of the chapter.

We know that opioids exert their mechanism of action through stimulation of G protein-coupled opioid receptors. The major opioid receptors include mu (μ), delta (δ), and kappa (Κ) receptors. Each is located primarily within the CNS and, to a lesser degree, in the peripheral nervous system (Feng et al., 2012). In neonates, the affinity of μ receptors to opioids is as strong as in the adult; δ and Κ receptors are less developed in neonates.

Neurons found within the locus coeruleus, located within the pons, are abundantly affixed with μ receptors. Given the volume of μ receptors in the locus coeruleus, and the fact that they are mature in neonates, this region of the brain is known to be most sensitive to opioids. Normally, neurons in the locus coeruleus modulate the synthesis and secretion of enzymes (e.g., adenylyl cyclase [AC]), which elicits the production of various neurotransmitters (Figure 9.1). However, consistent maternal ingestion of opioids induces chronic downregulation and desensitization of μ receptors, which suppresses enzymatic activity necessary for normal neurotransmitter production. As a consequence, norepinephrine release is upregulated (as a compensatory mechanism; Woodward et al., 2018).

FIGURE 9.1 Neurotransmitter release.

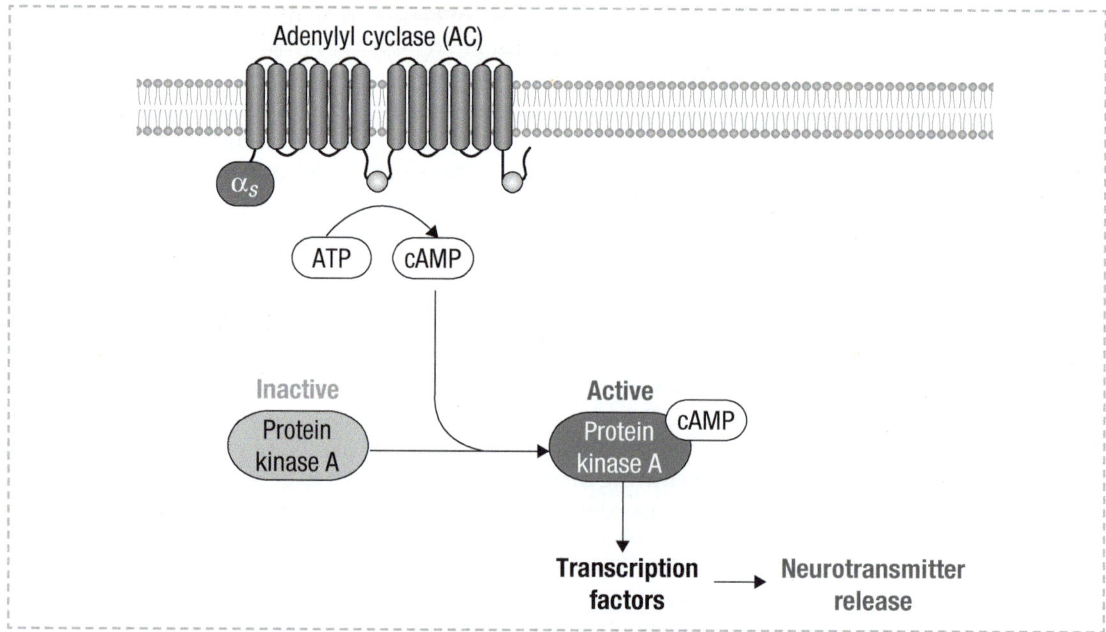

ATP, adenosine triphosphate; cAMP, cyclic adenosine monophosphate.
Design credit: Amy J. Jnah.

Abrupt cessation of opioid intake, which occurs after birth, induces neuronal upregulation, particularly at μ receptors, through hyperstimulation of the AC enzymatic cascade. The upregulation of AC activity elicits an abnormal release of neurotransmitters (Figure 9.2; Rehni et al., 2013). This activation is responsible for most of the signs of NAS (Anbalagan & Mendez, 2021; Little et al., 1996).

FIGURE 9.2 Pathogenesis of abnormal neurotransmission with neonatal abstinence syndrome.

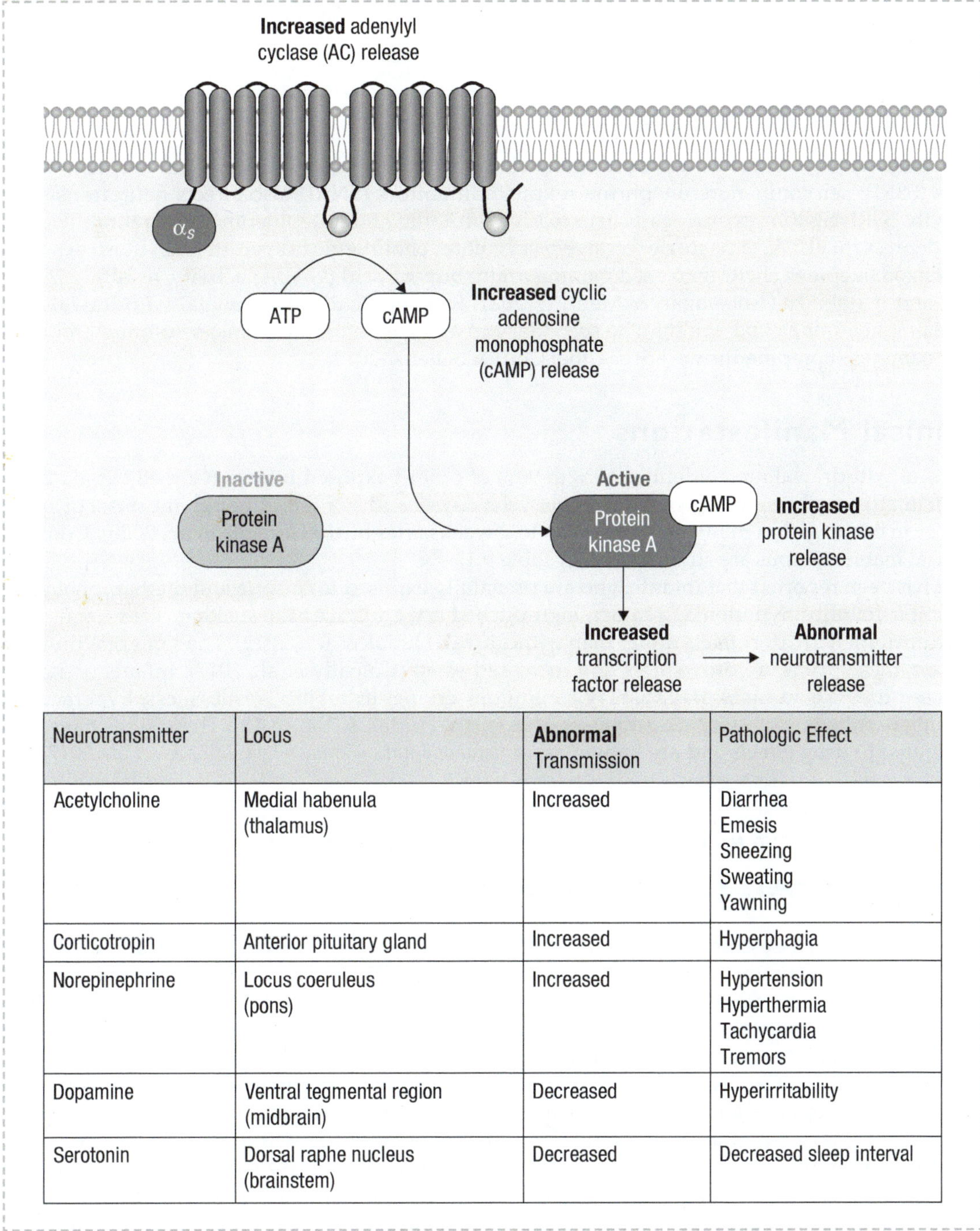

Neurotransmitter	Locus	**Abnormal** Transmission	Pathologic Effect
Acetylcholine	Medial habenula (thalamus)	Increased	Diarrhea Emesis Sneezing Sweating Yawning
Corticotropin	Anterior pituitary gland	Increased	Hyperphagia
Norepinephrine	Locus coeruleus (pons)	Increased	Hypertension Hyperthermia Tachycardia Tremors
Dopamine	Ventral tegmental region (midbrain)	Decreased	Hyperirritability
Serotonin	Dorsal raphe nucleus (brainstem)	Decreased	Decreased sleep interval

ATP, adenosine triphosphate; cAMP, cyclic adenosine monophosphate.
Design credit: Amy J. Jnah.
Sources: From Kocherlakota, P. (2014). Neonatal abstinence syndrome. *Pediatrics, 134*(2), e547–e561. https://doi.org/10.1542/peds.2013-3524; Kocherlakota, P. (2019). Pharmacologic therapy for neonatal abstinence syndrome. In W. Benitz & P. Smith (Eds.), *Infectious disease and pharmacology* (pp. 243–259). Elsevier.

The production of other neurotransmitters (e.g., dopamine, serotonin) is also altered and believed to cause other common clinical signs of NAS. Decreased dopamine from the ventral tegmental area of the midbrain, the storage center of dopamine, elicits hyperirritability. Decreased serotonin from the dorsal raphe nucleus, located on the brainstem, causes sleep deprivation. Increased acetylcholine causes cholinergic signs, such as sneezing and diarrhea, in babies with NAS (Anbalagan & Mendez, 2021; Radke et al., 2011). Increased corticotropin release from activation of the hypothalamic–pituitary–adrenocortical axis has been reported to cause stress and hyperphagia during the opioid withdrawal process in neonates (Anbalagan & Mendez, 2021; Nunez et al., 2007).

Nonopioid Withdrawal

To a lesser extent, withdrawal from intrauterine exposure to selective serotonin reuptake inhibitors (SSRI)/serotonin–norepinephrine reuptake inhibitors (SNRI) also affects neurotransmitter activity. SSRI/SNRI exposure leads to excessive serotonin and norepinephrine secretion. Tricyclic antidepressant (TCA) exposure excessively stimulates cholinergic transmitters. In utero exposure to benzodiazepines elicits increased gamma-aminobutyric acid (GABA) activity, resulting in anxiety and irritability (Anbalagan & Mendez, 2021; Sanz et al., 2005). Neonatal withdrawal from methamphetamine exposure may be secondary to a decrease in dopamine, serotonin, and other monoamines (norepinephrine, adrenaline; Chiu & Schenk, 2012).

Clinical Manifestations

Signs of withdrawal are evident in 60% to 90% of opioid-exposed infants (Gomella et al., 2020). Most infants exhibit signs of withdrawal between days 2 and 3 of life, although the onset of symptoms can occur within minutes of life or up to 2 weeks after birth (Gomella et al., 2020). Common clinical manifestations are summarized in Table 9.1.

It has been reported that infants who are prenatally exposed to cocaine and methamphetamine exhibit irritability, hypertonia, tremors, high-pitched cry, and excessive sucking. These signs have been attributed to drug effects rather than withdrawal (Hudak & Tan, 2012). The signs of withdrawal from these drugs are drowsiness and increased sleep (Galbally et al., 2017). Infants prenatally exposed to SSRIs in utero may display continuous crying, irritability, restlessness, hyperactivity, feeding problems, and sleep disturbances after birth (Hudak & Tan, 2012). These signs have been attributed to drug effects and are known as *neonatal adaptation syndrome* (Galbally et al., 2017).

THE FINNEGAN NEONATAL ASSESSMENT SCORING TOOL AND THE EAT, SLEEP, CONSOLE METHOD

There are several assessment tools that have been used to determine the presence and severity of NAS. The most common tool, which has been used since 1975 and is considered the gold standard, is the Finnegan Neonatal Abstinence Scoring Tool (FNAST; Orlando, 2014). Other tools that have been found to have nearly 100% correlation to the FNAST include the Neonatal Narcotic Withdrawal Inventory, Neonatal Narcotic Withdrawal Index, and the FNAST—Short Form (Grossman & Berkwitt, 2019). The FNAST is designed to quantify the most common clinical signs of drug withdrawal in opioid- and non-opioid-exposed infants (Kocherlakota, 2014). The tool contains 21 clinical signs of withdrawal that range from moderate to severe within the CNS, as well as the metabolic, vasomotor, respiratory, and GI systems (Finnegan et al., 1975). Some publications refer to the *modified* Finnegan tool. This suggests that the original tool was changed; however, in the early stages of tool development, items were refined and combined to reduce redundancy. For example, excoriation was scored according to three separate items with one point assigned to each site (nose, chin, and knees). These three items were combined into one item that correlates with a score of 1 if excoriation is present (Figure 9.3; Finnegan, 1990).

TABLE 9.1 Common Signs of Neonatal Abstinence Syndrome by Drug

	DRUGS						
	HEROIN	METHADONE	COCAINE	ALCOHOL	MARIJUANA	BARBITURATES	PHENYLCYCLOHEXYL PIPERIDINE (PCP)
PHYSIOLOGIC SIGNS							
Sneezing		*					*
Stuffy nose	*	*					
Spitting/drooling		*					
Diarrhea	*	*		*			*
Vomiting	*	*		*			*
Poor feeding	*	*		*			*
Sweating	*	*		*			
Tachycardia							
Fever	*	*					
Tachypnea	*	*		*			
NEUROBEHAVIORAL SIGNS							
Fist sucking		*					*
Irritability	*	*		*	*	*	
Restlessness	*	*		*	*	*	
Tremors	*	*		*	*	*	
High-pitched cry	*	*		*			
Seizures	*	*		*			
Yawning		*					
Disturbed sleep	*	*	*	*	*	*	
Increased crying		*		*		*	*
Hypertonicity	*	*		*			*
Drowsiness			*				
Increased sleep			*				

Source: From D'Apolito, K. (1996). Symptoms of withdrawal in drug-exposed infants. *Mother Baby Journal, 1*(2), 7–14.

FIGURE 9.3 Finnegan Neonatal Abstinence Scoring Tool.

Finnegan Neonatal Abstinence Scoring Tool (FNAST)

Patient ID: Name: Today's Weight: DOB: Date:

Signs and Symptoms	Time	Score	AM	PM	Comments
Central Nervous System Disturbances					
Crying: Excessive High Pitched		2			
Crying: Cont. High Pitched		3			
Sleeps <1 Hr After Feeding		3			
Sleeps <2 Hr After Feeding		2			
Sleeps <3 Hr After Feeding		1			
Hyperactive Moro Reflex		2			
Markedly Hyperactive Moro Reflex		3			
Mild Tremors: Disturbed		1			
Mod-Severe Tremors: Disturbed		2			
Mild Tremors: Undisturbed		3			
Mod-Severe Tremors: Undisturbed		4			
Increased Muscle Tone		2			
Excoriation (Specific Area)		1			
Myoclonic Jerk		3			
Generalized Convulsions		5			
Metabolic, Vasomotor, and Respiratory Disturbance					
Sweating		1			
Fever <101°F (37.2°C–38.3°C)		1			
Fever >101°F (38.4°C)		2			
Frequent Yawning (>3)		1			
Mottling		1			
Nasal Stuffiness		1			
Sneezing (>3)		1			
Nasal Flaring		2			
Respiratory Rate (>60/Min)		1			
Respiratory Rate (>60/Min With Retractions		2			
Gastrointestinal Disturbances					
Excessive Sucking		1			
Poor Feeding		2			
Regurgitation		2			
Projectile Vomiting		3			
Loose Stools		2			
Watery Stools		3			
Score					
Total Score					
Average Daily Score					
Inter-Observer Reliability %					
Initials of Scorer 1					
Initials of Scorer 2					

Note: The Finnegan Neonatal Abstinence score is used for the assessment of infants exposed in utero to psychoactive drugs, particularly opioids/opiates. The evaluator should check signs or symptoms observed at various time intervals and add the score to obtain a total score. Observation of the scores over time intervals provides the progression/diminution of symptoms.

Source: Adapted from Finnegan, L. P., & Kaltenbach, K. K. (1992). The assessment and management of neonatal abstinence syndrome. In R. A. Hoekelman & N. M. Nelson (Eds.), *Primary care* (3rd ed., pp. 1367–1378). C.V. Mosby.

Reliability of Tool

The FNAST has documented reliability. Initial clinical evaluation of the tool demonstrated an average interobserver reliability of 0.82 before minor tool refinements were made to reduce ambiguity (Finnegan et al., 1975). Assessment and scoring are completed every 3 to 4 hours. Scoring is dynamic, meaning that signs, such as yawning or sneezing, observed between scoring intervals are documented. Treatment is recommended for a score of 8 or higher on three consecutive assessments (Finnegan, 1990; Orlando, 2014). It has been demonstrated that when staff members are trained in the use of the tool (e.g., items defined and followed), interobserver reliability can be increased to 90% or greater (D'Apolito, 2014; Lucas & Knobel, 2021).

Protocol Consistency and Compliance

A standardized pharmacologic and nonpharmacologic treatment plan does not exist for the care of infants with NAS (Walsh et al., 2018). In 2014, the Ohio Perinatal Collaborative conducted a study with six regional children's hospitals in the state of Ohio to test the implementation of a standardized weaning protocol for infants hospitalized with NAS. The intervention group (n = 417) received the NAS weaning treatment protocol and the control group received standard care without the weaning protocol (n = 130). The findings suggest that regardless of treatment drug (morphine or methadone), infants who received the weaning protocol had fewer days of treatment (17 days vs. 32 days; p = .0001 [47%↓]) and shorter hospital stays (23 vs. 32 days; p = .004 [28%↓]; Hall et al., 2014).

An additional study in 2018 implemented both a standardized nonpharmacologic (swaddling, skin-to-skin contact, breastfeeding, rooming-in) and pharmacologic treatment (either morphine or methadone; when to treat, escalate, wean, add adjunctive medication) protocol in 3,300 infants with NAS. All infants received nonpharmacologic treatment. Of these infants, 48% (n = 157) required pharmacologic treatment with either methadone or morphine; morphine was used 99% of the time. Compliance with implementation of the nonpharmacologic protocol increased from 37% to 59% (60%↑) and the increase in compliance for implementation of the pharmacologic protocol was 59% to 68% (15%↑). The infants who received care from providers who were compliant with the protocols required fewer days of pharmacologic treatment (12 vs. 13.4 days; 10% ↓) and were discharged earlier (17 vs. 18.3 days; 7%↓; Walsh et al., 2018). Following a specific protocol for the management of infants with NAS can be beneficial.

Eat, Sleep, Console Method

Another more recent method used to assess for signs of withdrawal in opioid-exposed infants is Eat, Sleep, Console (ESC; Table 9.2). In this method, infants are assessed for their ability to eat one or more ounces of formula/breast milk per feeding, sleep undisturbed for longer than 1 hour, and be consoled from crying within 10 minutes (Grossman et al., 2018). The ESC method was developed based on observations of infants with NAS. It was determined that if an infant could eat and sleep, which were considered essential newborn behaviors, then the infant's withdrawal was well managed. If infants ate less than 1 ounce of formula/breast milk, slept less than 1 hour, and/or were not consolable within the allotted time frame, a nonpharmacologic measure would be augmented (placement in a quiet room, rooming in with the parents) and pharmacologic treatment with one dose of morphine (0.05 mg/kg/dose) was given. Infants are reassessed every 3 hours. If the infant could eat, sleep, and be consoled at this time, additional doses of morphine were not given. Using this method, length of hospitalization was reduced from 22 to 6 days (p >.001) and morphine use decreased from 98% to 14% (p <.001; Grossman et al., 2017). It is expected that parents will be present and participate in the care of their infant 24 hours a day, 7 days a week (Grossman et al., 2017). The ESC method may be an alternative to specifically examining the common signs of withdrawal in infants with NAS; however, more research is needed.

Confirmatory Diagnosis

In 2019, a distinction was made between the terms *NAS* and *neonatal opioid withdrawal syndrome* (*NOWS*). NOWS is being considered as the appropriate diagnosis for neonatal abstinence in infants who have only had intrauterine exposure to opioids. As a result of this differentiation, NAS is now considered a generalized term for the mild/moderate and transient signs of withdrawal present in infants exposed to drugs other than opioids (SSRI, nicotine, cocaine, methamphetamine, etc.); however, the term *NAS* can be used if an infant has had intrauterine polydrug exposure in

TABLE 9.2 Eat, Sleep, Console Scoring Sheet

TIME		
Eating		
Poor eating due to NAS: Yes? No?		
Sleeping		
Sleeps <1 hour due to NAS: Yes? No?		
Consoling		
Unable to console within 10 min due to NAS: Yes? No?		
Soothing support used to console infant: Soothes with little support: 1 Soothes with some support: 2 Soothes with much support or does not sooth in 10 minutes: 3		
Parental presence since last assessment: No parent present: 0 1–59 minutes: 1 1 h to 1 h, 59 min: 2 2 h to 2 h, 59 min: 3 3+ h: 4		
Team huddle called: Yes? No?		
Team huddle treatment decision: Optimize nonpharmacologic care further: 1 Initiate medication treatment: 2		

NAS, neonatal abstinence syndrome.
Source: From All Things Neonatal. (2017, June 8). *Is it time to (ESC)cape from neonatal abstinence?* https://www.allthingsneonatal.com/2017/06/08/is-it-time-to-escape-from-neonatal-abstinence

addition to opioids, and requires pharmacologic treatment (Mangat et al., 2019). A urine and/or meconium toxicity screen can confirm the presence of drugs known to precipitate symptoms of intoxication or withdrawal, assisting in diagnosis and treatment decision-making. The confirmatory diagnosis of NAS or NOWS is then conferred in the presence of physiologic and neurobehavioral signs indicative of infant withdrawal from intrauterine drug exposure.

HISTORIC PERSPECTIVE: SEMINAL AND OTHER NOTEWORTHY STUDIES

Opium, the first narcotic drug linked to addictive behaviors, was initially cultivated centuries ago in Mesopotamia. Although it is certainly likely that the genesis of opium addiction dates back to these early years, opium was brought to the United States in the early 1800s and the first report of opium-induced addiction was published shortly thereafter. Next, morphine, an opium derivative, was isolated in 1804 and commercially manufactured in 1827 for opium addiction and pain control. At the time, opium use was considered socially acceptable to the extent that women sought out and openly consumed opium for any type of routine physical ailment (e.g., headache). This was followed by heroin, another opium derivative, which was derived around 1874. These opioids quickly infiltrated the United States and addiction in women (and men) increased throughout the 19th century.

Before the mid-1800s, infants born to women who were opioid dependent were thought not to be affected because, at that time, morphine use was associated with sterility as well as a loss of sexual desire (Kocherlakota, 2014). This opinion quickly changed in 1875, when German women dependent on morphine gave birth to stillborn infants or full-term infants who demonstrated inconsolable crying beginning on the third day of life. Some newborns also developed generalized seizures. This poorly understood disease process was termed *congenital morphinism* and left untreated (Perlstein, 1947). As a result, NAS, the actual disease process, was frequently fatal to newborns (Perlstein, 1947; Pettey, 1912). Finally, in 1991, experts associated the symptomatology with withdrawal from the perinatal passive transfer of morphine. Next, experts hypothesized that providing infants with opioids would reduce the severity of symptomatology.

As early as 1892, infants were provided small doses of paregoric and tincture of opium, two drugs that decreased neuronal activity and mitigated withdrawal symptoms (Pettey, 1912; Siu & Robinson, 2014). Alternatively, addicted mothers would breastfeed their infants, which facilitated opioid transfer through breast milk. Use of paregoric and tincture of opium was later halted due to safety concerns (Siu & Robinson, 2014). Among other harmful additives, such as papaverine and benzoic acid, paregoric contained 44% ethanol (Siu & Robinson, 2014). Tincture of opium contained 19% ethanol (Siu & Robinson, 2014). These drugs were replaced with alternative opioid-based treatments, namely morphine (first used in 1903), methadone, and buprenorphine, which have remained the mainstays of primary treatment over the past 50 years. Adjunctive treatments, including phenobarbital and clonidine, were introduced in the 20th century.

A timeline of historic events that contributed to the NAS epidemic is provided in Box 9.1. Next, we offer an integrated review of current nonpharmacologic and pharmacologic therapies. Results of other seminal, noteworthy studies are woven throughout the next sections to establish historic context and help readers appreciate the evolution of science and our understanding of NAS over the years.

BOX 9.1 Noteworthy Events Contributing to the Neonatal Abstinence Syndrome Epidemic

Early 1800s: Opium import to the United States began.
1804: Morphine isolated from opium by German chemist.
1817: Morphine marketed publicly as an effective analgesic.
1827: Commercial manufacturing of morphine begins.
1827: Morphine gained social acceptance among middle/upper class women for the treatment of minor, recurring ailments (e.g., headaches).
1853: Hypodermic needle is invented by Scottish physician.
1875: First case of neonatal morphine withdrawal reported.
1892: First case of congenital morphinism in the United States reported.
1898: Commercial manufacturing of heroin as a "safe, non-addictive substitute for morphine" began.
Early 1900s: Heroin primarily prescribed as an antitussive agent.
1903: Morphine prescribed to neonates with withdrawal symptoms.
1910: Heroin use linked with chronic drug abusers.
1914: Harrison Narcotic Act of 1914 passed; heroin may only be obtained from a physician.
1924: Anti-Heroin Act of 1924 passed, banning all use of heroin in the United States.
1937: Methadone is developed by German scientists.
1966: Buprenorphine is developed by U.S. scientists.
1971: First report of neonatal methadone withdrawal.
1984: Vicodin marketed as effective opioid analgesic.
1989: Oxycontin marketed as effective opioid analgesic.
1997: First report of neonatal buprenorphine withdrawal.
1999: Percocet marketed as effective opioid analgesic.
2002: First report of neonatal oxycontin withdrawal.
2012: Neonatal abstinence syndrome declared an epidemic in the United States.

Sources: Campbell, N. D., & Lovell, A. M. (2012). The history of the development of buprenorphine as an addiction therapeutic. *Annals of the New York Academy of Sciences, 1248*(1), 124–139. https://doi.org/10.1111/j.1749-6632.2011.06352.x; Higby, G. J. (1986). Heroin and medical reasoning: The power of analogy. *New York State Journal of Medicine, 86*(3), 137–142; Kocherlakota, P. (2014). Neonatal abstinence syndrome. *Pediatrics, 134*(2), e547–e561. https://doi.org/10.1542/peds.2013-3524; Perlstein, M. A. (1947). Congenital morphinism: A rare cause of convulsions in the newborn. *Journal of the American Medical Association, 135*(10), 633. https://doi.org/10.1001/jama.1947.62890100006006c

CURRENT NONPHARMACOLOGIC TREATMENT MODALITIES FOR NEONATAL ABSTINENCE SYNDROME

All infants with a diagnosis of NAS or NOWS should be managed with nonpharmacologic interventions (NPI; Patrick et al., 2020). This should be the first line of treatment for infants exhibiting mild, moderate, and severe signs of drug withdrawal. In many cases, NPIs are sufficient for infants with mild to moderate signs of NAS (NFAST score <8). However, infants with severe signs will also require pharmacologic treatment.

NPIs used to manage NAS or NOWS focus on the reduction or elimination of treatment with opioids, promotion of family/infant bonding, and reduction of NICU admission. There are several NPIs that have improved outcomes for infants with NAS. These include controlling the environment by dimming the lighting and decreasing noise levels in the infant's room. These strategies decrease overstimulation of infants who are irritable or hyperaroused due to clinical signs of withdrawal (Mangat et al., 2019). Wrapping the infant snugly in a blanket (swaddling) has helped to decrease arousal and promote sleep. Nonnutritive sucking helps to decrease infant stress and calms erratic and uncoordinated movements as does holding and rocking (Velez & Jansson, 2008).

Placing infants in a prone versus supine position to improve quiet sleep, lower motor activity, enhance respiratory control, and decrease heart rate variability has also been suggested. Infants placed in a supine position demonstrated significantly higher NAS scores ($p = .0001$) but had higher caloric intake compared to infants lying prone (133 vs. 100 kcal/kg/d; Maichuk et al., 1999). If prone positioning is used, when parents room-in or visit, a discussion about safe sleeping recommendations should take place, indicating that supine positioning decreases the risk for sudden infant death syndrome in normal full-term infants (Mangat et al., 2019).

Other strategies include breastfeeding, skin-to-skin contact, rooming in, and weighted blankets (Sublett, 2013; Summe et al., 2020). Results of a study of breastfeeding versus use of a lactose-free formula in infants with NAS reported a significant decrease in length of treatment (LOT) by 11 days (95% CI: 6–16) and length of stay (LOS) by 10 days (95% CI: 6–15; Lembeck et al., 2020). Contraindications for breastfeeding or providing maternal breast milk to an infant diagnosed with NAS include maternal use of illicit drugs; polydrug use; or a positive hepatitis B, hepatitis C, or HIV maternal status (Anbalagan & Mendez, 2021; Kocherlakota, 2014). It is important to note that supporting the family in their attempts to bond with the infant, avoiding stigma, and decreasing other barriers to health-seeking behaviors promotes breastfeeding and decreases the effects of NAS (Recto et al., 2020).

Skin-to-skin contact has been studied among preterm infants but not specifically in infants with NAS. A few studies have reported outcomes related to respiratory rate and crying associated with skin-to-skin contact in preterm infants. In one study, preterm infants 34 to 36 weeks' gestation who were well received 1 hour of skin-to-skin contact on days 1, 3, 5, and 7 compared to similar infants who did not receive skin-to-skin contact. A statistically significant difference was seen between groups with a lower respiratory rate in those infants receiving 1 hour of skin-to-skin contact (day 1: 66 vs. 47 [$p = .001$]; day 3: 68 vs. 46 $p = .001$]; day 5: 67 vs. 46 [$p = .001$]; day 7: 67 vs. 46 [$p = .001$]). Significant differences in respiratory rate continued after the completion of skin-to-skin contact as well ($p = .001$; Parsa et al., 2018).

One study examined the effect of skin-to-skin contact on crying in full-term infants after cesarean birth. Infants in the intervention group received skin-to-skin contact three times daily for 60 minutes over 2 consecutive days compared to infants receiving standard care. Infants in the intervention group had significantly fewer episodes of severe crying (6 vs. 12.3; $p = .05$) than infants in the control group that received standard care. As increased respiratory rate and crying are among the common signs of withdrawal in neonates, the use of skin-to-skin contact for as little as 1 hour per day and up to 3 hours per day could potentially decrease FNAST scores in infants with NAS (Keshavarz & Haghighi, 2010).

A meta-analysis of randomized, clinical trials was performed comparing six studies that evaluated the effectiveness of mother/infant rooming-in versus infants with NAS cared for in the NICU. The outcome variables included the use of pharmacologic management and LOS. Results suggest that rooming-in is preferable to NICU for reducing both pharmacologic management (risk ratio [RR]: 0.37; 95% CI: 0.19–0.7) and LOS (weighted mean difference −10.4 days; 95% CI:

−17 to −4 days). The strength of this analysis included strict adherence to the Cochrane Library and PRISMA guidelines for systematic review and meta-analysis testing and reporting. Limitations include a lack of knowledge regarding whether there was any publication bias favoring rooming-in because researchers typically do not publish negative results and the studies reviewed may not have had sufficient power to fully evaluate published outcomes. The authors do recommend that rooming-in be considered in the management of infants with NAS. However, the results of this systematic review and meta-analysis should be interpreted with careful consideration (MacMillan et al., 2018).

A pilot study was conducted to examine the use of weighted blankets to decrease signs of withdrawal in infants with NAS (n = 16). Infants were used as their own controls. A blanket was designed to hold 1 pound of nonmolding polypellet stuffing beads. Infants were supine and swaddled. The weighted blankets were placed over the swaddled infant from their shoulders to feet for 30 minutes. This was alternated with 30 minutes using a nonweighted blanket. This alternating procedure occurred at the time of feeding or sleeping. The weighted and nonweighted blankets were applied four times (two sessions with weighted blanket and two sessions without) for 24 hours. This procedure occurred until the infant was discharged from the hospital. The study was conducted for a 7-month period. A total of 67 weighted-blanket sessions occurred during the study period. The results indicated a significant decrease in FNAST scores from preintervention to 30 minutes after blanket placement when the weighted blanket was used compared to when the nonweighted blanket was used (mean decrease of 1.5 vs. −0.18; p = .016). There was also a significant decrease in heart rate while the weighted blanket was in place (p = .011). There was no significant difference in body temperature between the use of the weighted blanket or nonweighted blanket (p = 0.233) nor with the infants' respiratory rate (p = .307). Further study is needed; however, a weighted blanket may be beneficial to decreasing signs of withdrawal (lowering FNAST scores and decreasing heart rate) in infants with NAS (Summe et al., 2020).

Acupressure and Laser Acupuncture

Acupuncture originated in China over 3,000 years ago and has been used to treat medical conditions. The treatment is grounded in meridian theory, which describes lines throughout the body that correspond with specific body organs. Stimulation of these lines using acupuncture (needle) or acupressure to specific acupuncture points relieves conditions or decreases symptoms (H. Jackson et al., 2020). Acupressure and acupuncture have been used in term and preterm infants for pain management prior to heel-stick. Results of a study (n = 42) that used laser acupuncture in the Yintang area (between the eyebrows) prior to heel-stick reported a significant decrease in procedure time (p = .008), but an increase in crying time ($p \leq .001$; Abbasoglu et al., 2015). A second study (n = 40) implemented auricular acupuncture at the Battlefield Acupuncture points of the ear (Cingulate Gyrus, Thalmus, Omega 2, Point Zero, and Shen Men) 2 hours prior to a heel-stick. These infants had significantly lower pain scores on the Premature Infant Pain Profile (PIPP; p = .04; Chen et al., 2017).

Three studies have specifically examined the use of acupressure or laser acupuncture to relieve signs of NAS. One study (n = 54) used acupressure at various pressure sites on the ear and top of the head, between the base of the thumb and index finger, on the inner arm near the wrist, along the sides of the stomach, on the dorsal part of the leg, and on the bottom of the foot (Yintang, Baihui, Hegu, Neiguan, Zusanli, Sanyingio, and Yongquan, respectively). Stimulation of these pressure points improved sleep, decreased agitation, and promoted better feeding after the treatment. Limitations of the study include a lack of discussion regarding statistics or time of treatment (Filippelli et al., 2012).

Schwartz and colleagues (2011) conducted a randomized trial with two groups of infants to determine whether acupressure would decrease LOS in infants with NAS. The intervention group received acupressure (n = 32) and the control group (n = 32) received standard care. The National Acupuncture Detoxification Association (NADA) protocol for acupressure was used, which included the following pressure points: wrist with palm facing up, upper third part of the ear, inner ankle, between the big toe and second toe, and tip of thumb downside of hand (sympathetic,

Shen Men, kidney, liver, and lung, respectively). No statistical differences were found between the groups regarding LOS (p=.95).

The final study in this discussion involves a randomized controlled trial (RCT) that sought to determine whether laser acupuncture could decrease the duration of oral morphine therapy and decrease LOS. Infants were randomized into the laser acupuncture intervention (n = 14) or control group (n = 14; Raith et al., 2015). The NADA acupuncture protocol was used with a laser device daily, 1 hour after feeding and oral morphine administration in the intervention group. Ear acupuncture points were treated for 30 seconds, and body acupuncture points were treated for 60 seconds. The duration of oral morphine in the intervention group was significantly decreased (28 days vs. 39 days; p = .019) and hospital stay was decreased from 50 days to 35 days (p = .048). The results of these studies suggest that acupressure or laser acupuncture may help promote sleep and feeding and reduce agitation and LOS in infants with NAS; however, more research is needed in this area.

CURRENT PHARMACOLOGIC TREATMENT MODALITIES FOR NEONATAL ABSTINENCE SYNDROME

The goal of pharmacologic treatment of NAS is to stabilize the clinical manifestations of withdrawal and restore normal newborn behavior (Bio et al., 2011). The current medications used to treat NAS include oral morphine, methadone, clonidine, and phenobarbital and, more recently, sublingual buprenorphine (Patrick et al., 2020). This section addresses the use of these medications in the treatment of NAS along with essential pharmacokinetic, pharmacodynamic, administration, and monitoring principles related to these medications.

Morphine

MECHANISM OF ACTION/PHARMACOKINETIC PRINCIPLES

As noted earlier, increased AC activity results in an immediate increase in norepinephrine after the in utero opioid exposure is eliminated at birth (Kraft & van den Anker, 2012). Morphine, a synthetic endorphin, is the standard first-line treatment for NAS (Kocherlakota, 2014). The mechanism of action of morphine involves mitigating the effect of upregulated norepinephrine neurotransmission, which occurs during withdrawal. Morphine is an opioid agonist; it binds at μ, δ, and K receptors in order to elicit physiologic responses. Morphine metabolites, especially morphine-6-glucuronide (M6G), are more selective for the μ receptor than the δ or K receptors (Christrup, 1997). Agonism of the μ and δ receptors increases potassium influx. Kappa receptor agonism reduces calcium influx. Activation of the various μ receptors helps to reduce the severity of specific signs of withdrawal in infants with NAS. Activation of the μ1 receptor is responsible for analgesia. Stimulation of this receptor can help to decrease the agitation seen in infants with NAS. Activation of the μ2 receptor can help to decrease tachypnea as well as decrease gastric motility, thereby helping to decrease the loose stools seen in infants with NAS. Activation of the δ opioid receptor also plays a role in promoting analgesia and decreasing gastric motility (Dhaliwal & Gupta, 2021).

Orally, morphine is absorbed in the alkaline environment of the upper GI tract and rectal mucosa (Hoskin & Hawkins, 1990). Morphine is soluble in water with poor solubility in lipids. It has a bioavailability of 20% to 50% when administered orally. Examination of 43 neonates with NAS receiving diluted tincture of opium (0.04 mg morphine equivalent/mL) reported a bioavailability of 46.3%, which is higher than the 23.9% bioavailability seen in adults (Liu et al., 2016). Morphine undergoes first-pass metabolism, specifically when administered orally, through absorption by the liver and gut wall before reaching systemic circulation (Herman & Santos, 2021). Higher bioavailability in neonates may be due to lower expression of UGT2B7 per unit of hepatocyte as well as smaller liver size (Pacifici, 2016).

The onset of morphine analgesia is relatively slow (6 to 30 minutes) due to the limited lipid solubility and its slow penetration through the blood–brain barrier. The half-life of morphine in adults is 3 to 4 hours; half-life is estimated to be 6 to 6.5 hours in term infants, 9 hours in ventilated preterm infants, and 2 hours in infants beyond 11 days of age (Farrington et al., 2013; Kart et al., 1997). Steady-state concentrations of morphine are reached by 24 to 48 hours. The half-life can be highly variable and is inversely related to gestational age. Tissue accumulation occurs with continued use with a volume of distribution of 21 L/kg.

Morphine is metabolized by various pathways with 70% of the drug metabolized via glucuronidation producing two metabolites: morphine-3-glucuronide (M3G) and M6G, with M6G being the major metabolite. Transport proteins, including organic cation transporter 1 (OCT1) and ATP-binding cassette (ABC) B1, ABCB2, and ABCB3, play a significant role in the disposition and metabolism of morphine in animal models (Thigpen et al., 2019). The ABC transporters, especially P-glycoprotein (P-gp), participates in the efflux of morphine across the blood–brain barrier; upregulation of P-gp after prolonged opioid exposure contributes to the development of tolerance to these drugs (Chaves et al., 2017). Morphine metabolites are excreted in the bile and urine (Christrup, 1997).

DOSING RECOMMENDATIONS

Typical initial dosing for the treatment of NAS ranges from 0.03 to 0.1 mg/kg per dose orally every 3 to 4 hours, depending on the specific protocol. Doses should be weaned by 10% to 20% every 1 to 3 days based on abstinence score. A 0.4-mg/mL dilution should be made from a concentrated oral morphine sulfate solution to facilitate accurate administration of low doses (Young & Mangum, 2021).

CLINICAL-MONITORING PEARLS

The reported side effects of morphine include respiratory depression, hypotension, bradycardia, transient hypertonia, ileus, and delayed gastric emptying. Therefore, it is important to monitor respiratory and cardiovascular status closely and observe the infant's abdomen for distension and loss of bowel sounds. Urine retention can occur and should be suspected if urine output is decreased (Pacifici, 2016).

Methadone

Methadone has been used to treat NAS. A few studies have compared the efficacy of treatment with morphine versus methadone. One multisite study (n = 33, United States and Puerto Rico) compared LOS among 7,667 infants who were divided into either a group receiving oral morphine (n = 1,167) or methadone (n = 6,480). The FNAST scoring tool was used to assess for the severity of withdrawal signs. No information regarding dosage was presented; physicians determined which drug was used to treat NAS. This decision was based on the drug used to treat signs of withdrawal within the first 7 days of life. Results reported a significantly shorter LOS for those infants treated with methadone versus morphine (18 days vs. 21 days, $p \leq .001$). One important limitation of the study is that a dosing protocol was not followed among the various sites (Tolia et al., 2018).

Two RCTs examined the efficacy of using either morphine or methadone to treat infants with NAS. Both studies stratified the sample based on maternal use of either methadone or buprenorphine. Brown and colleagues (2015) randomized 31 infants; LOT was significantly shorter in infants receiving methadone compared to morphine (14 days vs. 21 days, $p = .008$). The significant decrease in LOT was driven by infants prenatally exposed to methadone (15 vs. 22 days, $p = .004$), with no difference detected in infants prenatally exposed to buprenorphine (14 vs. 18 days, $p = .29$). Better response to methadone treatment in infants prenatally exposed to methadone may be due to subtle differences in mechanism of action compared to morphine and buprenorphine, detailed later in the chapter (Brown et al., 2015).

Davis and colleagues (2018) conducted a multisite study (eight hospitals in the United States). This randomized trial had a larger sample size (n = 116). The infants in this study were also prenatally exposed to methadone or buprenorphine. This study also reported a significant reduction in LOT in infants treated with methadone (12 vs. 15 days, $p = .009$). The infants treated with methadone also had a significant decrease in LOS (16 days vs. 20 days, $p = .005$), compared to infants in the morphine group. It is important to mention that the methadone used for this study was an alcohol-free, compounded solution, required by the U.S. Food and Drug Administration (FDA) specifically for this study.

There are, however, a number of analyses that have not demonstrated a preference for either morphine or methadone in the treatment of NAS. One analysis of eight studies (two RCTs and six cohort studies; $n = 8{,}876$) found no significant differences in either LOT (weighted mean difference [WMD] −1.39 days, $I^2 = 82\%$) or LOS (WMD −1.48 days, $I^2 = 92\%$, $p = .54$, and $p = .50$, respectively) between infants treated with morphine or methadone to alleviate signs of NAS. However, adjunct therapy was required significantly more often ($p = .0001$) among infants treated with morphine (RR: 1.5, $I^2 = 0\%$; Lee et al., 2019).

MECHANISM OF ACTION/PHARMACOKINETIC PRINCIPLES

Methadone, like morphine, is a μ and K receptor agonist, and also acts as an N-methyl-D-aspartate (NMDA) receptor antagonist. It is believed that agonist activity at the NMDA receptor blocks glutamate, a major excitatory neurotransmitter, and helps to suppress NAS symptoms. In addition, methadone is proposed to decrease tolerance to opioids (Lugo et al., 2005).

Methadone absorption follows first-order kinetics from the GI tract. It has a reported oral bioavailability of 86%, which is the same in neonates, children, and adults (Ward et al., 2014). Methadone has higher lipid solubility (distributing into fatty tissue and the CNS) and protein binding than morphine, which may explain the large volume of distribution and slower clearance rate (Chana et al., 2001; Grassin-Delyle et al., 2012).

Methadone binds to albumin (16%) and alpha 1-acid glycoprotein (AAG). AAG is responsible for the unbound free fraction of methadone found in humans (Yang et al., 2006). Plasma drug concentrations are variable. One study reported the volume of distribution in term neonates to be 2.53 L/kg (177 L/70 kg) and clearance 8.4 L/hr/70 kg (determination is standardized to a 70-kg adult; Wiles et al., 2015). Others reported a volume of distribution of 581 L/70 kg in neonates and clearance of 9.1 L/hr/70 kg (Stemland et al., 2013; Ward et al., 2014).

There is some variability regarding the half-life of methadone. The published mean half-life in late preterm and term neonates ranges from 14 to 25 hours, with a range of 3 to 62 hours (Chana et al., 2001; Lugo et al., 2005; Tang et al., 2021). It is important to note that the variable half-life is not associated with the maternal dose of methadone and that neonates with a plasma level greater than 0.06 μg/mL did not show signs of opioid withdrawal (Chana et al., 2001).

Methadone is metabolized in the liver by CYP2B6 into two metabolites: EDDP (2-ethylidene-1,5-dimethyl-3,3-diphenylpyrrolidine) and EMDP (2-ethyl-5-methyl-3,3-diphenyl-1-pyrroline). Both metabolites are excreted by the kidney and through the bile. Of the two, EDDP is the major metabolite found in the urine (Ward et al., 2014). Urine pH may contribute to the variability of methadone pharmacokinetics. Methadone is lipid soluble and has a pKa of greater than 9.2. When urine pH is less than 6, renal clearance of the drug accounts for 30% of total body clearance. When the urine pH is 7, renal clearance contributes little to the total body clearance (Yang et al., 2006).

DOSING RECOMMENDATIONS

The historic dosing of methadone for NAS was 0.05 to 0.2 mg/kg/d every 12 to 24 hours or 0.05 mg/kg/d divided into three doses and administered every 8 hours (Gomella et al., 2013). Wiles and colleagues (2015; $n = 20$) examined the pharmacokinetic properties of oral methadone to optimize the dosing regimen for NAS. Based on their data, the authors suggest two potential dosing regimens with a starting dose of 0.1 mg/kg/dose every 4 or 6 hours, followed by an expedited weaning phase to reduce the cumulative dose of methadone and shorten the LOS (Tables 9.3 and 9.4). The efficacy of these novel approaches has been validated in a large cohort of infants ($N = 360$) treated for NAS at six nurseries in southwest Ohio (Hall et al., 2015).

CLINICAL-MONITORING PEARLS

Oral methadone is available in 1 and 2 mg/mL concentrations that contain 8% alcohol (Mangat et al., 2019). Adverse effects of methadone treatment can include sedation, respiratory depression,

TABLE 9.3 Recommended Eight-Step Methadone Dosing for Neonatal Abstinence Syndrome

DOSE	FREQUENCY
0.1 mg/kg	Q6h x4
0.075 mg/kg	Q12h x2
0.05 mg/kg	Q12h x2
0.04 mg/kg	Q12h x2
0.03 mg/kg	Q12h x2
0.02 mg/kg	Q12h x2
0.01 mg/kg	Q12h x2
0.01 mg/kg	Q24h x1

Source: From Wiles, J. R., Isemann, B., Mizuno, T., Tabangin, M. E., Ward, L. P., Akinbi, H., & Vinks, A. A. (2015). Pharmacokinetics of oral methadone in the treatment of neonatal abstinence syndrome: A pilot study. *Journal of Pediatrics, 167*(6), 1214–1220. https://doi.org/10.1016/j.jpeds.2015.08.032

TABLE 9.4 Recommended 10-Step Methadone Dosing for Neonatal Abstinence Syndrome

DOSE	FREQUENCY
0.1 mg/kg	Q4h x6
0.1 mg/kg	Q8h x3
0.1 mg/kg	Q12h x2
0.075 mg/kg	Q12h x2
0.05 mg/kg	Q12h x2
0.04 mg/kg	Q12h x2
0.03 mg/kg	Q12h x2
0.02 mg/kg	Q12h x2
0.01 mg/kg	Q12h x2
0.01 mg/kg	Q24h x1

Source: From Wiles, J. R., Isemann, B., Mizuno, T., Tabangin, M. E., Ward, L. P., Akinbi, H., & Vinks, A. A. (2015). Pharmacokinetics of oral methadone in the treatment of neonatal abstinence syndrome: A pilot study. *Journal of Pediatrics, 167*(6), 1214–1220. https://doi.org/10.1016/j.jpeds.2015.08.032

and corrected QT interval (QTc) prolongation, which can lead to ventricular dysrhythmias (Schwinghammer et al., 2018; Thigpen et al., 2019). Little is known about the occurrence of methadone-induced QTc prolongation in the pediatric population. A retrospective study was conducted that included 89 patients from birth to 18 years of age who were treated with methadone at a tertiary pediatric hospital. Among the sample were six infants younger than 1 month of age. Of these six infants, three were reported to have a prolonged QTc. Prolongation of the QTc was defined as a QTc of 450 ms or greater. No specific data were provided regarding the dose of methadone the infants with prolonged QTc interval received. In patients with QTc prolongation, the longest mean QTc was 496 ± 43 ms, compared to 410 ms in patients without prolongation. The QTc prolongation was seen more frequently in patients with cardiac disease. Methadone was not used to treat NAS in this study (Schwinghammer et al., 2018).

An additional retrospective study examined prolongation of the QTc in infants treated with methadone with a mean gestational age of 32 ± 5.5 weeks (n = 44). The mean methadone equivalent oral dose was 0.52 mg/kg/d (range = 0.03 to 20.96 mg/kg/d in oral methadone equivalents). Nine infants received a dose of greater than 1 mg/kg/d. Electrocardiography (ECG) data were available prior to methadone treatment and at 8 days and 17 days during treatment for 38 infants. Prolongation of the QTc was defined as a QTc greater than 500 ms, or greater than 460 ms with an increase from baseline greater than 40 ms. The median baseline QTc was 426 ms, and 424 ms after methadone. These changes were not significant (p = .39). Only one patient had an increased QTc of 79 ms from baseline (388 to 467) on a dose of 0.58 mg/kg/d oral morphine equivalent; however, when the dose was decreased to 0.42 mg/kg/d, the QTc value decreased to 433 ms (Snyder et al.,

2021). These studies suggest that methadone use is safe in infants; however, it is recommended that a baseline ECG be obtained prior to starting methadone, followed by an additional ECG when steady state of the drug is reached (Snyder et al., 2021). In addition, the inclusion of ECG monitoring in RCTs would help to confirm the results of these two studies.

Buprenorphine

Buprenorphine has demonstrated shorter LOS and duration of medication use compared to morphine (Frazier et al., 2020; Kraft et al., 2008, 2011, 2017), which is the first-line medication in the majority of U.S. locations (Byerley et al., 2021; Kocherlakota, 2014). Hall and colleagues (2016) retrospectively compared buprenorphine to methadone ($N = 201$) and patients in the buprenorphine group had less opioid exposure and shorter LOS. Subsequently, a small RCT ($N = 63$) documented significantly fewer days of opioid treatment (15 vs. 28 days, $p < .001$) and a shorter LOS (21 vs. 33 days, $p < .001$) in neonates randomized to buprenorphine compared to morphine (Kraft et al., 2017). Adjunct phenobarbital use was also similar between the groups (15% vs. 23%, $p = .36$). Buprenorphine represents an emerging treatment for NAS with the potential to decrease LOS and duration of treatment; however, unique pharmacokinetic properties and an enticing adverse effect profile require further study (Frazier et al., 2020).

MECHANISM OF ACTION/PHARMACOKINETIC PRINCIPLES

Buprenorphine is a partial opioid agonist that binds to CNS μ opioid receptors. A partial agonist is a medication that binds to a receptor and activates it but results only in a percentage of the maximum possible effect (A. Jackson, 2010). Mu opioid receptor agonism is considered the primary mechanism for reducing withdrawal signs and symptoms (Kraft, 2018). Buprenorphine binds at μ receptors but dissociates more slowly than morphine, a full μ receptor agonist. Slower dissociation of a partial agonist means that buprenorphine remains bound to a receptor for a longer period of time, which results in sustained, less-than-maximal effects and prevents other substances from binding to a receptor. This results in antagonism at the receptor (Indivior, 2021).

The oral bioavailability of a 30% ethanol-containing solution has been estimated at 7% due to first-pass metabolism (Ng et al., 2015). Buprenorphine is lipophilic, which allows for increased bioavailability with sublingual administration. However, administering a sublingual dose of medication to a neonate is difficult. Practical processes include administering the buprenorphine under the tongue and inserting a pacifier to increase mucosal contact time. Interpatient and intrapatient variabilities may be due to the percentage of medication absorbed in the sublingual space relative to the percentage swallowed with each dose (Kraft et al., 2008). Buprenorphine is primarily metabolized by CYP3A4 to the active metabolite norbuprenorphine, which subsequently undergoes glucuronidation via UGT1A3. Buprenorphine is excreted as unchanged drug and metabolites in both feces (~70%) and urine (~30%). The half-life was estimated at 11 hours and clearance was estimated at 3.5 L/kg/hr in neonates at approximately 5 days of age and weighing approximately 3 kg. Clearance was impacted by body weight and postnatal age and was not affected by concomitant phenobarbital administration (Ng et al., 2015).

DOSING RECOMMENDATIONS

Buprenorphine is administered sublingually when treating NAS. Initial buprenorphine dosing strategies range from 13.2 to 15.9 mcg/kg/d divided every 8 hours (4.4 to 5.3 mcg/kg/dose; Kraft et al., 2008, 2011, 2017). Kraft and colleagues (2008) evaluated plasma concentrations of the parent medication, buprenorphine, and metabolite, norbuprenorphine, after 13.2 mcg/kg/d dosing, which identified patient variation hypothesized to be due to swallowing differences, subtherapeutic dosing, or variable metabolism. Buprenorphine plasma concentrations were less than the adult accepted minimal therapeutic concentration and norbuprenorphine plasma concentrations were undetectable in over two-thirds of samples (Kraft et al., 2008). Lower-than-anticipated plasma concentrations of parent medication suggested subtherapeutic dosing strategies or insufficient absorption, and undetectable metabolite concentrations suggested altered metabolism

(Bio et al., 2011). In order to optimize buprenorphine use, Kraft and colleagues (2011) increased the standard initial dose to 15.9 mcg/kg/d, which has subsequently been evaluated in two clinical trials. Buprenorphine can be titrated up to a maximum of 60 mcg/kg/d (Kraft et al., 2011, 2017). Dose escalations occurred when a modified FNAST score was 12 or greater or when two or three scores exceeded 24 in aggregate. One protocol escalated doses by 20% (Kraft et al., 2008) and the other two increased doses by 25% (Kraft et al., 2011, 2017). After 3 days, stable regimens were weaned once daily by 10% when modified FNAST scores were below 8 (Kraft et al., 2008, 2011). Kraft and colleagues (2017) adjusted the weaning protocol to start after 48 hours of stable scores and to continue once daily as long as the sum of three consecutive modified FNAST scores was below 18.

Buprenorphine is not available as a manufactured solution. An extemporaneous compound is required. The compounded concentration is 75 mcg/mL, which is made using an injectable manufactured product, alcohol, and simple syrup (Anagnostis et al., 2011). The resulting extemporaneous compound is 30% alcohol, which has caused apprehension in some studies (Hall et al., 2016). However, the volume of each dose is small, minimizing alcohol exposure. Alcohol exposure from the compounded product does not exceed the ethanol serum concentration threshold of 25 mg/dL established by the American Academy of Pediatrics (Committee on Drugs, 1984). No patient in the Kraft and colleagues (2017) study exceeded ethanol concentrations of 7 mg/dL. Of note, the percentage of alcohol of the product exceeds the over-the-counter recommendation of 0.5% alcohol content in formulations for patients under 6 years of age (*Code of Federal Regulations*, 2020). Expiration dating varies based on the product storage container (e.g., oral syringe, amber via; Taketomo, 2023).

CLINICAL-MONITORING PEARLS

Compared to morphine and methadone, buprenorphine does not have depressive respiratory effects due to its partial agonism and antagonism. Cardiovascular effects are also minimized compared to other opioids. In the RCT comparing buprenorphine to morphine (Kraft et al., 2017), adverse event profiles were similar between the groups. Buprenorphine is an emerging possible first-line agent with minimal adverse events. If a reduced or no-alcohol content formulation is developed, use may be adopted more broadly (Kraft, 2018).

Adjunctive Pharmacotherapies

Phenobarbital and clonidine are considered to be most effective as adjunctive or secondary pharmacotherapies for infants whose withdrawal is uncontrolled with NPI and primary therapies have reached maximum dosing. Although safety profiles for phenobarbital and clonidine for use in the neonatal population have not been adequately established and side effects, including hypotension, bradycardia, and oversedation, are a major concern, the literature is supportive of use in mitigating the effects of withdrawal (Wachman et al., 2018). According to Anbalagan and Mendez (2021), in the United States, phenobarbital is used more frequently than clonidine for nonopioid or polydrug-exposed infants. There is a lack of consensus in the literature regarding which medication is more effective (Burgos & Burke, 2009; Finnegan et al., 1979, 1984).

PHENOBARBITAL

A long-lasting barbiturate, phenobarbital is one of the oldest anticonvulsants in use. A high concentration of alcohol (13.5%–15% in the oral and 10% in the IV solutions) and side effects that include global oversedation, plus a potential impact on long-term neurodevelopmental outcomes, are major concerns in the neonatal population (Anbalagan & Mendez, 2021; Nahata et al., 1986; Roberts, 1984). From a historical perspective, phenobarbital has been shown to result in a significant decrease in hospitalization days from 79 to 38 days ($p < .001$) when used as an adjunct to tincture of opium in the treatment of NAS (Coyle et al., 2002). We refer readers to Chapter 12, "Neonatal Seizures," for an expanded discussion of phenobarbital.

Mechanism of Action/Pharmacokinetic Principles

Phenobarbital is a GABA agonist and CNS depressant that decreases seizure activity (and symptoms of NAS) by promoting inhibitory neurotransmission (Mangat et al., 2019). The volume of distribution in neonates (0.64 to 1.17 L/kg) is larger than in the adult population (Donovan et al., 2016; Roberts, 1984). The half-life of phenobarbital is 73.9 to 154.5 hours, with maximum serum concentrations occurring at 2 and 2 to 4 hours following intramuscular and oral administration, respectively (Donovan et al., 2016; Roberts, 1984). It is largely protein bound (30%), metabolized predominantly in the liver, and excreted in the urine. Renal clearance is affected by changes in the urine pH; neonates with acidic urine may have decreased clearance, leading to accumulation of the medication and subsequent toxicity (Roberts, 1984).

Dosing Recommendations

For the treatment of NAS, a loading dose of 16 mg/kg, with maintenance dosing of 1 to 4 mg/kg/dose every 12 hours, with a serum concentration goal of 20 to 30 mcg/mL, is appropriate (Burgos & Burke, 2009; Finnegan et al., 1979, 1984). Serum concentrations of 40 and 60 mcg/mL or greater are associated with sedation and respiratory depression, respectively. Avoid arterial infusion related to concerns for extravasation, necrosis, and gangrene (Cameron Pharmaceuticals, 2019). Although a variety of weaning schedules exist among various institutions, weaning the original dose by 10% to 20% every other day based on withdrawal scoring is advisable (Anbalagan & Mendez, 2021).

Clinical-Monitoring Pearls

Although it is not uncommon for neonates to be discharged from the hospital to receive continued treatment with phenobarbital as an outpatient, this results in a much longer exposure due to a slower weaning regimen and increased visits to the emergency room within the first 6 months of life (Murphy-Oikonen, 2018).

CLONIDINE

Clonidine has emerged as a potential primary or secondary treatment for NAS. A small RCT (N = 31) comparing clonidine to morphine as monotherapy documented decreased medication duration in the clonidine group (Bada et al., 2015). However, the consideration of clonidine as monotherapy has been overshadowed by the emergence of buprenorphine, a potentially safer opioid compared to morphine or methadone (Frazier et al., 2020). In modern practice, clonidine represents an appealing second-line option with superior short-term and long-term safety to phenobarbital. Clonidine reduced morphine duration by a mean of 27% in a placebo-controlled trial (N = 80; Agthe et al., 2009). In an RCT (N = 68) comparing clonidine to phenobarbital as second-line therapy to morphine, phenobarbital was superior at reducing opioid duration (−4.6 days, p = .037; Surran et al., 2013). However, phenobarbital was continued for an average of 3.8 months, resulting in substantially longer exposure to pharmacotherapy. This finding has been reaffirmed in a smaller randomized trial (N = 25), as well (Brusseau et al., 2020). On balance, the moderate reduction in length of therapy of clonidine is preferable given the expected short-term and long-term safety benefits compared to phenobarbital.

Mechanism of Action/Pharmacokinetic Principles

Clonidine, a centrally and peripherally acting α_2-adrenergic agonist, activates α_2 receptors of an inhibitory neuron in the brainstem, decreasing sympathetic outflow. Clonidine's inhibition of sympathetic outflow allows for effective treatment of NAS and other opioid withdrawal syndromes. Blood pressure may also be decreased due to suppression of adenosine triphosphate and norepinephrine of sympathetic nerves at the presynaptic α_2 receptor. Heart rate may decrease due to parasympathetic stimulation (Upsher-Smith Laboratories, 2018). Clonidine is an imidazoline, a compound containing a 5-member ring structure with three carbons and two nonadjacent nitrogens (Upsher-Smith Laboratories, 2018). Clonidine also agonizes the imidazole receptors centrally. The effects of imidazole receptor agonism are unknown in NAS.

Orally administered clonidine has a bioavailability of 75% to 95%; 20% to 40% is protein bound (Bio et al., 2011; Taketomo, 2023). Clonidine is hepatically metabolized, primarily by CYP2D6, prior to renal elimination as both inactive metabolites and unchanged drug. Neonatal half-life ranges from 44 to 72 hours and clearance is 0.16 L/kg/hr in neonates, which is approximately 5 times more and 2 times less than adult populations, respectively (Bio et al., 2011; Taketomo, 2023; Xie et al., 2011; Young & Mangum, 2021). Enteral nutrition does not impact the bioavailability or half-life of clonidine (Upsher-Smith Laboratories, 2018). However, renal dysfunction prolongs the half-life of the medication. Xie and colleagues (2011) modeled oral clonidine clearance during the newborn period. As neonatal renal function improved, clonidine clearance also improved to nearly 70% of adult clearance at 1 month of life. Xie and colleagues (2011) concluded higher weight-based clonidine dosing strategies may be needed starting in the second week of life.

Dosing Recommendations

Oral clonidine dosing strategies vary in the literature. Most regimens initiate clonidine at 0.5 to 1 mcg/kg/dose every 3, 4, or 6 hours (Agthe et al., 2009; Bada et al., 2015; Leikin et al., 2009). Doses were titrated to a maximum of 12 mcg/kg/d (Bada et al., 2015; Brusseau et al., 2020; Surran et al., 2013). Titration and tapering approaches also vary in the literature depending on their use as monotherapy or adjunct therapy. Bada and colleagues (2015), using clonidine as monotherapy, increased clonidine by 25% daily until symptoms were controlled and tapered by 10% every other day. When used as adjunctive therapy with morphine, clonidine was titrated by 1.5 mcg/kg/d every 24 hours until symptoms were controlled and tapered (after discontinuation of morphine) by 25% of the maximum dose per day (Brusseau et al., 2020). Another approach initiated morphine and clonidine at doses proportional to initial Finnegan scoring, and decreased clonidine after morphine discontinuation by 50% daily in a two-step process (e.g., 6 to 3 to 1.5 mcg/kg/d to 0; Surran et al., 2013).

A commercial oral liquid formulation of clonidine is not available, which requires a suspension to be compounded. Extemporaneous preparations may be compounded in different concentrations: 10 mcg/mL (Ma et al., 2014), 20 mcg/mL (Sauberan et al., 2016), or 100 mcg/mL (Levinson & Johnson, 1992). Through a Standardize-4-Safety initiative undertaken by the American Society of Health-System Pharmacists (ASHP) via an FDA grant, standard concentrations for compounded medications used in neonatal and pediatric populations were recommended. The recommended standard suspension concentration for clonidine is 20 mcg/mL (ASHP, n.d.).

Clinical-Monitoring Pearls

Clonidine has a relatively benign adverse effect profile, including hypotension and rebound hypertension. A case series describing clonidine use as monotherapy noted no bradycardia, excessive sedation, hypotension, or oxygen desaturations (Leikin at al., 2009). When patients who received morphine monotherapy were compared to those who received clonidine monotherapy after 1 year, neurobehavioral performance in cognitive, language, and motor skills did not vary between the groups (Bada at al., 2015). When clonidine was compared to phenobarbital as adjunctive treatment with morphine, no arrhythmias, hypotension, or hypertension were experienced in one study (Surran et al., 2013). In another study comparing the two agents, seven total doses were held for three different patients due to hypotension and one patient experienced rebound hypertension (Brusseau et al., 2020). Rebound tachycardia and hypertension risk increases with abrupt discontinuation or quick weaning (Taketomo, 2023).

CONCLUSIONS

There is a wide range of literature that supports a myriad of NPI and pharmacotherapeutic approaches for the treatment of NAS. Most studies are based on empiric regimen creation using withdrawal symptoms as a guide. However, one approach that needs further research is a weight-based versus symptom-based approach, as it is likely that withdrawal manifests itself differently for each individual. This approach may help illuminate a patient-specific ideal dose that could have impacts on length of hospitalization and exposure to medications. Although morphine and methadone remain the preferred first-line pharmacotherapeutic agents, buprenorphine may evoke superior short- and long-term outcomes. Once more data are published around buprenorphine, the partial agonist, including long-term outcomes, the medication may become the mainstay of therapy. Respiratory depression is minimized compared to other opioids and barbiturates, and cardiovascular fluctuations in blood pressure and heart rate are also minimized compared to opioids, barbiturates, and α-agonists. The barriers to use currently include the aforementioned alcohol content and the processes required for compounding. Once a manufactured, alcohol-free formulation is available, buprenorphine adoption should increase. Phenobarbital has traditionally been used as adjunctive therapy; however, concerns over long-term impact discourage widespread use in neonates with NAS. Adjunctive therapy with clonidine requires further research, representing a promising alternative with the potential to further optimize long-term outcome. In conclusion, we cannot emphasize enough the importance of developing a protocol and adhering to it, selecting a primary and adjunct medication, and educating all members of the healthcare team on the protocol.

LEARNING TOOLS AND RESOURCES

Advice From the Authors

Tiffany Gwartney, DNP, APRN, NNP-BC

Depending on what area of the world you practice in and the duration of your career, you will observe a menagerie of ways in which NAS is treated. The literature is largely supportive of nonpharmacologic methods of initial and ongoing treatment. Remember that involving the parents and families of this patient population in decision-making, hands-on care, and cuddling will lead to best outcomes. There is a major practice gap among these patients; do not be afraid to think outside the box or use technology to maintain a supportive, professional relationship with the families while the patient is undergoing treatment for NAS.

Karen D'Apolito, PhD, NNP-BC, FAAN

I encourage all healthcare providers to not use the term drug addicted baby. *That language has a negative connotation. The babies are not addicted. Infants don't crave drugs and seek them out. It would be better to use* drug-exposed infant. *These infants experience drug withdrawal from intrauterine drug exposure, not from drug addiction.*

John Brock Harris, PharmD, BCPS, BCPPS, FCCP

Neonatal abstinence syndrome outcomes are improved with standardized approaches within the unit. Pharmacotherapeutic treatment has decreased due to the emergence of effective nonpharmacologic approaches and use of standardized protocols. The first approach should be nonpharmacologic, adding medications if needed. Choice of treatment and adjunctive treatment will change over the course of your career and vary from institution to institution. However, following a standard initiation, titration, and weaning protocol will improve your patients' outcomes, decreasing lengths of stay and durations of treatment. One logistical thought from a pharmacist: When titrating and weaning your treatment of choice, please be mindful of what can actually be measured in an oral syringe.

Discussion Prompts

1. How does standardization of treatment, both nonpharmacologic and pharmacologic, as well as valid patient assessments between healthcare providers impact quality patient care?
2. What nonpharmacologic measures should be implemented when developing treatment protocols? Why?
3. List the evidence-based pros and cons of your unit's first-line and second-line medication of choice for NAS. If you feel a practice change is warranted, what barriers exist to such a change?

Mind Map

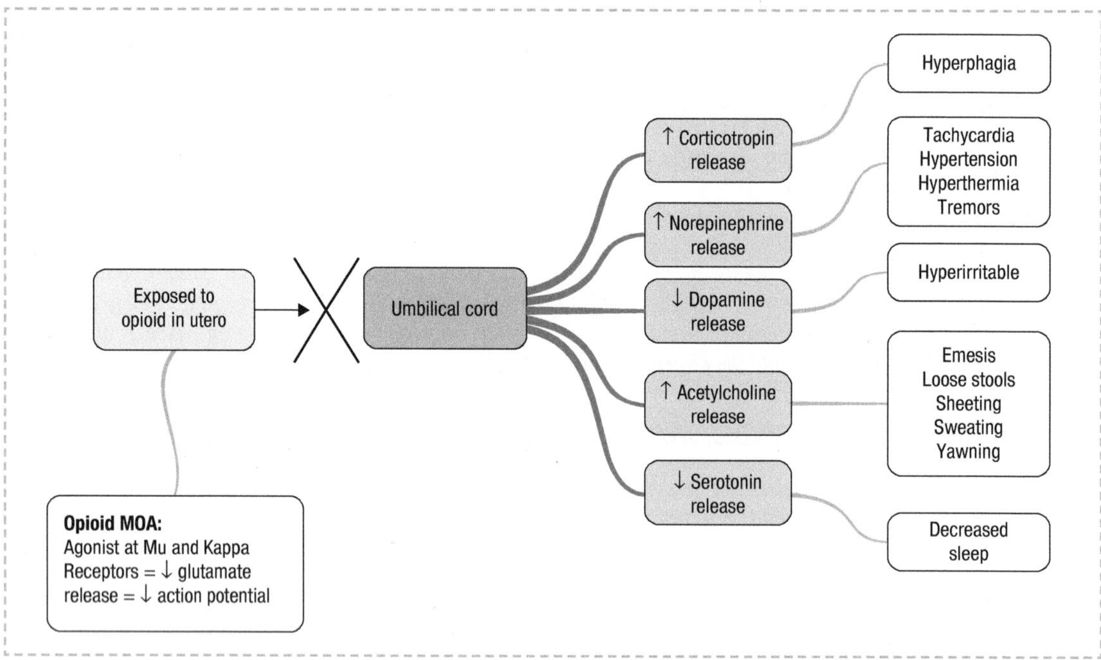

Design credit: Courtney Kitchen, MSN, APRN, NNP-BC, and Edythe Oliver, MSN, RNC-NIC, C-ONQS, East Carolina University College of Nursing.

REFERENCES

References for this chapter are online and available at https://connect.springerpub.com/content/book/978-0-8261-5884-0/part/partII/toc-part/ch9.

chapter 10

Apnea of Prematurity

Jodi Amador, John Brock Harris, Lisa Clevenger, and Andrew Heling

LEARNING OBJECTIVES

After completing this chapter, the reader should be able to:

- Define *apnea of prematurity (AoP)* and identify the epidemiology of the disease process.
- Explain the physiology of breathing.
- Correlate the pathophysiology of AoP with the need for pharmacologic treatment.
- Appraise the historical evolution of pharmacologic management for AoP.
- Evaluate current pharmacologic therapies for treatment of AoP.

INTRODUCTION

A well-established definition of *apnea of prematurity* (*AoP*) is a cessation of breathing for at least 20 seconds in preterm infants, or for a shorter duration if accompanied by hypoxemia and/or bradycardia (Eichenwald & American Academy of Pediatrics [AAP] Committee on Fetus and Newborn [COFN], 2016). However, there is no consensus on the duration or severity of what constitutes a significant bradycardia or hypoxemia event. Schoen et al. (2014) and Zhao et al. (2011) attempted to refine the definition, offering that AoP is a pause in breathing for at least 15 to 20 seconds, or shorter if accompanied by both an oxygen saturation level of 80% or less and a decrease in heart rate to lower than 67% of baseline levels for at least 4 seconds in infants born less than 37 weeks' gestational age (GA). Their definition has not been universally accepted.

The incidence of AoP is inversely related to GA at birth (Bakewell-Sachs et al., 2009; Darnall et al., 1997; Eichenwald & AAP COFN, 2016; Eichenwald et al., 1997; Fairchild et al., 2016; Henderson-Smart, 1981; Pillekamp et al., 2007). AoP is diagnosed nearly universally in infants born less than 29 weeks' GA, in greater than 50% of infants born at 30 to 31 weeks' GA, and in approximately 10% of infants born at 34 to 35 weeks' GA; rates of diagnosis vary across hospitals (Eichenwald et al., 1997, 2011; Henderson-Smart, 1981; Hofstetter et al., 2008).

Among nonventilated neonates, initial episodes of apnea and bradycardia most often occur within 36 hours after delivery, increase in frequency and severity before peaking by the end of the second postnatal week, and then continuously decrease in frequency and severity with advancing postmenstrual age (PMA; Fairchild et al., 2016; Pillekamp et al., 2007). Respiratory control maturation exists on a continuum, and maturity is increasingly achieved with advancing GA in utero and PMA (Patrinos, 2019). Infants born at GA less than 29 weeks often continue to experience apnea and bradycardia events until reaching 36 to 40 weeks' PMA. Some infants born at fewer than 29 weeks' GA may even continue to demonstrate events with decreasing frequency until reaching 43 to 44 weeks' PMA, at which time rates of apnea and bradycardia events decrease to levels that approximate those of term infants (Darnall et al., 1997; Hofstetter et al., 2008; Ramanathan et al., 2001). Conversely, premature infants born at 29 weeks' GA or greater who develop AoP routinely cease displaying apnea and bradycardia events before reaching 37 weeks' PMA (Bakewell-Sachs et al., 2009; Darnall et al., 1997; Henderson-Smart, 1981; Pillekamp et al., 2007). Infants born at term rarely experience apnea (Henderson-Smart, 1981; Ramanathan et al., 2001), and those who do should be evaluated for etiologies other than AoP (e.g., infection, metabolic disorders, neurologic pathologies; Patrinos, 2019; Patrinos & Martin, 2017).

A history of AoP may exist among infants who manifest with brief resolved unexplained events (BRUEs), sleep disordered breathing, and sudden infant death syndrome (SIDS; Erickson et al., 2021; Patrinos, 2019). However, AoP has not been proven to play a causative role in BRUEs or sleep disordered breathing, nor is AoP temporally associated with the timing of SIDS (Eichenwald & AAP COFN, 2016; Erickson et al., 2021; Patrinos, 2019; Ramanathan et al., 2001). Even further, there are no data to support that premature infants with a history of AoP who continue to experience clinically undetected apnea, bradycardia, or hypoxemia events after discharge incur increased risk of SIDS or hospital readmission (Eichenwald & AAP COFN, 2016).

Being diagnosed with a comorbid condition (e.g., bronchopulmonary dysplasia [BPD], necrotizing enterocolitis [NEC], retinopathy of prematurity [ROP]) is associated with delayed resolution of clinically apparent apnea and bradycardia events (Bakewell-Sachs et al., 2009; Eichenwald et al., 1997). Infants born less than 32 weeks' GA and who develop BPD may manifest with apnea and bradycardia events for 2 to 3 weeks longer than infants without BPD (Bakewell-Sachs et al., 2009; Eichenwald et al., 1997). Infants who are diagnosed with NEC or severe ROP may display apnea and bradycardia events for up to 1 week longer than would otherwise be expected (Bakewell-Sachs et al., 2009).

Given the incidence of AoP, its clinical significance, and the need for pharmacotherapy in treating it, neonatal clinicians must be prepared to identify the at-risk neonate, initiate and customize therapy to meet the needs of the affected infant, and monitor the infant for complications until respiratory maturation is achieved. Therefore, this chapter is structured to provide a brief overview of the definition and pathophysiology of AoP, its incidence and adverse effects, and a historical review of the evolution of its treatment. A thorough examination of the current treatment options, including nonpharmacotherapy and pharmacotherapy, is discussed.

PHYSIOLOGY REVIEW: BREATHING

The acts of inhalation and exhalation are modulated by a negative feedback system that is sensitive to changes in arterial pH, partial pressure of carbon dioxide (PCO_2), and partial pressure of oxygen (PO_2) levels. Under normal circumstances, afferent chemical receptors, located centrally in the brainstem and peripherally in the carotid artery, react to changes in PO_2 and PCO_2. More specifically, central chemoreceptors respond to changes in the pH and PCO_2 within the brain, and peripheral chemoreceptors respond to changes in pH, PCO_2, and arterial oxygenation in the carotid bodies (Prasad et al., 2021). Efferent outputs are thereby sent to muscles that affect respiratory control (Erickson et al., 2021). For example, decreased cerebral blood flow gives rise to hypercapnia, stimulation of the brainstem, and an increased respiratory rate. On the contrary, increased blood flow or a persistently elevated respiratory rate depletes cerebral carbon dioxide load and elicits a compensatory decrease in the rate of breathing.

Mechanical forces also implicate breathing. The primary muscles that affect respiratory control include the upper airway muscles, chest wall musculature, and lower respiratory muscles. For example, upper airway muscles located in the nose, mouth, pharynx, larynx, and trachea must maintain adequate tone to open and permit air exchange. Muscles in the diaphragm, external intercostal, and scalene muscles, as well as accessory muscles (e.g., sternocleidomastoid, pectoralis muscles), must function properly for inhalation to occur. As the act of inhalation stretches the bronchial smooth muscle, pulmonary stretch receptors must be activated to elicit the switch from inhalation to exhalation. Finally, internal intercostal and oblique muscle tone is necessary for exhalation and maintenance of proper functional residual capacity (FRC; Erickson et al., 2021; Patrinos, 2019).

The establishment of postnatal, continuous, and rhythmic breathing requires a functional brainstem capable of recognizing multiple afferent inputs from different receptors, appropriate chest wall compliance, and muscle tone. Preterm birth interrupts the normal maturational processes necessary for control of breathing and predisposes the neonate to AoP.

Types of Apnea of Prematurity

Before examining the pathophysiology of AoP, it is important to identify and define the three primary types of AoP: central apnea, obstructive apnea, and mixed apnea events. *Central apnea* involves an absence of inspiratory effort and chest wall motion without evidence of airflow obstruction. Central apnea is associated with physiologic immaturity of the central nervous system, including decreased myelination of the brainstem, lower chemosensitivity, fewer neuronal connections, and upregulation of inhibitory neurotransmitters (Kesavan & Parga, 2017; Rostas & McPherson, 2019). *Obstructive apnea* occurs when there is respiratory drive and chest wall movement, but an upper airway obstruction prevents airflow during the event. Obstructive apnea is caused by impaired neuromuscular upper airway control, with the obstruction most commonly happening at the pharynx, but it may also occur at the larynx (Erickson et al., 2021; Martin & Abu-Shaweesh, 2005; Martin & Wilson, 2012), and is particularly difficult to diagnose as commonly used chest impedance respiratory monitors do not detect such events (Eichenwald & AAP COFN, 2016; Erickson et al., 2021; Kesavan & Parga, 2017; Martin & Wilson, 2012; Martin et al., 2011; Patrinos, 2019; Soltau & Carlo, 2014). *Mixed apnea* involves both central and obstructive apnea, and typically occurs when airflow is obstructed following a centrally mediated pause in respiratory effort (Patrinos, 2019). In mixed apnea, respiratory effort will begin to resume following recovery from central apnea, but resistance is encountered from a closed upper airway, thereby extending the length of the apneic event (Erickson et al., 2021; Kesavan & Parga, 2017). Approximately 10% to 40% of AoP episodes are due to central apnea, 10% to 25% are due to obstructive apnea, and 50% to 75% are due to mixed apnea (Barrington & Finer, 1990; Zhao et al., 2011).

PATHOPHYSIOLOGY REVIEW: APNEA OF PREMATURITY

Altered chemical and mechanical responsiveness is associated with the pathophysiology of AoP. Premature infants have incompletely developed chemical receptors, immature brain development, and decreased neuromuscular control of respiratory muscles (Patrinos, 2019). This global immaturity results in diminished respiratory control and increased susceptibility to airway collapse, which clinically manifests as central, obstructive, and/or mixed apnea events, in addition to periodic breathing (Figure 10.1; Erickson et al., 2021). These factors are discussed in the following text.

Impaired Oxygenation Responses

Altered peripheral chemoreceptor function can contribute to AoP. As mentioned above, peripheral chemoreceptors are found within the carotid bodies and mediate the respiratory response to hypoxia (and hypercapnia). In older children and adults, a hypoxic state elicits an increase in minute ventilation (calculated as respiratory rate x tidal volume) in order to take in additional oxygen for transfer across the alveolar membrane. Among preterm infants, a transient compensatory state, referred to as *hypoxic ventilatory depression*, is observed. This involves a brief (2–3 minutes) period of compensatory tachypnea followed by a decline in spontaneous breathing effort, at times below baseline levels (Martin & Abu-Shaweesh, 2005; Martin & Wilson, 2012; Zhao et al., 2011). Incidentally, a hyperoxic state is associated with decreased minute ventilation, which in some cases leads to apnea.

Impaired Ventilatory Responses

Altered central and peripheral chemoreceptor function can also contribute to AoP. Recall that both receptors modulate the respiratory response to metabolic acidosis and hypercapnia. Older infants, children, and adults respond to hypercapnia with increased minute ventilation in order to expel excess carbon dioxide (Patrinos, 2019). However, this compensatory response is blunted in premature infants, who adapt by prolonging the expiratory time without a significant increase in the respiratory rate (Martin & Abu-Shaweesh, 2005). It remains unclear whether preterm infants elicit

FIGURE 10.1 A schematic showing how immature neuromuscular control, respiratory control centers, and receptors result in apnea and periodic breathing.

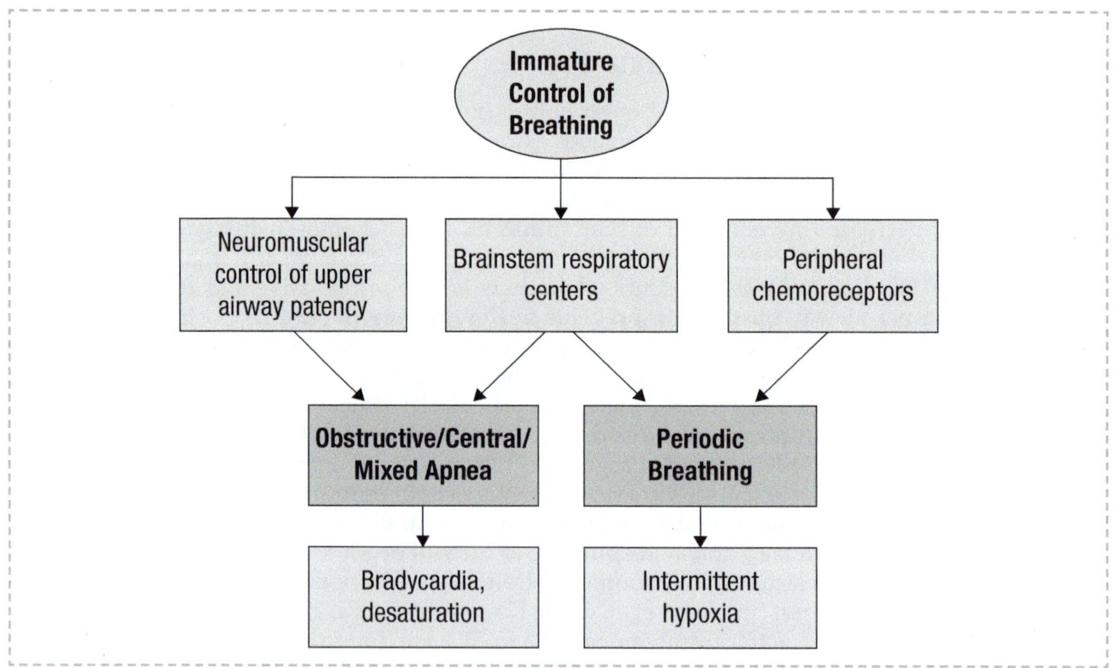

Note: Periodic breathing is another manifestation of respiratory immaturity; the incidence is inversely proportional to gestational age at birth (Barrington & Finer, 1990; Erickson et al., 2021; Richards et al., 1984). However, term infants may experience periodic breathing with decreasing frequency until 6 months of age (Richards et al., 1984). Periodic breathing generally does not lead to significant apnea or bradycardia events in premature infants (Barrington & Finer, 1990; Erickson et al., 2021).
Source: From Erickson, G., Dobson, N. R., & Hunt, C. E. (2021). Immature control of breathing and apnea of prematurity: The known and unknown. *Journal of Perinatology, 41*(9), 2111–2123. https://doi.org/10.1038/s41372-021-01010-z.

a change in tidal volume during hypercapnic episodes; some research shows an initial increase in tidal volume and others show minimal to no change (Kesavan & Parga, 2017; Martin & Abu-Shaweesh, 2005; Martin & Wilson, 2012; Zhao et al., 2011).

Furthermore, hypocapnia may also result in apnea. The lower carbon dioxide (CO_2) threshold at which premature infants will experience apnea is only marginally below baseline partial pressure CO_2 levels in premature infants, which can predispose these infants to having more apneic events with short periods of hyperventilation or irregular breathing patterns during sleep cycles (Alvaro, 2018; Kesavan & Parga, 2017; Martin & Wilson, 2012).

Impaired Neurotransmitter Responses

Multiple neurotransmitters, including adenosine, gamma aminobutyric acid (GABA), prostaglandins, endorphins, and serotonin, have also been implicated in respiratory control dysfunction (Abu-Shaweesh & Martin, 2008). Adenosine is known to depress respiratory function and is of particular significance as methylxanthines are believed to inhibit central adenosine receptors (Patrinos, 2019).

Exaggerated Laryngeal Chemoreflex

Altered laryngeal chemoreceptor function is often exaggerated in preterm infants and attributed to apnea and bradycardia events during enteral feedings and with gastroesophageal reflux. The *laryngeal chemoreflex* refers to activation of the laryngeal mucosa via the superior laryngeal nerve as a means to protect the airway from aspiration during feedings (Abu-Shaweesh & Martin, 2008; Kesavan & Parga, 2017; Martin & Abu-Shaweesh, 2005; Martin & Wilson, 2012; Zhao et al., 2011). Swallowing movements and protectively closing off the upper airway are responses seen with this type of reflex, but it can also lead to apnea, bradycardia, and hypotension (Kesavan & Parga, 2017; Martin & Abu-Shaweesh, 2005; Martin & Wilson, 2012).

Differential Diagnosis

AoP is considered a diagnosis of exclusion (Rostas & McPherson, 2019). Additional potentially modifiable etiologies are known to cause or potentiate apnea in premature infants and must be considered, particularly when the frequency or severity of apneic events acutely increases or escalation of care is required (Patrinos, 2019). Such etiologies include infection, hypoxemia, anemia, patent ductus arteriosus (PDA), metabolic derangements, upper airway anomalies or obstruction, medications (including opioids, benzodiazepines, magnesium sulfate, and alprostadil), temperature instability, hypoglycemia, and neurologic abnormalities (including seizures, intraventricular hemorrhage, and bilirubin-induced neurologic dysfunction; Crowley & Martin, 2020; Patrinos, 2019; Rostas & McPherson, 2019; Soltau & Carlo, 2014; Zhao et al., 2011).

HISTORICAL PERSPECTIVE: SEMINAL AND OTHER NOTEWORTHY STUDIES

It has been known for more than half a century that premature infants experience apnea, and during this time both the definition of AoP and its pharmacologic treatments have continued to evolve. Selected landmark studies that have had a significant influence on the management of AoP over the past 50 years are highlighted in Table 10.1.

By the 1970s, aminophylline, a methylxanthine, was a pharmacologic mainstay for treatment of respiratory disorders in adult populations, but its use had not yet been studied in preterm infants. Kuzemko and Paala (1973) were the first to study aminophylline as a treatment for apnea in preterm infants in a seminal study which included 10 infants born at 26 to 34 weeks' gestation with respiratory distress syndrome (RDS) who developed apnea. *Apnea* was defined as "a period of nonbreathing, usually lasting more than 30 seconds, during which cyanosis and slowing of the heart rate occurred" (p. 404). Aminophylline was used due to its known "direct action on the respiratory and vasomotor centres and on the myocardium" (p. 404) and because it was determined to have a wide safety margin and easy administration. The study involved administering 5 mg of aminophylline every 6 hours per rectum for three doses, and then as needed every 6 hours until the frequency of apnea was considered controlled. The authors showed that infants who received aminophylline demonstrated a decrease in apneic events, and apnea resolved in half of the patients, revealing aminophylline to be an effective treatment for what was ultimately to be defined as AoP (Kuzemko & Paala, 1973).

A more modern definition of AoP originated from Bednarek and Roloff (1976), who defined *apnea* as the "absence of spontaneous breathing for more than 20 seconds or less if associated with bradycardia or cyanosis" (p. 336). Bednarek and Roloff (1976) performed a similar study as Kuzemko and Paala (1973) and administered aminophylline to infants born at 25 to 33 weeks' GA who developed apnea. The authors' findings were similar to Kuzemko and Paala's, further demonstrating aminophylline to be an effective treatment for apnea in premature infants.

During the 1970s, additional methylxanthines were evaluated for their efficacy and safety in treating what would come to be defined as AoP, including theophylline and caffeine. In 1977, Aranda et al. studied caffeine for treatment of AoP and showed that infants who received caffeine demonstrated a reduction in the frequency and severity of apneic events, as well as a reduction in carbon dioxide levels, a significant increase in respiratory rate, and no change in heart rate as was previously witnessed with theophylline use. The results of this study suggested that caffeine was both effective and the preferred methylxanthine to use for treatment of apnea in preterm infants. The authors were also the first to publish recommended caffeine citrate dosing, which included a loading dose of 20 mg/kg followed by 5 to 10 mg/kg daily or twice daily caffeine citrate, and proposed that infants who received more than this dose may have an increased risk for toxicity (Aranda et al., 1977). Following this study, caffeine increasingly became the primary methylxanthine used to treat AoP.

In 1999, caffeine citrate became the first and only methylxanthine to be approved by the U.S. Food and Drug Administration for treatment of AoP despite limited data on short-term and long-term effects. This led to the Caffeine for Apnea of Prematurity (CAP) trial, which was a large international, multicenter, randomized, placebo-controlled trial conducted to identify the short-term and long-term effects of caffeine when used to prevent or treat apnea or facilitate endotracheal tube (ETT) removal in premature infants born with a birth weight of 500 to 1,250 grams, but notably did

TABLE 10.1 Seminal Findings Associated With Apnea of Prematurity

STUDY	MEDICATION STUDIED	STUDY POPULATION	MAJOR FINDING(S)
Kuzemko & Paala (1973)	Aminophylline	10 preterm infants born at 26–34 weeks' GA with a mean birth weight of 1,479 ± 484 grams	• Aminophylline decreased the frequency of apneic episodes in preterm infants.
Aranda et al. (1977)	Caffeine citrate	18 preterm infants with a mean GA of 27.5 ± 0.6 weeks and mean birth weight of 1,065.0 ± 72 grams	• Caffeine was demonstrated to be efficacious in treating infants with AoP. • The first recommended caffeine dosing was published.
Eyal et al. (1985)	Doxapram and aminophylline	Part 1: 16 preterm infants with a mean GA of 30.1 ± 2.2 weeks and mean birth weight of 1,289 ± 460 grams Part 2: 10 preterm infants with a mean GA of 27.5 ± 1.8 weeks and mean birth weight of 808 ± 200 grams	• Doxapram was equally as efficacious in treating AoP as aminophylline. • Dual therapy using both doxapram and aminophylline was more efficacious than monotherapy using either drug. • The safety profile of doxapram was not established.
Schmidt et al. (2006; CAP trial)	Caffeine citrate versus placebo	2,006 preterm infants with a birth weight of 500–1,250 grams, with a mean GA of 27 ± 2 weeks	• Short-term effects of caffeine administration included reduced rates of BPD, earlier discontinuation of positive pressure, and a temporary decrease in weight gain with no difference after 4 weeks. • No major adverse side effects were identified, including no difference in rates of death, NEC, or brain injury as identified by ultrasound.
Schmidt et al. (2007; CAP trial)	Caffeine citrate versus placebo	1,869 of original 2,006 preterm infants with a birth weight of 500–1,250 grams, assessed at 18–21 months corrected age	• Caffeine use resulted in an improved rate of the primary composite outcome of death or survival with neurodevelopmental disability at 18–21 months corrected age. • No major adverse side effects were identified.
Schmidt et al. (2012; CAP trial)	Caffeine citrate versus placebo	1,640 of original 2,006 preterm infants with a birth weight of 500–1,250 grams, assessed at 5 years corrected age	• Caffeine use did not result in a statistically significant difference in the rate of the composite outcome of death or survival with neurodevelopmental disability at 5 years corrected age, but did result in improved outcomes of gross motor function, motor coordination, and visual perception. • No long-term adverse effects were identified.
Schmidt et al. (2017; CAP trial)	Caffeine citrate versus placebo	1,202 of original 2,006 preterm infants with a birth weight of 500–1,250 grams, assessed at 11 years corrected age	• Caffeine use did not result in a statistically significant difference in the rate of the composite outcome of academic, motor, and behavioral impairments at 11 years corrected age, but did result in reduced rates of motor impairment. • No long-term adverse effects were identified.

AoP, apnea of prematurity; BPD, bronchopulmonary dysplasia; CAP, Caffeine for Apnea of Prematurity; GA, gestational age; NEC, necrotizing enterocolitis.

not directly assess caffeine's effect on reducing the frequency of apneic events. In the CAP trial, AoP was defined as a "cessation of breathing that lasts for more than 15 seconds and is accompanied by hypoxia or bradycardia" (Schmidt et al., 2006, p. 2113). The dosing of caffeine citrate used in the CAP trial was a loading dose of 20 mg/kg of caffeine, followed by maintenance dosing of 5 mg/kg/d, which could be increased to 10 mg/kg/d if apnea continued (Schmidt et al., 2006).

The short-term outcomes of the CAP trial were published first (Schmidt et al., 2006). Infants in the CAP trial who received caffeine compared with placebo had lower rates of BPD, had positive pressure discontinued 1 week earlier, and experienced a temporary decrease in weight gain velocity, with differences in weight resolving within 4 weeks of receiving pharmacotherapy. Infants who received caffeine demonstrated no difference in rates of death, NEC, head circumference growth, or brain injury as identified by ultrasound compared with infants who received placebo. The authors determined that the caffeine dose used in the study was safe with a low risk of toxicity (Schmidt et al., 2006).

The primary outcome of the CAP trial was a composite of death or survival with neurodevelopmental disability, including cerebral palsy, cognitive delay, deafness, or blindness, at 18 to 21 months corrected age (Schmidt et al., 2006, 2007). At 18 to 21 months corrected age, infants who received caffeine were found to have an improved rate of survival without neurodevelopmental disability, and specifically had a lower risk of cerebral palsy, cognitive delay, and severe ROP (Schmidt et al., 2007).

Study participants from the CAP trial were followed through 5 and 11 years corrected age to assess long-term outcomes. At 5 years corrected age, caffeine was not shown to significantly improve a composite outcome of death or survival with neurodevelopmental disability, but did result in improved gross motor function, motor coordination, and visual perception (Schmidt et al., 2012). At 11 years of age, children treated with caffeine did not have statistically different combined rates of academic, motor, and behavioral impairments, but continued to demonstrate reduced motor impairment compared with those who received placebo (Schmidt et al., 2017). No adverse long-term effects were noted at either 5 years or 11 years corrected age, including no difference in risk of developing behavioral problems (Schmidt et al., 2012, 2017).

Doxapram, a respiratory stimulant, is another drug that has been studied for its efficacy in the treatment of AoP. Some infants continue to demonstrate frequent apneic episodes despite implementation of methylxanthine therapy. Eyal et al. (1985) performed a double-blinded study involving 26 premature infants to assess whether doxapram used individually or as an adjunct to aminophylline would be efficacious in treating AoP. Eyal et al. (1985) showed no significant difference in efficacy between doxapram and aminophylline when the medications were used separately, but noted a greater reduction in apnea frequency when the two drugs were used in conjunction. There have since been limited studies involving doxapram as an adjunctive therapy. Vliegenthart et al. (2017) performed a systematic review of existing trials involving doxapram and suggested that doxapram monotherapy may have similar efficacy in treating AoP as methylxanthines, but noted that short-term and long-term side effects have not been adequately studied. Further research is needed before doxapram therapy should be clinically introduced.

CURRENT NONPHARMACOLOGIC TREATMENT MODALITIES FOR APNEA OF PREMATURITY

Noninvasive measures that are associated with a reduction in apneic episodes include provision of adequate thermal and respiratory support. Hypothermia is associated with apnea; therefore, maintaining euthermia with the use of a double-walled isolette or proper bundling with use of an open crib is essential. Nasal continuous positive airway pressure (CPAP) is known to reduce the incidence of apnea in preterm infants by stenting open airways and maintaining adequate FRC (Erickson et al., 2021; Patrinos, 2019). Heated, humidified, high-flow nasal cannula (HFNC), nasal intermittent positive pressure ventilation (NIPPV), and noninvasive neurally adjusted ventilatory assistance (NI-NAVA) are alternatives to CPAP which also provide a mechanical stimulus for breathing. A new method that may reduce the incidence of apnea events involves the provision of vibratory stimuli. This therapy has shown promise in reducing the frequency of apnea, bradycardia, and hypoxemia events, but long-term effects of vibratory stimuli have not been studied and therefore this method cannot be recommended (Cramer et al., 2018).

CURRENT PHARMACOLOGIC TREATMENT MODALITIES FOR APNEA OF PREMATURITY

Caffeine

Caffeine is efficacious in reducing the frequency and severity of apnea in premature infants. It also has a superior safety profile and a more favorable pharmacokinetic profile compared with other methylxanthines (e.g., aminophylline, theophylline; Henderson-Smart & De Paoli, 2010; Henderson-Smart & Steer, 2010; Skouroliakou et al., 2009). Therefore, caffeine, a trimethylxanthine, is currently the drug of choice for AoP.

MECHANISM OF ACTION/PHARMACOKINETIC PRINCIPLES

Caffeine has several mechanisms of action when treating or preventing AoP (Figures 10.2 and 10.3), which include (Taketomo, 2023; Schoen et al., 2014) the following:

- antagonism of adenosine A1 and A2A receptors
- inhibition of phosphodiesterase, resulting in increased 3′5′ cyclic adenosine monophosphate concentrations (cAMP)
- stimulation of the central nervous system, resulting in increased diaphragm contractility, medullary respiratory center carbon dioxide sensitivity, and central inspiratory drive

Adenosine receptors are located in the cardiovascular, central nervous, gastrointestinal, pulmonary, and renal systems. Adenosine A1 receptor antagonism results in an increased respiratory

FIGURE 10.2 Schematic of caffeine's mechanism of action on receptors (antagonism of adenosine A1 and A2A receptors).

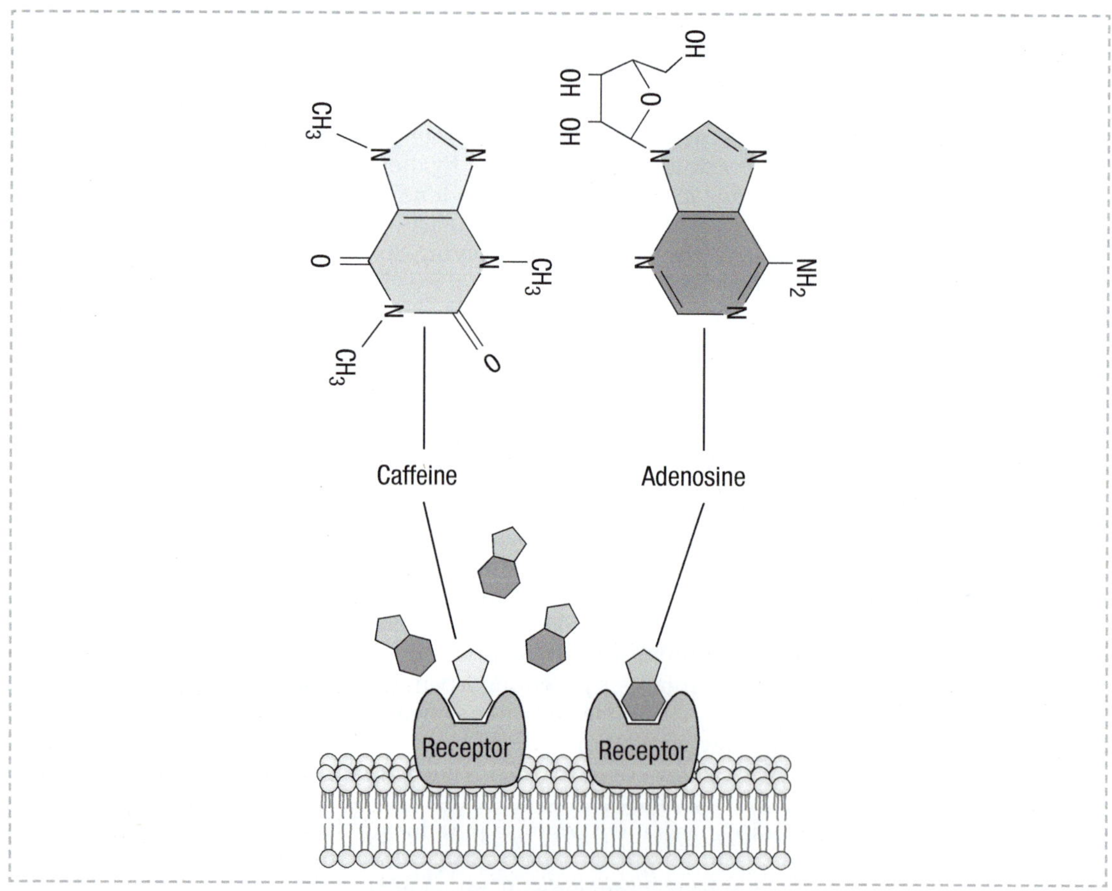

drive. Adenosine A2A receptor antagonism results in downstream inhibition of GABA neurons, ultimately suppressing inhibitory pathways in the pulmonary system (Schoen et al., 2014). Adenosine receptor genes have known polymorphisms, which may predispose some neonates to AoP and impact the efficacy of methylxanthine therapy (Kumral et al., 2012).

Pharmacokinetics in neonates differ compared with children and adults. Neonates have a greater volume of distribution compared with adults, at 0.8 to 0.9 L/kg versus 0.6 L/kg, respectively (Taketomo, 2023), which results in neonates requiring a larger weight-based loading dose to achieve therapeutic serum concentrations. Caffeine citrate is completely absorbed when administered enterally via a gastric feeding tube as well as intravenously (Charles et al., 2008). In preterm neonates, peak serum concentrations are achieved between 30 and 120 minutes when given orally (Taketomo, 2023). Therefore, clinical effects should be recognized relatively soon after administration, regardless of route of administration (Taketomo, 2023).

Caffeine is metabolized by CYP1A2, an enzyme not expressed adequately in the neonatal liver until approximately 4 months of life (Taketomo, 2023). This results in significantly reduced drug metabolism at a time when neonates and infants are subject to caffeine therapy; 86% of caffeine is excreted unchanged in the urine compared with 1% in infants older than 9 months of age (Sonnier & Crestell, 1998). In addition, the half-life of caffeine is approximately 15 to 20 times longer in neonates/infants (72–96 hours) compared with infants older than 9 months of age (5 hours; Taketomo, 2023). These principles explain less frequent (every 24 hours) neonatal dosing administration compared with older patient populations.

DOSING RECOMMENDATIONS

Dosing recommendations are identical for both intravenous and enteral routes of administration. Manufacturer labeling recommends a loading dose of caffeine citrate of 20 mg/kg followed by a 5 mg/kg daily maintenance dose beginning 24 hours after the loading dose (Ben Venue Laboratories, Inc., 2000). Note all dosing strategies are presented as caffeine citrate and not caffeine base. Dosing using caffeine base is half of the caffeine citrate dosing (i.e., caffeine citrate 10 mg/kg = caffeine base 5 mg/kg).

Other dosing strategies have been described in the literature. Maintenance dosing of caffeine citrate typically starts at 5 to 8 mg/kg/dose and may be increased to 10 mg/kg/dose daily if needed, a strategy similar to the one used in the CAP trial (Dobson & Hunt, 2013; Schmidt et al., 2006). Francart et al. (2013) demonstrated in a retrospective review of infants less than 28 weeks' PMA that infants who received less than 8 mg/kg/dose were more likely to need therapeutic intervention compared with those who received 8 mg/kg/dose or higher (94% vs. 76%, respectively). Another retrospective review compared caffeine citrate maintenance dosing of 10 mg/kg/dose every 24 hours and 5 mg/kg/dose every 12 hours, with no observable difference in the frequency of apneic or bradycardia events between the two groups, suggesting a lack of benefit in dividing maintenance dosing into twice-daily doses for preterm infants (Rebentisch et al., 2021).

A proposed alternative dosing strategy for using caffeine citrate for the purpose of facilitating extubation involves administering a loading dose of up to 80 mg/kg once, followed by maintenance dosing of up to 20 mg/kg/dose daily starting 24 hours later (Steer et al., 2004). However, loading doses of caffeine citrate of up to 80 mg/kg divided over 36 hours starting during the first 24 hours of life have been shown to result in an increased risk of cerebellar hemorrhages in a randomized, double-blinded trial (McPherson et al., 2015). Long-term safety and efficacy have not been evaluated when using high loading or maintenance dosing. Until more robust data are available on high-dose caffeine regimens, a lower, more traditional dosing strategy is recommended.

CLINICAL-MONITORING PEARLS

Therapeutic Drug Monitoring

Caffeine has a wide therapeutic index compared with theophylline. The therapeutic serum concentration range for caffeine is 8 to 40 mg/L, with data to support improved response in the higher therapeutic range, compared with 6 to 12 mg/L for theophylline (Ben Venue Laboratories, Inc., 2000; Gal, 2007; Taketomo, 2023). A pharmacokinetic study by Gorodischer and Karplus (1982) determined an effective caffeine serum concentration ranged from 12 to 36 mg/L, with infants demonstrating apnea with serum concentrations of up to 24 mg/L. Francart et al. (2013) retrospectively evaluated caffeine for dose optimization and found efficacious serum concentrations to

FIGURE 10.3 Methylxanthine mechanisms of action.

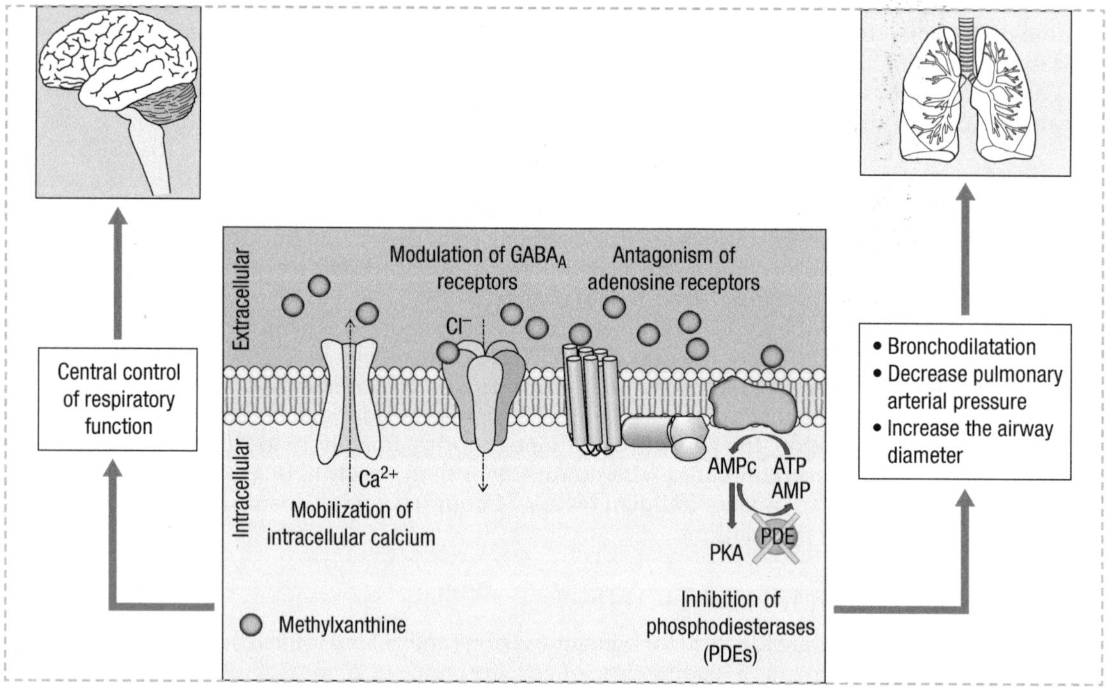

AMP, adenosine monophosphate; ATP, adenosine triphosphate; GABA, gamma aminobutyric acid; PDE, phosphodiesterase; PKA, protein kinase A.
Source: From Oñatibia-Astibia, A., Martínez-Pinilla, E., & Franco, R. (2016). The potential of methylxanthine-based therapies in pediatric respiratory tract diseases. *Respiratory Medicine, 112*, 1–9. https://doi.org/10.1016/j.rmed.2016.01.022.

be between 16.6 and 34.4 mg/L. A retrospective chart review completed by Alur et al. (2015) determined serum concentrations greater than 14.5 mg/L resulted in improved outcomes in infants 29 weeks' GA or less. These findings were similar to experiences reported at other institutions, as Kahn and Godin (2016) reported an improved response when caffeine serum concentrations were between 15 and 20 mg/L and Gal (2007) demonstrated that infants who had a serum concentration of 10 mg/L had 35% less clinical response compared with infants who had a serum concentration of 20 mg/L, with negligible differences in toxicity risk (Figure 10.4).

Caffeine also has a wider safety index compared with theophylline. Serum theophylline concentrations greater than 20 mg/L are considered toxic, whereas caffeine toxicity is associated with serum concentrations greater than 50 mg/L (Taketomo, 2023). One randomized dose–response trial of caffeine dosing strategies (3 mg/kg/d, 15 mg/kg/d, and 30 mg/kg/d) starting 24 hours prior to planned extubation did not find any significant differences in adverse events of tachycardia, jitteriness, or feeding intolerance at steady-state serum concentrations of 6.7, 31.4, and 59.9 mg/L, respectively (Steer et al., 2003). These ranges are not absolute, as individual patient characteristics may impact serum concentrations, efficacy, and toxicity, and adverse events may occur with serum concentrations below the expected range for toxicity.

Routine caffeine dosing strategies result in serum caffeine concentrations in the lower half of the therapeutic range. In a study performed by Skouroliakou et al. (2009), premature infants who received a loading dose of caffeine citrate of 20 mg/kg followed by maintenance dosing ranging from 5 to 10 mg/kg/dose had serum concentrations of 5.5 to 23.7 mg/L. A study by Natarajan et al. (2007) revealed similar findings, with infants who received maintenance dosing of caffeine citrate ranging from 2.5 to 10.9 mg/kg/dose having serum concentrations of 3 to 23.8 mg/L.

Because of caffeine's wide therapeutic index and favorable safety profile relative to other methylxanthines, routine monitoring of caffeine drug levels may not be warranted when traditional dosing strategies are used in infants younger than 33 to 34 weeks' PMA (Eichenwald & AAP COFN, 2016; Natarajan et al., 2007; Skouroliakou et al., 2009). There may be instances for which therapeutic drug monitoring is warranted. Obtaining serum caffeine concentrations may be useful for infants who are not responding clinically to caffeine or who may be experiencing potential toxicity. In addition,

FIGURE 10.4 Pharmacodynamic curves comparing caffeine efficacy (defined as acceptable or optimal response) versus toxicity (defined as tachycardia) based on 268 infants at a single institution.

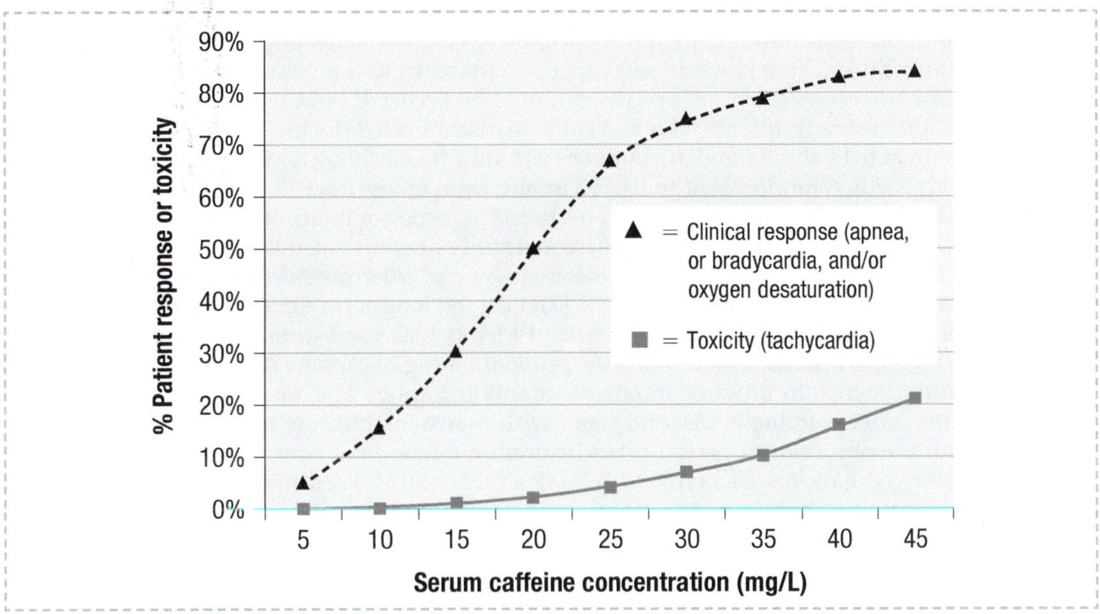

Source: From Gal, P. (2007). Caffeine therapeutic drug monitoring is necessary and cost-effective. *Journal of Pediatric Pharmacology and Therapeutics*, *12*(4), 212–215. https://doi.org/10.5863/1551-6776-12.4.212.

because efficacy is improved when serum caffeine concentrations are in the upper end of the therapeutic window, therapeutic drug monitoring may improve outcomes. Caffeine pharmacokinetics and patient characteristics change as patients age. Dobson and Hunt (2013) suggested obtaining serum concentrations may be beneficial in infants 33 weeks' PMA or greater as pharmacokinetic data are lacking for patients in this age group. Overall, the approach to caffeine therapeutic drug monitoring is institution-specific, with most practices obtaining caffeine serum concentrations only as needed.

Caffeine Citrate Initiation and Discontinuation

Caffeine initiation is classified as early (within 48–72 hours of life) or late (after 72 hours of life) administration. There have been conflicting data about the benefits and risks of early administration. In a retrospective study of neonates born at less than 29 weeks' GA initiated on caffeine for AoP, neonates who received early caffeine administration (<48 hours of life) had a lower risk of cognitive and neurodevelopmental impairment compared with late administration (adjusted odds ratio [aOR]: 0.67, 95% confidence interval [CI]: 0.47–0.95 and aOR: 0.68, 95% CI: 0.5–0.94, respectively) at 18 to 24 months corrected age (Lodha et al., 2019). Dobson et al. (2014) performed a separate retrospective study involving very-low-birth-weight (VLBW) neonates comparing early (within 72 hours of life) versus late administration of caffeine to determine differences in BPD and death between the two groups. They found the composite outcome of death or BPD was lower in the early administration group (odds ratio [OR]: 0.74, 95% CI: 0.69–0.8). The incidence of BPD was lower in the early administration group compared with the late group (OR: 0.68, 95% CI: 0.63–0.73), as was the incidence of PDA treatment and duration of mechanical ventilation. However, death was higher in the early administration group (OR: 1.23, 95% CI: 1.05–1.43; Dobson et al., 2014). A placebo-controlled, randomized trial of infants born between 23 and 30 weeks' GA who required mechanical ventilation was stopped early due to a trend in increased mortality in those who received loading and maintenance caffeine in the first 5 days of life versus a placebo (22% vs. 12%, $p = .22$; Amaro et al., 2018). Long-term outcomes of infants receiving early caffeine are lacking. Inherent biases in existing cohort studies and a lack of large, randomized controlled trials prevent a clear recommendation of optimal timing of caffeine initiation (Vujovic et al., 2020). Early caffeine initiation should be used with caution.

The AAP proposes discontinuing caffeine at 33 to 34 weeks' PMA or after 5 to 7 days of no apnea or bradycardia events while not receiving positive pressure, whichever comes first (Eichenwald

& AAP COFN, 2016). The PMA at which apnea and bradycardia episodes are expected to resolve should be considered. As described earlier, those who are born at 29 weeks' GA or greater typically resolve apneic and bradycardic episodes by 37 weeks' PMA. Those born before 29 weeks' GA often resolve apnea and bradycardia by 40 weeks' PMA, but in some cases not until 43 to 44 weeks' PMA. Typically, institutions discontinue caffeine at 33 to 34 weeks' PMA, reflecting practice in the CAP trial (Dobson & Hunt, 2013). There is significant practice variability, as a review of discharges from 2001 to 2016 from 304 NICUs revealed caffeine discontinuation occurred between 32 and 37 weeks' PMA (Ji et al., 2020). Interestingly, infants who had caffeine discontinued during the week of hospital discharge were shown to be discharged at younger PMA despite receiving a longer duration of caffeine therapy (Ji et al., 2020). A randomized trial of 95 infants born at less than 32 weeks' GA who received caffeine after 34 weeks' PMA demonstrated a reduced frequency of intermittent hypoxemia through 36 weeks' PMA (Rhein et al., 2014), and an additional study demonstrated that when similar patients were treated with increased caffeine doses the frequency of intermittent hypoxemia was reduced through 38 weeks' PMA (Dobson et al., 2017). Data on the long-term effects of prolonged caffeine administration, beyond approximately 34 weeks' PMA as was used in the CAP trial, are lacking. Additional studies are needed to determine the optimal timing of caffeine discontinuation.

It is common practice to monitor inpatient infants for apnea and bradycardia recurrence for a period of time after caffeine is discontinued, with many institutions monitoring for at least 5 to 7 days, with the observation period often beginning a few days after caffeine is discontinued due to its prolonged half-life (Eichenwald & AAP COFN, 2016). Feeding-related events are often considered separately when evaluating discharge readiness (Eichenwald & AAP COFN, 2016). The optimal time period needed to observe infants for subsequent events prior to hospital discharge remains unknown, as does when this observation period should begin following caffeine discontinuation, but a conservative approach is recommended. Therapeutic serum caffeine levels can persist for days after caffeine is discontinued. In a retrospective study, 29% of VLBW preterm infants demonstrated serum caffeine concentrations of 5 mg/L or greater 5 days after caffeine discontinuation (Chung et al., 2020), and a prospective study suggested that some preterm infants may continue to have serum caffeine concentrations on the lower end of the therapeutic range for as long as 11 to 12 days after caffeine discontinuation (Doyle et al., 2016). In addition, the risk of apnea and bradycardia recurrence is variable. In a retrospective study performed by Lorch et al. (2011), a 7-day apnea and bradycardia-free observation period was demonstrated to result in a greater than 95% success rate in predicting the resolution of apnea and bradycardia events in all preterm patients overall. However, the duration of the observation period required to achieve a 95% success rate in predicting apnea and bradycardia resolution varied by GA and was 13 days for infants born at 25 weeks' GA or lower, 9 days for infants born between 27 and 28 weeks' GA, and 1 to 3 days for infants born at 30 weeks' GA or greater (Lorch et al., 2011). The inpatient observation period need not be uniform for all preterm infants. Infants born at 25 weeks' GA or less in particular may require a longer observation period, and the event-free observation period may be individualized based on the severity of events (Eichenwald & AAP COFN, 2016).

OTHER NOTEWORTHY EFFECTS OF CAFFEINE THERAPY

In addition to treating apnea, caffeine has been shown to have other effects as well. We present these data and encourage readers to refer to Chapter 16, "Bronchopulmonary Dysplasia," and Chapter 17, "Patent Ductus Arteriosus," for additional disease-specific information.

Neurologic Effects

The CAP trial showed that premature infants with a birth weight of 500 to 1,250 grams who received caffeine demonstrated improved long-term neurodevelopmental outcomes compared with infants who received placebo (Schmidt et al., 2007, 2012, 2017). At 18 to 21 months corrected age, the risk of the primary combined outcome of death or survival with neurodevelopmental disability was decreased in infants who received caffeine (aOR: 0.77, 95% CI: 0.64–0.93), with the risks of cognitive delay and cerebral palsy specifically being reduced in infants who received caffeine (aOR: 0.81, 95% CI: 0.66–0.99 and aOR: 0.58, 95% CI: 0.39–0.87, respectively; Schmidt et al., 2007). At 5 years corrected age, there was no difference in risk in a composite outcome of death or neurologic outcomes, including motor impairment, behavior issues, deafness, or blindness ($p > .05$), but infants who received caffeine specifically demonstrated decreased gross motor impairment (Schmidt et al., 2012). At 11 years of age, some neurobehavioral outcomes were improved in patients who received caffeine for treatment of AoP. Although the rates of the composite outcome of impairment in attention, behavior, and intelligence were not different between groups, patients who received caffeine as infants demonstrated improved fine motor coordination, visual perception, visuomotor integration, and visuospatial organization at 11 years of age compared with those who received placebo (Mürner-Lavanchy et al., 2018; Schmidt et al., 2017). Notably, infants who received caffeine did not have increased risk of adverse neurologic outcomes, including specifically having no differences in the rates of brain injury as assessed via ultrasound (aOR: 0.97, 95% CI: 0.74–1.28), death prior to hospital discharge (aOR: 0.96, 95% CI: 0.64–1.44), or in rates of behavioral abnormalities at 11 years of age (Schmidt et al., 2006, 2017).

Davis et al. (2010) performed a post-hoc subgroup analysis of patients within the CAP trial and assessed outcomes based on both the original indication for initiating caffeine therapy (to treat apnea, prevent apnea, or facilitate extubation) as well as the mode of respiratory support infants received at the time of initial caffeine administration. The composite outcome of death or survival with a major disability at 18 to 21 months corrected age was decreased for all indications of caffeine use combined, with pre-extubation use specifically being associated with decreased risk (OR: 0.73, 95% CI: 0.54–0.99). Caffeine use in aggregate reduced the risk of cerebral palsy compared with placebo (OR: 0.6, 95% CI: 0.4–0.9), with caffeine use for the indication of facilitating extubation specifically being associated with decreased risk (OR: 0.51, 95% CI: 0.29–0.91). In addition, infants who received respiratory support via ETT at the time of receiving caffeine had a reduced risk of the composite outcome of death or survival with neurodevelopmental disability (OR: 0.73, 95% CI: 0.57–0.94), cognitive delay (OR: 0.74, 95% CI: 0.57–0.97), and cerebral palsy (OR: 0.59, 95% CI: 0.37–0.95) at 18 to 21 months corrected age compared with infants who received respiratory support via ETT and received placebo (Davis et al., 2010).

Pulmonary Effects

In premature infants born with a birth weight of 500 to 1,250 grams, Schmidt et al. (2006) demonstrated that caffeine administration for AoP resulted in a decreased risk of BPD, defined as supplemental oxygen required at 36 weeks' PMA. In addition, infants who received caffeine had positive pressure discontinued 1 week earlier than infants who received placebo ($p < .001$; Schmidt et al., 2006). In post-hoc subgroup analysis by indication for caffeine use, BPD risk was specifically decreased in infants who received caffeine for the purpose of treating apnea and facilitating extubation (OR: 0.62, 95% CI: 0.46–0.84 and OR: 0.63, 95% CI: 0.46–0.85, respectively; Davis et al., 2010). BPD risk was also decreased in infants who received caffeine and positive pressure ventilation (PPV) support via either ETT or noninvasive methods versus those who received placebo (OR: 0.6, 95% CI: 0.47–0.78 and OR: 0.58, 95% CI: 0.41–0.83, respectively; Davis et al., 2010).

Cardiovascular Effects

When compared with placebo, caffeine use for infants in the CAP trial decreased the risk of having surgical or pharmacotherapeutic closure of PDA (aOR: 0.32, 95% CI: 0.22–0.45 and aOR: 0.67, 95% CI: 0.55–0.81, respectively; Schmidt et al., 2006). In subgroup analyses, all indications for caffeine use decreased the risk of PDA ligation in the caffeine group compared with placebo, and the risk of PDA ligation was also decreased in the caffeine group for neonates who received PPV support via ETT or noninvasive methods compared with those who received placebo (OR: 0.33, 95% CI: 0.22–0.49 and OR: 0.33, 95% CI: 0.14–0.75, respectively; Davis et al., 2010). In a separate retrospective study involving premature infants born at less than 29 weeks' GA, infants who received larger doses of caffeine were shown to have lower odds of having PDA ligation (Puia-Dumitrescu et al., 2019). Note that the impact of caffeine on the need for PDA ligation is relational and not causative. During the time frames of the aforementioned studies, PDA closure was a treatment option for patients with persistent positive pressure and supplemental oxygen requirements.

Gastrointestinal and Ocular Effects

Infants in the CAP trial who were treated with caffeine or placebo for AoP did not differ in risk of developing ROP (aOR: 0.84, 95% CI: 0.68–1.03) or NEC (aOR: 0.93, 95% CI: 0.65–1.33) prior to hospital discharge (Schmidt et al., 2006). Interestingly, Puia-Dumitrescu et al. (2019) demonstrated that infants exposed to larger caffeine doses had lower odds of developing NEC.

Growth and Development

Infants in the CAP trial who were administered caffeine gained significantly less weight compared with those in the placebo group over the first 3 weeks of life ($p < .05$ for weeks 1, 2, and 3), but this difference was negated by week 4 of life (Schmidt et al., 2006) and there were no differences in weight gain between the two groups at 18 to 21 months corrected age (Schmidt et al., 2007). There was also no difference in head circumference growth (Schmidt et al., 2006). In a separate study, Philip et al. (2018) retrospectively reviewed the weight gain of infants treated with either 5 mg/kg or 10 mg/kg daily of caffeine citrate over 15 years at a single center. In their study, Philip et al. (2018) found that infants who received a maintenance caffeine dose of 5 mg/kg/d had an approximately 4 g per day greater growth velocity compared with the 10 mg/kg/d group during weeks 3 and 4 of life ($p = .04$) and 5.5 g per day greater growth velocity from weeks 5 to 8 ($p = .011$), suggesting an inverse relationship between caffeine dosing and short-term weight gain.

CONCLUSIONS

AoP is a developmental disorder resulting from an immature control of respiratory drive and function and is commonly observed in premature infants in the NICU. Other causes of apnea must always be considered, including neurologic, infectious, metabolic, hematologic, pharmacologic, and physiologic etiologies, particularly for premature infants who develop an acute worsening of symptoms and for infants who are born at term. The incidence, severity, and duration of AoP is inversely related to infants' GA. Extremely premature infants may continue to display apnea and bradycardia events until 43 to 44 weeks' PMA, at which time the frequency of apnea and bradycardia events equals that of term newborns. Premature infants born closer to term typically cease displaying apnea and bradycardia events before reaching 37 weeks' PMA. Wide individual and site variations exist, and premature infants with comorbid conditions, particularly BPD, typically display apnea and bradycardia events at a greater PMA compared with infants without comorbid conditions.

Despite biological plausibility, it remains unproven as to whether the frequency, severity, and duration of apnea, bradycardia, and desaturation events are markers of underlying pathology or are proximate causes of long-term neurodevelopmental impairment. It remains equally unclear whether a certain frequency, severity, or duration of apnea, bradycardia, and desaturation events is harmless (Di Fiore et al., 2016). There is no validated operational threshold of frequency or severity of events where escalation of therapy has been shown to result in improved outcomes (Di Fiore et al., 2016). As a result, there remains significant practice variability as to when and how to initiate, escalate, and discontinue therapy for treatment of AoP (Di Fiore et al., 2016; Erickson et al., 2021). However, it is clinically prudent for clinicians to aim to limit the frequency and severity of events infants experience as it is not known at what threshold apnea, bradycardia, and desaturation events are considered harmless. Providing appropriate respiratory support and maintaining homeostasis are considerations that should be given to all premature infants but particularly those with AoP. Caffeine is the primary pharmacotherapy used to treat AoP, as it is the methylxanthine with the greatest safety profile and has been shown to result in improved outcomes. Caffeine citrate is routinely administered to premature infants born at less than 1,250 grams until at least 33 to 34 weeks' PMA. Loading dosing of 20 mg/kg and maintenance dosing of 5 to 10 mg/kg/d are used to prevent or treat apnea or to facilitate removal of an ETT, although wide practice variation exists.

The questions as to the optimal PMA at which to discontinue caffeine therapy and how long to monitor infants after caffeine and positive pressure are discontinued remain unresolved, although the answers are not likely to be uniform for all infants and instead should be tailored based on individual patient characteristics, including GA at birth. A reasonable approach has been suggested by the AAP, which is to trial discontinuing caffeine after a 5- to 7-day apnea-free period while off positive pressure, or at 33 to 34 weeks' PMA, whichever is earlier. Infants should then be monitored for a period of time once off caffeine therapy, with many providers observing for 5 to 7 days, with the observation time period typically starting a few days after caffeine therapy is discontinued due to caffeine's extended half-life in preterm infants. The observation period may be increased for premature infants born at the youngest GAs and for those with a history of having more frequent and severe events. Many clinicians separate feeding-related apnea and bradycardia events from events that occur at rest when determining discharge readiness. Infants otherwise ready for discharge may continue to have clinically undetected apnea, bradycardia, and/or desaturation events, but these are of unclear significance as such events are not shown to be predictive of significant events after discharge or the need for readmission. AoP and SIDS are both associated with prematurity, but AoP itself is not a risk factor for SIDS.

LEARNING TOOLS AND RESOURCES

Advice From the Authors

Jodi Amador, DNP, APRN, NNP-BC

Throughout your career, you will encounter a multitude of patients. Many of them will have the diagnosis of apnea of prematurity, though each patient will be unique. Always take the time to assess the patient, know your patient, and listen to their parents. Often, they recognize the change in their child. Dedicate time to stay up to date on research, current practice, and recommendations. In the end, you will develop your own practice with the confidence to care for our special population.

John Brock Harris, PharmD, BCPS, BCPPS, FCCP

There are a variety of dosing approaches for caffeine. However, most use a loading approach of 20 mg/kg followed by 8 to 10 mg/kg of caffeine citrate, which equals 10 mg/kg followed by 4 to 5 mg/kg of caffeine base. With a wide therapeutic window, caffeine dosing adjustments can be made with limited to no therapeutic drug monitoring based on continued events. When determining when to discontinue caffeine, there are two schools of thought. (a) prove the patient needs it or (b) prove the patient does not need it. A patient proves to you they need caffeine by continuing to have events after discontinuing therapy at a predetermined postmenstrual age (e.g., 34 weeks) based on the institution practice. Proving a patient does not need therapy consists of waiting for the patient to not have events while on therapy and then stopping the caffeine. Anecdotally, option (b) tends to treat patients to greater postmenstrual ages than option (a). The duration of therapy and the watchful waiting after discontinuation contribute to patient length of stay impacting discharge.

Lisa Clevenger, MSN, APRN, NNP-BC

Reading, education, and understanding physiology are the best ways to learn normal and abnormal findings for patients. Apnea is a common diagnosis in the NICU, and if you invest the time in learning the physiology knowing how to treat it will become clearer.

Andrew Heling, MD

Apnea of prematurity is a frequently encountered condition in the NICU but remains a diagnosis of exclusion. Other causes of apnea should be considered, particularly when premature infants display an acute worsening in the frequency or severity of apnea and bradycardia events. Institutions should have standardized approaches to discharge management, including when to routinely discontinue caffeine pharmacotherapy and how long to monitor infants while inpatient for apnea and bradycardia events following caffeine discontinuation.

Discussion Prompts

1. Which patient populations should receive prophylactic caffeine therapy?
2. What frequency or severity of apnea, bradycardia, and desaturation events warrants an escalation of therapy?
3. At what PMA should infants routinely be trialed off methylxanthine pharmacotherapy when used for treatment of AoP, and should this PMA be different for infants born at different gestational ages?
4. How long should infants be monitored as inpatients following discontinuation of caffeine and positive pressure? How long should infants be monitored as inpatients if they have a subsequent apnea or bradycardia event, and should this PMA be different for infants born at different gestational ages?

Mind Map

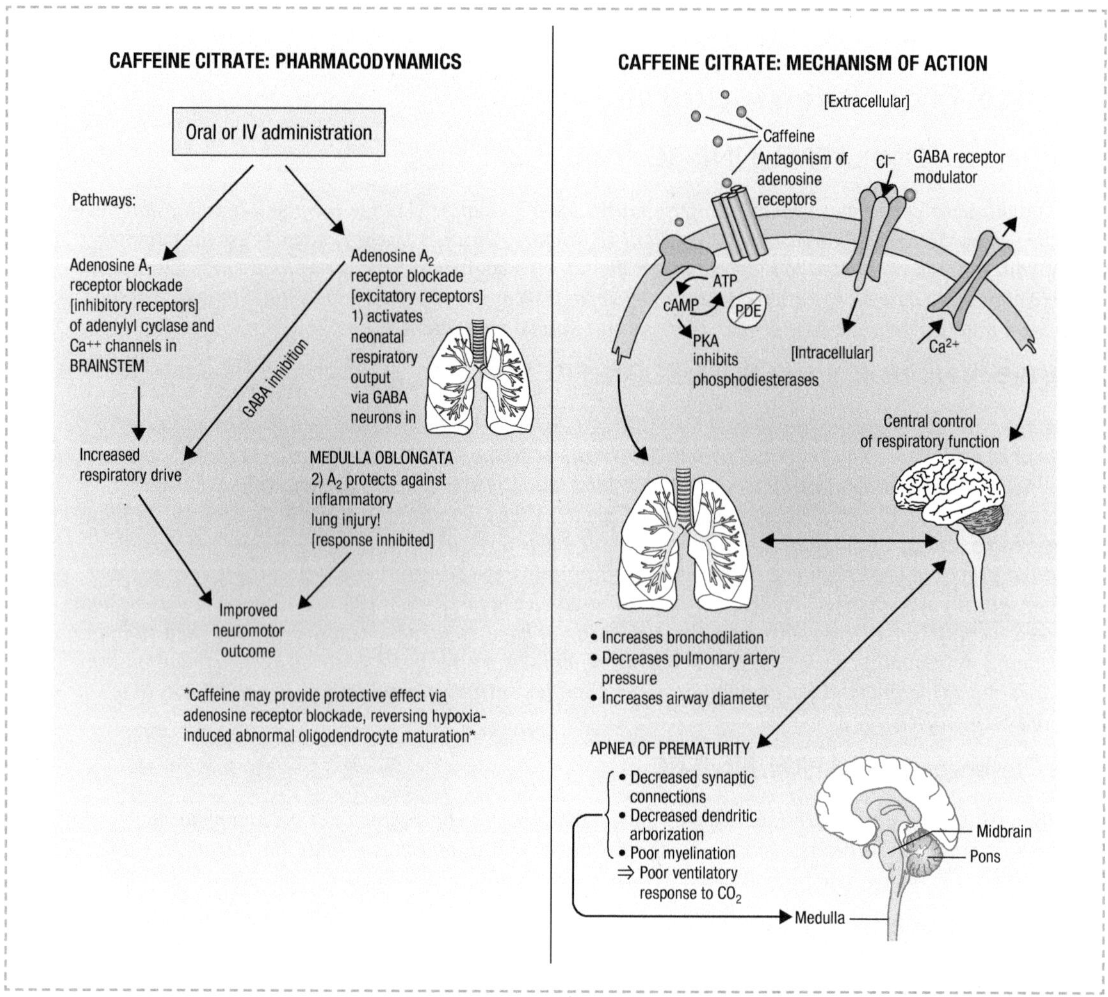

Note: This mind map reflects the design team's interpretation of a portion of one or more concepts addressed in this chapter. Readers should regard the mind maps woven throughout this textbook as examples of multisensory study tools that can be developed to encourage conceptual understanding. Readers are encouraged to develop their own unique mind maps in consultation with academic faculty or clinical preceptors.
ATP, adenosine triphosphate; cAMP, cyclic adeonside monophosphate; GABA, gamma aminobutyric acid; IV, intravenous; PDE, phosphodiesterase; PKA, protein kinase A.
Design credit: Lara Golden, PhD, MSN, RN, East Carolina University Neonatal Nurse Practitioner Program.

REFERENCES

References for this chapter are online and available at https://connect.springerpub.com/content/book/978-0-8261-5884-0/part/partII/toc-part/ch10.

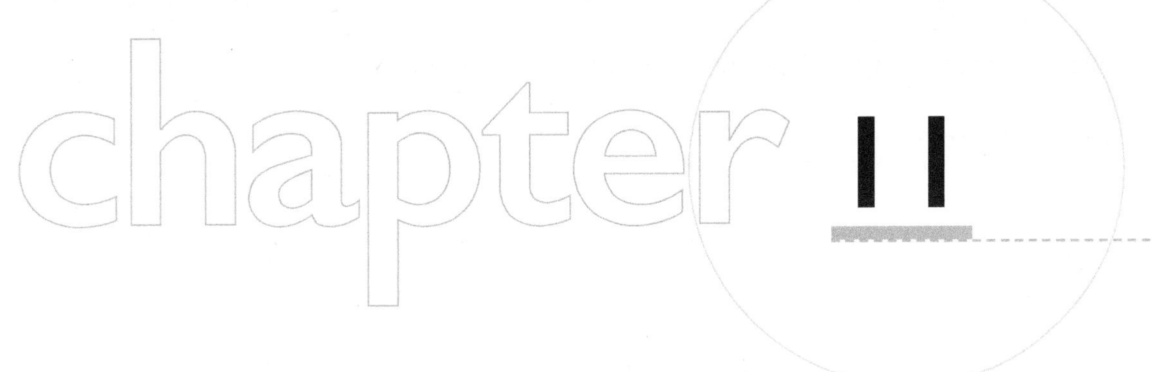

Analgesia and Sedation

Leanne Nantais-Smith, Carolyn J. Herrington, and Mirjana Lulic-Botica

LEARNING OBJECTIVES

After completing this chapter, the reader should be able to:

- Define *pain* and *analgesia*, and identify the epidemiology of the disease process.
- Explain the physiology of pain.
- Correlate the pathophysiology of pain with the need for pharmacologic treatment.
- Appraise the historical evolution of pharmacologic management for pain and sedation.
- Evaluate current pharmacologic therapies for the treatment of pain and sedation.

INTRODUCTION

Ten percent of all pregnancies in the United States ended prematurely in 2021 (Centers for Disease Control and Prevention, n.d.). Most preterm infants required hospitalization in NICUs, where they were exposed to multiple stressors, many of which involved painful procedural exposure. Historically, preterm infants between 27 and 31 weeks' gestational age (GA) average more than 100 painful procedures in the first 2 weeks of life (Stevens & Franck, 1995). More recent research confirms that although efforts to reduce procedures have decreased this burden, infants admitted to an NICU experience between 6,832 and 42,413 painful procedures throughout the birth hospitalization, with an average of 7.5 to 14 painful procedures per day during the first 2 weeks of life (Carbajal et al., 2008; Johnston et al., 2011; Roofthooft et al., 2014; Simons, van Dijk, Anand, et al., 2003).

A long-standing, traditional, and unscientific belief that minimized the need for attention to analgesia in the neonatal population was that an immature or underdeveloped nervous system protected the newborn, especially the preterm infant, from experiencing pain. In addition, pain was (and still is) usually described as subjective. This led to a misconception that a neonate's inability to definitively express pain meant that pain was neither perceived nor experienced. This perceived ambiguity left experts with the following question: *How does the somatosensory component of the nervous system process pain information from the periphery via neurons, to the thalamus, and to the sensory cortex* (Bautista & Grossman, 2019)?

Anand and Hickey (1987) suggested that focus be placed on nociceptive activity rather than on the notion of perceptions of pain (Anand & Hickey, 1987). We explore their work in a later section of this chapter. More recently, Puchalski and Hummel (2002) reviewed development of the nociceptive sensory pathways and summarized key evidence supporting the reality of neonatal pain:

- Sensory cutaneous receptors are present in the fetus beginning at 7 weeks of gestation (face), then 11 weeks of gestation (hands and feet), 15 weeks of gestation (trunk and proximal arms and legs), and by 20 weeks of gestation all cutaneous and mucous surfaces contain receptors.
- Synapse development between sensory fibers and interneurons appears as early as 6 weeks of gestation and neurotransmitter vesicles as early as 13 weeks, with completion by 30 weeks of gestation.
- Neural pathways for pain can be traced from sensory receptors in skin to spinal dorsal horn cells as early as 12 weeks of gestation, allowing autonomic reflex withdrawal from noxious stimuli, and to sensory areas in the brain by 24 to 26 weeks of gestation.
- By 20 weeks of gestation, density of nociceptive nerve endings peripherally may be higher in the newborn than the adult.
- Myelination of nociceptive neurons in the brainstem and thalamic tract is complete by 30 weeks of gestation; the entire nociceptive tract is complete by 37 weeks of gestation. Incomplete myelination results in slower, not absent, conduction; impulse has shorter interneuron and total distance to travel.
- Neonates (preterm) may have a decreased ability to modulate pain as a result of decreased inhibitory neuromodulators.

Thanks to the early work of Anand and Hickey (1987) and later work from Puchalski and Hummel (2002), clinicians widely agree that all infants, including viable preterm infants, have a nervous system capable of nociceptive activity and somatosensory processing. Infants can, in fact, feel pain by week 24 of gestation. In addition, descending inhibitory pathways are not mature until after birth, leaving preterm infants vulnerable to hypersensitivity to pain, or hyperalgesia, resulting from the inability to modulate, or block, painful stimuli (Perry et al., 2018). Hyperalgesia in preterm infants is exacerbated by local inflammation triggered by the initial injury and proliferation of new nerve endings (hyperinnervation), resulting in pain that may persist after healing of the initial injury (Puchalski & Hummel, 2002).

Although strides have been made toward purposeful assessment of pain and evidence-based pain management in the NICU, no research documents an overall improvement in neurologic outcomes among these infants, and, in fact, there is data to support that analgesia, in particular, may not ameliorate the neurologic sequelae. Thus, the use of sedatives and analgesics must be judiciously tempered between risk and benefit. Pain is harmful. However, zealous use of analgesia is also linked to the risk for harm, such as abnormalities in somatic and brain growth as well as neurodevelopmental outcomes (Chau et al., 2019; Ferguson et al., 2012; van den Bosch et al., 2015).

Caregiver knowledge deficits, attitudes about both assessment and management of pain, and gaps between knowledge and clinical practice in the neonatal population continue despite 30 years of research and education (Byrd et al., 2009; Cong et al., 2014). Despite significant research in understanding the physiology of pain, and efforts to reduce neonatal exposure, there is no consensus about safe and effective strategies for the management of pain and agitation in the neonate (McPherson, Ortinau, & Vesoulis, 2021). But it is now recognized that neonatal pain is real. Multiple pain scales are available for clinical use, but none are appropriate in all circumstances. These scales lack the specificity required to quickly quantify pain response in all GAs, and between acute and chronic pain. All pain scales use a rating scale, but there is still subjectivity involved in scoring neonatal pain. More objective tools available to measure pain include near-infrared spectroscopy (NIRS), skin conductance, and salivary cortisol levels. Additional research is indicated before these tools can be adopted for use in NICUs.

This chapter provides readers with a timely refresher of the physiology of pain and pain pathways. From there, we identify and discuss the effects of pain on the neonate. Next, we identify seminal and other noteworthy studies specific to pain scales and pharmacotherapies used to treat neonatal pain and agitation. Last, we present the current state of the science specific to pharmacologic treatment of pain and agitation. Learning tools and resources provided at the end of this chapter are offered to stimulate additional scholarly conversation both in the classroom and clinical settings, as well as encourage active learning habits for those preparing for clinical rotations or a board certification examination.

Definitions: Pain and Agitation

Pain is described as "an unpleasant sensory and emotional experience associated with actual or potential tissue damage or described in terms of such damage" (Raja et al., 2020, p. 1976). Heart rate and oxygen consumption are the most widely used indicators to appraise pain in infants, followed by respiratory rate, body temperature, and salivary or plasma cortisol levels (Stevens et al., 2013). Behavioral manifestations of pain include crying; grimacing; limb and trunk extension; squirming; startling; jerking of extremities; tremors; and finger, fist, or foot splaying (Yin et al., 2015). Crying is the most widely used indicator for pain intensity in preterm and term infants. However, crying may be reduced by up to 50% in premature infants as a consequence of hyperalgesia (Stevens et al., 2013).

Agitation is customarily regarded as a clinical manifestation of chronic neonatal stress (McPherson et al., 2020). Common precipitating factors include untreated, chronic pain; overstimulation from excessive noise; bright lights; chronic disruption of sleep–wake cycles; and the need for long-term ventilatory support (Noerr, 2000). Differentiating agitation from pain is challenging and this complicates prescribing decisions. Clinicians are often left to decide whether a sedative or analgesic is most appropriate in a given circumstance. As previously stated, the effect of sedatives on the developing brain remains unclear and they require judicious use in neonates (Duerden et al., 2016; Durrmeyer et al., 2010).

PHYSIOLOGY REVIEW: THE PAIN PATHWAY

A brief review of the nervous system and the mechanism of pain provides a basis from which to review evidence of neonatal pain in the developing nervous system. Students and clinicians should review this pathway before progressing to the latter discussions specific to physiologic consequences of pain and current pharmacotherapies. Specifically, the pain pathway works as follows in the nervous system (Bautista & Grossman, 2019; Huether, 2009):

- Pain receptors (nociceptors), which are bare unspecialized sensory nerve endings, are stimulated by noxious stimuli from the periphery (skin, viscera) caused by tissue damage.
- Noxious stimuli cause release of chemical mediators that translate information (transduction) into impulses; action potentials generated by excitation of the nociceptors propagate along specific nerve fibers, called axons (transmission), which are insulated by a myelin sheath that plays a role in conduction speed of the impulse.
- Cell bodies of the primary order pain-transmitting neurons located in the dorsal root ganglia lateral to the spine penetrate the posterior spine, terminate in the gray matter, and synapse with second-order afferent neurons (projection, excitatory, and inhibitory interneurons) in the dorsal horn.
- Nociceptive impulses are modulated by neurotransmitters (NTs), which are either excitatory (i.e., glutamate) or inhibitory (i.e., gamma-aminobutyric acid [GABA]) and bind to receptors in dorsal horn neurons in the spinal column. Excitatory NTs promote generation of the action potential in the receiving neurons; inhibitory NTs decrease the action potential.
- Impulses decussate and travel to the thalamus, the major relay station of sensory information. Third-order neurons in the thalamus relay the information to the cerebral cortex for further processing and interpretation of pain.
- Impulses can travel back to the periphery with an autonomic reflexive message to respond/withdraw.
- The body is capable of producing endogenous substances to relieve pain that inhibit the pain impulse via the ascending pathway (endorphins and opioid neuropeptides) and also via mechanisms of the descending pathway.
- Modulation of the nociceptive impulses produces analgesia.

HISTORICAL PERSPECTIVE: SEMINAL AND OTHER NOTEWORTHY STUDIES

Recall that prior to 1987, infants were generally thought not to have the ability to feel pain due to their immature central nervous development, and for those who thought infants might feel pain, the risks of anesthesia and analgesia were thought to be too great. Rationales offered for withholding anesthesia and analgesia centered on the belief that neonates were often too physiologically unstable, that anesthesia itself had a greater risk than benefit for infants, and that nerve pathways themselves were immature and not capable of transmitting pain impulses (Committee on Fetus and Newborn et al., 1987).

In a critical review of the pain literature, Rodkey and Pillai Riddell (2013) provide four views of infant pain that predominated in the 19th and 20th centuries: "the Darwinian view of the child as a lower being, extreme experimental caution, the mechanistic behaviorist perspective, and an increasing emphasis on brain and nervous system development" (p. 338). Rodkey and Pillai Riddell (2013) also provide historical insight about pain based on cultural and religious beliefs that prioritized pain as beneficial and necessary. They reviewed 20 publications from 1848 to 1974 refuting the ability of infants and children to feel pain. They remind us as well that anesthetic agents were limited to ether and chloroform in the late 1800s and early 1900s, which were difficult to administer safely and efficaciously.

All that changed rapidly in 1985, when Jill Lawson learned that her son, Jeffrey, born at 26 weeks of gestation, had undergone a patent ductus ligation without any anesthesia or analgesia (Rovner, 1986). As a result of Lawson's and other parents' investigation of the standard of care regarding use of anesthesia and analgesia for the preterm infant, the science of pain, pain assessment, and pain management changed quickly and dramatically.

Lawson's challenge resulted in a rapid response from the American Academy of Pediatrics (AAP). After reviewing extant literature on the state of knowledge related to pain in infants, the first official recommendation for the provision of anesthesia and analgesia was published in 1987 (Committee on Fetus and Newborn et al., 1987). See Table 11.1 for a brief review of the literature that influenced this seminal statement and launched what has become an extensive research trajectory on the phenomenon of pain and pain management in the fetus and neonate.

Following the AAP's official statement in support of appropriate anesthesia and analgesia for newborns in 1987, Anand and Hickey (1987) published their review of the effects of pain on the neonate, focusing on anatomy of the nervous system in the fetus and measurable effects that could be documented in the hormonal system. At that time, the focus was on short-term, measurable hormonal factors associated with the stress response.

The first studies published after the AAP official statement detailed the development of the central nervous system (CNS), peripheral nervous system, hormonal and physiologic changes associated with pain, and observable physical symptoms (cry, facial expression) and behavioral responses associated with pain (Anand & Hickey, 1987). Some of the early pain literature reported on pain responses in rat pups and studied the preterm infant's response to pain using the cutaneous flexor response. They noted that the response increases with GA, and that repeated exposure to heel prick can cause sensitization or habituation, depending again on GA; the most preterm responded with sensitization and increased response, whereas the more mature infant (>32 weeks' GA) responded with habituation (Fitzgerald and colleagues 1988). Fitzgerald and colleagues (1989) demonstrated the ability to reverse hyperalgesia from heel prick in preterm infants ranging in age from 27 to 32 completed weeks' gestation with the use of a topical anesthetic. This was one of the first double-blind studies to be conducted on pain reduction with local anesthetic.

In 1990, just 3 years after the AAP statement was published, Anand (1990) published a review of the literature describing the stress response in neonates and differentiated responses as they are impacted by GA, types of surgery, and variations in anesthesia. By the late 1990s, it was clear that there were long-term consequences of exposure to the multiple stressors present in the NICU, including maternal separation, handling, infection, and pain (Porter et al., 1999). These include lower pain thresholds, which lead to "windup" phenomenon, hyperalgesia, cognitive deficits, learning disorders, increased perceptions of somatic pain, increased likelihood of inappropriate social adaptation, sleep disturbances, feeding problems, and inabilities to self-regulate (Hack et al., 1994; Mitchell & Boss, 2002; Whitfield et al., 1997). These findings prompted the study of

TABLE 11.1 Seminal Literature Leading to American Academy of Pediatrics Statement on Pain in the Neonate

YEAR OF PUBLICATION	AUTHOR(S)	TITLE	MAJOR FINDINGS
1975	**Richards** et al.	Early Behavior Differences: Gender or Circumcision?	Circumcision has direct and indirect effects of unknown duration in male infants who have been circumcised. Future pain studies should include circumcision as a variable in analysis to better inform analysis of gender differences in pain response.
1979	**Brazelton**	Behavioral Competence of the Newborn Infant	Support for competence in the newborn to adapt to surroundings if secure. Presents the concept that newborns are capable of purposeful interaction with providers. This paper introduced the key elements of the Brazelton Neonatal Assessment Tool, which remains the gold standard for neonatal behavioral assessment.
1981	**Robinson & Gregory**	Fentanyl–Air–Oxygen Anesthesia for Ligation of Patent Ductus Arteriosus in Preterm Infants	This study reported on surgical stability in a group of 10 preterm infants undergoing PDA ligation with fentanyl, air, and oxygen anesthesia. Physiologic stability was demonstrated, supporting the use of fentanyl for safe and effective anesthesia in the preterm infant.
1983	**Williamson & Williamson**	Physiologic Stress Reduction by a Local Anesthetic During Newborn Circumcision	RCT of 30 newborns undergoing circumcision (20 received dorsal penile block, 10 received no anesthesia). Less stress was noted in the treatment group as measured by changes in transcutaneous oxygen pressure levels, decreased duration of cry, and smaller decreases in heart rate intraprocedure. No adverse effects were noted in the treatment group.
1984	**Owens**	Pain in Infancy: Conceptual and Methodological Issues	Brief historical review of the concept of pain in humans, discussion of applicability of the definition of pain, recommendation that there is ample opportunity to study pain response in neonates utilizing medically indicated procedures that are known to cause pain (particularly heel stick), and descriptions of multiple factors that can be used to assess pain in the neonate, including facial expression, body movement, cry, heart rate, and endocrine changes.
1984	**Vacanti et al.**	The Pulmonary Hemodynamic Response to Perioperative Anesthesia in the Treatment of High-Risk Infants With Congenital Diaphragmatic Hernia	This study reported outcomes of 14 infants who underwent repair of congenital diaphragmatic hernia under a prescribed anesthesia routine (fentanyl and pancuronium) and continued to receive continuous general anesthesia with those same agents during postop recovery. Results were compared with 19 historical controls who received anesthesia for surgery but did not receive general anesthesia postoperatively. The continuous-anesthesia group achieved significant improvement in intrapulmonary shunting within 24 hours of surgery, whereas the historical controls failed to reach half of the same level of improvement at 72 hours postop. Infants in the treatment group did not require use of vasoactive medication to maintain hemodynamic stability. This study supported continuous use of sedation and analgesia in the postoperative period for this critically ill newborn population.

(*continued*)

TABLE 11.1 Seminal Literature Leading to American Academy of Pediatrics Statement on Pain in the Neonate (*continued*)

YEAR OF PUBLICATION	AUTHOR(S)	TITLE	MAJOR FINDINGS
1984	**Dixon et al.**	Behavioral Effects of Circumcision With and Without Anesthesia	Infant behavioral responses were evaluated using the Brazelton Neonatal Assessment Scale (NBAS) 24 hours after circumcision. Three groups of term male infants were compared; one group received dorsal penile block, one group saline injection, and one group no anesthesia. Infants who received the dorsal penile block with lidocaine prior to circumcision were more attentive to stimuli and showed a better ability to self-quiet when disturbed the following day, in comparison to the infants who underwent circumcision after saline injection, or no treatment the preceding day. Support for use of dorsal penile block is provided.
1985	**Schechter**	Pain and Pain Control in Children	This is an extensive monograph discussing the complexities of pain from formulation of meaningful definitions of pain, mapping neuroanatomy, neurochemistry, pain transmission theories, and challenges with pain assessment in both adults and children. The author provided information about commonly used analgesics including both narcotic and nonnarcotic therapies, as well as some nonpharmacologic therapies. He closed with the acknowledgment that the current knowledge about pain and pain management in children was inadequate, and urged researchers to study a multitude of factors that impact pain recognition and management in children and recommended that the best approach regarding pain in infants and young children: (a) should involve close attention to physiologic factors (increase in heart rate, palmar sweating, rapid respirations), and use of visual analogue scales when age appropriate; (b) adequate analgesia should be provided and as-needed dosing should be avoided; and (c) importance of inclusion of adjunct therapies such as distraction techniques as well as inclusion of parents in pain treatment.
1987	**Anand et al.**	Randomized Trial of Fentanyl Anaesthesia in Preterm Babies Undergoing Surgery: Effects on the Stress Response	This study compared two groups: the treatment group underwent surgery with fentanyl, nitrous oxide, and curare, whereas the control group was given nitrous oxide and curare only. They used multiple hormonal levels to reflect the stress effect, including blood glucose, lactate, pyruvate, plasma insulin, adrenalin, noradrenalin, aldosterone, corticosterone, and cortisone. The samples were collected preoperatively, at induction, intraoperatively, and postoperatively at intervals during the first 24 hours postop. The results of this study noted that there were significant differences between the stress responses measured through hormonal response between these two groups, with the group receiving fentanyl having significantly less stress response to surgery and during the postop recovery. In addition, the nonfentanyl group was more likely to require increased ventilatory support and have circulatory and/or metabolic complications postoperatively compared with the infants who received the fentanyl regimen. They also noted that there were no "clinical signs" of pain in either group intraoperatively.

PDA, patent ductus arteriosis; RCT, randomized controlled trial.

the effects of early and repetitive pain on growth (both physiologic and neuronal) and brain function (Vinall et al., 2012). The earlier the gestation at birth (<28 weeks of gestation) and higher the number of skin-breaking procedures, the more likely the infant is to have alterations in thalamic, hippocampal, and amygdala growth, and to have decreases in brain volume; all changes associated with poorer cognitive, visual, and behavioral outcomes. These changes in brain volume persisted through early childhood in the infants they studied (Brummelte et al., 2012; Chau et al., 2019; Duerden et al., 2018). It is important to remember that pain is not the only stressor infants are exposed to while being cared for in the NICU, but it is one factor that can be readily addressed with appropriate pain management.

As we learned more about procedural pain, new frontiers arose and challenged us. In 2010, the AAP published a statement supporting premedication for nonemergent intubation in neonates (Kumar et al., 2010), which was reaffirmed in May 2018. However, no regimen of medications was universally adopted, and the range of possibilities was very large.

The use of analgesics and sedatives in ventilated infants has risen significantly without evidence to support clear benefit and lack of morbidity in infants in the NICU (Hall et al., 2007). Meta-analyses exist of randomized controlled trials (RCTs) comparing morphine or fentanyl with placebo, morphine with fentanyl, and midazolam with placebo. Primary findings include lower behavioral and physiologic indicators of pain in infants treated with opioids who need prolonged ventilatory support (Anand et al., 2004; Bhandari et al., 2005; Simons, van Dijk, van Lingen et al., 2003). Infants treated with midazolam had significantly more adverse effects compared with infants treated with morphine or placebo, including more days on the ventilator and increased risk for intraventricular hemorrhage (IVH), periventricular leukomalacia (PVL), or death (Anand et al., 1999). Zimmerman and colleagues (2017) conducted a large, multisite, retrospective study on analgesic, sedative, and paralytic use that included 85,911 mechanically ventilated infants in 348 NICUs between the years of 1997 and 2012. The study results showed a dramatic increase in medication use over the time period studied; opioid use rose from 5% to 32%, benzodiazepine use from 5% to 24%, and paralytics and other drug use remained unchanged at 1% or less. They did not find that increases were correlated with severity of illness overall, but rather varied by institution. They suggest that The Joint Commission standards regarding assessment and treatment of pain, including the use of continuous opioid infusions for the mechanically ventilated infant and availability of pain scales, were a major factor in the increased use of these medications, despite studies that now recommend judicious use of analgesics, sedatives, and paralytics due to the increased risk for poorer neurodevelopmental outcomes. Safety and efficacy of analgesics and sedatives remains elusive with our current methods of assessment, and to date, there are no studies comparing effects of untreated repetitive pain/stress with exposure to analgesics and sedatives in the neonatal period on long-term outcomes.

Therapeutic Hypothermia

The use of whole-body cooling as a therapeutic intervention for infants with hypoxic-ischemic encephalopathy (HIE) presents additional challenges to both pain assessment and pain management (McPherson, Frymoyer, et al., 2021). Treatment with therapeutic hypothermia (TH) is a stress-inducing event for the infant in and of itself, and concurrent therapies required for overall survival provide additive stressors. The provision of comfort measures is critical, yet ideal approaches remain elusive. Further, there is insufficient knowledge regarding the effect of sedation and analgesia on the already compromised brain of the asphyxiated infant, although there is growing evidence that general anesthesia is associated with undesirable long-term neurologic effects in young animal models (Vutskits & Xie, 2016).

TH reduces the metabolic rate, which alters pharmacokinetics, but these changes may be associated with both subtherapeutic levels as well as toxic drug levels (Wildschut et al., 2013). Other factors significantly confound efforts to understand drug metabolism, absorption, and elimination, including the degree of specific organ damage (kidneys and liver) as well as the rate of recovery during therapy, fluid shifts, and physiologic organ maturational changes that begin at birth (McPherson, Frymoyer, et al., 2021).

The use of sedatives and analgesics during TH varies widely from practice to practice (Natarajan et al., 2018). Natarajan and colleagues conducted a secondary analysis of the Eunice Kennedy Shriver National Institute of Child Health and Human Development (NICHD) TH RCT of infants with moderate or severe HIE. The focus of their secondary analysis was to improve knowledge about the effects of sedatives, analgesics, anticonvulsants, and neuromuscular blocking agents on neurodevelopmental outcomes of infants treated with TH. Their findings noted that of 208 participants, 18% received no sedatives, analgesics, or anticonvulsants during their TH; 10% received sedation or analgesics with no anticonvulsants; 39% received anticonvulsants only; and 33% received all three during TH. Thus, 57% of these infants did not receive sedation or analgesics during TH. They did not find an association between exposure to sedatives and analgesics and death or disability at 18 months; however, they also were not able to find an association between other outcomes and exposure or abstinence. Thus, they recommended systematic investigations into risk/benefits of exposure to sedatives and analgesics during TH.

Only one TH trial included continuous or scheduled opioids (morphine or fentanyl) for sedation, and this group demonstrated a larger effect size for reducing neurodevelopmental impairments or death when compared with historical trials (Simbruner et al., 2010). Interpretation of these results must be cautious, considering the high rate of neurodevelopmental impairments or death in the control group compared to previous RCTs. A secondary analysis of the Magnetic Resonance Biomarkers in Neonatal Encephalopathy (MARBLE) study found no neuroprotective effect of morphine infusion compared with infants who did not receive morphine infusion at 22 months of age in survivors, whereas there were significant increases in hypotension and length of hospital stay in the group receiving morphine (Liow et al., 2020). Could it be that the doses of morphine used (10–20 mcg/kg/h) resulted in higher concentrations due to the metabolic challenges of cooling and reduced clearance due to organ damage? The answer is not clear, and again reminds us that there is insufficient evidence at this time to inform best practice protocols for analgesia and sedation in this highly vulnerable population. Although many questions remain in the quest to provide comfort to this vulnerable population, one of the overarching demands is to continue to systematically assess the impact of all interventions on long-term outcomes in an effort to provide comfort without inadvertently compromising outcomes to a greater extent than the disease itself.

Delirium and State Regulation

An emerging concern in the newborn ICU is increasing reports of delirium in neonates. Delirium has been noted for some time in adult and pediatric ICU populations, and more recently, case reports of delirium in the NICU have been published (Liviskie & McPherson, 2021). Given that infants cannot describe their symptoms, diagnosis is contingent upon recognition by providers. However, many of the symptoms are associated with pain and agitation, which can complicate diagnostic reasoning (Figure 11.1).

Careful examination of the behaviors noted in the infants described in the aforementioned case reports reveals that delirium is not a new phenomenon, but rather a new realization of an extant problem. Symptoms include hyperactivity, hypoactivity, and mixed behaviors. Hyperactive behaviors include increased psychomotor activity, agitation, restlessness, and aggressive behavior, whereas hypoactive symptoms include lethargy, unresponsiveness, or decreased attention (Liviskie & McPherson, 2021). Although some symptoms are difficult to recognize or differentiate from adverse effects of therapies or pain, clinicians experienced in care of the infant in the NICU recognize these behaviors and are well positioned to note changes in infant behaviors. Unfortunately, symptoms of delirium can result from the nature of an invasive treatment, insufficient comfort measures, or as a result of medications used to provide sedation and analgesia. As clinicians become more aware of this phenomenon, they must begin to assess for delirium in the NICU, just as pain is regularly assessed.

Tools for screening delirium in pediatrics are available, including the Pediatric Anesthesia Emergence Delirium Scale (PAED) and the Cornell Assessment of Pediatric Delirium (CAPD). A point prevalence study conducted in a single NICU evaluated the prevalence of delirium using the CAPD (Siegel et al., 2021). Of 149 infants screened over an 8-day period, 22.4% screened positive for delirium; most of these infants were being mechanically ventilated and/or had underlying neurologic disorders, both of which the study determined were independently associated with positive screens. The need to regularly assess for delirium, as well as evidence on best practice for treatment, is critically needed.

Several medications used in the NICU are associated with increased risk for delirium, including corticosteroids, vasopressors, anticholinergics, opioids, and benzodiazepines (Liviskie & McPherson, 2021). Opioids and benzodiazepines are deliriogenic medications and are the most commonly prescribed analgesic/sedative medications for ventilated infants, as noted earlier. In the current

FIGURE 11.1 Overlap of behavioral cues in pain, sedation, withdrawal syndrome, and delirium.

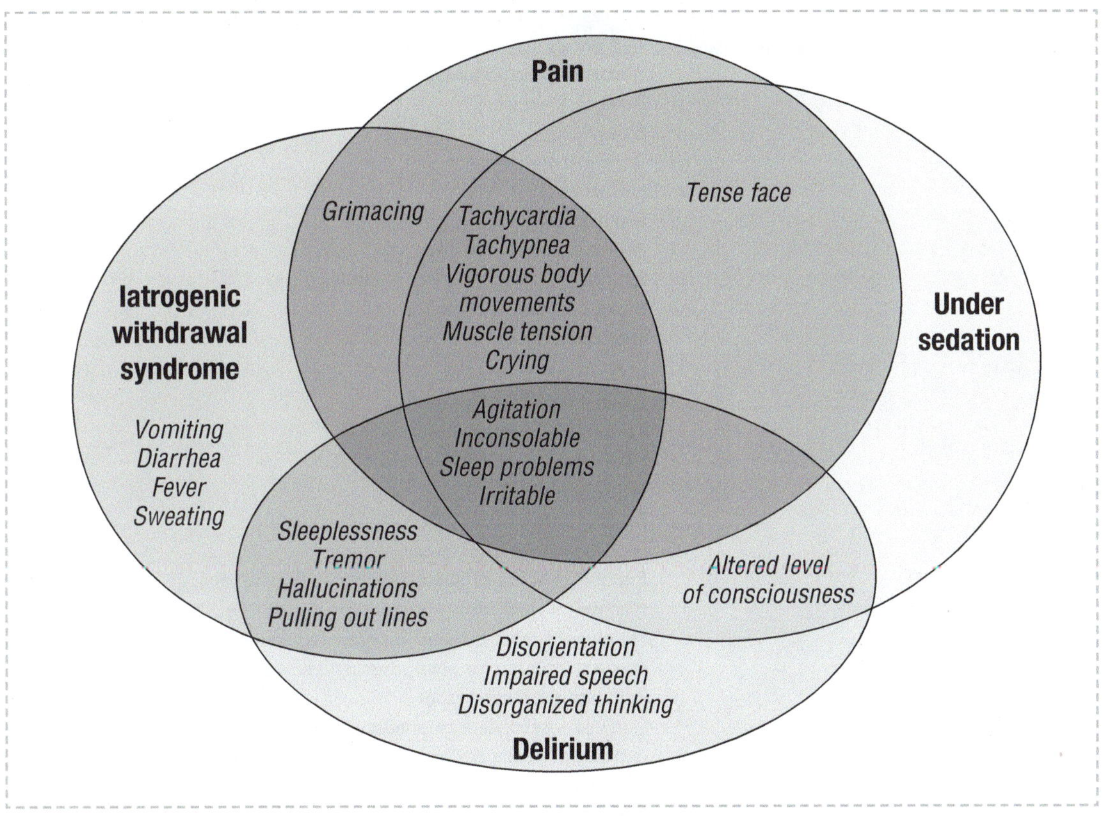

Source: From Harris, J., Ramelet, A.-S., van Dijk, M., Pokorna, P., Wielenga, J., Tume, L., Tibboel, D., & Ista, E. (2016). Clinical recommendations for pain, sedation, withdrawal and delirium assessment in critically ill infants and children: An ESPNIC position statement for healthcare professionals. *Intensive Care Medicine, 42*, 972–986. https://doi.org/10.1007/s00134-016-4344-1

case reports of delirium in the NICU, those infants demonstrated behaviors associated with pediatric patients with delirium with persistent agitation, lack of eye contact, and inconsolability not responsive to a heavy analgesic and sedation regimen that was initiated to reduce the initial signs of pain and agitation. When these infants were treated with antipsychotic medications and removed from the opioids and benzodiazepines, the symptoms of delirium resolved within 48 hours.

PAIN ASSESSMENT TOOLS

As the recognition of pain in the neonate increased, and studies providing support for the need to assess and treat pain grew, our perception of what constituted painful procedures broadened. Table 11.2 provides an overview of procedures now considered to be painful in the NICU.

Scales

Once the phenomenon of pain in newborns was validated, researchers began to study pain response in the neonate in an effort to capture characteristics that could be used to create pain scoring systems. Most pain tools are multidimensional in that biobehavioral changes in vital signs (heart rate, respiratory rate, oxygen saturation) and facial action correlated with cry, audible cry, and behavioral state are considered (Table 11.3). There are several problems associated with exclusive reliance on these biobehavioral indicators to assess pain. Although these signs may be seen during pain exposure, sick premature infants often do not demonstrate these signs (Craig et al., 2002; Johnston et al., 1999). GA, acuity of illness, and postnatal age all complicate the challenge of pain recognition and management; each may alter the infant's ability to demonstrate these biobehavioral patterns associated with the pain experience in infants (Evans et al., 2005). In addition, the

TABLE 11.2 Common Neonatal Procedures Identified as Painful or Uncomfortable

CATEGORY OF PROCEDURE	TYPE OF PROCEDURE
Diagnostic	• Abscess incision-drainage • Arterial puncture • Biopsy • Bone marrow sampling • Heel stick • Lumbar puncture • Paracentesis/thoracentesis • Retinopathy of prematurity screening exam • Suprapubic bladder taps • Venipuncture
Clinical	• Bladder catheterization • Central-line insertion/removal • Chest tube insertions/removal • Dressing changes of IV sloughs • Fractures • Feeding tube insertion/Replogle tube insertion • Iatrogenic drug withdrawal • Intramuscular/subcutaneous injections (e.g., vaccines) • Mechanical ventilation—agitation or asynchronous respirations • Peripheral venous catheterization/percutaneous venous catheter • Postural drainage (or physiotherapy)/Penrose drainage • Removal of adhesive tape • Skin injury secondary to prematurity, nasal excoriation, IV catheter extravasation, diaper dermatitis • Tracheal intubation/extubation • Tracheal suctioning • Ventricular reservoir tap
Surgical	• Circumcision • Dialysis • ECMO • Retinopathy of prematurity photocoagulation, cryopexy, or vitrectomy • Suture insertion • Suture removal (if embedded into skin)

ECMO, extracorporeal membrane oxygenation; IV, intravenous.

more often the premature infant is exposed to pain, the more varied the response may be. After just 2 weeks in the NICU, most infants display fewer of these biobehavioral signs of pain during heel sticks (Johnston & Stevens, 1996). Infants also cry for many reasons other than pain and heart rates will increase as a direct response to crying.

Pain scales that measure both physiologic and behavioral responses to pain, versus exclusively behavioral scales, are best suited for neonatal units imbedded within community-based hospitals, which manage infants greater than 34 weeks' gestation. A recent review by Olsson and colleagues (2021) indicated there are currently 22 neonatal pain scales in popular use; however, no universal tool has been identified, which continues to complicate clinician choice. It must be noted, as well, that there continues to be an element of subjectivity with these tools.

Objective Measures of Pain

NIRS is an objective tool that can be used to assess pain in neonates by measuring neocortical activation to noxious stimulation that provides a continuous, real-time, noninvasive measure of regional cerebral, renal, and mesenteric oxygenation. Exploration with NIRS for pain evaluation remains mostly in the research arena at the time of this publication (Benoit et al., 2017).

TABLE 11.3 Neonatal/Infant Pain and Agitation Scales

SCALE	YEAR OF INCEPTION	INDICATION FOR USE (TYPE OF PAIN)	ELIGIBILITY FOR USE (GESTATIONAL AGE)	ASSESSMENT DIMENSION(S)
Neonatal Pain, Agitation, and Sedation Scale (N-PASS)	2003	Acute pain Chronic pain Agitation	23–40 weeks of gestation	Biobehavioral Physiologic
Neonatal Infant Pain Scale (NIPS)	1993	Acute pain	26–47 weeks of gestation	Biobehavioral Physiologic
Bernese Pain Scale Neonates (BPN)	1996	Acute pain	27–41 weeks of gestation	Biobehavioral Physiologic
Premature Infant Pain Profile Revised (PIPP-R)	2014	Acute pain	25–40 weeks of gestation	Biobehavioral Physiologic
Neonatal Facial Coding System Revised (NFCS-R)	2010	Acute pain	25–40 weeks of gestation	Biobehavioral
COMFORTNeo	2009	Chronic pain Agitation	25–43 weeks of gestation	Biobehavioral

Skin-conductance monitors measure changes in palmar and plantar sweat glands and have been used successfully in pain research in neonates. These tools offer a noninvasive method of objectifying pain levels but are not commonly used in clinical practice (van der Lee et al., 2016).

Automated facial analysis of infant pain is a new component currently being used in clinical research. These tools are designed to recognize key facial movements that are the backbone of the Neonatal Facial Coding System (NFCS) designed by Grunau and Craig in 1987 and the facial changes used in many pain scales. In addition, some of these systems also include changes in physiologic parameters.

Although these tools offer hope that there may be easy-to-use, objective tools to assist with pain recognition in the neonate, they are not ready for clinical use as yet. Also, we must remember that cry, in and of itself, is not specific for pain in this population (Oster, 2021).

CONSEQUENCES OF NEONATAL PAIN AND USE OF ANALGESICS

Prolonged neonatal exposure to pain may cause adverse physiologic effects in all systems (Anand & Hickey, 1987). In response to pain, infants experience an increase in heart and respiratory rates, blood pressure, oxygen consumption, and intracranial pressure. In addition, there is increased release of cortisol, catecholamines, growth hormone, and a decreased release of insulin. These physiologic responses can have long-term effects on neurobehavioral development (Perry et al., 2018). This includes negative impact on sensorimotor and cognitive development, alteration in pain responses, attention deficit disorders, anxiety/depressive behaviors, and more (Vinall et al., 2014).

Analgesia leads to loss of sensation of pain resulting from the interruption in the pain pathway between the sense organ and brain and serves as the mechanism by which pharmacologic analgesic agents work. Analgesics may relieve pain by acting as an agonist and exerting effects on the pain pathway. For example, opioid analgesia results from activation of μ opioid receptors on the presynaptic neuron, blocking voltage-gated calcium channels and decreasing excitatory neurotransmitter release (glutamate), decreasing transmission of excitatory signals, thus inhibiting ascending neuronal pathways and altering perception of pain.

Risks associated with short-term use of opioids for analgesia include hypoventilation, apnea, hypotension, decreased gastrointestinal (GI) mobility, and urinary retention (McPherson, Ortinau, & Vesoulis, 2021). In addition to risks associated with episodic exposures, prolonged exposure to analgesics (greater than 7 days) may risk additional physiologic alterations, tolerance, and iatrogenic withdrawal sequence (Roze et al., 2008). There are neurodevelopmental concerns following the use of long-term analgesia, but, to date, the research is not clear (McPherson et al., 2020).

In summary, results from numerous studies support that repetitive pain is bad for infants' growth and development with both short-term and long-term effects, some of which are permanent. A preponderance of evidence from multiple studies underlines the detrimental effects of anesthesia, analgesics, and sedatives on neuronal growth. Systematic studies are needed to evaluate the relative risks and benefits of both untreated pain and aggressive use of analgesics and sedatives, but RCTs of that nature would not be ethical.

CURRENT PHARMACOLOGIC TREATMENT MODALITIES FOR MINIMALLY INVASIVE PROCEDURES

Several studies have demonstrated reduced pain reactivity with the use of nonpharmacologic pain management strategies. Skin-to-skin contact, or kangaroo care, during which the infant is positioned directly on a mother or father's chest, decreases pain responses in premature and term infants (Pillai Riddell et al., 2015). Sucking, mouthing, hand holding, grasping, and hand-to-mouth positioning can mitigate noxious overstimulation, conserve energy output, and promote optimal neurodevelopment (Yin et al., 2015). Swaddling, or facilitated tucking, in which the extremities are flexed and close to the trunk, is regarded as effective in reducing pain reactivity in infants. A meta-analysis of available RCTs found that facilitated tucking in combination with sucrose water achieves sensorial saturation and synergistic pain relief in infants undergoing painful procedures (Pillai Riddell et al., 2015).

Nonnutritive sucking is another pain management strategy: A pacifier induces sucking activity that invokes nociception through orotactile stimulation and the release of endogenous nonopioids (Yin et al., 2015). Studies consistently report decreased crying times and pain scores in term infants provided a pacifier for nonnutritive sucking during painful procedures. Available data conclude that nonnutritive sucking is a promising adjunct to pain management in term infants, with inconclusive evidence supporting its use with premature infants, if provided approximately 3 minutes prior to the painful intervention (Pillai Riddell et al., 2015).

Sucrose

When heel-stick sampling, venipuncture, or intramuscular injection is indicated, clinicians may synergistically pair nonpharmacologic interventions with oral sucrose administration. The use of 12% to 50% oral sucrose for pain prophylaxis is well documented and regarded as the most widely used pharmacologic intervention for pain management in infants exposed to painful procedures (Stevens et al., 2016). Available data consistently report decreased crying times among infants provided sucrose water with pacifier use prior to heel stick and venipuncture, with a similar magnitude of effect to nonpharmacologic interventions (e.g., facilitated tucking, skin-to-skin care).

MECHANISM OF ACTION

The mechanism of action for sucrose is not well understood. As discussed in Chapter 7, "Common Medications Prescribed in the Newborn Nursery," it is possible that sucrose alleviates pain via activation of endogenous opioid receptors at the tongue, which weakens nociceptive input at the level of the dorsal horn (Holsti & Grunau, 2010; Thakkar et al., 2016). More recent research suggests alternative hormone and amine pathways may be related to sucrose processing in neonates and infants (e.g., cholinergic, dopaminergic, or serotonergic pathways).

DOSING RECOMMENDATIONS/CORE PHARMACOKINETIC PRINCIPLES

The greatest analgesic effect from sucrose is observed when it is administered on the anterior aspect of the tongue, 2 minutes prior to a painful procedure, as the maximum effectiveness is 2 minutes with a duration of 3 to 5 minutes (Stevens et al., 2016). Oral sucrose may also be administered inside the cheek or a pacifier may be dipped into the sucrose solution to coat the pacifier, noting that a dip is approximately 0.1 mL. Combining the benefits of sucrose with pacifier use (nonnutritive sucking) appears to maximize impact (Stevens et al., 2016). Gavage or oral administration has not been shown to be effective and efficacy beyond 12 months of age has not been established.

The lowest effective dose of sucrose should be used to balance benefit and risk. Stevens and colleagues (2018) reported a significant reduction in behavioral responses to pain among preterm and term neonates with a dose of 0.1 mL (24% sucrose solution). These findings underpin current recommendations (Taketomo, 2023):

- less than 1 kg: 0.1 mL/dose
- 1 to 2 kg: 0.1 to 0.2 mL/dose
- greater than 2 kg: 0.1 to 0.5 mL/dose

Alternatively, currently recommended maximum dosages per GA and procedure are (Taketomo, 2023):

- 27 to 31 weeks of gestation: 0.5 mL/procedure
- 32 to 36 weeks of gestation: 1 mL/procedure
- greater than 37 weeks of gestation: 2 mL/procedure

Of note, objective physiologic pain indices (e.g., oxygen consumption, cortisol levels) do not significantly change with the administration of sucrose (Bauer et al., 2004; Slater et al., 2010). Further, sucrose has not been shown to prevent infants from developing an abnormally heightened sensitivity to pain (hyperalgesia; Taddio et al., 2009). An extensive variability in specific dosing guidelines among units is reported, with limited data on long-term safety and neurodevelopmental outcomes (Johnston et al., 2002, 2007).

CLINICAL-MONITORING PEARLS

Sucrose is effective for reducing pain from single-event procedures (heel stick, intramuscular injection, and venipuncture) in preterm and term infants (Stevens et al., 2016). Moderate-quality evidence has shown that sucrose in combination with nonnutritive sucking or other nonpharmacologic interventions is more effective than sucrose alone. Optimal dosing, duration, and concentration of sucrose have been inconsistent among published studies. Repeat doses in preterm infants, especially extremely low-birth-weight infants, require further investigation and long-term neurodevelopmental follow-up. An increased risk for poor attention and motor delay is associated with greater than 10 doses of sucrose administered within a 24-hour period (Johnston et al., 2002, 2007).

CURRENT PHARMACOLOGIC TREATMENT MODALITIES FOR INVASIVE PROCEDURES

Invasive procedures, including endotracheal intubation, surgical interventions, and TH, often require scheduled administration of intermittently dosed or continuously infused analgesics or sedatives. Here, we discuss the most commonly prescribed analgesics and sedatives used in the NICU.

Nonopioid Analgesics

ACETAMINOPHEN/PARACETAMOL

Acetaminophen (also known as *paracetamol*), N-acetyl-p-aminophenol, is classified as an aniline analog and commonly used for analgesic and antipyretic purposes. In fact, 95% of all infants receive at least one dose of acetaminophen by 9 months of life (Morton et al., 2013). Acetaminophen does not significantly reduce pain associated with heel stick or eye examinations but may reduce the total amount of morphine required in the first 48 hours following an invasive abdominal or thoracic procedure (Ceelie et al., 2013; Ohlsson & Shah, 2016).

Mechanism of Action/Core Pharmacokinetic Principles

Acetaminophen inhibits the synthesis of the prostaglandin cyclooxygenase (COX), predominantly COX-2, in the CNS and peripherally blocks pain impulses. This inhibition prevents the metabolism of arachidonic acid to prostaglandin H_2, an intermediate by-product that is converted to proinflammatory compounds. In the CNS, the inhibition of COX enzymes reduces the concentrations of prostaglandin E_2, which produces antipyresis from inhibition of the hypothalamic heat-regulating center. Unlike aspirin and other nonsteroidal anti-inflammatory drugs (NSAIDs), acetaminophen does not have anti-inflammatory properties, does not inhibit thromboxane, and does not alter platelet aggregation. It has been used in neonates for mild to moderate pain and for fevers. Additional and newer indications include its use as an adjuvant in severe pain to decrease overall opioid exposure and to treat neonatal patent ductus arteriosus (PDA).

Acetaminophen has good oral absorption, variable rectal absorption (absorption occurs primarily in the small intestine), and a larger volume of distribution and proportionally lower peak concentration in early infancy, which may warrant the use of a higher intravenous (IV) loading dose. Among infants born preterm, the estimated volume distribution is 0.64 L/kg at 27 weeks of gestation compared to 0.4 to 0.45 L/kg at 6 months' postnatal age (Allegaert et al., 2011). In addition, acetaminophen is weakly protein bound (10%–25%). The time to peak concentration is 15 minutes for IV administration and 10 to 60 minutes for oral administration with a duration of action of 4 to 6 hours (Pacifici & Allegaert, 2015).

The liver is primarily involved in the metabolism of acetaminophen, and, to a lesser extent, the kidney and intestine. Acetaminophen undergoes sulfation and glucuronidation by uridine 5′-diphospho-glucuronosyltransferase (UDP; Pacifici & Allegaert, 2015). Acetaminophen is mostly converted to pharmacologically inactive glucuronide (47%–62%) and sulfate conjugates (25%–36%; Miller et al., 1976). A minor fraction (8%–10%) of acetaminophen is oxidized by CYP2E1 to N-acetyl-p-benzoquinone imine (NAPQI), a toxic metabolite that can induce hepatotoxicity. With supratherapeutic doses of acetaminophen, NAPQI depletes the liver of the antioxidant glutathione and directly damages hepatic cells, which leads to liver failure and oxidative stress (Bunchorntavakul & Reddy, 2013). Fortunately, the NAPQI isoenzyme is less active in early infancy.

Acetaminophen follows first-order elimination, which as introduced in Chapter 3, "Pharmacokinetics and Pharmacodynamics," involves a linear, exponential elimination of drug over time. In other words, the rate (or speed) of elimination depends on the plasma drug concentration. However, with prolonged exposure or use of supratherapeutic doses of acetaminophen, mechanisms that eliminate the drug can become saturated. This results in a change from first-order to zero-order elimination. Recall from Chapter 3 that *zero-order elimination* is defined as the elimination of a constant quantity of drug per unit of time, regardless of the drug serum concentration. This mode of elimination increases the risk for dose accumulation and toxicity (Bunchorntavakul & Reddy, 2013). Clearance increases with advancing GA, from 0.138 L/kg/hour at 28 weeks of gestation to 0.167 L/kg/hour by 42 weeks of gestation (33% of adult values), with weight determined to be the primary covariate of clearance (Allegaert et al., 2011). The half-life is reported as 7 hours in neonates and decreases to 4 hours in infants. Recent reports suggest that once a steady state is achieved with use of an interval dose of 7.5 mg/kg (every 6 hours), the median acetaminophen concentration is 10 mg/L (van Ganzewinkel et al., 2014).

Dosing Recommendations

Acetaminophen can be administered IV, orally, or rectally. For the purpose of pain control, current IV dosing recommendations call for one loading dose of 20 mg/kg followed by interval dosages of 10 mg/kg every 6 hours. A summary of current dosing recommendations for all routes is provided in Table 11.4, which accounts for rapid postmenstrual age maturational changes. Readers are encouraged to note that pediatric labeling information includes the unique provision of a *maximum* cumulative dose for neonates.

Clinical-Monitoring Pearls

Clinical monitoring of renal and hepatic function is indicated with prolonged use. Dosage changes may be indicated with a glomerular filtration rate less than 10 mL/min/1.73 m^2. Among infants with evidence of liver impairment, including physiologic or pathologic jaundice, the lowest therapeutic dose with longest frequency is recommended. The total bilirubin concentration is inversely proportional to acetaminophen clearance (Cook et al., 2016; Palmer et al., 2008).

Prolonged or excessive consumption can increase the risk for GI bleeding. In these circumstances, the diagnostic workup will include review of a complete blood count. In addition, higher dosages of acetaminophen risk toxicity; the analysis of serum acetaminophen levels is indicated if toxicity is suspected (Ghanem et al., 2016).

TABLE 11.4 Dosing Recommendations and Daily Maximums for Acetaminophen (Paracetamol)

ADMINISTRATION METHOD	POSTMENSTRUAL AGE	LOADING DOSE	INTERVAL DOSE	MAXIMUM DAILY DOSE
Intravenous	28–32 weeks	20 mg/kg/dose	7.5–10 mg/kg/dose every 8–12 hours	22.5 mg/kg/day
	33–36 weeks		7.5–10 mg/kg/dose every 6 hours	40 mg/kg/day
	≥37 weeks		10 mg/kg/dose every 6 hours	40 mg/kg/day
Oral	28–32 weeks	N/A	10–12 mg/kg/dose every 6–8 hours	40 mg/kg/day
	33–37 weeks, term <10 days of age		10–15 mg/kg/dose every 6 hours	60 mg/kg/day
	Term ≥10 days of age		10–15 mg/kg/dose every 4–6 hours	75 mg/kg/day
Rectal	28–32 weeks	N/A	20 mg/kg/dose every 12 hours	40 mg/kg/day
	33–37 weeks, term <10 days of age	30 mg/kg/dose	15 mg/kg/dose every 8 hours	60 mg/kg/day
	Term ≥10 days of age	30 mg/kg/dose	20 mg/kg/dose every 6–8 hours	75 mg/kg/day; five-dose maximum in 24 hours

Note: The information in this table is intended for teaching purposes only. Clinicians should refer to the most current dosage handbook when prescribing this drug in neonates and infants.
Source: From Taketomo, C.K. (Ed.). (2023). *Pediatric & neonatal dosage handbook: An extensive resource for clinicians treating pediatric and neonatal patients* (29th ed.). Lexicomp/Wolters Kluwer.

N-acetylcysteine (NAC) has been shown to be an effective antidote for acetaminophen overdose in humans. NAC replenishes glutathione (GSH) stores, scavenges reactive oxygen species in mitochondria, and enhances the sulfation metabolic pathway. It is the treatment of choice for acetaminophen poisoning (Bunchorntavakul & Reddy, 2013).

NONSELECTIVE NONSTEROIDAL ANTI-INFLAMMATORY DRUGS (IBUPROFEN)

NSAIDs offer anti-inflammatory, analgesic, and antipyretic properties. In the United States, ibuprofen is not recommended for analgesia or antipyresis in infants less than 6 months of age; however, clinicians often prescribe IV ibuprofen lysine for treatment of a PDA (Aranda et al., 2017). Other countries, such as the United Kingdom and New Zealand, endorse the use of ibuprofen for pain and fever in infants older than 1 month of age (Tan et al., 2020).

Mechanism of Action/Pharmacokinetic Principles

The mechanism of action of ibuprofen involves nonselective competitive binding to COX-1 and COX-2 receptors. Binding to COX-2 receptors, in particular, prevents the conversion of arachidonic acid to proinflammatory prostaglandins. In doing so, ibuprofen peripherally blocks pain impulses, and inhibits the hypothalamic heat-regulating center, eliciting the antipyretic effect. Separately and simultaneously, binding to COX-1 receptors prevents the conversion of arachidonic acid to prostaglandin H_2 and thromboxane A_2, which permits platelet aggregation. Therefore, due to noncompetitive binding, ibuprofen elicits three primary effects: analgesia, antipyresis, and anti-inflammation.

NSAIDs are highly protein bound and, when administered orally, absorbed in the small intestine. The mean volume of distribution is 0.2 L/kg and half-life is 42 hours in preterm infants treated for a PDA (Padrini et al., 2021). Ibuprofen is hepatically metabolized through oxidation and conjugation. Renal excretion is slower than in adults and estimated at 0.007 L/kg/hour (Padrini et al., 2021). Based on outcomes of recent reports involving term neonates, ibuprofen clearance matures to 90% of adult values by 1 month of postnatal life (Anderson & Hannam, 2019).

Dosing Recommendations

NSAIDs are administered orally or via IV. In neonates, the IV route is typically reserved for PDA therapy. Currently, no recommended daily doses are provided for the treatment of pain in preterm or term infants. Among infants born at term and who reach 44 weeks postmenstrual age, the recommended dose is 10 mg/kg every 6 to 8 hours (Anderson & Hannam, 2019). Use is contraindicated among neonates or infants with hepatic failure.

Clinical-Monitoring Pearls

Clinicians customarily monitor serum electrolytes, renal function indices, the complete blood count, and liver enzymes; however, this is typically limited to use with a PDA and not for pain or fever. Urine output should be monitored, given that prostaglandins are synthesized near the afferent arteriole. Prostaglandin inhibition may elicit constriction of the afferent arteriole, reduce blood flow to Bowman capsule, and predispose the infant to acute renal failure. Dosage changes may be indicated with a glomerular filtration rate less than 10 mL/min/1.73 m^2. In addition, signs of bleeding warrant further evaluation.

Opioid Agonists

MORPHINE

Morphine ($C_{17}H_{19}NO_3$) is the main alkaloid isolated from the opium poppy (*Papaver somniferum*). The common indications for use in neonates, specific to analgesia, include invasive procedural pain, postoperative surgical pain, and chronic pain.

Mechanism of Action/Pharmacokinetic Principles

The mechanism of action of morphine involves the binding of drug molecules to opioid receptors (μ, κ, Δ) coupled to G proteins, which inhibit adenyl cyclase. Once bound to μ and κ receptors, voltage-gated calcium channels are inhibited, and potassium channels are activated. This decreases the transmission of nociceptive signals and inhibits ascending pain pathways in the spinal cord. This sequence of events elicits the desired analgesic effect (Thigpen et al., 2019).

The pharmacokinetics of morphine vary considerably in neonates, especially preterm neonates, which reflects immature hepatic glucuronidation and altered hepatic blood flow. Morphine is highly lipophilic, highly protein bound primarily to alpha-1 acid glycoprotein, and well absorbed by the GI tract. The volume of distribution of intravenously administered morphine is higher in preterm infants compared to term counterparts, in particular over the first few days of life, secondary to factors including fluid balance, renal function, fat/muscle content, protein binding affinity, and organ size (Thigpen et al., 2019). The half-life decreases with advancing age as hepatic metabolic pathways mature (Pacifici, 2016). The majority of morphine (70%) is metabolized via CYP3A4-modulated glucuronidation to morphine-3-glucuronide (M3G) and the more potent morphine-6-glucuronide (M6G) metabolites (Thigpen et al., 2019). M3G is known to elicit side effects, whereas M6G is an opioid agonist. Among those subject to morphine therapy, M3G is detected in the serum of preterm and term neonates and infants as early as 2 hours of life; concentrations decrease with advancing birth weight and GA (Pacifici, 2016). M6G is not detected in the plasma until 48 hours of life; among critically ill preterm neonates less than 32 weeks' GA, the M6G concentration comprises 20% to 25% of the total morphine plasma concentration. In addition, the available complement of hepatic uptake and efflux transporters may also affect morphine metabolism (Brouwer et al., 2015). Renal clearance is significantly correlated with advancing GA and weight; comorbid conditions that impair renal function will prolong drug clearance, increase half-life, and potentially increase the risk for dose accumulation and toxicity (Pacifici, 2016).

Dosing Recommendations

Morphine is administered IV or orally. Most clinicians agree that continuous IV dosing offers the most desirable analgesic effect; therefore, we focus this discussion on IV pharmacodynamic data. Olkkola and colleagues (1988) reported achievement of analgesia in neonates subject to cardiothoracic surgery with a continuous infusion of 5 mcg/kg/hour; infants 1 to 3 months of age required 10 mcg/kg/hour, infants 3 to 6 months of age required 15 mcg/kg/hr, and infants older than 6 months of life required 25 mcg/kg/hour. A more recent study published by Lynn and colleagues (2000) concluded that neonates required 10 to 15 mcg/kg/hour, whereas all other infants (1–3 months,

3–6 months, >6 months of age) required the same dosing regimen as published by Olkkola. Intramuscular and subcutaneous administration is no longer recommended in neonates secondary to localized adverse effects (e.g., tissue erythema, induration; Thigpen et al., 2019). Oral dosing is usually reserved for the management of neonatal abstinence syndrome or iatrogenic opioid withdrawal.

Clinical-Monitoring Pearls

To assess for oversedation, vital-sign trends should be carefully followed during therapy. Caution should be exercised when prescribing morphine to neonates with hepatic impairment and/or acute renal failure, as these infants incur increased risk for respiratory depression when plasma concentrations are greater than 20 ng/mL, secondary to dose accumulation (Lynn et al., 2000). Acute adverse effects reported in preterm infants include hypotension, tachyphylaxis, prolonged need for mechanical ventilation, and delayed tolerance of enteral feedings (McPherson, Ortinau, & Vesoulis, 2021). Clinicians should also be cognizant of the association between cumulative opioid exposure during neonatal intensive care and brain growth and development (McPherson et al., 2020).

In cases of suspected or confirmed intoxication or overdose, naloxone may be prescribed as a full reversal agent. IV administration is preferred in these situations. Customary naloxone dosing for opioid intoxication or overdose (full reversal) is 0.1 mg/kg/dose; repeat doses may be required. Lower doses of 0.01 mg/kg/dose are indicated for opioid-induced depression. Caution and clinical judgment must be used in order not to precipitate a withdrawal, especially in infants with prolonged exposure to an opiate (Moe-Byrne et al., 2018).

When formulating a plan for weaning and discontinuation of therapy, clinicians should consider the dose of morphine required for analgesia and duration of therapy. Readers are referred to the end of this chapter for example approaches to iatrogenic withdrawal and to Chapter 9, "Neonatal Abstinence Syndrome," for information related to morphine weaning in the setting of neonatal abstinence syndrome.

FENTANYL

Fentanyl ($C_{22}H_{28}N_2O$) is a potent synthetic lipophilic opioid agonist first synthesized by Dr. Paul Janssen in 1960 in his laboratories (Janssen Pharmaceutica, Belgium). His research interest focused on creating a potent, rapid-acting, and effective analgesic to treat the many different pain conditions of the time. His desire was to formulate a potent and more lipid-soluble compound compared to morphine or meperidine, with good CNS penetration and fewer unwanted side effects. Current indications for use in neonates include intermittent doses for invasive procedural pain, sedation in critically ill neonates, postoperative surgical pain, chronic pain, and anesthesia. Fentanyl provides rapid analgesia or sedation while maintaining hemodynamic stability.

Mechanism of Action/Pharmacokinetic Principles

Similar to morphine, fentanyl acts as an agonist and binds to μ and κ opioid receptors to elicit analgesic, anesthetic, and sedative effects. Fentanyl is 50 to 100 times more potent than morphine on a dose-per-weight basis (Thigpen et al., 2019).

We present a summary of pharmacokinetic principles specific to IV and intranasal fentanyl use. Fentanyl is highly protein bound. The volume of distribution is larger in neonates compared to adults, which is possibly attributed to the fact that fentanyl is readily distributed to both fat and muscle tissue after administration. Fentanyl crosses the blood-brain barrier by simple diffusion as well as active transport (Thigpen et al., 2019). Recall from Chapter 3, "Pharmacokinetics and Pharmacodynamics," and Chapter 5, "Perinatal Pharmacology," that simple transport involves the influx of a substance from a higher to lower concentration until equilibrium is achieved. Given the ease of entry into the cerebral vasculature, the time to peak effect is short (1 to 1.7 minutes after administration) and duration of action is approximately 30 to 60 minutes. Fentanyl is hepatically metabolized by CYP3A4, primarily by dealkylation and, to a lesser degree, by hydroxylation, to norfentanyl (inactive metabolite). Clearance is primarily dependent on hepatic perfusion.

Relatively robust data describes the pharmacokinetics and efficacy of intranasal fentanyl in pediatric and adult patients (Mudd, 2011; Thompson & Thompson, 2016). Transmucosal fentanyl administration is relatively novel in neonates. In older patients, intranasal fentanyl absorption is equivalent to IV absorption, although time to maximum concentration is significantly longer (4 to 9 minutes for intranasal compared to 2 to 4 minutes for IV; Thompson & Thompson, 2016). Pharmacokinetic data have not been reported in neonates. Studies describing safety and efficacy are emerging.

Dosing Recommendations

Fentanyl can be administered by way of IV or intranasal routes. IV dosing parameters typically range between 0.5 and 3 mcg/kg/dose (intermittent) every 2 to 4 hours or 0.5 and 2 mcg/kg/hour (continuous) for infants not subject to opioid exposure in utero. Intranasal dosing is typically comparable to intermittent IV dosing. Reported benefits of intranasal administration include the noninvasive ease of administration, rapid onset of action, and favorable safety profile compared to morphine (Harlos et al., 2013; Orge et al., 2013). Additional research is needed to discern optimal dosing parameters for infants.

Sindhur and associates (2020) published results of the seminal RCT, which compared intranasal fentanyl (2 mcg/kg) to intranasal saline during retinopathy of prematurity screening examinations. The authors reported a significant reduction in pain scores (using the Premature Infant Pain Profile Revised [PIPP-R] scale) with intranasal fentanyl use (8.3 vs. 11.5, mean difference: 3.2, $p < .001$).

Clinical-Monitoring Pearls

Clinicians commonly monitor vital-sign trends, level of sedation, chest wall mobility, and for signs of neuroexcitation (associated with excessive doses). Like morphine, caution should be exercised when prescribing fentanyl to neonates with acute renal failure or rapidly changing renal or hepatic function; a theoretical risk for hepatic accumulation of drug metabolites increases in these situations (Ziesenitz et al., 2018). Further, the half-life of fentanyl may be prolonged in cases of intra-abdominal infection and distention if blood flow from the splanchnic vein to the portal venous system is restricted.

Compared to morphine, fentanyl use is associated with reduced risk for hemodynamic instability, GI motility impairment (delayed passage of meconium), and urinary retention (Saarenmaa et al., 1999). In addition, reduced histamine release is observed compared to morphine, which is favorable among infants with bronchopulmonary dysplasia or congenital heart disease. Disadvantages linked to fentanyl therapy include transient chest wall rigidity with rapid intermittent doses or doses administered over less than a 3- to 5-minute period of time (Coruh et al., 2013). Tachyphylaxis and prolongation of intubation are associated with continuous therapy (Ancora et al., 2013); in addition, concern exists regarding the developmental outcome of neonates with prolonged fentanyl exposure during intensive care (McPherson et al., 2020).

In cases of rapid administration with chest wall rigidity, reversal may be required and can be accomplished with IV muscle relaxation (e.g., rocuronium) or naloxone. Customary naloxone dosing for full reversal is 0.1 mg/kg/dose; repeat doses may be required. Lower doses of 0.01 mg/kg/dose are indicated for opioid-induced depression. Caution and clinical judgment must be used when prescribing naloxone in order to avoid precipitating a withdrawal, especially in infants with prolonged exposure to an opiate (Moe-Byrne et al., 2018).

The process for weaning fentanyl is dependent on the dose of fentanyl given, indication for use, and duration of therapy. Typically, therapy greater than 5 days requires a slow, dosing taper prior to discontinuation (refer to "Tapering of Sedation (After Prolonged Use)" section of this chapter). Due to the current opioid epidemic, parental education may be warranted to alleviate fears specific to fentanyl dependence and withdrawal.

Alpha-2 Adrenergic Agonists

DEXMEDETOMIDINE

Dexmedetomidine ($C_{13}H_{16}N_2$) is a highly selective and potent alpha-2 adrenergic agonist with significant sedative, anxiolytic, sympatholytic, and analgesic effects. Off-label dexmedetomidine use is increasing both as a primary sedative and as an adjuvant in infants not achieving sedation goals.

Mechanism of Action/Core Pharmacokinetic Principles

Given its classification as an alpha-2 adrenergic agonist, dexmedetomidine has a selectivity ratio of 1600:1 for alpha-2 versus alpha-1 receptors. Alpha-2 adrenergic receptors are located throughout the central and peripheral nervous systems but specifically in the pontine locus coeruleus, ventrolateral medulla, and dorsal horn of the spinal cord. Alpha-2 agonists neuromodulate these centers causing sedation and analgesia, vasodilatation, and bradycardia, but, unlike opioids, elicit little effect on respiratory drive (Nguyen et al., 2017).

Greenberg and associates (2017) reported population pharmacokinetic parameters among a cohort of 20 neonates (range 27–40 weeks of gestation). The estimated volume of distribution was 1.5 L/kg. Dexmedetomidine is hepatically metabolized by way of oxidation via CYP2A6 (phase-1 reaction, see Chapter 3, "Pharmacokinetics and Pharmacodynamics"), glucuronidation, and methylation (phase-2 reaction). The majority of metabolized dexmedetomidine is excreted in the urine (~95%); clearance increases by approximately 4.5% per week of postnatal life except in cases involving cardiothoracic surgery. Neonates subject to cardiac surgery demonstrated a 40% reduction in clearance.

Dosing Recommendations

Dexmedetomidine is typically administered via IV in neonates. Loading doses of dexmedetomidine (0.1–0.5 mcg/kg/dose over 10 to 20 minutes) should be administered cautiously, as rapid infusions can precipitate bradycardia and hypotension. Use in preterm neonates should be cautious due to the decreased plasma clearance and longer elimination half-life (Greenberg et al., 2017). However, continuous infusions of 0.1 to 0.6 mcg/kg/hour have been reported in both preterm and term neonates (Chrysostomou et al., 2014; O'Mara et al., 2012).

Clinical-Monitoring Pearls

Clinicians customarily monitor blood pressure, vital-sign trends, level of sedation, and pain scores. Dexmedetomidine should be used cautiously in patients with hepatic impairment. Respiratory depression is unlikely when used alone but the risk increases with the use of concomitant sedatives. Rapid weaning of dexmedetomidine may precipitate withdrawal.

There is limited data in neonates specific to safety, efficacy, and long-term neurodevelopmental outcomes (van Hoorn et al., 2019). Among preterm intubated infants, dexmedetomidine therapy is associated with an increased risk for hypotension requiring vasopressor support when used in conjunction with opioids and/or benzodiazepines (Greenberg et al., 2017). When compared to alternative therapies (fentanyl, morphine, midazolam), dexmedetomidine use is associated with a decrease in adjunctive sedation, delirium, respiratory depression, and GI dysmotility (McPherson et al., 2020).

Benzodiazepines

MIDAZOLAM

Midazolam ($C_{18}H_{14}C_{12}FN_3$), the most commonly prescribed benzodiazepine in the NICU, is short acting with rapid onset of action. It is used as an anxiolytic, anticonvulsant, and sedative.

Mechanism of Action/Pharmacokinetic Principles

Benzodiazepines bind to stereospecific GABA-A receptors on the postsynaptic GABA neuron at several sites within the CNS. Benzodiazepines enhance the inhibitory effect of GABA on neuronal excitability, which results in increased neuronal membrane permeability to chloride ions. This shift in chloride ions elicits hyperpolarization (a less excitable state) and stabilization.

Midazolam is rapidly absorbed, highly protein bound, and widely distributed in fat and muscle tissue. The volume of distribution is higher in neonates compared to adults (de Wildt et al., 2001). Drug molecules are hepatically metabolized by CYP3A4 enzymes into active and inactive metabolites. The active metabolite of midazolam is 1-hydroxymidazolam, which is rapidly conjugated to 1-hydroxymidazolam glucuronide and accounts for 60% to 70% of drug metabolites. Other minor metabolites include 4-hydroxymidazolam and 1,4-dihydroxymidazolam. The pharmacokinetics of midazolam are significantly affected by reduced renal clearance among preterm and critically ill infants, as well as decreased hepatic CYP3A4/3A5 activity in early life (de Wildt et al., 2001).

Dosing Recommendations

Benzodiazepines can be administered by way of IV, oral, or intranasal routes. Just recently, labeling information for preterm infants was added by the U.S. Food and Drug Administration (FDA). Approved dosing is 0.03 mg/kg/hour (<32 weeks of gestation) and 0.06 mg/kg/hour (>32 weeks of gestation; Jacqz-Aigrain et al., 1992). Intermittent IV dosing is typically 0.05 to 0.2 mg/kg/dose, although the former generally produces subtherapeutic concentrations, whereas the latter confers a high risk of hypotension (Treluyer et al., 2005). Intranasal dosing is typically comparable to IV dosing (Milesi et al., 2018). Midazolam is 40% to 50% bioavailable after oral administration in adults, with IV doses typically doubled (Kanto, 1985); this dosing approach has not been validated in neonates.

Clinical-Monitoring Pearls

Clinicians customarily monitor liver enzymes and renal function prior to initiation of midazolam as a continuous infusion; during therapy, vital-sign trends (with special attention to blood pressure) and the level of sedation should be carefully evaluated. Given that midazolam is hepatically metabolized and renally excreted, hepatic and/or renal impairment can provoke dose accumulation, prolonging both the drug half-life and period of sedation. Other disadvantages linked to midazolam therapy, in particular among mechanically ventilated preterm infants, include an increased risk for hypotension, myoclonus, delirium, and the composite of severe IVH, PVL, and death (Anand et al., 1999; McPherson et al., 2020).

In cases of suspected or confirmed intoxication or overdose, flumazenil has been used as a reversal agent. The customary dose is 0.01 mg/kg IV over 15 seconds. The 0.01 mg/kg dose may be repeated after 45 seconds and then every minute to a maximum total dose of 0.05 mg/kg. Myoclonic jerking and evidence of delirium from midazolam require dose adjustment, discontinuation, or reversal. In these situations, the customary reversal dose of flumazenil is 0.0078 mg/kg IV once (Zaw et al., 2001). Incremental weaning of midazolam after long-term continuous IV infusion is required. Rapid weaning or discontinuation can precipitate withdrawal and/or seizures.

Despite being the most frequently used benzodiazepine in the NICU, there is little data on pharmacodynamics, efficacy, and safety, as well as long-term neurodevelopmental outcomes of neonates treated with midazolam. The FDA has issued warnings regarding the repeated use or lengthy exposure to sedatives and anesthetics on the developing brain of the newborn infant (FDA, 2017). These therapies may have detrimental effects on brain development and may cause cognitive and behavioral problems (Duerden et al., 2016). Animal models have shown adverse effects on brain maturation and neuronal apoptosis (Durrmeyer et al., 2010); further studies are required to elucidate the safety and efficacy of these agents in the newborn.

TAPERING OF SEDATION (AFTER PROLONGED USE)

As more liberal treatment of pain in neonates increased, the unanticipated consequences of iatrogenic neonatal abstinence were identified (Cramton & Gruchala, 2013). Iatrogenic withdrawal can occur after as little as 72 hours of analgesic or sedative use, and many neonates are treated with both analgesics (most often morphine or fentanyl) and benzodiazepines concurrently. Infants with more complex medical needs (extensive operations, extracorporeal membrane oxygenation [ECMO]) often require medication for longer periods of time. The AAP published guidelines in a clinical report in 2012 to guide NICUs in developing protocols to appropriately, but judiciously, manage withdrawal in this group of neonates (Hudak et al., 2012). The need for weaning and duration of the weaning period depend on total dose exposure, duration of exposure, and concomitant medications (Tables 11.5 and 11.6). Various tapering regimens have been suggested. The following suggested regimens are based on duration of therapy (Hudak et al., 2012):

- **If duration of therapy is less than or equal to 4 days:** Taper over 1 to 2 days beginning with an initial dosage reduction of 30% to 50% followed by 20% to 30% dosage reductions every 6 to 8 hours; monitor closely for signs and symptoms of withdrawal with each reduction in dose.
- **If duration of therapy is greater than 4 days:** Decrease infusion rate by 25% to 50% every 12 hours, then convert to an intermittent dose every 4 hours and then every 6 hours and then every 8 hours; monitor closely for signs and symptoms of withdrawal with each reduction in dose.

See Chapter 9, "Neonatal Abstinence Syndrome," for additional information.

CONCLUSIONS

Prolonged exposure to pain and agitation and the medications used to treat them may have far-reaching adverse effects on ongoing neonatal development and also impact future health outcomes. Best treatment options include a combination of nonpharmacologic interventions and pharmacologic agents. Assessment of pain and finding a balance between adequate alleviation of pain and agitation but judicious use of analgesics and sedatives are warranted and are ongoing challenges in the provision of evidence-based best treatment of neonatal pain and agitation.

TABLE 11.5 Sample Weaning Protocol of Continuous Intravenous Fentanyl Infusion

<5 DAYS' INFUSION	5–9 DAYS' INFUSION	10–27 DAYS' INFUSION	≥28 DAYS' INFUSION
Wean: Decrease by 1 mcg/kg/hr every 6–12 hours.	**Wean:** Decrease by 0.5–1 mcg/kg/hr every 12 to 24 hours. (Total daily dose reduced by **20%–25% daily** of the original starting wean dose.)	**Wean:** Decrease by 0.5 mcg/kg/hr every 24 hours. (Total daily dose reduced by **10% daily** of the original starting wean dose.)	**Wean:** Decrease by 0.5 mcg/kg/hr every 48 hours. (Total daily dose reduced by **10% every other day** of the original starting wean dose.)
Discontinue: Discontinue when dose weaned to 1 mcg/kg/hr.	**Discontinue:** Discontinue when dose weaned to 0.5 mcg/kg/hr. **Transition:** Consider fentanyl 0.5–1 mcg/kg IV q2–4h PRN if rescue intermittent doses are needed during transition.	**Discontinue:** Discontinue when dose weaned to 0.5 mcg/kg/hr. **Transition:** Continue long-course dose wean with fentanyl intermittent doses; fentanyl 0.5–1 mcg/kg IV q2h around the clock. Extend interval every 24 hours as tolerated and IV access available.	**Discontinue:** Discontinue when dose weaned to 0.5 mcg/kg/hr. **Transition:** Continue long-course dose wean with fentanyl intermittent doses; fentanyl 0.5–1 mcg/kg IV q2h around the clock. Extend interval every 24–48 hours as tolerated and IV access available.
Goal: Patients are at a **very low risk** of dependence/withdrawal. Transitioning to intermittent medications is NOT needed. Fentanyl continuous infusion should be rapidly tapered off and then discontinued in 24–48 hours. Monitor for signs of withdrawal and initiate withdrawal monitoring.	**Goal:** Patients are at a **low risk** of dependence/withdrawal. Consider a transition to intermittent doses only if needed to facilitate weaning. Goal is to wean off in 4–5 days. Monitor for signs of withdrawal and initiate withdrawal monitoring.	**Goal:** Patients are at a **moderate risk** for developing dependence/withdrawal. Goal is to wean off in 10 days. Monitor for signs of withdrawal and initiate withdrawal monitoring.	**Goal:** Patients are at a **high risk** for developing dependence/withdrawal. Goal is to wean off in 20 days. Monitor for signs of withdrawal and initiate withdrawal monitoring. **High-risk** patients will require a long-course wean plan with transition from around-the-clock intermittent doses of **IV** fentanyl and then convert to **oral** morphine. Consult clinical pharmacist for assistance with dose conversion.

Note: The information in this table is intended for teaching purposes only, to help student learners achieve conceptual understanding of considerations applicable to tapering of sedation.
IV, intravenous, PRN, pro re nata.

TABLE 11.6 Sample Weaning Protocol From Continuous Intravenous Fentanyl or Morphine Infusion to Oral Morphine

General Considerations for Learners

Consult clinical pharmacist to discuss weaning plan and initial dose conversion before initiating a treatment plan.

The IV fentanyl to IV morphine conversion is 1:100 (acute exposure) and 1:25–50 (chronic exposure). Consider using 1:25 conversion from IV fentanyl to IV morphine to account for incomplete cross tolerance.

IV morphine to oral morphine conversion is 1:3. Consider using 1:2 conversion from IV to oral morphine based on immature first-pass metabolism.

Consider a transition to oral morphine when IV morphine infusion is <15 mcg/kg/hr or IV fentanyl infusion is <1.5 mcg/kg/hr and duration of infusion exceeds 10 days. Thirty to 60 minutes after the first oral dose of morphine is administered, wean the IV infusion by 50%. Then, considering weaning the IV infusion by another 50% (or discontinue) 30–60 minutes after the second oral dose of morphine is administered.

Conversion of IV fentanyl to PO morphine:

1. Calculate the total daily dose of IV fentanyl in 24 hours (total mcg in 24 hours).
2. Divide by 1000 to convert to mg of fentanyl in 24 hours.
3. Multiply total daily dose of IV fentanyl by 25 to convert to total daily dose of IV morphine in mg.
4. Multiply total daily dose of IV morphine by 2 to give total daily dose of PO morphine in 24 hours (ODD in mg).
5. Divide total daily dose of PO morphine by 8 (total daily dose divided q3 hours).
6. Determine appropriate weaning schedule based on duration of continuous infusion.

Conversion of IV morphine to PO morphine:

1. Calculate the total daily dose of IV morphine in 24 hours.
2. Multiply the total daily dose of IV morphine by 2 to give total daily dose of PO morphine (ODD).
3. Divide total daily dose of PO morphine by 8 (total daily dose divided q3h).
4. Determine appropriate weaning schedule based on duration of continuous infusion.

FENTANYL OR MORPHINE CONTINUOUS INFUSION SPANNING 10–27 DAYS	FENTANYL OR MORPHINE CONTINUOUS INFUSION SPANNING ≥28 DAYS
10-day oral morphine wean	**20-day oral morphine wean**
ODD reduced by **10% daily** of the **original** starting wean dose.	ODD reduced by **10% every other day** of the **original** starting wean dose.
Day 1. Divide ODD q3 Day 2. Decrease to 90% of ODD and divide q3 Day 3. Decrease to 80% of ODD and divide q3 Day 4. Decrease to 70% of ODD and divide q3 Day 5. Decrease to 60% of ODD and divide q3 Day 6. Decrease to 50% of ODD and divide q4 Day 7. Decrease to 40% of ODD and divide q6 Day 8. Decrease to 30% of ODD and divide q8 Day 9. Decrease to 20% of ODD and divide q12 Day 10. Decrease to 10% of ODD and divide q24 Day 11. Discontinue morphine	Day 1. Divide ODD q3 Day 2. No change Day 3. Decrease to 90% of ODD and divide q3 Day 4. No change Day 5. Decrease to 80% of ODD and divide q3 Day 6. No change Day 7. Decrease to 70% of ODD and divide q3 Day 8. No change Day 9. Decrease to 60% of ODD and divide q3 Day 10. No change Day 11. Decrease to 50% of ODD and divide q4 Day 12. No change Day 13. Decrease to 40% of ODD and divide q6 Day 14. No change Day 15. Decrease to 30% of ODD and divide q8 Day 16. No change Day 17. Decrease to 20% of ODD and divide q12 Day 18. No change Day 19. Decrease to 10% of ODD and divide q24 Day 20. No change Day 21. Discontinue morphine

Note: The information in this table is intended for teaching purposes only, to help student learners achieve conceptual understanding of considerations applicable to tapering of sedation.
IV, intravenous; ODD, oral daily dose; PO, by mouth.

LEARNING TOOLS AND RESOURCES

Advice From the Authors

Leanne Nantais-Smith, PhD, RN, NNP-BC

I am a visual learner, so a mind map provides a clear illustration of the mechanism of action of any drug in the context of anatomy and physiology. "Map" the mechanism of action of other drugs to better "see" or understand how each drug exerts its effect.

Carolyn J. Herrington, PhD, RN, NNP-BC

I am an intuitive and reflective learner. I focus on the overall topic to study and review the chapter headings to develop an overall "map" of the materials. Once I have the overall map, I focus on the main issues (definitions, timelines, landmark studies, or societal shifts) that have influenced the science surrounding the topic. However, as an intuitive, reflective learner, I know that for every action, there must be a reaction, and in recognizing this fact, I move forward cautiously, always looking for newer information with which I can maintain an evidence-based practice within a rapidly changing knowledge environment.

Mirjana Lulic-Botica, PharmD, BCPS

I am a visual learner and so illustrations, such as graphs, charts, maps, and diagrams, help me to effectively interpret information.

Discussion Prompts

1. It is important to first understand normal physiology in order to make sense of pain and how medications that modulate pain work. Investigate how the nociceptive signal is transmitted and how endogenous opioids act to modulate (decrease) pain. Think about how opioid agonists mimic endogenous pain relief. Then think about how other medications that modulate pain produce their pharmacologic effects.
2. The study of pain in the neonate has made huge strides in the past 35 years, from denial of the existence of pain in infants to a well-established recognition of pain pathways and short- and long- term outcomes for the neonate exposed to painful procedures. Newer studies suggest that aggressive pain management in this vulnerable population may not provide improved outcomes for neonates and may be contributing to worse neurologic outcomes. Reflect on what history has revealed to us about infant pain, and what the newer evidence is suggesting about more judicious use of sedatives and analgesics. Be prepared to discuss how you might formulate your approach to pain management based on the early evidence tempered by the newer evidence, which recommends caution.
3. It is important to understand the pharmacology of a drug and the mechanisms of action of the drug classes used for pain and sedation in neonates. A review of the pharmacokinetics of any given drug, including its absorption, distribution, metabolism, and excretion properties, will assist you as the clinician to appropriately use these medications in your population safely and effectively. It is imperative as well to keep updated with the most recent literature so as to provide up-to-date care. Identify an article published in the last year on pharmacotherapy for neonatal pain and discuss why it does or does not warrant a practice change in your unit.

Mind Map

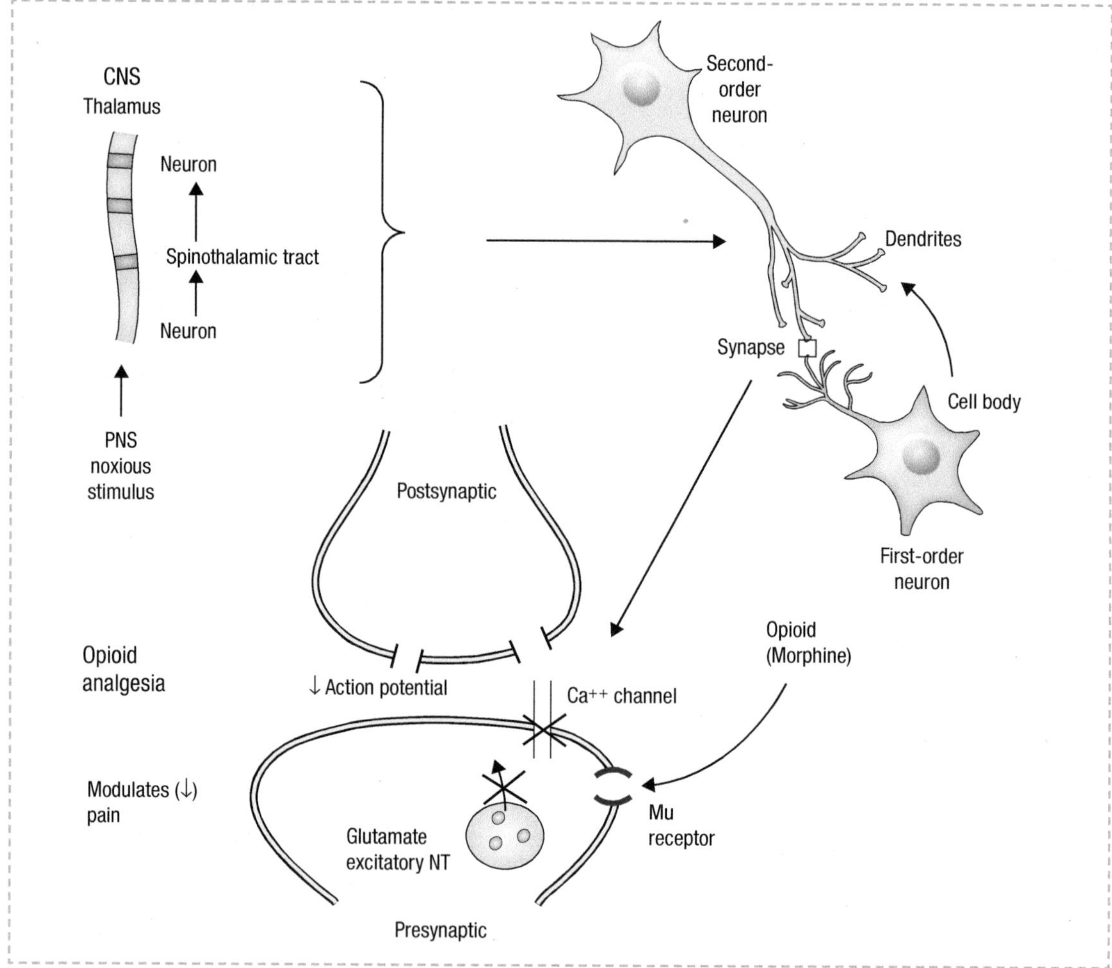

Note: This mind map reflects the design team's interpretation of a portion of one or more concepts addressed in this chapter. Readers should regard the mind maps woven throughout this textbook as examples of multisensory study tools that can be developed to encourage conceptual understanding. Readers are encouraged to develop their own unique mind maps in consultation with academic faculty or clinical preceptors. CNS, central nervous system; NT, neurotransmitter; PNS, peripheral nervous system.

REFERENCES

References for this chapter are online and available at https://connect.springerpub.com/content/book/978-0-8261-5884-0/part/partII/toc-part/ch11.

chapter 12

Neonatal Seizures

Allison Jones Guider and Christopher McPherson

LEARNING OBJECTIVES

After completing this chapter, the reader should be able to:

- Define the types of seizures and identify the epidemiology of the disease process.
- Enumerate the most common risk factors for seizures.
- Explain the physiology of neurotransmission.
- Correlate the pathophysiology of seizure activity with the need for pharmacologic treatment.
- Appraise the historical evolution of pharmacologic management of seizures.
- Evaluate the role of pharmacotherapeutic regimens with respect to pharmacodynamic and pharmacokinetic properties in relation to management/prevention of seizures.

INTRODUCTION

The highest risk for seizures during life occurs in the first month after birth, making treatment of this disorder relatively common in neonatal intensive care. Neonatal seizures occur in approximately 1 to 3.5 per 1,000 live, term births, most commonly precipitated by acute brain injury (Vasudevan & Levene, 2013). Seizures in early life alter synaptogenesis, myelination, and overall brain development, resulting in potential long-term functional and cognitive deficits (Holmes, 2009). Despite ongoing efforts to improve detection and treatment, mortality remains high (35% in preterm and 15% in term infants; Glass et al., 2017). Nearly one in three survivors suffer from long-term neurologic impairments, including cerebral palsy, intellectual disabilities, and/or prolonged epilepsy (Uria-Avellanal et al., 2013). Early identification and treatment of neonatal seizures is essential to optimize outcomes (McBride et al., 2000). Neonatal seizures may be challenging to identify, with subtle or absent clinical manifestations, highlighting the importance of targeted electrographic monitoring in neonates with symptoms concerning for seizures and those at high risk. Appropriate pharmacologic treatment is vital to minimize both acute and long-term consequences of prolonged seizures; however, antiseizure medications generally have unfavorable adverse effect profiles and limited data exist to guide selection of the optimal antiepileptic cocktail. In this chapter, we discuss the pathophysiology of neonatal seizures, the methods of diagnosing seizures in the newborn period, and the evolution of antiepileptic pharmacotherapy supporting current pharmacologic treatment algorithms.

PHYSIOLOGY REVIEW: NEUROTRANSMISSION

A neuron is an electrically excitable cell that communicates with other cells over synapses. Electrical signals from sensory nerves or other neurons, called *action potentials,* are received by dendrites on the neuron and then travel along the axon. Neurons translate these electrical signals into chemical signals in the form of neurotransmitter release at the axon terminal. Neurotransmitters cross the synapse and illicit a specific response in the receiving neuron or muscle cell.

Resting Membrane Potential and the Action Potential

At resting state, neurons have a negative charge (–70 mV). Neurons maintain a baseline negative charge through a higher intracellular concentration of negatively charged organic anions (primarily amino acids) compared with positively charged cations (primarily sodium). Resting state is maintained by adenosine triphosphate (ATP)-dependent pumps, which move charged ions across the cellular membrane against osmotic gradients.

Action potentials open voltage-gated ion channels, allowing positive ions (generally sodium or calcium) to enter the neuron by osmosis, depolarizing the cell from its resting negative state. Depolarization to the action potential threshold (–55 mV) results in the release of neurotransmitters. Other positively charged cations play a vital role in maintaining homeostasis. Calcium, a predominantly extracellular cation, transiently blocks voltage-gated sodium channels as a regulatory mechanism to prevent excessive depolarization. Potassium, a predominantly intracellular cation, exits the neuronal cell after depolarization to reestablish a resting negative charge.

Major Neurotransmitters: Glutamate and Gamma-Aminobutyric Acid

Neurotransmitters (e.g., glutamate, gamma-aminobutyric acid [GABA]) in the brain transmit chemical messages between neurons. Glutamate is an amino acid that stimulates a diverse array of postsynaptic neuronal receptors, including many ligand-gated ion channels like N-methyl-D-aspartate (NMDA) and G-protein-coupled receptors like alpha and beta receptors in the central nervous and cardiovascular systems. Glutamate generally makes the receiving neuron more likely to fire an action potential. Hence, glutamate is the major excitatory neurotransmitter in the central nervous system (CNS). On the contrary, GABA is an amino acid that targets GABA receptors, including $GABA_A$ (a ligand-gated ion channel complex) and $GABA_B$ (a G-protein-coupled receptor). GABA generally makes the target neuron less likely to fire an action potential in the mature CNS. Therefore, GABA functions as the primary inhibitory neurotransmitter in the mature CNS. It is important to note that glutamate is the metabolic precursor of GABA; conversely, GABA can be recycled to glutamate through the tricarboxylic acid cycle.

The immature neonatal brain is structurally and functionally susceptible to seizures due to excess neuronal excitation and reduced inhibition. Structurally, the fetal and neonatal brain is populated with the highest density of dendritic spines and synapses at any stage of life, which are necessary to facilitate neurogenesis and use-dependent synaptogenesis. Functionally, glutamate exhibits exaggerated activity due to increased expression of the GluN2B subunit of the NMDA receptor while paradoxical GABA functionality is observed (Carrasco & Stafstrom, 2018). Normally, the binding of GABA to the $GABA_a$ receptor permits an influx of negatively charged chloride ions, which hyperpolarizes the neuronal membrane and inhibits transmission of action potentials across the neuron. In neonates, exaggerated expression of sodium-potassium-chloride cotransporter 1 (NKCC1; responsible for chloride influx) and delayed expression of potassium-chloride cotransporter 2 (KCC2; responsible for chloride efflux) lead to a state of hyperchloremia within the neuronal membrane (Dzhala et al., 2005; Rivera et al., 1999). In this setting, opening of the $GABA_a$ receptor results in (paradoxical) chloride efflux, which depolarizes the neuronal membrane and increases the likelihood of action potential transmission. These factors make the neonatal brain highly vulnerable to acute symptomatic seizures following brain injury (e.g., birth asphyxia) or other CNS insults (e.g., hemorrhage, meningitis). After birth, incremental maturation of KCC2 expression normalizes intracellular chloride concentrations in neurons and standard GABA-mediated inhibition of action potentials.

PATHOPHYSIOLOGY: SEIZURES

Brain electrical activity is typically nonsynchronous. Seizures occur when abnormally excessive and/or synchronous depolarization of neurons occurs in the brain. The vast majority of neonatal seizures are considered acute, symptomatic events that manifest following brain injury due to hypoxic-ischemic encephalopathy (~40%), ischemic stroke (~20%), or intracranial hemorrhage (~10%; Glass et al., 2016). Seizures secondary to hemorrhage are most often observed in preterm neonates (45% of all cases; Vasudevan & Levene, 2013). These injuries lead to decreases in cellular energy production and may result in failure of ATP-dependent ion pumps, preventing active transport of ions that maintain the negative resting membrane potential of the neuron. In addition, cellular injury (secondary to apoptosis) can result in the excessive release of glutamate. Given that the newborn brain already demonstrates an exaggerated responsiveness to glutamate with intrinsically lower concentrations (and paradoxical activity) of GABA, excess glutamate release exacerbates seizure activity.

The minority of seizures are considered unprovoked and caused by genetic syndromes (e.g., pyridoxine-dependent epilepsy), infection, brain malformations (or cerebral dysgenesis), and metabolic abnormalities (Glass et al., 2016). For example, pyridoxal-5-phosphate, the active form of pyridoxine, is a required cofactor in the conversion of glutamate to GABA. Genetic disorders that disrupt pyridoxine metabolism or pyridoxal-5-phosphate synthesis result in rarer, yet severe epileptic seizures due to excessive glutamate and deficient GABA.

CNS infection, or meningitis, may elicit seizure activity due to inflammatory responses and the accumulation of bacterial toxins in the subpial space. Pathogens commonly linked to meningitis and seizures include the gram-positive pathogens group B *Streptococcus* and *Listeria monocytogenes*; the gram-negative pathogens *Citrobacter*, *Enterobacter*, *Pseudomonas*, *Proteus*, and *Serratia marcescens*; and the virus herpes simplex. Any of the aforementioned pathogens may elicit the inflammatory cascade, which begins in the choroid plexus. This is followed by infiltration of the ventricular fluid and lining, arachnoid matter, and vasculature, culminating in cerebral edema and potential infarction. Severe cerebral edema and/or diffuse infarction produce seizures by a similar mechanism to the brain injuries described in the previous paragraph.

Various potential mechanisms may contribute to the development of seizures in neonates with cerebral dysgenesis. Loss of interneurons and decreased functionality of inhibitory pathways, dysfunction of neuronal receptors resulting in intrinsic excitability, and alterations in the development of neuronal networks may contribute, depending on the specific genotype and developmental phenotype.

Electrolyte abnormalities, namely sodium and calcium deficiencies, and hypoglycemia are linked to the onset of severe seizures. Acute serum hyponatremia may produce cerebral edema as free water flows across the blood–brain barrier by osmosis. Given that calcium ions are necessary for sodium homeostasis in that they inhibit the movement of sodium across neuronal membranes, a deficiency of calcium ions permits excessive activity of sodium and neuronal hyperexcitability. Finally, hypoglycemia may produce seizures by several mechanisms. Acute serum hypoglycemia may produce cerebral edema in a fashion similar to hyponatremia. In an attempt to maintain homeostatic functions, the brain releases glutamate as an alternative fuel source, with resultant neuronal hyperexcitability. In the setting of total energy failure, the glucose-dependent production of ATP is lost, resulting in dysfunction of the ATP-dependent pumps required to maintain neuronal electrolyte homeostasis. Preterm neonates and those with brain injuries as previously described are at increased risk of electrolyte abnormalities; therefore, interval surveillance is customary to facilitate early identification. These etiologies may not respond to traditional antiepileptic medications and often require treatment of the underlying cause of the electrolyte imbalance.

Clinical Manifestations

Abnormal movements in neonates may raise concern for seizures, including focal clonic or tonic movements, intermittent forced gaze deviation, myoclonus, and/or oral-motor stereotypical movements (Shellhaas et al., 2011). Preterm infants are known to display uncoordinated movements, which may be described as subtle seizures. However, these symptoms often do not correlate with electrographic seizures on electroencephalography (Malone et al., 2009).

Of note, the vast majority of neonatal seizures identified by electroencephalography are focal or multifocal in electrical onset and localized to one hemisphere; generalized tonic-clonic seizures are rare in newborns due to the common etiology of brain injury and the status of neuroanatomic and neurophysiologic development at this maturity. All newborns with suspected or proven seizures should receive a thorough physical examination, as well as review of family history, antenatal records, and postnatal course. Neonatal APRNs should anticipate the need for pediatric neurology involvement and electroencephalographic studies as part of the diagnostic process.

Diagnosis

Initial laboratory studies for neonates with suspected or proven seizures include a comprehensive serum chemistry panel and blood glucose. Neonates considered eligible for invasive procedures should undergo a lumbar tap for cerebrospinal fluid (CSF) studies, ideally prior to the initiation of antibiotic and/or antiviral therapy. Head ultrasound should be utilized to screen for structural brain abnormalities or intracranial hemorrhage. Additional laboratory and imaging studies may be warranted in specific clinical scenarios.

More than half of electrographic neonatal seizures are subclinical, with no identifiable clinical symptomatology. Therefore, continuous electroencephalography (cEEG) is the gold standard for diagnosis of neonatal seizures. cEEG should be utilized to identify subclinical seizures in high-risk populations described in the Pathophysiology section (Box 12.1), who should be screened for a minimum of 24 hours (Shellhaas et al., 2011). cEEG should also be used to capture electrographic activity during periods of abnormal movements described previously, determining the need for pharmacologic treatment.

When cEEG is not feasible, pediatric neurology teams may resort to amplitude-integrated electroencephalography (aEEG), a less invasive monitoring tool capable of detecting extended seizure activity but less sensitive in detecting focal seizures. In addition, aEEG is not recommended for use in preterm infants, who often manifest with low-amplitude seizures (Mastrangelo et al., 2013).

HISTORICAL PERSPECTIVE: SEMINAL AND NOTEWORTHY STUDIES

Despite the overall frequency of neonatal seizures and high associated mortality, robust clinical data and evidence-based guidelines are lacking (El-Dib & Soul, 2017). Currently, there are no antiepileptics approved by the U.S. Food and Drug Administration (FDA) for use in neonates (Sharpe et al., 2020). Despite the known differences in the immature neonatal CNS and varying pharmacokinetics/pharmacodynamics, evidence for treatment has largely been extrapolated from studies in older children and adults (Mruk et al., 2015).

BOX 12.1 Clinical Scenarios With High Risk of Neonatal Seizures

Provoked

Hypoxic-ischemic encephalopathy
Ischemic stroke
Intracranial, subdural, or intraventricular hemorrhage
Perinatal stroke
Sinovenous thrombosis

Unprovoked

Meningitis
Inborn errors of metabolism
Cerebral dysgenesis
Acute electrolyte or glucose abnormalities

Much of the available published studies of antiepileptics in neonates report a wide range of efficacy and often conflicting data. The variability may be explained by a multitude of different reasons, including (but not limited to) the study's definition of seizure cessation, duration of effective seizure cessation, order of medication therapy initiation (first-line vs. second-line or third-line therapy), and underlying seizure etiology (El-Dib & Soul, 2017). Despite these limitations, careful review of historical and modern pharmacokinetic and clinical trials informs modern seizure treatment algorithms and ongoing research efforts.

Phenobarbital

The first barbiturate drug, barbital, was synthesized in Germany in 1902. Phenobarbital, a GABA agonist, was identified as an early derivative in 1904 and first marketed in 1912 (Table 12.1). Phenobarbital's antiepileptic effects were discovered that same year by chance; a young German clinician, Alfred Hauptmann, administered phenobarbital as a tranquilizer to adult patients with nocturnal epileptic attacks to achieve quiet in his sleeping quarters above the ward (when residents were truly residents of the hospital); the patients slept but also experienced a dramatic reduction or complete abolition of their seizures.

Phenobarbital is the oldest antiepileptic currently in clinical use in neonatal intensive care. A case series exists describing phenobarbital for treatment of newborns with spasms from tetanus beginning in the late 1950s (Box, 1964). Focused research in neonates peaked in the latter half of the 20th century, with initial research focused on pharmacokinetic studies in the late 1970s. Following a small pilot trial, investigators from the University of Pittsburgh and Columbia University collaborated to evaluate phenobarbital concentrations after loading and maintenance dosing in 59 neonates with clinical seizures (Painter et al., 1978). The authors established that phenobarbital has a mean volume of distribution of 1 L/kg in neonates, so a 20 mg/kg loading dose results in a mean phenobarbital concentration of 20 mcg/mL. Maintenance dosing of 3 to 4 mg/kg/d results in achievement of a similar steady-state concentration while avoiding drug accumulation (Painter et al., 1981). Subsequent studies focused on pharmacodynamics, initially defining efficacy as the cessation of clinical seizures. The likelihood of seizure cessation increased with escalating serum concentrations of phenobarbital; 40% to 60% of clinical seizures are controlled at a phenobarbital concentration of 20 mcg/mL; 70% to 85% of clinical seizures are controlled at 40 mcg/mL (Gilman et al., 1989). Modern cohort studies suggest a similar efficacy rate for electrographic seizures, although response rate is variable based on the underlying etiology of seizures (Spagnoli et al., 2016).

Phenytoin

Phenytoin was also synthesized as a derivative of barbital in 1908 by German chemists. Little use for phenytoin was recognized; it was a dramatically inferior sedative to phenobarbital and possessed a novel mechanism of action as a sodium channel blocker (see Table 12.1). However, in 1938, scientists searching for effective agents with less sedative effects evaluated its antiepileptic activity in animals. Phenytoin was approved by the FDA for treatment of seizures in adults in 1953. Although unlabeled for use in neonates, phenytoin has a long history of utilization for neonatal seizures, with anecdotal reports as a second-line therapy to phenobarbital dating to the early 1970s (Volpe, 1973).

Pharmacokinetic studies of phenytoin in neonates were conducted in parallel to studies of phenobarbital, but the complex and challenging nature of this drug was not fully appreciated until the early 1990s (Painter et al., 1994). First, scientists discovered that phenytoin was highly

TABLE 12.1 Antiepileptics by Mechanism of Action

MECHANISM OF ACTION	MEDICATION
Sodium channel blockade	Fosphenytoin/phenytoin, lacosamide, lidocaine, topiramate
GABA potentiation	Midazolam, phenobarbital, topiramate
Synaptic vesicle protein (SV2A) modifier	Levetiracetam

GABA, gamma-aminobutyric acid.

protein-bound (90% in adults), with efficacy and toxicity dependent mainly on the free fraction of the total phenytoin concentration. Neonates were observed to have an increased and highly variable free fraction of drug (generally about half the protein binding of adults but with fourfold variability between individual neonates), with some dependence on gestational age and albumin concentrations. Second, phenytoin was metabolized via oxidation at a rate determined by dose-dependent (Michaelis–Menten) pharmacokinetics. Therefore, the drug accumulated linearly until the metabolic pathway approached saturation, at which point accumulation occurred exponentially. In other words, as the concentration of drug increased, clearance decreased, and the half-life became longer. In the setting of dramatic variability in protein binding and clearance among individual neonates, experts concluded that personalized dosing was required (Takeoka et al., 1998). Finally, phenytoin in intravenous (IV) solution had a pH of 11. At this highly basic pH, rapid IV administration of phenytoin carried intrinsic risk of cardiovascular adverse effects and tissue necrosis. In 2% to 6% of patients, IV administration in an upper extremity resulted in "purple glove syndrome," with discoloration and edema of the affected hand resolving within days to weeks, or progressing to vascular compression, compartment syndrome, and amputation (Chokshi et al., 2007). To decrease risk of purple glove syndrome, fosphenytoin was developed, a phosphorylated prodrug of phenytoin with a pH in solution of 8.6. Despite these limitations, phenytoin/fosphenytoin has historically been and remains the second most commonly prescribed agent for neonatal seizures (Boer & Gal, 1982; Glass et al., 2012).

Concurrent with careful pharmacokinetic studies of phenobarbital and phenytoin at the University of Pittsburgh, investigators conducted a randomized controlled trial (RCT) comparing the two agents to determine the most appropriate first-line therapy for neonatal seizures ($N = 59$). Note that efficacy was determined by electrographic cessation of seizures. Doses were titrated to achieve free plasma concentration of 25 mcg/mL for phenobarbital (total concentration of 40 mcg/mL) and 3 mcg/mL for phenytoin (total concentration of 15 mcg/mL). Seizure control was similar between groups (43% vs. 45%, $p = 1$); utilization of both agents resulted in a cumulative rate of control of 59% (Painter et al., 1999). However, a similar trial in a larger population of exclusively late preterm or term infants with clinical seizures ($N = 109$) documented a higher response rate to a single 20 mg/kg loading dose of phenobarbital compared with phenytoin (72% vs. 15%, $p < .001$; Pathak et al., 2013). Overall, seizure cessation occurred more frequently in neonates initially randomized to phenobarbital (91% vs. 80%, $p = .014$), confirming the historical preference for phenobarbital as first-line therapy for neonatal seizures.

Concern about the neurotoxic effects of GABA agonism and sodium channel blockade has existed since initial reports in 1975 of fetal hydantoin syndrome, a constellation of craniofacial anomalies, nail and digital hypoplasia, growth failure, and developmental delay (Hanson & Smith, 1975). Concern about the clinical effects of long-term exposure to phenobarbital peaked in the early 1990s with the publication of an RCT ($N = 217$) documenting an 8-point IQ deficit after 2 years of maintenance phenobarbital in infants treated for febrile seizures (Farwell et al., 1990). In this setting, the decision to continue maintenance phenobarbital after neonatal or infantile seizures remains controversial and requires consultation with an experienced pediatric neurologist (Glass et al., 2021). In the acute setting, the balance of evidence suggests that the benefits of seizure control far outweigh the toxicities of available pharmacotherapies. However, the quest continued for antiepileptic agents (and therapies) with more appealing short- and long-term safety profiles.

Therapeutic Hypothermia

Induced hypothermia to reduce the long-term consequences of acute brain injury was described over 2,000 years ago by ancient medical providers, including Greek physician Hippocrates (Gunn et al., 2017). Small, uncontrolled studies published in the late 1950s describe immersion in cold water of newborns with no respiratory effort until the onset of respirations. Controlled, preclinical studies of modern, newborn therapeutic hypothermia began in the late 1990s. Clear benefit in term-born animals with induced hypoxic-ischemic encephalopathy prompted RCTs in human neonates. In a meta-analysis of 11 RCTs including 1,505 late preterm and term neonates with moderate or severe encephalopathy and evidence of intrapartum asphyxia conducted between 1998 and 2011, therapeutic hypothermia dramatically reduced the risk of both death (risk ratio [RR]: 0.75, 95% CI: 0.64–0.88, number needed to treat [NNT] to prevent one death = 11) and major disability in survivors (RR: 0.67, 95% CI: 0.55–0.80, NNT = 8; Jacobs et al., 2013). Therapeutic hypothermia also reduces seizure burden in neonates after hypoxic-ischemic injury (Glass, Nash, et al., 2011; Srinivasakumar et al., 2013). However, as previously described, hypoxic-ischemic encephalopathy remains the leading cause of neonatal seizures, with approximately one-third of neonates with moderate or severe encephalopathy still experiencing electrographic seizures in the era of therapeutic hypothermia, highlighting the continuing role of pharmacologic antiepileptics. In addition, therapeutic hypothermia and hypoxic-ischemic organ injury have important impacts on the pharmacokinetics of multiple agents used in neonatal intensive care (Lutz et al., 2020). Recognition of this fact has prompted pharmacokinetic studies of both historical and novel antiepileptic agents.

Levetiracetam

Piracetam was discovered in the early 1960s through experiments designed to develop lipophilic, synthetic GABA derivatives to treat insomnia. Piracetam was initially thought to be an inactive compound, with neither sedative nor stimulant properties and virtually no toxicity. However, serial experiments documented its efficacy for nystagmus and myoclonus and suggested some level of cognitive enhancement in children with epilepsy and adults with postconcussion syndrome. Piracetam is currently a prescription medication in the United Kingdom and Japan, but viewed as a dietary supplement in the United States. Levetiracetam was discovered in the early 1990s through serial screening of derivatives of piracetam against audiogenic seizures in susceptible mice. Levetiracetam was approved by the FDA for use in adults with seizures in 1999 and as adjunctive therapy in pediatric patients (1 month of age and older) in 2012. Levetiracetam rapidly gained popularity in neonates due to its favorable side effect profile, wide therapeutic window, and neuroprotective properties seen in animal models (Mruk et al., 2015). Small case series reporting use as adjunctive therapy for neonatal seizures refractory to conventional agents emerged in the late 2000s (Shoemaker & Rotenberg, 2007). The early 2010s brought small RCTs and large case series reporting its efficacy as first-line therapy (Furwentsches et al., 2010; Ramantani et al., 2011). Clinical enthusiasm outpaced robust RCTs. From 2012 through 2019, a randomized, blinded, phase IIb trial (NEOLEV2) was conducted to compare the efficacy of levetiracetam with phenobarbital as first-line therapy in neonates with electrographic seizures (Sharpe et al., 2020). Patients randomly assigned to phenobarbital ($n = 30$) received a loading dose of 20 mg/kg IV, which was repeated for persistent seizure activity to a cumulative loading dose of phenobarbital 40 mg/kg prior to the addition of levetiracetam. The levetiracetam group ($n = 53$) received 40 mg/kg IV, which was followed by 20 mg/kg for persistent electrographic seizures prior to crossover to phenobarbital. In this study, 80% of patients receiving phenobarbital responded and remained seizure-free at 24 hours as compared with 28% receiving levetiracetam ($p <. 001$). Hypotension was more common with phenobarbital therapy (10% vs. 2%). Given the reassuring safety profile of levetiracetam, investigators remain interested in exploring higher dose therapy. However, at this time, phenobarbital remains the evidence-based primary agent to control neonatal seizures, with little evidence to guide the sequence of use of subsequent agents.

Lidocaine and Midazolam

With limited available options to control refractory seizures, agents with a long history of use in neonates for other indications were repurposed. The most prevalent of these medications were lidocaine and midazolam. Lidocaine infusions were used for sodium channel blockade (see Table 12.1). Detailed pharmacokinetic studies have been conducted in neonates, both before and after the advent of therapeutic hypothermia for neonatal encephalopathy (van den Broek et al., 2011). Several case series describe robust efficacy as second-line therapy after phenobarbital (76%–92% in 13–25 patients; Hellstrom-Westas et al., 1988; Malingre et al., 2006; Rey et al., 1990; Shany et al., 2007). Despite these encouraging data, lidocaine use in the United States remains rare, most likely due to concerns for cardiac adverse effects despite relatively robust safety data (Weeke et al., 2015).

Available literature evaluating the efficacy of midazolam, a potent GABA agonist, is also limited to usage as second- or third-line therapy, treating seizures refractory to phenobarbital and/or phenytoin or lidocaine. The largest published report of midazolam for neonatal seizures included 15 full-term neonates with seizures refractory to phenobarbital and lidocaine after hypoxic-ischemic encephalopathy (van Leuven et al., 2004). The neonates received midazolam 0.1 mg/kg followed by 0.15 mg/kg/hr, with 73% achieving electrographic cessation of seizures.

CURRENT PHARMACOLOGIC TREATMENT MODALITIES FOR SEIZURES

Suspicion for neonatal seizures should initiate a careful diagnostic evaluation to identify reversible causes. Potential CNS infections require prompt treatment with broad-spectrum antibiotics with sufficient CSF penetration (see Chapter 28, "Neonatal Sepsis and Meningitis"). Hypoglycemia should be treated with a bolus of IV dextrose 10% at a dose of 2 mL/kg, followed by maintenance dextrose containing IV fluids, with careful monitoring of evolution of blood glucoses. Hypocalcemia is treated with calcium gluconate 100 mg/kg IV or calcium chloride 20 mg/kg IV. Hypomagnesemia is treated with magnesium sulfate 125 mg/kg IV.

Once the diagnosis of seizures is confirmed and any reversible causes for seizures are corrected, antiepileptic therapy should be initiated in a timely fashion to help reduce the severity of brain injury (Soul, 2018). Current prescribing practices are largely driven by clinical experience given the lack of robust data and clinical practice guidelines (Soul, 2018). Figure 12.1 describes a proposed treatment pathway. The most frequently used antiepileptics in neonates are described in detail in this chapter, with a summary available in Table 12.2.

Phenobarbital

Phenobarbital has long been the mainstay of therapy for neonatal seizures despite the varying reports of its efficacy as monotherapy and known adverse effects (Donovan et al., 2016). This is likely explained by the extensive history of usage, provider familiarity, ease of administration, predictable pharmacokinetics, and generally favorable bioavailability.

MECHANISM OF ACTION/PHARMACOKINETIC PRINCIPLES

Phenobarbital is a long-acting barbiturate that binds to and activates $GABA_A$ receptors, ultimately inhibiting neuronal excitability (Figure 12.2). As previously stated, however, the neonatal brain is known to have a paradoxical effect of $GABA_A$ activation. With the overall mixture of both immature and mature neurons, efficacy is achieved through overall net inhibition in the majority of patients (Soul, 2018).

Phenobarbital is metabolized predominantly by the hepatic cytochrome CYP2C9; thus, the prescriber should be cognizant of drug interactions and monitor accordingly (Pacifici, 2016). The pharmacokinetic parameters are not altered significantly by therapeutic hypothermia, but caution and likely dose reduction should occur in the setting of profound hepatic dysfunction (El-Dib & Soul, 2017). The half-life of phenobarbital in neonates ranges from approximately 100 hours in term infants to 140 hours in preterm infants.

DOSING RECOMMENDATIONS

Given the prolonged half-life of phenobarbital, dosing recommendations include a loading dose of 20 mg/kg IV, followed by a maintenance regimen ranging from 3 to 4 mg/kg/d starting 12 to 24 hours after the loading dose (either IV or oral). Additional bolus doses may be administered, 5 to 10 mg/kg, up to a maximum 40 mg/kg cumulative loading dose. IV and oral dosing recommendations are equivalent, allowing a one-to-one conversion.

CLINICAL-MONITORING PEARLS

Serum drug concentrations of 15 to 40 mcg/mL are generally accepted as therapeutic concentrations of phenobarbital; however, concentration does not always predict therapeutic efficacy in an individual patient (Pacifici, 2016). Notably, animal models have shown that phenobarbital can cause neuronal apoptosis at concentrations within the recommended therapeutic concentrations, around 25 to 35 mcg/mL, raising concern for poorer neurodevelopmental outcomes (Mruk et al., 2015). The net effect of this risk with the benefit of controlling seizures remains unclear, although available data suggest a net benefit in neurodevelopmental outcome in settings where

FIGURE 12.1 Suggested treatment algorithm for recurrent neonatal seizures.

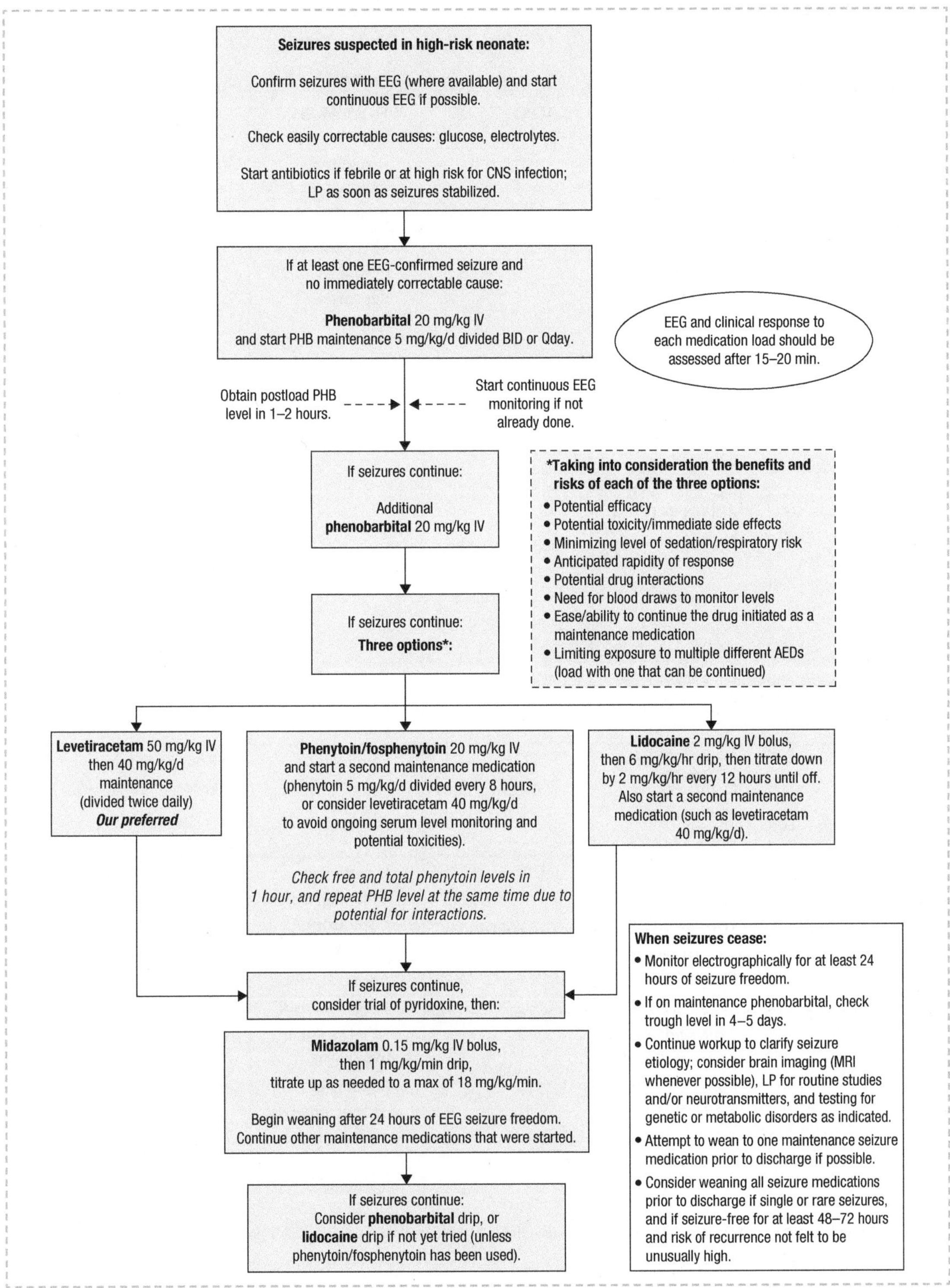

Note: Solid arrow indicates the next step if electrographically confirmed seizures are continuing (clinical or subclinical). Subtle dosing differences between this algorithm and chapter highlight gaps in the literature and the importance of individualized institutional consensus.

AED, antiepileptic drug; CNS, central nervous system; CSF, cerebrospinal fluid; IV, intravenous; LP, lumbar puncture; PHB, phenobarbital.

Source: From Slaughter, L. A., Patel, A. D., & Slaughter, J. L. (2013). Pharmacological treatment of neonatal seizures: A systematic review. *Journal of Child Neurology*, 28(3), 351–364. https://doi.org/10.1177/0883073812470734.

TABLE 12.2 Most Commonly Prescribed Antiepileptics in Neonatology

MEDICATION	DOSING	ROUTES	ADVERSE EFFECTS	THERAPEUTIC DRUG MONITORING GOAL
Phenobarbital	D_L: 20 mg/kg; up to 40 mg/kg total D_M: 3–5 mg/kg/d	IV, PO (1:1 conversion)	Hypotension, CNS depression, respiratory depression, bradycardia	15–40 mcg/mL
Fosphenytoin	D_L: 20 mg/kg; may repeat 5 mg/kg D_M: 4–8 mg/kg/d divided every 12 hours Dosing expressed as mg of phenytoin sodium equivalents	IV	Hypotension, arrhythmias, CNS depression	Total drug concentration: 8–15 mcg/mL Free drug concentration: 1–2 mcg/mL
Phenytoin	D_M: 4–8 mg/kg/d divided 8–12 hours	PO Oral bioavailability variable: may require dose increase when converting to PO		
Lidocaine	D_L: 2 mg/kg D_M: 5–7 mg/kg/hr	IV	Cardiac arrhythmias, hypotension	6–7 mcg/mL, <9 mcg/mL recommended
Levetiracetam	D_L: 40–60 mg/kg D_M: 10–80 mg/kg/d divided every 12 hr	IV, PO (1:1 conversion)	Somnolence	Routine monitoring not recommended
Midazolam	D_L: 0.1 mg/kg D_M: 0.1–1 mg/kg/hr	IN, IV	Hypotension, CNS depression, respiratory depression	Not applicable
Topiramate	Optimal dosing not established 1 mg/kg/d; may titrate to 8 mg/kg/d	PO	Anorexia, metabolic acidosis, lethargy, cognitive dulling Reports of necrotizing enterocolitis at higher doses in preterm neonates	Routine monitoring not recommended

CNS, central nervous system; D_L, loading dose; D_M, maintenance dose; IN, intranasal; IV, intravenous; PO, per os.

phenobarbital reduces seizure burden (El-Dib & Soul, 2017; Meyn et al., 2010). The lowest effective dose should be used and treatment duration should be continually evaluated. In addition, CNS depression and respiratory depression are known adverse effects of main concern in the acute management of seizures, which may result in the requirement for additional respiratory support. Hypotension and bradycardia are other potential side effects (Soul, 2018).

FIGURE 12.2 Mechanism of action of common antiepileptics used for treatment of neonatal seizures.

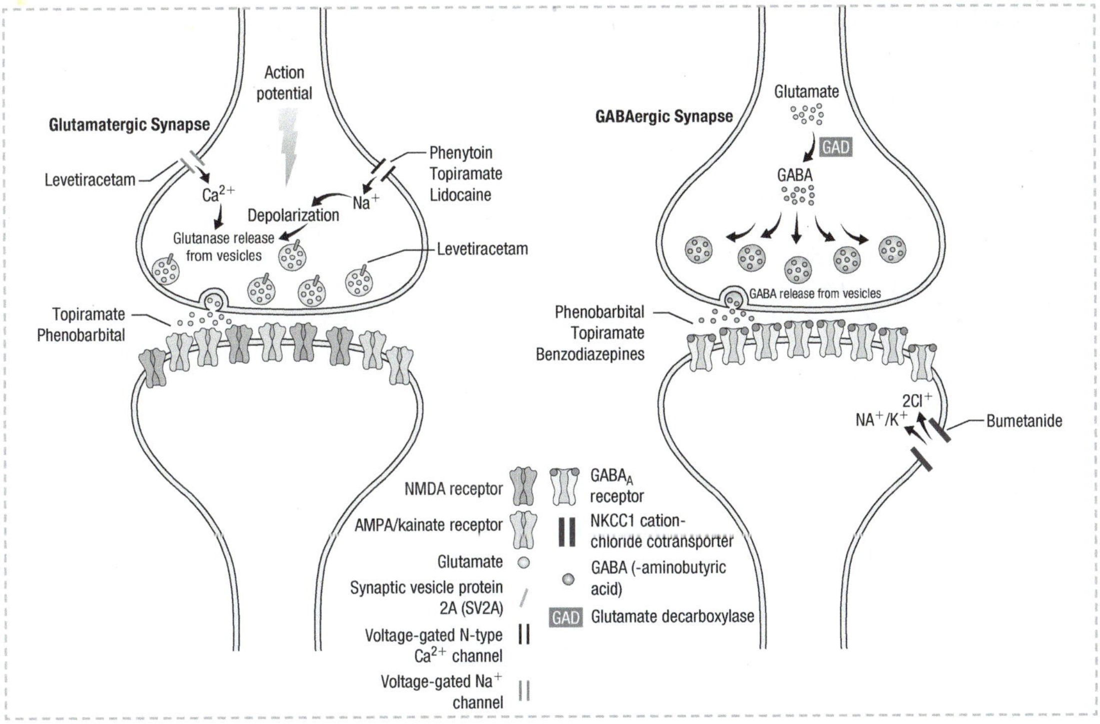

AMPA, α-amino-3-hydroxy-5-methyl-4-isoxazolepropionic acid; GABA, gamma-aminobutyric acid; NKCC1, sodium-potassium-chloride cotransporter 1; NMDA, N-methyl-D-aspartate.

Source: From Donovan, M. D., Griffin, B. T., Kharoshankaya, L., Cryan, J. F., & Boylan, G. B. (2016). Pharmacotherapy for neonatal seizures: Current knowledge and future perspectives. *Drugs*, 76(6), 647–661. https://doi.org/10.1007/s40265-016-0554-7.

Phenytoin

Historically, phenytoin/fosphenytoin has been the most common second-line therapy to phenobarbital for neonatal seizures in the United States. Complex pharmacokinetics, along with the proepileptic effects at toxic concentrations of free drug, have reduced the enthusiasm for this agent in modern neonatal seizure treatment algorithms, with consideration of emerging alternatives.

MECHANISM OF ACTION/PHARMACOKINETIC PARAMETERS

Phenytoin prevents the depolarization of voltage-dependent sodium channel membranes, preventing the release of glutamate in the presynaptic terminal, as shown in Figure 12.2. Fosphenytoin is a water-soluble prodrug of phenytoin that is quickly converted to phenytoin (and phosphate) by plasma esterases.

As previously described, phenytoin has several pharmacokinetic and pharmacodynamic challenges in the neonatal population. Recall that phenytoin follows saturable Michaelis–Menten pharmacokinetics, meaning that at a certain concentration, increasing doses result in a much greater increase in serum concentration, increasing the risk of adverse effects. Metabolism primarily occurs via oxidation followed by enterohepatic recycling and renal elimination. Like phenobarbital, metabolism also occurs through the CYP2C9 enzyme, resulting in variations of clearance and potential drug interactions (Mruk et al., 2015). Specific data regarding metabolism and concentrations in the setting of therapeutic hypothermia are lacking; thus, close monitoring is warranted given the known effect on CYP2C9 metabolism (El-Dib & Soul, 2017). Also remember that neonates have low serum albumin concentrations, and phenytoin has been shown to have significantly less protein binding compared with adults (Painter et al., 1999). Combining these pharmacokinetic complexities with poor enteral bioavailability, maintenance therapy with phenytoin is generally not used in modern practice (El-Dib & Soul, 2017; Mruk et al., 2015).

DOSING RECOMMENDATIONS

Dosing recommendations for phenytoin include an IV loading dose of fosphenytoin 20 mg/kg (expressed as phenytoin sodium equivalents), with additional doses of 5 mg/kg if needed for seizure cessation after careful consideration of phenytoin level, protein stores, and alternative pharmacotherapeutic options. Historically, maintenance phenytoin therapy ranged from 4 to 8 mg/kg/d divided every 8 to 12 hours, depending on infant maturity. Serum drug concentration monitoring is recommended given the narrow therapeutic window and wide variability in unbound drug concentrations and clearance. Free phenytoin trough concentrations are recommended, with a reference range of 1 to 2 mcg/mL (El-Dib & Soul, 2017). However, obtaining a free phenytoin concentration from a serum sample is more labor-intensive and costly than a total phenytoin concentration; thus, many centers do not conduct free phenytoin sampling in house, leading to a significant delay in the availability of results (Kiang & Ensom, 2016). Total phenytoin concentrations may be used as a surrogate (which includes free phenytoin concentration in addition to protein-bound phenytoin) with a recommended concentration of 8 to 15 mcg/mL in neonates; however, this reference range should be utilized with caution considering known variations in protein binding.

CLINICAL MONITORING PEARLS

Adverse effects of phenytoin/fosphenytoin include cardiac arrhythmias, CNS depression, and hypotension. Despite a lower risk of injection site reactions with fosphenytoin compared with phenytoin, extravasation may occur, warranting careful monitoring of line patency before and during infusion. Like phenobarbital, phenytoin has been shown to cause neuronal apoptosis in the developing brain (Forcelli et al., 2011).

Levetiracetam

As described previously, levetiracetam has tremendous appeal for treatment of neonatal seizures due to a very mild toxicity profile compared with historical standards of care. However, its efficacy as monotherapy for a subset of pediatric and adult seizure disorders cannot be extrapolated to neonates, with a recent RCT documenting dramatic inferiority to phenobarbital as first-line therapy. Considering this result, levetiracetam may be considered for refractory neonatal seizures and/or as maintenance therapy in a subset of patients, although RCTs are urgently needed to interrogate these indications.

MECHANISM OF ACTION/PHARMACOKINETIC PARAMETERS

The exact mechanism of levetiracetam in treating seizures is unknown. Unlike other antiepileptics, levetiracetam binds to the synaptic vesicle protein, SV2A, blocking its binding to the SV2A receptors, thus preventing the release of neurotransmitters (as shown in Figure 12.2; El-Dib & Soul, 2017). In stark contrast to historical antiepileptic agents, levetiracetam has an appealing and straightforward pharmacokinetic profile. Levetiracetam has high oral bioavailability, with one-to-one conversion between IV and oral doses. Levetiracetam is minimally protein-bound. Levetiracetam is not extensively metabolized, with roughly one-quarter of the dose undergoing enzymatic hydrolysis to an inactive metabolite that is renally excreted. The vast majority of drug is excreted unchanged in the urine after glomerular filtration. Therefore, dose adjustment is required in the setting of renal dysfunction.

DOSING RECOMMENDATIONS

Despite published pharmacokinetic data, there is considerable variability in both the loading dose and maintenance dose recommendation of levetiracetam in published studies. Loading doses of up to 60 mg/kg may be warranted based on the NEOLEV2 study (Sharpe et al., 2020). Maintenance therapy recommendations range from 10 mg/kg/d up to 80 mg/kg/d, divided into two doses (Mruk et al., 2015).

CLINICAL-MONITORING PEARLS

Levetiracetam is associated with few major adverse effects. Headaches and somnolence are among the most prominent, but are challenging to discern in the neonatal population (El-Dib & Soul, 2017). At this time in clinical practice, clear correlation between serum drug concentrations and therapeutic efficacy is lacking, limiting the applicability of serum therapeutic drug monitoring.

Lidocaine

Lidocaine is widely used in Europe as second-line therapy for neonatal seizures, but use is limited in the United States, likely related to the concern for cardiac adverse effects (Soul, 2018; Vento et al., 2010).

MECHANISM OF ACTION/PHARMACOKINETIC PARAMETERS

Like phenytoin, lidocaine acts on voltage-gated sodium channels preventing depolarization (see Figure 12.2). Note that the risk of adverse effects is substantially higher when lidocaine is used in conjunction with phenytoin/fosphenytoin, given the similar mechanism of actions. Lidocaine rapidly crosses the blood–brain barrier after IV administration. Metabolism occurs predominantly via hepatic CYP1A2 and CYP3A4 to active metabolites. Excretion occurs in the urine. Therefore, premature newborns and neonates receiving therapeutic hypothermia have a high risk of drug accumulation and subsequent toxicity.

DOSING RECOMMENDATIONS

Lidocaine is administered as a loading dose (2 mg/kg) followed by a continuous infusion (generally initiated at 5–7 mg/kg/hr, with dosing reduced over 24–36 hours to avoid accumulation and toxicity). Detailed dosing algorithms have been established in neonates with and without concurrent therapeutic hypothermia (Donovan et al., 2016; Malingre et al., 2006; van den Broek et al., 2013).

CLINICAL-MONITORING PEARLS

As previously described, lidocaine has the potential to produce significant cardiac adverse effects, including arrhythmias or bradycardia. The incidence in neonates appears to be relatively low with appropriate dosing and diligent monitoring. Risk factors for cardiac adverse effects include unstable serum potassium levels, baseline cardiac dysfunction, and concurrent phenytoin utilization (Weeke et al., 2015).

Benzodiazepines (Midazolam)

Normally the first-line therapy for the acute treatment of seizures in pediatric and adult patients, benzodiazepines are not routinely used as first-line therapy in neonates (Donovan et al., 2016). Midazolam is commonly used as third-line therapy for refractory neonatal seizures, with a high rate of efficacy in the setting of dose-limiting adverse effects (most prominently, hypotension). Efficacy and safety data utilizing other benzodiazepines, specifically lorazepam and clonazepam, in neonates are scarce (Slaughter et al., 2013). Benzodiazepine use carries significant concern regarding long-term neurodevelopmental impact in neonates, reenforcing this agent's place in therapy as last in line.

MECHANISM OF ACTION/PHARMACOKINETIC PARAMETERS

Benzodiazepines bind to postsynaptic $GABA_A$ receptors, resulting in activation of the inhibitory neurotransmitters (see Figure 12.2). Although benzodiazepines are generally well absorbed via the enteral route, these agents are not used as maintenance therapy and the enteral route is not relevant in the treatment of acute neonatal seizures. Midazolam has high intranasal bioavailability and this route may be used for acute symptomatic seizures, although IV access should be prioritized. Midazolam is highly protein-bound and extensively hepatically metabolized by CYP3A4 primarily to an active metabolite. Neonates have a longer elimination half-life than older pediatric patients and adults, with excretion occurring renally.

DOSING RECOMMENDATIONS

Midazolam is generally administered as an IV bolus dose (0.05–0.2 mg/kg) followed by a continuous infusion, ranging from 0.05 to 0.5 mg/kg/hr, with careful titration to effect or toxicity.

CLINICAL-MONITORING PEARLS

Hypotension is a common adverse effect, with a 10% incidence found in a study using midazolam as first-line therapy (Dao et al., 2018). The risk and severity of hypotension increase with increasing doses. Utilizing midazolam as third-line therapy for neonatal seizures, respiratory depression is a near certainty; a stable airway and mechanical ventilation should be utilized during titration if they are not already in place.

Alternate Agents

Multiple antiepileptic agents have emerged in the 21st century. All have limited data in neonates, but a subset have demonstrated utility, generally as maintenance therapy for refractory neonatal seizures.

TOPIRAMATE

Topiramate is a newer antiepileptic with multiple mechanisms of blocking seizures. These include modulation of GABA activity at GABA receptors, blocking α-amino-3-hydroxy-5-methyl-4-isoxazolepropionic acid (AMPA) glutamate receptors and blocking voltage-gated sodium channels (Donovan et al., 2016). Limited efficacy data have been published in neonates. A retrospective study of six neonates with seizures refractory to phenobarbital found that four of the six patients responded to topiramate with no reported side effects (Glass, Poulin, et al., 2011). Nuñez-Ramiro and colleagues studied the impact of prophylactic topiramate versus placebo on the incidence of seizure development in neonatal patients undergoing whole-body cooling for treatment of hypoxic-ischemic encephalopathy but did not find statistically significant decrease overall. A small subset of patients who achieved therapeutic topiramate serum concentrations within a few hours of cooling did experience reduced seizure burden ($p < .016$; Nuñez-Ramiro et al., 2019).

Topiramate is only available as an enteral formulation, greatly limiting its usefulness in the acute setting. Pharmacokinetic data in neonates have been published, showing favorable concentration and safety profiles. Side effects in older pediatric patients include irritability, cognitive dulling, anorexia, and metabolic acidosis (El-Dib & Soul, 2017). Topiramate has shown promising neuroprotective potential in animal models, but further study is warranted in neonates (El-Dib & Soul, 2017).

CONCLUSIONS

Seizures occur more commonly in the neonatal period and are often subtle, making diagnosis and treatment a challenge to practitioners. Continuous electroencephalography is the gold standard for seizure diagnosis and should be used in high-risk patients to ensure subclinical seizures are detected. Pharmacologic management should be initiated promptly once any reversible causes are ruled out. Phenobarbital remains the first-line pharmacologic treatment for neonatal seizures. There is no consensus among providers as to second- and third-line options for treatment, but multiple viable therapeutic options are available.

LEARNING TOOLS AND RESOURCES

Advice From the Authors

Allison Jones Guider, PharmD, BCPPS

With the lack of evidence-based guidelines for the management of neonatal seizures, institutional treatment algorithms require routine evaluation to ensure appropriateness with emerging literature. Attention should be paid to accessibility and availability to ensure a pharmacologic treatment algorithm can be rapidly followed in a real-case scenario. Lastly, close attention to necessary clinical monitoring for antiepileptic agents may help decrease the risk for known adverse effects.

Christopher McPherson, PharmD, BCPPS

Neonatal seizures represent a unique and challenging opportunity to protect the neonatal brain. A nurse practitioner must master both basic and complex aspects of care to optimize outcomes for the baby. Carefully and consistently evaluate historic and emerging primary literature and collaborate with colleagues specializing in pediatric neurology to develop a clear treatment algorithm for your unit. Ensure that basic aspects of care are also streamlined, including rapid acquisition of critical laboratory tests and easy access to appropriate dosage forms of medication in your algorithm to treat when indicated.

Discussion Prompts

1. In your clinical practice, are the first-, second-, and third-line medications discussed in this chapter used as presented? Why or why not? What is the evidence base for your NICU practice?
2. Benzodiazepines are the gold standard for acute management of seizures in pediatric and adult patients. Why does this differ in neonates?
3. Which of the commonly used maintenance antiepileptics require therapeutic drug monitoring?

Mind Map

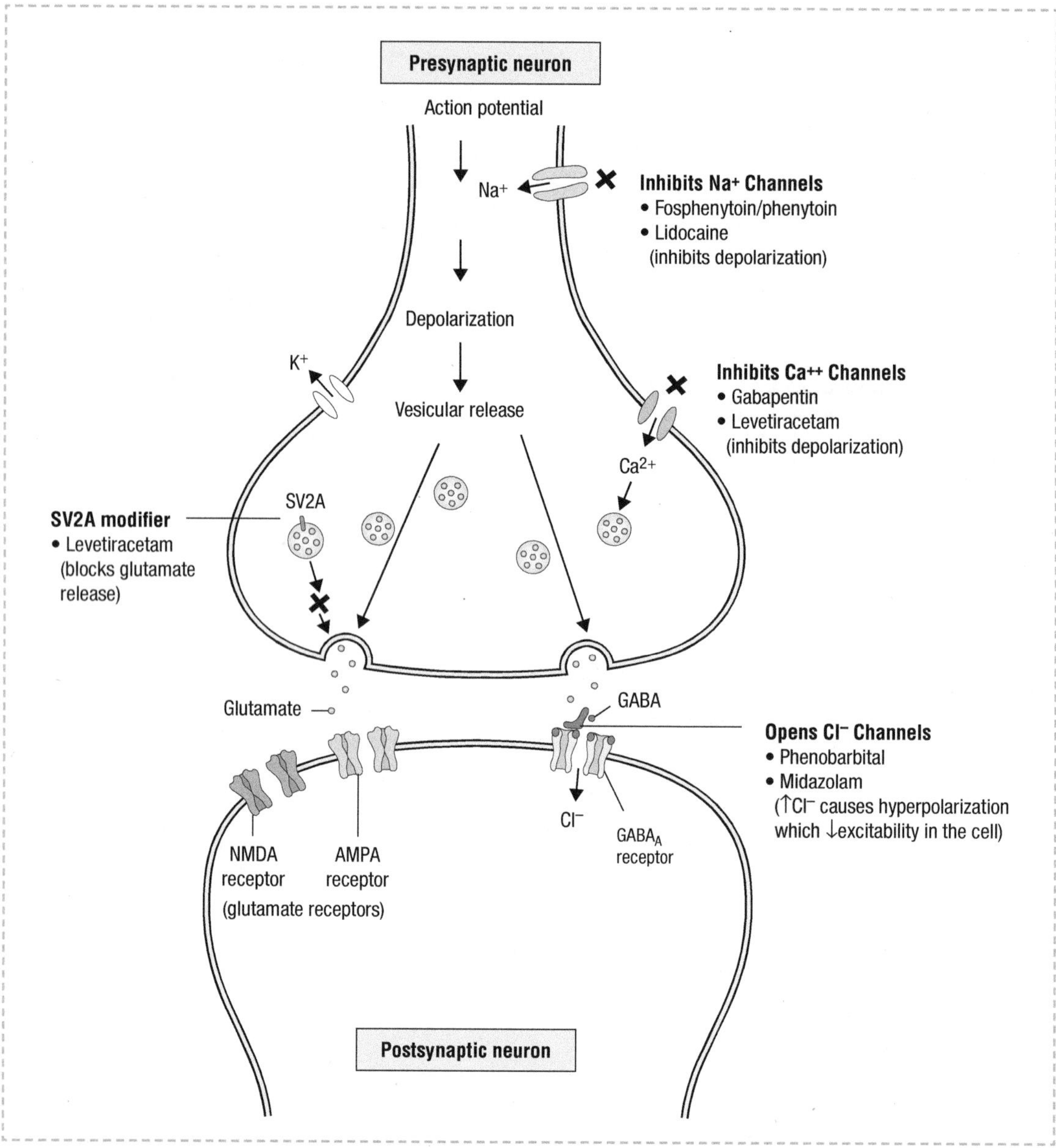

Note: This mind map reflects the design team's interpretation of a portion of one or more concepts addressed in this chapter. Readers should regard the mind maps woven throughout this textbook as examples of multisensory study tools that can be developed to encourage conceptual understanding. Readers are encouraged to develop their own unique mind maps in consultation with academic faculty or clinical preceptors. Design credit: Meghan Whelan, MSN, APRN, NNP, and Jamie Johnson, BSN, RN, CCRN, East Carolina University Neonatal Nurse Practitioner and Neonatal Clinical Nurse Specialist Programs.

REFERENCES

References for this chapter are online and available at https://connect.springerpub.com/content/book/978-0-8261-5884-0/part/partII/toc-part/ch12.

PART III

Common Respiratory Problems

chapter 13

Respiratory Distress Syndrome

Ryan Moore, Meredith Chanas, Amy J. Jnah, and Alexander Berwick

LEARNING OBJECTIVES

After completing this chapter, the reader should be able to:

- Define *respiratory distress syndrome (RDS)* and identify the epidemiology of the disease process.
- Explain the physiology of pulmonary function in utero and during the transition to extrauterine life.
- Correlate the pathophysiology of RDS with the need for pharmacologic treatment.
- Appraise the historical evolution of pharmacologic management for RDS.
- Evaluate current pharmacologic therapies for the treatment of RDS.

INTRODUCTION

Respiratory distress syndrome (RDS) of the neonate is characterized by hypoxic respiratory failure secondary to an insufficient quantity and quality of surfactant production, decreased pulmonary compliance, atelectasis, hypercapnia, and acidosis (Jnah & Trembath, 2019). A poorly understood but likely contributing factor is insufficient activation of epithelial sodium channels (ENaC) and retained fetal lung fluid, which is tightly linked to the absence of spontaneous labor and cesarean delivery (Helve et al., 2004).

RDS was an unrelenting cause of death in preterm neonates until the late 1980s, when antenatal steroids and surfactant replacement therapy were introduced. These therapies led to a significant reduction in neonatal death, RDS, air leak syndrome, and the combined outcome of death or bronchopulmonary dysplasia (BPD; Crowley, 1995; Engle & Committee on Fetus and Newborn, 2008). However, as the cusp of viability decreased and life-sustaining technologies were enhanced, the incidence of RDS rebounded. More recent data suggest that an average of 260 per 1,000 premature neonates (<37 weeks' gestation) are diagnosed with RDS each year, an increase in prevalence with decreased all-cause mortality (Donda et al., 2019). Neonates at highest risk for RDS are those born less than 24 weeks of gestation (95%–98% incidence) compared to infants born less than 28 weeks (60%–80%), between 32 to 36 weeks (15%–30%), and after 37 weeks of gestation (1%; Hibbard et al., 2010; Holme & Chetcuti, 2012). A slight predominance among White males is reported (Anadkat et al., 2012; Fanaroff, 2007; Stoll et al., 2010).

Risk factors for RDS include maternal chorioamnionitis, cesarean delivery in the absence of labor, and preterm birth (Table 13.1; Vitaliti & Falsaperia, 2021). Protective factors include African ethnicity, maternal hypertension, prolonged rupture of membranes, and antenatal corticosteroid use. When preterm birth (<37 weeks) is imminent within 7 days, the American College of Obstetricians

TABLE 13.1 Risk Factors for RDS: Historic Versus Current

HISTORIC RISK FACTORS	CURRENT RISK FACTORS
Family history of respiratory distress	Advanced maternal age
Gestational diabetes	Caesarean delivery
Intrapartum asphyxia	Caucasian ethnicity
Prematurity	Congenital diaphragmatic hernia
	Family history of respiratory distress
	Gestational diabetes
	Hypothermia
	Intrapartum asphyxia
	Male gender
	Meconium aspiration
	Multiple gestation
	Prematurity
	Pulmonary hypoplasia, pneumonia, hemorrhage

Sources: From Rudolph, A. J., & Smith, C. A. (1960). Idiopathic respiratory distress syndrome of the newborn: An international exploration. *Journal of Pediatrics, 57*, 905–921. https://doi.org/10.1016/S0022-3476(60)80143-6; Holme, N., & Chetcuti, P. (2012). The pathophysiology of respiratory distress syndrome in neonates. *Paediatrics and Child Health, 22*(12), 507–512. https://doi.org/10.1016/j.paed.2012.09.001

and Gynecologists (ACOG) Committee on Obstetric Practice (2017) and World Health Organization (WHO) Reproductive Health Library (2015) recommend the provision of a single course of antenatal steroids; repeat dosing is indicated when more than 2 weeks have elapsed since the single course of treatment was provided and preterm birth less than 34 weeks of gestation is imminent (Committee on Obstetric Practice, 2017; WHO Reproductive Health Library, 2015). Betamethasone (BMZ) and dexamethasone (DMZ), corticosteroids prescribed to eligible pregnant patients, are known to upregulate growth factor synthesis and structural maturation of the respiratory system by expediting thinning of the walls surrounding the double capillary loops within the alveoli (to facilitate gas exchange) and enhance surfactant production within the fetal lung (to resist atelectasis; Vafaei et al., 2021). In addition, antenatal steroids decrease the risk for postnatal air leak syndrome.

Globally, RDS remains a major cause of morbidity and mortality for premature infants (Stoll et al., 2010). RDS is the leading cause of neonatal death in the United States, with a mortality rate of 13.4 per 100,000 live births (Dyer, 2019). The most notable long-term consequence of RDS is BPD, which results from lung damage secondary to inflammation provoked by conditions including severe RDS. We encourage readers to consult Chapter 16, "Bronchopulmonary Dysplasia," for a detailed discussion of this disease process.

Exogenous surfactant is the primary pharmacotherapy prescribed to premature infants who manifest with severe RDS. Although associated with a promising increase in lung compliance, ventilation-perfusion matching, and reduced supplemental oxygen administration, multiple doses of surfactant may increase the risk for air leak (Coshal et al., 2021). As noted in most chapters of this textbook, no pharmacotherapy is risk free. We explore the available data and long-term outcomes specific to increased survival with and without disabilities in infants born preterm later in this chapter (Engle & Committee on Fetus and Newborn, 2008).

Given the prevalence of RDS and mortality risk, neonatal APRNs must enter the clinical arena with a strong understanding of respiratory embryology, physiology, the pathogenesis of RDS, and postnatal treatment strategies. We seek to help the trainee, preceptor, and novice clinician crystallize core concepts and apply this information in clinical practice. Therefore, this chapter has been constructed to review core physiologic and pathophysiologic concepts. Next, we provide readers with a historic overview of seminal works that guided our understanding of the efficacy of antenatal steroids and the pharmacodynamics and pharmacokinetics of exogenous surfactant therapy. Last, we offer a detailed discussion of antenatal steroids and exogenous surfactant, the mainstays of pharmacotherapy for RDS.

REVIEW OF PULMONARY PHYSIOLOGY

We begin this chapter with an abbreviated overview of respiratory embryology, which will lead us into a deeper discussion of the anatomy and function of the alveoli. Lung development begins during week 4 of gestation, with the embryonic phase of development. This phase involves the formation, elongation, and septation of the lung bud into the trachea and esophagus; failed septation is associated with tracheoesophageal fistula (Jnah & Trembath, 2019). Next, airway branching occurs, which gives the bronchial tree a glandular-like appearance. Likewise, this phase of development is termed the *pseudoglandular phase*, which spans from week 6 to 17 of gestation (Wilson & Fitzgerald, 2019). Columnar cells form, which will participate in later gas exchange. Glucocorticoid receptors (GR) develop and are found within the alveolar wall, bronchial vessels, and epithelium of the conducting airways. These receptors bind cortisol as well as maintain homeostasis by synthesizing 11-beta-hydroxysteroid dehydrogenase (11β-HSD-2), an enzyme that inactivates cortisol. Low 11β-HSD-2 production is observed during early development and levels increase closer to term gestation. Readers will come to understand that this gradual enzymatic maturational process is likely protective for preterm infants, as reduced 11β-HSD-2 permits optimal glucocorticoid binding when antenatal steroids are administered secondary to threatened preterm labor. Additional changes observed toward the end of this period of development that extend into the canalicular phase include the production of antioxidant enzymes, increasing lung tissue growth factor signaling, and inflammatory mediators.

The canalicular phase spans weeks 16 to 26 of gestation (Jnah & Trembath, 2019). Precursors to type I pneumocytes, which modulate gas exchange, and type II pneumocytes, which synthesize and secrete surfactant, appear. Lamellar bodies (LB) develop within the type II pneumocytes, which fill with phospholipid precursors to pulmonary surfactant, and acini give rise to primitive alveoli. These developments establish the air–fluid interface. By approximately the 22nd week of gestation, the fetus may be able to survive outside the womb (with life support).

The saccular phase (weeks 24–36) partially overlaps the preceding phase and most notably involves continued maturation of type II pneumocytes. Some type II pneumocytes will differentiate into type I pneumocytes, whereas the rest remain unchanged. In addition, acini begin to undergo several generations of differentiation (saccules to alveolar ducts to sacs; Jnah & Trembath, 2019). Toward the end of this phase, the endothelial walls of the double capillary loops lining the exterior of each alveolus thin. This thinning process facilitates an optimal exchange of gases and other substances (e.g., drugs). Finally, during the alveolar phase, which begins around week 32 of gestation, alveolar sacs develop at the ends of terminal bronchioles and septate. The result is an ever-increasing number of alveolar sacs (Jnah & Trembath, 2019). This permits increased production of surfactant, which prepares the fetus for postnatal life.

The developmental changes summarized here are influenced by the synthesis and activity of several growth factors. A delicate balance is required for normal lung development. For example, normal morphogenesis during early lung formation is contingent on adequate fibroblast growth factor (FGF) and bone morphogenic protein (BMP) signaling (Bellusci et al., 1997; Weaver et al., 2000). Proliferation and differentiation of alveoli during the alveolar phase is contingent upon adequate FGF and platelet-derived growth factor (PDGF) signaling (Boström et al., 1996; Weinstein et al., 1998). Although a detailed discussion is beyond the scope of this chapter, it is prudent to mention that some of the aforementioned growth factors stimulate proliferation and maturation of cells, whereas others inhibit these processes in order to maintain equilibrium. A summary of growth factors and their effect on the developing lung is summarized in Table 13.2.

Let's now turn our attention to the anatomy of the alveoli, which appear in primitive form around week 16 of gestation and mature over the following 5 months of fetal development. Alveoli are polygonal structures that are tightly linked to one another. They share flat epithelial walls, which are in part composed of phospholipid multilamellar bodies, giving them a "frothy" appearance under the microscope (Figure 13.1; Levitzky, 2013). The wall of each alveolus contains sublayers, including the (a) endothelium, a fluid-filled layer consisting of collagen and elastin; and (b) a surface epithelial layer composed of type I and type II pneumocytes and the overlying double capillary plexus. Mechanically, the wall of the alveolus separates its air-filled interior from the plexus of double capillaries. The thicker the alveolar wall, the more difficult it is to exchange gases and other substances. Further limiting the exchange of gases and substances is the thickness of the endothelial lining of each capillary wall. It is here that the movement of water, macromolecules, drugs (e.g., nitric oxide), and hormones into the systemic circulation occurs (Haschek et al., 2022). From a clinical standpoint, injury to this endothelial layer increases the risk for acquired disease (e.g., excess water leakage from the capillaries into the interstitium, resulting in pulmonary edema).

Recall that type I and type II pneumocytes reside within the surface epithelial layer of the alveoli. As such, it is here, within this fluid-filled layer, that surface tension is generated. Surface tension

TABLE 13.2 Commonly Investigated Growth Factors That Influence Pulmonary Development

GROWTH FACTOR	INFLUENCE ON PULMONARY DEVELOPMENT
Bone morphogenic protein	Extracellular matrix Vascularization
Epidermal GF	Airway branching, elongation, and differentiation
Fibroblast GF	Alveolarization Airway branching, elongation, and differentiation
Granulocyte-macrophage colony stimulating factor	Macrophage differentiation
Platelet-derived GF	Alveolarization
Transforming GF	Airway branching, elongation, and differentiation Extracellular matrix formation
Vascular endothelial GF	Vascularization

GF, growth factor.

Sources: From Boström, H., Willetts, K., Pekny, M., Levéen, P., Lindahl, P., Hedstrand, H., Pekna, M., Hellström, M., Gebre-Medhin, S., Schalling, M., Nilsson, M., Kurland, S., Törnell, J., Heath, J. K., & Betsholtz, C. (1996). PDGF-A signaling is a critical event in lung alveolar myofibroblast development and alveogenesis. *Cell, 85*(6), 863–873. https://doi.org/10.1016/s0092-8674(00)81270-2; Weaver, M., Dunn, N. R., & Hogan, B. L. (2000). Bmp4 and Fgf10 play opposing roles during lung bud morphogenesis. *Development, 127*(12), 2695–2704. https://doi.org/10.1242/dev.127.12.2695; Weinstein, M., Xu, X., Ohyama, K., & Deng, C. X. (1998). FGFR-3 and FGFR-4 function cooperatively to direct alveogenesis in the murine lung. *Development, 125*(18), 3615–3623. https://doi.org/10.1242/dev.125.18.3615

FIGURE 13.1 Surface epithelium of alveoli.

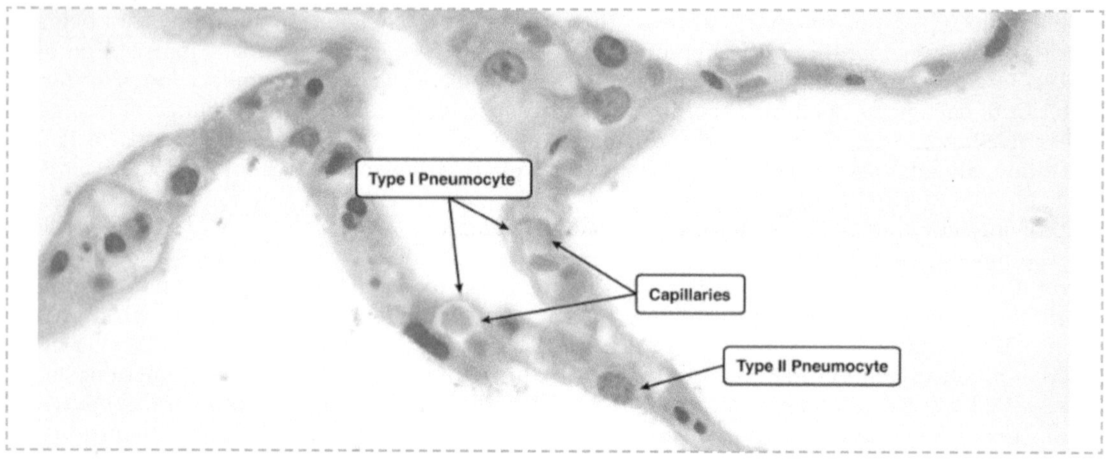

Source: Image courtesy of Peter Takizawa, Yale University, School of Medicine. Reprinted with permission.

plays a major role in the mechanics of inhalation (lung inflation), which is a dynamic process occurring immediately after birth, particularly among preterm neonates. Beginning with the initial cry (or initiation of positive pressure ventilation) after birth, alveoli must fill with air and exchange gases (Figure 13.2). The tension imposed on each alveolus, by virtue of size and complement of available surfactant, makes that process inefficient or difficult.

Consider the following relationship: Tension increases as the radius of an object (e.g., alveolus) decreases (e.g., expiration) when surface tension is constant. This relationship is supported by LaPlace's Law (of physics), which states the distending pressure (P) is directly proportional to the surface tension (T) and inversely proportional to the radius (r) of the alveoli, or $P = 2T/r$. Simply stated, the pressure inside an alveolus (to keep it open) is inversely proportional to its radius. The smaller the radius, as occurs during exhalation when air is expelled from inside the alveolus, the higher the pressure needed to keep the alveolus open. Again, this assumes that surface tension remains unchanged throughout inhalation and exhalation (which is not practical). We know that postnatal surfactant synthesis and secretion is anything but constant. It is a dynamic process that can be accentuated (e.g., antenatal corticosteroid exposure) or inhibited (e.g., extreme prematurity, meconium aspiration). Therefore, in neonatal intensive care, surface tension is affected by the maturity (size) of each alveolus and presence or deficiency of surfactant. In addition, the overall

FIGURE 13.2 The alveolus and blood flow.

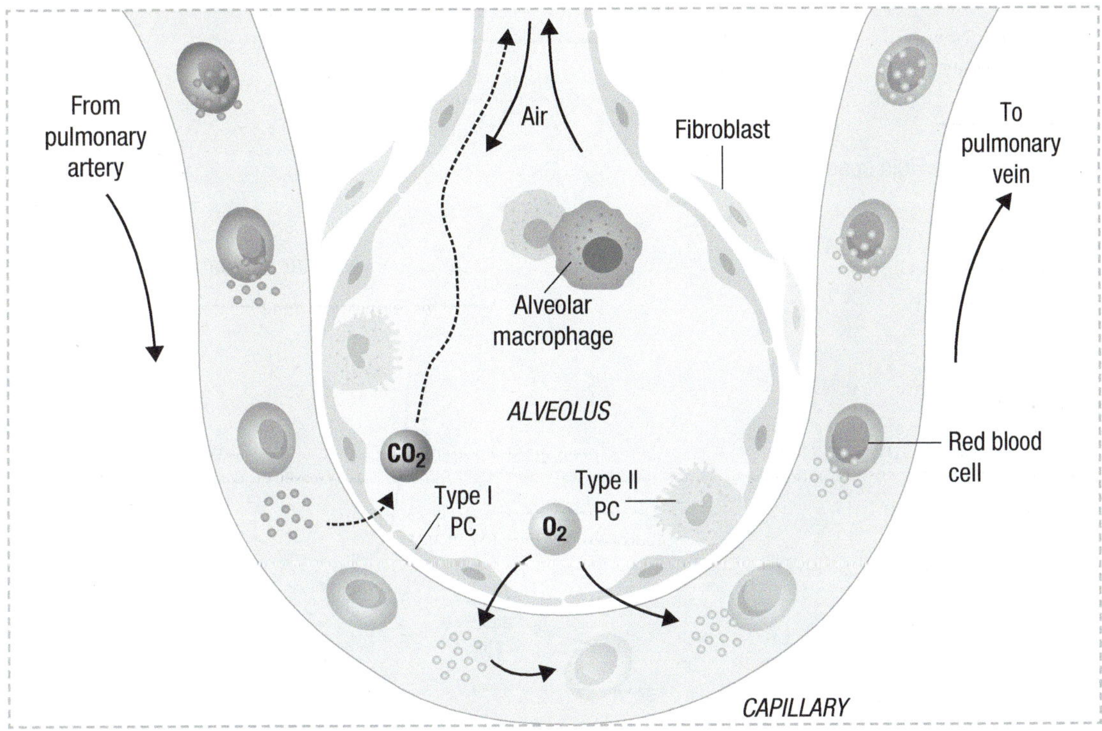

PC, pneumocyte.
Design credit: Amy J. Jnah. Created in BioRender.com.

complement of alveoli available for gas exchange decreases with gestational age, which limits the mechanics of inhalation and gas exchange.

Pulmonary Surfactant

Pulmonary surfactant is primarily (80%) composed of a blend of phospholipids, proteins (10%), and neutral lipids (10%; Jnah & Trembath, 2019). The most prevalent phospholipids are phosphatidylcholine (PC), phosphatidylglycerol (PG), and phosphatidylinositol (Whittle et al., 1983). As surfactant matures, phosphatidylinositol concentrations decrease in exchange for increased PG; mature surfactant contains approximately 10% PG, whereas fetal (immature) surfactant contains less than 1% (Hallman et al., 1976; Plauché et al., 1982). Although proteins account for only 10% of surfactant, their function is critical. Four pulmonary surfactant proteins (SP) are known, labeled A to D, and hold different key roles in surfactant production and function.

Surfactant proteins A (SP-A) and D (SP-D) are hydrophilic proteins with a collagen domain. Both proteins are primarily involved with host defenses (modulation of lung inflammation) and, to a lesser extent, surfactant stabilization and phospholipid absorption (Kingma & Whitsett, 2006; Whitsett & Weaver, 2002). In addition, SP-A and SP-D protect against oxidative stress (Bridges et al., 2000). SP-A polymorphisms, which cause abnormal SP-A function, increase the risk for RDS, BPD, and viral infections (Bersani et al., 2012; Hallman & Haataja, 2006; King & Chen, 2020). There is no known correlation with SP-D polymorphisms and RDS. Surfactant protein B (SP-B) and C (SP-C) are hydrophobic proteins involved in the absorption and incorporation of phospholipids at the air-alveolar interface. The effect is an increased rate of spreading of surfactant, which decreases surface tension. SP-B also stabilizes the phospholipid layers during alveolar expansion (inhalation) and collapse (exhalation) as well as regulates surfactant metabolism. Deficient SP-B concentrations increase the risk for increased surface tension and the development of RDS and lung inflammation (Ikegami et al., 2005; Whitsett & Weaver, 2002). Mutations in SP-C have been shown to contribute to interstitial lung disease and BPD (Nogee, 2004). The role of SP-C deficiency in neonatal RDS remains unclear. Surfactant metabolism is summarized in Figure 13.3.

FIGURE 13.3 Surfactant metabolism.

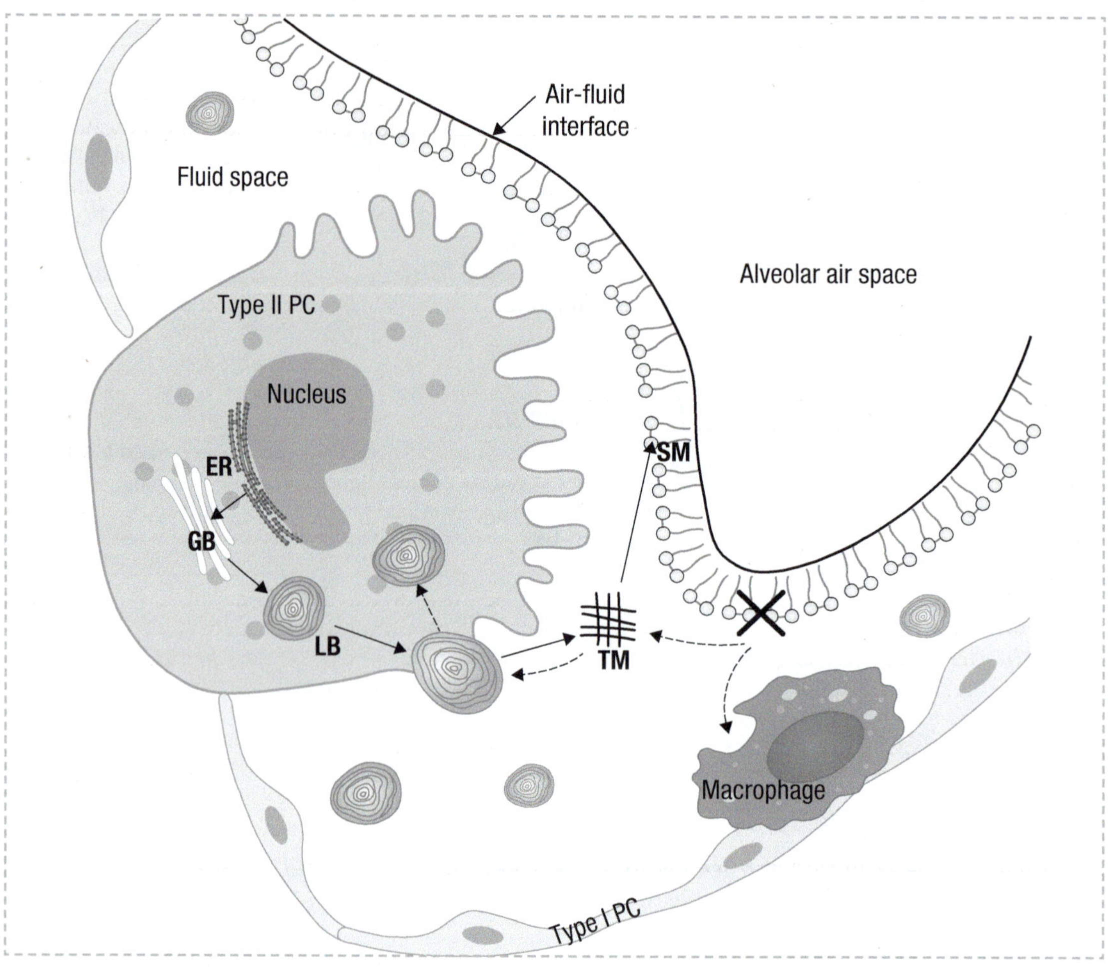

Note: Surfactant protein-B precursor protein and surfactant protein-C, as well as phospholipids from the circulation, enter the lipid vesicles within the type II PC. These substances undergo proteolytic processing in the ER and GB before being assembled and stored in LBs. LB leave the type II PC and enter the alveolar fluid space, where they interact with SP-A to form TM. Surfactant molecules then leave TM and line up to create the SM biofilm at the air-liquid interface, which acts to reduce alveolar surface tension. Surfactant remnants (denoted by the X) are then taken up by endocytosis (dotted lines) and recycled. Recycling involves transport back to TM, a LB, and into the type II PC. Most of surfactant is recycled (~95%). Remaining remnants are ingested by alveolar macrophages and cleared.
ER, endoplasmic reticulum; GB, Golgi bodies; LB, lamellar bodies; PC, pneumocyte; SM, surfactant monolayer; TM, tubular myelin.
Image credit: Amy J. Jnah. Created in Biorender.com.

Physiology of Gas Exchange

Recall from Chapter 5, "Perinatal Pharmacology," that, at a cellular level, oxygen and carbon dioxide move across the placental membrane by way of passive diffusion. This is also true within the lung. Gas exchange in the lung is further enhanced with inspiration and expiration, which forces a continued back-and-forth movement of air through the anatomic and conducting airways. In keeping with the concept of diffusion from a higher to lower gradient, the partial pressure of carbon dioxide in the airways is higher than the environment, favoring elimination through exhalation. The partial pressure of oxygen is higher in the environment compared to the airways (excluding the provision of supplemental oxygen, of course), favoring diffusion from the airspaces and into the circulation. Preterm neonates have an overly compliant chest wall and low complement of alveoli. Therefore, many preterm neonates struggle to establish adequate gas exchange immediately after birth and manifest with RDS.

PATHOPHYSIOLOGY OF RESPIRATORY DISTRESS SYNDROME

Many neonates, both term and premature, present with a degree of respiratory distress after birth. Etiologies range from an occluded nare to a spontaneous tension pneumothorax, pulmonary hypoplasia, or surfactant deficiency with atelectasis. The pathogenesis of RDS, however, directly corresponds with hypoxic respiratory failure secondary to an insufficient quantity and quality of surfactant production, decreased lung compliance, atelectasis, hypoxia, hypercapnia, and acidosis (Figure 13.4).

Impaired clearance of fetal lung fluid also contributes to the pathogenesis of RDS. Immaturity of the ENaC channels favors sodium and water retention in the alveoli. Zelenina and colleagues (2005) added to our understanding of this phenomenon by noting that activity from one particular water channel, the aquaporin 4 channel, is increased after the administration of antenatal corticosteroids. Immaturity of this channel in combination with increased permeability of both the alveolar wall and delayed clearance of fluid in the lymphatic system, observed in animal models, accentuates pulmonary fluid overload (Egan et al., 1980, 1984; Jackson et al., 1990). The effect of decreased fluid clearance is reduced compliance and suboptimal gas exchange.

Surfactant serves three primary functions in the neonatal lung: (a) reduces surface tension and improves compliance, (b) recruits atelectatic alveoli, and (c) resists new or worsening atelectasis. Deficient surfactant, observed in preterm neonates with RDS, increases surface tension in the fluid layer of the alveolus, which makes the recruitment of these airways more difficult. Excess inspiratory pressure, greater than what is normally required to inflate the lungs, may be required to aerate the alveoli. Excess end expiratory pressure, beyond what is customarily needed to maintain functional residual capacity (FRC), may be necessary to splint the airways and resist atelectasis (Figure 13.5; Warren & Anderson, 2009).

Poor lung compliance and function customarily extend across the first 3 to 4 days after birth. Decreased compliance is attributed to the fact that preterm neonates have fewer viable alveoli for gas exchange and, of those that are available, fewer are recruited and ventilated. In addition, recruited alveoli may be overdistended and exhibit increased elastic recoil (Ainsworth, 2005). Lung compliance usually improves after the first 3 to 4 days after birth, once surfactant storage pools reach 100 mg/kg and surface tension lowers to that of mature lung tissue (Jackson et al., 1986).

FIGURE 13.4 Pathogenesis of respiratory distress syndrome.

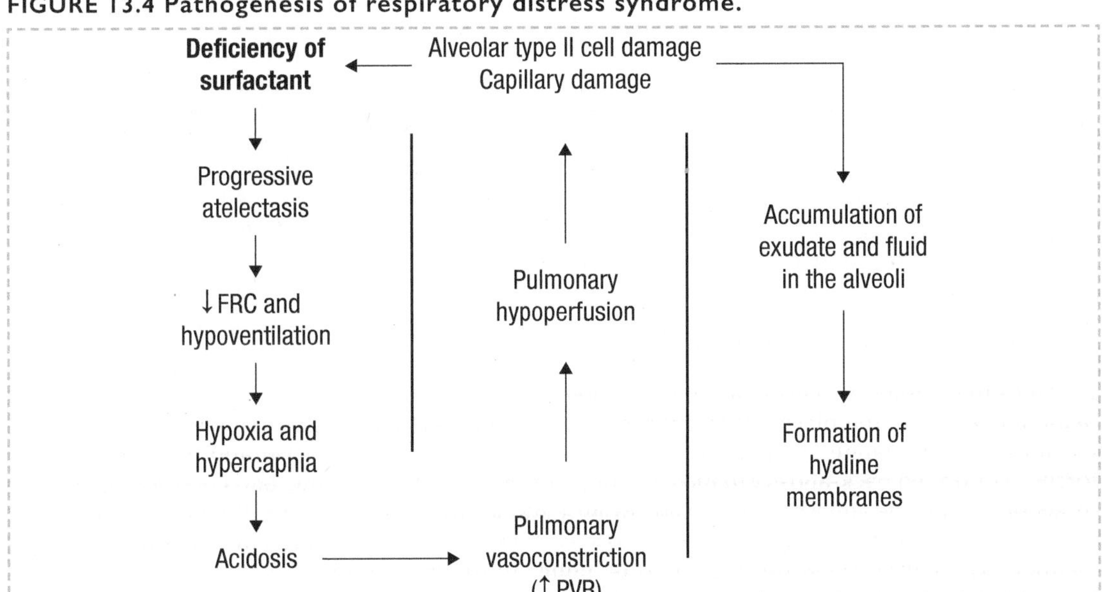

FRC, functional residual capacity; PVR, pulmonary vascular resistance.

Source: From Rubarth, L. B., & Quinn, J. (2015). Respiratory development and respiratory distress syndrome. *Neonatal Network, 34*(4), 231–238. https://doi.org/10.1891/0730-0832.34.4.231

FIGURE 13.5 Comparison of lung compliance in normal lung and lung affected by respiratory distress syndrome.

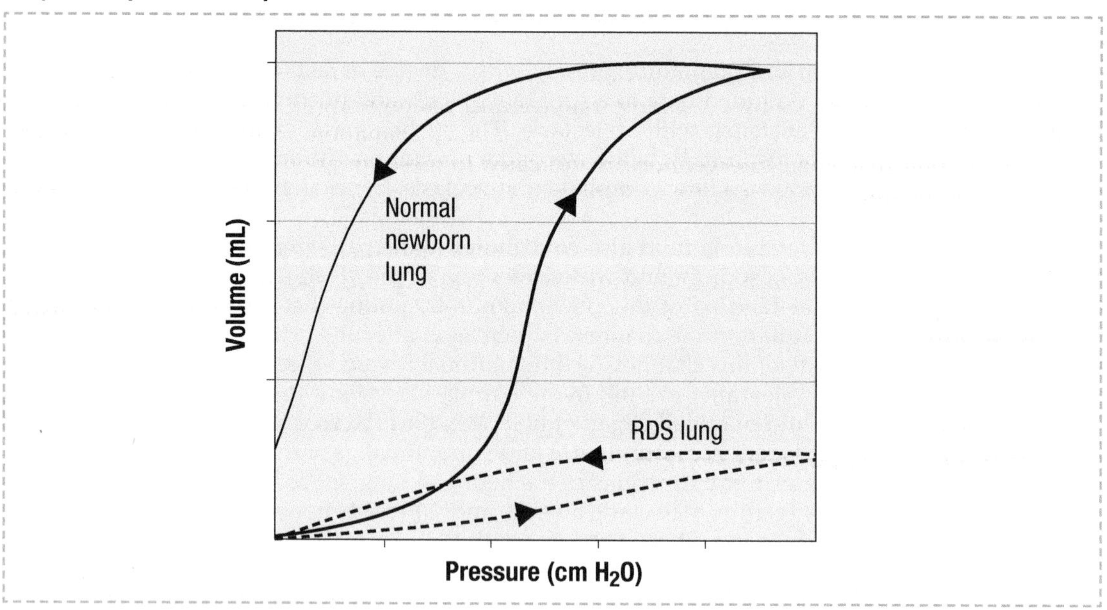

RDS, respiratory distress syndrome.

Studies have also shown that the composition of surfactant in preterm neonates is immature and therefore less functional compared to adults, making the gradual state of improvement and stabilization after the first days after birth less robust (Ueda et al., 1994). Further, shearing forces imposed on the alveolar epithelium may exacerbate and prolong resolution of the disease process as well as increase the likelihood for respiratory morbidities.

Recall that optimal gas exchange requires adequate ventilation-perfusion matching. Preterm newborns often struggle with establishing optimal ventilation-perfusion matching after birth. This occurs because the partial pressure of oxygen in the blood is low, chest wall compliance is high, FRC is low (favoring atelectasis), metabolic demands are high, and respiratory drive is low or even absent. Hypoxia encourages pulmonary vasoconstriction to poorly inflated or hypoventilated lung segments with compensatory intrapulmonary shunting of blood to well aerated lung spaces (Rubarth & Quinn, 2015). Over time, larger and larger areas of atelectasis may develop, leading to a significant ventilation-perfusion mismatch and resultant hypoxemia and hypercarbia (Ainsworth, 2005). Should this worsen, acidosis will develop and pulmonary vascular resistance increases, encouraging right to left shunting across the foramen ovale and ductus arteriosus (further exacerbating hypoxemia). Among preterm infants, this may be deleteriously enhanced by reduced synthesis of endogenous vasodilators, including prostacyclin and nitric oxide (NO). Condò and associates (2003) reported that preterm infants have little to no endogenous NO production immediately after birth; NO synthesis increases, albeit slowly, over the first 24 hours after birth.

Clinical Presentation

Alveolar collapse results in ventilation/perfusion mismatch and hypoventilation. This, in turn, results in hypoxemia and hypercarbia, and thus metabolic acidosis and respiratory acidosis. The atelectasis as well as acidosis cause pulmonary vasoconstriction. These events further lead to impaired endothelial and epithelial injury, proteinaceous exudate, and further impaired surfactant production, resulting in worsening RDS and clinical course in the preterm neonate.

Clinical manifestations present early after birth, usually within the first 6 hours. Affected neonates may present with any combination of the following common manifestations: grunting, retractions, nasal flaring, cyanosis, and increased FiO_2 requirement. Apnea is observed with severe cases and is considered a sign of impending respiratory failure. Grunting is a compensatory action meant to generate increased positive end-expiratory pressure (PEEP) and preserve FRC.

Retractions are elicited in an attempt to generate large, negative intrathoracic pressures and expand atelectatic lung tissue. Cyanosis manifests with right-to-left shunting across the foramen ovale and ductus arteriosus, as the pulmonary vascular resistance is heightened secondary to alveolar collapse and resultant capillary bed collapse (Jnah & Trembath, 2019).

A more life-threatening manifestation of RDS is air leak. The relative immaturity of the alveolar epithelium increases the risk for shearing damage and pneumothorax or pneumomediastinum, with or without pulmonary hemorrhage. Prompt transillumination, radiographic studies, and medical and pharmacologic intervention are indicated in these situations.

Radiographic findings of RDS are well described. Neonates demonstrate decreased lung volumes secondary to atelectasis. Atelectatic alveoli are radiopaque, diffuse, and reticulogranular ("ground glass") in appearance. Bronchi appear as radiolucent (air-filled "bronchograms") circles or lines that take on the appearance of branches of a tree. Air bronchograms are typically easily noticed on account of the air-filled bronchi situated on a background of collapsed alveoli (Jnah & Trembath, 2019).

HISTORICAL PERSPECTIVE: SEMINAL AND OTHER NOTEWORTHY STUDIES

Here we present seminal and other noteworthy studies that helped advance our understanding of the use of antenatal steroids and exogenous surfactant. In addition, we offer readers an abbreviated history of the nomenclature that characterized the disease process currently referred to as *RDS*.

Surfactant

In 1929, Kurt Von Neergaard first conducted experiments on pigs during which he removed air from the lung and administered an isotonic gum solution in order to "eliminate surface tension" at the air–lung interface. His research led to three seminal conclusions, which were accurate and insightful:

1. "Surface tension is responsible for the greater part of total lung recoil compared to tissue elasticity";
2. "A lower surface tension would be useful for the respiratory mechanisms because without it, pulmonary retraction might become so great as to interfere with adequate expansion"; and
3. "Surface tension as a force counteracting the first breath of the newly born should be investigated further." (Von Neergaard, 1929, as cited in Halliday, 2008, p. S47)

Peter Gruenwald (1947) repeated Von Neergaard's experiments, using stillborn infants, and reported similar findings. He concluded that "the resistance to aeration is due to surface tension which counteracts the entrance of air," another accurate and insightful finding (Halliday, 2008, p. S48). He also demonstrated that surface active substances reduced the distending pressure for aeration of the lung. Charles Macklin, a Canadian pathologist, was able to conclude through his research on the effects of nerve gas on lung physiology that there is a mucoid film present within the lung (Macklin, 1954). In 1955, a physicist by the name of Richard Pattle published a finding of foam and bubbles arising from the lung parenchyma that differed in composition and behavior compared to lung mucus. This foam was noted to have resistance to degradation from antifoaming agents used at that time (Pattle, 1955). Around the same time, a physiologist by the name of John Clements was working to find out how nerve gas affects lung physiology. In 1957, he published the surface tension values of films extracted from rats, cats, and dogs. Of interest, he reported smaller surface tension measurements at lower surface areas (Clements, 1956, 1957).

Two physicians, Jere Mead and Mary Ellen Avery (a former student of Dr. Gruenwald), surmised that Clement's findings of decreased surface tension at smaller surface areas were due to this lung film. Mead and Avery used similar techniques described by Pattle and Clements to measure surface tension of the lungs of demised neonates. They observed higher surface tension in neonates who died from hyaline membrane disease (HMD; alternative terminology for RDS) compared to neonates who died from other pathologies. They concluded HMD is associated with the absence or the late appearance of some substances, which in the normal subject renders the internal surface capable of attaining a low surface tension when the lung volume is decreased (Avery & Mead, 1959).

Patrick Bouvier Kennedy, the son of President John F. Kennedy, was born at Otis Air Force Base Hospital on August 7, 1963, at 1,860 grams and an estimated gestational age of 34 to 35 weeks. He died 2 days later from HMD. This event promptly resulted in increased awareness of RDS and there were clinical trials of synthetic surfactant that ensued shortly thereafter. In 1964 and 1967, two clinical trials administered synthetic dipalmitoylphosphatidylcholine (DPPC), without proteins, via nebulization to patients with HMD; no beneficial clinical effect was observed (Halliday, 2008, 2017). In 1972, Goran Enhörning (obstetrician) and Bengt Robertson (pediatric pathologist) administered surfactant extracted from adult rabbit lungs to premature rabbit neonates (Enhörning & Robertson, 1972). They found that the premature rabbits did not die as soon as expected and that the lung parenchyma of surfactant-treated rabbits had moderate to prominent air expansion compared to controls. One year later, Enhörning and Robertson demonstrated similar findings when surfactant was given via the pharynx (Enhörning et al., 1973). Five years later, in 1978, Dr. Forrest Adams administered natural surfactant to premature lambs; he reported 100% survival over the duration of the study as well as improved lung compliance with "generally well aerated lungs on autopsy" (Adams et al., 1978, p. 841). In 1980, Tetsuro Fujiwara administered artificial surfactant to 10 preterm neonates (28–33 weeks' gestation) with severe RDS. He reported significant improvements in oxygenation with less supplemental oxygen, respiratory acidosis, and hypotension, along with improvement in radiographic findings in these 10 patients (Fujiwara et al., 1980).

Between the 1980s and early 2000s, synthetic and natural surfactants were refined and subjected to randomized controlled trials (RCTs; Table 13.3). These trials examined numerous important issues, including the efficacy of natural versus synthetic surfactant, the relative efficacy of various natural surfactants, optimal timing of administration, optimal doses, and single versus multiple doses. Both older synthetic and natural surfactants have been shown to reduce pulmonary air leaks and mortality in RDS-affected neonates. It is important to note that the trials of surfactant showed the most benefit on neonates younger than 30 weeks and less than 1,250 grams. Currently, there is no evidence that surfactant administration decreases the rate of other comorbidities like intraventricular hemorrhage (IVH), retinopathy of prematurity, necrotizing enterocolitis, sepsis, BPD, or patent ductus arteriosus.

Nomenclature

As we are certain you have ascertained by reading the preceding information in this chapter, no standard vernacular for respiratory distress in the newborn prevailed throughout the 1950s. The IX International Congress of Pediatrics convened in 1959 with the intent to establish definitive biochemical, pathologic, physiologic, clinical, and physical manifestations of the disease as well as to settle on one title for the disease process. It is interesting to note that, despite seminal findings

TABLE 13.3 Surfactants Used in Clinical Trials

OLD SYNTHETIC (PROTEIN FREE)	NEW SYNTHETIC (PROTEIN ANALOGUES)	NATURAL (MINCED LUNG EXTRACTS)	NATURAL (LUNG LAVAGE EXTRACTS)	NATURAL (AMNIOTIC FLUID EXTRACT)
Pumactant (ALEC, ~1980)	Lucinactant (Surfaxin, 2012)	Surfactant TA (Surfacten, 1980)	CLSE (bLES, 1993)	Human surfactant (1983)
Colfosceril palmitate (Exosurf, ~1980)	rSP-C surfactant (Venticute, 2015)	Beractant (Survanta, 1991)	Calfactant (Infasurf, 1999)	
Turfsurf (Belfast surfactant, ~1980)		Poractant alfa (Curosurf, 1983)	SF-RI1 (Alveofact, 1992)	

Source: Modified from Halliday, H. L. (2008). Surfactants: Past, present, and future. *Journal of Perinatology: Official Journal of the California Perinatal Association, 28*(Suppl. 1), S47–S56. https://doi.org/10.1038/jp.2008.50

published by Avery and Mead (1959) that linked surfactant deficiency with the disease process and affirmed that infants who succumbed to the disease seldom had hyaline membranes at autopsy, attendees did not consider these data. The Congress ultimately settled on HMD as the name for the disease; however, of the 34 voting members, none voted to adopt HMD into the vernacular. Fifteen favored *idiopathic respiratory distress syndrome of the newborn*, four favored *pulmonary syndrome of the newborn*, and three voted in favor of *hyaline membrane syndrome*. For readers who noticed that 12 participant votes went uncounted, historians believe that those members retired to their rooms for the evening, opting not to vote, as the meeting went on until close to midnight (Jobe, 2010). The complete story behind the adoption of HMD as the official disease title will likely remain a mystery.

Since that time, scientists developed increasing discomfort with the term *HMD*, given that it was a pathologic diagnosis discoverable only on autopsy. As therapies advanced and the disease process became survivable, scientists were unable to determine whether surviving infants developed the pathology. Further, as reported by Avery and Meade (1959), hyaline membranes were not present in all infants who died of the disease soon after birth. These noteworthy findings and subsequent discussions nudged clinicians away from using the term *HMD*. By the turn of the century, most clinicians had adopted RDS as the vernacular for the disease.

Antenatal Steroids

The discussion of the historical events leading to the use of antenatal steroids, a preventative strategy for RDS, begins with the work of G. C. Liggins in 1969. As Dr. Liggins was researching the effects of antenatal DMZ on the incidence of preterm delivery in fetal sheep, he noticed lung inflation in preterm lambs' lungs when it was not expected. His preclinical work informed an RCT with R. N. Howie in 1972 (Liggins & Howie, 1972). They administered BMZ in the antepartum period and found that when administered 2 to 7 days prior to a preterm delivery at less than 32 weeks of gestation, there was a significant reduction in RDS and neonatal mortality.

Then, in 1981, Liggins's findings were replicated with DMZ (Collaborative Group on Antenatal Steroid Therapy, 1981). From there, 12 RCTs that included over 3,000 patients were executed between 1972 and 1990. Each trial consistently yielded the same outcome: Antenatal steroid administration reduced the incidence of RDS as well as IVH, necrotizing enterocolitis, and death. The most benefit was observed when steroids were given 24 hours to 7 days prior to delivery (Briceño-Pérez et al., 2019). These findings prompted an NIH Consensus Conference in 1994 that would spark increased use of antenatal corticosteroids for the prevention of perinatal morbidity and mortality (Wapner & Waters, 2003). Two steroid regimens were accepted as there was evidence that they were both effective in reducing neonatal morbidity and mortality. These regimens included: (a) DMZ phosphate 6 mg every 12 hours for a total of four doses and (b) BMZ phosphate/acetate 12 mg every 24 hours for two doses.

Later studies were conducted to investigate the efficacy of rescue or repeated dosing of corticosteroids. These studies yielded favorable outcomes (as those previously mentioned) when steroids were administered at less than 32 6/7 weeks' gestation and when delivery was anticipated within the following 7 days (Briceño-Pérez, 2019). Peering through the looking glass of history, it becomes clear that surfactant replacement therapy as well as antenatal corticosteroid therapy have significantly reduced the incidence and severity of neonatal RDS as well as neonatal mortality.

CURRENT PHARMACOLOGIC TREATMENT MODALITIES FOR RESPIRATORY DISTRESS SYNDROME

Recall that structural differentiation in the lungs, phospholipid development, and the production of antioxidant enzymes, lung tissue growth factors, and inflammatory mediators occur to a large degree during the pseudoglandular and canalicular phases of development. The exact timing of these developments varies in the literature but tends to substantively increase near the cusp of viability. Antenatal corticosteroids and exogenous pulmonary surfactant are often prescribed prior to and immediately after preterm birth of less than 34 weeks to stimulate and upregulate these processes.

Antenatal Corticosteroids

Use of antenatal corticosteroids in cases of imminent preterm delivery has led to an overall reduction in mortality associated with neonatal RDS (McPherson & Wombach, 2018). A recent Cochrane review, published in 2020, analyzed numerous studies and concluded that antenatal corticosteroids are associated with a reduced risk of (a) perinatal death (relative risk [RR]: 0.85, 95% confidence interval [CI]: 0.77–0.93), (b) neonatal death (RR: 0.73, 95% CI: 0.7–0.87), and (c) RDS (RR: 0.71, 95% CI: 0.65–0.78) in neonates born less than 34 weeks of gestation (McGoldrick et al., 2020). Another meta-analysis published the same year found antenatal corticosteroids reduced neonatal mortality (OR: 0.63, 95% CI: 0.46–0.86) specifically in preterm small-for-gestational age infants, with no effect on morbidity (Blankenship et al., 2020).

The use of antenatal corticosteroids in late preterm infants (34 0/7–36 6/7 weeks of gestation) remains controversial. It is true that late preterm neonates incur risk for RDS after birth; however, studies using antenatal steroids have produced mixed results (Dixon et al., 2018). For example, the Antenatal Late Preterm Steroids Study (ALPSS), a randomized, double-blind, placebo-controlled study, investigated outcomes among late preterm neonates exposed to either BMZ or placebo (Gyamfi-Bannerman et al., 2016). Their composite primary outcome included the use of continuous positive airway pressure (CPAP) or high-flow nasal cannula for 2 or more hours within the first 72 hours of life, fraction of inspired oxygen (FiO_2) of 30% or more for 4 or more hours within the first 72 hours of life, mechanical ventilation or extracorporeal membrane oxygenation (ECMO) at any time, stillbirth, or neonatal death. Neonates exposed to BMZ manifested with a reduced incidence of the primary outcome (RR: 0.80, 95% CI: 0.66–0.97; $p = .02$), driven by a less frequent need for CPAP or high-flow nasal cannula. BMZ exposure was also associated with less surfactant use, transient tachypnea of the newborn, and BPD. The most common postnatal adverse reaction to BMZ exposure was hypoglycemia (RR: 1.60, 95% CI: 1.37–1.87; $p < .001$). Next, consider a retrospective cohort study published by Bitar and colleagues (2020). These authors also evaluated the use of antenatal corticosteroids in late preterm pregnancies and with growth-restricted fetuses using a similar composite primary outcome to the ALPSS study. Outcomes did not differ between groups in this study (16.2% vs. 12.5%, $p = .41$; Bitar et al., 2020). Similar to the ALPSS study, the most common postnatal adverse reaction was hypoglycemia (40.4% vs. 25.2%, $p = .012$).

At present, the American Academy of Pediatrics (AAP) recommends consideration of glucocorticoid therapy for late preterm neonates (AAP, 2017), endorsing the ACOG, Committee on Obstetric Practice, Antenatal Corticosteroid Therapy for Fetal Maturation, Committee Opinion No. 713 (2017). Important caveats exist. Antenatal corticosteroids in women at risk for late preterm delivery should be avoided in the setting of clinical chorioamnionitis. Tocolysis should not be used to delay delivery to administer antenatal corticosteroids in the late preterm period, nor should delivery for significant maternal indications be delayed for this reason (ACOG Committee on Practice Bulletin-Obstetrics, 2016). Additional research is required before this position statement may be considered for revision, including investigation of women with multiple gestations and women with pregestational diabetes.

MECHANISM OF ACTION/PHARMACOKINETIC PRINCIPLES

Although the exact mechanism of action is not fully understood, experts hypothesize that corticosteroids induce RNA coding for proteins involved in the biosynthesis of phospholipids, structural maturation of the epithelium, antioxidant synthesis, and the inhibition of edema and inflammation (Table 13.4; Ballard & Ballard, 1995; Bolt et al., 2001; Roberts et al., 2017). The acceleration of fetal lung maturation and augmentation is attributed to the activity of enzymes responsible for

TABLE 13.4 Proposed Effects of Antenatal Corticosteroids on Fetal Lungs

BENEFICIAL	UNDESIRABLE
• Antioxidant enzyme synthesis • Alveolar epithelial wall thinning • Inhibition of pulmonary edema • Lung epithelial wall matrix maturation • Phospholipid synthesis	• Decrease in lung growth • Reduced alveolar proliferation with hypertrophy among new and existing alveoli

surfactant biosynthesis. Increased surfactant phospholipid synthesis, particularly PC, is thought to occur because glucocorticoids enhance the activity of phosphocholine cytidylyltransferase, the enzyme that elicits the production pathway for PC. This ultimately increases the rate of production of pulmonary surfactant. Glucocorticoids also upregulate structural lung maturation at the pulmonary epithelium, possibly due to inhibition of DNA synthesis, which inhibits cellular proliferation in exchange for increased differentiation (maturation) of these epithelial cells (Schittny et al., 1998; Wang et al., 1995; Whitsett & Stahlman, 1998). However, experiments using animal models suggest that several growth factors (summarized earlier in this chapter) are upregulated during this process, which can shift the composition of the epithelial–interstitial tissue interface or lung parenchyma.

Fetal glucocorticoid exposure is also associated with protective benefits. For example, antioxidant enzyme synthesis is upregulated, which can offer a degree of protection during periods of hyperoxia (Walther et al., 1991, 1998). In addition, postnatal pulmonary edema is diminished in fetuses exposed to antenatal corticosteroids compared to untreated fetuses. Experts propose that steroids upregulate aquaporin-1 water channels, beta-adrenergic channels, and ENaC channels in the lung tissues, which modulate lung fluid reabsorption.

In addition to postnatal hypoglycemia, other undesirable effects associated with glucocorticoid exposure include a decrease in postnatal lung differentiation (growth), which precipitates a decrease in alveolar septation. This effect may be attributed to steroid-induced inhibition of DNA synthesis, which is proposed to inhibit proliferation (septation, or branching) of alveoli (Schittny et al., 1998). A reduced total complement of alveoli is also observed compared to babies born at term. Based on studies using rat models, alveoli present at birth and that develop postnatally are customarily larger than normal (Tschanz et al., 1995). This may be a compensatory response to decreased postnatal alveolar proliferation.

BMZ and DMZ are fluorinated glucocorticoids with nearly identical chemical structures. These agents are preferred over other steroids because they are less susceptible to enzymatic metabolism by 11β-HSD-2, which, as readers may recall, converts bioactive cortisol to cortisone. Decreased susceptibility to 11β-HSD-2 allows active drug molecules to cross the placenta, reach the fetus, and elicit the desired biologic activity (Kemp et al., 2016).

A rapid onset of action is observed with both drugs, making them ideal in the face of threatened preterm birth. The most significant difference between the two agents is the shorter duration of action of DMZ compared to BMZ. The shorter duration of action necessitates a narrower dosing interval and increased number of doses over the 48-hour dosing period. BMZ, in contrast, has a larger volume of distribution, longer half-life, and decreased clearance compared to DMZ. Given these differences, some obstetric providers prescribe BMZ as dosing requires fewer painful intramuscular (IM) injections and theoretically less risk for medication error.

DOSING RECOMMENDATIONS

Recall that the ACOG recommends routine administration of antenatal corticosteroids for pregnant women between 24 0/7 and 33 6/7 weeks of gestation who are at risk of preterm delivery within 7 days (Committee on Obstetric Practice, 2017). They also recommend that obstetric clinicians consider the use of antenatal corticosteroids among pregnant women at risk of preterm birth within 7 days starting at 23 0/7 weeks' gestation or between 34 0/7 and 36 6/7 weeks of gestation who have not received a previous course of steroids. In women who are less than 34 0/7 weeks of gestation, at risk of preterm delivery within 7 days, and whose prior course of steroids was given more than 14 days previous, a single repeat course of antenatal steroids should be considered. Regularly scheduled repeat steroid courses for more than two repeat courses are not recommended (Committee on Obstetric Practice, 2017).

The only method of administration that has been studied and shown to provide clinical benefit is IM injection. Oral and intravenous doses are not recommended nor prescribed. The dosing recommendation for one course of BMZ is 12 mg IM, every 24 hours, for two total doses. In contrast, the DMZ dose is 6 mg IM every 12 hours, for four total doses. Each 12-mg dose of BMZ consists of 6 mg of BMZ sodium phosphate (for a rapid onset) and 6 mg of BMZ acetate (for sustained exposure), whereas DMZ involves four individual 6-mg doses. Despite the existence of these standard approaches, there is currently no consensus in the literature supporting one formulation or dosing regimen over any other, highlighting the importance of attention to emerging primary literature and updated tertiary references (Williams et al., 2022).

Timing of therapy is particularly important to maximize benefits to the vulnerable fetus. Experts believe that drug efficacy is maximized when a full course of steroids is completed, and the neonate is born at least 24 hours after therapy is completed or within 7 days of therapy. Norman and colleagues (2017) investigated outcomes stratified by timing of therapy in 4,594 singleton live-births between 24 and 31 weeks of gestation. Forty-one percent of women received antenatal corticosteroids 24 hours to 7 days before delivery and 24% of women were treated within 24 hours of delivery (Norman et al., 2017). Decreased neonatal mortality was associated with steroid use at any time compared to no steroids. For example, steroids administered 3 hours prior to delivery were associated with a 26% reduction in mortality risk. However, the largest reduction in mortality risk (50%) was observed among neonates born 24 hours to 7 days after completed therapy (Norman et al., 2017).

The total number of full courses of antenatal steroids is also a topic of interest. Limited data are available specific to this inquiry. Readers should consider current AAP/ACOG guidance in the setting of existing and ongoing research regarding the impact of antenatal corticosteroids on neurodevelopmental outcome, discussed in the next section of this chapter.

CLINICAL-MONITORING PEARLS

A well-described adverse effect of antenatal steroids is postnatal hypoglycemia. For example, a retrospective cohort study of 6,675 preterm deliveries found that BMZ-exposed neonates were 1.6 times more likely to develop hypoglycemia compared to nonexposed neonates (Pettit et al., 2014). Given the available data, blood glucose levels should be monitored closely during the first 60 to 90 minutes after birth and periodically thereafter, until a consistent euglycemic state is confirmed.

Concerns have been raised that antenatal corticosteroid exposure may increase the risk for postnatal infection. However, no data have corroborated this theory. Further, a relatively recent Cochrane review found no increased risk for chorioamnionitis or endometritis with antenatal corticosteroid use (Roberts et al., 2017).

Recall that BMZ and DMZ are both fluorinated glucocorticoids, drugs that may increase the risk for IVH and poor neurodevelopment in exposed infants (Scott & Rose, 2018). More recent data suggest this theory may be flawed. McGoldrick and colleagues (2020) reported a reduced risk for IVH and long-term developmental delay among neonates exposed to antenatal steroids in a meta-analysis of 27 studies, including 11,272 women and 11,925 neonates (McGoldrick et al., 2020). At present, the benefits of antenatal steroid exposure outweigh possible risks and underpin the ACOG recommendations for use (Committee on Obstetric Practice, 2017). These recommendations are endorsed by the AAP (2017). We encourage readers to explore Chapter 16, "Bronchopulmonary Dysplasia," and compare the proposed long-term outcomes of antenatal steroid exposure to prolonged postnatal glucocorticoid (e.g., hydrocortisone, DMZ) therapy.

Exogenous Surfactant

In 1990, the Food and Drug Administration (FDA) declared pulmonary surfactant safe and effective for the treatment of surfactant deficiency of prematurity (Polin et al., 2014). The AAP initially published guidance in favor of the use of surfactant in 1999 and subsequently updated and reaffirmed this position in 2008 and 2014. Over the past 3 decades, numerous RCTs have confirmed that mortality risk, the incidence of pulmonary air leak, and BPD are reduced with the use of surfactant in preterm infants less than 34 weeks (Bahadue & Soll, 2012; Pfister et al., 2009; Rojas-Reyes et al., 2012; Seger & Soll, 2009; Soll, 1998; Soll & Blanco, 2001; Soll & Özek, 1997, 2009, 2010; Stevens et al., 2007; Suresh & Soll, 2005). More recently, Ramaswamy and colleagues (2022) published a systematic review of studies using surfactant in late preterm and term infants with RDS. They reported with moderate certainty that mortality risk decreased with the use of surfactant among neonates requiring noninvasive respiratory support or conventional mechanical ventilatory support (odds ratio [OR]: 0.45, 95% CI: 0.32–0.64).

Currently, there are both natural (animal-derived) and synthetic surfactants that are FDA approved for use in the United States. Animal-derived products, either porcine or bovine, are the only surfactants available at this time. Beractant (Survanta), a bovine surfactant, was the first animal-derived surfactant approved by the FDA in 1991. In 1998, calfactant (Infasurf), another bovine surfactant, was approved for use. Beractant and calfactant are extracted from cow lungs using bronchoalveolar lavage. The first porcine surfactant derived from minced pig lungs, poractant alfa

TABLE 13.5 Phospholipid Concentration of Commonly Prescribed Pulmonary Surfactants

	BERACTANT	CALFACTANT	PORACTANT ALFA
Phospholipid concentration (mg/mL)	25	35	76

(Curosurf), was approved in 1999. The concentration of phospholipid, per brand of surfactant, is summarized in Table 13.5.

All animal-derived surfactant preparations have been shown to be effective in clinical trials. Therefore, no preparation is specifically recommended or considered superior to others. For the benefit of trainees, we offer a summary of outcomes from key trials in the text that follows. We encourage clinicians to keep abreast of the state of the science as new trials always have the potential to yield new findings. Singh and colleagues (2015) published a meta-analysis comparing the three animal-derived surfactants for the treatment and prevention of RDS in premature neonates for the outcomes of mortality, BPD, and other morbidities. They did not find any difference in death or BPD in trials comparing calfactant to beractant (RR: 0.95, 95% CI: 0.86–1.06). They did, however, find a significant increase in the risk of mortality prior to hospital discharge (RR: 1.44, 95% CI: 1.04–2.00), death or oxygen requirement at 36 weeks' postmenstrual age (RR: 1.30, 95% CI: 1.04–1.64), need for more than one dose of surfactant (RR: 1.57, 95% CI: 1.29–1.92), and patent ductus arteriosus requiring treatment (RR: 1.86, 95% CI: 1.28–2.70) in infants treated with beractant compared to poractant alfa. Of note, the differences that were found were limited to studies that used the higher initial dose of poractant alfa (2.5 mL/kg), so they could not definitively say whether the difference was due to the surfactant source or due to the inequivalent doses used.

Retrospective studies have produced mixed results regarding the superiority of high-dose poractant alfa compared to other natural surfactants. A retrospective cohort study compared the incidence of all-cause in-hospital mortality in preterm infants treated with natural surfactant preparations (beractant, calfactant, and poractant alfa; Ramanathan et al., 2013). The study included a total of 14,173 infants from 236 different hospitals. Calfactant was associated with increased mortality risk compared to poractant alfa (OR: 1.496, 95% CI: 1.014–2.209). No statistically significant difference in mortality risk was observed between beractant and poractant alfa use (OR: 1.37, 95% CI: 0.996–1.885) or beractant and calfactant use (OR: 1.092, 95% CI: 0.765–1.559). However, an even larger retrospective study conducted by Trembath and colleagues (2013) compared effectiveness of the three natural surfactant preparations in 51,282 premature neonates in 322 U.S. hospitals. The investigators compared the individual agents for the incidence of air leak, death, and a composite of BPD or death, with adjustments made for gestational age, antenatal steroids, discharge year, and small-for-gestational-age status. The authors found no statistically significant differences among any of the agents for any outcomes. The individual results of the different comparisons are given in Table 13.6.

MECHANISM OF ACTION/PHARMACOKINETIC PRINCIPLES

The mechanism of action of pulmonary surfactants is reduction in surface tension at the alveolar air–liquid interface in order to prevent atelectasis in preterm infants with RDS. Surfactant also exhibits antioxidant activity against oxygen radicals, anti-inflammatory activity, and inhibition of microbial invasion, and also aids in the removal of microorganisms and inflammatory agents.

TABLE 13.6 Results From a Large Retrospective Analysis Comparing Three Natural Surfactants

OUTCOME	CALFACTANT VS. BERACTANT OR (95% CI)	CALFACTANT VS. PORACTANT ALFA OR (95% CI)	BERACTANT VS. PORACTANT ALFA OR (95% CI)
Air leak	1.17 (0.95–1.43)	1.23 (0.98–1.56)	1.06 (0.87–1.29)
Death	1.14 (0.93–1.39)	0.98 (0.78–1.23)	1.19 (1.00–1.41)
BPD or death	1.08 (0.93–1.26)	1.19 (1.00–1.41)	1.10 (0.96–1.27)

BPD, bronchopulmonary dysplasia; OR, odds ratio.

Source: From Trembath, A. N., Hornik, C. P., Clark, R., Smith, P. B., Daniels, J., & Laughon, M. (2013). Comparative effectiveness of three surfactant preparations in premature infants. *Journal of Pediatrics, 163*(4), 955–960. https://doi.org/10.1016/j.jpeds.2013.04.053

Pharmacokinetic studies using beractant, calfactant, or poractant alfa are limited to animal models. Drug absorption and distribution are rapid at the surface of the alveolar air–liquid interface. Studies of calfactant using rabbit models suggest that drug metabolism is also rapid; 50% to 75% of the drug is metabolized within 24 hours of administration (https://infasurf.com/prescribing-information). However, a long effective half-life is observed, which corresponds with the recommended 12-hour interval between doses (except in cases of infection, meconium aspiration, or hemorrhage, diseases associated with surfactant inactivation).

DOSING RECOMMENDATIONS

The recommended dose for each surfactant product is listed in Table 13.7. All natural surfactant products should be stored in a refrigerator and protected from light until ready for use. The contents of the vial should be gently swirled, but not shaken, to disperse the suspension prior to use. Manufacturers of beractant and poractant alfa recommend slowly warming the vial contents to room temperature prior to use. Conversely, warming of calfactant prior to administration is not necessary. Any surfactant product that has warmed to room temperature may be returned to the refrigerator once within 24 hours. Vials should not be returned to the refrigerator more than once. Finally, the vials are intended for single use and should not be entered more than once. Any unused suspension left in the vial after use should be discarded.

Surfactant is typically administered through an endotracheal tube as a single bolus or in smaller aliquots, or through an adaptor port on the end of an endotracheal tube. There is insufficient evidence from clinical trials to recommend one administration technique or body position over others (Polin et al., 2014). Prior to administration, clinicians must verify appropriate endotracheal tube placement by noting color return on CO_2 detector, bilateral breath sounds (with tube at appropriate depth), and/or chest radiograph.

Preferences for timing of administration of surfactant have changed as clinicians have gained more knowledge and experience. Prophylactic surfactant replacement involves the administration of preemptive surfactant within 10 to 30 minutes after birth to avoid worsening RDS. Another earlier approach consisted of intubation followed by rescue surfactant administration should the patient show signs of decompensation secondary to RDS. In historic trials, prophylactic surfactant therapy compared to rescue therapy for intubated patients was associated with a lower incidence of mechanical ventilation (RR: 0.67, 95% CI: 0.57–0.79), air leak (RR: 0.52, 95% CI: 0.28–0.96), and BPD (RR: 0.51, 95% CI: 0.26–0.99; Stevens et al., 2007). However, more recent trials compare prophylactic surfactant to early CPAP support. Rojas-Reyes and colleagues (2012) considered data from trials that compared prophylactic surfactant and routine CPAP in neonates with RDS. The meta-analysis concluded that prophylactic surfactant use was associated with a *higher* risk of death or BPD compared to early stabilization with CPAP and rescue surfactant administration (three trials, 1,866 infants; typical RR: 1.13, 95% CI: 1.02–1.25 [I^2 0%]; typical RD: 0.06, 95% CI: 0.01–0.10 [I^2 0%]). When looking at the combined outcome of BPD or death, the number needed to harm (NNTH) was calculated at 17 (95%, 10–100). In other words, for every 17 neonates who were exposed to prophylactic surfactant, one experienced BPD or death. Clearly, clinicians should consider these data when determining whether prophylactic surfactant is in the best interest of the neonate. The AAP recommends that clinicians provide CPAP immediately after birth as an alternative to routine intubation with prophylactic surfactant administration (Polin et al., 2014).

TABLE 13.7 Surfactant Type and Dose

TYPE	DOSE	INTERVAL
Natural (animal-derived)		
Beractant (Survanta)	4 mL/kg	Every 6 hours; maximum of four doses in 48 hours
Calfactant (Infasurf)	3 mL/kg	Every 12 hours; maximum of three doses
Poractant alfa (Curosurf)	Initial dose: 2.5 mL/kg Repeat dose: 1.25 mL/kg	Every 12 hours; maximum of three doses

Sources: From AbbVie Inc. (2020, October). *Survanta* [Package insert]. https://www.rxabbvie.com/pdf/survanta_pi.pdf; Chiesi (2021). *Curosurf: full prescribing information*. https://resources.chiesiusa.com/Curosurf/CUROSURF_PI.pdf; ONY Biotech Inc. (2018). *Infasurf* [Package insert]. https://infasurf.com/prescribing-information

Early rescue therapy is defined as the initiation of surfactant replacement between 30 minutes and 2 hours of life, after the diagnosis of RDS is confirmed by radiographic studies and blood gas analysis. *Late rescue therapy* involves the initiation of surfactant replacement 2 or more hours after birth. A meta-analysis of studies comparing the different times of administration reported that early rescue surfactant therapy (compared to late rescue therapy) was associated with a significant decrease in risk for mortality (RR: 0.84, 95% CI: 0.74–0.95), BPD (RR: 0.69, 95% CI: 0.55–0.86), and a combined endpoint of BPD or death (RR: 0.83, 95% CI: 0.75–0.91; Bahadue & Soll, 2012). In addition, the risk for pneumothorax (RR: 0.69, 95% CI: 0.59–0.82) and pulmonary interstitial emphysema (RR: 0.60, 95% CI: 0.41–0.89) decreased among intubated infants who received early surfactant (compared to late administration). In concert, these data support an approach of early CPAP followed by surfactant administration as soon as possible after intubation is required.

Emerging data regarding surfactant administration have the potential to alter this paradigm by making therapy feasible without traditional, invasive endotracheal intubation. Invasive techniques include prolonged endotracheal intubation and the INtubation-SURfactant-Extubation (INSURE) technique. Minimally invasive surfactant administration (MISA) or less invasive surfactant administration (LISA) techniques involve the use of a laryngeal mask airway (LMA), pharyngeal surfactant administration, or the use of thin intratracheal catheters. When intubated or receiving nasal CPAP, a small (5 French) feeding tube is inserted into the trachea by way of direct laryngoscopy and surfactant is administered through that feeding tube. Isayama and colleagues (2016) investigated seven ventilation strategies: nasal CPAP alone, mechanical ventilation alone, noninvasive intermittent positive pressure alone, INSURE, nebulized surfactant, LISA, and surfactant administration with an LMA. The LISA technique was superior to mechanical ventilation and nasal CPAP alone. Compared to mechanical ventilation, LISA was associated with lower odds of acquiring BPD or death (OR: 0.49, 95% CI: 0.30–0.79). When compared to nasal CPAP, LISA was also associated with lower odds of BPD or death (*OR*: 0.58, 95% CI, 0.35–0.93) and air leak (*OR*: 0.24, 95% CI, 0.05–0.96).

CLINICAL-MONITORING PEARLS

Administration-related adverse events reported by the manufacturers of surfactant include endotracheal tube reflux or obstruction, cyanosis, bradycardia, the need for dose interruption, and reintubation. Right mainstem endotracheal tube placement is associated with uneven distribution of surfactant, which precipitates atelectasis among untreated lung fields. In these circumstances, subsequent doses tend to follow the "path of least resistance" and re-enter the airspaces previously treated with surfactant. Significant cardiopulmonary decompensation warrants immediate discontinuation of surfactant administration and stabilization of the neonate, which may require insertion of a new, patent endotracheal tube. It is essential that clinicians with expertise in endotracheal intubation and ventilatory management are present throughout the duration of drug administration. Clinicians are encouraged to note the neonate's baseline vital signs and ensure that continuous pulse oximetry and cardiorespiratory monitoring are established preprocedure.

Surfactant delivery is also associated with a dynamic improvement in lung volume, FRC, and compliance. To minimize the risk of lung injury and air leak, prompt titration of mechanical respiratory support settings, to minimize the risk of lung injury and air leak, is indicated.

CONCLUSIONS

RDS secondary to surfactant deficiency represents a clinically significant and common problem diagnosed in the NICU. A tragedy, the death of President Kennedy's son, helped catapult this disease to the forefront of attention around the world. If he had been born in an age where surfactant was available, Patrick Bouvier Kennedy might still be alive. This observation highlights the vast progress made in the field of treating premature neonates and surfactant deficiency. Antenatal steroids and exogenous surfactant are cornerstone therapies prescribed for the prevention and mitigation of RDS in NICUs around the world. These therapies successfully took a life-limiting process and transitioned it to a survivable disease.

Work in this field is still needed, though. Despite significant gains, preterm neonates with RDS often succumb long term to BPD and recurrent respiratory infections. Future research efforts have the potential to elucidate risk factors and mechanisms for short- and long-term disease and to identify management strategies that reduce or eliminate the long-term consequence of RDS altogether. For example, researchers are currently investigating outcomes (e.g., duration of mechanical ventilation, short-term respiratory outcomes, BPD) after combination surfactant–budesonide therapy. Some studies suggest that direct intratracheal administration of the budesonide (a corticosteroid) offers anti-inflammatory and diuretic activity that may reduce the burden of BPD or recurrent admissions for pulmonary infections, whereas other studies report no significant difference in outcomes with this combined therapy compared to surfactant alone (Hillman et al., 2020; Kothe et al., 2020; Moschino et al., 2021; Ricci et al., 2017; Yeh et al., 2008). Studies like these are invaluable to neonatologists, neonatal APRNs, pharmacists, and neonates and families.

We encourage trainees as well as novice and experienced clinicians to maintain awareness of the evolving state of the science. Thanks to the Best Pharmaceuticals Act of 2002, resultant prioritization of neonatal-specific pharmaceutical research, and the efforts of scores of nurse and physician scientists, novel discoveries are likely on the horizon.

LEARNING TOOLS AND RESOURCES

Advice From the Authors

Ryan Moore, MD

Mistakes are valuable opportunities. Do not fear being wrong and admitting it. When you are wrong, learn from it and move forward so that you don't repeat it in the future.

Meredith Chanas, PharmD, MSCR, BCPPS

A team-based approach is necessary when caring for neonatal patients. Make sure to always include all members of the team, if possible, when making decisions in the care of your patients in order to provide the best possible evidence-based care, as well as continuing to learn from each other along the way.

Amy J. Jnah, DNP, APRN, NNP-BC

Prepare yourself for the urgency associated with some cases of RDS. Stable hands and a calm head are necessary to work efficiently and effectively. Study the pathogenesis of the disease and pharmacologic data linked to each common medication prescribed to affected neonates. Teach others. This will help you crystalize the information. And last but certainly not least, remember that any stress you feel as a novice pales in comparison to that felt by the family. Talk with them, support them, and help them find glimmers of hope amid their despair.

Alexander Berwick, DO, FAAP

There are subtle differences among the various pathologies that cause respiratory distress in the neonate. Take the time to develop a solid understanding of alveolar and surfactant physiology, as well as the pathophysiology of RDS. This is key in applying therapies in clinical practice when it comes to treating RDS.

Discussion Prompts

1. Discuss the evidence supporting the various timing methods for exogenous surfactant administration; prophylactic, early (<2 hours of life), and late (>2 hours of life). Then compare the data to the current practice of your unit.
2. Describe the challenges a neonate will face when born at 23 weeks in terms of lung development. Describe the stage of development for the lungs and how this will provide challenges to resuscitation and stabilization.
3. Compare the risks and benefits for antenatal corticosteroids in women at risk of preterm delivery. Discuss different patient populations and scenarios for which the answer to when and how to administer antenatal corticosteroids may not be as clear, and what recommendations you would make in these situations.

Mind Map

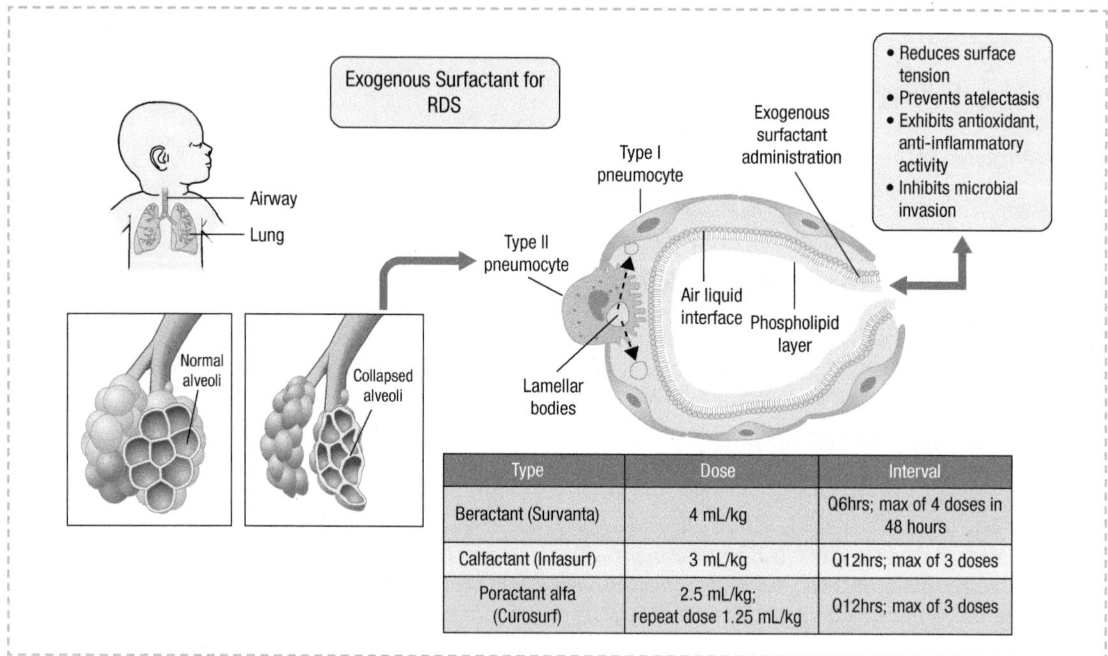

Type	Dose	Interval
Beractant (Survanta)	4 mL/kg	Q6hrs; max of 4 doses in 48 hours
Calfactant (Infasurf)	3 mL/kg	Q12hrs; max of 3 doses
Poractant alfa (Curosurf)	2.5 mL/kg; repeat dose 1.25 mL/kg	Q12hrs; max of 3 doses

Note: This mind map reflects the design team's interpretation of a portion of one or more concepts addressed in this chapter. Readers should regard the mind maps woven throughout this textbook as examples of multisensory study tools that can be developed to encourage conceptual understanding. Readers are encouraged to develop their own unique mind maps in consultation with academic faculty or clinical preceptors. RDS, respiratory distress syndrome.
Design credit: Kristen Landis, MSN, APRN, NNP, RNC-NIC, and Sarah Byler, MSN, APRN, NNP-BC.

REFERENCES

References for this chapter are online and available at https://connect.springerpub.com/content/book/978-0-8261-5884-0/part/partIII/toc-part/ch13.

chapter 14

Pulmonary Hemorrhage

Amy Williford, Meredith Chanas, Erica Davenport, and Amy J. Jnah

LEARNING OBJECTIVES

After completing this chapter, the reader should be able to:

- Define *pulmonary hemorrhage (PH)* and identify the epidemiology of the disease process.
- Explain the physiology of the cardiopulmonary transition to extrauterine life.
- Correlate the pathophysiology of PH with the need for pharmacologic treatment.
- Appraise the historical evolution of pharmacologic management for PH.
- Evaluate current pharmacologic therapies for treatment of PH.

INTRODUCTION

Neonatal pulmonary hemorrhage (PH), first described in the 1950s, is an acute and potentially life-limiting respiratory emergency (Ahvenainen & Call, 1952a; Landing, 1957). PH is customarily described as acute blood loss within the respiratory tract, which when severe leads to an acute clinical decompensation (Plosa, 2017). The pathogenesis of PH, which is explored later in this chapter, is largely (but not always exclusively) attributed to increased pulmonary blood flow from persistent left-to-right shunting across the patent ductus arteriosus (PDA; Aziz & Ohlsson, 2020; Plosa, 2017).

From the 1970s through the 1990s, PH was considered universally fatal (St. John & Carlo, 2015). However, as scientists explored and reported outcomes associated with treatment strategies (e.g., pulmonary surfactant), the disease became survivable. Currently, the risk of developing a PH is inversely proportional to gestational age (GA). Among neonates born preterm, 10.2% of extremely low-birth-weight (ELBW) and 3% to 5% of very-low-birth-weight (VLBW) neonates with respiratory distress syndrome (RDS) develop a PH (Agarwal & Ernst, 2020; Ahmad et al., 2019; Aziz & Ohlsson, 2020; Crowley, 2020). In aggregate, 1 to 12 per 1,000 neonates and infants are affected by PH each year (Wang et al., 2019).

The majority (80%) of PHs develop within the first 72 hours after birth (Agarwal & Ernst, 2020; Crowley, 2020). Among ELBW neonates, 24% of PHs develop on the first day of life and 33% on the second day of life. GA less than 28 weeks, birth weight <1,500 grams, a persistent PDA with left-to-right shunting, and exposure to exogenous pulmonary surfactant therapy are considered primary risks for PH (Table 14.1; St. John & Carlo, 2015; Welde et al., 2021; Zahr et al., 2012). In contrast to these aforementioned risks, antenatal corticosteroids reduce the risk of neonatal PH (Ferreira et al., 2014).

The mortality risk, which is based on outcomes of published studies, ranges between 38% and 85% (Ahmad et al., 2019; Crowley, 2020; Ferreira et al., 2014; Narasimhan & Papworth, 2009; Plosa, 2017). Of those who survive PH, short-term comorbidities include RDS, pneumothorax,

TABLE 14.1 Risk Factors for Pulmonary Hemorrhage: Past and Present

TIME FRAME	RISK FACTORS (1950s–1970s)	RISK FACTORS (1980s–PRESENT; WELDE ET AL., 2021)
Prenatal/ Intrapartum	• Asphyxia (Rowe & Avery, 1966)	• Asphyxia • Cocaine exposure • Maternal hypertension • Intrapartum antibiotic use • Placental abruption
Postnatal	• Coagulopathy (Chessells & Wigglesworth, 1971) • Congenital heart disease (Esterly & Oppenheimer, 1966) • Hemolytic disease of the newborn (Chessels & Wiggleswprth, 1971) • Hypothermia (Mann & Elliott, 1957) • Small for gestational age (Frederick & Butler, 1971)	• Birth weight <1,500 grams • Coagulopathy • Congenital heart disease • Disseminated intravascular coagulation • Extreme prematurity (GA <28 weeks) • Hemodynamically significant PDA with left-to-right shunt • Hypothermia • Intrauterine growth restriction • Intubation and positive pressure ventilation in the delivery room • Low Apgar scores • Low birth weight • Male gender • Mechanical ventilation • Meconium aspiration • Multiple birth • Neutrophil activation in cord blood in the setting of RDS • Polycythemia • Sepsis • Surfactant administration • Urea cycle defects with hyperammonemia

GA, gestational age; PDA, patent ductus arteriosus; RDS, respiratory distress syndrome.

Sources: From Rowe, S., & Avery, M. E. (1966). Massive pulmonary hemorrhage in the newborn. *Journal of Pediatrics*, *69*(1), 12–20. https://doi.org/10.1016/S0022-3476(66)80355-4; Chessells & Wigglesworth, 1971; Esterly & Oppenheimer, 1966; Mann & Elliott, 1957; Fedrick & Butler, 1971; Welde, M. A., Sanford, C. B., Mangum, M., Paschal, C., & Jnah, A. J. (2021). Pulmonary hemorrhage in the neonate. *Neonatal Network*, *40*(5), 295–304. http://doi.org/10.1891/11-T-696.

hypotension, and prolonged oxygen requirement. Long-term comorbidities include bronchopulmonary dysplasia (BPD), intraventricular hemorrhage (IVH), periventricular leukomalacia (PVL), and retinopathy of prematurity (ROP; Ahmad et al., 2019; Crowley, 2020; Ferreira et al., 2014; Lee et al., 2017; Narasimhan & Papworth, 2009; Plosa, 2017; Welde et al., 2021; Zahr et al., 2012).

It is without question that PH is a medical emergency, and because of this it is absolutely necessary that neonatal APRNs understand the pathogenesis of the disease and the evidence specific to current pharmacologic and adjunctive treatment strategies. Therefore, this chapter has been crafted to offer a comprehensive discussion of PH. We begin with a concise review of the normal cardiopulmonary transition to extrauterine life. This leads to a discussion of the pathogenesis of PH as well as common clinical and radiographic manifestations. Before we transition to a discussion of current pharmacologic treatment regimens, we offer a historical look-back to seminal and noteworthy studies of drug therapies used to treat PH. This information will help readers recognize when PH became a topic of interest in the scientific community, when seminal studies were published, and how those data prompted decades of subsequent scientific inquiries. In fact, data from high-fidelity trials and systematic reviews took a once-fatal diagnosis and turned it into a survivable one. We end the chapter with a thorough discussion of current treatment options, including adjunctive therapies and pharmacotherapeutics.

PATHOPHYSIOLOGY OF PULMONARY HEMORRHAGE

PH is considered a complication of other diseases, most notably RDS. Ahvenainen and Call (1952b) were among the first to investigate the pathogenesis of PH, followed by Rowe and Avery (1966), who analyzed autopsy results of 135 neonates who succumbed to PH. Early theories pointed to asphyxia, hypoxia, and pulmonary congestion as the root causes of PH. Asphyxia and hypoxia were considered predecessors to left ventricular failure, pulmonary venous engorgement, and rupture of the pulmonary microcirculation (Cole et al., 1973).

Although the pathophysiology of PH remains incompletely understood, research over the years has helped clinicians understand causal relationships that precipitate a PH. Before we discuss these relationships, we offer readers a review of the transitional circulatory adaptations that begin immediately after birth. A solid understanding of these normal postnatal cardiorespiratory changes is necessary before studying pathologic changes. Trainees are encouraged to consult *Fetal and Neonatal Physiology for the Advanced Practice Nurse* (Jnah & Trembath, 2019) for an expanded discussion of the cardiopulmonary transition to extrauterine life, as needed.

Let us begin with the physiologic response to clamping of the umbilical cord. Once the umbilical cord is clamped, systemic vascular resistance (SVR) in the neonate exceeds pulmonary vascular resistance (PVR). This is a normal physiologic adaptation to extrauterine life, which encourages blood to flow into the right ventricle, main pulmonary artery, and right or left pulmonary artery branches and into the pulmonary microvasculature. This is vital for gas exchange and survival. Oxygenated blood thereby drains from the pulmonary capillaries and into one of the four pulmonary veins (two per lung), to the left atrium, through the mitral valve, and into the left ventricle. The blood is then ejected into the aorta and takes one of two pathways: (a) toward the upper extremities and brain; or (b) toward the adrenal glands, lower extremities, and other nearby vital organs. Under normal circumstances, as these transitional changes are occurring, the PDA, connected to the left pulmonary artery (on one side) and descending aorta (on the other side), functionally (and later, anatomically) closes.

Notice that closure of the ductus arteriosus is necessary for normal postnatal cardiorespiratory function. When the ductus arteriosus remains patent, several pathologic problems, including PH, may develop. In these situations, the PDA becomes a conduit for left-to-right blood flow. A portion of blood flowing through the descending aorta and toward the adrenal glands and lower extremities is enticed to take the path of least resistance (given that SVR is greater than PVR) and move in a left-to-right direction across the PDA and back into the pulmonary circulation. The proportion of blood that traverses the PDA in this pathologic direction depends on cardiac output and the diameter of the PDA (small, moderate, or large).

As blood flow persists in a left-to-rightward direction, the pulmonary microvasculature engorges. This increases the risk of capillary leakage and pulmonary edema. Should this persist or worsen, capillary pressure may increase and affected capillaries shear. As a result, fluid and blood leak from vasculature and into the interstitial spaces and alveoli. This marks the onset of a PH (Figure 14.1; Crowley, 2020). This hemorrhagic state may be mild (subclinical), moderate, or severe (visible blood in endotracheal tube, mouth, and/or nares).

Clinical Manifestations and Diagnosis

PH can present as a focal, regional, or diffuse hemorrhage with concurrent alveolar injury, and in some cases injure the anatomic space situated between the epithelial lining of the alveoli and the endothelium of the pulmonary capillaries (lung interstitium). Mild cases of PH may involve rupture of few, isolated red blood cells within the intra-alveolar and intraparenchymal areas and little or no visible bleeding (Tonse, 2017). Moderate cases of PH may involve more extensive hemorrhage into the alveoli and main airways; pink-tinged, frothy secretions may be observed from the endotracheal tube or during oral suctioning. If uncontrolled bleeding develops, a severe PH may result. Frank hemorrhage and hypovolemic shock (e.g., apnea, bradycardia, cyanosis with pallor, hypotension) are common manifestations. Similar to moderate hemorrhages, blood migrates from the alveoli and bronchioles and toward the main bronchi. However, the volume of hemorrhagic fluid in the trachea obstructs the flow of air and oxygen. This impairs the acid–base balance, precipitates a ventilation-perfusion mismatch, and promotes lung consolidation (Crowley, 2020; Plosa, 2017; Tonse, 2017; Zahr et al., 2012). In addition, endogenously synthesized surfactant is inactivated in the presence of blood and plasma proteins, further impairing respiratory function (Tonse, 2017). Radiographic findings may include one or more lung fields, which take on a tissue-like density, which suggests consolidation distal to fluid-blood-filled bronchioles (fluid bronchograms). Air bronchograms (gas-filled bronchi surrounded by alveoli composed of fluid or blood) have also been reported.

FIGURE 14.1 Pathophysiology of pulmonary hemorrhage.

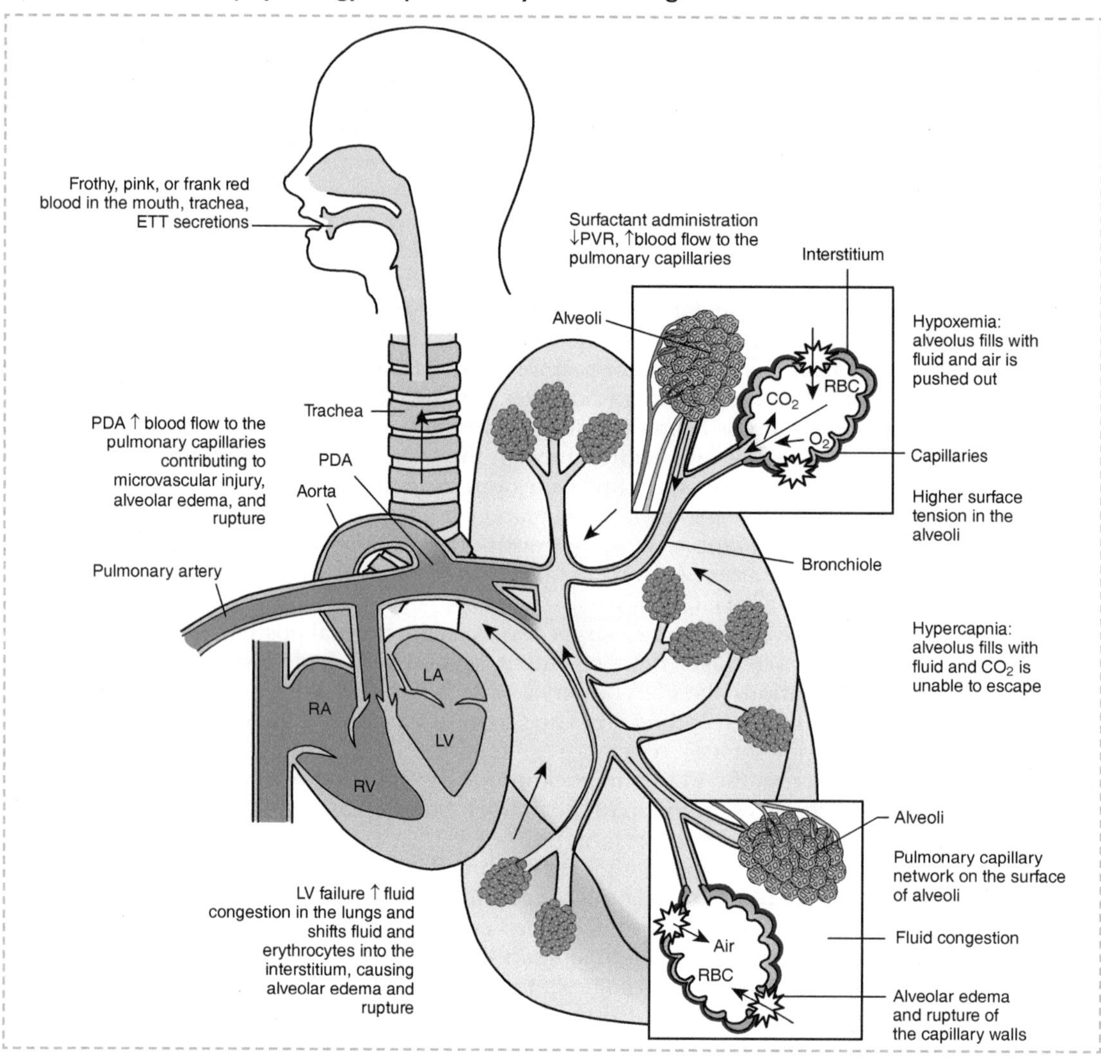

ETT, endotracheal tube; LA, left atrium; LV, left ventricle; PDA, patent ductus arteriosus; PVR, pulmonary vascular resistance; RA, right atrium; RBC, red blood cells; RV, right ventricle.
Source: From Welde, M. A., Sanford, C. B., Mangum, M., Paschal, C., & Jnah, A. J. (2021). Pulmonary hemorrhage in the neonate. *Neonatal Network, 40*(5), 295–304. http://doi.org/10.1891/11-T-696.
Design credit: Cassidy Sanford, MSN, APRN, NNP-BC.

HISTORICAL PERSPECTIVE: SEMINAL AND OTHER NOTEWORTHY STUDIES

Prior to the late 20th century, neonatal PH was almost always a fatal condition primarily affecting infants who were either asphyxiated or small for GA. In fact, Avery and Fletcher (1974) noted that there was no established treatment regimen for PH throughout this era. Blood products, inotropic agents, and even cocaine were prescribed to try to rectify the disease process. Some infants survived, but most did not. Physicians then trialed the use of surfactant into hemorrhaging lungs. This therapy proved to be both counterintuitive and therapeutic.

Blood Products

Reports of use of blood products as a treatment adjunct for PH, namely packed red blood cells (PRBC), vitamin K, hemocoagulase, and factor VII, were published beginning in the mid-1970s. As readers will come to recognize, these blood products were (and still are) useful but not curative.

We summarize the outcomes of a small number of case reports that used PRBC as a primary intervention in the treatment of PH.

Trompeter and colleagues (1975) reported the outcomes associated with the administration of PRBC among six neonates with PH. Four of the infants were between 28 and 32 weeks of gestation and two infants were term; the PH manifested between 7 and 144 hours of life. The researchers resuscitated the neonates with intermittent positive-pressure ventilation (IPPV) and 10 mL/kg of PRBC. Adjuncts included tris-hydroxymethyl aminomethane (THAM), an alkali buffer, digoxin, morphine, and furosemide. Two of the six infants survived. Markestad and Finne (1980) also reported clinical improvement associated with resuscitating one term neonate with endotracheal intubation and mechanical ventilatory support, followed by one PRBC transfusion (unspecified volume) and tolazoline. Of note, tolazoline is a nonselective alpha-adrenergic antagonist and pulmonary vasodilator. No additional reports using this drug for management of PH are found in the literature likely due to advancements in the treatment of conditions causing constriction of pulmonary arterioles and central right-to-left shunting of blood. Currently, tolazoline is only marketed in the United States for use in veterinary medicine.

The use of vitamin K as part of the treatment regimen for PH was first reported by Amizuka and colleagues (2003). Of the 27 neonates enrolled in the study, 26 were endotracheally intubated and mechanically ventilated. These 26 neonates also received standardized parenteral fluids, vasopressors, and bovine pulmonary surfactant at the onset of PH. One of the 26 neonates received a PRBC transfusion as additional adjunctive therapy. All neonates recovered from PH, although the researchers did not specifically investigate the effect of vitamin K or PRBC therapy in this cohort. From this date forward, clinicians have prescribed vitamin K when a coagulopathy was suspected or confirmed, but not necessarily as a standardized component of a study protocol (given that the provision of intramuscular vitamin K within the first hour of life was standard of care for all neonates in the United States).

The investigation of potential new treatments to stop PH and achieve hemostasis led to the evaluation of therapies, including hemocoagulase and recombinant activated factor VIIa (rFVIIa), which are discussed in more detail later in this chapter. Hemocoagulase is a newer agent that has been investigated outside the United States to achieve hemostasis in neonates with PH. It is a purified mixture of two enzymes derived from the venom of the Brazilian snake *Bothrops atrox* and used clinically in plastic and abdominal surgery and human vitrectomy (Shi et al., 2005; Zahr et al., 2012). The activity of the first enzyme is similar to thrombin, which cleaves fibrinogen to form active fibrin and allow clot formation. The second enzyme is similar to thromboplastin, which activates factor X to factor Xa. Factor Xa leads to the conversion of prothrombin to thrombin, leading to platelet aggregation, activation of further plasma factors, and fibrin formation. One Klobusitzky unit (KU) of enzyme coagulates human plasma in about 60 seconds (Zahr et al., 2012). Therefore, a therapeutic effect involves a prompt decrease in bleeding time with enhanced coagulation at the site of injury (Zahr et al., 2012).

The seminal work of Shi and associates (2005) is summarized for historical context. Readers are advised that both studies were limited by design flaws, which in turn limited their external validity. The first prospective randomized study measured time to hemostasis in neonates randomized to receive either 0.5 KU of hemocoagulase endotracheally every 4 to 6 hours or mechanical ventilation alone. The patients treated with hemocoagulase had a significant reduction in duration of PH, duration of mechanical ventilation, and mortality ($p < .05$).

Two years later, the same group of investigators performed a second randomized trial that evaluated the use of hemocoagulase prophylaxis to *prevent* PH in premature neonates. Neonates randomized to the interventional group were prescribed 0.25 KU of hemocoagulase, endotracheally, every 4 to 6 hours, for 3 to 5 days. A significant decrease in incidence of PH, duration of PH, total days of mechanical ventilation, and death was associated with hemocoagulase use ($p < .05$; Shi et al., 2008). This drug is not currently marketed in the United States. Well-powered, randomized trials are necessary for this drug to be adopted for routine use in neonatal patients with PH.

To date, there have been no published prospective clinical studies evaluating the safety or efficacy of rFVIIa use in neonates for treatment of PH. Olomu and associates (2002) were among the first to investigate the outcomes linked to this therapy among infants with PH. Their report included two infants, each received 50 mcg/kg/dose, twice daily, for a total of 2 to 3 days. Hemostasis was achieved within 7 days of therapy. Cetin and colleagues (2006) reported hemostasis after rFVII therapy in a 31-week GA male neonate with sepsis, PH, and a coagulopathy. Treatments, including parenteral vitamin K, fresh frozen plasma (FFP; 60mL/kg), and PRBC transfusions, were ineffective. Therefore, rFVII (120 mcg/kg) was administered three times and hemostasis was achieved. Dang and associates (2011) were the first to publish a larger case series of five preterm neonates (28–32 weeks of gestation) who were treated with rFVIIa (1–3 doses of 90 mcg/kg) for PH. Hemostasis was achieved in all cases. Given the lack of prospective studies and variable dosages reported in these case reports, no standardized regimen has been established to date.

Epinephrine and Cocaine

Historical efforts to induce vasoconstriction at the site of the pulmonary capillaries with epinephrine or cocaine via the endotracheal tube are described as both a primary treatment and in combination with mechanical ventilation. Bhandari and associates (1999) were the first to report the outcomes of neonates (<35 weeks of gestation) treated with 4 mg/kg of cocaine (this is not a typo) and/or 0.1 mL/kg of epinephrine. Standard ventilatory support involved an increase in mean airway pressure (MAP). Less than half of the study population survived (12 of 34 neonates).

Later, Yen et al. (2013) reported that 0.5 mL epinephrine 0.1 mg/mL with 1 mL of air, sprayed via the endotracheal tube three to five times, was successful in stopping a majority of PH. Epinephrine also reduced the need for repetitive (and unnecessary) endotracheal suctioning.

Pulmonary Surfactant

Holm and Notter (1987) found excised rat lung compliance was decreased after introducing hemoglobin, membrane lipids, or albumin. This was especially true for those lungs already partially surfactant deficient. However, exogenous surfactant reversed this process and improved compliance. Fibrinogen, then human serum, and last albumin produced the highest surface tension in an experiment performed by Fuchimukai and colleagues (1987). Thus, it was concluded these proteins may negatively impact exogenous surfactant activity. The rationale for the use of exogenous surfactant to treat PH is predicated on the previously described pathology. Available surfactant is inactivated by the presence of blood and surface tension is increased within the alveoli and surrounding airways. This results in a clinical picture of secondary surfactant dysfunction (Yen et al., 2013).

Pandit et al. (1995) were among the first to investigate the use of bovine surfactant in 15 neonates (median GA of 28 weeks) who developed PH between 1 and 62 hours of life. The authors reported a prompt improvement in respiratory status, as defined by a decrease in the oxygenation index (mean [M] = from 24.6 to 8.6), after surfactant was administered to treat the PH ($p < .001$). Amizuka and colleagues (2003) also investigated the use of bovine surfactant in 26 neonates with PH. Neonates with a mean GA of 31.5 weeks or birth weight <1,500 grams exhibited a favorable response to surfactant therapy. Eighty-one percent of the neonates experienced rapid resolution of PH after a single dose of surfactant, whereas the remaining five neonates recovered slowly, with resolution as late as 96 hours of age. Including these noteworthy studies, all other reports (involving neonates as subjects) published between 1975 and 2014 were retrospective in design.

Finally, in 2015, Bozdağ and colleagues published the first prospective, randomized controlled trial (RCT) comparing the use of two animal-derived (natural) surfactants for treatment of PH: poractant alfa (porcine surfactant) and beractant (bovine surfactant). Similar to the aforementioned studies, the mean GA of neonates randomized in the study was 27.9 weeks, with birth weight of <1,500 grams (M = 1,051 grams), and onset of PH of between 46 and 96 hours of life. The administration of poractant alfa and beractant reduced the oxygenation index at 1 hour post-therapy (from 22.7 to 14.6 and from 17.9 to 12.8, respectively). A summary of outcomes and limitations of these studies is provided in Table 14.2.

EMERGENT STABILIZATION

Given the paucity of randomized trials of therapies and drugs used to treat PH, neonatal clinicians must make individualized decisions based on limited (or no) evidence. For this reason, no single standardized treatment regimen exists. Between 1980 and 1992, 33 different treatment regimens were reported in the literature alone (Raju & Langenberg, 1993). Presently, regimens still vary among institutions and clinicians.

TABLE 14.2 Seminal and Noteworthy Studies Using Surfactant to Treat Pulmonary Hemorrhage

STUDY	OBJECTIVE	STUDY DESIGN	POPULATION	OUTCOME	LIMITATIONS
Pandit et al. (1995)	Evaluate the effect of exogenous bovine surfactant on oxygen/ventilatory needs with respiratory deterioration due to PH.	Retrospective case series Time period: July 1991–December 1993	15 neonates Median birth weight: 960 grams Mean GA: 28 weeks Median age at PH: 24.4 hours Mean interval between PH and surfactant therapy: 10 hours	Mean OI improved post surfactant ($p < .001$) No patients deteriorated following surfactant therapy	Lack of comparable control group Small sample size
Amizuka et al. (2003)	Evaluate the clinical and biochemical factors associated with surfactant dysfunction and response to exogenous surfactant.	Observational Time period: May 1991–March 1998	27 neonates Admitted to 2 NICUs 33% were VLBW (<1,500 grams) 96% were preterm (<37 weeks' gestation) 70% delivered via Cesarean section 44% were intubated in the delivery room	Post surfactant (1 hour): Improved respiratory failure No recurrence of hemorrhagic pulmonary edema No chronic lung disease No deaths	No comparable control group
Neumayr et al. (2008)	Describe the clinical effect of surfactant in a patient with PH.	Case report	1 PICU patient Age: 4 weeks old Unilateral PH after iatrogenic lung injury during corrective surgery for a congenital heart defect	Post surfactant (2 hours): Reduction in both ventilation and oxygenation needs Improved chest radiograph	Single patient
Bozdağ et al. (2015)	Compare the efficacy of two surfactant products for treatment of PH in VLBW infants.	Prospective, randomized, controlled trial Poractant 100 mg/kg versus beractant 100 mg/kg after the second hour of PH	42 VLBW infants with pulmonary hemorrhage in the first 2 weeks of life <32 weeks' GA Birth weight <1,500 grams	Mean OI decreased after surfactant in both groups, without significant difference	Not blinded No placebo control Small sample size

GA, gestational age; OI, oxygenation index; PH, pulmonary hemorrhage; PICU, pediatric intensive care unit; VLBW, very-low-birth-weight.

Clinicians agree that the onset of PH is often abrupt, and moderate to severe hemorrhage requires a multisystem approach to stabilization (Chen et al., 2012; Welde et al., 2021). Most clinicians prioritize the establishment of a patent airway and high-frequency ventilatory support with adequate MAP before pursuing adjunctive therapies. Other pharmacotherapies include the provision of pulmonary surfactant and correction of cardiac output and acidosis with inotropic agents and blood products. RCTs are necessary to refine this multisystem approach.

This section of the chapter offers a detailed discussion of common medications used to treat neonatal PH. We explore the mechanism of action, available neonatal-specific pharmacokinetic data, dosages, and clinical-monitoring pearls specific to each drug. The drugs are organized based on frequency of inclusion in published reports. In the absence of a position statement by the American Academy of Pediatrics, one therapy cannot be considered superior to others.

Ventilatory Support

In cases of moderate to severe hemorrhage, the airway is customarily cleared to establish and maintain patency for air flow and gas exchange (Table 14.3). Gentle suctioning may remove obstructive clots and hemorrhagic fluid. Ventilatory support maneuvers include increasing baseline positive end-expiratory pressure (PEEP) as a means to increase MAP and tamponade hemorrhaging pulmonary capillaries (Zahr et al., 2012). High-frequency oscillatory ventilation (HFOV) may be used to effectively increase MAP; numerous studies indicate HFOV is safe and effective in treating PH (Alkharfy, 2004). As an alternative, IPPV is also effective in controlling PH. Supplemental oxygen is often provided to achieve target oxygen saturation parameters.

Laboratory Studies

A chest radiograph and laboratory tests (arterial blood gas [ABG], complete blood count [CBC], blood culture, coagulation panel, metabolic panel) are ordered to appraise the severity of the PH and the need for pharmacologic therapies. ABG can quickly inform the acid–base balance as well as the hemodynamic status. CBC and blood culture help clinicians determine whether sepsis is an underlying cause of the hemorrhage. These studies are often paired with coagulation studies. Recall that sepsis may cause disseminated intravascular coagulation (DIC), which can precipitate a hemorrhage; affected infants manifest with increased prothrombin (PT) and partial thromboplastin (PTT) times and thrombocytopenia. Likewise, an underlying coagulation disorder (e.g., von Willebrand) may be a contributing factor to the hemorrhage; infants with von Willebrand disease commonly manifest with normal PT, markedly elevated PTT, and normal platelet count. Given that bleeding removes blood and components from the systemic circulation, electrolyte imbalances are common. Most clinicians repeat metabolic panels to closely monitor electrolyte status as well as glucose levels, which can decrease with sepsis or shock. Last, it is important to consider the risk of bleeding in other regions of the body, namely the germinal matrix and the intraventricular spaces. For this reason, a screening head ultrasound is often pursued; in rarer and severe cases, head ultrasound is a necessary prerequisite to extracorporeal membrane oxygenation (ECMO) therapy.

TABLE 14.3 Emergency Stabilization With Pulmonary Hemorrhage: A Multisystem Approach

1. Gentle airway clearance (avoiding repetitive/unnecessary suctioning)
2. Endotracheal intubation
3. Mechanical ventilation: HFOV versus IPPV
    - ⇨ Increase peak end expiratory pressure
    - ⇨ Increase mean airway pressure
4. Chest radiograph
5. Hematologic studies (ABG, CBC, blood culture, coagulation panel, metabolic panel)
6. Fluid and nutritional support
7. Analgesia and sedation

Note: Most stabilization steps can be executed simultaneously when clinicians communicate using an evidence-based teamwork system.
ABG, arterial blood gas; CBC, complete blood count; HFOV, high-frequency oscillatory ventilation; IPPV, intermittent positive-pressure ventilation.

CURRENT PRIMARY PHARMACOLOGIC TREATMENT

Primary therapies include pulmonary surfactant and inotropic agents, which may be prescribed to reestablish surface tension and optimize cardiac output and blood pressure, respectively. Adjunctive therapies include PRBC, FFP, epinephrine, rFVIIa, or hemocoagulase. These drugs may be necessary to replace blood volume lost to the hemorrhagic state and achieve hemostasis; their use remains controversial, largely due to the lack of controlled trials that demonstrate clear benefits (Barnes et al., 2021).

Pulmonary Surfactant

Although it may seem counterintuitive, given that multiple doses of surfactant are associated with an increased risk of hemorrhage, single-dose surfactant may be prescribed in cases of hemorrhage to reestablish surface tension. In fact, several studies presented in the historical section of this chapter, including one randomized trial, concluded that surfactant (poractant alfa or beractant) is effective in the treatment of PH (Amizuka et al., 2003; Bozdağ et al., 2015; Neumayr et al., 2008; Pandit et al., 1995; Trompeter et al., 1975). That said, surfactant alone is not sufficient to stop PH; a multisystem treatment strategy is necessary and has been reported in each of these studies.

MECHANISM OF ACTION/PHARMACOKINETIC PRINCIPLES

As discussed in Chapter 13, "Respiratory Distress Syndrome," pulmonary surfactants act to reduce surface tension at the alveolar air–liquid interface as well as exhibit antioxidant activity. The reduction in surface tension induces a decrease in intrapulmonary pressure, which encourages left-to-right shunting across the PDA. This increases pulmonary blood flow.

One particular pharmacokinetic difference between data presented in the RDS chapter relates to the half-life of surfactant when exposed to blood products (and meconium). Red blood cells, hemoglobin, plasma proteins, and lipids that migrate into the alveolus and interact with surfactant inactivate it, decreasing its half-life (Holm & Notter, 1987). Therefore, when surfactant is prescribed *after* a PH, it is with the intent to reverse the effect of surfactant inactivation that occurred during the hemorrhage. Single-dose surfactant may decrease surface tension and improve ventilation-perfusion matching and oxygenation index.

DOSING RECOMMENDATIONS

Currently, one supplemental dose of surfactant may be considered after PH is diagnosed. Supplemental beractant dosing is 4 mL/kg/dose, calfactant dosing is 3 mL/kg/dose, and poractant alfa dosing is 1.25 mL/kg/dose (Taketomo, 2023). Randomized trials are needed to properly evaluate this therapy in the setting of a multisystem approach to the treatment of PH.

CLINICAL-MONITORING PEARLS

Administration-related adverse events, as discussed in Chapter 13, "Respiratory Distress Syndrome," and that also apply to PH, include endotracheal tube reflux of surfactant, cyanosis, bradycardia, the need for dose interruption, and the need for reintubation secondary to obstruction. In situations that require the insertion of a new endotracheal tube, clinicians should be mindful that right mainstem endotracheal tube placement is associated with uneven distribution of surfactant.

CURRENT ADJUNCTIVE PHARMACOLOGIC TREATMENT

Adjunctive therapies, including fluid and nutritional support, use of analgesics and/or sedatives, and inotropic agents, are presented in complementary chapters within this textbook. We have focused this discussion of adjunctive therapies to endotracheal epinephrine and blood products, two therapies customized based on the severity of PH and suspicion for a preexisting coagulation disorder.

Epinephrine

Given the vasoconstrictive and inotropic effects associated with epinephrine therapy, this drug may be prescribed as an adjunctive therapy to treat PH.

MECHANISM OF ACTION/PHARMACOKINETIC PRINCIPLES

The mechanism of action of epinephrine, as discussed in Chapter 20, "Hypotension and Shock," is elicited with dose-dependent binding to alpha-adrenergic and beta-adrenergic receptors. Endotracheal administration is associated with activation of alpha-1-adrenergic receptors (vasoconstriction), and to a lesser extent beta-1-adrenergic receptors (chronotropy, inotropy, and lusitropy) and beta-2 receptors (myocardial contractility and vascular smooth muscle relaxation). The activation of beta receptors is desirable when left ventricular failure is suspected (Chen et al., 2012). It is believed that the combination of increased strength and rate of cardiac contraction, airway smooth muscle relaxation, and arteriolar smooth muscle contraction within the bronchioles leads to cessation of PH.

DOSING RECOMMENDATIONS

Epinephrine is typically administered through the endotracheal tube. The customary endotracheal dosage for epinephrine, which is standardized for use in neonates regardless of indication for use, is 1 mL/kg (drug concentration = 0.1 mg/mL), given as a rapid push; three to five repeat doses may be administered, as needed.

CLINICAL-MONITORING PEARLS

Clinicians should monitor the neonate for signs of decreased bleeding or lack of response to therapy. Side effects associated with repeat dosing include tachycardia, hyperglycemia, hypokalemia, lactic acidosis, and myocardial ischemia (Valverde et al., 2006).

Blood Products

The use of blood products in neonatal PH has been described in the literature for decades for treatment of a suspected coagulopathy or for replacement of blood volume lost via PH (Amizuka et al., 2003; Barnes et al., 2021; Trompeter et al., 1975; Yen et al., 2013). Blood products are often a necessary adjunctive therapy, which are transfused, as indicated, based on lab indices and clinical stability (Tonse, 2017). Although the precedent for the use of blood products to manage PH is well documented, replacing large volumes of blood may exacerbate underlying hemorrhagic edema (Shi et al., 2005; St. John & Carlo, 2015). Thus, clinicians must consider the primary pathophysiology when attempting to restore hemodynamic stability.

PACKED RED BLOOD CELLS

Transfusion of PRBCs may be considered to correct the anemia and/or hypovolemia due to the loss of blood via the respiratory tract (or elsewhere). If necessary, transfusion should be done slowly (St. John & Carlo, 2015). Table 14.4 offers a blood type compatibility chart; neonates traditionally receive leukoreduced, irradiated, O-negative blood.

Dosing Recommendations

Most of the literature describing the use of PRBCs in PH does not specify the volume administered, although the aforementioned retrospective study by Trompeter et al. (1975) used 10 mL/kg. The usual volume range to correct anemia or hypovolemia is 5 to 20 mL/kg transfused over 1 to 4 hours (approximately 5 mL/kg/hr).

To minimize the risk of complications, neonates are assigned a dedicated unit of PRBC; each unit customarily expires 42 days after being opened (American Red Cross, 2022). The ordered dose and transfusion time may be tailored depending on GA, severity of hemorrhage and hypovolemia/hypotension, preexisting comorbidities, and real-time assessment of the integrity of intravenous catheter access (Sloan, 2017). The maximum window for infusing PRBC is 4 hours.

TABLE 14.4 PRBC Compatibility Chart

NEONATE BLOOD TYPE	COMPATIBLE PRBC
O	O
A	A or O
B	B or O
AB	Any type

Note: O-negative, leukoreduced, irradiated PRBCs are commonly prepared by hospital blood banks for use in neonatal intensive care. PRBC, packed red blood cells.

Clinical-Monitoring Pearls

Clinicians should make every effort to obtain a sample for blood typing (ABO/Rh) and screening (type and screen) prior to the transfusion of blood products; life-threatening circumstances may require emergent transfusion of uncrossmatched units of group O red blood cells. The type and screen are valid for 4 consecutive months; therefore, clinicians should verify the expiration date of the most recent type and screen before ordering blood products.

Informed consent from the parent or legal guardian should be obtained except in cases of life-threatening emergency, which require immediate transfusion. The risk for transfusion-related disease should be reviewed as part of the informed consent process, to include the risk for bacteremia (1/6,000), parvovirus B19 (1/20,000–50,000), hepatitis B (1/843,000–2,008,000), hepatitis C (1/1,149,000), and HIV (1/1,467,000; Cohn et al., 2020). The risk for cytomegalovirus infection with leukoreduced blood has never been studied; experts estimate the risk to be less than 1/1,000,000 (Bianchi et al., 2020). PRBCs are leukocyte-reduced to minimize the concentration of white blood cells, a process known to decrease the risk of febrile reactions, immunization against human leukocyte antigen (HLA) and human platelet antigen (HPA), and the transmission of cytomegalovirus (Lasky et al., 2021).

Clinicians should anticipate the need for one staff member to leave the unit and retrieve the blood product. In addition, the hospital protocol should be reviewed by all participating clinicians to ensure proper analysis and documentation of pretransfusion vital signs, blood product verification, as well as continuous patient monitoring by at least one clinician. Bedside clinicians must ensure patency of the intravenous catheter that will be used to administer the blood product. Transfusion reactions (e.g., hyperthermia, respiratory distress, hypoxemia, hypotension or hypertension, and hemoglobinuria) are rare and usually present within the first 15 minutes of transfusion.

FRESH FROZEN PLASMA

FFP contains proteins, clotting factors, immunoglobins, and vitamin K-dependent factors. Indications for use include refractory hypotension and for treatment of a coagulopathy in the presence of factor deficiencies with evidence of laboratory abnormality or bleeding. Omansky (2019) presented a case report of a term infant with PH who was treated with two doses of FFP and dopamine. Although the coagulation studies (PT and activated partial thromboplastin time [aPTT]) remained abnormal after FFP transfusion, bleeding via the endotracheal tube decreased (Omansky, 2019). Table 14.5 offers an FFP compatibility chart; most hospitals provide AB plasma; Rh is not taken into consideration when transfusing this blood product.

Dosing Recommendations

FFP is customarily irradiated for use in infants younger than 4 months of age. The dosing range is 10 to 20 mL/kg, which may be repeated every 8 to 12 hours (Sloan, 2017). Once prepared, FFP is considered fresh for a total of 6 consecutive hours and must be infused within a maximum 4-hour window.

Clinical-Monitoring Pearls

Pulmonary congestion may worsen with empiric transfusion of FFP (St. John & Carlo, 2015). Interval monitoring of ABG, lung dynamics as reported in real time on conventional ventilator dashboards, as well as radiographic studies may be indicated.

CRYOPRECIPITATE

Cryoprecipitate is indicated for correction of factor VIII, XIII, and von Willebrand factor deficiencies, and is considered the most effective source of fibrinogen for neonates (Croteau, 2017). Its usefulness in neonates with PH is in the treatment of associated coagulopathies or DIC. It is not indicated for volume expansion in the treatment of hypotension (Poterjoy & Josephson, 2009). Table 14.6 offers a cryoprecipitate compatibility chart; Rh is not taken into consideration when transfusing this blood product.

Dosing Recommendations

Dosing recommendations may vary depending on the underlying condition. A single unit of cryoprecipitate contains 15 to 20 mL. The literature suggests a transfusion range of 2 mL/kg to 1 unit/7 kg (Poterjoy & Josephson, 2009). Dosing may even be as much as 1 to 2 units/10 kg for hypofibrinogenemia (Croteau, 2017). Although the half-life of fibrinogen is approximately 3 to 5 days, the primary cause of the coagulopathy also determines the dosing frequency (e.g., consumptive vs. congenital causes). The need for additional transfusion may vary from every 8 to 12 hours to every several days (Poterjoy & Josephson, 2009).

Clinical-Monitoring Pearls

As with the use of other blood products, pulmonary congestion may worsen with empiric transfusion of plasma products (St. John & Carlo, 2015). Interval monitoring of ABG, lung dynamics as reported in real time on conventional ventilator dashboards, as well as radiographic studies may be indicated.

ACTIVATED RECOMBINANT FACTOR VIIA

At this time, rFVIIa is Food and Drug Administration-approved only for treatment and prevention of bleeding in surgical interventions or procedures in patients with acquired hemophilia. Nevertheless, rFVIIa is an attractive therapeutic option for treatment of neonatal PH for several reasons, including the rapid onset of action and the low volume needed for administration (Cosar et al., 2017; Dang et al., 2011; Fischer et al., 2008; Hunseler et al., 2006; Lindley et al., 1994; Lisman et al., 2003).

Mechanism of Action/Pharmacokinetic Principles

Intravenous rFVIIa is a vitamin K-dependent glycoprotein and an effective hemostatic agent. It activates the extrinsic pathway of the coagulation cascade by binding to tissue factor in locally injured endothelial areas, leading to the formation of a fibrin clot.

TABLE 14.5 Fresh Frozen Plasma Compatibility Chart

NEONATE BLOOD TYPE	COMPATIBLE FFP
O	Any type
A	A or AB
B	B or AB
AB	AB

Note: Type AB FFP is commonly prepared by hospital blood banks for use in neonatal intensive care.
FFP, fresh frozen plasma.

TABLE 14.6 Cryoprecipitate Compatibility Chart

NEONATE BLOOD TYPE	COMPATIBLE CRYOPRECIPITATE
O	Any type
A	
B	
AB	

Note: Type AB cryoprecipitate is commonly prepared by hospital blood banks for use in neonatal intensive care.

There are two proposed mechanisms for rFVIIa in clot formation. First, rFVIIa binds to tissue factor, forming a complex that activates factor X. Factor Xa, along with other factors, converts prothrombin to thrombin, which then converts fibrinogen to fibrin, thus forming a seal at the vascular injury site. Second, rFVIIa and tissue factor complex activate platelets at the site of the endothelial injury. At high doses, rFVIIa can bind directly to activated platelets, stimulating factor X and factor II to form a localized fibrin clot (Cosar et al., 2017; Dang et al., 2011; Fischer et al., 2008; Hunseler et al., 2006; Lindley et al., 1994; Lisman et al., 2003). Due to the platelet activity associated with rFVIIa activity, it is usually recommended to replenish platelets prior to rFVIIa administration in the setting of thrombocytopenia.

Although the mechanism of action of rFVIIa should lead to localized thrombin formation at the site of injury, the risk of thromboembolism persists, especially in neonates with DIC or sepsis, due to diffusely circulating activated platelets (Brady et al., 2006). Puetz et al. (2009) conducted a systematic review of all published literature and data submitted to the SeveN Bleep registry to compare the rate of thromboses in 134 neonates who received rFVIIa for refractory bleeding versus 100 neonates who received only FFP transfusions. No statistically significant difference was found in the incidence of thrombotic events between the groups (7.5% vs. 7%). However, the same year, a retrospective cohort study was published of 139 pediatric patients with nonhemophilia bleeding treated with rFVIIa. Although the study showed 72% of patients had complete or partial response, they did find an overall thrombosis rate of 4.3%, with the highest rate in neonates (17.3%; Young et al., 2009). Therefore, at this time, use of rFVIIa in neonates should be limited to life-threatening bleeding that is refractory to blood products.

Dosing Recommendations

Given the lack of randomized trials, there is no recommended dose for rFVIIa with neonatal PH. Doses reported in the literature, specific to the treatment of PH, range from 50 to 100 mcg/kg/dose every 2 to 8 hours. In comparison, hemophilia A- or B-related bleeding is treated with 90 mcg/kg/dose every 2 hours until hemostasis is achieved.

The smallest vial size for rFVIIa is 1,000 mcg, and vials are stable for up to 2 hours after reconstitution. Given that the majority of neonates affected by PH weigh <1,500 grams at birth, a significant portion of the vial will be wasted when treating one neonate.

Clinical-Monitoring Pearls

Clinical evaluation of hemostasis should be used as a means of evaluating the effectiveness of rFVIIa therapy. There is no direct correlation between laboratory coagulation parameters and achievement of hemostasis; however, they may be used as an adjunct to clinical evaluation in practice. Patients should also be monitored for signs or symptoms of thrombosis.

CONCLUSIONS

PH remains a catastrophic problem associated with a high mortality rate affecting neonates. Prematurity represents the largest risk factor for developing PH and the incidence is inversely related to GA. The presence of a PDA and surfactant therapy are other risk factors for preterm infants, whereas sepsis, asphyxia, and meconium aspiration increase the probability of developing PH in the term population. Most PH develops within the first 72 hours of life, with overall survival approximately 50% in infants less than 28 weeks' gestation. A multisystem approach is crucial to the management of PH and involves adequate ventilation and use of different pharmacotherapies.

PH should always be considered in a mechanically ventilated stable infant with worsening hypoxia, hypercapnia, and acidosis. Serious PH occurs very abruptly, and aggressive management is crucial to the neonate's survival. Initial stabilization should be aimed at preventing exsanguination from blood loss and optimizing gas exchange. Ventilatory strategies include raising the PEEP and switching to HFOV to increase the MAP to provide tamponade of the pulmonary capillaries. Blood products can be given for volume resuscitation and correction of blood pH should be aggressive. Pharmacotherapies include the use of endotracheal epinephrine, although controversial, for its vasoconstrictive and inotropic effects; rFVIIa for its activation of the extrinsic coagulation pathway which helps in the formation of a fibrin clot; and surfactant therapy (also controversial), which can overcome the secondary surfactant dysfunction from the presence of hemoglobin. Understanding the etiology of PH and using a multisystem approach to its management are vital to improve the outcomes of neonates affected by PH.

LEARNING TOOLS AND RESOURCES

Advice From the Authors

Amy Williford, MSN, APRN, NNP-BC

Try never to become complacent in your practice; always work to be the best version of you. Keep yourself in the open mind-set of a learner.

Meredith Chanas, PharmD, MSCR, BCPPS

There is a constant influx of new literature and medications, making it impossible to keep up with everything. Neonatal pharmacology is an ever-changing field, so those in practice need to be continually open to new ideas and information. However, it can be easy to fall into the trap of wanting to try anything and everything for critically ill patients, with a significant risk of causing further harm with some therapies. It is important to always know your limitations in these high-risk situations and seek help from others, when necessary, in order to provide the best care for our vulnerable patients.

Erica Davenport, DO

Neonatology is a fascinating specialty in that it is fairly new and there are still so many things to learn about it. Keep being curious and ask questions.

Amy J. Jnah, DNP, APRN, NNP-BC

Life-threatening emergencies, like pulmonary hemorrhage, require immediate diagnosis and triage. This can be intimidating to novice clinicians. I suggest dedicating time to the study of the pathogenesis of the disease first, followed by intent study of the multisystems approach to stabilizing and pharmacologically managing a hemorrhage. Some of my students develop catchy acronyms that help elicit quick recall during emergencies. Always seek a multidisciplinary team effort, think out loud to help your learning curve, and listen to your senior colleagues. In time, you will become an adept and empathetic teacher to new learners like yourself.

Discussion Prompts

1. Available data from retrospective and prospective uncontrolled studies show promise of benefit regarding therapeutic use of surfactant for neonatal PH. With a paucity of current evidence based on RCTs, how is the most at-risk neonatal population (<1,500 grams) addressed concerning the safety and efficacy of surfactant administration for PH?
2. Compare and contrast the mechanisms of action of the individual agents to treat coagulopathy, including rFVIIa, cryoprecipitate, and hemocoagulase. When, if ever, would you consider using these agents in a neonate with PH, and which agent would you choose? What are the risks and benefits of each agent?
3. Discuss blood volume in the neonate and how blood loss through PH can be significant, especially for the ELBW infant. Weigh the risks and benefits of obtaining additional blood from the neonate to check coagulation factors versus preemptively giving blood products like FFP.

Mind Map

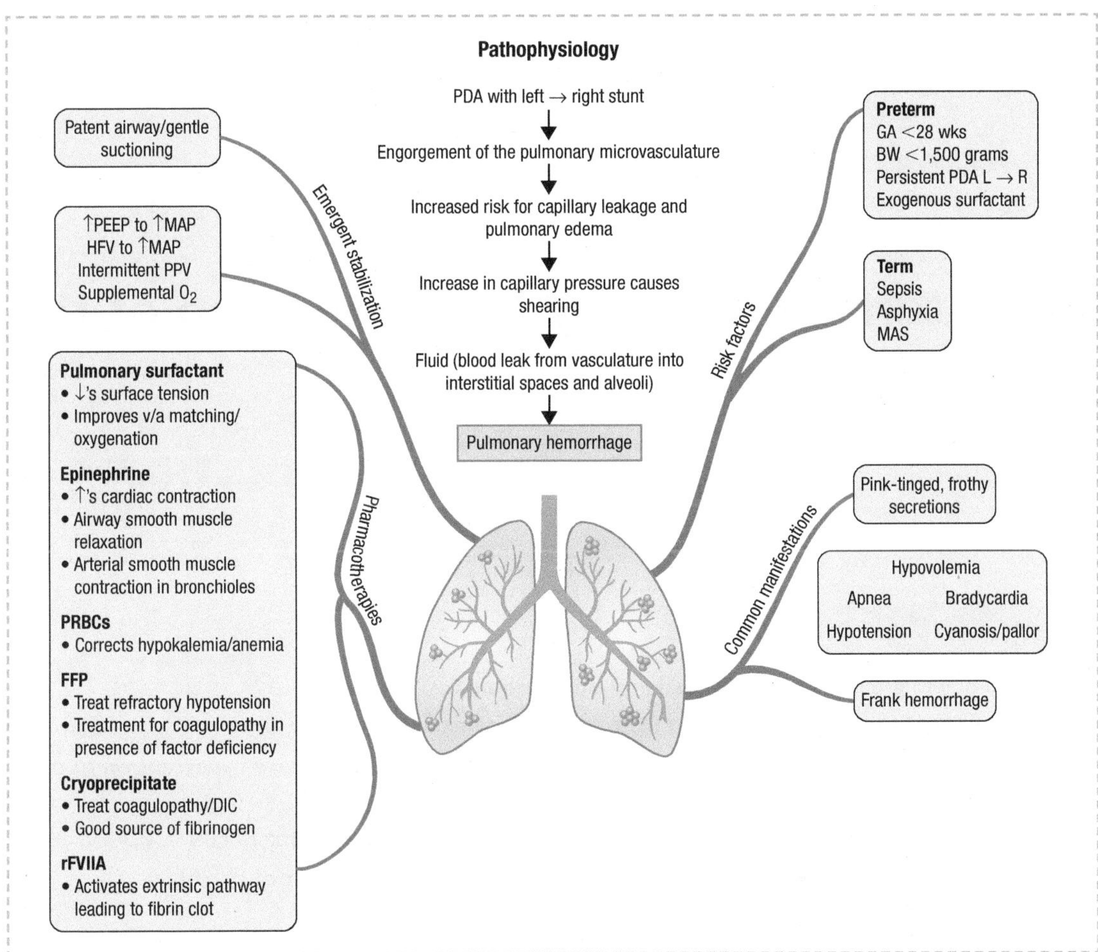

Note: This mind map reflects the design team's interpretation of a portion of one or more concepts addressed in this chapter. Readers should regard the mind maps woven throughout this textbook as examples of multisensory study tools that can be developed to encourage conceptual understanding. Readers are encouraged to develop their own unique mind maps in consultation with academic faculty or clinical preceptors.
BW, birth weight; DIC, disseminated intravascular coagulation; FFP, fresh frozen plasma; GA, gestational age; HFV, high frequency ventilation; MAP, mean airway pressure; MAS, meconium aspiration syndrome; PDA, patent ductus arteriosus; PEEP, positive end-expiratory pressure; PPV, positive-pressure ventilation; PRBCs, packed red blood cells; rFVIIa, recombinant activated factor VIIa.
Design credit: Heather Myers, MSN, APRN, NNP, East Carolina University Neonatal Nurse Practitioner Program.

REFERENCES

References for this chapter are online and available at https://connect.springerpub.com/content/book/978-0-8261-5884-0/part/partIII/toc-part/ch14.

chapter 15

Persistent Pulmonary Hypertension of the Newborn

Deborah S. Bondi and Mary Hurley

LEARNING OBJECTIVES

After completing this chapter, the reader should be able to:

- Understand the normal transition from fetal to postnatal circulation.
- Describe the pathophysiology and risk factors for persistent pulmonary hypertension of the newborn (PPHN).
- Review ventilator therapy and other respiratory support strategies for PPHN.
- Evaluate the current pharmacologic agents used for the management of PPHN.

INTRODUCTION

Persistent pulmonary hypertension of the newborn (PPHN) is defined as a syndrome of failed circulatory adaptation at birth. Each year, nearly two of every 1,000 newborns (0.4–6.8 per 1,000 live births) in the United States are affected by this disease (Lakshminrusimha & Keszler, 2015; Walsh-Sukys et al., 2000). A recent analysis of a California birth cohort database reported a mortality risk of 7.6% to 32% among newborns with PPHN; newborns with congenital anomalies of the respiratory tract incur a higher mortality risk (Steurer et al., 2017).

Morbidity risks include feeding issues and short-term respiratory issues, two problems that affect 25% of infants who survive the disease process. Long-term outcomes vary and depend on the pathophysiologic type of PPHN as well as what therapies were provided at birth. One major concern is for neurodevelopmental impairment, including cognitive delays and hearing deficits, which has been reported in 6.4% of survivors (Rosenberg et al., 2010). Eriksen and colleagues (2009) found that sensorineural hearing loss, chronic health problems, need for bronchodilator therapy, and need for remedial education were common among 5- and 10-year-old children formerly treated for PPHN in the newborn period (Eriksen et al., 2009). The need for extracorporeal membrane oxygenation (ECMO) was associated with increased risk for long-term disability.

Beginning in the early 1990s, endogenous nitric oxide (NO) was identified as a key signaling molecule synthesized at the vascular endothelial layer, which selectively modulates pulmonary vascular tone. This piqued the interest of numerous scientists and prompted decades of critical research into the safety and efficacy of inhaled nitric oxide (iNO), first among adults and later among newborns. As a result of several seminal and noteworthy studies, which will be discussed in this chapter, the Food and Drug Administration (FDA) approved iNO for use in term and near-term newborns greater than 34 weeks of gestation (for up to 14 consecutive days) in 1999. Labeling has not been expanded to include preterm infants less than 34 weeks of gestation; however, numerous reports indicate that off-label prescribing persists despite significant morbidity risks (e.g., 20% incidence of intraventricular hemorrhage; Barrington, Finer, & Pennaforte, 2017).

Clearly, newborns who manifest with hypoxic respiratory failure (HRF) at birth and evidence of PPHN require prompt identification and diagnostics. For neonatal APRNs, manifestations of PPHN may present immediately after birth, particularly when associated with early-onset sepsis or meconium aspiration, or become apparent later into the birth hospitalization, when a clinician is called to examine a newborn exhibiting mild or moderate signs of distress. Early dysfunction, customarily involving the heart, lungs, or pulmonary vasculature, can quickly worsen to secondary organ failure. Therefore, it is imperative that advanced practice clinicians are well versed in the signs and symptoms, diagnostic criteria, and management of PPHN. Several principles of the management of PPHN can be considered the gold standard, whereas others are still being investigated and require further study to standardize practice.

This chapter has been designed to provide the reader with the ability to develop a pathophysiologic understanding of PPHN and understand the history of PPHN management to better approach the current therapeutic options in these patients. We begin with an explanation of fetal and transitional circulation, review the different etiologies and risk factors for PPHN, and then detail the diagnostic approach to PPHN. Next, we identify seminal and other noteworthy studies that have led to our current management strategies for PPHN. Last, we present the current state of the science specific to nonpharmacologic and pharmacologic treatment of PPHN. Learning tools and resources, provided at the end of this chapter, are offered to stimulate additional scholarly conversation both in the classroom and clinical setting, as well as to encourage active learning habits for those preparing for a board certification examination.

PHYSIOLOGY REVIEW: FETAL AND POSTNATAL CIRCULATION

The physiology of the fetus fundamentally differs greatly from that of the newborn both structurally and functionally. Transitioning from intrauterine life to extrauterine life requires rapid and complex steps to ensure neonatal survival. Here we offer a brief review of fetal and neonatal circulation and the pathophysiology of PPHN. This review establishes a foundation for the subsequent discussion of nonpharmacologic and pharmacologic management strategies for this disease.

Fetal Circulation

Blood flow from the fetal ductus venosus, carrying freshly oxygenated blood from the placenta, preferentially shunts across the foramen ovale and to the left side of the heart (Figure 15.1). This left-ventricular output provides blood flow to the preductal vessels that supply the brain, coronary arteries, and the upper body. This accounts for 25% of fetal cardiac output with an oxygen content 65% higher than the postductal area (Remien & Majmundar, 2021). Blood flow from the fetal inferior vena cava (IVC) and superior vena cava (SVC) supplies the right side of the heart. This results in a differential in oxygenation in pre- and postductal aortic vessels. Blood flow from the IVC enters the right atrium of the heart and mixes with poorly oxygenated blood flow entering the heart via the SVC. Oxygen content of the IVC/SVC is lower than that of the ductus venosus due to shunting (40%–45%). This oxygen content increases slightly due to mixing with ductus venosus blood flow in the right atrium. IVC/SVC blood flow is mainly directed into the right ventricle. Right ventricular output is directed across the ductus arteriosus (DA) to the descending aorta with an approximate oxygen content of 60% to provide blood flow to the lower body before returning to the placenta. About 5% to 10% of this blood flow will go into the lungs. These fluid-filled lungs do not participate in gas exchange and maintain a high resistance to blood flow.

Fetal circulation essentially bypasses fetal lungs due to the persistence of several right-to-left intrauterine shunts. Recall that deoxygenated blood traversing the SVC and IVC preferentially shunts to the right atrium and then to the right ventricle, whereas more well-oxygenated blood from the ductus venosus preferentially crosses the foramen ovale and enters the left atrium.

It is important to note that this normal state of reduced fetal pulmonary blood flow suppresses the production of pulmonary vasodilators, including NO and prostaglandins. This encourages

FIGURE 15.1 Fetal circulation.

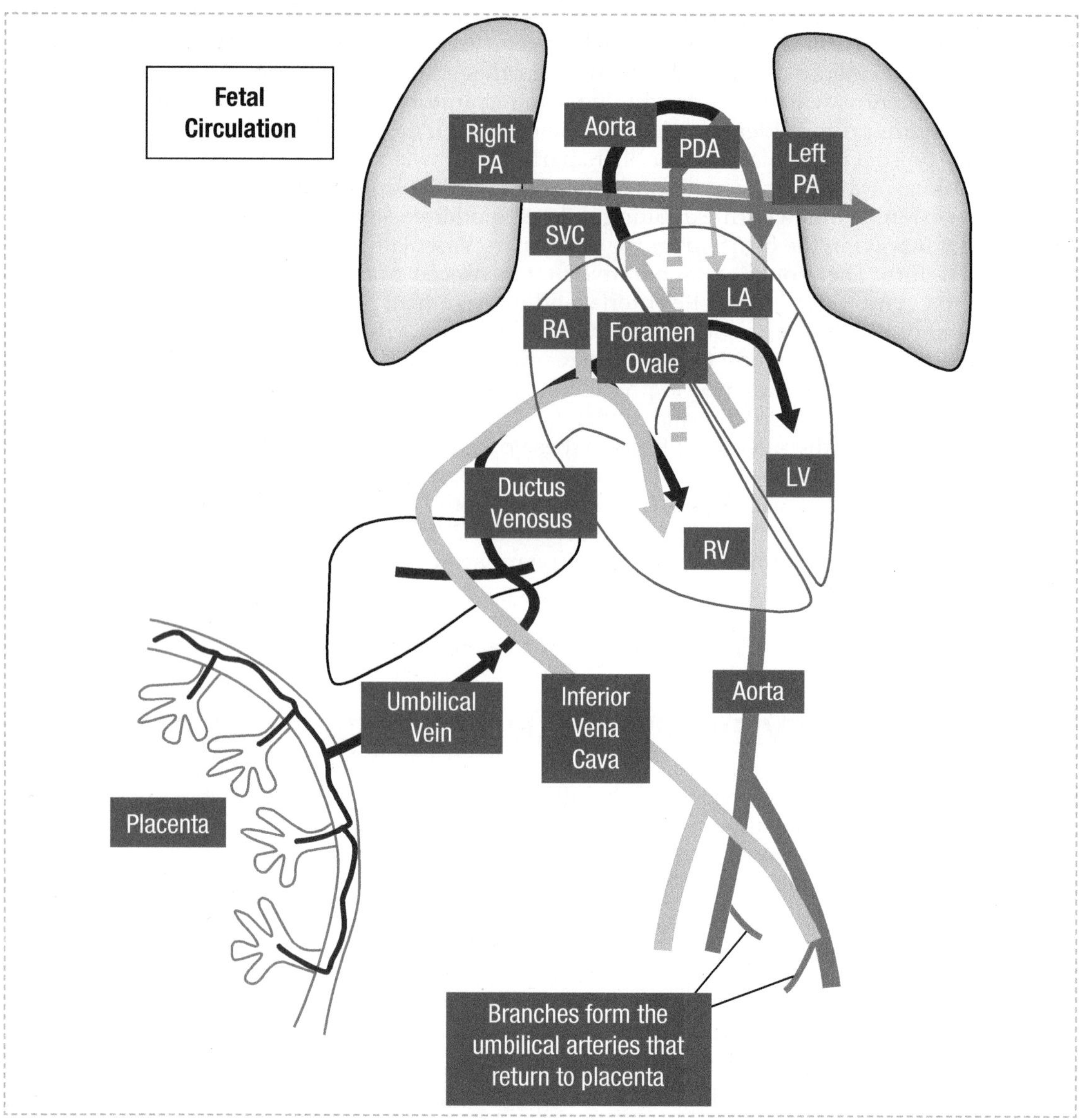

Note: This schematic summarizes the fetal circulation. The placenta provides oxygen and nutrients to the fetus via the umbilical vein (UV). The UV splits at the level of the liver with some blood perfusing the hepatic circulation and the remainder entering the ductus venosus. Although most of the blood from the ductus venosus is directed across the foramen ovale to the left atrium, the inferior and superior vena caval blood preferentially enters the right atrium. Right ventricular output is directed across the patent ductus arteriosus (PDA) into the descending aorta, whereas left ventricular output provides blood flow to the preductal vessels supplying the brain, coronary arteries, and upper body. Intrauterine pulmonary blood flow is initially limited because of high pulmonary vascular resistance and the right-to-left shunting across the patent foramen ovale and PDA.

LA, left atrium; LV, left ventricle; PA, pulmonary artery; PDA, patent ductus arteriosus; RA, right atrium; RV, right ventricle; SVC, superior vena cava.

Source: Adapted from Morton, S. U., & Brodsky, D. (2016). Fetal physiology and the transition to extrauterine life. *Clinics in Perinatology, 43*(3), 395–407. https://doi.org/10.1016/j.clp.2016.04.001

a high, sustained pulmonary vascular resistance (PVR) with low oxygen tension. Reduced oxygen tension perpetuates the normal in utero release of endogenous vasoconstrictors, specifically endothelium-1 and thromboxane. The net result is high PVR with persistent right-to-left shunting of blood across the foramen ovale and DA.

Transitioning From Intrauterine Circulation to Extrauterine Circulation

Important physiologic changes must occur for a successful transition to extrauterine life. Most of these changes happen concurrently but are discussed individually here, beginning with the first breath. The first inspiration after birth distends the lung cavities and dilates the capillary network, causing an eight-fold increase in pulmonary blood flow (Figure 15.2; Lloyd & Smith, 2016). These events induce a transient state of sheer stress. In response, endothelial NO synthase (eNOS) production is upregulated.

The amino acid L-arginine is stimulated by eNOS to produce NO. Upon release from the vascular endothelium, NO elicits the release of other endothelium-derived pulmonary vasodilatory mediators, including substance P, vasopressin, angiotensin II, and histamine. Next, NO and prostaglandin I_2 (PGI_2) diffuse through the endothelium, enter the vascular smooth muscle, and activate soluble guanylyl cyclase. This elicits increased production of cyclic guanosine monophosphate (cGMP), and activation of the cGMP-dependent protein kinase G (PKG). PKG stimulates

FIGURE 15.2 Estimated intrauterine oxygen saturations.

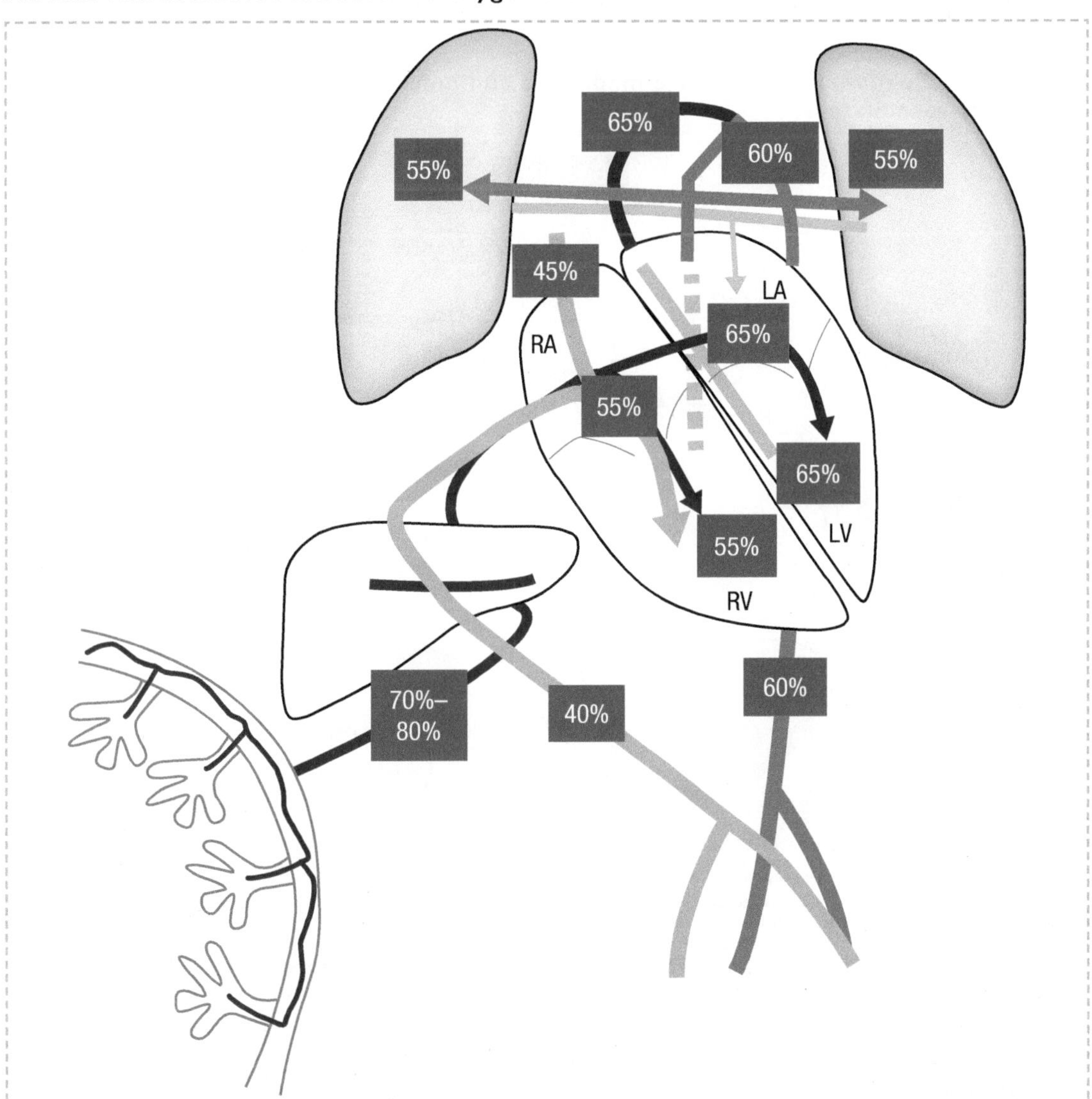

Blood within the umbilical vein has the highest oxygen saturation (70%–80%, estimated PO_2 = 32–35 torr) compared with the rest of the fetal circulation. Because of the preferential shunting of ductus venosus blood into the left atrium, and the poorly oxygenated inferior and superior vena caval blood (40%–45%, estimated PO_2 = 12–14) preferentially entering the right atrium, the left side of the heart has a slightly higher oxygen saturation (65%, estimated PO_2 = 26–28 torr) compared with the right side of the heart (55%, estimated PO_2= 20–22 torr). As a result, the left ventricular output to the brain, coronary arteries, and the upper body has a slightly higher oxygen saturation/oxygen content compared with the lower body, which is mostly provided by the right ventricular output.

LA, left artery; LV, left ventricle; RA, right atrium; RV, right ventricle.

Source: Adapted from Morton, S. U., & Brodsky, D. (2016). Fetal physiology and the transition to extrauterine life. *Clinics in Perinatology, 43*(3), 395–407. https://doi.org/10.1016/j.clp.2016.04.001

the myosin phosphatase enzyme, which activates potassium channels. The result is hyperpolarization, a reduction of the influx of calcium, and vasodilation (Figure 15.3; Konduri, & Kim 2009). Prostaglandin synthesis also increases, but imposes a reduced effect on vascular relaxation compared to NO.

Pulmonary artery pressure decreases by 50%, permitting pulmonary blood flow to increase 10-fold. With each subsequent breath, the partial pressure of carbon dioxide ($PaCO_2$) decreases, and blood pH normalizes. Meanwhile, clamping of the umbilical cord increases systemic vascular resistance (SVR) and left atrial pressure. This encourages the initial functional closure of the foramen ovale; anatomic closure is observed toward the end of the second month of life (Hoffman et al., 2018).

With a rise in SVR after clamping the umbilical cord, the pressure in the aorta is now higher than in the truncus pulmonalis. Thus, the right-to-left shunting that was present before birth changes to a left-to-right shunt. In addition, clamping of the umbilical cord leads to a loss of prostaglandins,

FIGURE 15.3 Pulmonary vasculature mediators and mechanism of action targets of pulmonary vasodilators.

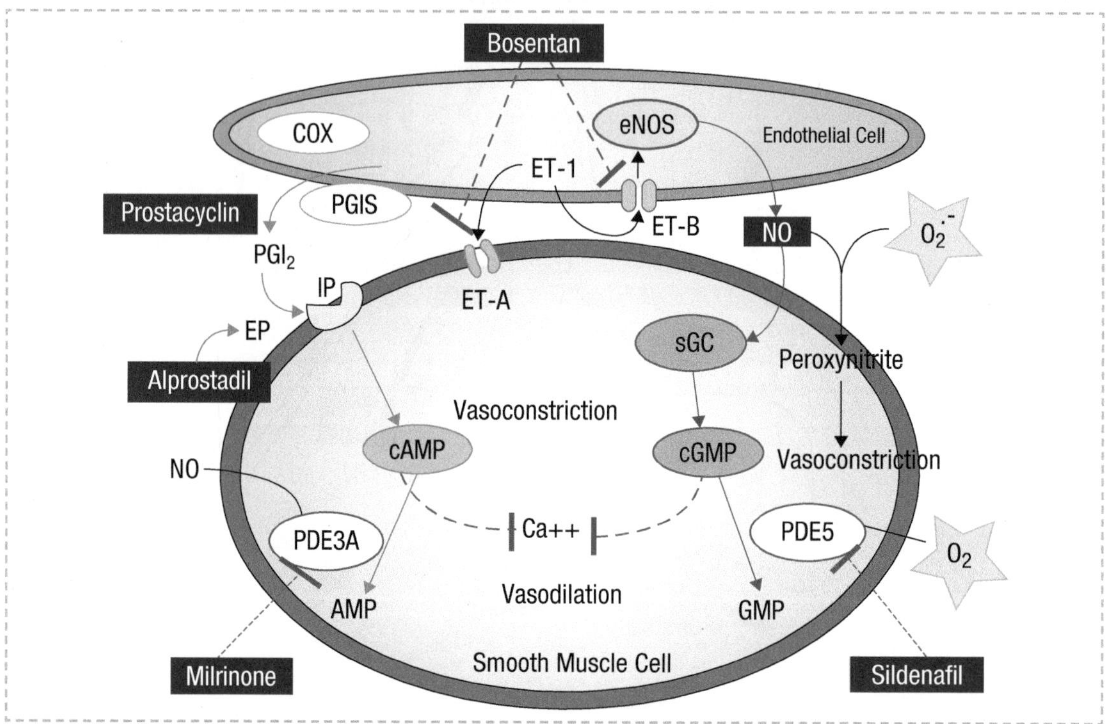

Endothelium-derived vasodilators include PGI2 and NO, while endothelin (ET-1) is a vasoconstrictor. COX and PGIS are involved in the production of prostacyclin. Prostacyclin acts on its receptor (IP) in the smooth muscle cell and stimulates AC to produce cAMP. Cyclic AMP is broken down by PDE3A (the enzyme most prevalent in vasculature) in the smooth muscle cell. Milrinone inhibits PDE3A and increases cAMP levels in arterial smooth muscle cells and cardiac myocytes, resulting in pulmonary (and systemic) vasodilation and inotropy. NO stimulates PDE3A. Endothelin is a powerful vasoconstrictor and acts on ET-A receptors in the smooth muscle cell and increases ionic calcium concentration. A second endothelin receptor (ET-B) on the endothelial cell stimulates NO release and vasodilation. eNOS produces NO, which diffuses from the endothelium to the smooth muscle cell and stimulates sGC enzyme to produce cGMP. Cyclic GMP is broken down by PDE5 enzyme in the smooth muscle cell. Sildenafil inhibits PDE5 and increases cGMP levels in pulmonary arterial smooth muscle cells. Natriuretic peptides stimulate pGC to produce cGMP. Cyclic AMP and cGMP reduce cytosolic ionic calcium concentrations and induce smooth muscle cell relaxation and pulmonary vasodilation. NO is a free radical and can avidly combine with superoxide anions to form a toxic vasoconstrictor, peroxynitrite. Hence, the bioavailability of NO in a tissue is determined by the local concentration of superoxide anions. Hyperoxic ventilation with 100% oxygen can increase the risk of formation of superoxide anions in the pulmonary arterial smooth muscle cells and limit the bioavailability of NO and stimulate PDE5 activity. Medications used in PPHN are shown in black boxes.

AC, adenylate cyclase; AMP, adenosine monophosphate; cAMP, cyclic adenosine monophosphate; cGMP, cyclic guanosine monophosphate; COX, cyclooxygenase; eNOS, endothelial nitric oxide synthase; EP, prostaglandin E1 receptor; ET-A, endothelin-receptor A; ET-B, endothelin-receptor B; ET-1, endothelin-1; GMP, guanosine monophosphate; IP, PGI_2 receptor; NO, nitric oxide; PDE3A, phosphodiesterase 3A; PDE5, phosphodiesterase type 5; pGC, particulate guanylate cyclase; PGIS, prostacyclin synthase; PGI_2, prostacyclin; PPHN, persistent pulmonary hypertension of the newborn; sGC, soluble guanylate cyclase.

Source: Adapted from Sharma, V., Berkelhamer, S., & Lakshminrusimha, S. (2015). Persistent pulmonary hypertension of the newborn. *Maternal Health, Neonatology and Perinatology, 1*, 14. https://doi.org/10.1186/s40748-015-0015-4

which previously helped keep the right-to-left fetal shunts open. PaO_2 in the aorta increases since the blood is now oxygenated by the newborn's lungs. This increase in PaO_2 results in smooth muscle contraction in the wall of the DA, thus resulting in a functional seal. After a few weeks to months, there is complete resolution of this shunt via the DA, and the remnant is known as the *ligamentum arteriosus* (Quaye & Kummer, 2020).

A failed transition to extrauterine life, which may be precipitated by etiologies including sepsis-induced endothelial injury, is associated with the development of PPHN.

RISK FACTORS AND ETIOLOGIES FOR PERSISTENT PULMONARY HYPERTENSION OF THE NEWBORN

Numerous single and multicenter studies have identified risk factors for PPHN over the years (Bearer et al., 1997; Hernández-Diaz et al., 2007; Reece et al., 1987; Storme et al., 2013; Van Marter et al., 1996; Walsh-Sukys et al., 2000; Wilson et al., 2011; Winovitch et al., 2011). In comparison to these data, Steurer and colleagues (2017) published a seminal large-scale population-based epidemiologic study. A comparison of findings is provided in Table 15.1. Common etiologies for PPHN are provided in Table 15.2, organized by type of PPHN, which is discussed in the next section of this chapter.

TABLE 15.1 Risk Factors for the Development of Persistent Pulmonary Hypertension of the Newborn

RISK FACTORS FROM SINGLE AND MULTICENTER STUDIES (1987–2007)	RISK FACTORS FROM SEMINAL POPULATION-BASED STUDY (2017)
Birth weight	Birth weight (SGA & LGA > AGA)
Cesarean delivery	Cesarean delivery
Ethnicity	Ethnicity[a]
Gender	Gender (male > female)
Gestational age	Gestational age (late preterm > term)
Maternal age (advanced)	Maternal age (advanced)
Maternal asthma	Maternal diabetes
Maternal chorioamnionitis	Maternal obesity
Maternal diabetes	Maternal smoking
Maternal hypertension	
Maternal illicit drug use	
Maternal obesity	
Maternal preeclampsia	
Maternal smoking	
Mode of delivery	
Oligohydramnios	
Premature rupture of membranes	
Prenatal care	
Socioeconomic status	

[a]Black race was associated with an increased risk for PPHN (adjusted relative risk [RR]: 1.3, 95% CI: 1.1–1.5) whereas Hispanic race was protective against PPHN (adjusted RR 0.8, 95% CI: 0.7–0.9).

AGA, adjusted gestational age; LGA, large for gestational age; SGA, small for gestational age.

Sources: From Bearer, C., Emerson, R. K., O'Riordan, M.A., Roitman, E., & Shackleton, C. (1997). Maternal tobacco smoke exposure and persistent pulmonary hypertension of the newborn. *Environmental Health Perspectives, 105*(2), 202–206. https://doi.org/10.1289/ehp.97105202; Hernández-Díaz, S., Van Marter, L. J., Werler, M. M., Louik, C., & Mitchell, A. A. (2007). Risk factors for persistent pulmonary hypertension of the newborn. *Pediatrics, 120*(2), e272–e282. https://doi.org/10.1542/peds.2006-3037; Reece, E. A., Moya, F., Yazigi, R., Holford, T., Duncan, C., & Ehrenkranz, R. A. (1987). Persistent pulmonary hypertension: Assessment of perinatal risk factors. *Obstetrics & Gynecology, 70*(5), 696–700; Steurer, M. A., Jelliffe-Pawlowski, L. J., Baer, R. J., Partridge, J. C., Rogers, E. E., & Keller, R. L. (2017). Persistent pulmonary hypertension of the newborn in late preterm and term infants in California. *Pediatrics, 139*(1), e20161165. https://doi.org/10.1542/peds.2016-1165; Van Marter, L. J., Leviton, A., Allred, E. N., Pagano, M., Sullivan, K. F., Cohen, A, & Epstein, M. F. (1996). Persistent pulmonary hypertension of the newborn and smoking and aspirin and nonsteroidal antiinflammatory drug consumption during pregnancy. *Pediatrics*, 97(5), 658–663. https://doi.org/10.1542/peds.97.5.658; Walsh-Sukys, M. C., Tyson, J. E., Wright, L. L., Bauer, C. R., Korones, S. B., Stevenson, D. K., Verter, J., Stoll, B. J., Lemons, J. A., Papile, L. A., Shankaran, S., Donovan, E. F., Oh, W., Ehrenkranz, R. A., & Fanaroff, A. A. (2000). Persistent pulmonary hypertension of the newborn in the era before nitric oxide: Practice variation and outcomes. *Pediatrics, 105*(1 Pt 1), 14–20. https://doi.org/10.1542/peds.105.1.14

TABLE 15.2 Types of Persistent Pulmonary Hypertension of the Newborn

PPHN TYPE	DEFINITION	COMMON ETIOLOGIES
Maladaptation	Hypoxia-induced pulmonary vasospasm with normally formed pulmonary vasculature	Asphyxia MAS Pneumonia RDS Sepsis
Maldevelopment	Abnormally remodeled pulmonary vasculature, in particular at the alveolar membrane	Chronic fetal hypoxia Fetal anemia Idiopathic causes Premature closure of the PDA Fetal exposure to SSRI
Underdevelopment	Reduced maturation of the pulmonary vasculature	Alveolar capillary dysplasia CDH Oligohydramnios
Intrinsic obstruction	Increased viscosity which partially obstructs the pulmonary arteries	Polycythemia

CDH, congenital diaphragmatic hernia; MAS, meconium aspiration syndrome; PDA, patent ductus arteriosus; RDS, respiratory distress syndrome; SSRI, selective serotonin reuptake inhibitor.

PATHOPHYSIOLOGY OF PERSISTENT PULMONARY HYPERTENSION OF THE NEWBORN

PPHN develops as a consequence of an impaired circulatory adaptation to postnatal life or secondary to a comorbid condition. Thus, PVR remains elevated above SVR after birth (Singh & Lakshminrusimha, 2021). Four types of PPHN (maladaptation, maldevelopment, underdevelopment, intrinsic obstruction) have been identified and reported throughout the literature (Table 15.2). *Maladaptive* PPHN is characterized by abnormal remodeling of the pulmonary vasculature. This leads to hyperplasia and thickening of vessel walls, impairing blood flow and gas exchange. Sepsis currently accounts for approximately 30% of maladaptation-related cases (Steurer et al., 2017). Bacterial infiltration (e.g., Group B *Streptococcus*) at the vascular endothelium upregulates the production of cytokines, chemokines, and adhesion molecules. Leukocytes and platelets migrate to the site of infection and elicit the release of vasoactive cells, including endothelin (vasoconstrictor), thromboxane (vasoconstrictor), platelet-activating factor, NO (vasodilator), prostaglandin (vasodilator), and histamine (vasodilator; Wynn & Wong, 2010). Overproduction of endothelin and thromboxane, secondary to bacteria-induced endothelial damage, contributes to the development of PPHN. To a lesser degree, approximately 2% to 10% of newborns with meconium-stained fluid aspirate meconium and develop maladaptive PPHN (Lee et al., 2016; Whitfield et al., 2009). The pathophysiology of maladaptation in these cases involves surfactant inactivation and the release of proinflammatory mediators, which increase PVR through the release of potent endothelial vasoconstrictors (e.g., thromboxane; Nair & Lakshminrusimha, 2014).

Maldevelopment-specific PPHN is characterized by remodeling of the pulmonary vasculature in the presence of normal lung parenchyma. This is often idiopathic but has also been associated with chronic fetal hypoxia, fetal anemia, and in utero closure of the DA secondary to maternal nonsteroidal anti-inflammatory drug (NSAID) use (Lakshminrusimha & Kezler, 2015). Fetal exposure to selective serotonin reuptake inhibitors (SSRIs) late in pregnancy is associated with a modest increased risk for PPHN; the number needed to harm (NNH) with one postnatal case of PPHN is between 286 and 351 women (Grigoriadis et al., 2014). These disease processes force excess blood flow through the constricted fetal pulmonary blood vessels and impose a persistent state of shear stress. The capillary vascular bed, namely around the alveoli, remodels in response to the shear stress.

Underdevelopment-specific PPHN from lung hypoplasia is not as common as the other types of PPHN; however, it is associated with worse outcomes. This type of PPHN is associated with alveolar capillary dysplasia, congenital diaphragmatic hernia (CDH), and oligohydramnios. CDH is often associated with intractable PPHN because it frequently presents with impaired cardiac development and function, further complicating the clinical outcomes of these patients. Resultant pulmonary arterial hypertension, hypertrophy or failure of the right ventricle, and hypoplasia of the left ventricle with pulmonary venous hypertension precipitates a severe form of PPHN that is frequently not responsive to medical treatment (Nair & Lakshminrusimha, 2014).

Intrinsic obstruction of the pulmonary arteries, due to hyperviscosity, is also associated with PPHN. This type of obstruction increases PVR. Newborns born to diabetic mothers are at increased risk of polycythemia and should be monitored for this potential complication.

Regardless of the type of PPHN, the end result is persistence of fetal cardiovascular circulation. This sustained elevated PVR decreases the flow of blood to the lungs, as blood always takes the path of least resistance. Instead, blood is preferentially shunted to the systemic circulation through the patent foramen ovale (PFO) or patent ductus arteriosus (PDA). The resultant ventilation-perfusion (V/Q) mismatch permits the persistent return of deoxygenated blood to the systemic circulation, bypassing the lungs. A summary of the pathophysiology types of PPHN can be found in Table 15.2 and additionally visualized in Figure 15.4.

FIGURE 15.4 Pathophysiologic mechanisms of persistent pulmonary hypertension of the newborn.

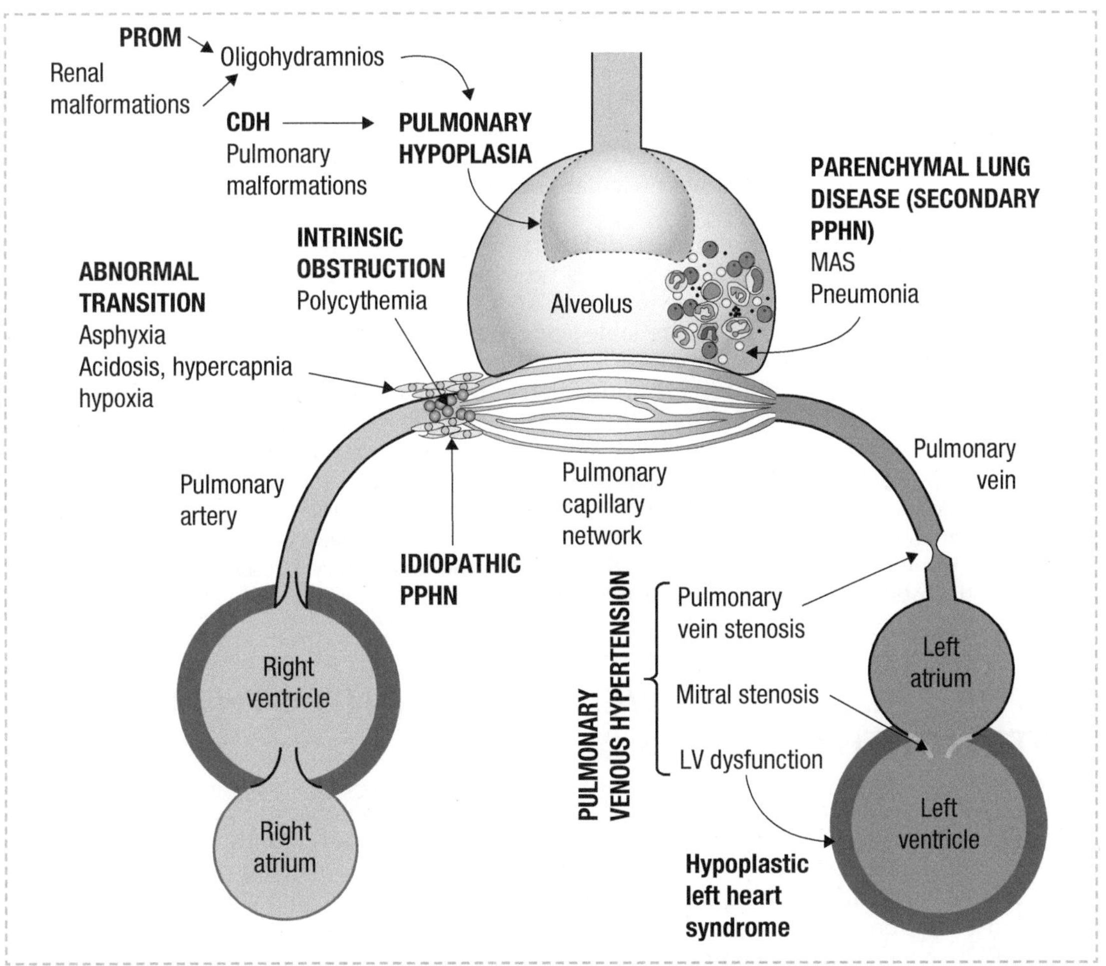

CDH, congenital diaphragmatic hernia; LV, left ventricle; MAS, meconium aspiration syndrome; PPHN, persistent pulmonary hypertension of the newborn; PROM, premature rupture of membranes.

Source: Adapted from Mathew, B., & Lakshminrusimha, S. (2017). Persistent pulmonary hypertension in the newborn. *Children, 4*(8), Article 63. https://doi.org/10.3390/children4080063

Differential Diagnosis

Clinicians should consider cyanotic congenital heart disease as the most likely diagnosis until proven otherwise.

Diagnostic Pathway

A systematic approach is necessary to efficiently and accurately diagnose PPHN. Physical exam findings, including tachypnea, grunting, cyanosis, systolic murmur (tricuspid regurgitation), or prominent S2, may be present but are not diagnostic. Rather, the initial studies that are performed while awaiting arrival of the pediatric cardiology team include the chest radiograph and arterial blood gas, followed by Doppler echocardiogram (ECHO). Radiographic findings may reflect the proximate cause for PPHN (e.g., parenchymal disease), diminished pulmonary vascular markings, or appear normal. Lung ultrasound is a newer tool that has been shown in a recent pilot study to be useful at diagnosing the underlying cause of PPHN in a more timely and effective way in comparison to chest radiograph (del Rey Hurtado de Mendoza et al., 2019).

Umbilical or peripheral arterial access is indicated due to the need for frequent blood sampling. Interval assessment of arterial blood gases permits close monitoring of the oxygenation index (OI), one index used to appraise the severity of HRF and PPHN in newborns. The formula is as follows:

$$\text{Mean airway pressure } (cmH_2O) \times \text{fraction of inspired oxygen } (FiO_2)$$

$$\div$$

$$\text{Partial pressure of oxygen } (PaO_2).$$

Newborns with an OI greater than 25 may benefit from iNO, which reduces the combined risk for death or need for ECMO (Barrington, Finer, Pennaforte, & Altit, 2017). Those with an OI greater than 40 incur a 60% to 80% mortality risk and an indication for ECMO. The cranial ultrasound is obtained to assess for intraventricular hemorrhage, as bleeding is an exclusionary factor for ECMO.

Given that clinical manifestations of PPHN overlap with cyanotic heart disease, clinicians should pursue the Doppler ECHO as soon as possible. ECHO is the gold standard test for the assessment of congenital heart disease (e.g., total anomalous pulmonary venous return, left-sided defects) and PPHN (Figure 15.5). It is reliable, convenient, and offers a noninvasive assessment of right and left ventricular systolic and diastolic function, right ventricular pressure and pulmonary artery pressure, the PDA, atrial-level shunting, left-ventricular outflow/systemic blood flow, and the presence or absence of a pericardial effusion. In cases of suspected PPHN, additional measurements specific to tricuspid valve peak velocity and pulmonary regurgitation (diastolic velocity) are included (Mertens et al., 2011). Findings suggestive of PPHN include right-to-left shunting across the DA and/or foramen ovale, right ventricular dilatation and high systolic time interval (>0.5), shortened pulmonary blood flow velocity (ratio of time to peak velocity at pulmonary valve to right ventricular ejection time <0.34) with high pulmonary artery pressure, and flattening or bowing of the intraventricular septum (Ostrea et al., 2006).

HISTORICAL PERSPECTIVE: SEMINAL AND OTHER NOTEWORTHY STUDIES

The association of respiratory distress syndrome (RDS) with pulmonary hypertension and right-to-left ductal shunting was first identified by Rudolph and colleagues (1961) and later described by Stahlman (1964). The first published report of term hypoxic newborns with right-to-left shunting in the absence of significant lung disease was likely that of Roberton and colleagues (1967). They described 13 newborns at or near term who had significant hypoxemia but did not have clinical signs of RDS or reduced lung compliance. Their speculation was that the cause of hypoxemia was right-to-left shunting, although they did not comment on increased PVR as the cause. Gersony and colleagues (1969) were the first to accurately describe the pathophysiology of PPHN (as it is currently understood). These authors labeled the disease process "persistence of fetal circulation."

FIGURE 15.5 Cardiopulmonary changes on echocardiogram in neonates with and without persistent pulmonary hypertension of the newborn.

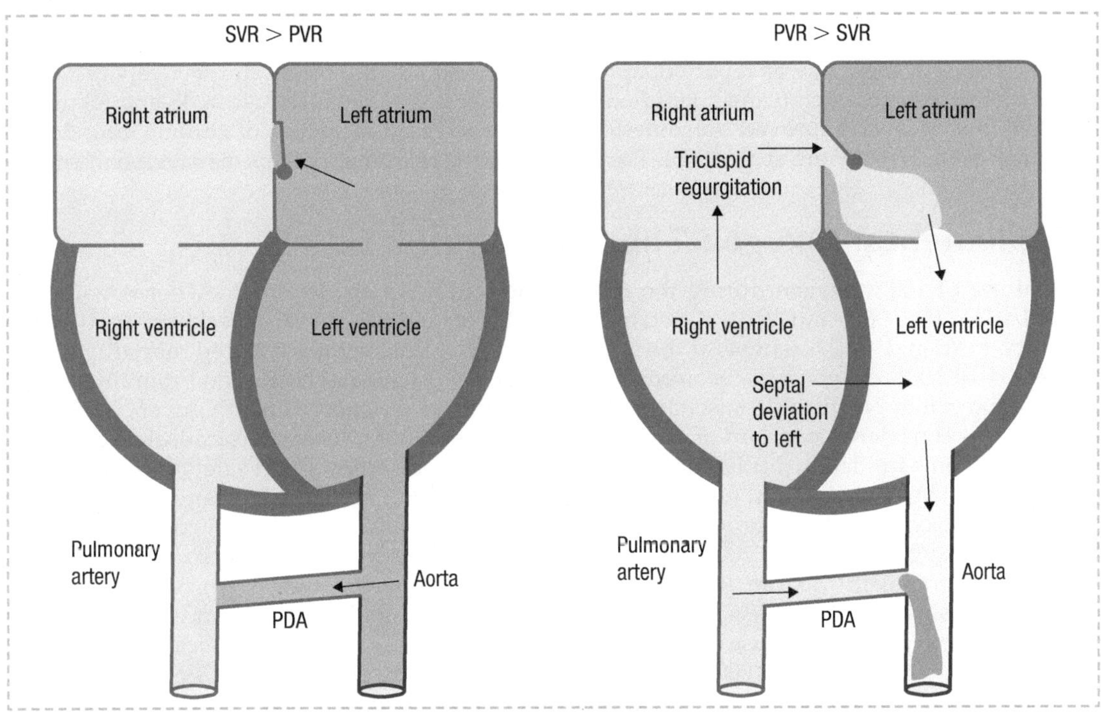

Note: Echocardiographic findings in normal infants (*left*) and in PPHN (*right*). Soon after birth the pressures within the left-sided chambers of the heart are higher than in the right and the fetal shunts are reversed. The interatrial shunt and the shunt across the PDA are left to right. In infants with PPHN the pressures remain elevated in the right atrium and ventricle with right to left shunt at the atrial level and at the PDA causing desaturation (due to interatrial shunt) and differential cyanosis (due to PDA). There is right ventricular hypertrophy with bulging of the interventricular septum to the left and tricuspid regurgitation.

PDA, patent ductus arteriosis; PPHN, persistent pulmonary hypertension of the newborn; PVR, pulmonary vascular resistance; SVR, systemic vascular resistance.

Source: Adapted from Mathew, B., & Lakshminrusimha, S. (2017). Persistent pulmonary hypertension in the newborn. *Children, 4*(8), Article 63. https://doi.org/10.3390/children4080063

Use of this term continued until Levin and colleagues (1976) introduced "persistent pulmonary hypertension of the newborn" and it was adopted into the vernacular (Levin et al., 1976).

Several seminal and noteworthy studies shaped our current understanding of pharmacologic treatment regimens for PPHN. Identification of these studies allows us to evaluate the genesis of key scientific questions, timing of dissemination of outcomes data, and retirement of certain treatments in exchange for the implementation of new therapies, namely iNO. We present an overview of this research in this section of the chapter.

Alkali Infusions and Hyperventilation

Two of the earliest therapies used in the treatment of PPHN included alkali infusions and hyperventilation. Reports of use date back to the 1960s and 1970s (Goetzman et al., 1976; Levin et al., 1976; Peckham & Fox, 1978; Rudolph & Yuan, 1966). Alkali infusions were adopted to correct a pH less than 7.25, as clinicians believed acidosis elicited exaggerated hypoxic pulmonary vasoconstriction (Rudolph & Yuan, 1966). However, alkali infusions increased the need for ECMO and oxygen at 28 days of life (Walsh-Sukys et al., 2000). These findings led to the retirement of alkali infusions as a primary treatment modality. Although most centers currently avoid significant acidosis, judicious use of alkali is observed.

The use of hyperventilation was also retired as investigators rather quickly realized that this therapy was associated with barotrauma, volutrauma, air leaks, and lung disease. Prolonged hyperventilation elicits hypocapnia and alkalosis, two proximate causes for physical, neuromuscular, psychomotor, and mental disability as well as sensorineural deafness in children (Bifano &

Pfannenstiel, 1988; Hendricks-Munoz & Walton, 1988). Bifano and Pfannenstiel (1988) reported long-term outcomes of 21 newborns subject to prolonged hyperventilation therapy for PPHN. Newborns demonstrated decreased head growth and failure to thrive, followed by spastic diplegia, hemiplegia, and spastic quadriplegia. Severe and mild/moderate neurodevelopmental disability (physical and/or mental) was reported among 19% and 33% of the cohort, respectively ($p < 0.05$). Meanwhile, other research teams identified that maintaining a $PaCO_2$ between 45 and 60 mmHg resulted in similar or improved outcomes, and with a reduced incidence of chronic lung disease (Dworetz et al., 1989; Wung et al., 1985). The data led to the retirement of this management strategy.

Supplemental Oxygen Therapy

Liberal use of 100% oxygen during the resuscitation and management of newborns with HRF dates back to the 1960s and 1970s (Goetzman et al., 1976; Levin et al., 1976; Peckham & Fox, 1978; Rudolph & Yuan, 1966). Scientists at the time believed that this therapy reduced mortality risk, so much so that 100% oxygen was recommended as part of the neonatal education program and was later adopted into Neonatal Resuscitation Program (NRP) curricula (Kim & Nguyen, 2019). This therapy was considered standard of care between 1987 and 2010. Meanwhile, critical research was underway, some funded by NRP grant monies, to examine the efficacy and safety of 100% oxygen versus 21% oxygen on cerebral function (Hoffman et al., 1996). Between 1980 and 1990, scientists learned that oxygen radicals produced after a period of hypoxia were associated with increased PVR and reoxygenation with 100% oxygen elicited increased formation of free oxygen radicals compared to room air (McCord, 1985; Saugstad, 1990; Saugstad & Aasen, 1980). Several noteworthy studies using bovine models concluded that resuscitation with 21% oxygen was just as effective as 100% oxygen, and the use of 21% oxygen reduced the risk of oxygen radical formation and cellular damage (Kondo et al., 2000; Kutzsche et al., 2001; Rootwelt et al., 1992, 1993).

Next, Temesvári and colleagues (2001) reported that room air and 100% oxygen offered similar efficacy in the treatment of cardiorespiratory, blood gas, and acid–base abnormalities among piglet models. The safety profile differed. Use of 100% oxygen during the reoxygenation period was associated with lower neurologic examination scores (9.5 ± 4.1) compared to reoxygenation with room air (13.5 ± 3.1); a neurologic score greater than 20 was considered normal and a score of 5 or less designated brain death ($p < .05$; Temesvári et al., 2001). The results of these and other studies led the NRP Steering Committee to include the following statement in the fifth edition of their textbook: "research suggests that resuscitation with something less than 100% may be just as successful" (American Academy of Pediatrics [AAP], 2006, p. 3–33).

The next year, Lakshminrusimha and colleagues (2007) discovered that, after a period of hypoxia, use of 21% oxygen elicited a near immediate decrease in PVR and did not impede the mechanism of action (selective pulmonary vascular dilatation) of iNO. More specifically, optimal pulmonary vasodilation occurred when oxygen tension remained between 60 and 80 mmHg. Lakshminrusimha and colleagues (2009) went on to evaluate the effect of supplemental oxygen (21% vs. 50% vs. 100%) on the efficacy of iNO in a cohort of lambs with PPHN. The team concluded that 21% to 50% oxygen decreased PVR, whereas use of 100% oxygen during the initial resuscitation after birth did not decrease PVR and impeded the efficacy of iNO-mediated vasodilation, permitting persistent vasoconstriction (Lakshminrusimha et al., 2009). The analysis of these studies prompted a permanent change of practice, involving the initial provision of 21% oxygen to term newborns, with the launch of the sixth edition NRP textbook (Kattwinkel et al., 2010). Lakshminrusimha and colleagues (2011) went on to investigate the hemodynamic effects of prolonged hyperoxia (≥30 minutes). The authors concluded that prolonged hyperoxia induced pulmonary vascular contraction, the formation of superoxide anions, and free radicals (Lakshminrusimha et al., 2011). These seminal and noteworthy findings led to the prioritization of judicious use (minimum effective dose) of supplemental oxygen after birth and throughout the birth hospitalization.

Surfactant

Surfactant replacement was first introduced in the mid-1960s as a therapy for meconium aspiration. Findlay and associates (1996) reported that newborns subject to surfactant therapy exhibited disease resolution by 24 hours of age (19/20 surfactant vs. 0/20 control subjects; $p < 0.001$), a reduced need for ECMO (1/20 surfactant vs. 6/20 control subjects; $p = 0.037$), shorter duration of mechanical ventilation (p <0.05), shorter duration of oxygen (p <0.05), and shorter length of stay (p <0.05). Additional studies confirmed a reduction in the need for ECMO with the use of surfactant in newborns with PPHN or HRF with moderate OI of approximately 15 to 25 (Konduri et al., 2013; Lotze et al., 1998).

More recently, results of a seminal randomized trial compared the use of surfactant replacement in newborns with maladaptive PPHN and those who received iNO (González et al., 2021). Similar to results published by Lotze and colleagues (1998), surfactant replacement significantly reduced the combined outcome of death or ECMO from 36% in the placebo group to 16% in the surfactant group (p <0.05). Readers are cautioned against extrapolating these data to patients with nonparenchymal types of PPHN.

Pulmonary Vasodilators (Tolazoline and Inhaled Nitric Oxide)

TOLAZOLINE

Tolazoline was the seminal pulmonary vasodilator prescribed to newborns with PPHN during the 1960s and 1970s (Cotton, 1965; Gersony et al., 1969). Levin and colleagues (1976) reported outcomes of one of the first cohorts treated with tolazoline. Four of 11 newborns received tolazoline injections of 1 mg/kg, with improvement in PaO_2 noted in two of the four newborns. Curare, a plant-derived skeletal muscle relaxant that is not FDA approved, was also prescribed to three newborns supported by mechanical ventilation. Two of the three newborns showed marked improvement in their PaO_2, whereas the third newborn failed to respond to curare or tolazoline and eventually died. Over the years, adverse effects, including systemic hypotension, were reported, and use was discontinued (Goetzman et al., 1976; Korones & Eyal, 1975; Stevenson et al., 1979). Currently, tolazoline is not approved by the FDA for use in newborns.

INHALED NITRIC OXIDE

Prior to the 1980s, NO gas was regarded as an atmospheric pollutant that, when combined with oxygen, produced smog (Williams et al., 2004). However, by the 1980s, scientists discovered that endogenously produced NO exerted a significant vasodilatory effect on the pulmonary circulation of newborn animal models (Furchgott & Zawadzki, 1980; Ignarro et al., 1987; Palmer et al., 1987). Additional animal studies, published in the 1990s, demonstrated that deliberate pharmacologic inhibition of NO synthesis altered the transition to extrauterine life. The normal drop in PVR and consequential rise in pulmonary blood flow at delivery was not observed; the lack of adequate NO modulation created a favorable environment for PPHN (Abman et al., 1990; McQueston et al., 1993; Tiktinsky et al., 1993).

Human use of iNO was first described in 1991 in adults with severe pulmonary hypertension (Pepke-Zaba et al., 1991). This seminal study confirmed the theory that iNO was a selective pulmonary vasodilator. Next, Roberts and colleagues (1992) reported outcomes of a small trial involving seven full-term newborns with PPHN who received iNO (20, 40, and 80 ppm). They concluded that a median dose of 20 ppm of iNO was necessary to maintain arterial oxygen concentrations between 65 and 80 mmHg and a dose of up to 80 ppm could be safely tolerated in newborns (Roberts et al., 1992). Shortly after, Kinsella and Neish (1992) published results of a study, funded (in part) by the National Institutes of Health (NIH), using low-dose (10 and 20 ppm) iNO in nine newborns between 35 and 40 weeks of gestation. The authors concluded that low-dose iNO increased pulmonary artery blood flow, lowered the oxygenation index by 66%, and eliminated the need for ECMO (Kinsella & Neish, 1992).

Although research specific to dosing continued, scientists realized that cessation of therapy also demanded closer scrutiny. Several case reports presented evidence of life-threatening hypoxia with abrupt discontinuation of therapy, in particular when a dose of 10 ppm or more was being continuously administered (Lavoie et al., 1996). Few studies included weaning parameters, usually decreasing therapy from 20 ppm to 5 ppm to zero, which was not considered part of the study design (Demirakça et al., 1996).

Outcomes of the first large-scale randomized trial (Neonatal Inhaled Nitric Oxide Study, or NINOS), funded by the National Institute of Child Health and Human Development (NICHD), were published in 1997. Newborns greater than 34 weeks of gestation were initially randomized to receive 20 ppm iNO or 100% oxygen. Newborns randomized to the interventional arm and who did not respond to 20 ppm were subject to 80 ppm iNO therapy. The maximum duration of therapy was 24 hours and therapy was abruptly discontinued with a failed response or at the end of the treatment window. Newborns subject to iNO demonstrated (a) less need for ECMO (46% vs. 64%, respectively, $p = 0.006$), (b) a lower OI ($p < 0.001$), and (c) a significant increase in arterial oxygen levels (mean increase ± *SD*, 58.2 ± 85.2 mmHg vs. 9.7 ± 51.7 mmHg, $p < 0.001$). Of the newborns who received 80 ppm iNO, 65% manifested with methemoglobinopathy and required dose titration to 20 ppm. These data refuted Roberts and colleagues' (1992) claim that high-dose (80 ppm) iNO was safe. In addition, 17 newborns randomized to the iNO arm of the study died, and although the authors did not quantify the number of infants who exhibited hypoxic failure after cessation of therapy, given that 46% of these newborns went on to require ECMO, it is likely that abrupt discontinuation of therapy was a contributing factor.

Research regarding safe weaning of iNO culminated with the publication of an industry-sponsored dose-finding study in 1998 and 1999. Davidson and colleagues (1998) randomized 155 near-term or term newborns with HRF to an iNO dose of 5 ppm, 20 ppm, 80 ppm, or placebo. The trial confirmed previous findings, in that improved oxygenation was observed at all doses compared to placebo and methemoglobinemia was only observed with use of the 80 ppm dose. It is important to note that iNO was weaned in 20% decrements, every 4 hours or less, regardless of randomized dose. In other words, newborns randomized to 80 ppm were weaned in increments of 16 ppm, whereas newborns randomized to 5 ppm were weaned in increments of 1 ppm. In newborns who achieved treatment success at any dose, the mean duration of therapy was 88 hours, and no rebound hypoxia was observed in any group until the final step of withdrawal (Davidson et al., 1999). Upon cessation of therapy, from 1, 4, or 16 ppm, patients experienced dose-related rebound hypoxia (PaO_2 −11 ± 23, −28 ± 24, and −50 ± 48 mmHg, respectively). These findings clearly reinforced the current standard of care for weaning iNO; decreasing therapy by 4 ppm or more was deemed safe *until* the final step of discontinuation of therapy, when even cessation from 1 ppm elicited mild rebound hypoxia.

Subsequently, a large industry-sponsored study (the Clinical Inhaled Nitric Oxide Research Group Investigation, or CINRGI) combined lessons regarding dosing and weaning of iNO from previous trials. Near-term or term newborns with HRF ($N = 248$) were randomized to receive 20 ppm iNO or supplemental oxygen for a median duration of 44 hours. If newborns met criteria for weaning at 4 hours of therapy (PaO_2 ≥60 mmHg, pH ≥7.55), iNO was weaned to 5 ppm. For all other newborns who did not meet criteria for weaning within the first 24 hours of life, a standardized wean to 5 ppm was imposed at 24 hours of life. Then, therapy was discontinued once supplemental oxygen demand fell below 70%, or treatment spanned 96 hours, or at 7 days of life (whichever occurred first). The trial demonstrated that a max dose of 20 ppm iNO in newborns with PPHN significantly reduced the need for ECMO (38% iNO vs. 64% standard treatment; Clark et al., 2000). Further, the research team identified that newborns subject to iNO therapy demonstrated a reduced need for oxygen at 30 days of life (7% vs. 20%).

On the basis of data from the NINOS and CINRGI studies, the FDA approved iNO for use in term and near-term (> 34 weeks' gestational age) newborns (INO Therapeutics, 2013). The maximum approved dose was 20 ppm and product labeling discouraged abrupt discontinuation. The approved indication for use was the treatment of HRF associated with clinical or echocardiographic evidence of pulmonary hypertension. iNO was approved for use in conjunction with ventilator support and other cardiotonic agents to improve oxygenation and reduce the need for ECMO. This approval was met with relief from practicing clinicians, as dosing was now properly defined and prescribing practices were supported by adequate data.

In 2000, the AAP formally recommended iNO use among near-term and term newborns with HRF, excluding those with CDH (AAP, 2000). Since that time, several other organizations have published guidelines for the use of iNO in newborns (AAP, 2000; Abman et al., 2015; Hansmann et al., 2019).

ADJUNCTIVE VENTILATOR MANAGEMENT

Pharmacologic management alone is inadequate to achieve disease resolution in newborns with PPHN. Nonpharmacologic management involves the provision of noninvasive or invasive ventilation support. Newborns with mild disease are more likely to require less invasive respiratory support, whereas newborns with moderate to severe disease usually require endotracheal intubation and mechanical ventilation.

Conventional or high-frequency ventilators are useful when the recruitment of collapsed alveoli and maintenance of adequate lung volumes are necessary. Clinicians should target ventilator settings that reduce PVR. Strategies to reduce PVR include:

- Maintain judicious use of supplemental oxygen to achieve PaO_2 between 60 and 80 mmHg.
- Titrate peak inspiratory pressure to achieve $PaCO_2$ between 35 and 55 mmHg.
- Titrate mean airway pressure to gently recruit atelectatic alveoli.
- Maintain lung volume at functional residual capacity (FRC).

Given that FRC is the volume of air present at the end of exhalation, this is the point of maximum lung compliance, when PVR is lowest (Weiz & McNamara, 2017). Increasing the tidal volume beyond FRC distends adjoining alveoli, compresses the capillary network, and impedes optimal gas exchange.

Surfactant

Exogenous surfactant therapy has been shown to improve oxygenation and reduce the need for ECMO when PPHN is secondary to parenchymal lung disease (e.g., RDS, MAS, pneumonia, sepsis). This includes both studies with lower OI of 15 to 20 (Findlay et al., 1996; Konduri et al., 2013; Lotze et al., 1998), as well as patients with OI in the upper 30s who are already on iNO (González et al., 2021). There are currently three FDA-approved surfactant products: beractant, calfactant, and poractant alfa. Readers should refer to Chapter 13, "Respiratory Distress Syndrome," for additional information on the available pulmonary surfactants.

MECHANISM OF ACTION

Exogenous pulmonary surfactant serves as a replacement for endogenous surfactant in patients with surfactant deficiency or inactivation. Surfactant (endogenous or exogenous) reduces surface tension at the air–liquid interface of the alveoli during ventilation and stabilizes the alveoli against collapse at resting transpulmonary pressures. Exogenous surfactant restores surface activity to the newborn's lungs.

DOSING RECOMMENDATIONS

Surfactant therapies are available in varying vial sizes and are administered endotracheally or intratracheally. Ensure that the vials are warmed to room temperature prior to using through slow rolling or swirling in the hands. Do not shake the vials.

Dosing has varied, but some studies have used poractant alfa at a dosing of 100 to 200 mg/kg (1.25 to 2.5 mL/kg poractant alfa; Chinese Collaborative, 2005; González et al., 2021) or beractant at a dosing of 100 to 150 mg/kg (4 to 6 mL/kg beractant; Findlay et al., 1996; Lotze et al., 1998), with the ability to repeat doses at the recommended dosing interval (up to three doses for poractant alfa and up to four doses for beractant). One expert suggests reducing the dose by 50% in patients with CDH with evidence of surfactant deficiency due to pulmonary hypoplasia (Lakshminrusimha & Keszler, 2015).

CLINICAL-MONITORING PEARLS

Frequent monitoring of oxygen saturations and arterial blood gases is necessary to prevent any hyperoxia or hypocarbia that could occur after administration of the surfactant dose. Close clinical monitoring is indicated to ensure early identification of complications including endotracheal tube obstruction and pulmonary hemorrhage.

CURRENT PHARMACOLOGIC TREATMENT MODALITIES FOR PERSISTENT PULMONARY HYPERTENSION OF THE NEWBORN

The primary indication for pharmacologic management in PPHN is to reduce PVR. However, newborns with PPHN may concurrently demonstrate compromised systemic vascular tone and cardiac performance, which may progress to systemic hypotension. Because PPHN is associated with numerous diseases, there is no single management strategy for all patients. Generally speaking, in cadence with optimizing ventilatory support, clinicians aim to minimize systemic oxygen demands (e.g., maintaining euthermia, minimize stimulation), correct metabolic abnormalities (e.g., hypoglycemia, hypocalcemia, acidosis), treat any underlying pulmonary parenchymal or hematologic disease (e.g., polycythemia), and sustain cardiac performance and systemic hemodynamic stability. Most newborns with moderate to severe PPHN require sedation with opioids (e.g., morphine or fentanyl) and the addition of benzodiazepines or dexmedetomidine may be required.

In addition, some centers prescribe paralytics to further reduce oxygen demand. Although a single retrospective study initially demonstrated a significant association between the use of paralytics and death in the setting of PPHN, the association was no longer significant after patients with CDH were removed from the analysis (Walsh-Sukys et al., 2000). Given that this was a retrospective review, it is possible that subjects who received paralytics had more severe disease at baseline. Regardless, clinicians should be judicious in their use of paralytics and reserve their use to cases in which conventional sedation with opioids +/- benzodiazepines/dexmedetomidine is inadequate.

The drugs presented in this section of the chapter include those most commonly prescribed to newborns with PPHN (Table 15.3). A sample protocol for a combined approach to the treatment of PPHN and hypotension/shock is provided in Figure 15.6.

Nitric Oxide

The use of iNO therapy is currently the gold standard for term and near-term newborns with severe HRF, and it is currently the only FDA-approved vasodilator specifically for the treatment of PPHN. Studies have demonstrated that iNO improves oxygenation and decreases the need for ECMO therapy in newborns greater than 34 weeks of gestation with diverse causes of PPHN (Davidson et al., 1998; Kinsella et al., 1997; Neonatal Inhaled Nitric Oxide Study Group, 1997; Roberts et al., 1997; Wessel et al., 1997). Use in preterm newborns under 34 weeks of gestation is still under investigation, with conflicting results.

MECHANISM OF ACTION/PHARMACOKINETIC PRINCIPLES

To begin the process, iNO enters well-recruited alveoli and diffuses into the smooth muscle of the pulmonary arteriole. From there, iNO binds to the heme moiety of cytosolic guanylate cyclase (GC), activating GC and increasing intracellular levels of cGMP, which leads to smooth muscle relaxation. Dilation of pulmonary vessels in well-ventilated lung areas redistributes blood flow away from lung areas where V/Q ratios are poor. From there, NO molecules react with lung water, oxygen-containing heme molecules, or hypoxic blood. This oxidation reaction reduces heme iron to the ferric state, forming *met*hemoglobin and nitrate. Methemoglobin exhibits a higher affinity for oxygen but is composed of fewer heme moieties to bind with oxygen. Given the reduced oxygen-carrying capacity, the oxyhemoglobin dissociation curve shifts leftward. When methemoglobin levels remain less than 2% of the total proportion of hemoglobin in the body, no toxic effect is observed. Rather, methemoglobin is metabolized by the enzyme methemoglobin reductase back to normal hemoglobin. When iNO is administered at dosages of more than 80 ppm for longer than 8 hours, or a deficiency of methemoglobin reductase is present, toxic accumulation of methemoglobin may occur (Davidson et al., 1998). Renal clearance is observed.

DOSING RECOMMENDATIONS

When initiated, the recommended starting dose of iNO is 20 ppm in term and near-term newborns greater than 34 weeks of gestation with PPHN (Davidson et al., 1998; Kinsella et al., 1997; Neonatal Inhaled Nitric Oxide Study Group, 1997; Roberts et al., 1997; Wessel et al., 1997). Generally, patients who fail to respond to iNO at 20 ppm will not demonstrate an improvement at higher doses of 40 to 80 ppm. Brief exposure to these higher doses does appear to be generally safe (with the exception of a higher risk of methemoglobinemia with a sustained treatment of 80 ppm), so dose escalation may be considered in refractory cases (Davidson et al., 1998). Davidson and colleagues (1998) reported that the average time frame required to achieve the peak methemoglobin concentration in newborns treated with 80 ppm of iNO was 19.6 ± 27.5 hours (median time frame = 8 hours). The peak methemoglobin level reported was 11.9% (after 8 hours of therapy at 80 ppm; Davidson et al., 1998).

TABLE 15.3 Medication and Therapeutic Classes for Persistent Pulmonary Hypertension of the Newborn

MEDICATION OR THERAPEUTIC CLASS	DOSING	EVIDENCE	PLACE IN THERAPY
Surfactant	100–200 mg/kg endotracheal or intratracheal May give repeat doses per package insert	RCTs showing reduced need for ECMO in the setting of parenchymal disease both with and without iNO	For PPHN secondary to parenchymal lung disease (e.g., RDS, MAS, pneumonia, sepsis) to reduce the need for ECMO or death
Beractant	4–6 mL/kg (100–150 mg/kg)		
Poractant alfa	1.25–2.5 mL/kg (100–200 mg/kg)		
Calfactant	3 mL/kg (100 mg/kg)		
iNO	20 ppm inhaled May be titrated up to 40 to 80 ppm Requires weaning as PPHN resolves	Meta-analysis (including 17 RCT) showing a decreased need for ECMO and improvement in oxygenation (high quality of evidence)	Gold standard first-line treatment after oxygen and supportive care
PDE3 inhibitors Milrinone	Optional: IV Loading dose 50 mcg/kg over 60 minutes (many experts avoid loading doses due to hypotension) Initial: IV 0.25–0.5 mcg/kg/min May be titrated up to 1 mcg/kg/min	Case series	Refractory to iNO May be especially beneficial in patients showing ventricular dysfunction
PDE5 inhibitors Sildenafil	PO 0.5–3 mg/kg/dose every 6 to 12 hours IV 0.4 mg/kg followed by 0.067 mg/kg/hour (1.6 mg/kg/day) Some centers utilize intermittent IV sildenafil at 50% of the PO dose and administer each dose over 1–3 hours	Meta-analysis (including five RCTs) showing a reduction in mortality (low quality of evidence)	Refractory to iNO May also be beneficial for chronic pulmonary hypertension
Prostaglandins (PGE_1) Alprostadil	IV Initial 0.01 mcg/kg/min and maintained at 0.01 to 0.05 mcg/kg/min Nebulized 150 to 300 ng/kg/min (diluted to run at 4 mL/hour)	RCTs and case series	Refractory to iNO with constricting PDA and signs of RV failure
Prostaglandins (PGI_2)	IV and inhaled/nebulized routes (varies by product)	Case series and case reports showing improvements in oxygenation	Refractory to iNO
Epoprostenol	IV Initial: 4 ng/kg/min titrated up to 20 ng/kg/min Inhaled/nebulized initial: 50 ng/kg/min (minimum 10 ng/kg/min and maximum 100 ng/kg/min)		
Iloprost	IV Initial: 0.5–3 ng/kg/min titrated up to a maximum of 10 ng/kg/min Inhaled/nebulized 1–2.5 mcg/kg q2-6h		
Treprostinil	IV Initial: 4–6 ng/kg/min titrated up to a maximum of 20–30 ng/kg/min (up to 52 ng/kg/min has been reported)		
Endothelin receptor antagonists Bosentan	PO 1–2 mg/kg q12h	RCTs and case series	Likely more beneficial for chronic pulmonary hypertension than acutely for PPHN

ECMO, extracorporeal membrane oxygenation; iNO, inhaled nitric oxide; IV, intravenous; MAS, meconium aspiration syndrome; PDA, patent ductus arteriosus; PDE, phosphodiesterase; PO, by mouth; PPHN, persistent pulmonary hypertension of the newborn; RCT, randomized controlled trial; RDS, respiratory distress syndrome; RV, right ventricular.

FIGURE 15.6 Sample approach to management of persistent pulmonary hypertension of the newborn in term and near-term infants.

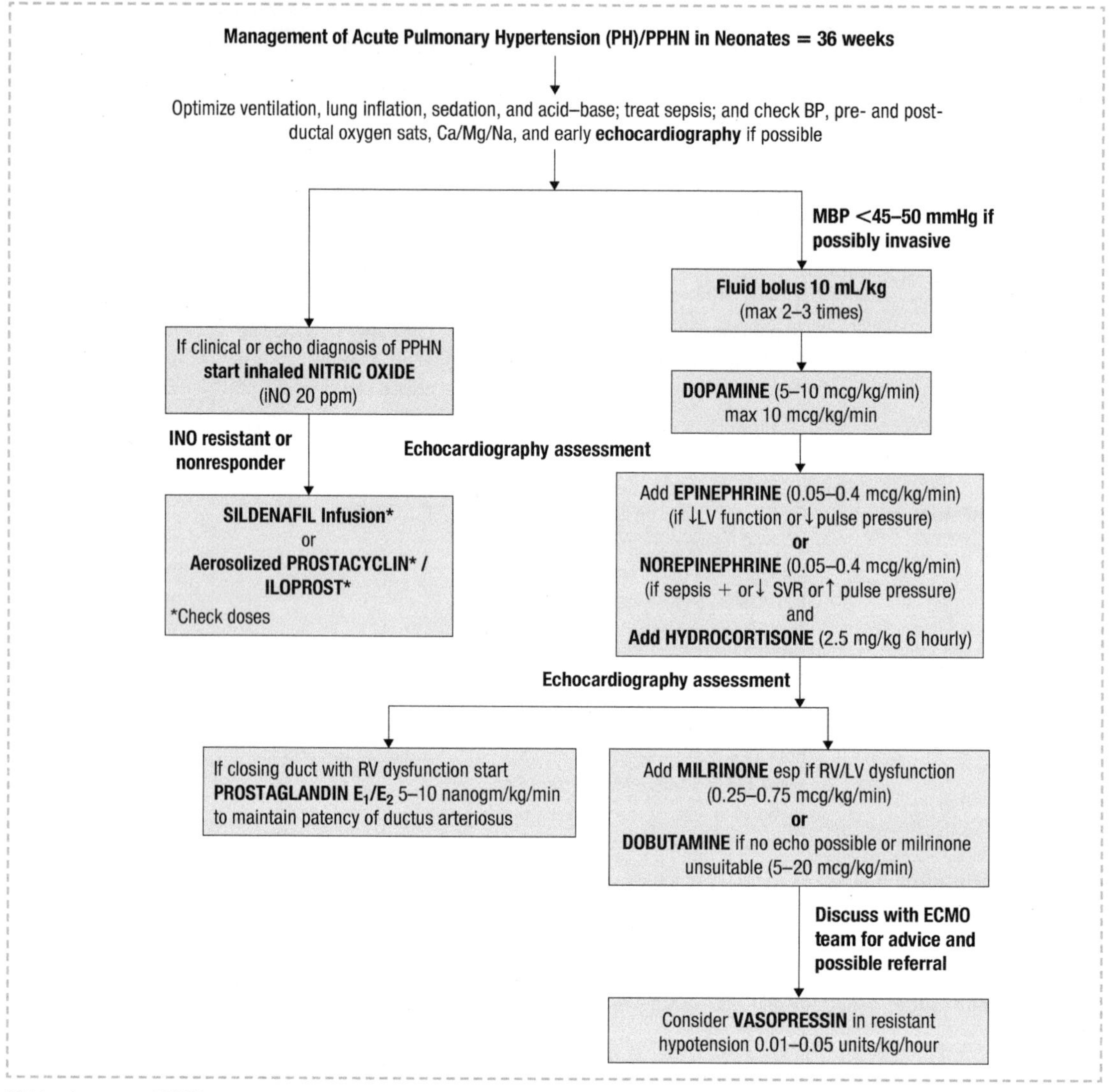

BP, blood pressure; ECMO, extracorporeal membrane oxygenation; LV, left ventricle; MBP, mean blood pressure; PPHN, persistent pulmonary hypertension of the newborn; RV, right ventricle.

Source: Adapted from Singh, Y., & Lakshminrusimha, S. (2021). Pathophysiology and management of persistent pulmonary hypertension of the newborn. *Clinics in Perinatology, 48*(3), 595–618. https://doi.org/10.1016/j.clp.2021.05.009

Institutions should develop criteria for gradual weaning of iNO therapy, once PPHN begins to resolve. Common thresholds used to determine appropriateness for iNO weaning include an FiO_2 of 60% or less, PaO_2 of 60 mmHg or more, and SpO_2 of 90% or more (Lakshminrusimha & Keszler, 2015). Dosages are usually decreased in intervals of 5 ppm, every 1 to 4 hours, until the continuous inhalational dose reaches 5 ppm. Then, clinicians carefully wean by only 1 ppm, every 2 to 4 hours, to reduce the risk for rebound PPHN. A sample weaning protocol is provided in Figure 15.7.

CLINICAL-MONITORING PEARLS

Although rare at standard iNO doses in newborns, methemoglobinemia is a potential side effect (Hamon et al., 2010). In newborns, this complication may arise secondary to a deficiency of methemoglobin reductase enzyme versus exposure to the ordered dose of iNO. Because enzyme deficiencies like this are not easily identified after birth, a serum methemoglobin level is customarily

FIGURE 15.7 Sample approach to weaning inhaled nitric oxide in term and near-term infants with persistent pulmonary hypertension of the newborn.

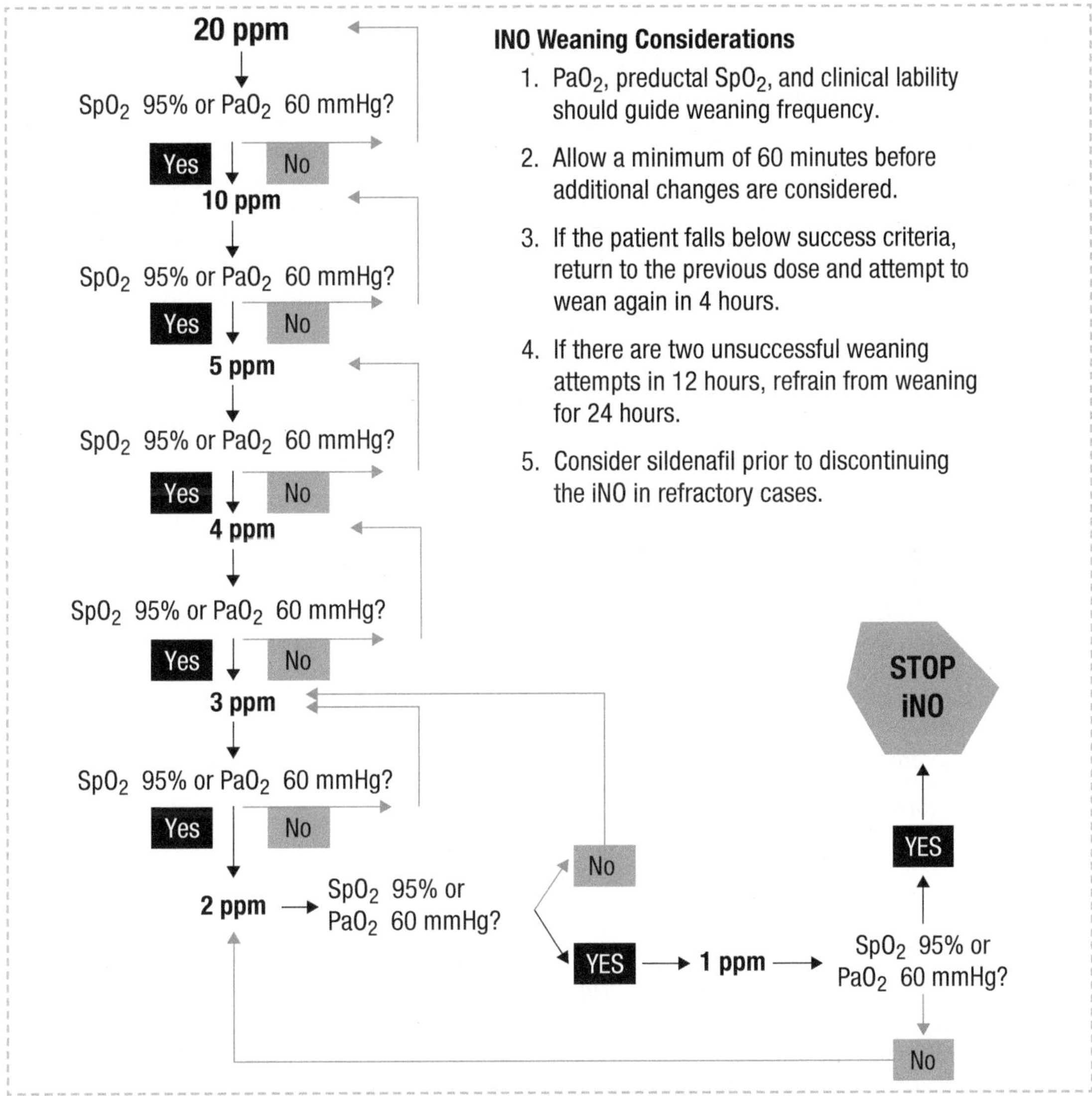

iNO, inhaled nitric oxide.

Source: From University of North Carolina Newborn Critical Care Center. (2018). *UNC health 2017 clinical practice guidelines*. UNC. Kelly, L. E., Ohlsson, A., & Shah, P. S. (2017). Sildenafil for pulmonary hypertension in neonates. *Cochrane Database of Systematic Reviews, (8)*, Article CD005494. https://doi.org/10.1002/14651858.CD005494.pub4

obtained before the initiation of therapy, 1 to 4 hours after therapy is initiated, and daily thereafter. Dose reductions or discontinuation of therapy should be considered in patients with elevated methemoglobin (>5%).

Other Pulmonary Vasodilators

In addition to iNO, other pulmonary vasodilators may be considered in patients who continue to worsen. These treatments include phosphodiesterase-5 (PDE5) inhibitors (sildenafil), phosphodiesterase-3 (PDE3) inhibitors (milrinone), prostaglandins (PGI_2 [prostacyclins] and PGE_1 [alprostadil]), and endothelin receptor antagonists (bosentan). A summary of each pulmonary vasodilator is provided in Figure 15.3.

SILDENAFIL

Mechanism of Action/Pharmacokinetic Principles

Of all PDE5 inhibitors, sildenafil is most commonly used for long-term treatment of PPHN. Inhibition of PDE5 in the smooth muscle of the pulmonary vasculature results in an increase in cGMP, because PDE5 normally degrades cGMP. Increased cGMP concentrations elicit pulmonary and systemic vascular relaxation and vasodilation.

The first PK study specific to sildenafil use in newborns was published in 2009. Mukherjee and colleagues (2009) reported a higher volume of distribution (22.4 L) and elimination half-life of 56 hours in 1-day-old newborns compared to 48 hours in 7-day-old newborns. Sildenafil is hepatically metabolized by CYP3A4 enzymes. Hepatic drug clearance increases over the first week of life, from 0.84 L/hour at 1 day of life to 2.58 L/hour by 7 days of life; results vary among newborns due to variable cytochrome P450 maturation and organ perfusion (Hornik et al., 2018). Excretion is primarily via the stool (80%) and, to a lesser degree, in the urine.

Dosing Recommendations

Sildenafil is available in both enteral and intravenous formulations in the United States. In addition to use during the acute phase of PPHN, some institutions will also use sildenafil to facilitate weaning off iNO.

Studies report that an oral dosage between 0.5 and 2 mg/kg administered every 6 hours offered similar exposure to therapeutic dosing in adults (Ahsman et al., 2010). Dosing in clinical practice is variable. Oral doses of sildenafil 1 to 3 mg/kg given every 6 hours improve oxygenation and mortality in resource limited settings without access to iNO (Baquero et al., 2006; Vargas-Origel et al., 2010).

Intravenous sildenafil has also been shown to be effective in improving oxygenation in newborns with PPHN with and without iNO exposure (Steinhorn et al., 2009). Intravenous sildenafil is commonly given as a loading dose of 0.4 mg/kg over 3 hours with a continuous infusion of 0.067 mg/kg/hour. However, due to issues with intravenous (IV) compatibility, some centers use an intermittent dosing strategy with a per os (PO; by mouth):IV conversion of sildenafil of 2:1 with IV doses administered over 1 to 3 hours (Stultz et al., 2013).

Clinical-Monitoring Pearls

The primary adverse event to monitor for with sildenafil is systemic hypotension due to systemic vasodilation (Steinhorn et al., 2009). It is otherwise generally well-tolerated.

MILRINONE

Mechanism of Action/Pharmacokinetic Principles

Milrinone is a PDE3 inhibitor and inotropic agent. As a result, milrinone is likely the pulmonary vasodilator of choice in patients with left ventricular dysfunction (Lakshminrusimha & Steinhorn, 2013). Its mechanism as a pulmonary vasodilator is through PDE3 inhibition, which results in increased concentrations of cyclic adenosine monophosphate (cAMP). Similar to cGMP, this results in pulmonary vasculature relaxation and therefore vasodilation. And again similarly, this effect notably occurs in both the pulmonary and systemic vasculature. Additional pharmacokinetic data can be found in Chapter 20, "Hypotension and Shock."

Dosing Recommendations

Milrinone is available as an intravenous medication and is given as a continuous infusion with or without a loading dose. If a loading dose is given, the dose is typically 0.05 mg/kg (50 mcg/kg) given over 1 hour; some centers do not use a loading dose due to concerns for hypotension. The continuous infusion dose range is typically initiated at 0.25 to 0.5 mcg/kg/min (titrated up to a maximum 1 mcg/kg/min), which has demonstrated an improvement in infants with PPHN who have been refractory to iNO (Bassler et al., 2006; McNamara et al., 2006, 2013). Doses should be reduced in the setting of renal dysfunction due to the potential for accumulation.

Clinical-Monitoring Pearls

Similar to PDE5 inhibitors, the primary adverse event to monitor with milrinone is systemic hypotension due to systemic vasodilation. In addition, since it is an inotropic agent, the potential for dysrhythmias is reported.

PROSTAGLANDINS

Prostaglandins have been used in patients with iNO-resistant PPHN due to their ability to cause pulmonary vasodilation. These include PGE_1 (alprostadil) and PGI_2, or prostacyclins (epoprostenol, iloprost, and treprostinil). We present a summary of the mechanism of action for prostaglandins, followed by an itemized discussion of dosage parameters for each individual drug. Clinical-monitoring pearls are summarized at the end of this section, with customized alerts for specific drugs, as indicated.

Mechanism of Action/Pharmacokinetic Principles

PGE_1 (alprostadil) causes vasodilation through a direct effect on vascular smooth muscle. In addition to pulmonary vasodilation, alprostadil may provide the additional benefit of maintaining an open PDA since it affects the smooth muscle in the DA as well. This can work as a "pop-off" valve in patients with very high PVR, which will result in decreasing right ventricular afterload through right-to-left shunting through the PDA (Gupta et al., 2013). In comparison, PGI_2 medications elicit pulmonary vasodilation by increasing the production of cAMP.

Alprostadil and epoprostenol are both direct mimetics of endogenous PGE_1 and PGI_2, respectively. Alprostadil metabolism occurs predominantly through oxidation in the first passage through the lungs with elimination primarily in the urine, with a half-life of 30 seconds to 10 minutes. Similarly, epoprostenol is metabolized by enzymatic hydrolysis in the blood and eliminated in the urine with a half-life of 3 minutes.

Iloprost and treprostinil are synthetic derivatives of PGI_2, manipulated primarily to prolong elimination half-life. Iloprost is metabolized by beta oxidation of a carboxyl side chain in the liver prior to renal elimination, prolonging the half-life to 20 to 30 minutes. Treprostinil is metabolized primarily by CYP2C8 in the liver before renal elimination, prolonging the half-life even further to approximately 4 hours.

The bioavailability of inhaled prostaglandins is highly variable based on the specific formulation, nebulizer, and mode of ventilation. Adults receiving treprostinil via the branded inhalation system in the outpatient setting achieve bioavailability of approximately 70%. However, delivery of nebulized epoprostenol (a highly basic solution intended for intravenous administration) to newborns via high-frequency ventilation is thought to be negligible. The formulation of iloprost mitigates this limitation to some degree, with 30% simulated bioavailability via neonatal high-frequency ventilation (DiBlasi et al., 2016).

Dosing Recommendations

Dosing for prostaglandins is mostly limited to case series and retrospective evaluations. PGE_1 (alprostadil) use in NICUs is more commonly given intravenously to maintain an open PDA, although studies have used the aerosolized route for PPHN (Sood et al., 2004, 2014). Both intravenous and aerosolized/inhaled routes have been used for various PGI_2 medications.

Alprostadil

Alprostadil is a reasonable consideration in patients with PPHN, a constricting PDA, and signs of right ventricular failure. One study assessing newborns with CDH dosed intravenous alprostadil with a goal to maintain an open PDA: initiation of 0.01 mcg/kg/min and maintained at 0.01 to 0.05 mcg/kg/min for the duration of therapy (Lawrence et al., 2019). Nebulized alprostadil was studied at 150 to 300 ng/kg/min diluted in saline to provide 4 mL/hour as a continuous nebulization (Sood et al., 2014) based on an earlier report finding this dose was safe and improved oxygenation (Sood et al., 2004).

Epoprostenol

Newborns with PPHN refractory to iNO may respond to epoprostenol therapy. Ahmad and colleagues (2018) reported use of an initial continuous intravenous infusion rate of 4 ng/kg/min; the dosage was increased, as needed, by 2 ng/kg/min to a maximum dose of 20 ng/kg/min. A therapeutic response was observed in 15 of the 36 newborns evaluated (Ahmad et al., 2018). Nebulized epoprostenol dosing typically ranges from 10 to 100 ng/kg/min (Berger-Caron et al., 2019). The initial dose has varied from 10 ng/kg/min (Berger-Caron et al., 2019) to 50 ng/kg/min (Brown et al., 2012; Kelly et al., 2002). The largest evaluation to date of 43 newborns demonstrated a significant improvement in OI after 12 hours of treatment with nebulized epoprostenol ($p = 0.047$; Berger-Caron et al., 2019).

Iloprost

Intravenous iloprost has been used as a rescue therapy among newborns with PPHN or primary therapy when iNO was unavailable for use. Janjindamai and colleagues (2013) demonstrated a significant reduction in the median OI and alveolar-arterial oxygen difference ($p < 0.05$) with an initial dosage of 0.5 to 3 ng/kg/min, titrated to a maintenance dose of 1 to 10 ng/kg/min (Janjindamai et al., 2013).

Inhaled iloprost has also been used among newborns with PPHN. Kahveci and colleagues (2014) were one of the first to retrospectively compare iloprost to sildenafil. Iloprost was administered via jet nebulizer at doses of 1 to 2.5 mcg/kg every 2 to 4 hours. When compared to sildenafil 0.5 to 3 mg/kg administered enterally every 6 hours, iloprost demonstrated faster response to treatment as well as an earlier ability to discontinue the study drug due to clinical improvement (Kahveci et al., 2014). Next, Kim and colleagues (2019) investigated inhaled iloprost as a first-line medication when iNO was unavailable. A dosage of 1 to 2 mcg/kg administered every 3 to 6 hours was associated with clinical improvement in eight of nine full-term newborns (Kim et al., 2019).

Treprostinil

Intravenous or subcutaneous treprostinil use has been mainly limited to patients with CDH and PPHN who are unable to wean from assisted ventilation, iNO, and other adjunctive therapies. Published studies and case reports indicate that a customary initial dose ranges between 4 to 6 ng/kg/min and can be titrated to a maximum dose of 20 to 52 ng/kg/min. Olson and colleagues (2015) reported the use of treprostinil in two term newborns with CDH with persistently elevated PVR refractory to iNO and prostaglandin. A continuous infusion of treprostinil was initiated between 2 and 20 ng/kg/min and titrated to a maximum dose of 48 to 52 ng/kg/min (Olson et al., 2015). Park and Chung (2017) reported an initial dose of 5 ng/kg/min, which was titrated up to a maximum of 20 ng/kg/min in two preterm newborns with sepsis and PPHN refractory to iNO; intravenous treprostinil use was associated with significant improvement and no systemic side effects (Park & Chung, 2017). A more recent retrospective review of 17 patients with CDH identified a typical intravenous initiation dose of 4 ng/kg/min with titration to a maximum dose between 20 to 30 ng/kg/min (Lawrence et al., 2018). A similar study also including 17 patients initiated at 6 ng/kg/min and titrated up to a maximum of 21 ng/kg/min (Jozefkowicz et al., 2020). Most newborns initially treated with continuous intravenous infusions were transitioned to continuous subcutaneous infusions in preparation for discharge; catheter replacement occurred approximately once monthly.

Clinical-Monitoring Pearls

Intravenous administration of prostaglandins infers a significant risk for hypotension due to systemic vasodilation. Alprostadil is associated with hyperthermia and apneic events, in particular, when a higher continuous infusion dose is prescribed. Bedside staff should be prepared to turn off overhead radiant heat to prevent overwarming. APRN clinicians should be prepared to endotracheally intubate patients who manifest with apnea.

Epoprostenol has an extremely short half-life (~3 minutes). Therefore, operational processes need to be in place to ensure that a replacement product is always available. This mitigates the risk for rebound pulmonary hypertension. In addition, subcutaneous injection sites should be monitored, as localized infections can occur and require treatment.

Iloprost and treprostinil mitigate this risk to some degree with longer half-lives, although careful attention to the injection site remains warranted given the life-sustaining nature of these therapies. Substantial multidisciplinary planning is required to optimize the preparation and administration of both intravenous and inhaled prostaglandins. Advanced practitioners should collaborate with physicians and allied healthcare clinicians to develop guidelines. Customized dilution of intravenous prostacyclins is required to deliver therapeutic doses at measurable rates through dedicated access while avoiding volume overload. Guidelines for delivery of inhaled prostacyclins must consider the relationship between desired dose and the parameters for specific nebulizers to define concentrations that allow both escalation and weaning of therapy.

BOSENTAN

Bosentan is a nonspecific endothelin-1 receptor blocker proven to be well tolerated (despite being available only as an enteral medication) in newborns. However, its use for PPHN has declined due to data demonstrating variable efficacy (Maneenil et al., 2018; W. A. Mohamed & Ismail, 2012; Steinhorn et al., 2016). Bosentan may be considered among patients who continue to demonstrate chronic pulmonary hypertension after the initial acute PPHN episode, since oral availability would be convenient for outpatient administration.

Mechanism of Action/Pharmacokinetic Principles

Stimulation of G protein-coupled endothelin-1 receptors in vascular smooth muscle produces vasoconstriction; bosentan antagonizes these receptors. The pharmacokinetics of bosentan have been described in pediatric patients, but limited description exists in newborns (Zisowsky et al., 2017). Enteral bosentan has approximately 50% bioavailability. Metabolism occurs in the liver through CYP2C9 and CYP3A4 prior to excretion in the feces. The half-life in children is approximately 5 hours.

Dosing Recommendations

Bosentan is only available as an enteral tablet that must be compounded into an oral suspension. The customary enteral dosage is 1 mg/kg/dose every 12 hours. Dose titration up to 2 mg/kg/dose every 12 hours may be considered (W. A. Mohamed & Ismail, 2012; Steinhorn et al., 2016).

Clinical-Monitoring Pearls

Serum transaminases (aspartate aminotransferase [AST] and alanine transaminase [ALT]) and bilirubin should be monitored for hepatotoxicity, ideally prior to initiation of therapy and periodically thereafter.

Inotropic and Blood Pressure Support

The American College of Critical Care Medicine (ACCM) provided guidelines in 2017 on the management of hemodynamic support of pediatric and neonatal shock (Davis et al., 2017).

Systemic hemodynamics should be optimized with volume and inotropic therapy to enhance cardiac output and systemic oxygen transport. Common agents used include dopamine, epinephrine, and milrinone. Vasopressin and norepinephrine have additionally become more appealing agents for the management of PPHN. Catecholamines produce cardiovascular effects through alpha-1, beta-1, and beta-2-receptors (Overgaard & Dzavík, 2008). Beta-1-adrenergic receptor stimulation increases myocardial contractility through calcium-mediated facilitation of the actin-myosin complex binding with troponin C and enhances chronicity through calcium channel activation. Beta-2-adrenergic receptor stimulation on vascular smooth muscle cells results in vasodilation through increased calcium uptake by the sarcoplasmic reticulum and vasodilation. Activation of alpha-1-adrenergic receptors on arterial vascular smooth muscle cells results in increased SVR through smooth muscle contraction. A brief overview of the mechanism of action of each agent is outlined in the text that follows (Siefkes & Lakshminrusimha, 2021). Additional information can be found in Chapter 20, "Hypotension and Shock."

DOPAMINE

Mechanism of Action

Dopamine has remained the mainstay first-line therapy for neonatal shock for many years (Davis et al., 2017). At low to moderate doses, dopamine predominantly focuses on the stimulation of beta-1-receptors, leading to cardiac stimulation and increased cardiac output. Doses in the higher range increase SVR through stimulation of alpha-1-receptors; however, this vasoconstrictive effect may also worsen pulmonary hypertension by increasing PVR (Liet et al., 2002). Dopamine directly stimulates D_1 and D_2 dopamine receptors in the kidney and splanchnic vasculature, leading to renal and mesenteric vasodilation. Dopamine is then metabolized to norepinephrine, which stimulates alpha-1 and beta-1-receptors.

Dosing Recommendations

When prescribed for use in newborns with PPHN, dosages between 5 to 10 mcg/kg/min are typically used to focus on the stimulation of beta-1-receptors (Davis et al., 2017). Doses in the higher range of 10 to 20 mcg/kg/min would increase stimulation alpha-1-receptors, which may worsen PVR.

Clinical-Monitoring Pearls

Heart rate and blood pressure should be monitored carefully and continuously during dopamine therapy. Clinicians should clearly define the acceptable mean arterial blood pressure range (see Chapter 20, "Hypotension and Shock") and titration parameters for bedside nurses. Although general guidance regarding dosing thresholds for cardiac and vascular effects are provided in this chapter and Chapter 20, "Hypotension and Shock," substantial interpatient variability exists and dosing must always be customized to the individual newborns and clinical goals. In newborns with PPHN, it is essential to avoid titrating the dopamine dose to a level that would elicit vasoconstriction and hypertension. In addition to monitoring the heart rate and blood pressure, all patients receiving vasopressors should be monitored for signs of reduced perfusion to the kidneys, liver, intestines, and digits. Interval assessments of urinary output, blood urea nitrogen and creatinine levels, gastrointestinal function, and capillary refill are indicated. Finally, clinicians should visually inspect and palpate over the intravenous access site, at least hourly, to prevent extravasation.

DOBUTAMINE

Mechanism of Action

After initiating dopamine, addition of dobutamine would further increase cardiac output through its inotropic effect from stimulation of beta-1-receptors while remaining relatively SVR neutral. It also has a chronotropic effect, demonstrating an increase in neonatal heart rate after initiation, especially at higher doses (Mahoney et al., 2016).

Dosing Recommendations

Dobutamine is typically initiated at 5 mcg/kg/min and may be titrated up to 20 mcg/kg/min (Davis et al., 2017). It should be noted that doses greater than 10 mcg/kg/min are likely to produce a greater chronotropic effect (Siefkes & Lakshminrusimha, 2021).

Clinical-Monitoring Pearls

Heart rate (to avoid tachycardia) and blood pressure (to avoid hypotension) must be monitored carefully during dobutamine therapy. Detection of improved cardiac output may require echocardiography, although interval improvement in oxygenation is reassuring.

EPINEPHRINE

Mechanism of Action

Similar to dopamine, epinephrine at low to moderate doses predominantly focuses on the stimulation of beta-1-receptors, leading to cardiac stimulation and increased cardiac output. This may be especially beneficial for a newborn with depressed myocardial function. Again, like dopamine, doses in the higher range would increase SVR through stimulation of α_1-receptors; however, this vasoconstrictive effect could worsen pulmonary hypertension by also increasing PVR.

Dosing Recommendations

Per the ACCM guidelines, epinephrine may be dosed between 0.05 to 0.3 mcg/kg/min. However, some experts suggest that epinephrine should ideally be dosed between 0.05 to 0.1 mcg/kg/min to focus on the stimulation of beta-1-receptors in newborns. Doses higher than 0.1 mcg/kg/min increase stimulation of alpha-receptors, which may increase PVR. As evidence of this, one study of neonatal septic shock found that epinephrine doses of 0.2 mcg/kg/min were equivalent to doses of dopamine at 10 mcg/kg/min (Baske et al., 2018).

Clinical-Monitoring Pearls

Like dopamine, monitoring for epinephrine consists primarily of careful attention to heart rate and blood pressure. As with dopamine, the dosing threshold between cardiac and vascular effects varies among patients, and hypertension should be avoided in the setting of PPHN. In addition, epinephrine produces tachycardia to a greater degree than dopamine, which should be strictly avoided in the setting of compromised cardiac function to allow adequate ventricular filling (Valverde et al., 2006).

NOREPINEPHRINE

Pharmacokinetic Principles

The addition of norepinephrine may further increase SVR through stimulation of α_1-receptors. It has minimal effect on inotropy through beta-1-receptors. Although vasoconstriction through stimulation of alpha-1-receptors may also increase PVR, evidence has suggested that the ratio of pulmonary/systemic arterial pressure actually decreases following norepinephrine infusion (Tourneux et al., 2008), which would be ideal in newborns with PPHN.

Dosing Recommendations

Norepinephrine may be initiated at 0.05 to 0.1 mcg/kg/min and titrated up as tolerated to a usual maximum dose of 0.5 to 1 mcg/kg/min (Tourneux et al., 2008).

Clinical-Monitoring Pearls

In PPHN, norepinephrine functions as a focused vasopressor for newborns with significant hypotension, with preferential action on SVR as compared to PVR. It is important to note that norepinephrine should only be utilized to maintain *normotension* and avoid end-organ hypoperfusion. Utilizing any vasopressor to induce systemic hypertension in an effort to reverse right-to-left ductal shunting dramatically compromises ventricular function and risks cardiac collapse (Reller et al., 1987).

VASOPRESSIN

Mechanism of Action

Vasopressin does not act via alpha- or beta-receptors, but rather via three subtypes of vasopressin receptors. V_1 vasopressin receptors have potent vasoconstrictor properties on the systemic vasculature with minimal effect on PVR, leading to a decreased pulmonary/systemic arterial pressure ratio. In addition, vasopressin is thought to produce pulmonary vasodilation via stimulation of oxytocin endothelial receptors and subsequent NO pathway activation (Thibonnier et al., 1999), potentially making this an ideal agent for PPHN.

Dosing Recommendations

Vasopressin may be dosed as units/kg/hour, units/kg/min, or milliunits/kg/min depending on the reference. Close attention should be paid to the units used to prevent medication errors. Dosing is typically initiated at 0.1 to 0.2 milliunits/kg/min (0.0001 to 0.0002 units/kg/min) and may be titrated up as tolerated. One study demonstrated titrations up to 1 milliunit/kg/min (0.001 units/kg/min) (Acker et al., 2014), whereas another study titrated up to 1.2 milliunits/kg/min (0.0012 units/kg/min; A. Mohamed et al., 2014). Much higher doses of up to 10 milliunits/kg/min (0.01 units/kg/min) have been reported for the management of vasodilatory shock in patients without PPHN, although most patients do not require doses this high.

Clinical-Monitoring Pearls

Monitoring parameters for vasopressin match those for norepinephrine, with utilization strictly focused on maintenance of normotension and end-organ perfusion while avoiding hypertension and cardiac compromise. For vasopressin specifically, urine output and sodium levels should be closely monitored after initiation, as hyponatremia and reduced urine output have been reported.

Extracorporeal Life Support

ECMO has been used as rescue therapy in newborns with severe PPHN since 1982 (Ford, 2006). ECMO offers a modified cardiopulmonary bypass system that provides oxygenation and gas exchange while allowing the newborn's lungs to rest to facilitate repair while avoiding barotrauma and volutrauma associated with mechanical ventilation. Because of the invasiveness of ECMO, it is reserved for those who meet the Bartlett criteria (OI >40), which is indicative of a greater than 60% to 80% risk of death if not performed (Ostrea et al., 2006). The Extracorporeal Life Support Organization (ELSO) has set guidelines for ECMO in newborns with respiratory failure. Ventilator management while on ECMO differs due to the fact that the ECMO pump essentially does the work of the lungs and allows the lungs to rest. However, it is essential to maintain some ventilation to the lungs to prevent collapse.

One of the reasons ECMO is saved as the last rescue therapy for PPHN is that it comes with many of its own complications and risks (Table 15.4). For example, newborns must remain in an anticoagulated state. Bleeding is considered one of the major risks of ECMO and the most commonly reported adverse effect. On the opposite side, clotting is also a significant risk while on ECMO. Fortunately, due to the introduction of iNO and other therapies, use of ECMO in newborns with PPHN has decreased.

PERSISTENT PULMONARY HYPERTENSION OF THE NEWBORN AND PREMATURITY

The vast majority of newborns with PPHN are born term and near term; however, nearly 2% of cases occur in preterm newborns (V. H. Kumar et al., 2007). The effectiveness of iNO for pulmonary vasodilation for term and near-term newborns has been proven and accepted as a standard

TABLE 15.4 Potential Complications of Extracorporeal Membrane Oxygenation

HEMOLYSIS	BLEEDING	CLOTTING
Hemolysis: Free hemoglobin in the blood plasma is present in concentrations exceeding >50 mg/dL (normal <10 mg/dL). **Suspect** hemolysis if the urine is dark and urinalysis shows large blood, but no red cells. **Verify** hemolysis with an elevated plasma hemoglobin level. There may also be increased conjugated bilirubin, anemia, and increased haptoglobin. **Higher plasma hemoglobin** can be caused by negative pressure generated by centrifugal pumps, partial circuit or component thrombosis, malocclusion of the roller pump, high shear stresses related to turbulent flow, and chattering of the venous lines. **Hemolysis** results in increased free circulating hemoglobin that causes nephrotoxicity, increased vascular resistance, increased thrombin generation, platelet dysfunction, and clotting disorders.	**Bleeding** at the ECMO cannula site, surgical site bleeding, and CNS hemorrhage rates have shown an increased frequency since 2000. **Bleeding into the head or brain parenchyma** is the most serious ECMO complication. It can be extensive and fatal. **Bleeding post chest tube placement** is a common complication even if all appropriate steps are taken during tube placement. It may occur early or after several days. **Mucous membranes:** Bleeding from the nasopharynx, mouth, trachea, rectum, or bladder commonly occurs with patient care. Patients should not have rectal temperatures, rectal suppositories, or receive intramuscular medications. Bladder catheterizations should be avoided if possible. **GI bleeding** can occur from gastritis from sump placement/local irritation. Acid suppression medication is often adequate, although gastric lavage with saline may be indicated to evaluate for ongoing bleeding. Topical agents, such as Carafate and Mylanta, should be avoided due to an unacceptably high aluminum content.	**Clots** in the circuit (oxygenator, bridge, bladder, hemofilter, or other) are the most common mechanical complications. They are common with respiratory than cardiac ECMO runs. **Detection** requires careful visual examination of the circuit using a strong light source. **Clots are dark** (red, brown, black) nonmoving areas seen on the circuit, typically in areas of alterations in flow (reservoir, oxygenator, and connectors). Small preoxygenator clots may not require intervention other than continuing observation and monitoring. **Light-colored thrombi** (white, cream) consisting of platelets and fibrin are often observed in areas of turbulent flow such as at tubing/connector ends. Typically, no intervention is required unless a significant change is observed in color, size, or mobility causing concern for dislodgement. **Intervention** ranges from isolated component changes versus consideration to change the entire circuit.

CNS, central nervous system; ECMO, extracorporeal membrane oxygenation; GI, gastrointestinal.

Source: Adapted from Wild, K.T., Rintoul, N., Kattan, J., & Gray, B. (2020). Extracorporeal Life Support Organization (ELSO): Guidelines for neonatal respiratory failure. *ASAIO Journal, 66*(5), 463–470. https://doi.org/10.1097/MAT.0000000000001153

of care. However, iNO has shown other benefits in laboratory studies, such as reducing oxidative stress, decreasing lung inflammation, and enhancing alveolarization and lung growth. It is for these reasons that studies on reducing bronchopulmonary dysplasia (BPD) in preterm newborns have been done. There have been several randomized controlled trials (RCTs) that have been completed over the last 2 decades. Initial results were promising, demonstrating a reduction in BPD in subsets of preterm newborns; however, subsequent trials failed to confirm these benefits. Thereafter, the AAP, NIH, and Pediatric Pulmonary Hypertension Network published statements that the use of iNO to prevent BPD is not supported by the available evidence (Table 15.5; AAP, 2000; Cole et al., 2011; Kinsella et al., 2016; P. Kumar & Committee on Fetus and Newborn, 2014; Hansmann et al., 2019). One important positive result from these clinical trials was that iNO was not found to be associated with any increased risks to preterm newborns. However, iNO is still an expensive therapy and judicious use only in patients with the highest likelihood of benefit is prudent.

Consequently, there are some clinical case reports that have demonstrated benefits for preterm newborns who have HRF with PPHN due to prolonged oligohydramnios and pulmonary hypoplasia. The pathophysiology of HRF with PPHN from prolonged oligohydramnios and pulmonary hypoplasia is similar to that of the PPHN in term/near-term newborns in the clinical trials that initially led to FDA approval of iNO. Neonates who are affected by prolonged oligohydramnios and pulmonary hypoplasia have HRF and PPHN in their first days of life, much like term and near-term newborns with PPHN from failed transition to extrauterine life. Several of these case reports have described preterm newborns with severe HRF and PPHN in their first few days of life that were treated with iNO resulting in improvement in oxygenation and PPHN. The recent AAP statement fails to address iNO use in preterm newborns with PPHN from prolonged oligohydramnios or pulmonary hypoplasia; however, the NIH has concluded that "there are rare clinical situations, including pulmonary hypertension and pulmonary hypoplasia, that have been inadequately studied in which iNO may have benefit in newborns born < 34 weeks of gestation" and that "use in this population should be left to the clinical discretion" (Kinsella et al., 2016, p. 313). Currently there are substantial barriers to large RCTs for preterm newborns with prolonged oligohydramnios or pulmonary hypoplasia due to study design concerns. Because preterm newborns are not ECMO candidates, the only primary outcome measure for a preterm newborn would be mortality, unlike the term studies that use a combined outcome of mortality and ECMO. Future retrospective studies may not provide enough detail to be informative either. Thus, prospective registry may provide outcome comparisons that would aid in the debate of iNO use in preterm newborns.

TABLE 15.5 Guideline Recommendations for Nitric Oxide in Neonates

GUIDELINE	KEY RECOMMENDATIONS REGARDING INDICATIONS FOR iNO
AAP (2000)	• iNO should only be used for FDA-approved indications (≥34 weeks' gestation with PPHN). • All other uses are considered "experimental."
NIH (2011)	• Do not recommend iNO use for routine or rescue treatment for <34 weeks' gestation neonates. • In rare clinical situations (e.g., pulmonary hypertension or hypoplasia), iNO can be considered.
AAP (2014)	• Do not recommend routine or rescue iNO treatment for <34 weeks' (no benefit on survival, BPD, or neurodevelopmental outcomes).
AHA/ATS (2016)	• iNO may be beneficial for preterm infants with PPHN, especially if associated with PPROM or oligohydramnios.
EPPVDN/AEPC/ESPR/ISHLT (2019)	• iNO may be considered for <34 weeks' with respiratory failure and confirmed pulmonary hypertension.

AAP, American Academy of Pediatrics; AEPC, Association for European Pediatric and Congenital Cardiology; AHA, American Heart Association; ATS, American Thoracic Society; BPD, bronchopulmonary dysplasia; EPPVDN, Europenia Pediatric Pulmonary Vascular Disease Network; ESPR, European Society for Pediatric Research; FDA, U.S. Food and Drug Administration; iNO, inhaled nitric oxide; ISHLT, International Society of Heart and Lung Transplantation; NIH, National Institutes of Health; PPROM, preterm premature rupture of membranes.

CHRONIC PULMONARY HYPERTENSION (COR PULMONALE)

Concerns have been raised regarding long-term pulmonary morbidity in newborns who experience PPHN, particularly those who develop a persistent, chronic state of PPHN. Consider, for example, former preterm infants who develop BPD-associated PPHN. While the corrected gestational age at which BPD-associated PPHN develops is typically at or near term, an age commensurate with eligibility for iNO therapy, the associated pathophysiology may preclude this therapy. Affected infants usually manifest with arteriovenous maldevelopment, vascular remodeling, and increased vasoreactivity. In these cases, pulmonary vasodilators may be ineffective or cause pulmonary wedge pressures to deteriorate.

The overall goals of pharmacologic management of chronic pulmonary hypertension are to (a) increase pulmonary arterial vasodilation, (b) unload pressure to support the right ventricle, (c) avoid coronary artery ischemia and heart failure, (d) improve clinical outcomes and quality of life, and (e) improve signs and symptoms to reduce aggravation of pulmonary hypertension. Bosentan is the only FDA-approved therapy for infants and children with pulmonary hypertension. However, clinicians also prescribe oral sildenafil to manage affected infants. For patients with very severe disease, escalation to chronic prostaglandins (subcutaneous, inhaled, or more recently oral routes) may be required.

CONCLUSIONS

Our understanding of the pathophysiology and management of PPHN has greatly improved over the past 50 years. This includes the biochemical pathways leading to vasoconstriction of pulmonary vasculature, differentiation between different etiologies of PPHN, the use of pulmonary vasodilators, and more. The gold standard for prompt diagnosis of PPHN includes the use of bedside ECHO, which also provides continued monitoring of the disease process and response to treatments. The gold standard pulmonary vasodilator of choice for PPHN is iNO. Ventilation strategies have evolved over time from previously utilizing hyperoxygenation-hyperventilation-alkalosis to the current methods of gentle ventilation strategies. Overall, there has been a dramatic reduction in the need for ECMO with all these interventions and others that have been highlighted in this chapter. All clinical practitioners should be aware of the first-line recommendations for the management of the newborn with PPHN as well as which additional newer agents may be considered in those with refractory PPHN in order to improve outcomes.

LEARNING TOOLS AND RESOURCES

Advice From the Authors

Deborah S. Bondi, PharmD, FCCP, BCPS, BCPPS

The best way to understand the pathophysiology and treatment algorithm of a disease is to explain them out loud in your own words. Trying to simply memorize and recite these processes do not generally result in fundamental understanding. Break it down into simple terms and work your own way through it.

Mary Hurley, DNP, APRN, NNP-BC

There are two very important pieces of information for readers. The first is when managing a neonate with PPHN, early transfer to an ECMO center is crucial. Survival rates are significantly lower for outborn infants compared to inborn infants. This is likely from the delay in initiating ECMO. Second, early intervention with iNO can improve PPHN mortality. Studies have shown that infants treated with iNO earlier than the control groups responded more favorably to iNO.

Discussion Prompts

1. Describe the pathophysiology of transitioning from fetal to extrauterine circulation and where this breakdown can occur, resulting in PPHN. Connect risk factors for PPHN and how many of them tie back to interfering with the transition from normal fetal to extrauterine circulation.
2. Compare the different types of PPHN. Why would maladaptation be the most common but also have the highest rate of survival?
3. Which clinical features of PPHN overlap with other respiratory and cardiac diseases in newborns? What diagnostic criteria would help you in differentiating these diseases?
4. Discuss the various nonpharmacologic and pharmacologic methods available to manage PPHN. Walk through your management strategy and treatment algorithm for the newborn who presents in PPHN. When would you consider iNO? ECMO?

Mind Map

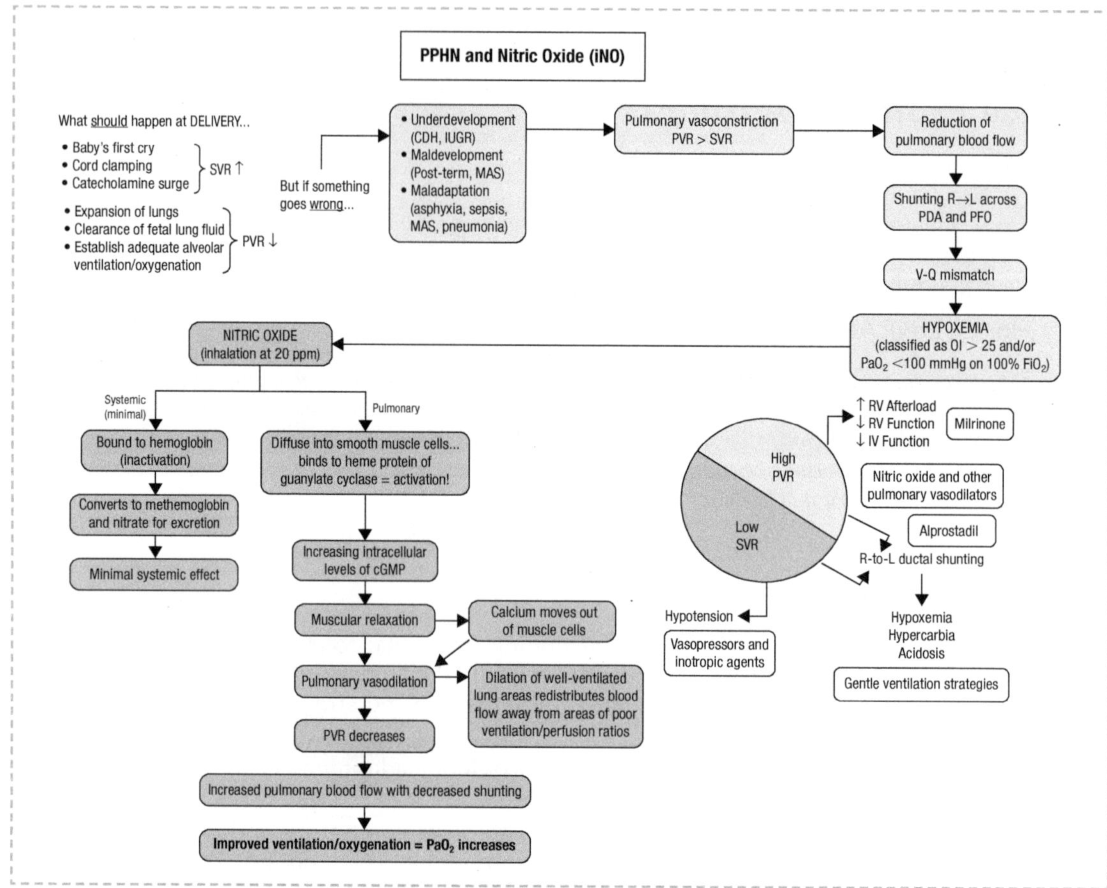

Note: This mind map reflects the design team's interpretation of a portion of one or more concepts addressed in this chapter. Readers should regard the mind maps woven throughout this textbook as examples of multisensory study tools that can be developed to encourage conceptual understanding. Readers are encouraged to develop their own unique mind maps in consultation with academic faculty or clinical preceptors.
CDH, congenital diaphragmatic hernia; cGMP, cyclic guanosine monophosphate; IUGR, intrauterine growth restriction; LV, left ventricle; MAS, meconium aspiration syndrome; OI, oxygenation index; PDA, patent ductus arteriosus; PFO, patent foramen ovale; PPHN, persistent pulmonary hypertension of the newborn; PVR, pulmonary vascular resistance; RV, right ventricle; SVR, systemic vascular resistance.
Design credit: Elizabeth Jones, MSN, APRN, NNP, RNC-NIC, East Carolina University Neonatal Nurse Practitioner Program.

REFERENCES

References for this chapter are online and available at https://connect.springerpub.com/content/book/978-0-8261-5884-0/part/partIII/toc-part/ch15.

chapter 16

Bronchopulmonary Dysplasia

Macrina Liguori, Sarah Croop, and Andrea N. Trembath

LEARNING OBJECTIVES

After completing this chapter, the reader should be able to:

- Define *bronchopulmonary dysplasia* (*BPD*) and identify the epidemiology of the disease process.
- Review the physiology of fetal lung development.
- Examine the pathophysiology of BPD.
- Appraise the historical evolution of pharmacologic management of BPD.
- Investigate current pharmacologic therapies for treatment of BPD.

INTRODUCTION

Bronchopulmonary dysplasia (BPD) is the most common morbidity of prematurity and yet its causes and outcomes are often hard to define. From a pathologic perspective, it is a developmental disruption in lung growth and maturation that can be seen on microscopy. From a clinical perspective, it manifests with decreased oxygenation, as well as increased work of breathing and susceptibility to pathogens and environmental factors.

Depending on the severity of BPD, the impact of the disease can be lifelong. Infants with BPD have longer initial hospitalizations, higher rates of readmission, lower health-related quality-of-life measures, and higher costs of healthcare (Gough et al., 2012; Katz-Salamon et al., 2000; McAleese et al., 1993). In the United States, 10,000 to 15,000 new diagnoses of BPD are made annually. However, the incidence varies widely between centers (ranging from 32% to 74%) for infants born between 22 and 24 weeks' gestation (Ambalavanan et al., 2011). The risk of BPD and severity increase with decreasing gestational age (GA); surviving infants born at 22 weeks' GA have the highest risk. In this chapter, we explore how the pharmacologic and nonpharmacologic therapies aimed at reducing BPD point to a complex and likely "multihit" pathway.

DEFINITION

The preferred term for chronic lung disease (CLD) of prematurity is *BPD*; however, it is also commonly referred to as *CLD* in the clinical setting. Use of this clinical terminology has several disadvantages: (a) CLD is very nonspecific and does not indicate the etiology of the disease, allowing confusion with other childhood and adult lung diseases such as cystic fibrosis and pulmonary fibrosis; and (b) CLD does not distinguish the unique and important role prematurity plays in the etiology. In 2001, the National Institute of Child Health and Human Development (NICHD) held a workshop to develop a consensus on the diagnostic criteria for BPD and to distinguish this disease from other CLDs with the creation of a severity-based definition (Jobe & Bancalari, 2001).

Although there is no universal definition of BPD, the three most commonly used definitions all have specific limitations in clinical practice (Table 16.1). The challenges related to defining BPD include that the current definitions all measure a single point in time and a waiting period must occur, making early identification and targeted therapies (pharmacologic and nonpharmacologic) challenging (Ehrenkranz et al., 2005). In addition, although BPD may be categorized as mild, moderate, or severe, the diagnosis alone is not informative of the functional outcomes for the infant and the family (Gough et al., 2012).

The most common definition of BPD used in clinical practice is the receipt of supplemental oxygen at 28 days of life (Figure 16.1). Although this definition is simple and easy to assess, with the

TABLE 16.1 National Institute of Child Health and Human Development Severity-Based Definition of Bronchopulmonary Dysplasia

GESTATIONAL AGE AT BIRTH	MILD BPD	MODERATE BPD	SEVERE BPD
<32 weeks	Room air at 36 weeks' PMA or discharge	<30% oxygen at 36 weeks' PMA or discharge	≥30% oxygen and/or positive pressure at 36 weeks' PMA
≥32 weeks	Room air by 56 days' postnatal age or discharge	<30% oxygen at 56 days' postnatal age or discharge	≥30% oxygen and/or positive pressure at 56 days' postnatal age or discharge

Note: All categories require treatment with more than 21% oxygen for at least 28 days, then assessment at PMA/postnatal day or discharge, whichever comes first.

BPD, bronchopulmonary dysplasia; PMA, postmenstrual age.

Source: From Jobe, A. H., & Bancalari, E. (2001). Bronchopulmonary dysplasia. *American Journal of Respiratory and Critical Care Medicine, 163*(7), 1723–1729. https://doi.org/10.1164/ajrccm.163.7.2011060.

FIGURE 16.1 History of bronchopulmonary dysplasia.

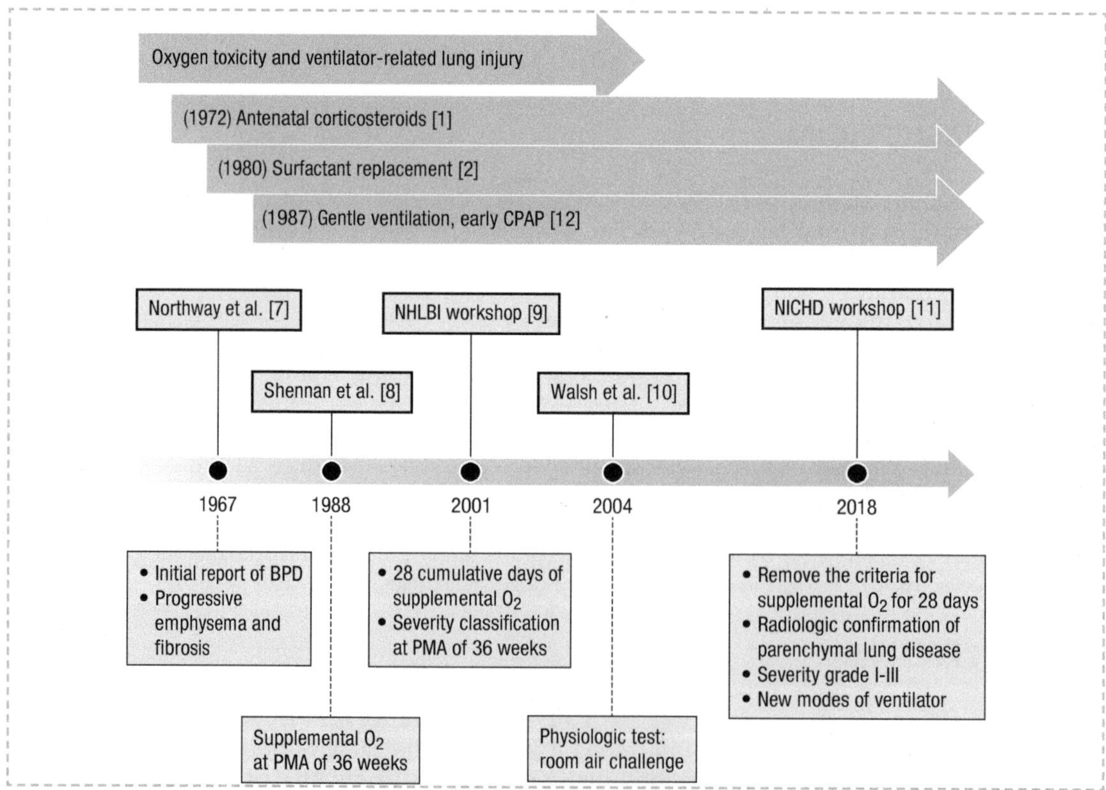

BPD, bronchopulmonary dysplasia; CPAP, continuous positive airway pressure; NHLBI, National Heart, Lung, and Blood Institute; NICHD, National Institute of Child Health and Human Development; PMA, postmenstrual age.

Source: From Wang, S-H., & Tsao, P-N. (2020). Phenotypes of bronchopulmonary dysplasia. *International Journal of Molecular Sciences, 21*, 6112. https://doi.org/10.3390/ijms21176112.

survival of smaller and more gestationally immature infants (e.g., 22- and 23-week postmenstrual age [PMA]), it does not take into account the developmental maturity and degree of interruption that may occur at the extremes of prematurity. In addition, it remains unclear what optimal oxygen saturation target ranges may be for each level of maturity and what the clinical practices are across different NICUs. An alternative definition of BPD is the need for supplemental oxygen at 36 weeks' PMA. However, this definition also suffers from the same limitations as the receipt of oxygen at 28 days. To address these issues, the *physiologic definition* for BPD was developed by Walsh and colleagues (2004) in an attempt to consider developmental maturation and standardize practices. In this definition, BPD is diagnosed by a failure to maintain oxygen saturations greater than 90% when given a room-air trial at 36 weeks' PMA. This physiologic definition was shown to reduce intercenter variability, as well as reduce the diagnosis of BPD by as much as 10%. Yet this definition has still not been fully adopted at many centers due to the more labor-intensive nature of making this diagnosis (Natarajan et al., 2012).

PHYSIOLOGY REVIEW: FETAL LUNG DEVELOPMENT

Lung development, growth, structure, and function are dependent on a variety of key factors occurring at the precise moment in fetal development. During the early embryonic phases of lung development (weeks 0–7), the large airways, such as the trachea and the mainstem bronchi, are formed (Figure 16.2). In the pseudoglandular stage (weeks 8–17), the terminal bronchioles and primary blood supply are formed. The extremely low GA neonates (22–27 weeks) are typically in the canalicular phase of development during which the respiratory bronchioles and primitive alveoli are formed. Preterm birth during this GA window, therefore, arrests the normal developmental pathway and contributes to the physiology of early respiratory distress syndrome (RDS) and later BPD (A. J. Jobe, 1999). With only primitive alveoli, there is little or inefficient gas exchange possible. After 27 weeks,

FIGURE 16.2 Stages of fetal lung development.

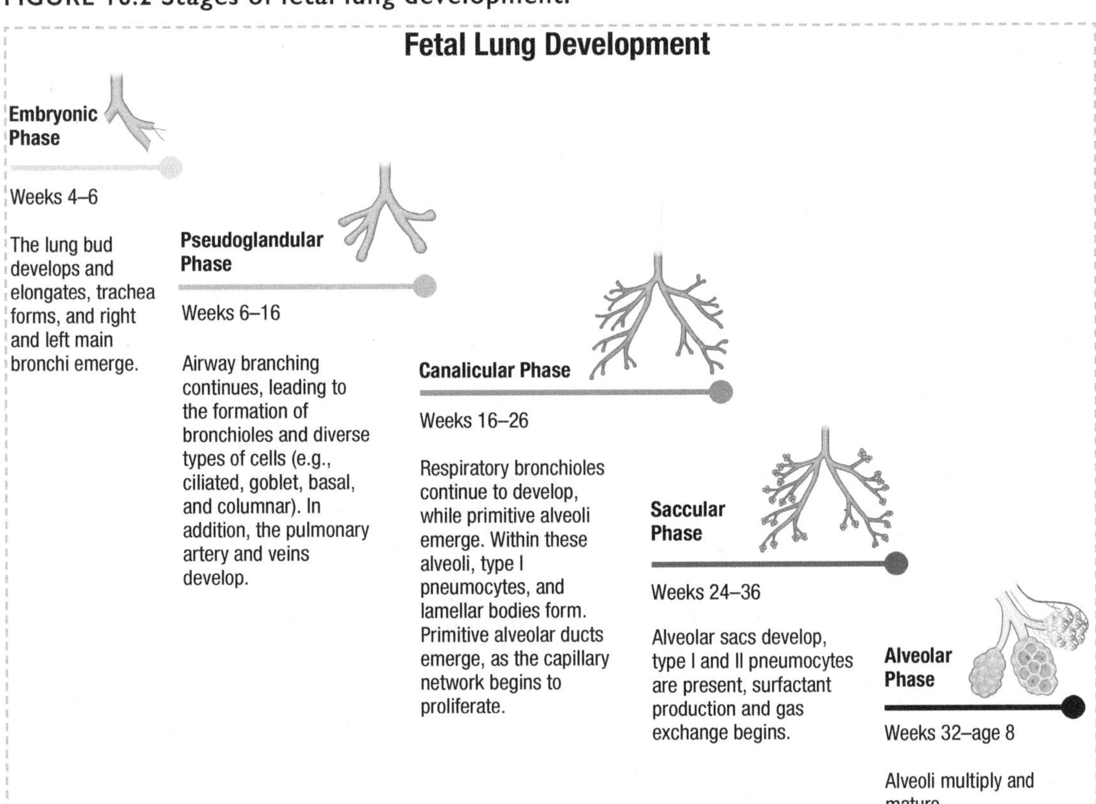

during the saccular stage of development, further expansion of the alveoli and more efficient gas exchange can occur. However, the absence of surfactant until about 28 weeks' gestation leads to the need for supplemental oxygen and positive pressure, both of which influence the incidence of BPD.

PATHOPHYSIOLOGY OF BRONCHOPULMONARY DYSPLASIA

The pathogenesis of BPD is complex and multifactorial, challenging the clinician's ability to accurately predict who will develop BPD, as well as disease severity. It is widely accepted that the development of BPD occurs amid a complex interplay between risk factors and protective effects (Trembath & Laughon, 2012). Although a single risk factor may lead to BPD, the disease most often manifests secondary to multiple hits. This interrupts the customary balance between risk and protection and normally increases the likelihood of developing a disease. We present these hits in the following paragraphs.

Often, the reasons for premature birth (e.g., chorioamnionitis, placental insufficiency/maternal preeclampsia, smoking, medication exposure) precipitate interrupted and abnormal lung development secondary to fetal exposure to inflammatory mediators, such as cytokines (Been & Zimmerman, 2009; Bose et al., 2009). This incomplete lung development at birth sets the stage for BPD in multiple ways.

Although gentle fetal breathing movements (which generate negligible tidal volume) are detected prenatally, this does not infer that preterm lungs are equipped to deal with the stretch created by the inhalation of air after birth. Premature lungs are stiff and noncompliant. They require high ventilatory support pressures to maintain functional residual capacity. Positive airway pressure, although necessary to permit gas exchange, subjects the lungs to direct barotrauma. In addition, to protect against atelectotrauma, positive end-expiratory pressures are often applied to lungs not yet ready to be stretched or exposed to air and oxygen.

Neonatal ventilation, although lifesaving, induces mechanical stretch injury, provocation of an exaggerated inflammatory response, and disruption of the normal developmental architecture of the lungs. This stretch injury ultimately leads to a disruption in alveolarization, even among well-appearing late-preterm infants (McEvoy et al., 2013). On histologic examination, altered alveolar number and capillary development can be seen, suggesting both mechanical injury as well as an increased inflammatory response due to mechanical ventilation are to blame. This pathology can develop rapidly. In animal models, altered elastin has been observed within 1 day of birth. Alterations in structure, cell death pathways, and proliferation have been observed at 3 days' PMA (Ogihara et al., 1999).

One of the most challenging aspects of preventing BPD is that diagnosis occurs *after* the disease state is already present and nonmodifiable. Several models have been developed in an attempt to pinpoint infants early in their clinical course and allow mitigation. However, although these models have low negative predictive values, they also have low positive predictive values, which limit their clinical utility. Today, the most frequently used predictive model in clinical practice and for research purposes was created by Laughon et al. (2011). The web-based calculator was developed using data from the Neonatal Research Network, a large multicenter collaborative, and can be used to determine the risk of a diagnosis of BPD (and severity) at a number of time points throughout the first month of life. The calculator is available at https://neonatal.rti.org and uses data based on GA, sex, race/ethnicity, respiratory support, and oxygen requirement. We encourage students and trainees to explore this calculator and discuss ways clinicians may use data in the hospital setting.

HISTORICAL PERSPECTIVE: SEMINAL AND OTHER NOTEWORTHY STUDIES

In this section, we discuss the evolution of the diagnosis of BPD, along with several key studies and their impact on clinical practices. The pharmacotherapeutics used in the management of BPD, their mechanisms of action, dosing, monitoring, and relative impacts on the disease are discussed later in the chapter.

The first case descriptions of BPD were written by Dr. William Northway, a radiologist at Stanford University Medical Center. Dr. Northway described the clinical and radiologic evidence of a new disease in a series of 32 preterm infants born between 1962 and 1965. All of these preterm infants had recovered from severe RDS with the assistance of mechanical ventilation and oxygen therapy, which were relatively new advances in neonatal care at the time (Northway, 1990;

Northway et al., 1976). Prior to the availability of mechanical ventilation and oxygen therapy, the standard treatment of RDS consisted of supportive care, including thermoregulation and nutritional support. Infants who survived RDS recovered by day 3 of life without radiographic or clinical sequela of pulmonary disease. The BPD initially described by Northway, now known as "old" BPD, reflected the surviving patient population and therapies available at that time. Infants with "old" BPD were generally born between 30 and 36 weeks' PMA and exposed to prolonged courses of mechanical ventilation and large amounts of oxygen. On chest radiographs, diffuse heterogeneity of the lung fields was described with coarse reticular areas of hyperlucent lung tissue that represented emphysematous alveoli. Histologic examination further demonstrated areas of hyperinflation alternating with areas of focal collapse, hyperplasia of the bronchial epithelium, and fibrosis.

Following the initial descriptions of BPD, questions arose regarding the role of oxygen and barotrauma in the pathogenesis of this disease. Attempts to limit these exposures led to significant advances in neonatal care, and the availability of exogenous surfactant led to the survival of more premature infants. As a result, premature infants (<28 weeks of gestation) in the modern era are exposed to less oxygen and fewer days of positive pressure. These infants develop what is now known as "new" BPD. Radiographically, "new" BPD involves more diffuse, scattered, and course opacities compared with the "old" BPD (Figure 16.3). However, the areas of hyperinflation due to the emphysematous alveoli are less obvious. On histologic examination, a reduced number of alveoli are seen as is a minimal amount of fibrosis.

Since the first description of BPD by Northway, thousands of studies have investigated the antecedents and mitigating actions for BPD development (see Table 16.2 for landmark studies). Unfortunately, predictive factors are easy to identify but difficult to modify (Table 16.3). Many of the strongest predictors of BPD are nonmodifiable, including GA, birth weight, gender, and race/ethnicity. Pharmacologic and nonpharmacologic interventions have had mixed evidence to support their use as prevention for BPD, such as treating patent ductus arteriosus (PDA) or gentle ventilation strategies intended to limit exposure to barotrauma. In the case of reducing barotrauma with positive pressure or direct oxygen toxicity of oxygen exposure, the balancing factor may be in survival of the smallest infants, and generally the development of BPD has been an accepted trade-off.

FIGURE 16.3 Pathologic features of "old," "new," and severe bronchopulmonary dysplasia; severe bronchopulmonary dysplasia demonstrates mixed pathologic features of both "old" and "new" bronchopulmonary dysplasia, with arrest in lung development as well as significant lung injury.

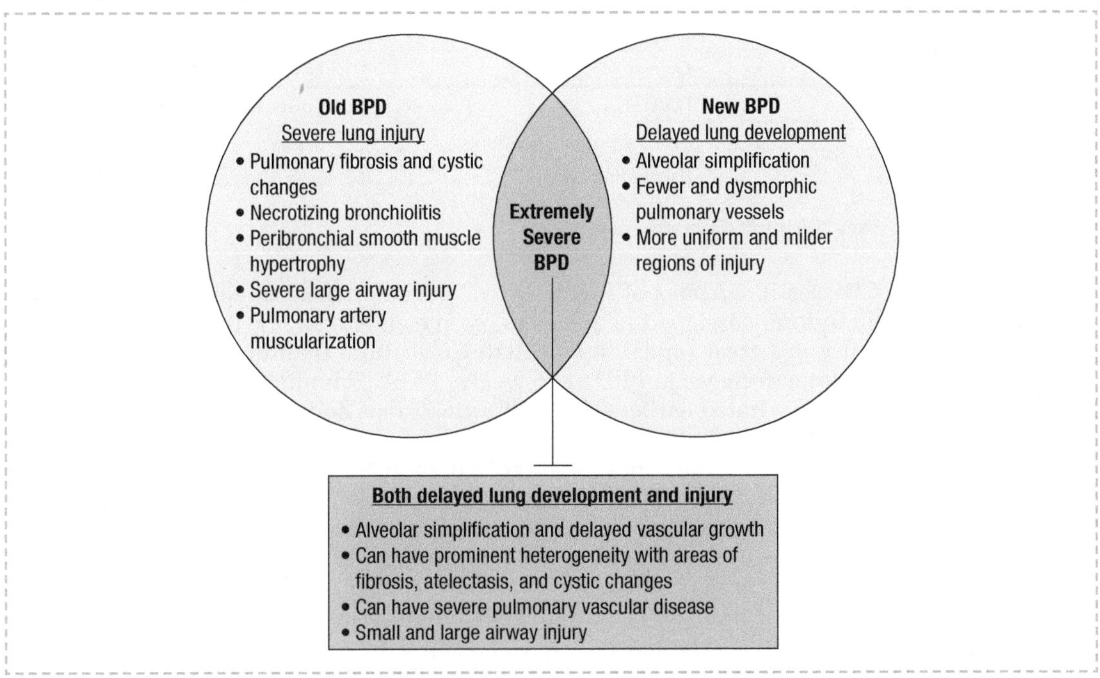

BPD, bronchopulmonary dysplasia.

Source: From Obgyn Key. (n.d.). *Management of the infant with bronchopulmonary dysplasia.* https://obgynkey.com/management-of-the-infant-with-bronchopulmonary-dysplasia.

TABLE 16.2 Landmark Studies for Bronchopulmonary Dysplasia

STUDY NAME	INVESTIGATOR	YEAR	KEY FINDINGS	RISK CHANGE	NNT
	Northway	1967	The study provides the first description of BPD in former preterm infants exposed to oxygen and mechanical ventilation.		
Caffeine for Apnea of Prematurity trial	Schmidt et al.	2006	Caffeine citrate used for treatment of apnea of prematurity reduces the incidence of BPD.	OR: 0.64, 95% CI: 0.52–0.78	9
Vitamin A	Tyson	1999	Vitamin A supplementation for infants <1,000 grams decreases the incidence of BPD.	RR: 0.89, 95% CI: 0.80–0.99	14
Dexamethasone: A Randomized Trial	L. W. Doyle et al.	2006	Low-dose dexamethasone did not reduce the incidence of BPD.	OR: 0.58, 95% CI: 0.13–2.66	
SUPPORT	Carlo	2010	Limiting oxygen exposure did not decrease the incidence of BPD.	RR: 0.91, 95% CI: 0.83–1.01	

BPD, bronchopulmonary dysplasia; NNT, number needed to treat; OR, odds ratio; RR, relative risk; SUPPORT, Surfactant Positive Airway Pressure and Pulse Oximetry Trial.

TABLE 16.3 Risk Factors for Bronchopulmonary Dysplasia

DECREASES RISK OF BPD	NO OR UNCLEAR EFFECT ON BPD	INCREASES RISK OF BPD
Caffeine	Antenatal Steroids	Chorioamnionitis
Dexamethasone	Exogenous surfactant	Small for gestational age
Vitamin A	Oxygen	Lower gestational age
Female Sex	PDA	Lower birth weight
	Limiting positive pressure	Sepsis
	Race/ethnicity	

BPD, bronchopulmonary dysplasia; PDA, patent ductus arteriosus.

As discussed in Chapter 10, "Apnea of Prematurity," the landmark Caffeine for Apnea of Prematurity (CAP) trial randomly assigned neonates to receive either caffeine or placebo during the first 10 days to prevent apnea, treat apnea, and facilitate extubation. Treatment with caffeine in this trial led to an 11% absolute decrease in BPD at 36 weeks' PMA (Schmidt et al., 2006). The infants treated with caffeine demonstrated earlier successful extubations and discontinuation of positive airway pressure by 1 week. They were also weaned to room air earlier than the infants in the control group. Other studies, although not necessarily demonstrating a difference in BPD, have observed significant decreases in the need for invasive ventilation and/or use of supplemental oxygen, as well as a reduction in extubation failure (Henderson-Smart & Davis, 2010).

The seminal studies on the use of vitamin A (VA) to prevent BPD were published in the 1980s and 1990s. One of the largest trials comparing VA with a control, an NICHD-sponsored multicenter, randomized controlled trial (RCT), enrolled 807 infants. This study demonstrated that for extremely low-birth-weight (ELBW) infants, there was a slight decrease in the risk of death or BPD in the group treated with VA (55% vs. 62%; relative risk [RR]: 0.89, 95% CI: 0.80–0.99). Further, researchers identified that the number needed to treat (NNT) to prevent one case of BPD was 14 infants, a relatively low NNT (Tyson et al., 1999). These formative studies, 11 in total, including the work of Tyson et al., are well summarized in the Cochrane Database of Systematic Reviews. The Cochrane review reports an overall "modest" reduction in the incidence of BPD with intramuscular (IM) administration of VA for very-low-birth-weight (VLBW) infants (Darlow et al., 2016). More recently, a systematic review and meta-analysis of four trials found that VA supplementation for ELBW infants is potentially effective in decreasing oxygen dependency at 36 weeks' PMA (Araki et al., 2018).

The association between improved respiratory outcomes and corticosteroids has been established; however, the ideal corticosteroid, dosing, and timing of administration has not been clearly demonstrated. Prolonged, high-dose courses of dexamethasone were used in the late 1990s and 2000s to decrease respiratory support; however, they came with a detriment of neurodevelopmental impairment (NDI) in surviving infants and subsequently fell out of favor (Doyle et al., 2021a, and Doyle et al., 2021b). In 2006, L. W. Doyle et al. examined the role of a short course (10 days) of dexamethasone in Dexamethasone: A Randomized Trial (DART; L. W. Doyle et al., 2006). The multicenter trial examined the outcomes of infants known to be at high risk of BPD (<28 weeks' PMA or <1,000 grams) who remained on mechanical ventilation after 7 days of life. The infants were randomized to receive either a tapering dose of dexamethasone over 10 days or placebo. Infants who received dexamethasone were more likely to be extubated by the last dose of dexamethasone compared with placebo (60% vs. 12%), without a difference in rates of NDI. Of note, 85% of infants exposed to dexamethasone had BPD at 36 weeks as compared with 91% among the placebo-exposed infants. Although this is a modest reduction in BPD rate and not found to be statistically significant (OR: 0.58, 95% CI: 0.13–2.66), dexamethasone may elicit a risk reduction in infants at highest risk for BPD or NDI (L. W. Doyle et al., 2007; Watterberg et al., 2010). It should be noted that these findings may be the result of a true relationship between dexamethasone and BPD; however, they may also be due to a lack of statistical power to detect a causal relationship as the trial was stopped early due to low recruitment.

Recent clinical trials have examined the role of hydrocortisone for BPD prevention. As a corticosteroid with balanced glucocorticoid and mineralocorticoid activity, hydrocortisone may have a superior safety profile to dexamethasone; however, as a much less potent glucocorticoid, relative efficacy remains an area of active concern for clinicians. In 2016, the Early Prevention of Bronchopulmonary Dysplasia and Neonatal Mortality in Very Preterm Infants Using Low Dose of Hydrocortisone (PREMILOC) trial (N = 523) documented improved BPD-free survival in premature neonates treated with low-dose, prophylactic hydrocortisone initiated on the first day after birth and continued for 10 days compared with placebo (60% vs. 51%, p = .04; Baud et al., 2016). Prophylactic hydrocortisone did not increase the risk of spontaneous intestinal perforation in this trial, possibly due to prohibition of nonsteroidal anti-inflammatory drugs (NSAIDs) within the first 24 hours of life. Prophylactic hydrocortisone also did not increase the risk of long-term NDI, including cerebral palsy (CP), at 2 years of age (Baud et al., 2017). Late hydrocortisone therapy also holds some promise. In 2019, the Systemic Hydrocortisone to Prevent Bronchopulmonary Dysplasia in preterm infants (STOP-BPD) trial (N = 372) documented a significant reduction in mortality among ventilator-dependent premature neonates randomized to hydrocortisone compared with placebo between 7 and 14 days of life (15.5% vs. 23.7%, p = .048; Onland et al., 2019). Although the intervention did facilitate earlier extubation, hydrocortisone did not alter the incidence of BPD. As with prophylactic therapy, no differences were detected in the incidence of NDIs at 2 years of age (Halbmeijer et al., 2021). In the setting of outstanding questions regarding the anti-inflammatory potency of hydrocortisone, and thus its role in the prevention of BPD, dexamethasone remains the standard corticosteroid used for BPD prevention in most units. However, trainees should continue to monitor emerging literature regarding the relative efficacy and safety of alternative corticosteroids.

CURRENT NONPHARMACOLOGIC PREVENTIVE STRATEGIES

As BPD is a result of complex interactions, few therapies have been shown to dramatically increase or decrease the risk of developing the disease. From a statistical perspective, the nonpharmacologic strategies in particular have little evidence to strongly support their use in clinical practice. However, both nonpharmacologic and pharmacologic management concepts related to the mitigation of BPD pathogenesis are covered here.

Limiting Mechanical Ventilation

Mechanical ventilation is an essential part of the care of the extremely premature infant. Lung injury, however, is an established complication of prolonged mechanical ventilation. As previously discussed, damage can be caused by barotrauma, volutrauma, or atelectotrauma. Preventing lung injury begins in the delivery room, by limiting pressures and volume delivered and preventing atelectasis, and continues into NICU management (Leone et al., 2006) Recommendations for delivery room management include avoiding "hand bagging" by using a pressure-limited device and transitioning as soon as feasibly possible to a ventilator on which tidal volumes can be both measured and displayed (Finer et al., 2004). In the delivery room, this can be accomplished by limiting chest wall expansion by using the minimal necessary volume and pressure. The Neonatal Resuscitation Program (NRP) now recognizes the benefits of preserving functional residual capacity using continuous positive airway pressure (CPAP) for infants not requiring intubation (American Heart Association [AHA] NRP, 2021).

Early strategies related to the timing and administration of surfactant have not demonstrated a direct reduction in BPD risk; however, the administration of surfactant significantly reduces the risk of mortality due to severe RDS (Carlo et al., 2010). In the Surfactant Positive Airway Pressure and Pulse Oximetry Trial (SUPPORT), two strategies related to surfactant administration were examined: (a) early prophylactic surfactant administration and (b) initial management with CPAP and administration of surfactant if/when endotracheal intubation occurred. The hypothesis was that early prophylactic surfactant administration would lead to an improvement in the primary outcome of death or BPD; however, no association was seen (RR with CPAP: 0.95, 95% CI: 0.85–1.05). Several secondary outcomes, including reduced need for postnatal corticosteroids and fewer days of mechanical ventilation, were seen in infants initially managed with CPAP ($p < .001$, $p = .03$), suggesting that it may be beneficial toward reducing BPD risk (Carlo et al., 2010).

Judicious Use of Supplemental Oxygen

A link between oxygen supplementation and BPD has been established since the original descriptions were created by Northway; however, whether oxygen is directly responsible for the cascade of lung damage resulting in BPD is unclear. In laboratory studies, oxygen exposure to lung tissues results in the production of superoxides, hydrogen peroxide, and free radicals that can damage developing alveoli (Delacourt et al., 1996). These by-products lead to inactivation of key enzymes needed in protein synthesis and metabolism and alter cell membranes through lipid peroxidation. In animal models, exposure to high fractional inspired oxygen concentrations results in DNA breakage and triggers apoptosis pathways (Ogihara et al., 1999). Among studies of neonates, the deleterious effects of oxygen may be less direct. Oxygen may be a marker of severity of illness, which leads to its association with BPD. In the SUPPORT trial, infants who received higher amounts of supplemental oxygen therapy to maintain higher target oxygen saturation levels had similar rates of death or BPD when compared with the lower oxygen saturation target group (48.5% vs. 54.2%, RR: 0.91, 95% CI: 0.83–1.01). These findings along with a lower risk of death in the higher oxygen-exposed groups suggest oxygen's association with BPD is as a surrogate marker of illness (Carlo et al., 2010).

Optimizing Enteral Nutrition

Early, aggressive nutritional support in premature infants has become a mainstay of neonatal intensive care management. Few studies exist to directly link either carbohydrate, protein, or fat supplementation and BPD. In addition, little evidence suggests the ideal amounts of essential nutritional components, yet a total daily energy intake during the first 7 days of life in ill neonates significantly influences the rates of BPD. For each increase of 1 kcal/kg/d of total energy intake, there is ~2% decrease in the outcomes of necrotizing enterocolitis (NEC), length of stay (LOS), and BPD (Ehrenkranz et al., 2011). In general, providing adequate macro/micronutrients and calories to see weight gain and linear and head growth has been the goal, as they may not only influence the rates of BPD, but are more clearly linked to improvements in NDI.

CURRENT PHARMACOLOGIC PREVENTIVE AND TREATMENT STRATEGIES

Caffeine Citrate

Caffeine citrate is routinely used in the NICU for both treatment of apnea of prematurity (AOP) and prevention of BPD. It is specifically approved by the U.S. Food and Drug Administration (FDA) for treatment of AOP in infants at 28 to 33 weeks' gestation. Although its use is off-label, caffeine is in fact one of the best evaluated treatments for reducing the risk of BPD (Thébaud et al., 2019). Given the frequency with which caffeine is prescribed in the NICU, we provide a summary of data explored in Chapter 10, "Apnea of Prematurity," to offer readers additional opportunity to apply core concepts to disease management.

MECHANISM OF ACTION/CORE PHARMACOKINETIC PRINCIPLES

Caffeine is a methylxanthine that acts as an adenosine receptor antagonist by competitively binding to adenosine receptors at the cell surface. Specifically, regarding the respiratory system, the pharmacologic effects of caffeine include stimulation of the respiratory center in the medulla; improved chemoreceptor sensitivity to carbon dioxide (CO_2); enhanced diaphragmatic contractility; as well as increased minute ventilation, tidal volume, and lung compliance. Caffeine also possesses mild bronchodilator, diuretic, and anti-inflammatory properties (Abdel-Hady et al., 2015; Dekker et al., 2017; Hennelly et al., 2021; Micromedex Neofax Online, n.d.-a; Picone et al., 2012).

The exact mechanism of action for reducing the risk of BPD is unknown. However, it has been suggested that the anti-inflammatory properties of caffeine may play a role in reducing the pathogenic mechanisms of BPD development (Hwang & Rehan, 2018; Picone et al., 2012; Principi et al., 2018). This risk reduction may also be derived from the improvements in pulmonary function mentioned previously and a decrease in the need for assisted ventilation (Abdel-Hady et al., 2015; Principi et al., 2018; Schmidt et al., 2006).

Route of administration does not affect the pharmacokinetics of caffeine citrate as the bioavailability is the same whether the medication is administered enterally or intravenously (IV). Caffeine is completely absorbed, with almost no first-pass metabolism, and it is rapidly distributed in the body. Caffeine reaches peak blood concentration in less than 2 hours, with central nervous system (CNS) levels approximating plasma levels. In neonates, it is largely excreted unchanged in the urine (approximately 86%), and the remainder is metabolized via the CYP1A2 enzyme system (Micromedex Neofax Online, n.d.-a). The half-life of caffeine ranges from 40 to 230 hours and decreases with advancing PMA until 60 weeks, although it can be prolonged in infants with cholestatic hepatitis (Abdel-Hady et al., 2015; Micromedex Neofax Online, n.d.-a). In a pharmacokinetic study of preterm infants treated with caffeine, serum levels were evaluated following discontinuation of therapy (at approximately 35 weeks' PMA). The mean half-life was 87 ± 25 hours and the mean serum caffeine concentrations were 13.3 mg/L at 24 hours and 4.3 mg/L at 168 hours after the last dose was administered. Of note, the caffeine was dosed at 5 mg/kg/d for the majority of infants in the study and the remainder received between 6 and 8 mg/kg/d (J. Doyle et al., 2016).

One small, observational study of infants less than 30 weeks' gestation demonstrated a significant decrease in interleukin-10 (IL-10) levels approximately 24 hours after the caffeine loading dose was administered. At 1 week from the initial loading dose, caffeine serum concentrations on the lower end of the therapeutic range directly correlated with tumor necrosis factor (TNF), interleukin-1β (IL-1β), and interleukin-6 (IL-6) levels. However, an inverse correlation was noted with caffeine levels >20 mg/L. Although many studies suggest benefit from the anti-inflammatory properties of caffeine, this study implies that supratherapeutic levels could be associated with a proinflammatory pulmonary profile and the authors advise caution with use of high-dose caffeine (Valdez et al., 2011).

DOSING RECOMMENDATIONS

As previously mentioned, because the route of administration does not affect the pharmacokinetics of caffeine, the dosing recommendations are the same whether caffeine is administered orally or IV. The CAP trial used a loading dose of 20 mg/kg of caffeine citrate. Maintenance dosing should be initiated 24 hours after administration of the loading dose and a dose of 5 to 10 mg/kg is recommended every 24 hours. A recent retrospective analysis of 89 preterm infants demonstrated little benefit in twice-daily dosing of maintenance caffeine (Rebentisch et al., 2021).

Several studies have examined the hypothesis that administration of caffeine at higher dosing compared with standard dosing may result in a reduction in extubation failure. In one RCT, Steer and colleagues (2004) gave preterm infants, less than 30 weeks' gestation, a higher loading dose (80 mg/kg) of caffeine citrate 24 hours before planned extubation. Those infants were compared with a cohort given a lower loading dose (20 mg/kg). The higher dosing group not only had a significant reduction in the rate of extubation failure (15.0% vs. 29.8%; RR: 0.51, 95% CI: 0.31–0.85; NNT: 7, 95% CI: 4–24), but also a significant reduction in the duration of mechanical ventilation for infants less than 28 weeks' gestation (mean [*SD*] days = 14.4 [11.1] vs. 22.1 [17.1], $p = .01$). No significant differences were noted between the cohorts in regard to mortality, major neonatal morbidity, death, or severe disability.

In a second randomized, double-blind study of 120 preterm infants less than 32 weeks' gestation, the use of higher loading doses (40 mg/kg caffeine citrate) and maintenance dosing (20 mg/kg caffeine citrate) was associated with a reduction in extubation failure (22% vs. 47%) in mechanically ventilated infants. The use of higher dosing was also associated with a decrease in the frequency of apnea (9 events vs. 16 events during caffeine therapy) and days of documented apnea (2.5 days vs. 5 days) without significant side effects compared with standard dose (20 mg/kg loading dose and 10 mg/kg/d maintenance dosing; Mohammed et al., 2015).

Given the benefits, an additional loading dose and/or higher maintenance doses could be considered, although several authors recommend monitoring the serum concentrations of caffeine in these cases (Eichenwald, 2016; Micromedex Neofax Online, n.d.-a; Schmidt et al., 2006). Caution should be used, giving consideration not only to the potential for a proinflammatory pulmonary profile associated with use of caffeine outside the therapeutic range, but also given two studies demonstrating slight increases in the risk of mortality for preterm infants treated with caffeine (Amaro et al., 2018; Dobson et al., 2014). These two studies are discussed in more detail later in the text.

Initiation of Therapy and Effect on Bronchopulmonary Dysplasia

The optimal time at which to initiate treatment with caffeine is uncertain. Early use of caffeine in the NICU is relatively common, not only as a prophylactic measure for AOP, but also based on the studies demonstrating improvements in the risk of BPD and neurodevelopmental outcomes demonstrated in follow-up to the CAP trial and more recently by Lodha and colleagues (2019). Early use (<3 days) of caffeine in infants who require mechanical ventilation compared with later use (≥3 days) has been studied. However, there are conflicting data on the subject.

Several observational studies have examined the question of early versus late initiation of prophylactic caffeine therapy. A post-hoc analysis of the CAP trial found a greater reduction in the duration of respiratory support among infants who received early caffeine therapy (<3 days of age) compared with later (≥3 days; Davis et al., 2010). In another analysis of 140 infants with birth weight less than 1250 grams, the initiation of early (<3 days) compared with late (≥3 days) caffeine therapy resulted in improved outcomes; 25% of infants in the early-caffeine group died or developed BPD compared with 53% of infants in the late-caffeine group (OR: 0.26, $p < .01$; Patel et al., 2013).

A retrospective analysis of a larger group of infants ($N = 2{,}951$) demonstrated a reduction in BPD with early initiation of caffeine compared with delayed initiation (reduction in BPD, OR: 0.69, $p < .001$); BPD and death, OR: 0.77, $p = .01$; Taha et al., 2014). In an even larger observational study ($N = 29{,}070$ propensity score-matched infants), early caffeine therapy (<3 days) was associated with a lower incidence of BPD in survivors (23% vs. 30%; OR: 0.68, $p < .001$), lower risk of BPD or death (27% vs. 34%; OR: 0.74, $p < .001$), and shorter duration of mechanical ventilation (11 days vs. 17 days) when compared with later dosing. However, a slightly higher mortality (4.5% vs. 3.7%; OR: 1.23, $p < .001$) was observed in the early therapy group as mentioned in the "Dosing Recommendations" section of this chapter. Of note, upon further examination (subgroup analysis by GA), early caffeine therapy was consistently associated with a decreased risk of BPD across all GA subgroups, whereas the increased risk of death was only noted in the subgroup of infants <24 weeks' gestation who received early caffeine therapy (Dobson et al., 2014). In 2015, a retrospective cohort study ($N = 5{,}101$) of infants less than 31 weeks' GA examined early (<3 days) versus late

(≥3 days) caffeine administration. Again, this study showed decreased odds of development of the outcome of death or BPD in the early caffeine group (OR: 0.81), as well as a decrease in the duration of both invasive and noninvasive respiratory support (Lodha et al., 2015).

More recently, an unblinded RCT by Dekker and colleagues (2017) demonstrated that initiation of caffeine immediately after birth (in the delivery room) was also effective at decreasing the need for invasive ventilation in ELBW infants. Around the same time, an observational study of premature infants less than 32 weeks' gestation ($N = 286$) demonstrated that caffeine administered within the first 24 hours of life was associated with a decreased need for mechanical ventilation (71.3% vs. 83.2%) and a shorter duration of mechanical ventilation than later caffeine initiation (mean 5 days vs. 10.8 days; Borszewska-Kornacka et al., 2017).

In another, retrospective study of infants less than 29 weeks' GA by Lodha and colleagues (2019), early caffeine administration (<48 hours of life) was associated with a lower risk of cognitive impairment and NDI when compared with late administration (OR: 0.67, 95% CI: 0.47–0.95 and OR: 0.68, 95% CI: 0.5–0.94, respectively) at 18 to 24 months corrected age.

Although retrospective studies appear to agree that earlier caffeine initiation is superior to late initiation, caution is warranted on the basis of a recent randomized, placebo-controlled trial. In the trial ($N = 83$), the age at first successful extubation did not differ between early caffeine use and placebo in preterm infants 23 to 30 weeks' gestation requiring mechanical ventilation on the first 5 days. The trial was terminated early (at 75% enrollment) due to a trend of higher mortality in one group; however, an unblinded analysis demonstrated an insignificant trend favoring placebo (12% vs. 22%, $p = .22$). In addition, no differences were noted between the groups in the secondary outcomes, including duration of mechanical ventilation and oxygen supplementation, BPD, or death. The standard dosage for caffeine was used in this study: 20 mg/kg, followed by 5 mg/kg/d (Amaro et al., 2018). Based on these results, the authors urge caution with the early use of caffeine until more efficacy and safety data become available.

Current evidence supports the cautious early use of caffeine as one of the few pharmacologic therapies proven to decrease the risk of development of BPD (Hennelly et al., 2021). However, further studies, specifically more RCTs, are needed to determine the safety and efficacy of this practice, especially in medically complex ELBW infants such as those requiring high-frequency ventilation, with agitation requiring pharmacologic sedation/analgesia, or with elevated risk of seizure (Dobson et al., 2014; Eichenwald, 2016).

Duration and Cessation of Therapy

The optimal duration of treatment with caffeine is also unknown. Eichenwald (2016) recommends considering a trial of caffeine in infants who have been free of clinically significant apnea/bradycardia events after 5 to 7 days off positive pressure or at 33 to 34 weeks' PMA, whichever comes first. In one RCT ($N = 95$) of caffeine versus placebo in infants 34 to 37 weeks' gestation, extending caffeine treatment beyond when it would normally be discontinued (for AOP) reduced the number and severity of intermittent hypoxia episodes in infants; however, the long-term benefits and risks to extended treatment are unknown (Rhein et al., 2014). More studies are needed before implementing extended caffeine treatment beyond apnea resolution (Eichenwald, 2016).

CLINICAL-MONITORING PEARLS

Caffeine is a pharmacotherapy often used for two concurrent purposes: prevention of BPD and postextubation management of AOP. Please refer to Chapter 10, "Apnea of Prematurity," for clinical-monitoring suggestions specific to the management of the disease process. Here we discuss monitoring priorities specific to BPD. Caffeine therapy is relatively safe in preterm infants, with few side effects noted in most studies. The most commonly seen in clinical practice are tachycardia, slowed growth, and irritability. However, even in the case of toxicity, supportive therapy is provided. Possible toxic effects are vomiting/gastroesophageal reflux disease (GERD)/feeding intolerance, and more rare complications include tachypnea, pulmonary edema, increased tone and opisthotonos, seizures, and metabolic disturbances such as hyperglycemia, hypokalemia, and hyperbilirubinemia (Abdel-Hady et al., 2015; Picone et al., 2012). Renal effects include diuresis and increased urinary calcium excretion (Harer et al., 2018; Micromedex Neofax Online, n.d.-b).

LONG-TERM OUTCOMES

As discussed in Chapter 10, "Apnea of Prematurity," a series of follow-up studies were carried out to examine the long-term neurodevelopmental outcomes of the infants in the original CAP trial. Initial follow-up at 18 months corrected age demonstrated a reduction in the risk of death or disability. At 5-year follow-up, there was no difference in death or disability between the caffeine and the placebo group. At 11-year follow-up, although the combined rate of academic, motor, and behavioral impairment did not differ, there was a reduced risk of motor impairment with caffeine compared with placebo (Schmidt et al., 2007, 2012, 2017). In addition to evaluation of neurodevelopmental outcomes, the CAP trial follow-up studies evaluated the children's respiratory function at 11 years of age. Children in the caffeine treatment group had improved expiratory flow rates compared with children treated with placebo by approximately 0.5 *SD* for most variables (e.g., forced expiratory volume in the first second (FEV_1); mean *z*-score, −1.00 vs. −1.53; mean difference, 0.54; 95% CI: 0.14–0.94, $p = .008$). Based on these results, caffeine treatment in the newborn period improves expiratory flow rates in childhood. However, when adjusted for BPD, the difference in flow rates between the groups diminished (L. W. Doyle et al., 2017).

Vitamin A

Supplementation with IM injections of VA is one of the only pharmacologic interventions that have demonstrated a reduction in BPD in RCTs (Araki et al., 2018; Beam et al., 2014; Darlow et al., 2016). This pharmacotherapy is FDA-approved for use in the NICU specifically to prevent/treat VA deficiency in high-risk, premature neonates. It is used off-label as an intervention to reduce the risk of BPD (Beam et al., 2014; Darlow et al., 2016; Laughon et al., 2009; Shenai, 1999; Tyson et al., 1999).

VA supplementation led to a reduction in evidence of deficiency in one RCT; 5% of infants in the control group had VA levels <0.35 µmol/L (indicating severe VA deficiency) versus none of the infants in the group supplemented with VA (at 28 days). Supplementation was also associated with a significant reduction in the duration of intubation (10.8 ± 3.1 days VA supplemented group vs. 26.1 ± 6.4 days control group, $p = .03$) and days on supplemental oxygen (29.8 ± 5.1 days VA supplemented group vs. 58.2 ± 9.1 days control group, $p = .01$; Kiatchoosakun et al., 2014).

A retrospective cohort study of preterm ELBW infants compared two time periods; the pre-VA group ($N = 76$) was routinely cared for with early nasal CPAP, and the post-VA group ($N = 102$) were cared for similar to pre-VA but with the addition of VA supplementation. A nonsignificant trend toward a reduction in the incidence of moderate to severe BPD was observed, from 33% to 22% ($p = .2$). No difference was found in the number of ventilator days or in the incidence of any other neonatal morbidities or mortality between the groups (Moreira et al., 2012).

In a more recent systematic review and meta-analysis of nine RCTs ($N = 1{,}409$ patients), Ding and colleagues (2021) showed that the incidence of BPD in the VA group was significantly less than that of the control group (OR = 0.67, 95% CI: 0.52–0.88). There was no significant difference noted in the incidence of any other evaluated morbidities or mortality between the two groups. The authors suggest that VA supplementation is beneficial to the prophylaxis of BPD in premature infants, but caution that further studies on the administration approaches and dosages of VA in premature infants are warranted (Ding et al., 2021).

MECHANISM OF ACTION/CORE PHARMACOKINETIC PRINCIPLES

VA is the generic name for a group of fat-soluble compounds, including retinol and its active metabolite, retinoic acid. VA is metabolized in the liver and then circulated as retinol-retinol binding protein (RBP) complex before being delivered to sites of action and storage, specifically in the liver, the eye, and the lung. Circulating concentrations of retinol and the response in those levels to VA supplementation are used as a surrogate for VA levels/stores; however, this does not provide a complete assessment of total body stores or the levels of biologically active metabolites in tissue; thus, there is little known about the precise pharmacokinetics in preterm infants (Mactier & Weaver, 2005). The precise mechanisms of intracellular activity are not completely understood or well defined in the literature, but it is clear that retinol metabolites exhibit potent and site-specific effects on gene expression and on lung growth and development (Mactier & Weaver, 2005; Shenai,

1999). Not only is VA vital to the normal growth and differentiation of the epithelial cells in the respiratory tract, it also plays an important role in surfactant synthesis (Mactier & Weaver, 2005).

It has been noted that the pulmonary histopathologic changes of BPD and VA deficiency are remarkably similar. When these changes (e.g., necrotizing tracheobronchitis and squamous metaplasia) are due to VA deficiency, they can be reversed by restoration of adequate VA status (Darlow et al., 2016). As a result of VA accretion largely occurring in the last trimester of pregnancy, preterm infants have low plasma levels of VA at birth, which is also reflective of reduced hepatic stores. This relative deficiency is hypothesized to be associated with an increased risk of developing BPD (Darlow et al., 2016; Mactier & Weaver, 2005).

DOSING RECOMMENDATIONS

Given the conflicting data regarding the amount of benefit derived from VA supplementation, several factors have been recommended for consideration prior to routine use in individual NICUs. We begin with a discussion of data specific to the timing for initiation of VA therapy.

Initiation of Therapy

Darlow et al. suggested, in a Cochrane review on the use of VA supplementation in VLBW infants, that the local incidence of BPD should be taken into consideration. The local incidence and value placed on "achieving a modest reduction" in BPD should be balanced with the acceptability of administration related to the pain of IM injection, fragile skin, and lack of muscle mass in this population (Darlow et al., 2016). As mentioned earlier, one of the major drawbacks to VA administration is the pain associated with IM injection. Although enteral VA supplementation increases plasma retinol levels, it does not seem to improve the severity of BPD in clinical trials (Rakshasbhuvankar et al., 2021). It should also be noted that several reviews on the treatment of BPD refer to one study demonstrating an increased risk of sepsis in VLBW given IM injections of VA; however, this was only in infants >1,000 grams (Uberos et al., 2014). No other studies have reported similar risks. Pooled data from three studies in the most recent Cochrane review (Darlow et al., 2016) actually showed a nonsignificant trend toward a reduction in sepsis in the groups receiving VA (typical RR: 0.89, 95% CI: 0.76 to 1.04; typical risk difference [RD]: –0.05, 95% CI: –0.11 to 0.01, 947 infants).

Standard Dosing

In 1999, Tyson and colleagues established that 5,000 units IM three times weekly for 4 weeks reduced the evidence of VA deficiency more effectively than lower dosing regimens used in previous trials in ELBW infants (Tyson et al., 1999). More recently, in an RCT comparing three dosing regimens, the standard dosing regimen of 5,000 IU three times weekly for 4 weeks appeared to be optimal for ELBW infants. Once-per-week dosing appeared to worsen VA deficiency and higher dosing was demonstrated to be no better than standard, although it should be noted that on the higher dose regimen 26% of infants still had plasma VA concentrations below 20 mcg/dL, which may indicate deficiency (Ambalavanan et al., 2003). An even higher dose of VA may be required to achieve sufficiency in very premature infants (Darlow et al., 2016).

CLINICAL-MONITORING PEARLS

Although routine monitoring of serum VA concentrations is not recommended, desired concentrations are approximately 30 to 60 mcg/dL. Concentrations less than 20 mcg/dL indicate deficiency, whereas those greater than 100 mcg/dL are potentially toxic (Shenai, 1999). Vomiting and increased intracranial pressure have been reported in infants, and high VA levels in children and adults can result in bone and joint pain, mucocutaneous lesions, and liver dysfunction, although this constellation of findings has not been recognized in studies of preterm infants (Darlow et al., 2016). Most studies report minimal to no signs of potential toxicity or adverse effects in preterm infants (Araki et al., 2018; Darlow et al., 2016).

LONG-TERM OUTCOMES

Only one trial investigated long-term neurodevelopmental outcomes after VA supplementation. In a follow-up study to the NICHD-sponsored trial originally conducted by Tyson et al., no significant difference in neurodevelopmental outcomes or mortality at 18 to 22 months corrected age was demonstrated between infants receiving VA and controls (Ambalavanan et al., 2005; Darlow et al., 2016). In addition, the study failed to demonstrate any significant difference in rates of bronchodilator or diuretic use at 18 to 22 months, home oxygen use, or rehospitalization rates in infants receiving VA versus controls, suggesting that long-term pulmonary effects of VA were negligible, although the study was underpowered to find statistically conclusive differences in outcomes (Ambalavanan et al., 2005).

Dexamethasone

Given the role of the inflammatory response in the pathogenesis of BPD, corticosteroids have long been studied as a potential therapeutic agent for treatment and prevention of BPD. Although corticosteroids are not FDA-approved for use in the prevention or management of BPD, many studies have demonstrated improved respiratory outcomes in infants treated with corticosteroids. Hydrocortisone represents an emerging corticosteroid option for the prevention of BPD; readers should refer to Chapter 20, "Hypotension and Shock," for a thorough description of pharmacology and recent review articles for emerging data regarding benefits and risk (Htun et al., 2021). Of the corticosteroids, dexamethasone remains one of the most widely studied and used steroids within the NICU, and is the primary focus of this chapter (Gupta et al., 2012).

MECHANISM OF ACTION/CORE PHARMACOKINETIC PRINCIPLES

Dexamethasone is a highly potent corticosteroid with exclusive glucocorticoid activity and long half-life that is used in infants at risk of developing BPD for its anti-inflammatory effects (Gupta et al., 2012). One of the primary mechanisms by which glucocorticoids exert an anti-inflammatory effect is via induction of annexin-1 synthesis, which in turn suppresses phospholipase A2 activity. Phospholipase A2 is needed for the production of eicosanoids, including prostaglandin, leukotriene, thromboxane, and prostacyclin; thus, dexamethasone reduces production of these inflammatory products. Annexin-1 also inhibits cyclooxygenase-1 and 2 (COX-1, COX-2), enzymes involved in prostaglandin synthesis; thus, dexamethasone-driven induction of annexin-1 inhibits production of potent inflammatory mediators on many levels. (Gupta et al., 2012). This downregulation of prostaglandins leads to a less inflammatory environment in the lung parenchyma, which is thought to mitigate the development of BPD. Dexamethasone also reduces the occurrence of pulmonary edema by stabilizing the alveolar–capillary barrier within the neonatal lung and inhibits the development of fibrosis after inflammation has occurred (Ballabh et al., 2003; Micromedex Neofax Online, n.d.-c).

Several studies have demonstrated changes in the inflammatory cytokine profile of infants with BPD who were treated with dexamethasone. Both in vitro and in vivo studies have demonstrated significant reduction in the proinflammatory IL-2 and IL-3 production from preterm polymorphonuclear (PMN) cells at lower doses/dexamethasone concentrations than were required to attain similar reductions in term infant and adult PMN cell cytokine production (Bessler et al., 1996). Other proinflammatory chemokines, such as IL-8 and macrophage inflammatory protein (MIP), have been isolated in pulmonary lavage samples of preterm infants who develop BPD (Munshi et al., 1997; Murch et al., 1996). In vitro studies by Irakam et al. in 2002 demonstrated the ability of corticosteroids to inhibit cord blood PMN production of both IL-8 and MIP at much lower drug concentrations than are observed in infants being treated with dexamethasone for BPD.

Ballabh and colleagues (2003) later studied the soluble adhesion molecules sL-selectin, sE-selectin, and soluble intercellular adhesion molecule-1 (sICAM-1) in 44 preterm infants <30 weeks' gestation with RDS over the first 28 days of life. In those who developed BPD, a pattern of decreased levels of sL-selectin and increased sE-selectin was observed, which was not seen in term infants or preterm infants without BPD. Dexamethasone treatment (given as a 6-day tapering course starting at 0.5 mg/kg/d divided every 12 hours) was noted to counteract the pattern of soluble adhesion molecules observed in BPD by increasing sL-selectin and decreasing sE-selectin (Ballabh et al., 2003).

In 2021, Yazdi and colleagues evaluated the T-cell population and cytokine profile in tracheal aspirates of preterm infants born at 23 to 28 weeks' gestation who were treated with the more contemporary 10-day tapered dosing regimen of dexamethasone. The study found that respiratory severity score (mean airway pressure multiplied by fractional inspired oxygen) was correlated to the percentage of CD4+IL-6+ cells in tracheal aspirates and treatment with dexamethasone significantly reduced the percentage of CD4+IL-6+ cells (Yazdi et al., 2021).

Dexamethasone is metabolized in the liver prior to being renally excreted (Lugo et al., 1996). As with many drugs, data are limited regarding the pharmacokinetics and dynamics of dexamethasone in preterm infants. It may be administered IV or orally and dosing recommendations are 1:1, although studies in adult populations have shown only 70% to 80% bioavailability after oral administration (Micromedex Neofax Online, n.d.-c). Half-life is long, with most sources reporting a half-life of 36 to 54 hours (Gupta et al., 2012; Micromedex Neofax Online, n.d.-c). One study of nine premature infants receiving IV dexamethasone demonstrated that the volume of distribution was smaller and renal clearance was lower with increasing prematurity; thus, the authors caution about the risk of reaching higher-than-intended plasma concentrations in preterm infants less than 27 weeks' gestation (Lugo et al., 1996).

DOSING RECOMMENDATIONS

At present, there is still a need for studies to investigate the ideal dose of dexamethasone for the prevention and treatment of BPD. As mentioned earlier, dexamethasone doses in the late 1990s were typically high, with dosing regimens ranging from 1.5 mg/kg in pulses every 10 days (Brozanski et al., 1995) up to 8 mg/kg cumulative dose attained with tapered daily dosing over 6 weeks (Cummings et al., 1989), with the majority of studies starting at 0.5 mg/kg/d dosing (Halliday et al., 2000a). These regimens had a clear benefit on pulmonary function, with a Cochrane meta-analysis demonstrating significant benefits, including earlier extubation, decreased risk of BPD at 28 days' and 36 weeks' PMA, decreased risk of the combined outcome of death or BPD at 28 days' and 36 weeks' PMA, as well as decreased risk of PDA and of severe retinopathy of prematurity (ROP; Halliday et al., 2000b). However, nine of the included trials reported on long-term neurologic outcomes and found increased incidence of developmental delay, CP, and abnormal neurologic exam (Halliday et al., 2000b). Notably, the studies that measured major neurosensory disability or combined outcomes of major disability or death did not find a significant increase in these outcomes in the dexamethasone-treated infants versus controls. However, the existing evidence of increased risk of CP (risk difference: 0.12 [95% CI: 0.06–0.18], number needed to harm [NNH]: 8.3 [95% CI: 5.5–16.7]) was sufficient for the American Academy of Pediatrics (AAP) to publish a recommendation that routine use of systemic dexamethasone could not be recommended and postnatal systemic dexamethasone use should be limited to well-designed RCTs that investigated long-term outcomes or exceptional clinical circumstances (Halliday, 2002).

Concurrently, the landmark DART had been recruiting infants to assess the effect of low-dose (<0.5 mg/kg/dose) dexamethasone on survival free of major neurologic disability, although the reports of adverse neurologic outcomes with systemic dexamethasone use led to low enrollment and early suspension of the trial (L. W. Doyle et al., 2006). Infants randomized to the interventional arm were prescribed a total cumulative dose of 0.89 mg/kg dexamethasone given twice daily in a tapered course over 10 days (0.15 mg/kg/d for 3 days, 0.1 mg/kg/d for 3 days, 0.05 mg/kg/d for 2 days, and 0.02 mg/kg/d for 2 days), initiated after the first week of life (L. W. Doyle et al., 2006). Analysis of short-term outcomes showed that low-dose dexamethasone facilitated extubation (OR: 11.2, 95% CI: 3.2–39.0) and decreased total duration of intubation (median 14 days, interquartile range [IQR]: 5.5–21.5 days vs. 21 days, IQR: 9–35 days; L. W. Doyle et al., 2006). Although the DART trial failed to detect any difference in mortality (OR: 0.52, 95% CI: 0.14–1.95) or BPD (OR: 0.58, 95% CI: 0.08–3.32) in dexamethasone-treated infants, the study was underpowered to detect important reductions in these outcomes (L. W. Doyle et al., 2006). Notably, with this lower dose of dexamethasone, the only significant adverse effect observed was a temporary slowing in growth, but other outcomes, such as gastrointestinal (GI) perforation, hypertension, and hyperglycemia, were not significantly increased in dexamethasone-treated infants (L. W. Doyle et al., 2006). In a long-term follow-up at 2 years, patients from the DART study did not show a difference in long-term morbidity, including death, CP, or hospital readmissions (L. W. Doyle et al., 2007). The promise of facilitating extubation and reducing time on mechanical ventilation without increasing the risk of short-term adverse events and without clear evidence of long-term detriment to health has made the DART protocol the most widely used contemporary regimen for administering systemic dexamethasone.

Subsequent studies have examined whether even lower doses of dexamethasone could be effective in facilitating improvement in respiratory outcomes. A small retrospective study of 16 infants treated with extremely low-dose dexamethasone (total dose of 0.24 mg/kg, starting with

0.05 mg/kg/d and tapering over 9 days) found a significant decrease in the median oxygenation index from 14.6 (range 5.1–27.1) on day 0 to 5.2 (range 1.4–9.9) on day 7, with 75% of the infants being extubated during their course (Tanney et al., 2011). However, evaluations of lower dosing have less consistently supported beneficial pulmonary effects. Most recently, a systematic review and network meta-analysis of postnatal corticosteroid use evaluated the outcomes of 14 different treatment regimens in 62 different studies, including a low (<2 mg/kg), medium (2–4 mg/kg), and high (>4 mg/kg) cumulative dose of dexamethasone initiated moderately early (8–14 days) or late (>14 days). Surface under the cumulative ranking curve (SUCRA) evaluation found high-dose dexamethasone (> 4mg/kg cumulative dose) initiated at either time and medium-dose dexamethasone (2–4 mg/kg cumulative dose) initiated at 8 to 14 days to be the most beneficial in decreasing the risk of BPD or death when compared with all studied corticosteroid regimens (Ramaswamy et al., 2021). Thus, this meta-analysis would suggest that further lowering of dexamethasone dosing is unlikely to provide much benefit in the prevention of BPD. In summary, further RCTs are needed to evaluate the lowest safe and effective dose of dexamethasone.

Initiation of Therapy

In addition to the debate surrounding optimal dosing of dexamethasone for BPD, the optimal timing has been thoroughly investigated and many questions remain, with the overall trend representing a movement toward later dosing of dexamethasone due to concerns about serious adverse events in early use.

Early initiation of dexamethasone therapy is defined as initiation within the first week of life, with only a few studies focusing on very early initiation within the first 72 hours of life. A Cochrane meta-analysis updated in 2021 that reviewed early use of corticosteroids (<7 days) found that dexamethasone probably reduced the risk of BPD at 36 weeks' PMA (RR: 0.72, 95% CI: 0.63–0.82) and reduced the combined outcome of mortality or BPD at 36 weeks' PMA (RR: 0.88, 95% CI: 0.81–0.95; L. W. Doyle et al., 2021a). However, this benefit was outweighed by the findings of increased GI perforation (RR: 1.73, 95% CI: 1.20–2.51) and increased incidence of CP (RR: 1.43, 95% CI: 1.07–1.92) and the combined risk of mortality or CP (RR: 1.18, 95% CI: 1.01–1.37; L. W. Doyle et al., 2021a). Within the analysis, the earliest trial to demonstrate the efficacy of dexamethasone was that by Yeh et al. in 1990, in which 57 preterm infants were randomized to a 12-day taper of dexamethasone or placebo and treated infants were significantly less likely to experience BPD or death (39% vs. 65%, $p < .05$). However, in the mid- to late 1990s, two large studies ($N = 248$ and $N = 262$) demonstrated increased risk of adverse neurologic outcomes with both a short six-dose course of dexamethasone and a prolonged 28-day taper (Shinwell et al., 1996; Yeh et al., 1997). The risk of adverse neurologic outcomes in addition to increased risk of GI perforation has led early courses of dexamethasone to fall out of favor.

Moderately early and late treatments, on the other hand, have been more promising. The Cochrane review of corticosteroid use beginning after 7 days of life reported that dexamethasone probably decreases the incidence of BPD (RR: 0.76, 95% CI: 0.66–0.87) or the combined outcome of BPD or death at 36 weeks' PMA (RR: 0.75, 95% CI: 0.67–0.84), without evidence of effect on CP or combined outcome of CP or mortality, although they note none of the studies are sufficiently powered to evaluate late neurodevelopmental outcomes (L. W. Doyle et al., 2021b). Within this meta-analysis, a study by Kothadia et al. raised concern for its findings of increased risk of abnormal neurologic examination or CP; however, the combined outcome of death or CP and long-term functional outcomes were not significantly different between the control and treated groups (Kothadia et al., 1999). Other studies within the meta-analysis did not replicate the findings of significantly increased risk of CP, and the authors emphasize that only the DART trial was designed with the intent of investigating long-term neurologic outcomes and that all of the studies available for review are underpowered to detect clinically important differences in neurosensory outcomes (L. W. Doyle et al., 2021b). Given this information, "it appears prudent to reserve the use of late dexamethasone to infants who cannot be weaned from mechanical ventilation, and to minimize the dose and duration of any course of treatment" (L. W. Doyle et al., 2010, p. 293).

There is, however, a limit to the timing of initiation of dexamethasone for beneficial effects to be observed. A cohort study of 951 infants in the NICHD Neonatal Research Network who received postnatal steroids between 8 days of life and 36 weeks' PMA found the adjusted odds ratio (aOR) for severe BPD was higher in infants treated between days 49 and 63 (aOR: 1.77, 95% CI: 1.03–3.06) and later than 64 days (aOR: 3.06, 95% CI: 1.44–6.48) compared with infants treated on days 8 to 49, with no difference in the aOR of NDI by age at treatment (Harmon et al., 2020).

Duration and Cessation of Therapy

As discussed earlier, the most widely used regimen is that reported in DART, which consists of a 10-day tapering course amounting to a total dose of 0.89 mg/kg (L. W. Doyle et al., 2006); however, many other durations have been studied, and even within the DART study population 29% of infants received a second course of open-label corticosteroids. In the 2021 Cochrane review of late (>7 days) corticosteroid use, there were 21 trials of dexamethasone and the initial treatment durations ranged from 3 days to 6 weeks (L. W. Doyle et al., 2021b). Given the lack of sufficient evidence of safety and concern for potential detrimental effects on long-term neurodevelopmental outcomes, current recommendations are to use the lowest dose and shortest course of dexamethasone to achieve desirable respiratory outcomes (L. W. Doyle et al., 2021b; Watterberg et al., 2010).

Repeat courses of dexamethasone for infants who remain intubated are common. Cuna et al. examined the efficacy of a second course of dexamethasone in facilitating a step-down in respiratory support and found that 38% of infants had a step-down in therapy following a second course of steroids, compared with 52% with the initial course (Cuna et al., 2021). Regarding the safety of the repeat course, there was no significant difference in growth parameters at discharge in infants treated with one versus two courses of steroids; however, the authors did not investigate any long-term outcomes (Cuna et al., 2021).

CLINICAL-MONITORING PEARLS

Although dexamethasone has utility as a potent anti-inflammatory agent in BPD, it is not without significant safety concerns. Dexamethasone is known to decrease cellular glucose uptake and glucokinase activity, leading to hyperglycemia, and increased acetyl-CoA carboxylase activity causes hypertriglyceridemia (Micromedex Neofax Online, n.d.-c). Although it is not a mineralocorticoid, dexamethasone increases responsiveness to catecholamines and can thus lead to hypertension (Micromedex Neofax Online, n.d.-c). As occurs with other glucocorticoids, it increases protein catabolism, increases bone resorption and thus increases urinary calcium excretion, and suppresses ACTH (Micromedex Neofax Online, n.d.-c). Clinically, the most prominent concerns have been related to acute increased risk of GI perforation or hemorrhage and long-term risk of impaired neurodevelopmental outcomes. A Cochrane review of early use (<7 days) of dexamethasone demonstrated increased risk of GI perforation (RR: 1.73, 95% CI: 1.20–2.51) in nine studies of 1,936 infants, whereas similar findings were not observed in the use of late (>7 days) dexamethasone (L. W. Doyle et al., 2021a, 2021b). Similarly, early use of dexamethasone was associated with increased risk of CP (RR: 1.77, 95% CI: 1.21–2.58) in seven studies of 921 infants, whereas there was little to no effect of late systemic corticosteroid use on CP (RR: 1.17, 95% CI: 0.84–1.61) in 17 studies of 1,290 infants, although none of the late corticosteroid studies have been sufficiently powered to detect rates of neurodevelopmental outcomes (L. W. Doyle et al., 2021a, 2021b). Given these safety concerns, the AAP has issued policy statements, first in 2002 stating that the routine use of dexamethasone for prevention or treatment of BPD could not be recommended, and then refined in 2010 to clarify that therapy with high-dose dexamethasone (≥0.5 mg/kg/dose) cannot be recommended, but there is insufficient evidence to make a recommendation regarding treatment with low-dose dexamethasone (Watterberg et al., 2010).

Hypertension

As dexamethasone enhances sensitivity to endogenous catecholamines (Micromedex Neofax Online, n.d.-c), hypertension has been a frequently reported side effect. In the DART trial, blood pressure was monitored and no significant increases in blood pressure were observed with the low dose used in that trial (L. W. Doyle et al., 2006). However, hypertension remains a concern. In the most recent Cochrane review, there was increased risk of hypertension with dexamethasone treatment (RR: 1.67, 95% CI: 1.19–2.33), although various doses and durations were used; thus, the maximal safe dose and duration of dexamethasone to avoid hypertension remains unclear (L. W. Doyle et al., 2021).

Hyperglycemia

Dexamethasone is known to decrease cellular glucose uptake and reduce glucokinase activity, resulting in hyperglycemia (Micromedex Neofax Online, n.d.-c). The DART trial did not observe any clinically significant differences in blood glucose (Doyle et al., 2006); however, the broader dosing and duration varieties of dexamethasone used in various studies in the 2021 Cochrane review did result in an increased risk of hyperglycemia (RR: 1.59, 95% CI: 1.34–1.89); L. W. Doyle et al., 2021b).

Postnatal Growth

Given the known effects of dexamethasone on metabolism and the importance of the role of nutrition in the development of BPD, growth has been closely monitored in studies of dexamethasone. In the 10-day dexamethasone regimen used in the DART trial, growth was impaired for the period of treatment, with significantly lower weight change among infants receiving dexamethasone; however, the *z*-scores of all growth parameters at discharge were not significantly different in the treated and control groups, as has been the case in other studies (Anttila et al., 2005; Cuna et al., 2021; L. W. Doyle et al., 2006).

Cardiovascular Function

An early, moderate dose of dexamethasone (2–4 mg/kg cumulative dose started <7 days of age) has been associated with left ventricular hypertrophic cardiomyopathy that may be symptomatic and was shown to resolve within 2 to 3 weeks of discontinuation of steroids (Zecca et al., 2001). In the use of late steroids (after 7 days of age), this appears to remain a concern. One study examining high-dose dexamethasone (>4 mg/kg cumulative dose) in the Cochrane review of late steroid use found an increase in hypertrophic cardiomyopathy in treated infants (RR: 2.76, 95% CI: 1.33–5.74) L. W. Doyle et al., 2021. This outcome was not specifically measured in the DART trial (L. W. Doyle et al., 2006).

LONG-TERM OUTCOMES

The uncertainty of long-term outcomes remains the primary concern for the use of dexamethasone in the prevention of BPD. Several studies in both animal models and human subjects have demonstrated potential harm to the developing brain (Wilson-Costello et al., 2009), and although dexamethasone decreases mortality in the immediate neonatal period (<28 days) L. W. Doyle et al. did not find that dexamethasone had any effect on long-term mortality (L. W. Doyle et al., 2021a, 2021b).

To date, the DART trial has been the only trial designed to assess long-term neurologic outcomes; however, recall that the trial's early suspension of enrollment has left it underpowered to detect clinically significant differences in long-term outcomes. Despite this, the trial cohort has been followed and several published reports on their outcomes offer speculations about late, low-dose dexamethasone's long-term effects. At the 2-year mark, there were no significant differences in the incidence of mortality, major disability, CP, or the combined outcome of death or CP in infants who had received dexamethasone compared with controls (L. W. Doyle et al., 2007). However, other studies have observed increases in CP with postnatal corticosteroid use. In a prospective cohort study investigating the effects of dose, timing, and BPD risk on neurodevelopment of infants treated with postnatal corticosteroids, the authors observed a 2.0-point reduction in Bayley Mental Developmental Index and a 40% increase in risk of disabling CP for each 1.0 mg/kg increase in dexamethasone dose (OR: 1.4, 95% CI: 1.2–1.6; Wilson-Costello et al., 2009).

A key meta-analysis in 2005 examined 20 RCTs and evaluated the impact of baseline BPD risk on response to corticosteroid therapy. The authors found that with BPD risk less than 35%, there was a significant increase in the outcomes of death or CP, whereas with BPD risk greater than 65% the risk of death or CP was significantly reduced (L. W. Doyle et al., 2005). This analysis led to the revision of the prior 2002 AAP policy statement recommending against systemic dexamethasone use to now recommend that clinicians use their judgment in determining appropriateness of corticosteroid treatment based on risk of BPD and of potential harm (Watterberg et al., 2010).

In addition to the concern about neurodevelopment, there have been concerns regarding the risk of severe ROP and blindness associated with dexamethasone. A retrospective cohort study sought to examine this and found a correlation between steroid exposure and severe ROP (incidence of 26% in no dexamethasone exposure compared with 61% in low cumulative exposure <1.8mg/kg and 85% in high cumulative exposure >1.8mg/kg); however, there was not a significant difference in the incidence of severe ROP when adjusted for the confounding variables of GA and severity of lung disease (Cuculich et al., 2001). Thus, the higher incidence of ROP in infants treated with dexamethasone may be more reflective of the severity of their lung disease, rather than an effect of the dexamethasone itself.

Inhaled Corticosteroids

Decreasing pulmonary inflammation using systemic corticosteroids has been shown to facilitate extubation and potentially reduce the incidence of BPD in preterm infants. However, use of systemic corticosteroids has been associated with adverse long-term neurodevelopmental outcomes. Theoretically, selective, local administration of steroids via inhalation could reduce the side effects associated with systemic distribution and absorption. Inhaled corticosteroids may improve oxygenation, increase airway compliance and functional residual capacity, and decrease airway resistance.

Data that point toward potential benefits of early inhaled corticosteroid use (within the first 2 weeks life) in VLBW infants are increasing. A Cochrane review of 10 trials (N = 1,644) of VLBW infants receiving early inhaled corticosteroid versus placebo beginning within the first 2 weeks of life did not find significant differences in rates of BPD at 28 days' or 36 weeks' PMA, but there was a significant reduction in the combined outcome of death or BPD (typical RR: 0.86, 95% CI: 0.75–0.99, p = .04; V. S. Shah et al., 2017). Within that meta-analysis is the key Neonatal European Study of Inhaled Steroids (NEUROSIS) trial, a large RCT of infants 23 to 27 weeks' gestation (N = 863) comparing early initiation (within the first 24 hours) of inhaled corticosteroids (specifically budesonide) with placebo, which reported a significant reduction in BPD at 36 weeks in infants receiving steroids (RR: 0.74, 95% CI: 0.60–0.91, p = .004; Bassler et al., 2015).

However, when inhaled corticosteroids are compared with systemic steroids, the benefits to survival and BPD reduction become less promising. A second Cochrane analysis compared inhaled corticosteroids with systemic corticosteroids rather than placebo (2 studies, N = 294) and found no evidence that inhaled steroids, started within the first week of life, offered an advantage over systemic steroids in preventing death or BPD, nor was there evidence to suggest a lessened adverse event profile (S. S. Shah et al., 2017a). Another Cochrane review of three studies (N = 431) comparing inhaled versus systemic corticosteroids after the first week of life also demonstrated no evidence of differences in effectiveness or adverse event profiles between the inhaled and systemic routes of delivery (S. S. Shah et al., 2017b).

With regard to the efficacy of late inhaled steroids (started ≥7 days), a Cochrane review by Onland and colleagues (2017) did not show a beneficial effect on death or BPD. This review included eight RCTs (N = 232) comparing in halation steroids with placebo in ventilated and nonventilated infants at risk of BPD. There was also no impact on the duration of mechanical ventilation or oxygen dependency. Based on the evidence, the authors conclude that routine use of inhaled corticosteroids at ≥7 days in preterm infants at risk of developing BPD cannot be recommended.

MECHANISM OF ACTION/CORE PHARMACOKINETIC PRINCIPLES

Inhaled corticosteroids are potent glucocorticoids with weak mineralocorticoid activity that exert an anti-inflammatory effect on lung tissue. The mechanism by which they exert this effect is multifaceted and includes depression of PMN cell and fibroblast migration, lysosomal stabilization, decreasing capillary permeability, and control of rates of protein synthesis (Taketomo, 2023). The two most frequently utilized inhaled corticosteroids in the neonatal setting are budesonide and beclomethasone. There are no data to suggest any difference in the mechanisms of action of specific agents, although there are differences in drug potency and commercially available doses. Pharmacokinetic studies have demonstrated that budesonide is 1.6 times more potent than beclomethasone; thus, it could be suspected that lower doses of budesonide may demonstrate comparable clinical efficacy (Raghuram et al., 2018).

There are no studies on the effect of inhaled corticosteroids on the pulmonary mechanics or inflammatory profile of neonatal lung, but direct application of a single dose of budesonide with surfactant in fetal sheep lung resulted in improved airway compliance, pulmonary edema, acute phase response, and surfactant production (Kothe et al., 2018). Neonatal data on bioavailability are not available, but pharmacokinetic and pharmacodynamic properties are extrapolated from studies in older children. Peak concentration is achieved in the lung within 20 minutes (Taketomo, 2023) and systemic absorption is likely low, with reported bioavailability of nebulized formulations in children ages 4 to 6 of around 6% (Taketomo, 2023). Half-life is short, about 1 to 2 hours (Taketomo, 2023). Although pulmonary concentrations reach a peak promptly following administration, in adult studies, peak effect is not observed until 4 to 6 weeks of nebulized therapy, or

1 to 2 weeks of orally inhaled therapy, likely due to the higher systemic absorption (up to 40%; Taketomo, 2023).

DOSING RECOMMENDATIONS

One nonrandomized study has investigated the dosing of inhaled beclomethasone in ventilator-dependent infants born less than 32 weeks' gestation or <1,250 grams (*N* = 41) and found that although none of the treatment groups were able to attain the primary goal of extubation or reduction in fraction of inspired oxygen (FiO_2) by >75% of baseline for more than 60% of infants, there was a significant reduction in FiO_2 requirement (from 0.37 to 0.30, p = .02) in infants receiving 800 mcg twice daily for as little as 1 week (Raghuram et al., 2018). The reduction in FiO_2 requirement was not significantly different between doses of 200 mcg, 400 mcg, and 600 mcg twice daily (Raghuram et al., 2018). In the NEUROSIS trial, which demonstrated reduction in the incidence of BPD at 36 weeks' PMA (NNT: 10, *p* = .04), patients received 400 mcg of budesonide twice daily for the first 14 days of life followed by 200 mcg twice daily until 32 weeks' PMA (Bassler et al., 2015).

Initiation of Therapy and Effect on Bronchopulmonary Dysplasia

As is the case with the use of systemic corticosteroids for BPD, much attention has focused on the ideal timing of initiation of inhaled corticosteroid therapy. Outcomes have been stratified by early versus late initiation of therapy, with early therapy beginning in the first week of life, very early therapy beginning within 24 hours as in the NEUROSIS trial, and late therapy beginning after 1 to 2 weeks of life.

There have been two Cochrane reviews evaluating the effects of early initiation of inhaled corticosteroid treatment, one examining inhaled corticosteroids versus placebo and the other comparing inhaled corticosteroids with systemic corticosteroids. Recall from our earlier discussion that only two studies are included in the review of inhaled versus systemic corticosteroids (*N* = 294) and it found no evidence that inhaled steroids, started within the first week of life, offered an advantage over systemic steroids in preventing death or BPD (S. S. Shah et al., 2017a). The Cochrane review that compared inhaled corticosteroids with placebo at less than 7 days was much larger (*N* = 1,644), examining 10 different trials, including the large NEUROSIS trial, and found significant reduction in the combined outcome of death or BPD at 36 weeks' PMA, although there was no significant difference in outcomes of BPD or death separately (V. S. Shah et al., 2017). The NEUROSIS trial, with therapy beginning in the first 24 hours and continued through 32 weeks' PMA, did show a significant decrease in the rates of BPD at 36 weeks (RR: 0.74, 95% CI: 0.60–0.91, *p* = .004); however, there was an increase in mortality (RR: 1.37, 95% CI: 1.01–1.86, *p* = .04; Bassler et al., 2018). Thus, early use of inhaled corticosteroids may help decrease the risk of BPD, but their routine use cannot be recommended until more information is obtained regarding the increased risk of mortality.

Late therapies have been less successful in demonstrating improvement in BPD outcomes. Trials comparing systemic and inhaled corticosteroids in ventilated infants older than 7 days failed to show any significant difference in BPD nor in duration of mechanical ventilation, supplemental oxygen, or hospital stay (S. S. Shah et al., 2017b). Similar outcomes were seen when compared with placebo, so authors concluded that until more data exist on the safety and efficacy, routine use of inhaled corticosteroids initiated after 7 days of life could not be recommended (Onland et al., 2017).

Duration and Cessation of Therapy

Little is known about the appropriate duration of therapy with inhaled corticosteroids. Although adult pharmacologic data would suggest that therapy must be for at least 1 to 2 weeks to reach maximal effect with orally inhaled steroids or 4 to 6 weeks with nebulized steroids (Taketomo, 2023), infant studies have shown beneficial clinical effect on FiO_2 requirement as early as 1 week of therapy (Raghuram et al., 2018). In the NEUROSIS trial, which demonstrated a reduction in the risk of BPD at 36 weeks' PMA, corticosteroids were initiated within the first 24 hours of life and continued until 32 weeks' PMA (Bassler et al., 2015). However, follow-up studies revealed that 24% of patients in that study from both treatment and placebo groups were prescribed inhaled corticosteroids at the discretion of their physician for at least 2 months following hospital discharge (Bassler et al., 2018).

CLINICAL-MONITORING PEARLS

The theorized advantage of inhaled corticosteroids over systemic corticosteroids is the reduction in systemic absorption and thus decreased systemic adverse effects. In existing studies of inhaled corticosteroid use in preterm infants, these advantages have shown to be true. In all four Cochrane reviews of inhaled corticosteroid use, there have been no significant differences in the risk of hypertension, hyperglycemia, GI bleeding, intraventricular hemorrhage (IVH), periventricular leukomalacia (PVL), severe ROP, NEC, or culture-negative sepsis (Onland et al., 2017; S. S. Shah et al., 2017a, 2017b; V. S. Shah et al., 2017). However, the NNT for budesonide in the NEUROSIS trial is ~10 and may expose premature infants to risk not yet elucidated. There are reports in pediatric populations of increased risk of oral candidiasis and adrenal insufficiency with chronic orally inhaled corticosteroid use (Micromedex Neofax Online, n.d.-a). Although Cochrane reviews have not found a significant increase in candidiasis, adrenal insufficiency, hyperglycemia, and hypertension in neonates, these should be considered during therapy.

LONG-TERM OUTCOMES

In most of the studies evaluating the use of inhalation steroids, there was a paucity of data on long-term adverse effects, especially for extremely premature infants at highest risk for development of BPD. The NEUROSIS trial demonstrated no difference in neurodevelopmental disability at 2 years, but there remained an increased mortality rate in infants receiving steroids (Bassler et al., 2018). The long-term effects of inhaled corticosteroids should be more thoroughly addressed in future studies, especially given the neurodevelopmental risks known to be associated with use of systemic steroids in this population.

Loop Diuretics

Furosemide, the most commonly used loop diuretic in the NICU, is an anthranilic acid derivative that works by inhibiting the Na^+-K^+-$2Cl^-$ symporter in the thick ascending limb of the loop of Henle, thus leading to increased excretion of Na^+ and water. This symporter is responsible for reabsorption of about 25% of luminal sodium load; therefore, loop diuretics have a potent effect on natriuresis. Other loop diuretics that have been used in U.S. NICUs include bumetanide and ethacrynic acid. We focus our discussion on furosemide, given its relatively widespread use in NICUs across the United States.

Despite the effect of furosemide on pulmonary mechanics, there is little evidence for its utility in the prevention or management of BPD. The 2011 Cochrane review of IV or enteral furosemide use found six studies examining the effect of furosemide and concluded that in preterm infants less than 3 weeks of age, furosemide had inconsistent or undetectable effect, and in infants older than 3 weeks of age furosemide use improved oxygenation and compliance; however, sufficient evidence regarding important outcomes was lacking and thus routine use of furosemide or other loop diuretics could not be recommended (Stewart & Brion, 2011).

MECHANISM OF ACTION/CORE PHARMACOKINETIC PRINCIPLES

It is postulated that furosemide has two major mechanisms by which it improves respiratory outcomes in infants with BPD: First, it has an immediate effect on urine output that leads to lung fluid resorption and thus improved pulmonary function, and second the diuresis leads to total body fluid redistribution and further lung fluid resorption. The immediate effect was demonstrated in a study of the pulmonary mechanics of 10 infants with chronic BPD following a single dose of IV furosemide or placebo, which found a significant, albeit transient, increase in urine output, airway conductance, and airway compliance, accompanied with a significant but transient decrease in airway resistance within hours of administration (Kao et al., 1983). The longer term effects are suggested in trials such as by McCann et al. in 1985, which found a sustained improvement in pulmonary function at 7 days of therapy that exceeded the duration of increased diuresis, which only lasted 48 to 72 hours (McCann et al., 1985).

The pharmacokinetics of furosemide vary greatly by PMA. In preterm infants less than 31 weeks' PMA, half-life is often greater than 24 hours (Mirochnick et al., 1988). This decreases to 12 hours by 33 weeks' PMA and approaches 4 hours (the half-life in term neonates) as preterm infants approach a term PMA (Mirochnick et al., 1988). Although the prolonged half-life of furosemide in preterm infants leads to higher plasma concentrations of the drug, the pharmacodynamic response to furosemide may be decreased at lower PMA. This is because the effect of furosemide is dependent on the renal tubular concentration of the drug, and tubular secretion of the drug is low at PMA less than 32 weeks (Mirochnick et al., 1988).

DOSING RECOMMENDATIONS

Furosemide may be given by the IV, IM, and enteral routes, all of which have been studied in neonates with BPD. The recommended initial IV dose is 1 mg/kg, which may be increased to a maximum dose of 2 mg/kg (Micromedex Neofax Online, n.d.-d). The dosing interval varies by age given the change in pharmacokinetics as described previously. In infants less than 32 weeks' PMA, it is recommended that dosing frequency not exceed every 24 hours; between 32 weeks' PMA and term, dosing may be as frequent as every 12 hours, given the prolonged half-life with lower PMA (Mirochnick et al., 1988).

Bioavailability of oral furosemide is highly variable in infants. In one study of 10 infants, oral bioavailability ranged from 56% to 106%, with a mean of 84.3% at a PMA of 39 weeks (Mirochnick et al., 1988). Although the range of bioavailability is broad, it is widely recommended that enteral dosing may need to be twice that of IV dosing to achieve similar effect, with a maximum enteral dose exceeding that of IV dosing at 6 mg/kg (Micromedex Neofax Online, n.d.-d).

Initiation of Therapy

There are no RCTs designed to evaluate the ideal timing of initiation of loop diuretics. In fact, there is only one trial that examined the effects of furosemide in 1-week-old infants with RDS, which found transient improvement in compliance and ventilation, but long-term outcomes were not evaluated (Najak et al., 1983). The majority of trials of furosemide for BPD have initiated therapy at more than 3 weeks of age.

Duration and Cessation of Therapy

Similarly, there are no clear guidelines on the appropriate duration of treatment with loop diuretics. Given that many of the adverse effects of furosemide have been linked to higher cumulative dose exposure, efforts are often made to limit chronic loop diuretic use. In addition, there is evidence that renal response to furosemide (determined by the logarithm of urinary furosemide excretion and diuretic/natriuretic response) decreases significantly over a 3-week course (Mirochnick et al., 1990), although the actual clinical impact of this remains to be determined. Although single doses have been shown to have a positive effect on pulmonary mechanics (Kao et al., 1983), clinically relevant parameters, such as decreased FiO_2 requirement or ability to wean respiratory support, were not seen at 24 to 48 hours of furosemide exposure but were observed at 7 days (McCann et al., 1985); thus, many studies use at least a 7-day course.

Potentially in favor of prolonging furosemide courses was the finding of decreased mortality and BPD with increasing percentage of furosemide exposure days in a large retrospective cohort study (N = 37,693) of preterm and ELBW infants (Greenberg et al., 2019). The study found that a 10% increase in furosemide exposure days was associated with a decrease in the incidence of BPD (4.6%, p = .001) and BPD or mortality (3.7%, p = .01; Greenberg et al., 2019). However, RCTs have not demonstrated the same beneficial effects in prolonged furosemide exposure (Stewart et al., 2011). When considering chronic use of furosemide, every-other-day dosing is suggested to minimize risk of toxicity and electrolyte disturbance (Micromedex Neofax Online, n.d.-d).

CLINICAL-MONITORING PEARLS

Cardiovascular Effects

As furosemide is known to increase renal prostaglandin production, there has been concern about the early use of furosemide increasing the incidence of PDA. However, in a study of infants receiving indomethacin for PDA, furosemide exposure led to increased likelihood of acute renal failure without affecting the rates of PDA closure (Lee et al., 2010).

Renal Effects

Furosemide use is contraindicated in infants with anuric renal failure and has been associated with acute renal injury, especially when given with other nephrotoxic medications (Micromedex Neofax Online, n.d.-d). In a study of factors associated with nephrocalcinosis in preterm infants, furosemide exposure had the strongest influence on the development of nephrocalcinosis, with a 10 mg/kg cumulative dose leading to a fourfold increase in odds of nephrocalcinosis (Gimpel et al., 2010).

Endocrinologic Effects

Electrolyte disturbances are among the most frequently reported adverse effects of loop diuretics. Furosemide has been associated with hyponatremia, hypochloremic alkalosis, hypokalemia, hypomagnesemia, and hypocalcemia (Micromedex Neofax Online, n.d.-d). Hyponatremia and hypochloremia may limit effectiveness of the drug. Hypocalcemia is due to increased renal excretion of calcium and can be associated with nephrolithiasis or nephrocalcinosis as described earlier. In addition, hypercalciuria can lead to dysregulation of parathyroid hormone (PTH) and thus contribute to metabolic bone disease. Severity of metabolic bone disease has been most closely associated with total cumulative dose of loop diuretics rather than the timing of initiation (Orth & O'Mara, 2018). Electrolytes should be monitored during loop diuretic therapy and supplementation may be necessary.

LONG-TERM OUTCOMES

There are no current studies investigating the effects of loop diuretic use on neurodevelopmental outcomes, nor are there any data on long-term pulmonary effects. There has been concern about furosemide exposure-related ototoxicity. Adult studies have demonstrated furosemide-associated ototoxicity at levels of 25 mcg/mL, and levels have been shown to accumulate near that in preterm infants receiving furosemide every 12 hours (Mirochnick et al., 1988). A 2018 retrospective cohort study of infants exposed to ≥28 days of furosemide prior to 36 weeks' PMA (N = 1,020) did not find any significant difference in the incidence of abnormal hearing screen ("refer" or "fail") versus control infants; however, the risk of ototoxicity should not be underestimated (Wang et al., 2018). Regarding other long-term outcomes, there are no randomized trials that examine important clinical outcomes such as survival, duration of ventilatory support or supplemental oxygen, or pulmonary disease at long-term follow-up; thus, current evidence is lacking to support the routine use of loop diuretics in the prevention of BPD (Stewart et al., 2011).

Thiazide Diuretics

As with other classes of diuretics, thiazides are suspected to improve lung function by both an immediate resorption of fluid due to diuresis and a more chronic fluid redistribution that occurs as diuresis leads to intravascular depletion (Stewart et al., 2011). Many studies have demonstrated the effect of thiazides on pulmonary mechanics. In a randomized, double-blind, crossover study of infants with grade 3 or 4 BPD (N = 10), there were significant decreases in pulmonary resistance with increases in mean airway conductance and dynamic pulmonary compliance following 1 week of treatment with chlorothiazide (20 mg/kg/dose) and spironolactone (1.5 mg/kg/dose) given twice daily (Kao et al., 1984). A later RCT of infants with BPD (N = 22) found that following 4 weeks of daily diuretic therapy (chlorothiazide 40 mg/kg/d and spironolactone 4 mg/kg/d), dynamic airway compliance improved by 46% ($p < .001$) and airway resistance decreased by 31% ($p < .05$); however, changes in pulmonary mechanics were reversed with discontinuation of therapy (Kao et al., 1994). Oxygen requirement improved over time for both the diuretic and placebo group, but the decrease in FiO_2 requirement at 4 weeks for the diuretic group was significantly larger (0.35 ± 0.1 to 0.23 ± 0.02 vs. 0.37 ± 0.16 to 0.29 ± 0.11, $p < .01$; Kao et al., 1994).

Only one trial has examined the effect of chlorothiazide alone versus chlorothiazide with spironolactone. The randomized, double-blind, placebo-controlled trial sought to examine the need for electrolyte repletion with use of spironolactone, but also followed pulmonary mechanics in infants treated with a 14-day course of chlorothiazide (40 mg/kg/d) alone or with the addition of spironolactone (3 mg/kg/d). The percentage of change in pulmonary compliance and airway resistance from day 0 to day 14 was not significantly different between the chlorothiazide-plus-spironolactone and the chlorothiazide-only groups (Hoffman et al., 2000).

A Cochrane review of six trials of infants receiving thiazides for BPD found that in preterm infants greater than 3 weeks of age, a 4-week course of thiazide and spironolactone increased airway compliance and decreased the need for furosemide, with one study of an 8-week course demonstrating reduced mortality; however, the authors advise caution given the paucity of trials available for review and the limited data on clinically relevant outcomes (Stewart et al., 2011).

MECHANISM OF ACTION/CORE PHARMACOKINETIC PRINCIPLES

Thiazide diuretics are sulfonamide derivatives that function in the distal convoluted tubule by inhibition of the Na^+/Cl^- channel, thus increasing natriuresis and diuresis (Chemtob et al., 1989). Thiazides prevent 5% to 8% of filtered sodium from being reabsorbed; thus, they are less potent than the loop diuretics (Chemtob et al., 1989). The increased distal sodium delivery increases the activity of the aldosterone-dependent Na/K pump, leading to increased potassium excretion; thus, thiazides are often used in conjunction with the aldosterone inhibitor spironolactone.

Thiazides are rapidly absorbed after enteral administration with about 65% to 75% bioavailability (Chemtob et al., 1989). Half-life has not been rigorously studied in neonates, but is estimated to be about 5 hours, with peak effect on urine and solute excretion from 2 to 6 hours (Chemtob et al., 1989; Micromedex Neofax Online, n.d.-b).

DOSING RECOMMENDATIONS

The two most common thiazides used in the neonatal population are chlorothiazide and hydrochlorothiazide. Chlorothiazide is given in doses of 10 to 20 mg/kg/dose enterally every 12 hours and hydrochlorothiazide 1 to 2 mg/kg/dose enterally every 12 hours (Micromedex Neofax Online, n.d.-b, n.d.-e). When coupled with spironolactone, the dose of spironolactone is 1 to 3 mg/kg/d; combined products of hydrochlorothiazide and spironolactone are available (Micromedex Neofax Online, n.d.-f, n.d.-g).

Initiation of Therapy

Few studies have examined the ideal timing of initiation of thiazide use in neonates. In the 2011 Cochrane review, all six controlled trials examined the effect of thiazide diuretics started after 3 weeks of life (Stewart et al., 2011).

Duration and Cessation of Therapy

Currently, there are trials examining the appropriate duration of thiazide use in BPD, but existing trials have demonstrated that the beneficial effects of thiazides on pulmonary mechanics dissipate when therapy is discontinued (Kao et al., 1984, 1994; Stewart et al., 2011). At least one study has failed to demonstrate a significant effect of hydrochlorothiazide and spironolactone on pulmonary function at 6 to 8 days (Engelhardt et al., 1989), and the study that demonstrated improved survival to hospital discharge used an 8-week course of diuretic therapy (Albersheim et al., 1989). Thus, the majority of studies have focused on a more chronic course, ranging from at least 4 to 8 weeks of therapy, if tolerated.

Thiazides are often prescribed on hospital discharge and the duration of thiazide therapy in the outpatient setting is highly variable. A single-center, retrospective, observational study found the range of diuretic duration for 59 infants following hospital discharge was 31 to 368 days, with a median duration of 94 days (Bhandari et al., 2010). The study noted that 58% of patients were taken off or had their thiazide dose actively tapered at the first follow-up visit, and only one patient required resumption of diuretics, suggesting that thiazides could be tapered or discontinued more aggressively than is current practice (Bhandari et al., 2010).

CLINICAL-MONITORING PEARLS

Electrolytes

Electrolyte derangements comprise the majority of adverse effects from thiazides in neonates. In theory, thiazide diuretics should be milder than loop diuretics, as the distal convoluted tubule is responsible for the resorption of a smaller percentage of filtered sodium, and the addition of spironolactone to a thiazide should prevent significant potassium wasting; however, this is not always the case. A retrospective cohort study that reviewed 127 chlorothiazide courses found the incidence of hyponatremia was 35.4%, with an average decrease in serum sodium concentration of 2.9%, reaching a nadir at 5 days of therapy (Harkin et al., 2022). In that study, enteral sodium supplementation was used in 41% of chlorothiazide courses and 13% of treatment courses were aborted within the first 2 weeks due to hyponatremia (Harkin et al., 2022). A much larger retrospective cohort study ($N = 3,252$) explored the relationship between various diuretic exposures and risk of enteral electrolyte repletion and found that infants exposed to loop diuretics, thiazides, thiazides plus spironolactone, and loop diuretics plus thiazides were all significantly more likely to require repletion with sodium chloride or potassium chloride than the control, and of those diuretic exposures thiazide monotherapy was associated with higher rates of electrolyte supplementation than loop monotherapy (Nelin et al., 2021). The addition of spironolactone to thiazide therapy provided some reduction in the need for potassium chloride supplementation, but the reduction was mild (from 20.5% to 16.5% risk-interval days; Nelin et al., 2021).

Lipid Profiles

Hyperlipidemia and hypertriglyceridemia have been reported as potential adverse effects of thiazide diuretics (Chemtob et al., 1989; Micromedex Neofax Online, n.d.-b) and have even been observed in infants on entirely enteral nutrition (Wareham et al., 1989). In a 1992 study of metabolic effects of thiazide diuretics in neonates with BPD, high-density lipoprotein (HDL) concentration was 33% higher in infants who had received 4 weeks of diuretic therapy compared with their control counterparts ($p < .05$) and the HDL concentration for those treated had increased 44% from their baseline prior to therapy ($p < .05$; Kazzi et al., 1992). Note that when diuretics were continued for a total of 8 weeks of therapy, the difference in lipid profiles was diminished. There was no significant difference in total cholesterol, triglycerides, HDL, or low-density lipoprotein (LDL) concentrations between those treated and the controls, although the sample size was smaller for the prolonged therapy ($N = 12$ in the treatment group; Kazzi et al., 1992).

LONG-TERM OUTCOMES

There are no studies examining the effects of thiazide use on BPD and long-term neurodevelopmental outcomes. One RCT of preterm infants ($N = 34$) requiring mechanical ventilation demonstrated improved survival to hospital discharge (87% vs. 47%, $p < .05$) following an 8-week course of hydrochlorothiazide (2 mg/kg every 12 hours) and spironolactone (1.5 mg/kg every 12 hours), although there was not a significant difference in total duration of ventilator days or hospital days (Albersheim et al., 1989). Of note, the infants studied in this trial did not have exposure to corticosteroids, bronchodilators, or aminophylline (Stewart et al., 2011). Thus, although the promise of thiazide usage in improving pulmonary mechanics is well established, their use in the prevention of BPD cannot be recommended given the limited evidence on long-term benefit (Stewart et al., 2011).

CONCLUSIONS

BPD is a complex disease with many antecedents and few modifiable factors. Nonpharmacologic measures aimed at improving the risk of development of BPD have little basis in evidence or statistical influence on the outcome. However, several key medications, including caffeine, VA, and dexamethasone, have been demonstrated to mitigate BPD risk. As with all medications, these pharmacotherapeutics each come with their own risks and may not be appropriate for all neonates, which requires the decision-making surrounding their use to be evaluated on an individual basis. Early identification of infants most at risk of BPD development may allow clinicians to tailor and target these interventions to those most likely to benefit, impacting the long-term morbidities and mortality associated with the most common outcome of prematurity.

LEARNING TOOLS AND RESOURCES

Advice From the Authors

Macrina Liguori, MD, FAAP

Bronchopulmonary dysplasia is a result of the complex interplay between interrupted fetal lung development and the physiologic response to modern medicine's effort to provide support for neonatal respiratory distress. While many pharmacologic and nonpharmacologic interventions have plausible mechanisms by which to improve pulmonary dynamics and minimize harm to the developing neonatal lung, few have been shown by RCTs to be effective in preventing clinically important long-term morbidities of prematurity, including BPD and neurodevelopmental impairment. The decision to treat an infant with therapies intended to prevent BPD should be carefully weighed against that individual infant's risk of BPD and other comorbidities.

Sarah Croop, DNP, APRN, NNP-BC

First and foremost, understand the fundamental pathophysiology of BPD and recognize the variations in presentation and approach to management for individual infants, which is frequently complicated by concomitant conditions such as structural airway anomalies, pneumonia, and pulmonary hypertension. Second, consider the mechanism of action of the pharmacologic agent and how it relates to the underlying pathology in each situation. Remember, the pharmacologic agents described in this chapter are largely adjuncts to mechanical ventilation and used with the ultimate goal of decreasing the need and/or the duration of use for this intervention. As the underlying pathology changes and evolves for each infant, so should the pharmacologic approach, always keeping in mind the ultimate goal. Finally, maintain an open mind to the empiric opinions and suggestions from experienced colleagues as I hope you have gleaned from this chapter, there are not always clear, evidence-based recommendations when considering pharmacologic interventions for BPD.

Andrea N. Trembath, MD, MPH, FAAP

Bronchopulmonary dysplasia is very common among premature infants and yet has few clear targets for prevention. Decision-making around the use of nonpharmacologic and pharmacologic agents therefore must involve a clear balancing of the risks and potential benefits to each. Gentle ventilation strategies must be balanced with providing adequate ventilation and oxygenation while supporting growth and neurodevelopment. When thinking about the prevention strategies for BPD, keep in mind no single therapy will be appropriate for every infant.

Discussion Prompts

1. What would the risk of severe BPD be for a 25-week, 700-gram, white male, intubated infant on 30% oxygen at 7 days of life? At 14? At 21? At 28?
2. At which point should dexamethasone be considered to facilitate extubation?
3. What are the risks to giving the dexamethasone at each time point and what might the benefits be?

Mind Map

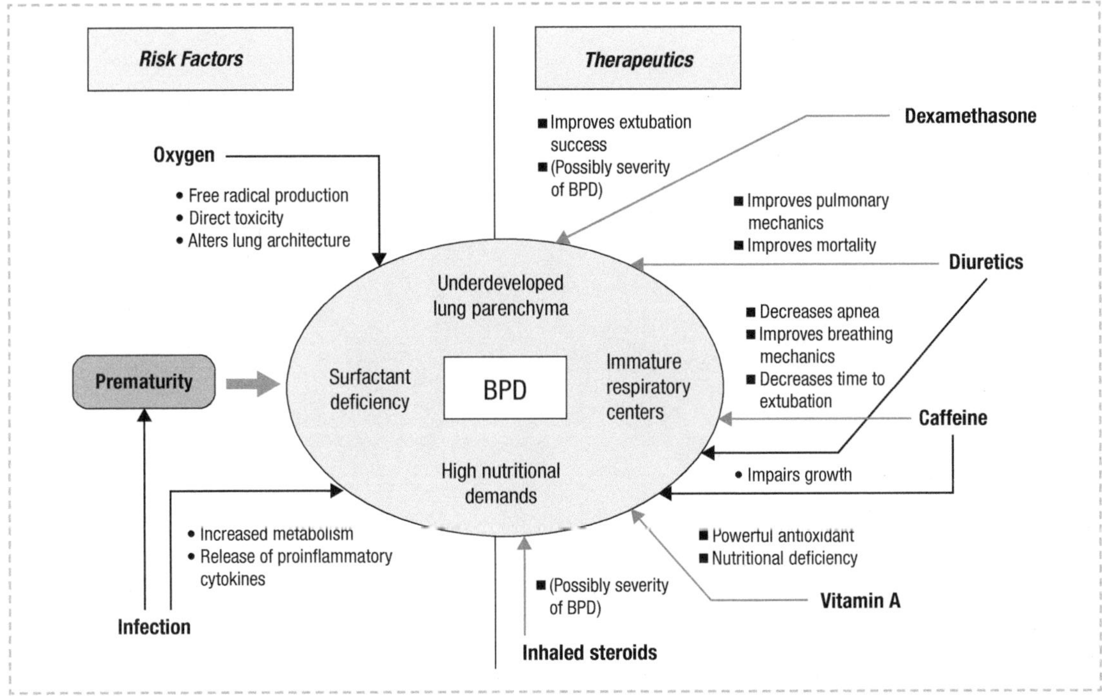

Note: This mind map reflects the design team's interpretation of a portion of one or more concepts addressed in this chapter. Readers should regard the mind maps woven throughout this textbook as examples of multisensory study tools that can be developed to encourage conceptual understanding. Readers are encouraged to develop their own unique mind maps in consultation with academic faculty or clinical preceptors.
BPD, bronchopulmonary dysplasia.
Design credit: Andrea N. Trembath, MD, MPH, FAAP.

REFERENCES

References for this chapter are online and available at https://connect.springerpub.com/content/book/978-0-8261-5884-0/part/partIII/toc-part/ch16.

PART IV

Common Cardiovascular Problems

chapter 17

Patent Ductus Arteriosus

Denise Kirsten

LEARNING OBJECTIVES

After completing this chapter, the reader should be able to:

- Define *patent ductus arteriosus (PDA)* and identify the epidemiology of the disease process.
- Explain the physiology of ductal regulation in utero and after birth.
- Correlate the pathophysiology of a PDA with the need for pharmacologic treatment.
- Appraise the historical evolution of pharmacologic management for a PDA.
- Evaluate current pharmacologic therapies for the treatment of a PDA.

INTRODUCTION

The patent ductus arteriosus (PDA) is the most common acyanotic cardiovascular abnormality diagnosed in preterm infants after 4 days of life. The incidence is estimated to be 70% among all neonates born at less than 28 weeks of gestation and 39% among infants weighing less than 1,500 grams at birth (Clyman, 2018; El-Khaffash et al., 2019; Vermont Oxford Network, 2016). Recent data suggest that 85% of PDAs in preterm neonates spontaneously close without pharmacologic treatment; however, natural closure may subject the infant to more than 60 postnatal days of retrograde shunting (Semberova et al., 2017).

Although the ductus arteriosus (DA) should functionally close within 3 days of birth, it often remains patent in preterm neonates (Hoffman et al., 2018). The pathology of a PDA involves retrograde left-to-right shunting with reduced renal blood flow, pulmonary overcirculation, and increased left ventricular stroke volume (Backer et al., 2016). This increases the risk for the onset of other acquired diseases, including intraventricular hemorrhage (IVH), renal disease, necrotizing enterocolitis (NEC), bronchopulmonary dysplasia (BPD), and periventricular leukomalacia (PVL; Dice & Bhatia, 2007; Mitra & McNamara, 2020; Schneider & Moore, 2006).

Pharmacologic, surgical, and interventional therapies may be prescribed to close a PDA; preferences vary widely among and across institutions in the United States. Pharmacologic therapy involves the use of indomethacin (INDO), ibuprofen (IBU), or acetaminophen. However, outcomes associated with pharmacologic therapies remain unclear, mainly due to design-related limitations (e.g., selection bias) of randomized trials. As a consequence, some clinicians aggressively seek pharmacologic closure of a PDA, whereas others advocate in favor of conservative treatment (Benitz, 2017).

This chapter begins with a review of fetal and postnatal physiologic blood flow. Given that ductal closure does not occur in 100% of neonates born preterm, we review the pathophysiology of the PDA, associated hemodynamic consequences, and common clinical manifestations. Next, we present noteworthy historic content specific to the genesis of understanding of the PDA and emergence of treatment regimens. Last, we present a comprehensive investigation of INDO, IBU, and acetaminophen, three available therapies used to elicit ductal closure.

PHYSIOLOGY REVIEW: THE DUCTUS ARTERIOSUS

We begin this section of the chapter with a detailed review of the structure, nomenclature, and metabolism of prostaglandins (PGs). This should help readers recognize the relationship between the structure of a PG and its tissue-specific physiologic function. Readers are referred to Chapter 18, "Critical Congenital Heart Defects," for a discussion of PG therapy for maintaining ductal patency.

Prostaglandin Formation and Metabolism

PGs, also referred to as *eicosanoids*, are potent vasodilators. Biochemically, each is composed of a unique cyclopentanone nucleus and two side chains. PGs are differentiated into three classes. The "1 class" (e.g., PGE_1) of PGs is derived from dihomo-linolenic acid. The "2 class" (e.g., PGE_2) is derived from arachidonic acid, and the "3 class" (e.g., PGE_3) is derived from eicosatetraenoic acid. Each PG is also assigned a group letter (e.g., PGE_1), which corresponds with the biochemical structure of the cyclopentanone nucleus. Of importance to this chapter, the PGs assigned to the "E" group maintain the patency of the DA in utero, as well as implicate vascular tone at the afferent renal arteriole.

A stepwise sequence of chemical reactions is required to form PGs. First, phospholipase enzymes hydrolyze (split) phospholipids. As a result, numerous polyunsaturated fatty acids (namely, arachidonic acid) are formed. Second, PG synthase-1 (cyclooxygenase or COX-1) and PG synthase-2 (COX-2), catalyze the biosynthesis (metabolism) of PG. In doing so, arachidonic acid is converted to an unstable endoperoxide, known as *PGG_2*, at the COX site. PGG_2 is further reduced to PGH_2 (peroxidase). Lastly, PGH_2 is hydrolyzed (split) into the stable, yet short-acting, eicosanoids (e.g., prostacyclin, thromboxane A_2, PGD_2, PGE_2, PGF_2). These eicosanoids exert a tissue-specific biochemical effect before being rapidly metabolized (Figure 17.1; Ovali, 2020; Takahashi et al., 2000).

FIGURE 17.1 The cyclooxygenase pathway.

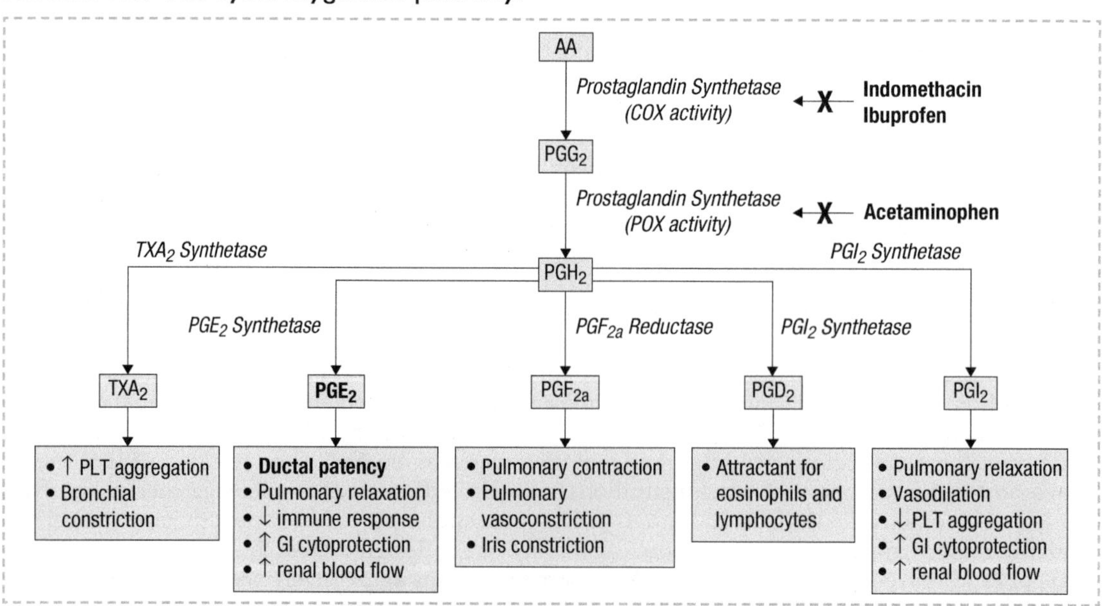

AA, arachidonic acid; COX, cyclooxygenase; GI, gastrointestinal; PLT, platelet; POX, peroxidase.

Source: Adapted from Rostas, S. E. & McPherson, C. C. (2016). Pharmacotherapy for patent ductus arteriosus: Current options and outstanding questions. *Current Pediatric Reviews, 12*(2), 110–119. https://doi.org/10.2174/1573396312021605060028.

Fetal Ductal Patency

The DA is derived from the distal portion of the sixth aortic arch and serves as a necessary in utero conduit for blood flow between the left pulmonary artery and descending aorta (Hoffman et al., 2018). By the eighth week of embryologic development, the internal diameter of the DA is equivalent to the pulmonary artery and the descending aorta. This establishes the DA as a bridge capable of shunting blood away from the developing lungs and toward the systemic fetal circulation (Benitz & Bhombal, 2020; Dice & Bhatia, 2007). Patency of the DA is maintained in utero through the combined effects of a low partial pressure of oxygen (PaO2) and a high level of circulating PGE_2 (Dice & Bhatia, 2007; Hung et al., 2018; Prescott & Keim-Malpass, 2017). Early in fetal development, PGE_2 is produced at the placenta and distributed to the DA. As the fetus matures, the vasa vasorum (microvasculature at the endothelial lining of the ductal smooth muscle wall) also contribute to PGE_2 production.

PGs are not the only substrates with a role in maintaining ductal patency. In fact, nitric oxide (NO) primarily modulates ductal patency early in gestational development. PGs overtake NO as the primary regulator of ductal tone closer to term gestation. NO production is catalyzed by the enzyme endothelial NO synthase and, like PGs, is synthesized at the vasa vasorum. This endogenously produced NO differs from exogenously inhaled NO, which does not regulate smooth muscle tone at the DA.

Postnatal Ductal Closure

Spontaneous closure of the DA in term infants begins with functional constriction and ends with anatomic obliteration. Among healthy term newborns, functional closure (constriction) of the lumen of the DA occurs within 72 hours after delivery. Clamping of the umbilical cord elicits an increase in systemic vascular resistance (SVR). The partial pressure of oxygen increases as the newborn cries and establishes a normal respiratory pattern; pulmonary vascular resistance (PVR) consequently decreases (Pacifici, 2013). As blood perfuses the lungs, circulating PGs are metabolized (Dice & Bhatia, 2007). In aggregate, these new postnatal changes favor smooth muscle contraction at the DA, ductal wall thickening, and functional closure. Anatomic closure is characterized by remodeling of the ductal tissue, fibrosis, and obliteration of the duct, which usually occurs by 4 months' postnatal age (Hoffman et al., 2018; Schneider & Moore, 2006).

PATHOPHYSIOLOGY REVIEW: THE PATENT DUCTUS ARTERIOSUS

As discussed, PGE_2 is the major PG that modulates ductal patency (Jasani et al., 2018; Sunil B et al., 2018). During fetal development, PGE_2 levels remain elevated because the placenta offers a continuous supply of PG. In addition, blood flow to the lungs (where PG is primarily metabolized) is reduced. After birth, PGs in the circulation are diverted to the lungs and metabolized by 15-hydroxyprostaglandin dehydrogenase. To a lesser extent, PGs are also metabolized in the spleen and kidneys. This significantly lowers the concentration of circulating PGs and should encourage functional closure of the DA.

However, biochemical and mechanical factors resist functional closure in preterm infants, which, in many cases, leads to persistent ductal patency. Biochemically, the circulating PGE_2 concentration remains elevated in premature infants. This may be due to functional immaturity of the lungs (reduced biosynthesis) or the presence of comorbid conditions, including sepsis and NEC (Clyman, 2018). In addition, the functionally immature smooth muscle wall of the DA is sensitive to the postnatal increase in the partial pressure of oxygen. Increased oxygen tension (e.g., mechanical ventilation with supplemental oxygen use) upregulates NO production and encourages persistent ductal patency.

Mechanically, failed closure of the intimal "cushion" (center of the endothelial smooth muscle arterial wall of the DA) resists functional closure of the DA. Normally, the intimal layer increases in thickness across gestation. After birth, under the influence of the biochemical factors mentioned in the prior paragraph, the thick intimal cushion merges and obliterates the lumen of the DA.

However, in preterm neonates, the intimal cushion is typically missing or too thin to facilitate obliteration, which favors persistent patency (Hamrick et al., 2020).

The pathology of a hemodynamically significant PDA remains under debate. Many experts believe that cause and effect (e.g., a hemodynamically significant PDA is associated with BPD) has not been proven to date. In fact, randomized trials have shown that early medical (pharmacologic) treatment does not reduce the incidence of BPD or death (Kluckow et al., 2014; Sosenko et al., 2012; Sung et al., 2020; Van Overmeire et al., 2001). Factors, including selection bias, confound some of these results and make it difficult to generalize findings and standardize approaches across institutions.

In contrast to human studies, results of animal studies suggest that a hemodynamically significant PDA does subject the heart and lungs to overcirculation. Therefore, in order to provide a complete discussion and explain the basis for which some clinicians choose medical treatment, we present the common pathophysiologic consequences of a hemodynamically significant PDA reported in the literature.

The pathology of a hemodynamically significant PDA depends on the size (internal diameter) and shape of the DA, vascular resistance, influences from chemical mediators, and blood viscosity (Benson et al., 2020; Park & Salamat, 2021). The most significant of all factors is the size and shape of the PDA. A large, short, and less torturous ductus permits a significant amount of retrograde (left-to-right) blood flow, whereas a small, S-shaped, or sharply angled ductus limits retrograde blood flow (Elsayed & Fraser, 2017). The second most important contributing factor to the pathogenesis of a PDA is vascular resistance, both systemic and pulmonary (Bernstein, 2020a; Hoffman et al., 2018). When the DA does not close within the first few days of life and SVR exceeds PVR, retrograde shunting of blood across the PDA may be observed. Retrograde flow across a moderate or large PDA may precipitate pulmonary overcirculation and edema, pulmonary vascular stress, and left atrial and ventricular dilatation (Ungerleider et al., 2019). If prolonged, left ventricular hypertrophy may develop (Schneider & Moore, 2006). Further, pulmonary overcirculation may impose shear stress on the vasculature and a compensatory increase in medial smooth muscle. This increases the risk for irreversible pulmonary vascular disease, pulmonary hypertension, and right-sided heart failure (Benson et al., 2020; Ungerleider et al., 2019). Chemical mediators, including oxygen, cytokines, and, of course, PGs, influence ductal patency. Finally, blood viscosity influences shunting. Viscous blood (e.g., polycythemia) is less capable of shunting across a PDA, whereas more dilute blood (e.g., anemia of prematurity) can readily shunt in a retrograde fashion across the PDA.

Clinical Manifestations

Clinical manifestations of a PDA develop as the PVR declines yet may not reflect the full hemodynamic significance of the persistent pathology. The symptomology of a PDA can involve the cardiovascular, renal, respiratory, and gastrointestinal (GI) systems (Conrad & Newberry, 2019; Gournay, 2010). Common manifestations are summarized in Table 17.1.

The classic cardiovascular manifestation is a holosystolic murmur heard best along the upper left sternal border. This murmur customarily radiates down the left side of the sternum and to the infant's back. However, infants with a large PDA and pulmonary overcirculation may exhibit no audible murmur; decreased turbulence is associated with reduced transmission of sound (Conrad & Newberry, 2019; Schneider & Moore, 2006). Additional cardiovascular-specific findings include a hyperactive precordium and tachycardia with or without gallop rhythm, bounding pulses, and a widened pulse pressure caused by runoff of blood into the pulmonary artery during diastole. The chest radiograph may reveal cardiomegaly or evidence of pulmonary edema or increased pulmonary vascular markings (Bernstein, 2020a; Park & Salamat, 2021).

Pulmonary, renal, and GI manifestations are also associated with a hemodynamically significant PDA. Should pulmonary overcirculation intensify, the risks for pulmonary edema, shear stress, and hemorrhage increase. Associated clinical manifestations include tachypnea, retractions, agitation, and blood-tinged secretions manifesting from the airway (Conrad & Newberry, 2019). Renal manifestations include oliguria and metabolic acidosis, which develop secondary to hypoperfusion from retrograde flow and reverse end-diastolic blood flow ("diastolic steal"). Reduced mesenteric blood flow increases the risk for feeding intolerance and NEC. In a study by Dollberg and colleagues (2005), the incidence of NEC was as high as 9.4% in infants with a PDA when compared to 4.3% of neonates without persistent ductal patency.

TABLE 17.1 Common Clinical Manifestations Associated With the Patent Ductus Arteriosus

Cardiovascular	• Active precordium • Bounding peripheral pulses • Cardiomegaly • Coarse systolic heart murmur • Diastolic hypotension • Holosystolic murmur • Tachycardia • Thrill • Wide pulse pressure
Gastrointestinal	• Feeding intolerance • Hepatomegaly • Increased risk for NEC • Poor weight gain
Renal	• Elevated creatinine level • Hyponatremia • Metabolic acidosis • Oliguria
Respiratory	• Apnea • Increased pulmonary vascular markings • Pulmonary edema • Pulmonary hemorrhage • Respiratory distress

NEC, necrotizng enterocolitis.
Sources: From Conrad, C., & Newberry, D. (2019). Understanding the pathophysiology, implications and treatment options in patent ductus arteriosus in the neonatal population. *Advances in Neonatal Care, 19*(3), 179–187. https://doi.org/10.1097/ANC.0000000000000590; Dice, J., & Bhatia, J. (2007). Patent ductus arteriosus: An overview. *Journal of Pediatric Pharmacology and Therapeutics, 12*(3), 138–146. https://doi.org/10.5863/1551-6776-12.3.138

HISTORICAL CONTEXT: SEMINAL AND OTHER NOTEWORTHY STUDIES

The evolution of understanding specific to the DA is fascinating. The initial description of a DA was made centuries ago by Claudius Galen (c 130–200 CE). Galen used cadavers and animal dissections to inspect the anatomy of the heart and, in doing so, identified distinct differences between fetal and adult lungs. He theorized that (a) breathing did not occur in utero; and (b) blood primarily flowed in a single direction through the foramen ovale and the DA, bypassing the fetal lungs (Raju, 2019). Although these discoveries were based almost entirely on the study of monkeys and dogs, Galen's work prompted additional inquiries into human anatomy and, specific to this chapter, the two conduits for oxygenation of blood from the placenta: the foramen ovale and DA.

Most other early anatomical discoveries occurred during the Renaissance and Reformation periods (14th to 17th centuries), when artists took an interest in human anatomy and physicians performed public dissections for all to see. Andreas Vesalius was one influential physician–surgeon who performed numerous human dissections during the 16th century. These were held in outdoor locations to facilitate viewing by medical students, clergy, artists, and the general public. In 1543, Vesalius published *De Humani Corporis Fabrica,* a collection of 227 wooden anatomical engravings based upon his direct observations. His engravings of the heart suggested that he believed that blood flowed from the vena cava to the right ventricle, impurities were routed to the lungs, and the remaining blood flowed through "invisible pores" in the ventricular septum and into the left ventricle. Here, impurities were routed to the lungs, combined again with the blood in the left ventricle forming a "vital spirit," routed to the aorta, and then moved to the general circulation (Steele, 2014). Clearly, Vesalius's findings were fraught with error, but his insistence on direct observation marked a seminal shift away from the subjective (conjecture) and toward objective investigations.

Next, Giulio Cesare Aranzi (c 1530–1589 CE), a student of scientist Leonardo Botallo, discovered that the DA and foramen ovale physiologically closed after birth (Kaemmerer et al., 2004). In honor of Leonardo Botallo (1519–1587 CE), his teacher, Aranzio named the structure the *ductus Botalli*. This term was then adapted to *ductus arteriosus apertus*, which persisted for 3 centuries until *patent ductus arteriosus* was adopted into the vernacular (Murshid & Elassal, 2021; Raju, 2019).

Given the high infant mortality rates during this era, this is no surprise that persistence of the DA went undiscovered until the 19th century. Finally, patency beyond the first days of life was recognized as a congenital malformation (Kaemmerer et al., 2004). Around this same time, heart sounds associated with the PDA were identified. In 1898, George Gibson was the first to classify the PDA as a systolic murmur heard loudest immediately after the second heart sound (Kaemmerer et al., 2004). Then, nearly 40 years later, cardiac catherizations facilitated more accurate descriptions of heart murmurs and their precise anatomic origins (Raju, 2019).

Given that a PDA was now considered a pathologic problem, early 19th-century physicians began to consider treatment options. John Cummings Munro was the first surgeon to propose surgical ligation of a PDA in 1907 but did not attempt the procedure. In 1920, Evarts Ambrose Graham lobbied to perform the procedure, but was provided an adult male (53 years of age) instead of a child (Brock, 1965). After all, pediatric surgery was not an established subspecialty at that time. It was not until 1938 that surgeon Robert Gross performed the first successful ligation of a DA in a 7-year-old girl. Preterm neonates were not yet recognized as an at-risk population potentially in need of treatment.

This perspective changed in 1958 when E. D. Burnard shared his seminal finding that prematurity was a risk for persistent ductal patency beyond the first few days of life. He also elucidated the relationship between the PDA and the manifestation of dyspnea (Burnard, 1958). His findings sparked decades of follow-up conversations, observational studies, and randomized trials, each of which associated the PDA to a pathologic finding in need of early treatment. Cotton and colleagues (1978) published the seminal randomized study, which investigated "early surgical closure" compared to "no treatment." Infants were randomized at 1 week of life to receive the intervention (surgical ligation) or no treatment. Early surgical ligation (within the first few weeks of life) was associated with reduced pulmonary morbidities compared to conservative management. Interestingly, current studies suggest the opposite; morbidity risks (e.g., vocal cord paralysis, BPD) are lower when surgical closure is avoided or delayed until late in the neonatal course (Jhaveri et al., 2010; Sung et al., 2016).

The next major breakthrough occurred in the mid-1970s and involved the introduction of INDO, a nonsteroidal anti-inflammatory drug (NSAID), specifically a COX-2 inhibitor, as an alternative to surgical closure (Raju, 2019). Physicians were quick to adopt this therapy, as aggressive management was favored (Benitz & Bhombal, 2020). Heymann and colleagues (1976) and Friedman and colleagues (1976) were the first to investigate the efficacy of INDO for PDA closure. Preterm infants with a large PDA with left-to-right shunting were provided one or two doses of oral or rectal INDO (0.1–5 mg/kg/dose). Of the 21 infants enrolled across these two landmark studies, 95% achieved ductal closure. Complications included renal failure (two infants) and death (two infants; Friedman et al., 1976; Heymann et al., 1976). Next, Friedman (1977) investigated intravenous INDO use and reported a 90% closure rate. Based on the results of these seminal studies, INDO use found favor among many neonatologists in the United States.

After the adoption of INDO came IBU, another NSAID COX-2 inhibitor. Van Overmeire and colleagues (1997) were the first to investigate the efficacy of INDO compared to IBU in preterm infants less than 30 weeks of gestation, to determine whether IBU use elicited fewer renal side effects (e.g., oliguria, anuria). No significant difference in treatment efficacy was reported; however, renal side effects were significantly reduced with IBU use. Urine output (within the first 48 hours) was higher in the IBU group ($p = .001$) and the rate of oliguria was 35% higher in the INDO group ($p = .02$). Shortly thereafter, IBU use gained favor over INDO (Van Overmeire et al., 1997). To date, over 30 randomized trials have been published comparing INDO and IBU, which have been analyzed in multiple meta-analyses (Ohlsson et al., 2020).

After INDO and IBU were adopted by neonatologists in the United States, and concerns increased specific to hematologic, GI, and renal complications, acetaminophen (paracetamol) was uncovered as a potential alternative. Hammerman and colleagues (2011) published the seminal case series of acetaminophen (15 mg/kg/dose every 6 hours) use. The authors noted ductal closure after administration of acetaminophen for an unrelated indication and subsequently reported five total preterm neonates who experienced efficacy without adverse effects within 72 hours of treatment. These data introduced acetaminophen, a drug that did not elicit a vasoconstrictive effect, as an alternative to INDO or IBU (Hammerman et al., 2011). To date, eight studies ($N = 916$) have been published that compare acetaminophen to IBU, acetaminophen to INDO, or acetaminophen to placebo, and suggest equal efficacy compared to NSAIDs with fewer adverse effects (Al-Lawama et al., 2018; Akbari Asbagh et al., 2015; Dang et al., 2013; El-Mashad et al., 2017; Härkin et al., 2016; Oncel et al., 2014, Yang et al., 2016).

These studies and others published between the inception of therapy and the present day helped advance the state of the science specific to the treatment of a PDA. However, an important consideration that leading experts call attention to is that the majority of all randomized trials enrolled neonates if a PDA was present, without considering the magnitude of shunting (Clyman & Liebowitz, 2017). This lack of specificity complicates the ability to determine whether morbidity risks reported in studies developed as a result of exposure to the pharmacologic treatment regimen or as a result of PDA-induced mitigation measures prescribed to treat the hemodynamic effects of the pathology. Long-term studies are needed to better understand the neurodevelopmental implications associated with PDA-targeted pharmacotherapy, surgical ligation, and conservative management.

CURRENT PHARMACOLOGIC TREATMENT MODALITIES FOR THE PATENT DUCTUS ARTERIOSUS

More recently, many clinicians consider the PDA to be an innocent physiologic bystander versus a pathologic condition (Abdel-Hady et al., 2013; Benitz, 2017; Benson et al., 2020). As a result, the management of a hemodynamically significant PDA in preterm infants varies among institutions. Some clinicians prefer to begin with fluid restriction, diuretic therapy, and ventilator support; however, the use of drugs that inhibit 15-hydroxyprostaglandin dehydrogenase activity (e.g., loop diuretics) inhibit PG metabolism and may encourage ductal patency. Practitioners must carefully review primary literature and guidelines examining the optimal timing of therapy for PDA, as active research continues in this area (Benitz & Committee on Fetus and Newborn, 2016; Clyman et al., 2019; Van Overmeire et al., 2001). The remainder of this chapter focuses on medical management of clinically symptomatic, persistent, and hemodynamically significant PDA. Medical (pharmacologic) management involves the use of INDO, IBU, or acetaminophen. INDO and IBU are U.S. Food and Drug Administration (FDA)-approved nonselective COX inhibitors (Dice & Bhatia, 2007). Although COX inhibitors remain the treatment of choice to treat a hemodynamically significant PDA, acetaminophen is becoming an attractive option when COX inhibitors are ineffective or contraindicated (Hamrick et al., 2020; Prescott & Keim-Malpass, 2017). Acetaminophen uniquely inhibits the production of PG H-synthase, an essential enzyme responsible for the biosynthesis of PGs from arachidonic acid. Other treatment modalities include surgical ligation and interventional cardiac catheterization, which extend beyond the scope of this chapter.

Indomethacin

INDO is the seminal NSAID. It has been prescribed for PDA closure since Heymann and colleagues (1976) reported successful ductal obliteration with INDO use in 18 preterm neonates.

MECHANISM OF ACTION/PHARMACOKINETIC PRINCIPLES

INDO is a potent and nonselective COX inhibitor (Shah, 2019). INDO promotes closure of the DA through reversible inhibition of COX-1 and COX-2 enzymes, key enzymes in the PG synthesis pathway discussed earlier in this chapter (see Figure 17.1; Pacifici, 2016). The vasoconstrictive effects of INDO on the ductus manifest as quickly as 30 minutes after administration and do not return to pretreatment levels until after 120 minutes (Corff & Sekar, 2007).

INDO is administered intravenously, which is associated with 100% bioavailability. Oral administration is associated with the risk for erratic absorption and reduced bioavailability as well as an increased risk of GI adverse effects. Once within the systemic circulation, a high volume of distribution is observed in preterm neonates compared to children or adults. Drug half-life is prolonged, particularly in preterm infants less than 1,500 grams. Hepatic metabolism is modulated primarily by CYP2C9 and INDO metabolites are eliminated in the urine (C. J. Smith et al., 2017).

DOSING RECOMMENDATIONS

The customary intravenous dose of INDO is 0.1 to 0.25 mg/kg/dose administered once or twice daily for 3 doses. Two courses of therapy have been reported in an attempt to achieve ductal closure (Pacifici, 2016).

Initiation of Treatment

The effectiveness of INDO in permanently closing the DA depends on the age of the infant at the beginning of treatment. INDO tends to be more effective when used during the first several days after birth, before the effect of PG on ductal patency wanes with advancing postnatal age (Narayanan-Sankar & Clyman, 2003). Overall, optimal timing of pharmacologic intervention remains controversial and may be delayed in the absence of hemodynamic compromise (Conrad & Newberry, 2019).

CLINICAL-MONITORING PEARLS

The use of COX inhibitors is associated with increased risk for alterations in cerebral, renal, GI, and hematologic function (Johnston et al., 2012). Contraindications to use and common side effects are summarized in Table 17.2.

Cerebral Function

INDO is relatively contraindicated for use in any infant with an IVH, as this drug is known to influence cerebral hemodynamics. Recall that 50% of germinal matrix (GM) hemorrhages present during the first 24 hours of life and 90% develop by 72 hours of life (Parodi et al., 2020). COX enzymes contribute to the maintenance of normal cerebral autoregulation by maintaining vascular tone (Leffler et al., 1985). INDO use can promote cerebral vasoconstriction and reduce cerebral blood flow, volume, cerebral oxygen delivery, and intracellular oxygenation (Corff & Sekar, 2007; Gournay, 2005).

It is interesting to note that prophylactic INDO use, when initiated within several hours after birth and in the absence of a preexisting GM hemorrhage, is associated with a decreased risk for IVH. No differences in neurodevelopmental outcomes have been reported to date (Fowlie et al., 2010; Gournay, 2005). In small trials examining INDO in the setting of existing IVH, therapy

TABLE 17.2 Contraindications or Risks Associated With Indomethacin Therapy

	CONTRAINDICATION FOR USE	RISKS WITH USE
CNS	Intraventricular hemorrhage	
Cardiovascular	Ductal-dependent lesion	
Gastrointestinal	Bleeding NEC Spontaneous intestinal perforation	Spontaneous intestinal perforation
Renal	Acute renal failure	Renal insufficiency or failure (oliguria) Elevated serum creatinine
Hematologic	Coagulopathy (thrombocytopenia)	Coagulopathy
Endocrine		Electrolyte disturbances (hyponatremia, hyperkalemia)
Other	Concomitant corticosteroid use[a]	

[a]Denotes increased risk for spontaneous intestinal perforation with concomitant use of a corticosteroid (e.g., hydrocortisone) and nonsteroidal anti-inflammatory drug.

CNS, central nervous system; NEC, necrotizing enterocolitis.

Sources: From Abdel-Hady, H., Nasef, N., Shabaan, A., & Nour, I. (2013). Patent ductus arteriosus in preterm infants: Do we have the right answers? *Biomedical Research International, 2013*, 676192. https://doi.org/10.1155/2013/676192; Allegaert, K., Anderson, B., Simons, S., & van Overmeire, B. (2013). Paracetamol to induce ductus arteriosus closure: Is it valid? *Archives of Disease in Childhood, 98*, 462–466. https://doi.org/10.1136/archdischild-2013-303688; Conrad, C., & Newberry, D. (2019). Understanding the pathophysiology, implications and treatment options in patent ductus arteriosus in the neonatal population. *Advances in Neonatal Care, 19*(3), 179–187. https://doi.org/10.1097/ANC.0000000000000590

did not promote reduction or extension of hemorrhage (Maher et al., 1985; Ment et al., 1994). Therefore, many clinicians obtain a baseline head ultrasound prior to initiation of INDO therapy; however, this should not delay initiation of prophylactic INDO for neonates with high risk of severe IVH.

Renal Function

Clinicians are encouraged to order baseline renal function testing prior to the initiation of therapy and daily throughout therapy. PGE_1 and PGE_2 are produced at the afferent arteriole and within the renal tubule. Both PGs are responsible for autoregulating renal blood flow and glomerular filtration rate (GFR). PGE_2 regulates sodium and water reabsorption through inhibition of the Na^+- K^+-$2Cl^-$ cotransporter in the ascending loop of Henle. In fact, PGE_2 is the major prostanoid excreted in the urine (F. Smith et al., 2012). This helps to maintain sodium homeostasis. Given that INDO enhances vasopressin action and increases renal vascular resistance, reduced renal perfusion and tubular function, as well as decreased urinary output, may develop (Akima et al., 2004).

A significant elevation in serum creatinine level warrants careful consideration for cessation of therapy, as this indicates that INDO is negatively affecting PG activity in the kidney and decreasing renal function (Shah, 2019). *Oliguria,* as defined as a urine output less than 1 mL/kg/hour, has been observed and is more common in immature infants, especially those with a birth weight less than 1,000 grams (Pacifici, 2014b). These side effects are usually transient and resolve with cessation of therapy (McIntyre et al., 2001).

Gastrointestinal Function

Clinical monitoring should include close observation of stooling pattern and consistency/color and physical examination findings (e.g., abdominal girth, abdominal distension). Frank GI bleeding (or hematuria) is a contraindication to the use of INDO (Narayanan-Sankar & Clyman, 2003).

INDO use is associated with an increased risk for spontaneous intestinal perforation (SIP) when given concomitantly with corticosteroids (Shah, 2019). Paquette and colleagues (2006) reported a 9.6-fold increase in the risk of SIP in very-low-birth-weight infants who received concomitant INDO and dexamethasone therapy during the first week of life (Paquette et al., 2006).

INDO use is also associated with an increased risk for GI bleeding and NEC. The association between INDO and NEC is less clear as there are conflicting data implicating COX therapy and PDA as a causative factor for NEC. Although the pathogenesis of NEC is multifactorial, alterations in intestinal perfusion leading to ischemia are thought to occur secondary to retrograde diastolic steal from left-to-right shunting through the PDA. This decreases mesenteric perfusion and increases the risk for bacterial translocation and sepsis. A complementary hypothesis involves the combined hits of INDO-induced vasoconstriction and diastolic steal on mesenteric perfusion, which may accentuate intestinal ischemia (Corff & Sekar, 2007; Gournay, 2005). Despite the potential for adverse effects on the GI tract, early prophylactic use of INDO in infants has not been associated with an increased risk of NEC in large randomized controlled trials (RCTs; Corff & Sekar, 2007).

Hematologic Function

It is essential to obtain a complete blood count and appraise the pretherapy platelet count prior to the initiation of INDO therapy. Most clinicians consider moderate to severe thrombocytopenia to be a contraindication for INDO therapy (Sallmon et al., 2018; Shah, 2019).

Platelet aggregation is modulated by thromboxane A_2, a potent vasoconstrictor and platelet activator produced through the PG biosynthesis pathway (Schafer, 1995). INDO inhibits COX-1 enzyme activity, which inhibits thromboxane synthesis and platelet aggregation. Delayed platelet aggregation may persist for 7 to 9 days after INDO therapy, or until platelets are replaced (Narayanan-Sankar & Clyman, 2003). Despite these effects, an increase in clinically significant bleeding has not been detected in RCTs of INDO. Recall that INDO reduces the risk of severe IVH and does not promote extension of existing IVH.

Ibuprofen

With the reported side effects associated with INDO and safety concerns related to its use, an alternative medication to treat a hemodynamically significant PDA was needed. IBU is a nonselective COX inhibitor that remains an alternative NSAID to INDO for the treatment of a PDA.

MECHANISM OF ACTION/PHARMACOKINETIC PRINCIPLES

The primary mechanism of action of IBU is inhibition of PG synthesis through nonselective and reversible inhibition of COX-1 and COX-2 enzymes. This prevents the conversion of arachidonic acid to the various PG types (Poon, 2007). By inhibiting COX activity, a reduction in the synthesis of vasodilating PGs, including PGE_2, occurs, thereby promoting constriction of the DA (Capparelli, 2007; Gournay, 2005).

The pharmacokinetic profile of IBU in preterm infants is unique secondary to hepatic and renal immaturity, in particular among preterm infants born less than 36 weeks of gestation. Absorption is rapid and complete with intravenous administration and slowed and slightly reduced with oral administration; oral dosing and subsequent absorption are not subject to first-pass hepatic metabolism. CYP2C9 and CYP2C8 modulate IBU metabolism; however, the complement of these enzymes is less than 5% of adult values during early postnatal life. This increases half-life, the circulating drug concentration, and efficacy. Enzymatic activity rapidly increases over the first week of life, to 33% of adult levels in all infants, independent of gestational age (Capparelli, 2007; van der Lugt et al., 2012).

Given the reduced state of hepatic metabolism, the half-life of IBU is approximately 10 times longer over the first several days of life compared to adults (Capparelli, 2007; Poon, 2007). However, as the hepatic system matures, drug half-life rapidly decreases as CYP2C9 and CYP2C8 concentrations increase and phase II glucuronidation matures (Capparelli, 2007; Pacifici, 2014a).

Renal clearance is observed. Nearly 80% of IBU is excreted as drug metabolites, and the balance is eliminated in its active form (Capparelli, 2007; Poon, 2007). Given that glomerular filtration in preterm infants less than 36 weeks of gestation is less than 30% of adult values, renal IBU clearance may be delayed (Bellflower et al., 2019). Clearance improves with advancing postnatal age and continued nephrogenesis; gestational age and birth weight are not associated with the efficiency of drug elimination (Aranda & Thomas, 2006).

DOSING RECOMMENDATIONS

The standard dose for IBU is based on pharmacokinetic and research studies. Intravenous IBU is ordered as three doses with an initial dose of 10 mg/kg followed by two doses of 5 mg/kg each at 24 and 48 hours after the initial dose (Capparelli, 2007; Pacifici, 2016). The efficacy of this regimen is equivalent to the efficacy of standard doses of INDO (Ohlsson et al., 2020). If the PDA does not close after three doses of IBU, a second course of therapy may be pursued at the discretion of the neonatology team.

To improve the efficacy of IBU, multiple pharmacokinetic and clinical studies have examined higher doses (Dani et al., 2012; Desfrere et al., 2005; Hirt et al., 2008). RCTs have consistently documented superior efficacy from 20 mg/kg followed by 10 mg/kg for two additional doses compared to standard dosing. Conflicting data suggest the potential for an increase in renal adverse effects from the higher dose regimen, although the impact is mild and transient.

Both intravenous and oral preparations of IBU are equally safe and well tolerated by preterm infants. Standard doses of oral IBU have been shown to be more effective in closing the PDA when compared to the intravenous (IV) route; oral dosing yields a sustained drug concentration with an area under the curve (AUC) equal to or even greater than IV dosing (Barzilay et al., 2012; Ohlsson et al., 2020; Pacifici, 2016). Oral absorption of IBU is slower and elimination prolonged, thus allowing the drug more time to interact with the PDA (Barzilay et al., 2012). Of note, investigators have also documented the superiority of high-dose oral IBU compared to standard-dose oral IBU (Pourarian et al., 2015). On this basis, some experts deem high-dose, oral IBU to be the pharmacologic treatment of choice for PDA (Mitra et al., 2018). However, clinicians must consider the high osmolality of the oral solution and only utilize this route in patients with some enteral feeding tolerance.

CLINICAL-MONITORING PEARLS

IBU consistently produces fewer and less severe renal adverse effects when compared with INDO (Table 17.3; Hamrick et al., 2020; Narayanan-Sankar & Clyman, 2003; Ovali, 2020). The relative impact on other organ systems is controversial.

TABLE 17.3 Contraindications and Risks Associated With Ibuprofen Therapy

	CONTRAINDICATION FOR USE	RISKS WITH USE
CNS	Intraventricular hemorrhage	
Cardiovascular	Ductal-dependent lesion	
Gastrointestinal	Bleeding NEC Spontaneous intestinal perforation	
Renal	Renal insufficiency or failure	Fluid retention Renal insufficiency or failure (oliguria)
Hematologic	Coagulopathy (thrombocytopenia)	Coagulopathy
Endocrine	Elevated liver enzymes	Adrenal insufficiency Electrolyte disturbances (hypoglycemia, hypocalcemia)
Other	Concomitant corticosteroid use[a]	

[a]Denotes increased risk for spontaneous intestinal perforation with concomitant use of a corticosteroid (e.g., hydrocortisone) Únd nonsteroidal anti-inflammatory drug.
CNS, central nervous system; NEC, necritizing enterocolitis.
Source: From Poon, G. (2007). Ibuprofen lysine (NeoProfen) for the treatment of patent ductus arteriosus. *Baylor University Medical Center Proceedings, 20*(1), 83–85. https://doi.org/10.1080/08998280.2007.11928244

Cerebral Function

Like INDO, a head ultrasound may be obtained to evaluate for the presence or absence of an IVH prior to beginning IBU therapy (Sivanandan & Agarwal, 2016). IBU minimally alters cerebrovascular perfusion and can even enhance cerebral vascular autoregulation after oxidative stress (Chemtob et al., 1990; Johnston et al., 2012). However, randomized trials have failed to confirm the efficacy of IBU as a protective therapy for IVH in preterm infants (Ohlsson et al., 2020).

Renal Function

Similar to INDO, clinicians are encouraged to order baseline renal function testing prior to the initiation of therapy and daily throughout therapy, as NSAIDs inhibit COX enzymes, PGE_2 synthesis, and interfere with renin-angiotensin-aldosterone activity (Gournay, 2005; Pacifici, 2014a). As PGE_2 is the main prostanoid synthesized in the nephron, inhibition of this PG may decrease glomerular filtration and increase the risk for oliguria, albeit to a lesser degree with IBU compared to INDO (Johnston et al., 2012; Vieux et al., 2010).

Gastrointestinal Function

Similar to INDO, clinical monitoring should include close observation of stooling pattern and consistency/color and physical examination findings (e.g., abdominal girth, abdominal distension). Rao and colleagues (2011) reported an 8% incidence of SIP among preterm neonates less than 7 days of life who were subject to IBU therapy. However, all neonates were hypotensive during treatment and three of the five were subject to concomitant hydrocortisone therapy (Rao et al., 2011). Like INDO, IBU therapy should be avoided when neonates are subject to corticosteroid therapy.

Hematologic Function

A baseline complete blood count should be obtained prior to the initiation of therapy to establish a pretherapy platelet and red blood cell count. Like INDO, IBU is known to inhibit platelet aggregation and IBU may suppress erythropoiesis (Aranda & Thomas, 2006; Poon, 2007). IBU inhibits platelet aggregation through the inhibition of COX-1 production. By blocking COX-1, thromboxane production is reduced, and normal platelet aggregation is inhibited (Knijff-Dutmer et al., 2002). Most clinicians consider moderate to severe thrombocytopenia to be a contraindication for IBU therapy.

Acetaminophen

Unlike nonselective COX inhibitors that inhibit the COX site, acetaminophen is believed to block the peroxidase (POX) segment, inhibiting PG synthetase activity, thereby facilitating ductal closure (see Figure 17.1; Hammerman et al., 2011) The success rate for PDA closure with the use of acetaminophen is the subject of active study, but appears to be comparable to INDO and IBU (Clyman, 2018; Ohlsson & Shah, 2020). In addition, acetaminophen avoids many of the adverse effects commonly associated with COX inhibition.

MECHANISM OF ACTION/PHARMACOKINETIC PRINCIPLES

The mechanism of action of acetaminophen involves the inhibition of PG H-synthase, an essential enzyme responsible for initiating the PG biosynthesis pathway (Manalastas et al., 2021; Oncel et al., 2017). This ultimately inhibits the production of the most potent PG, PGE_2. Given that the PDA is particularly sensitive to PGE_2, the reduced concentration of PGE_2 permits smooth muscle constriction and obliteration of the PDA (Allegaert et al., 2013).

The pharmacokinetics of acetaminophen are well described in the literature. Acetaminophen may be administered orally or intravenously. Absorption of oral acetaminophen occurs within the small intestine. Hepatic first-pass metabolism occurs primarily by sulfation, and to a lesser extent glucuronidation and oxidation, via CYP2E1 enzyme activity. Enzyme activity increases with advancing postnatal age (Jasani et al., 2018). Certain comorbid conditions that rely on hepatic metabolism, such as hyperbilirubinemia, may further reduce acetaminophen clearance. As reviewed in Chapter 11, "Analgesia and Sedation," a small fraction (8%–10%) of acetaminophen is oxidized by cytochrome P540 enzymes (CYP2E1) to N-acetyl-p-benzoquinone imine (NAPQI). This is a toxic metabolite, which, when excessive amounts accumulate, depletes the liver of the antioxidant glutathione and damages hepatic cells, which leads to hepatoxicity, liver failure, and oxidative stress. Fortunately, the NAPQI isoenzyme is less active in early infancy.

Once within the systemic circulation, active drug molecules are widely distributed and can penetrate most tissues with the exception of adipose tissue. The volume of distribution is inversely proportional to gestational age; a higher volume of distribution is observed in neonates less than 1,500 grams at birth. The low molecular weight and reduced binding with plasma proteins facilitate distribution into the central nervous system. Once inactivated and metabolized, drug metabolites are eliminated in the urine. Renal clearance tends to be reduced in preterm infants and increases with advancing postnatal age. The elimination half-life for neonates at 28 to 32 weeks of gestation, 32 to 36 weeks of gestation, and at term is 11 hours, 5 hours, and 3 hours, respectively (Manalastas et al., 2021).

DOSING RECOMMENDATIONS

Acetaminophen can be administered orally at the same dose and interval with similar efficacy as the intravenous route (Gillam-Krakauer & Reese, 2018). Given the high volume of distribution in very preterm neonates, a loading dose may be indicated in this population (Manalastas et al., 2021). Dosing regimens range from 7.5 to 15 mg/kg every 6 hours for a total of 3 to 7 days of therapy (Gillam-Krakauer & Reese, 2018; Manalastas et al., 2021). Differences in dosing recommendations, frequency, and length of treatment emphasizes the need for additional research.

Initiation of Therapy

Randomized trials have investigated early (<7 days of life), standard (0–14 days of life), and late (>14 days of life) therapy for PDA closure. A summary of studies that investigated dosages and duration of therapy between days 0 to 14 of life is provided in Tables 17.4 and 17.5.

CLINICAL-MONITORING PEARLS

Acetaminophen has fewer reported side effects as compared to NSAIDs. However, given the pharmacokinetic profile presented earlier in this section, clinicians are encouraged to monitor hepatic function, renal function, and GI function with its use.

Renal Function

No significant changes in renal function have been reported with acetaminophen use (Meena et al., 2020). However, it is reasonable to obtain baseline renal function testing prior to the initiation of therapy and daily until therapy ceases.

TABLE 17.4 Early Acetaminophen Therapy Versus Indomethacin or Ibuprofen (Day of Life 0–7)

STUDY AUTHORS	DRUGS INVESTIGATED	DRUG DOSAGE	DURATION OF THERAPY (DAYS)
Oncel et al. (2014)	ACE vs. IBU	ACE: 60 mg/kg/day PO IBU: 10 mg/kg PO day 1 5 mg/kg PO day 2 5 mg/kg PO day 3	ACE: 3 IBU: 3
Dash et al. (2015)	ACE vs. INDO	ACE: 60 mg/kg/day PO INDO: 0.2 mg/kg IV	ACE: 7 INDO: 3
Bagheri et al. (2016)	ACE vs. IBU	ACE: 60 mg/kg/day PO IBU: 20 mg/kg PO day 1 10 mg/kg PO day 2 10 mg/kg PO day 3	ACE: 3 IBU: 3
Härkin et al. (2016)	ACE vs. placebo (prophylaxis)	ACE: 20 mg/kg/dose IV (load) 7.5 mg/kg/dose IV every 6 hours	ACE: 4 Placebo: 4
Al-Lawama et al. (2018)	ACE vs. IBU	ACE: 40 mg/kg/day PO IBU: 10 mg/kg PO day 1 5 mg/kg PO day 2 5 mg/kg PO day 3	ACE: 3 IBU: 3
Dani et al. (2018)	ACE vs. IBU	ACE: 60 mg/kg/day IV IBU: 10 mg/kg IV day 1 5 mg/kg IV day 2 5 mg/kg IV day 3	ACE: 3 IBU: 3
Hochwald et al. (2018)	ACE+IBU vs. IBU	ACE: 20 mg/kg/dose IV (load) 10 mg/kg/dose IV every 6 hours IBU: 10 mg/kg IV day 1 5 mg/kg IV day 2 5 mg/kg IV day 3	ACE: 3 IBU: 3

Note: "Early" therapy is defined as occurring within the first week of postnatal life.
ACE, acetaminophen; IBU, ibuprofen; INDO, indomethacin; IV, intravenous; PO, by mouth.

Gastrointestinal Function

Although SIP is a known complication associated with INDO and IBU use, it is not associated with acetaminophen use (El-Mashad et al., 2017; Luecke et al., 2017). To date, one report of multiple intestinal perforations following oral acetaminophen therapy has been published involving a very-low-birth-weight infant (Tuteja et al., 2020). As previously discussed with oral IBU, clinicians should consider the osmolality of oral acetaminophen solution and enteral feeding volumes when selecting oral or intravenous therapy.

Hepatic Function

Although uncommon, increased aspartate aminotransferase (AST), alanine transaminase (ALT), and gamma-glutamyl transferase (GGT) levels have been reported in the literature. All elevations were transient and returned to baseline with cessation of therapy (Gillam-Krakauer et al., 2019; Shah, 2019). We recommend that clinicians order baseline hepatic function testing prior to therapy and monitor hepatic function during therapy. Elevated lab indices warrant interval surveillance until normal function is reestablished.

Long-Term Outcomes

Despite very few reported immediate side effects, several studies have raised concern for possible long-term neurotoxic effects secondary to prenatal or neonatal acetaminophen exposure. For example, Viberg and colleagues (2014) reported that neonatal mice exposed to acetaminophen during periods of critical brain development developed long-lasting cognitive impairment as well as alterations in locomotion and spatial learning in adulthood (p <.001; Viberg et al., 2014). Van den Anker and Allegaert (2018) provide a useful commentary on this topic and highlight the need for long-term neurodevelopmental follow-up in studies examining acetaminophen for pain or PDA in preterm infants.

TABLE 17.5 Acetaminophen Therapy Versus Indomethacin or Ibuprofen (Day of Life 0–14)

STUDY AUTHORS	DRUGS INVESTIGATED	DRUG DOSAGE	DURATION OF THERAPY (DAYS)
Dang et al. (2013)	ACE vs. IBU	ACE: 60 mg/kg/day IBU: 10 mg/kg IV day 1 5 mg/kg IV day 2 5 mg/kg IV day 3	ACE: 3 IBU: 3
Yang et al. (2016)	ACE vs. IBU	ACE: 60 mg/kg/day IBU: 10 mg/kg IV day 1 5 mg/kg IV day 2 5 mg/kg IV day 3	ACE: 3 IBU: 3
El-Mashad et al. (2017)	ACE vs. IBU vs. INDO	ACE: 60 mg/kg/day IBU: 10, 5, 5 mg/kg/dose (24 h apart) INDO: 0.2 mg/kg/dose q12h	ACE: 3 IBU: 3 INDO: 2 (three doses)
Clyman et al. (2019) Liebowitz et al. (2019)	ACE vs. IBU vs. INDO vs. no treatment	ACE: 20 mg/kg followed by 15 mg/kg q6h (trough on third dose), if >25 mgL decrease to 12.5 mg/kg q6h IBU: 10, 5, 5, 5 mg/kg/dose (24 h apart) INDO: 0.2 mg/kg 0, 12, 24, 48 h (four doses) Could get rescue course under specific criteria	ACE: 5 IBU: 3–4 INDO: 2 (four doses)
Meena et al. (2020)	ACE vs. IBU vs. INDO	ACE: 60 mg/kg/day IBU: 10, 5, 5 mg/kg/dose (24 h apart) INDO: 0.1–0.25 mg/kg/dose q12h	ACE: 3 IBU: 3 INDO: 2 (three doses)

ACE, acetaminophen; IBU, ibuprofen; INDO, indomethacin; IV, intravenous; PO, by mouth.

CONCLUSIONS

A hemodynamically symptomatic PDA, a well-known complication of prematurity, can be associated with many morbidities. Studies have been done over the past decade challenging PDA treatment based on beliefs that short-term morbidities and long-term outcomes may not be improved with closure of the ductus with potentially unnecessary exposure to harmful therapies that are not without adverse effects. The decision to treat a PDA is beyond the scope of this chapter. However, for providers who decide to treat a hemodynamically significant PDA with medications, options include INDO, IBU, and acetaminophen. All have reported efficacy in closing a PDA; however, significant effects on the renal, digestive, and cerebral systems related to both PG synthesis inhibition and COX-independent mechanisms have been documented (Gournay, 2005). INDO prophylaxis is useful to prevent severe IVH; high-dose oral IBU may be the most effective option for selective treatment of hemodynamically significant PDA; acetaminophen has the most favorable adverse effect profile; however, to date, there is insufficient evidence to recommend one pharmacologic therapy over another. Although a PDA is one of the more common acyanotic cardiac conditions affecting preterm infants and decades of publications describe pharmacologic treatment, the management of a PDA remains a challenge for providers in the NICU.

LEARNING TOOLS AND RESOURCES

Advice From the Author

Denise Kirsten, DNP, APRN, NNP-BC

A PDA is one of the most common acyanotic cardiac conditions seen in preterm infants. There are many documented morbidities associated with a PDA; however, adverse effects related to pharmacologic therapies may be more pronounced and severe. The risks versus benefits of using pharmacologic therapies to treat a hemodynamically significant PDA must be considered prior to beginning therapy.

Discussion Prompts

1. There are many possible consequences associated with a PDA. Discuss possible consequences of a PDA and the decision to treat this condition in preterm infants.
2. Compare and contrast the mechanism of action of acetaminophen with that of ibuprofen and indomethacin in facilitating ductal closure in the preterm infant.
3. Discuss the risks associated with indomethacin and ibuprofen use and situations in which they might not be used. Compare the decision to hold treatment with policies in your NICU.

Mind Map

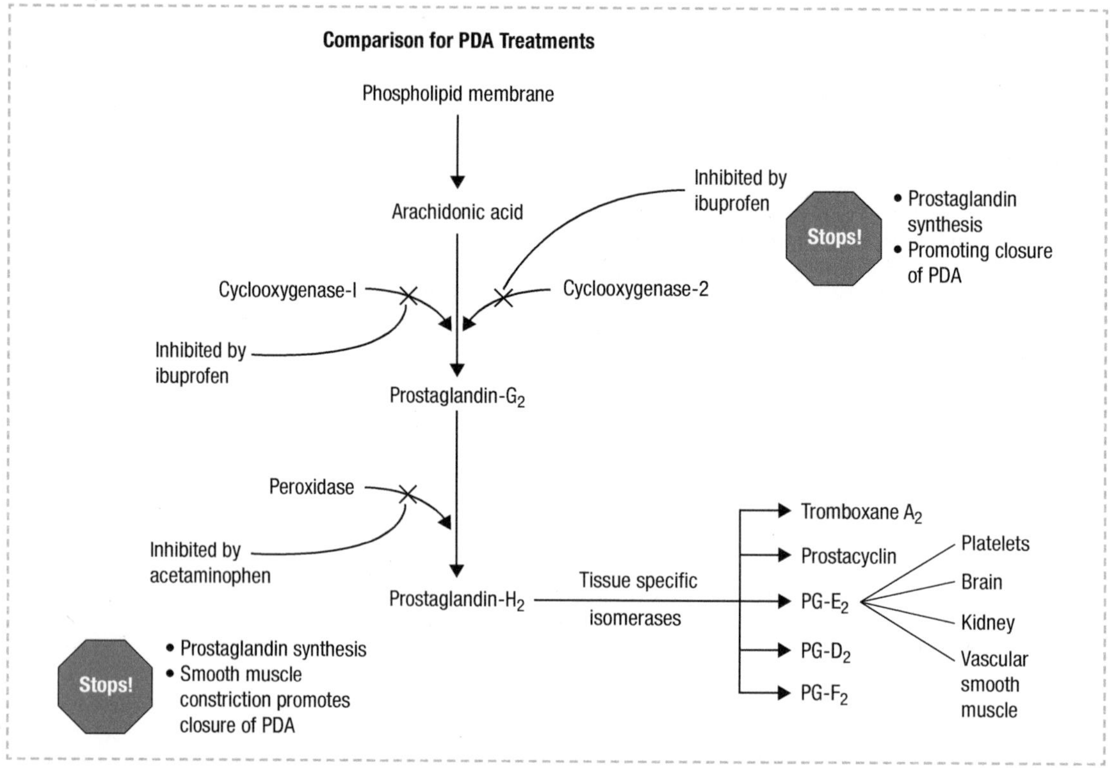

Note: This mind map reflects the design team's interpretation of a portion of one or more concepts addressed in this chapter. Readers should regard the mind maps woven throughout this textbook as examples of multisensory study tools that can be developed to encourage conceptual understanding. Readers are encouraged to develop their own unique mind maps in consultation with academic faculty or clinical preceptors.
PDA, patent ductus arteriosus.
Design credit: Sarah Tyson, MSN, APRN, NNP-BC, and Stephanie Church, MSN, APRN, NNP-BC, East Carolina University Neonatal Nurse Practitioner Program.

REFERENCES

References for this chapter are online and available at https://connect.springerpub.com/content/book/978-0-8261-5884-0/part/partIV/toc-part/ch17.

chapter 18

Critical Congenital Heart Defects

Karen Wright

LEARNING OBJECTIVES

After completing this chapter, the reader should be able to:

- Define *critical congenital heart defects* (*CCHDs*) and identify the epidemiology of the disease process.
- Enumerate the most common risk factors for CCHDs in the neonate.
- Explain the embryology and physiology of cardiac function.
- Correlate the pathophysiology of CCHDs with the need for pharmacologic treatment.
- Appraise the historical evolution of pharmacologic management for CCHDs in the neonate.
- Evaluate the current pharmacotherapy used with the initial stabilization and treatment of ductal-dependent CCHDs.

INTRODUCTION

The term *congenital heart defect (CHD)* is used to describe structural or vascular defects of the heart or great vessels that are present at birth. Although some CHDs develop between weeks 3 and 6 of embryonic development, the most vulnerable period of human development, other CHDs develop later in gestation. The incidence is 0.3% to 0.8% in developed countries (Dolk et al., 2011; van der Linde et al., 2011). More specifically, 1% or 40,000 live-born infants in the United States are diagnosed with a CHD each year (Centers for Disease Control and Prevention [CDC], 2021). Neonatal clinicians are likely to diagnose one or both of the following CHDs each year: (a) dextro-transposition of the great arteries (d-TGA), the most common cyanotic CHD diagnosed during the neonatal period; and (b) tetralogy of Fallot, the most common cyanotic CHD diagnosed during infancy (Hoffman et al., 2018).

CHDs are classified as acyanotic, obstructive, or cyanotic (Table 18.1). Obstructive and cyanotic lesions are considered critical congenital heart defects (CCHDs) because early postnatal survival depends on continued patency of the ductus arteriosus (DA). The presence of an extracardiac (e.g., total anomalous pulmonary venous return [TAPVR]) or intracardiac defect, which arises during embryonic development, prevents the normal flow of blood from the right heart to the lungs and the left heart for dissemination to the systemic circulation. Mortality risk is high, even when the DA remains patent after birth, and directly proportional to gestational age. Steurer and colleagues (2017) reported a mortality risk of 9% to 12% in United States born term newborns and 19% to 41% in preterm newborns. The combined mortality and morbidity risk for newborns less than 29 weeks of gestation was 83% (Steurer et al., 2017).

TABLE 18.1 Classification of Congenital Heart Defects

CLASSIFICATION	CONGENITAL HEART DEFECT
Acyanotic	Ventricular septal defect Atrial septal defect Atrioventricular canal defect Patent ductus arteriosus
Obstructive[a]	Aortic stenosis Coarctation of the aorta Hypoplastic left heart syndrome Pulmonary atresia
Cyanotic[a]	Tetralogy of Fallot Dextro-transposition of the great arteries Single ventricle Total anomalous pulmonary venous return

[a]Obstructive and cyanotic lesions are considered critical congenital heart diseases.

The prevalence of CHDs has increased in a nonlinear pattern over time; this trend is attributed to biologic and other factors. First, women are waiting longer to have children, linking advanced maternal age to some CHDs. In addition, the incidence of environmental exposures and maternal diseases (e.g., pregestational diabetes mellitus) has increased over the years and tightly linked to CHDs (van der Linde et al., 2011). Prenatal surveillance practices, including use of large prospective birth registries for tracking purposes, have been standardized and are capturing more CHDs during the prenatal period. Postnatally, infant survival has increased and the use of gold standard diagnostic tools, namely pediatric Doppler echocardiography with pediatric cardiology input, has enhanced the detection of CHDs. Further studies are warranted to evaluate the impact of socioeconomic status, racial differences, assisted reproduction, and epigenetics on the development of CHDs.

This chapter focuses on the pharmacologic management of infants with ductal-dependent CCHDs. We begin with a basic review of embryology and physiology. A brief overview of the evolution of knowledge of CCHDs is reviewed, as well as relevant pathophysiology and blood flow dynamics. Next, common clinical manifestations, diagnostic considerations, and the differential diagnosis are reviewed. This is followed by a comprehensive discussion of the pharmacotherapy of choice for the immediate treatment of CCHDs.

HISTORICAL REVIEW: CONGENITAL HEART DEFECTS

Since the second century CE, the common belief that blood had to be continuously produced in the liver and flow centrifugally to nourish the tissues was based on the opinions of Claudius Galen, a Greek physician and philosopher. His notion was that blood was not circulated or recycled; tissues consumed blood in a one-way direction and the liver replenished what was consumed (Aird, 2011). It was not until the 16th and 17th centuries that Galen's theory was questioned, and cardiology-specific inquiries flourished. We review some of the more noteworthy discoveries here.

We begin in 1489, when Leonardo da Vinci, a Renaissance painter, was gifted a human skull. This gift turned out to be a catalyst for years of increasingly complex anatomic inquiries. By 1513, da Vinci emerged as one of the greatest anatomists. He would spend countless hours observing and performing human dissections and illustrating many aspects of human anatomy, particularly of the heart and circulation (Clayton & Philo, 2012). Then, in 1628, William Harvey, an English physician, anatomist, and professor of anatomy and surgery, studied the state of the science at the time and elucidated a new theory: The pulmonary and systemic circulations worked together. He shared his theory in the publication *Exercitatio Anatomica de Motu Cordis et Sanguinis in Animalibus* (Harvey, 1975).

Next, scientists closely inspected hearts and identified structural anomalies, which would later be classified as CHDs. In 1665, Niels Stensen, a Danish scientist, described four cardiac defects present in a stillborn fetus that had never been reported before: (a) pulmonary stenosis (PS), (b) ventricular septal defect (VSD), (c) overriding aorta, and (d) right ventricular hypertrophy (Tubbs et al., 2019). He wrote:

> The unusual form of the arteries arising from the heart attracted the chief attention and called for admiration. In particular, the pulmonary artery, which was much narrower than the aorta, seemed to be suggestive of something new, and hence I opened this vessel from the right ventricle to the hilus pulmonum, and then I could plainly see that the communication between the pulmonary artery and the aorta [ductus arteriosus] which usually is quite distinct in any fetus, was completely absent. When I opened the right ventricle, however, the probe that was passed forward and upward along the interventricular septum entered directly into the aorta just as readily as the probe passed from the left ventricle into the aorta. Thus, no less than three openings led into the right ventricle: one from the right atrium, the other two being connected with the arteries. The same aortic canal that was common to both ventricles, found, together with the interventricular septum, a double opening. The auricles were normal. Although in this case the arteries were of uncommon structure, the resulting effect of this was in compliance with nature, like the circulation of the blood in any fetus occurs. Just as the vena cava empties into both atria [through the foramen ovale], the right ventricle empties into both arteries; just as the left ventricle receives blood from both auricles, thus the aorta receives blood from both ventricles at the same time. So, no matter whether the blood leaving the right ventricle first passes through the pulmonary artery and then is sent through its own channel [ductus arteriosus] into the aorta, or the aorta receives the blood directly as it partly straddles the right ventricle, without the blood first passing through any other channel, the movement of the blood will be the same from the right ventricle out into both arteries. As to the cause of this phenomenon, I have nothing to say. But, supposing that in the open thorax the pulmonary artery separates from the aorta, while in the closed thorax it receives the blood from the right ventricle and permits it to pass on to the aorta. There still remain two perplexities. It cannot be taken for granted that the arterial structure will remain obscure how an open thorax would contribute to a change in the arterial structures. There can be no doubt that the ductus arteriosus found in the infant gradually resolves itself into a ligament as the lungs expand with the establishment of respiration, and that this structure is patent only in the fetus, because all the blood coming from the right ventricle cannot pass through the pulmonary arteries. But why the blood in this case has not been able even to make its way into the pulmonary artery, but has made its way directly into the aorta, I am unable to explain. Still, no matter what the reason of this might be, I take it plainly to prove the wisdom of Nature, in as much as the effect is produced, if not in the same way, yet always somehow. Just as this fetus proves this point with regard to that part of the blood that has to be expelled from the right ventricle in the large artery [aorta], this fetus also illustrates that the formation of the solid parts of animals does not always proceed in the same manner even though the effect obtained remains the same. (Stensen, cited in Marr, 1948, pp. 317–320)

Stensen went on to describe the physiologic consequences of this complex cardiac defect, which 200 years later was named *tetralogy of Fallot* by Etienne-Louis Fallot. Some early reports and more modern publications refer to this defect as *Steno-Fallot tetralogy* in honor of Dr. Stensen's work.

This preintervention era, or period of time prior to the inception of invasive interventions for CHDs (e.g., cardiac surgery, catheterization), is hallmarked by the work of Thomas Bevill Peacock, a London physician of the mid-1800s. Dr. Peacock was the first to consider embryologic development and human anatomy in his description of CHDs. In doing so, he stratified CHDs into four different categories: (a) misplacements of the heart, (b) abnormalities of the pericardium, (c) cardiac malformations, and (d) distortion of the primary vessels. His findings were published in *On Malformations of the Human Heart*, where he attributed most CHDs to errors that occur during embryologic development but also proposed that environmental factors and hereditary predispositions could be associated with CHDs (Twite et al., 2018).

In the early 1900s, Maude Abbott, a pathologist, became the first global authority on CHDs by recognizing the link among inheritance, CHDs, and polydactyly. Dr. Abbott reported that CHDs exhibited a hereditary preference (were prevalent in families), a genetic preference (e.g., Down syndrome and CHD), and occurred in cases of consanguinity and among women of advanced maternal age (Gelb, 2015). These and other novel findings, which correspond with modern risk factors for CHD, were published by Dr. Abbott in 1936, in the well-known *Atlas of Congenital Cardiac Disease* (Abbott, 1936). The dissemination of these findings helped advance the state of the science and prompt further inquiries.

A shift from palliation to primary repair occurred in the mid-1930s, marking the beginning of the interventional era. The first cardiac surgery was performed in 1938 by Dr. Robert Gross, a physician at the Children's Hospital of Boston. He successfully ligated the patent DA in a 7-year-old girl (Gross & Hubbard, 1984). In 1952, Dr. John Lewis performed the first intracardiac surgery on an atrial septal defect (ASD). Around this same time, Dr. Helen Brooke Taussig published the first comprehensive textbook devoted to CHDs and began the first pediatric cardiology training program (Salmon & Barkley, 1947). Dr. Taussig is considered the founder of the subspecialty of pediatric cardiology (Neill, 1994). In 1961, pediatric cardiology became the *first* pediatric subspecialty. The first Blalock–Taussig–Thomas shunt (BT shunt) was performed in 1944. Then, in 1975, Dr. Adib Jatene performed the first successful arterial switch on a patient with d-TGA and a VSD (Morfaw et al., 2020).

Historical knowledge about the evolution of knowledge of CCHD has provided a path forward for present-day therapies. The genetic etiology and genotype/phenotype penetration of CHD is becoming more prevalent, allowing clinicians to forecast clinical care needs. Identifying the causality of CCHD by teratogens will reduce fetal exposure and may lead to either fetal interventions or informed postnatal methods for improvement of the outcome of infants with CCHD. This is in lockstep with the vision of Dr. Helen Taussig, printed in *Circulation* in 1965 (p. 774): "Our next great step forward will come in the field of cause and the prevention of malformations" (Gelb, 2015).

EMBRYOLOGY AND PHYSIOLOGY REVIEW

Given that CHDs are structural or vascular defects of the heart or great vessels, it is prudent to briefly review the embryologic development of the heart and great vessels. Readers who would benefit from a more complete discussion of embryologic development are referred to Chapter 5, "The Cardiovascular System," in the textbook, *Fetal and Neonatal Physiology for the Advanced Practice Nurse* (Hoffman et al., 2018).

Heart development begins with the formation of a primitive heart tube, which forms by day 22 of gestation in a cranial to caudal (top to bottom) direction (Hoffman et al., 2018). This primitive structure differentiates into the endocardium and the surrounding muscle layer, the myocardium. By day 23 of gestation, the heart tube can pump blood in an "ebb and flow" fashion. It is important to note that primitive cardiac function is essential to normal structural development of the heart and, without these early functions, cardiac development may be altered abnormally due to the result of abnormal fetal blood flow (Hoffman et al., 2018). By week 4 of gestation, dextral looping, septation, and partitioning of the four chambers of the heart have occurred; failed differentiation during this critical period of time may give rise to a CHD (Table 18.2). During this same time frame, the aortic arches form, giving rise to the great vessels of the heart. These vessels differentiate into their mature arrangement (carotid, subclavian, and pulmonary arteries) by week 8 of gestation. Simultaneously, the pulmonary vasculature forms, which includes the four pulmonary veins (PVs). Therefore, by week 8 of gestation, the fetal cardiovascular system is fully formed and functioning (Goble et al., 2020).

Recall that placental and systemic vascular resistance (SVR) are low and pulmonary vascular resistance (PVR) is high during fetal development. High PVR is protective of the fetus, as this discourages blood flow to the lungs to facilitate optimal pulmonary growth (expansion) and development. Rather, the majority of freshly oxygenated blood from the fetal umbilical vein moves through the ductus venosus and inferior vena cava (IVC), enters the right atrium (RA), and preferentially shunts across the foramen ovale. A smaller proportion of blood descends into the right ventricle (RV), ascends the main pulmonary artery, and preferentially moves across the DA (in a right-to-left direction). The blood thereby enters the systemic circulation and feeds the fetal tissues (Hoffman et al., 2018).

Significant pressure changes occur at birth, with the onset of crying, inhalation of oxygen (even in room air), and removal of the low-resistance placental circuit. These factors elicit a sharp increase in SVR and concurrent relaxation of the pulmonary microcirculation. In fact, SVR rises above PVR in healthy newborns. These changes contribute to a reversal of blood flow within the cardiopulmonary circuit. Now, blood entering the right side of the heart is preferentially diverted to the RV, main pulmonary artery, and right and left pulmonary arteries. Although some blood may slip across the DA in a right-to-left direction, the majority of blood flow enters the pulmonary

TABLE 18.2 Critical Congenital Heart Defects

LESION	COMMON ANATOMIC DEFECTS	SUMMARY OF PATHOPHYSIOLOGY	COMMON CLINICAL MANIFESTATIONS
d-TGA	• RV remains properly positioned on the right side of the heart. • LV remains properly positioned on the left side of the heart. • Aorta arises from the RV, is anterior and to the right of the PA. • PA arises from the LV, is posterior and to the left of the aorta. • Coronary arteries normally arise from the aorta.	• Deoxygenated blood returning to the RA flows into the RV, aorta, and vital organs without entering the pulmonary vasculature. • Oxygenated blood returning to the LA (from the pulmonary veins) flows into the PA and then the LA. • Requires a communication between the two parallel circuits (PFO). • Requires ductal patency for pulmonary blood flow.	• Cyanosis • Hypothermia • Anaerobic glycolysis and hypoglycemia leading to metabolic acidosis • Cardiomegaly • Increased pulmonary vascular markings • No murmur • Single S2 due to increased distance of pulmonary valve from the chest wall
Tetralogy of Fallot	• RV hypertrophy • Pulmonary stenosis • Overriding aorta • VSD	• Size of VSD may equalize ventricular pressures, encouraging right-to-left shunting. • Severe PS leads to RV hypertrophy and influences the magnitude of shunt through VSD. • Requires ductal patency for pulmonary blood flow.	• Cyanosis at birth • Normal cardiac silhouette • Decreased pulmonary vascular markings • Absent main pulmonary trunk "boot-shaped heart" • Ejection-type murmur or systolic murmur depending on the severity of PS and size of VSD
Truncus arteriosus	• Four-chamber heart • Large VSD • PA and branches innervate the truncus, which functions as the aorta	• Ventricular pressures equalize due to the large VSD. • Near-complete mixing occurs between the RV and LV. • As PVR decreases after birth, pulmonary blood flow increases. • May require ductal patency for pulmonary blood flow (contingent open difference between PVR and SVR).	• Degree of cyanosis depending on the difference between PVR and SVR • Cardiomegaly and/or signs of congestive heart failure if PVR < SVR • Increased pulmonary vascular markings if PVR < SVR • Systolic ejection murmur if pulmonary valve stenosis is present • Diastolic murmur with truncal valve regurgitation

(continued)

TABLE 18.2 Critical Congenital Heart Defects (*continued*)

LESION	COMMON ANATOMIC DEFECTS	SUMMARY OF PATHOPHYSIOLOGY	COMMON CLINICAL MANIFESTATIONS
Tricuspid atresia	• PFO or ASD • Absent tricuspid valve • RV hypoplasia • VSD (variable size; restrictive is most common) • Pulmonary stenosis (common) • Normally positioned great arteries (majority of cases)	• RA pressure exceeds LA pressure, leading to shunting of venous return across the PFO/ASD. This leads to RA, LA, and LV hypertrophy. • A VSD permits left-to-right shunting of a small proportion of blood from the LV to the hypoplastic RV and pulmonary vasculature for oxygenation. • Requires ductal patency for adequate pulmonary blood flow.	• Cyanosis at birth (normally positioned great vessels) or mild cyanosis (with transposed great vessels) • RA, LA, and LV enlargement • Decreased pulmonary vascular markings • Harsh murmur consistent with VSD • Hepatomegaly
TAPVR	• *Supracardiac type*: Right/left PV forms confluence behind the heart and drains through the vertical vein into the RA. • *Intracardiac type*: PV confluence drains into the RA through the coronary sinus. • *Infracardiac type:* PV confluence drains into a vertical vein and then into the portal vein, hepatic vein, or IVC. From there blood ascends into the RA.	• Pathology is contingent on the size of ASD and presence or absence of pulmonary obstruction to venous outflow. • Small ASD diverts venous return to the RV and pulmonary arteries. RV hypertrophy and pulmonary overload develop. Systemic output decreases. • Moderate to large ASD permits mixing of oxygenated and deoxygenated blood at the RA and flow to the LA, LV, aorta, DA (left-to-right shunt), and systemic circulation. • TAPVR with outflow obstruction does not benefit from maintaining ductal patency.	• Mild cyanosis • Small cardiac silhouette with RA and/or RV engorgement • Increased pulmonary vascular markings and pulmonary edema, particularly with outflow obstruction • Systolic ejection murmur and diastolic murmur • Split S2
Ebstein anomaly	• Septal and posterior leaflets of the tricuspid valve adhere to the underlying myocardium. • Anterior leaflets of the tricuspid valve are redundant, fenestrated, and/or tethered. • Annulus of the tricuspid valve is displaced downward. • Dilatation of the RA and right atrioventricular junction occurs.	• Stalled forward flow of blood from the RA to RV leads to RA enlargement. • Increased RA pressure induces a right-to-left shunt through the PFO, which over time leads to LV overload and congestive heart failure. • Persistent low RV pressure leads to RV hypoplasia and tricuspid valve regurgitation.	• Cyanosis • Congestive heart failure • Radiograph shows right-side cardiomegaly and decreased pulmonary vascular markings • Systolic murmur • Split, wide S2

Single ventricle	• Single right or left ventricle • Ventricular foramen between single ventricle and bulboventricular foramen • Pulmonary stenosis (some cases)	• Two atrioventricular valves drain into one ventricle. • One great vessel arises from the single ventricle. • One great vessel arises from a small ventricular chamber called the *bulboventricular foramen.* • Mixing of deoxygenated and oxygenated blood occurs in the single ventricle.	• Degree of cyanosis depending on the difference between PVR and SVR • Cardiomegaly and/or signs of congestive heart failure if PVR < SVR • Increased pulmonary vascular markings if PVR < SVR
Pulmonary atresia (with intact ventricular septum)	• Mechanical closure/obstruction at the pulmonary artery	• Reduced pulmonary blood flow secondary to atresia • Right-to-left shunting of venous return at PFO or VSD (if present) • Requires ductal patency for pulmonary blood flow	• Severe cyanosis at birth • Small cardiac silhouette • Reduced pulmonary vascular markings • No murmur (or soft ductal murmur)
Double-outlet right ventricle	• PA and aorta arise entirely or predominately from the RV • VSD • Arteriovenous connection (most cases)	• Pathophysiology is associated with the classification (multiple variants have been reported) and location of the VSD.	• Cyanosis develops with severe pulmonary outflow obstruction, transposition of the great vessels, with aortic coarctation or aortic arch interruption. • Radiograph may show RV enlargement. • Manifestations vary per classification of lesion.
Hypoplastic left heart syndrome	• Hypoplastic left ventricle • PFO/ASD or intact atrial septum	• Left side of the heart cannot support systemic circulation. • Pulmonary venous return must cross the PFO left to right to reach the systemic circulation. • Right ventricular output supports systemic circulation by way of right-to-left shunting across the DA. • Requires ductal patency for pulmonary blood flow.	• If the DA is initially open and large, there is minimal to no cyanosis, machine-like murmur, widened pulse pressure, cardiomegaly, tachypnea, increased pulmonary vascular markings, and hepatomegaly. • If intact atrial septum or small PFO, cyanosis at birth, cardiomegaly, tachypnea, and increased pulmonary vascular markings occur. • Possible coarctation with weak or absent femoral pulses and manifestations of heart failure are seen.

(*continued*)

TABLE 18.2 Critical Congenital Heart Defects (*continued*)

LESION	COMMON ANATOMIC DEFECTS	SUMMARY OF PATHOPHYSIOLOGY	COMMON CLINICAL MANIFESTATIONS
Coarctation of the aorta	• Abnormal narrowing of the aorta occurs, most often at the region where the DA interfaces with the aorta.	• *Ductal theory*: Ductal tissue surrounds the aorta during fetal development. After birth, as the DA constricts, the ductal tissue around the aorta also narrows and restricts blood flow. • *Developmental theory*: Hemodynamic changes during fetal development disrupt blood flow through the aortic arch, leading to abnormal formation (narrowing) of the aorta.	• Asymptomatic immediately after birth (if DA is open and/or aortic narrowing is minor). • After ductal closure, cyanosis, tachypnea, feeding difficulties, oliguria, and shock may occur.
Interrupted aortic arch	• Interrupted communication occurs between the ascending and the descending aorta. • VSD	• DA provides blood flow to the systemic circulation during fetal and early postnatal life. • Progressive functional closure of the DA obstructs systemic blood flow and quickly progresses to cardiopulmonary collapse. • Requires ductal patency for pulmonary blood flow.	• After ductal closure, cyanosis, tachypnea respiratory distress, mottling/gray appearance of the lower extremities, feeding difficulties, oliguria, shock, and upper/lower extremity discordant blood pressure measurements occur. • Chest radiograph is usually unremarkable. • Cardiomegaly occurs if ductal patency is maintained after birth.

ASD, atrial septal defect; d-TGA, dextro-transposition of the great arteries; DA, ductus arteriosus; IVC, inferior vena cava; LA, left atrium; LV, left ventricle; PA, pulmonary artery; PFO, patent foramen ovale; PS, pulmonary stenosis; PV, pulmonary vein; PVR, pulmonary vascular resistance; RA, right atrium; RV, right ventricle; SVR, systemic vascular resistance; TAPVR, total anomalous pulmonary venous return; VSD, ventricular septal defect.

Sources: From Balakrishnan, P. L., & Juraszek, A. L. (2012). Pathology of congenital heart disease. *Neoreviews (Elk Grove Village, Ill.), 13*(12), e703–e710. https://doi.org/10.1542/neo.13-12-e703; Barron, D. J., Kilby, M. D., Davies, B., Wright, J. G. C., Jones, T. J., & Brawn, W. J. (2009). Hypoplastic left heart syndrome. *The Lancet, 374*(9689), 551–564. http://doi.org/10.1016/S0140-6736(09)60563-8; Beck, A. E., & Hudgins, L. (2003). Congenital cardiac malformations in the neonate: Isolated or syndromic? *Neoreviews (Elk Grove Village, Ill.), 4*(4), 105. https://doi.org/10.1542/neo.4-4-e105; Hoffman, J., Thompson-Bowie, N., & Jnah, A. J. (2018). The cardiovascular system. In A. J. Jnah & A. N. Trembath (Eds.), *Fetal and neonatal physiology for the advanced practice nurse*. Springer Publishing Company; McCrindle, B. W., Shaffer, K. M., Kan, J. S., Zahka, K. G., Rowe, S. A., & Kidd, L. (1996). Cardinal clinical signs in the differentiation of heart murmurs in children. *Archives of Pediatrics & Adolescent Medicine, 150*(2), 169–174. https://doi.org/10.1001/archpedi.1996.02170270051007; Park, M. K. & Salamat, M. (2021). *Park's pediatric cardiology for practitioners* (7th ed.). Elsevier.

circulation. Gas exchange occurs and freshly oxygenated blood drains into the PVs and left atrium (LA). From there, blood is ejected into the left ventricle (LV), up the aorta, and toward the upper and lower extremities. Following these shifts in atrial and ventricular pressures, functional closure of the fetal shunts (foramen ovale, DA) is observed (Hoffman et al., 2018).

PATHOPHYSIOLOGY REVIEW

The pathophysiology associated with each CCHD is summarized in Table 18.2. More broadly, clinicians should recognize that the following pathologic states are considered "ductal dependent." In these circumstances, a continuous prostaglandin (PGE_1) is required to resist physiologic (functional) closure

- by restricting pulmonary blood flow,
- by assisting noncommunicating parallel cardiac circuit, and
- by inviting systemic blood flow dependent upon ductal patency.

Common Clinical Manifestations

The two most common clinical manifestations of CCHDs, often first detected by bedside nursing staff, are *cyanosis* and respiratory distress, particularly *tachypnea*. Loss of between 3 and 4 grams of reduced hemoglobin is sufficient to elicit noticeable cyanosis in the newborn. Tachypnea most often manifests secondary to pulmonary over circulation or pulmonary venous outflow obstruction. Clinical manifestations associated with each CCHD are summarized in Table 18.2.

Differential Diagnosis

To determine the underlying cause of cyanosis and respiratory distress in the newborn, with or without an audible cardiac murmur, clinicians must consider all mechanisms that may precipitate cyanosis. This includes the exclusion of malformations or dysmorphic findings that may be associated with a syndrome or sequence. We encourage novices to consult the information provided in Table 18.3 when formulating a differential diagnosis for a newborn.

Diagnostic Workup: Pearls for Novice Clinicians

We present a summary of pulse oximetry screening, performed on all well-appearing newborns prior to discharge. This intervention alone reduces CCHD-related deaths by 33% (Martin et al., 2020), which is a stark reminder that late preterm and term newborns with a CCHD are not always prenatally diagnosed nor clinically unwell, leading up to discharge to home. Next, we summarize the most common tests ordered when a high index of suspicion for a CCHD is present. In these more urgent situations, manifestations of cardiopulmonary disease are overt (or a prenatal diagnosis is available), yet clinicians often cannot differentiate between an underlying pulmonary disease and a cardiac disease without further diagnostic testing. Adjunctive tests that may be ordered during the initial cardiopulmonary diagnostic workup, based on the differential diagnosis, include complete blood count, blood culture, and metabolic panel.

Pulse Oximetry Screening

Well-appearing infants born in the United States are subject to an American Academy of Pediatrics (AAP) endorsed CCHD pulse oximetry screening prior to discharge. This AAP protocol began in 2011, and by 2018 all U.S. states passed legislation mandating CCHD screening prior to discharge. The false-positive rate is estimated at 0.035% among asymptomatic newborns screened after 24 hours of life (Mahle et al., 2009). The strategy for CCHD screening was recently revised; a summary of past and present criteria is provided in Table 18.4.

TABLE 18.3 Differential Diagnosis for Cyanosis in the Newborn

SYSTEM	MECHANISM FOR CYANOSIS	ASSOCIATED DIAGNOSIS
Cardiac	Intracardiac right-to-left shunt	d-TGA Tetralogy of Fallot Tricuspid atresia Total anomalous pulmonary venous return Truncus arteriosus Pulmonary atresia Ebstein anomaly Hypoplastic left heart syndrome
	Extracardiac right-to-left shunt	Persistent pulmonary hypertension of the newborn
	Intrapulmonary right-to-left shunt	Pulmonary arteriovenous malformation
	Impaired peripheral circulation	Hypothermia Meningitis Polycythemia Sepsis Shock
	Left-side obstruction	Aortic stenosis or atresia LV hypertrophy (cardiomyopathy)
	Reduced cardiac output	Cardiomyopathy Hypocalcemia
Respiratory	Ventilation/perfusion mismatch	Air leak Aspiration CPAM Pleural effusion Pneumonia Pulmonary hemorrhage Respiratory distress syndrome Transient tachypnea of the newborn
	Alveolar hypoventilation	Asphyxia IVH Meningitis Sedation Seizure
	Airway obstruction	Choanal atresia Pierre Robin sequence
	Neuromuscular injury	Brachial plexus injury (phrenic nerve)

CPAM, congenital pulmonary adenomatoid malformation; d-TGA, dextro-transposition of the great arteries; IVH, intraventricular hemorrhage; LV, left ventricle.

Chest Radiograph

Common radiographic findings associated with CCHDs are summarized in Table 18.2. Chest radiography is often quite informative while awaiting the results of an echocardiogram, as images can rule out air leaks and a congenital diaphragmatic hernia. Three CCHDs that present uniquely on radiographs include d-TGA, tetralogy of Fallot, and TAPVR. The anterior/posterior positioning of the great vessels that occurs with d-TGA creates the appearance of an "egg on a string." The right ventricular hypertrophy that develops in cases of tetralogy of Fallot creates the appearance of a "boot-shaped heart." Finally, cases of supracardiac TAPVR create the appearance of a "figure 8." The upper circle of the "figure 8" is created from the engorged superior vena cava (shadow on the right side of the trachea), engorged vertical vein (shadow on the left side of the trachea), and innominate vein. The cardiac silhouette creates the appearance of the lower circle of the "figure 8." Some clinicians also refer to this as a "snowman" sign (Kemper et al., 2011).

TABLE 18.4 Critical Congenital Heart Defect Screening: Past and Present

CRITERIA	2011–2018 RECOMMENDATION	CURRENT (2020–PRESENT) RECOMMENDATION
Timing of first screening	24–48 hours of life (or just prior to 24 hours of life if eligible for discharge at 24 hours)	24–48 hours of life (or just prior to 24 hours of life if eligible for discharge at 24 hours)
Criteria for passing result	≥95% in the right hand or foot **AND** ≤3% difference between the right hand and foot	≥95% in the right hand **AND** foot
Number of repeat screens permitted before further diagnostic evaluation is pursued	Two	One

Sources: From Kemper, A., Mahle, W., Martin, G., Cooley, W., Kumar, P., Morrow, W., Kelm, K., Pearson, G., Glidewell, J., Grosse, S., & Howell, R. (2011). Strategies for implementing screening for critical congenital heart disease. *Pediatrics*, *128*(5), e1259–e1267. https://doi.org/10.1542/peds.2011-1317; Martin, G. R., Ewer, A. K., Gaviglio, A., Hom, L. A., Saarinen, A., Sontag, M., Burns, K. M., Kemper, A. R., & Oster, M. E. (2020). Updated strategies for pulse oximetry screening for critical congenital heart disease. *Pediatrics*, *146*(1), e20191650. https://doi.org/10.1542/peds.2019-1650.

Hyperoxia Test

The hyperoxia test is helpful in differentiating CCHD from an underlying pulmonary disease and may be pursued while awaiting arrival of the echocardiography technician. Before the test is initiated, a baseline arterial blood gas should be obtained. Then, 100% oxygen is administered for at least 10 minutes and a repeat arterial blood gas is obtained. A partial pressure of oxygen (PaO_2) >100 mmHg after administration of 100% oxygen suggests the underlying cause for cyanosis and/or respiratory distress is of pulmonary etiology. However, some CCHDs are associated with a positive response to the hyperoxia test (e.g., truncus arteriosus with PVR < SVR, tricuspid atresia with a large VSD). Therefore, this test is not considered diagnostic and must be paired with an echocardiogram.

Doppler Echocardiography

Two- and three-dimensional echocardiography is the gold standard test in the assessment of suspected CHDs. Guidelines published by the American Society of Echocardiography (ASE) offer technicians a standardized approach to gathering images during the study. This aids in the assessment of pathologic findings and hemodynamics. Similar to concepts discussed in Chapter 22, "Enteral Nutrition and Gastrointestinal Problems: Formulas, Supplements, and Pharmacotherapeutics," pediatric cardiologists interpret cardiac measurements and other data relative to *z*-scores generated from normative data sets.

Neonatal clinicians should quickly initiate a pediatric cardiology consult into the diagnostic sequence. This reduces the length of time between the request for the echocardiogram, performance of the test, and interpretation of results.

HISTORICAL PERSPECTIVE: SEMINAL AND OTHER NOTEWORTHY STUDIES

Most forms of CCHD are ductal-dependent; therefore, maintaining ductal patency in the immediate newborn period is critical. This section of the chapter focuses on the fascinating history of prostaglandin use in NICUs.

We begin in 1930, when Raphael Kurzrok and Charles Lieb, obstetricians at Vanderbilt University, observed that uterine smooth muscle exhibited noteworthy responsiveness in the presence of seminal fluid. Ulf von Euler, a Swedish physiologist, documented similar results and hypothesized that the mysterious bioactive compound in seminal fluid must arise from the prostate gland. He named the compound *prostaglandin*.

At von Euler's request, biochemist Sune Bergstrom investigated the chemical structure of prostaglandin. He quickly isolated one particularly noteworthy fatty acid precursor (arachidonic acid).

Ten years later, Bergstrom isolated two complete and pure prostaglandin molecules and named them *prostaglandin* E_2 (PGE_2) and *prostaglandin* $F_{2\alpha}$. Bergstrom was awarded the Nobel Prize for this seminal and noteworthy discovery.

Over the following two decades, scientists incrementally identified prostaglandins in nearly all nucleated cells and human tissues. This led to the realization that prostaglandin modulated diverse physiologic actions. PGE_2 was identified as the most abundant prostaglandin in the human body. Prostaglandin I_2 produced bronchodilation and vasodilation in pulmonary tissue, whereas prostaglandin $F_{2\alpha}$ produced bronchoconstriction, vasoconstriction of cerebral vasculature, and reduced intraocular pressure (used pharmacologically to treat glaucoma). Next, prostaglandin E_1 (PGE_1), less robustly expressed, was isolated in 1957.

Now that many prostaglandins were identified and their mechanism of action explained, chemists focused on the synthesis of prostaglandin. In 1969, PGE_1 was synthesized by chemist William Paul Schneider; chemist E. J. Corey, in consultation with Pfizer, synthesized PGE_2 in 1970. This spurred a race to identify pharmacologic uses (and source of revenue) for both molecules.

Meanwhile, in the early 1970s, New Zealand-based physician Sir Robert Bartlett Elliott experimented with dilating the DA of fetal calves and newborn lambs with PGE_1. Within 5 years, Elliott successfully maintained ductal patency with a continuous infusion of PGE_1 (0.1 mcg/kg/min) in two infants with CCHDs whose parents had refused surgery. Concurrently, Toronto-based physician Peter Olley demonstrated similar outcomes using a continuous infusion of PGE_2 in animal models. In 1976, Olley and colleagues disseminated the results of an observational study of four infants with CCHD who received a continuous PGE_2 infusion for treatment of a right-side obstructive heart lesion prior to surgical intervention. The authors reported that PGE_2 "produced consistently an immediate and persistent rise in arterial oxygen saturation" (Olley, 1976, p. 728) and correctly attributed the change in clinical status to ductal patency. Despite the success with use of PGE_2, Olley hypothesized that PGE_1 may possess a superior safety profile because it is a weak vasodilator of the pulmonary microvasculature, whereas PGE_2 elicited pulmonary vasoconstriction. Subsequent to Olley's discoveries, numerous case reports were published, each confirming the efficacy of PGE_1.

Next, experts focused efforts on establishing a safety profile for prostaglandin, as this was a fundamental requirement for Food and Drug Administration (FDA) approval. Kensey and colleagues, in partnership with Upjohn Pharmaceuticals, reviewed 492 reports of infants treated at 56 United States based NICUs with PGE_1 with the intent of identifying and appraising adverse effects (Lewis et al., 1981). Cardiovascular-specific adverse effects were reported in 18% of subjects and included cutaneous vasodilation or edema, rhythm disturbances, and hypotension. These adverse effects were more prevalent with a continuous arterial versus venous infusion. Central nervous system-specific adverse effects were reported in 16% of subjects and included temperature elevation (currently the most common adverse effect associated with therapy) and seizure-like activity. Twelve percent of patients weighing less than 2 kg manifested with apnea, currently regarded as the second most common adverse effect associated with prostaglandin therapy. Ultimately, prostaglandin earned FDA approval in 1981 for use in neonates with CHDs; the generic name *alprostadil* was assigned to the drug at this time (Roehl & Townsend, 1982). Clinicians were advised to closely monitor temperature, respiratory activity, and blood pressure throughout alprostadil therapy. In addition, clinicians were encouraged to prescribe the lowest effective dose in order to reduce the risk of adverse effects.

Given the longstanding FDA approval, known efficacy linked to alprostadil use in neonates with CCHDs, and ethical implications associated with potentially treating a neonate with a subtherapeutic treatment regimen just for the purpose of obtaining blinded, randomized data, these higher fidelity trials cannot be pursued (Akkinapally et al., 2018). Therefore, observational data must be relied on when standardizing treatment protocols (dosing, duration of therapy) for ductal-dependent cardiac lesions.

CURRENT PHARMACOLOGIC TREATMENT MODALITIES

Alprostadil (Prostaglandin E_1)

As stated throughout this chapter, maintaining the patency of the DA is critical to postnatal survival when a CCHD is present. Clinicians may anticipate the need for alprostadil when the antenatal diagnosis of a ductal-dependent CCHD is known. In other circumstances, formerly well-appearing neonates may exhibit a rapid cardiopulmonary decompensation as the DA constricts. In these situations, alprostadil therapy should be considered and likely initiated based on this clinical index of suspicion, pending laboratory and echocardiographic data (Singh & Mikrou, 2018).

MECHANISM OF ACTION/CORE PHARMACOKINETIC PRINCIPLES

PGE_1 is a naturally occurring eicosanoid, or lipid compound. The mechanism of action involves smooth muscle vasodilation at the DA. Consequently, this facilitates pulmonary and/or systemic blood flow, a lifesaving hemodynamic shift for infants with ductal-dependent CCHDs who await surgical palliation or primary repair.

Alprostadil is intravenously administered; therefore, 100% bioavailability is observed. Alprostadil readily distributes to target tissues and is thereby metabolized (by oxidation) in the lungs. Approximately 75% of drug molecules are metabolized during a single circulation. The elimination half-life is estimated to be less than 1 minute in neonates. Clinicians should be aware of the extremely short half-life of this life-sustaining medication and administer alprostadil through a central venous catheter. Peripheral administration is effective when other alternatives do not exist, but requires meticulous monitoring of the infusion site. The maximum clinical effect should be observed within 30 minutes of initiating therapy when treating a CCHD. In comparison, the therapeutic effect is observed between 1.5 and 11 hours after the initiation of therapy with acyanotic lesions. Alprostadil is excreted primarily as metabolites in the urine (Taketomo, 2023).

DOSING RECOMMENDATIONS

Intravenous dosing ranges between 0.01 and 0.1 mcg/kg/min (Vari et al., 2021). Most clinicians initiate therapy at approximately 0.025 to 0.05 mcg/kg/min, particularly if Doppler echocardiography is pending. If the ductus is determined to be large, the dose may be titrated to a lower continuous infusion capable of maintaining patency (e.g., 0.01–0.025 mcg/kg/min). In contrast, if the ductus is closing or functionally closed, a high-dose continuous infusion may be necessary to dilate or reestablish patency (e.g., 0.05–0.1 mcg/kg/min; Vari et al., 2021). Pediatric cardiologists customarily guide dosing decisions; neonatal APRNs are encouraged to maintain open lines of communication during these emergency situations. Note that neonatal clinicians should remain at bedside during the first 30 minutes of treatment to observe for pharmacodynamic effects of drug therapy.

CLINICAL-MONITORING PEARLS

Close monitoring of PaO_2, respiratory status, thermoregulation, and mean arterial pressures is indicated. The two noteworthy side effects associated with alprostadil therapy that all neonatal clinicians must be mindful of are fever and apnea. Currently, the incidence of fever (14%) surpasses apnea (10%–12%), likely because the minimum effective dose is prescribed often at or below 0.05 mcg/kg/min and further customized to each neonate. Despite these low doses, it is commonplace to discontinue overhead radiant heat during therapy to maintain euthermia. The risk of fever and apnea increases as the dosage is increased. Other commonly reported adverse reactions include flushing (10%), bradycardia (7%), hypotension (4%), and tachycardia (3%). Less than 1% of neonates manifest with adverse respiratory, gastrointestinal, hematologic, or renal reactions (Pfizer, 2022).

Although rare, should alprostadil therapy extend beyond 120 hours, clinicians should monitor for feeding intolerance, which could be an early sign of gastric obstruction. In addition, the risk of cortical hyperostosis increases with long-term therapy lasting more than 9 days (Kaufman et al., 1996; Woo et al., 1994).

CONCLUSIONS

CCHDs represent one of the most emergent diseases identified during the neonatal period. Among well-appearing newborns, CCHDs often clinically manifest once the DA becomes significantly constricted. This may occur just prior to discharge to home if a short stay is requested by the family. Therefore, neonatal clinicians must uphold the highest standards when completing physical examinations and delay the CCHD screening until as close to 24 hours of life as possible. The recently revised AAP guidelines for CCHD screening simplify the diagnostic pathway and expedite the time frame from recognition of the at-risk newborn to confirmatory diagnosis. All clinicians responsible for hands-on neonatal care are responsible for complying with the AAP recommendations. In other circumstances, newborns may require direct admission to the NICU. Consistent with the convergent care model (Wei, 2022), a multidisciplinary team-based approach to the stabilization and treatment of the newborn optimizes outcomes. Simulation-based training focused on the steps required to stabilize the newborn with a CCHD may benefit new clinicians or those who staff units in rural areas without immediate pediatric cardiology support. Looking ahead, increased use of fetal and postnatal cardiac MRI (cMRI) may be on the horizon; these tests may aid obstetricians and midwives with prenatal counseling and coordination of care for the delivery of the newborn. Postnatally, cMRI offers a more granular assessment of cardiac structure, which may assist NICU providers and cardiothoracic surgeons.

LEARNING TOOLS AND RESOURCES

Advice From the Author

Karen Wright, PhD, APRN, NNP-BC

Cyanotic heart disease and PPHN have identical presentations. The initial approach to cyanosis is to treat as if the infant is experiencing a respiratory problem or sepsis. That said, if there is a delay in echocardiography and the patient is not improving despite adequate ventilation and the provision of 100% oxygen, begin PGE_1. PGE_1 will rarely cause a problem with newborns if the diagnosis is ultimately not CHD, but if it is, you are providing a lifesaving therapy. In addition, make certain that you are maximizing other therapies that may overlap with congenital heart disease such as sepsis.

Discussion Prompts

1. Identify and describe the ductal-dependent lesions.
2. Create a simulation-based training scenario focused on the stabilization of a newborn with a CCHD. Test your scenario with colleagues and debrief with the participants. Could this type of interval training benefit new hires, per diem staff, or others who may assist during emergencies?
3. Apply your understanding of the mechanism of action of alprostadil to each of the CCHDs mentioned in this chapter. Consider the function of the DA and how reestablishing patency would alter hemodynamics.

Mind Map

Ductal dependence involves

Three pathologic states

Restriction of pulmonary blood flow

- Pulmonary atresia
- TOF
- Interrupted aortic arch
- Truncus arteriosus
- Tricuspid atresia
- Ebstein anomaly

Noncommunicating parallel cardiac circuit

- d-TGA

Obstructed systemic blood flow

- Hypoplastic left heart
- TAPVR
- Single ventricle
- Coarctation of the aorta
- Interrupted aortic arch

Clinical manifestations

- Shock-like appearance when ductus arteriosus closes
- Profound cyanosis
- Tachypnea—respiratory distress
- Lactic acidosis—little to no systemic perfusion
- Upper/lower extremity BP differential
- Pre/post ductal SpO_2 differential

Diagnostic tools

- Pre/post SpO_2 monitoring
- All 4 extremity blood pressures
- Chest x-ray
- Echocardiogram

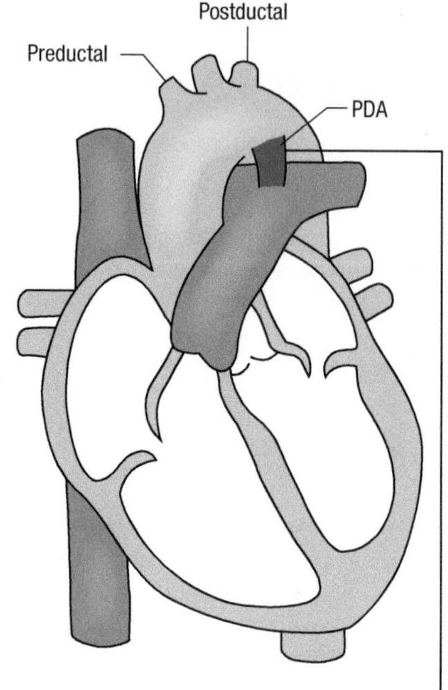

Maintaining ductal patency is key

Alprostadil

- Prostaglandin E_1
- Smooth muscle vasodilation at the ductus arteriosus
- Peak effect within 30 minutes of administration
- Half-life <1 minute
- Therapeutic effect within 1.5 to 11 hours of initiation

!! important to monitor for !!

- Fever
- Apnea

Note: This mind map reflects the design team's interpretation of a portion of one or more concepts addressed in this chapter. Readers should regard the mind maps woven throughout this textbook as examples of multisensory study tools that can be developed to encourage conceptual understanding. Readers are encouraged to develop their own unique mind maps in consultation with academic faculty or clinical preceptors.
BP, blood pressure; d-TGA, dextro-transposition of the great arteries; TAPVR, total anomalous pulmonary venous return; TOF, tetralogy of Fallot.
Design credit: Mary Thompson, MSN, APRN, NNP-BC, and MSN, APRN, NNP, RNC-NIC, East Carolina University Neonatal Nurse Practitioner Program.

REFERENCES

References for this chapter are online and available at https://connect.springerpub.com/content/book/978-0-8261-5884-0/part/partIV/toc-part/ch18.

chapter 19

Tachyarrhythmias

Jacqui Hoffman and Amy J. Jnah

LEARNING OBJECTIVES

After completing this chapter, the reader should be able to:

- Define *Wolff-Parkinson-White syndrome (WPW)*, *orthodromic reciprocating tachycardia (ORT)*, and *antidromic reciprocating tachycardia (ART)*, as well as identify the epidemiology of the disease process.
- Enumerate the most common risk factors for arrhythmias in the neonate.
- Explain the physiology of normal cardiac conduction.
- Correlate the pathophysiology of tachyarrhythmias with the need for pharmacologic treatment.
- Appraise the historical evolution of pharmacologic management for arrhythmias in the neonate.
- Evaluate the role of pharmacotherapeutic regimens with respect to pharmacodynamic and pharmacokinetic properties in relation to management/prevention of WPW, ORT, and ART.

INTRODUCTION

For centuries, clinicians have recognized the presence of irregular heart rhythms while palpating a patient's pulse. Some of the most interesting observations and discoveries include:

- **1839**: Czech physiologist Jan Purkinje identified a web of conductive fibers in the subendocardium.
- **1840s**: Italian physicist Carlo Matteucci demonstrated that an electric current accompanied each cardiac contraction and Emil Du Bois-Reymond, a German physiologist, described that an action potential accompanied each muscular contraction.
- **1880**: British physiologist Walter Gaskell identified the sinus venosus as the conductive area of the heart where impulses are first generated.
- **1892**: The first pediatric case of supraventricular tachycardia (SVT) was reported in a child with measles (Buckland, 1892).
- **1893**: Swiss anatomist Wilhelm His made the important discovery that a bundle of conductive fibers are situated between the atria and ventricles.
- **Early 1900s**: Scottish anatomist Arthur Keith and medical student Martin Flack identified the sinoatrial node (in a rodent) as the pacemaker of the heart. They wrote: "There is a remarkable remnant of primitive fibres persisting at the sino-auricular junction in all the mammalian hearts examined . . . in them the dominating rhythm of the heart is believed to normally arise" (Keith & Flack, 1907, p. 188).

Although these noteworthy, seminal findings advanced the state of the science, clinicians still struggled to differentiate between abnormal rhythms and to diagnose arrhythmias. The only tools available to appraise heart rhythm were the sphygmograph, which could pulse waves, and the capillary electrometer, which could record the heart's electrical current (Figure 19.1). These devices were rarely used in clinical practice.

Diagnostic accuracy improved significantly once the string galvanometer, now known as the *EKG*, was invented in 1902 by Dutch physiologist Dr. Willem Einthoven (Fye, 1994). The string galvanometer allowed the electrical activity of the heart to be recorded, offering the first opportunity to evaluate cardiac arrhythmias. Incidentally, Einthoven was awarded the Nobel Prize in 1924 for this invention. In 1910, the first American review on electrocardiography was published (James & Williams, 1910), followed by several illustrated books.

Electrocardiography was refined over the years, from direct-writing machines used in the 1930s (Fye, 1994) to the three-lead and later, in 1942, the 12-lead EKG (Goldberger, 1942). Postgraduate courses were incepted during the 1920s and 1930s as the field of electrocardiography continued to develop. Focus shifted to diagnostics versus the role of pharmacologic agents. As a result, digoxin and quinidine remained the two primary drugs used to treat arrhythmias until the 1950s (Fye, 1993). In the late 1970s, computer-analyzed EKGs were introduced into clinical practice (Fye, 1994). As the pediatric cardiology subspecialty flourished in the 20th century, many decades after the advent of pediatric cardiac surgeries and cardiac catherization, the study of fetal and neonatal arrhythmias began.

Arrhythmias, namely tachyarrhythmias, can be life-threatening and require immediate diagnosis and triage. Therefore, neonatal APRNs must remain familiar with normal cardiac conduction, understand the pathogenesis of abnormal conduction, and be adept at prescribing proper drugs to treat the affected neonate. This chapter offers readers a concise review of the normal cardiac conduction and the pathogenesis of common tachyarrhythmias. A historic look at seminal and noteworthy studies of drug therapies used to treat tachyarrhythmias precedes the evaluation of common pharmacologic treatment modalities. We present this information in a manner that facilitates knowledge acquisition and application of knowledge in the clinical setting.

FIGURE 19.1 The capillary electrometer and Einthoven's string galvanometer.

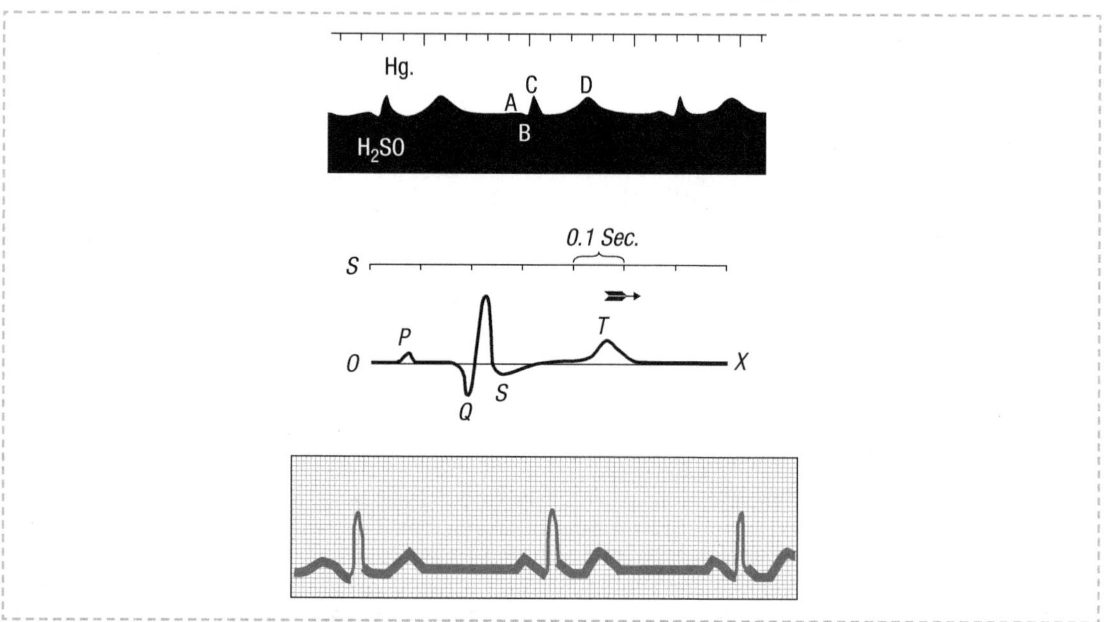

Note: Einthoven's string galvanometer (*bottom*) and the mathematically corrected curves (*middle*) obtained with the capillary electrometer (*top*).
Source: From Fleckenstein, K. (1984). The early ECG in medical practice. *Medical Instrumentation, 18*(3), 191–912.

FIGURE 19.2 Automaticity of cardiac cells.

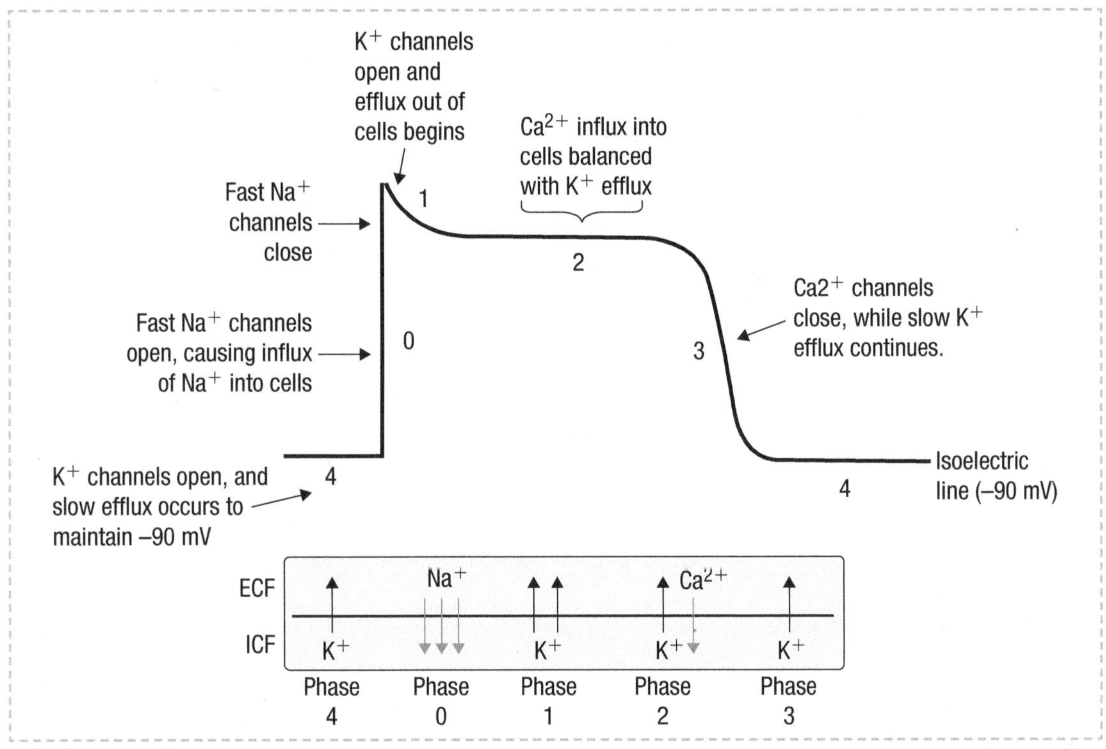

ECF, extracellular fluid; ICF, intracellular fluid.
Source: Design credit: Mya Jnah.

PHYSIOLOGY REVIEW: CARDIAC CONDUCTION

Here we offer an abbreviated review of cardiac conduction. A more detailed discussion of cardiac conduction can be found in *Fetal and Neonatal Physiology for the Advanced Practice Nurse* (Hoffman et al., 2018).

The sinoatrial (SA) node, found in the region of the right atrium, functions as the pacemaker, or "voltage clock," for the heart. Under normal conditions, an electrical impulse begins in the SA node. Voltage-gated ion channels, located within the sarcolemma, open to permit movement of sodium and calcium ions into cardiomyocytes and inactivation of potassium channels. This marks the beginning of depolarization, which yields spontaneous impulse initiation and the formation of an action potential (Figure 19.2; Bravo-Valenzuela et al., 2018). The impulse spreads rapidly through the atria to the atrioventricular (AV) node. Next, a brief delay occurs at the AV node, before the impulse conducts toward the bundle of His, down the right and left bundle branches, and to the Purkinje fibers found within the ventricular septum (Figure 19.3).

PATHOPHYSIOLOGY REVIEW: CARDIAC CONDUCTION

Any number of factors that impair normal generation of the impulse in the SA node may give rise to a bradyarrhythmia (in which the AV node functions as an escape pacemaker) or tachyarrhythmia (in which the impulse arrives when one of the pathways is refractory). Arrhythmias can also occur in isolation (idiopathic etiology). Common precipitating factors include gene disorders and structural heart defects. The conduction system may be abnormally displaced in infants with structural heart defects, resulting in abnormalities at impulse generation or across conduction pathways.

Arrhythmias are most commonly classified as premature complexes, bradycardia, or tachycardia. The focus here is specific to tachyarrhythmias, as these often require pharmacologic therapy to normalize the heart rhythm.

FIGURE 19.3 Normal conduction system.

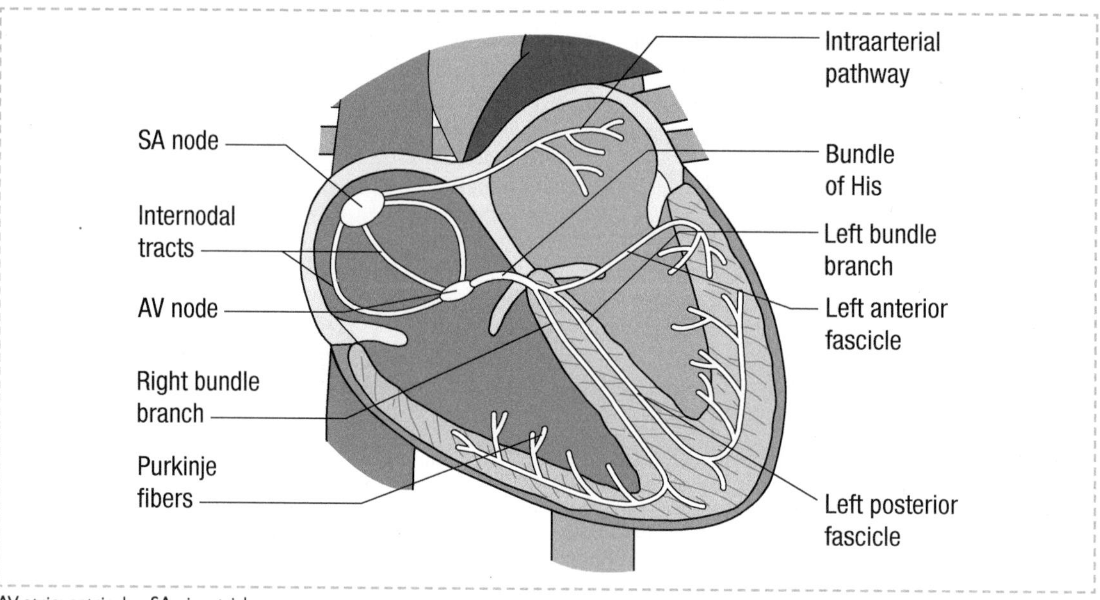

AV, atrioventricular; SA, sinoatrial.
Source: From Jnah, A. J., & Trembath, A. N. (Eds.). (2018). *Fetal and neonatal physiology for the advanced practice nurse*. Springer Publishing Company.

BOX 19.1 Conditions Associated With Sinus Tachycardia

Fever
Hypoxemia
Electrolyte disturbances
Anemia
Pain, agitation
Administration of sympathomimetic agents

Supraventricular Tachycardia

It is important to distinguish sinus tachycardia from reentrant forms of tachycardia. Sinus tachycardia manifests gradually. Common findings include a normal upright P-wave and a variable ventricular rate that is less than 220 beats per minute (Topijan et al., 2020). Management is usually abortive and nonpharmacologic. Focus is placed on resolving the proximate cause for the increase in heart rate (e.g., iatrogenic hyperthermia). When this occurs, return to normal sinus rhythm usually follows in a timely manner (Box 19.1).

In contrast, reentrant tachycardias develop from abnormal impulse conduction. SVT accounts for almost 85% of all cases of neonatal reentrant tachycardia and is the focus of this section of the chapter. SVT affects one in 200 to 250 neonates and a 2:1 male predominance pattern is reported. Over 70% of all cases of SVT present within the first 48 hours of life, with the rest presenting within the first few months of life (Begum & Sharker, 2020; Garson et al., 1981; Gilljam et al., 2008; Tortoriello et al., 2003). Nearly 50% of infants who exhibit SVT in the newborn period are not affected by recurrent events; however, those who are affected may require long-term pharmacologic therapy (Garson et al., 1981).

SVT is associated with several heart defects, including transposition of the great arteries (TGA), Ebstein anomaly, and hypertrophic cardiomyopathy (Weindling et al., 1996). A population-based study from a birth cohort database in Taiwan found 25% of significant arrhythmias were associated with congenital heart defects (CHDs), including (in descending order of occurrence) atrial septal defect, ventricular septal defect, patent ductus arteriosus, tetralogy of Fallot, pulmonary stenosis, and Ebstein anomaly (Wu et al., 2016). SVT can also be present after cardiac surgery (Park & Salamet, 2021).

The pathogenesis of SVT involves an abrupt start and stop (paroxysmal) of the rhythm disturbance, which arises at or above the bundle of His and manifests with a heart rate ranging from 220 to 300 beats per minute. While the pathogenesis of the disease should precipitate obvious clinical instability, many healthy-appearing newborns with SVT remain asymptomatic until the rhythm disturbance presents for a prolonged period of time. This leads to the onset of congestive heart failure and signs of illness (Bauersfeld et al., 2001; Gilljam et al., 2008).

At present, the congenital cyanotic heart screening is the only standardized cardiac screening test performed on all neonates prior to discharge to home. Therefore, it is essential that bedside nurses and APRNs include a full 60 seconds of cardiac auscultation as part of interval cardiovascular assessments. This helps promote the early identification and diagnosis of cardiac abnormalities in the newborn period. A stepwise approach to SVT management is utilized in neonatal intensive care. The approach begins with vagal maneuvers, procedures first described in 1977 by Whitman and colleagues. Vagal maneuvers include the placement of a bag of ice to the face, which should elicit the diving reflex, slow AV conduction, and terminate the tachycardia. When vagal maneuvers are unsuccessful, clinicians prescribe intravenous (IV) adenosine. When both vagal maneuvers and adenosine fail to restore a normal heart rhythm, low-voltage cardioversion may be required (Park & Salamet, 2021). In rarer cases, when SVT is refractory to all of the aforementioned therapies (recurrent episodes over a prolonged period of time), ablation is considered.

Long-term therapy (e.g., beta-blocker, antiarrhythmic agent, or calcium channel blocker) may be required to encourage normal conduction through the AV node, slow conduction through an accessory pathway (e.g., flecainide and procainamide), or provide a combination of both mitigation strategies (e.g., amiodarone and sotalol). When choosing a pharmacologic agent, it is imperative that clinicians consider the type of SVT, as some individuals are adenosine sensitive, whereas others are not. Clinicians should identify concomitant contributing factors (e.g., CHDs, myocardial dysfunction) and identify potential adverse effects associated with use of the selected pharmacologic agent. We discuss these therapies later in the chapter.

Importantly, approximately 75% of SVT cases involve an accessory pathway between the atrium and the ventricle, termed an atrioventricular reciprocating (back and forth) or reentry tachycardia (AVRT; Ko et al., 1992). Accessory pathways are abnormal tracts made of myocardial fibers that span the AV groove; this extra electrical conduction pathway bypasses the AV node, conducting impulses from the atrium to the ventricle in a forward-moving (antegrade) manner, or from the ventricle to the atrium in a backward-moving (retrograde) manner (Figure 19.4). Given the multitude of types of SVT, we will discuss the most common types (Wolff-Parkinson-White syndrome [WPW], orthodromic reciprocating tachycardia [ORT], and antidromic reciprocating tachycardia [ART]) that affect hospitalized preterm and term neonates.

WOLFF-PARKINSON-WHITE SYNDROME

WPW, first described by Wolff, Parkinson, and White (1930), is considered a reentrant form of SVT. The pathogenesis involves movement of an electrical impulse from the SA node to the AV node *and* an abnormal accessory pathway. As the impulse passes through the AV node, normal conduction is abnormally delayed, whereas the impulse through the accessory pathway is not delayed. The result is abnormal *antegrade* conduction through the accessory pathway with ventricular preexcitation (Figure 19.5). Ventricular preexcitation can lead to intraventricular dyssynchrony and left ventricular dysfunction. The EKG usually shows a short PR interval and classic delta wave (slurring of the upstroke of the QRS complex). WPW-related SVT is associated with a high risk of cardiac arrest or sudden death later in life.

ORTHODROMIC RECIPROCATING TACHYCARDIA

ORT accounts for approximately 90% of AVRT. Normal antegrade conduction is observed from the SA node to the AV node and to the ventricles. However, the presence of an accessory pathway encourages *retrograde* (reverse-moving) conduction, ventricular preexcitation, and tachycardia (Figure 19.6). A premature atrial contraction (PAC) is often responsible for initiating the abnormal,

FIGURE 19.4 Narrow and wide QRS-complex reentrant supraventricular tachycardias.

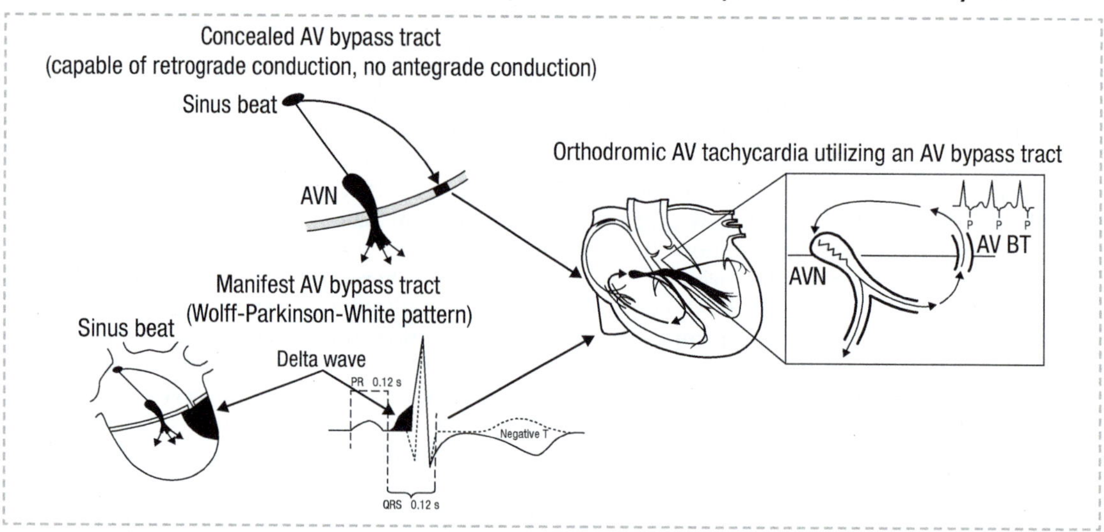

Note: The directions of the arrows reflect the direction of impulse generation within the reentrant circuit. The slow pathway within the circuit is represented by the "wavy" arrow. The lower image depicts the presence (ventricular preexcitation or Wolff-Parkinson-White syndrome) of antegrade conduction via the AV bypass pathway in sinus rhythm; the upper image depicts the absence (concealed pathway without ventricular preexcitation or orthodromic AV reentrant) of antegrade conduction via the AV bypass pathway in sinus rhythm.
AV, atrioventricular; AV BT, atrioventricular bypass tract; AVN, atrioventricular node.
Source: From Srinivasan, C., & Balaji, S. (2019). Neonatal supraventricular tachycardia. *Indian Pacing and Electrophysiology Journal, 19*(6), 222–231. https://doi.org/10.1016/j.ipej.2019.09.004

FIGURE 19.5 Abnormal conduction in Wolff-Parkinson-White syndrome.

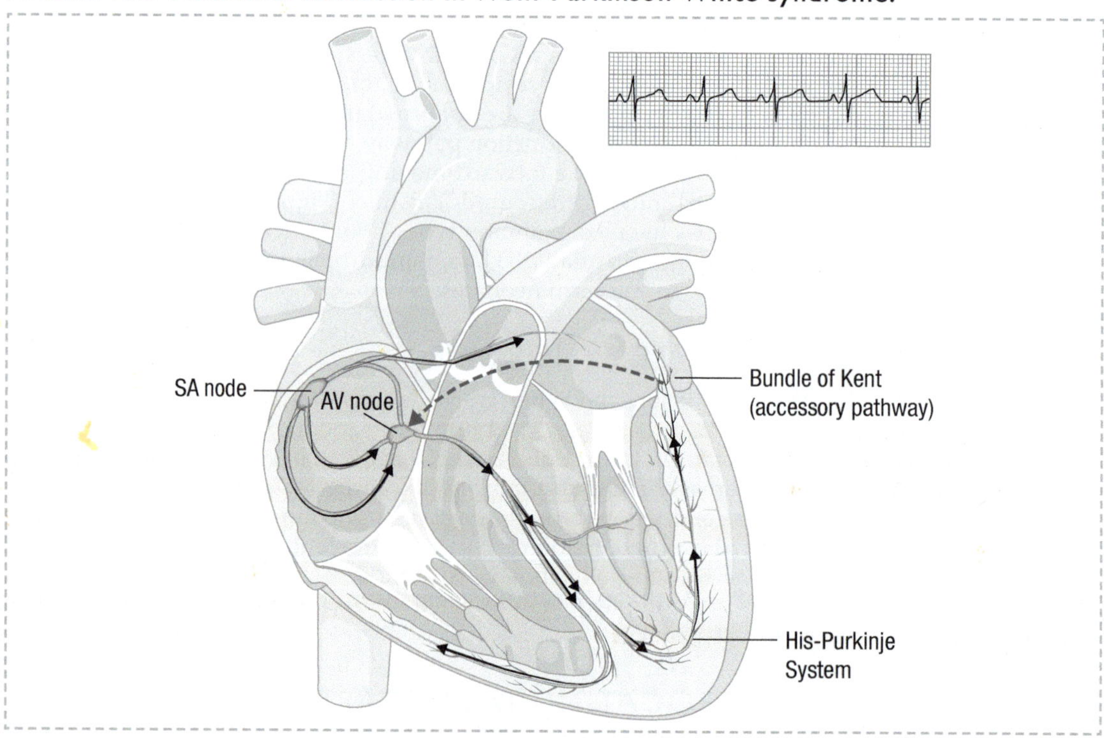

Note: In Wolff-Parkinson-White syndrome, electrical impulses form a continuous circuit capable of bypassing the AV node through the use of an accessory pathway that connects the ventricle and atria. One such accessory pathway is called the *bundle of Kent.* This leads to antegrade conduction, persistent ventricular preexcitation, and tachycardia. A short PR interval and abnormally long QRS are is observed on EKG.
AV, atrioventricular; SA, sinoatrial.
Source: Design credit: Amy J. Jnah.

FIGURE 19.6 Abnormal pathway in orthodromic reciprocating tachycardia.

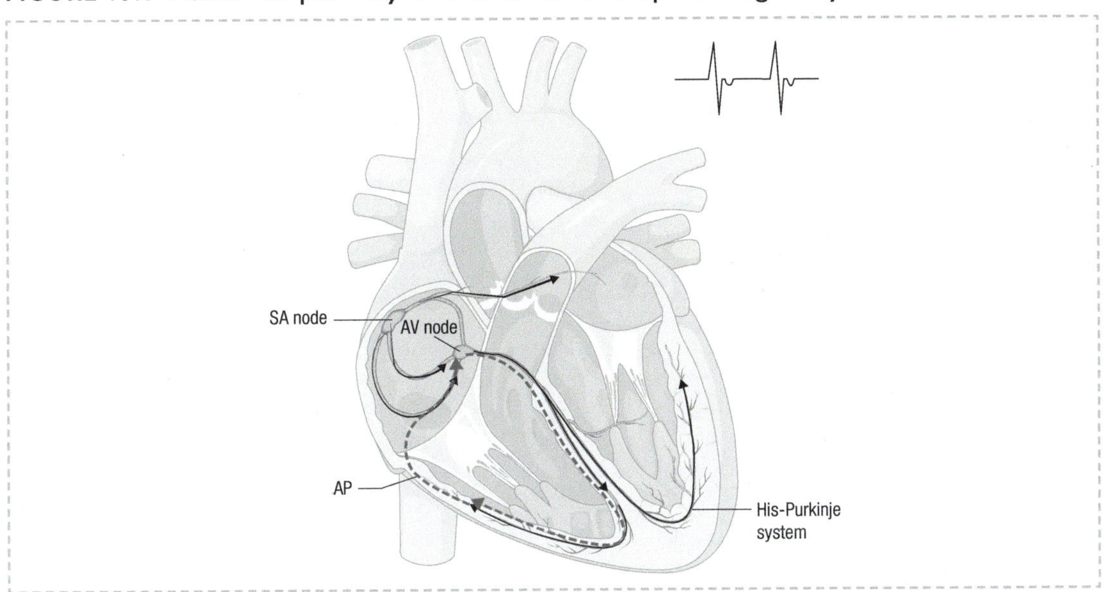

Note: The AV node and His-Purkinje system function as the antegrade limb (also known as the "ortho") while the accessory pathway functions as the retrograde limb.
AP, accessory pathway; AV, atrioventricular; SA, sinoatrial.
Sources: Design credit: Amy J. Jnah. Data from Mavroudis, C., Deal, B. J., Backer, C. L., & Tsao, S. (2008). Arrhythmia surgery in patients with and without congenital heart disease. *Annuals of Thoracic Surgery, 86*(3), 857–868. https://doi.org/10.1016/j.athoracsur.2008.04.087

reverse-moving circuit between the AV node and the accessory pathway. The result is retrograde conduction, which elicits atrial activation shortly after ventricular depolarization. The EKG usually shows a narrow QRS complex and retrograde P waves are often seen overtop the T wave.

When infants exhibit periods of normal sinus rhythm, no preexcitation is apparent. This conceals the accessory pathway and complicates early identification and diagnosis. This arrhythmia is typically well tolerated for a short time frame in the absence of other underlying structural heart defects. However, ORT that occurs over a prolonged period of time is associated with reduced cardiac output, thinning of the ventricular wall, and congestive heart failure.

ANTIDROMIC RECIPROCATING TACHYCARDIA

ART is unique in that a blockage at the AV node prevents normal movement of a retrograde impulse through the node and toward the His-Purkinje system. Rather, conduction originates in the SA node. The impulse does not repolarize and is thereby "blocked" at the AV node. This forces the impulse to move (backward) in an antegrade direction through the accessory pathway and into the outer wall of the affected ventricle(s). Once at the ventricle, retrograde conduction occurs from the ventricles and backward through the AV node (Figure 19.7). The EKG normally shows a wide QRS complex, a finding easily misinterpreted as ventricular tachycardia.

FOCAL ATRIAL TACHYCARDIA

Another type of tachycardia is focal atrial tachycardia (FAT). This type of tachycardia occurs when cells in the atria depolarize faster than cells in the SA node. Because of the ectopic nature of the atrial impulse, there is an abnormal P-wave morphology. This distinguishes FAT from sinus tachycardia. FAT has gradual onset and termination is variable, although it is typically gradual as well. Initially, infants appear asymptomatic, but as the arrhythmia persists, infants develop a dilated cardiomyopathy and congestive heart failure.

This arrhythmia is not adenosine sensitive nor responsive to cardioversion. For acute management, esmolol is used. Long-term management typically involves the use of an oral beta-adrenergic blocker (e.g., propranolol, atenolol, or sotalol). Amiodarone therapy is reserved for refractory cases. If pharmacologic therapy is unsuccessful, catheter ablation may be indicated.

FIGURE 19.7 Abnormal pathway in antidromic reciprocating tachycardia.

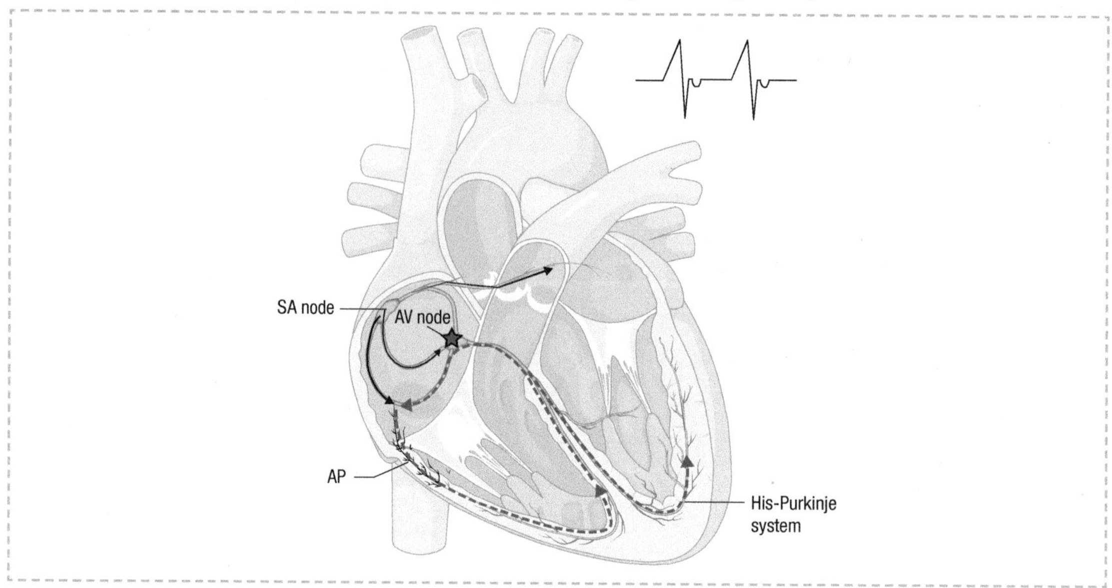

Note: The black star indicates block at AV node, preventing conduction. The impulse moves toward the AV node prior to repolarizing, which creates the blockage. In the presence of the accessory pathway, the impulse moves in a retrograde (backward) fashion, creating a recurring circuit of impulses (tachycardia), while current also travels down toward the His-Purkinje system in the opposing ventricle. The EKG wave displays a shortened PR interval and wide QRS axis.

AP, accessory pathway; AV, atrioventricular; SA, sinoatrial.

Sources: Design credit: Amy J. Jnah. Created using Biorender.com. Data from Mavroudis, C., Deal, B. J., Backer, C. L., & Tsao, S. (2008). Arrhythmia surgery in patients with and without congenital heart disease. *Annuals of Thoracic Surgery, 86*(3), 857–868. https://doi.org/10.1016/j.athoracsur.2008.04.087

Clinical Manifestations of Supraventricular Tachycardia

Among otherwise well-appearing late preterm and term newborns admitted to routine newborn nurseries, episodes of SVT may be subclinical at onset. Nonspecific symptoms include lethargy/irritability, emesis, poor feeding, and tachypnea (due to pulmonary venous congestion). In cases in which the SVT remains undetected over an extended period of time, impaired diastolic filling of the ventricles will lead to decreased cardiac output and negatively affect myocardial blood flow. Infants will develop hemodynamic instability and present with shock-like symptoms that may be confused with late-onset sepsis or with cardiovascular collapse; this presentation is associated with a 1% to 4% mortality (Salerno et al., 2011; Sanatani et al., 2002).

EVALUATION OF SUPRAVENTRICULAR TACHYCARDIA

SVT that is observed in utero will require further evaluation, namely by way of a fetal echocardiogram that is conducted by a maternal–fetal medicine expert. Fetal tachyarrhythmias, defined as a fetal heart rate exceeding 180 beats per minute, are considered a cardiac emergency.

Fetal SVT is initially managed with transplacental (maternal oral or IV) pharmacologic therapy in an attempt to return the fetus to normal sinus rhythm to avoid the risk of development of low cardiac output, fetal hydrops, or even fetal death (Bravo-Valenzuela et al., 2018). Mono- or combination drug therapy may include digoxin, flecainide, sotalol, or (less commonly) amiodarone. For additional information regarding fetal therapy, please refer to the Severin and colleagues (2013) reference.

Postnatal SVT is initially triaged by more than one clinician. It is essential to perform a complete physical exam and simultaneously establish or maintain hemodynamic stability. If the infant is hemodynamically stable, clinicians may have time to obtain a perinatal and family history. This informs clinicians whether the family has a history of heart disease, arrhythmias, or sudden unexplained death during infancy, childhood, or early adult life. A summary of the diagnostic evaluation is provided in Table 19.1. When possible, clinicians should obtain an EKG with rhythm strip before, during, and after pharmacologic therapy is rendered, as these data can assist the pediatric cardiology team.

TABLE 19.1 Diagnostic Evaluation of the Hemodynamically Stable Neonate With Tachycardia

TYPE OF STUDY	NAME	EVALUATES
Laboratory blood analysis	• Arterial blood gas • Lactate	• Hypoxia, metabolic and/or lactic acidosis
	• Blood culture • Complete blood count	• Sepsis • Red cell indices
	• Comprehensive metabolic panel	• Electrolyte (potassium) or mineral imbalance (calcium, phosphorus, and magnesium) and • Renal function
	• Glucose	• Hypoglycemia
	• TSH • T4	• Thyroid function
Radiographic	• Chest x-ray	• Heart size • Lung fields
Cardiac function	• 12-lead ECG	• Identify arrhythmia (imperative to have baseline as well as rhythm recording with any acute interventions)
	• Echocardiogram	• Heart anatomy • Heart function

ECG, electrocardiogram; T4, thyroxine; TSH, thyroid stimulating hormone.
Source: Begum, N.A., & Sharker, S. (2020). Neonatal supraventricular tachycardia—A review of literature. *Pediatric Research and Child Health, 4*(1), 1–7. https://www.sciaeon.org/articles/Neonatal-Supraventricular-Tachycardia-A-Review-of-Literature.pdf

HISTORICAL PERSPECTIVE: SEMINAL AND OTHER NOTEWORTHY STUDIES

Digoxin was the seminal drug used to treat SVT. Physicians preferred digoxin due to its negative inotropic properties, which were advantageous in newborns with arrhythmias that decreased cardiac output. However, clinicians realized over time that digoxin was not an ideal therapy for SVT. First, it was discovered that digoxin offers a slow onset of action, which meant a considerable delay (up to 10 hours!) from administration to termination of the arrhythmia (Greco et al., 1982; Sreeram & Wren, 1990). Second, numerous calculation and dosing errors occurred, leading to both subtherapeutic and toxic administrations. Third, clinicians realized that digoxin use was associated with a higher risk for proarrhythmias if cardioversion was required (Greco et al., 1982). Finally, the danger of digoxin-induced ventricular fibrillation came to light, particularly when ventricular tachycardia was the prevailing arrhythmia. This led researchers to explore further agents for acute management of SVT and paved the way for adenosine to become the preferred drug for the acute treatment of SVT. Adenosine proved to be safe and effective in terminating SVT with minimal to no side effects.

Adenosine was initially reported in the literature in the early 1900s, when scientists were using mammalian models to explore the efficacy of adenosine in slowing the sinus rate secondary to AV block (Drury & Szent-Gyorgyi, 1929). Several publications followed that explored the electrophysiologic effects of adenosine in restoring the normal cardiac rhythm in the human adult heart (Honey et al., 1930; Jezerm et al., 1933). However, many adults presented with recurrent SVT after adenosine therapy. This confused scientists and led many to believe that adenosine was a "failed therapy."

Adenosine was ignored for approximately 20 years, until Somló (1955) published the results of successful treatment of 214 episodes of SVT with adenosine triphosphate (ATP; a precursor of adenosine). By the 1980s, adenosine use increased while numerous preclinical and clinical studies were underway. For example, some research teams investigated adenosine use in the management of paroxysmal tachycardia in adults, followed by children and infants (DiMarco et al., 1983; Overholt et al., 1988; Till, Shinebourne, Rigby, et al., 1989). The advantage of the short half-life, with transient adverse effects even with repeated and increased dosages that do not result in toxic effect, made adenosine the preferred agent for acute management of SVT in people of all ages. The U.S. Food and Drug Administration (FDA) formally approved adenosine for use with SVT in 1991 (Greco et al., 1982; Till & Shinebourne, 1991; Till, Shinebourne, Rigby, et al., 1989).

ANTIARRHYTHMIC DRUG CLASSIFICATION SYSTEM

The Vaughan-Williams classification of antiarrhythmic medications breaks medications into four broad classes based on the drug's mechanism of action on ion movement, and a fifth group that includes digoxin and adenosine (Tables 19.2 and 19.3). Class I agents block sodium influx, slowing conduction in the atria, ventricles, and His-Purkinje system. Class II beta-blocking agents block calcium influx, slowing AV conduction. Class III agents block potassium efflux, delaying repolarization, which results in prolongation of both the duration of the action potential and the refractory period (Figure 19.8). Class IV agents are not used in infants younger than 1 year of age due to the high risk of electromechanical dissociation, so they are not discussed here. Digoxin and adenosine both decrease conduction through the AV node and reduce automaticity in the SA node (Burchum & Rosenthal, 2016). Keep in mind that some of the medications may have more than one effect, and some medications, such as adenosine and digoxin, do not act by mechanisms corresponding with the original four Vaughan-Williams classes, so they are in a group by themselves. It is important to note that the action of the medication does not predict efficacy. Please refer to Table 19.4, which summarizes outcomes of studies that evaluated safety and efficacy of the various antiarrhythmic agents discussed in this chapter.

CURRENT PHARMACOLOGIC MODALITIES FOR SUPRAVENTRICULAR TACHYCARDIA: ACUTE MANAGEMENT

Acute termination of SVT is targeted at blocking or slowing conduction at the AV node in order to terminate the tachycardia and restore normal sinus rhythm. This can be done as previously discussed with vagal maneuvers (ice to the face, gagging the infant), pharmacologic measures, and, if these fail or the infant is hemodynamically unstable, synchronized direct-current (DC) cardioversion starting at 0.5 joules/kg (Park & Salamet, 2021). Cardioversion causes depolarization and, due to the highest degree of automaticity, allows the sinus node to resume its role as the pacemaker (White & Humphries, 1967). Remember to provide sedation if cardioversion is required as it is painful. The other factor to keep in mind is that cardioversion can potentially cause myocardial damage, especially in the preterm infant. If pharmacologic management is required, cardiology consultation is imperative to assist in determining the best acute and chronic pharmacologic agents, as well as appropriate long-term follow-up. The most common pharmacologic management for emergent treatment of SVT is adenosine. If vagal maneuvers or administration of adenosine do not terminate the tachycardia, it may more likely be atrial in nature and other antiarrhythmic agents should be considered (Paret et al., 1996).

Adenosine

Adenosine is the first pharmacologic agent that is used in the acute management of the infant with SVT; an 85% to 100% success rate in restoring normal sinus rhythm is reported (Overholt et al., 1988; Paret et al., 1996; Sherwood et al., 1998; Till, Shinebourne, Rigby, et al., 1989). Administration of adenosine can be diagnostic if an underlying rhythm is not apparent, such as atrial fibrillation/flutter, as well as therapeutic. Adenosine is most effective in restoring normal sinus rhythm with AVRT using an accessory pathway as well as AV nodal reentrant tachycardia (DiMarco et al., 1983).

MECHANISM OF ACTION/PHARMACOKINETIC PRINCIPLES

Adenosine, found in every cell of the human body, is formed by the breakdown of the enzymes ATP or S-adenosyl-L-homocysteine. Endogenous adenosine appears to play a role in maintaining the balance between oxygen demand and delivery in the heart due to its actions of dilating coronary arteries, slowing the heart rate, and, in a hypoxemic state, decreasing the oxygen demand (Camm & Garratt, 1991). Exogenously administered adenosine acts via secondary messengers that block AV nodal conduction via A_1 receptors in the cardiac tissue (Figure 19.9). Adenosine binds to

TABLE 19.2 Vaughan-Williams Classification of Antiarrhythmic Medications (Classes I–IV)

CLASS	EXAMPLES OF PHARMACOLOGIC AGENTS	MECHANISM OF ACTION	CONTRAINDICATIONS/ CAUTIONS	MONITOR
Class IA	Procainamide	Sodium channel blocker Decreases (slows) conduction velocity and automaticity, increases refractory period (delays repolarization)	Widens QRS, prolongs QT. Contraindicated in infant with prolonged QTc interval or on medications that prolong QTc interval.	Hypotension during IV infusion; causes mild depression of myocardial function; moderate risk for proarrhythmia
Class IB	Lidocaine	Sodium channel blocker Decreases conduction velocity and automaticity. Decreases the refractory period (accelerates repolarization)	Toxicity associated with drowsiness, muscle twitching, and seizures—hold dose until level is checked.	Myocardial function depression with high serum levels; proarrhythmia is uncommon
Class IC	Flecainide	Sodium channel blocker leading to decreased conduction velocity and automaticity; has no effect on refractory period	Use with caution in infants with structural heart disease due to negative ionotropic effects. Widens QRS and prolongs PR interval.	High incidence of proarrhythmia
Class II	Atenolol Esmolol Metoprolol Nadolol Propranolol	Beta-adrenergic receptor blocker Calcium channel blocker Decreases conduction velocity in the AV node and reduces automaticity in the SA node, and increases the refractory period; decreases contractility in the atria and ventricles	Prolongs PR interval. Use with caution in infants with hypotension or who have decreased ventricular function. Use with caution if infant has reactive airway disease.	Risk for bronchial constriction varies among agents; can have central nervous system effects; monitor for hypotension, bradycardia, and hypoglycemia with propranolol
Class III	Amiodarone Sotalol (at high doses)	Potassium channel blocker; sotalol is a beta-blocker Increases refractory period; has no effect on conduction velocity or automaticity	Amiodarone prolongs QT and PR, widens QRS intervals; sotalol prolongs QT and PR. Use with caution in infants with prolonged QTc interval; avoid concurrent administration of medications that prolong QTc interval. Need to decrease dose of digoxin, phenytoin, or warfarin if taken concurrently with amiodarone.	Proarrhythmia less frequent with amiodarone; 10% risk with sotalol within a few days of treatment initiation; risk for hypotension with IV amiodarone dose; need baseline and monitoring every 6 months of liver, renal, and thyroid function as well as ophthalmologic exams and pulmonary function tests due to risk of multisystem problems (interstitial lung disease, abnormal thyroid function, and corneal pigmentation) with long-term amiodarone therapy.

(*continued*)

TABLE 19.2 Vaughan-Williams Classification of Antiarrhythmic Medications (Classes I–IV) (*continued*)

CLASS	EXAMPLES OF PHARMACOLOGIC AGENTS	MECHANISM OF ACTION	CONTRAINDICATIONS/ CAUTIONS	MONITOR
Class IV	Verapamil	Slows calcium influx across cell membrane Decreases conduction velocity and automaticity and increases refractory period	Prolongs PR. Contraindicated in infants younger than 1 year of age due to risk of electromechanical dissociation and cardiovascular collapse. Contraindicated in infant with WPW, increases conduction down the accessory pathway.	

AV, atrioventricular; IV, intravenous; SA, sinoatrial; WPW, Wolff-Parkinson-White syndrome.

TABLE 19.3 Vaughan-Williams Classification of Other Antiarrhythmic Medications

AGENT	MECHANISM OF ACTION	CONTRAINDICATIONS/CAUTIONS	MONITOR
Digoxin	Increases myocardial catecholamine levels at low doses; inhibits sodium-potassium ATPase activity at high doses. Increases vagal tone, prolonging SA node refractoriness and slows the AV nodal conductance.	Prolongs PR and depresses ST. Do not use in infant with WPW.	Avoid hypokalemia and hypercalcemia as they increase risk for cardiac toxicity effect. Monitor EKG for sinus bradycardia, AV block, or ventricular ectopy, which suggest cardiac toxicity.
Adenosine	Endogenous purine nucleoside that slows or blocks AV node conduction	Prolongs PR. Do not continue to use if the tachycardia is not interrupted after two or three doses or if there is rapid return of tachycardia.	Obtain EKG during administration of adenosine to help determine etiology of tachycardia. May have brief bradycardia before return to normal sinus rhythm or back into tachycardia rhythm.

AV, atrioventricular; SA, sinoatrial; WPW, Wolff-Parkinson-White syndrome.

FIGURE 19.8 Effect of antiarrhythmic agents on the cardiac action potential.

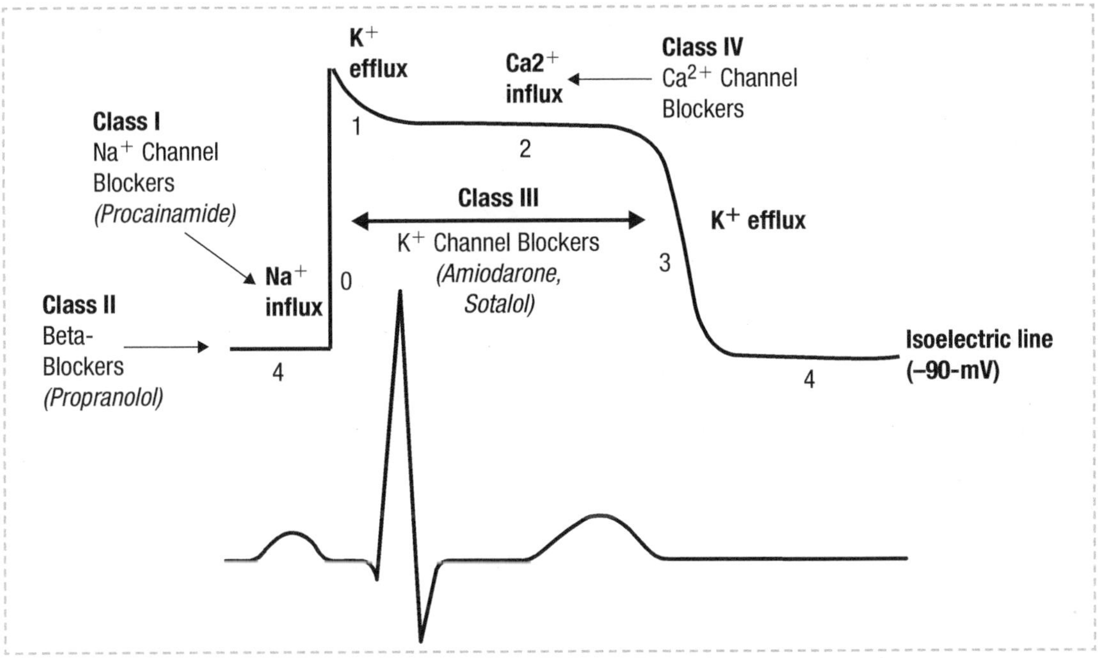

Note: Class I antiarrhythmics (e.g., procainamide, flecainide) decrease sodium influx into the cell to slow the onset of an action potential. Class II antiarrhythmics (e.g., propranolol) inhibit spontaneous depolarization. Class III (e.g., amiodarone, sotalol) and class IV (not routinely prescribed in infants younger than 1 year of life) antiarrhythmics slow the rate of calcium influx into the cell.
Source: Design credit: Mya Jnah. Created using Biorender.com.

A_1 receptors, leading to stimulation of potassium channels, which results in hyperpolarization of cardiac myocytes and slows conduction through the AV node (remember the AV node forms part of the reentrant circuit in AVRT). Cyclic adenosine monophosphate (cAMP) is decreased due to actions on G_i-proteins, resulting in blocking of calcium channels and calcium entry into the cells. Inhibition of the calcium channels leads to decreased conduction velocity (negative dromotropic effect). The duration of the action potential shortens, resulting in the negative chronotropic effect (lower spontaneous firing rate). There is decreased diastolic depolarization of the SA node (phase 4), resulting in inhibition of the pacemaker current of the SA node. The combination of these mechanisms results in blocking conduction at the AV node, which restores the heart rhythm to normal sinus rhythm (DiMarco et al., 1983; FDA, 2005; McDowell et al., 2020; Shryock & Belardinelli, 1997).

The first reports in the neonatal/infant population described the rapid onset of action within 20 seconds (Komor & Garas, 1955; Somló, 1955); subsequent studies found that administration into a central vein rather than peripheral site resulted in much shorter onset of action (within 10 seconds of administration; Till, Shinebourne, Rigby, et al., 1989). Adenosine has an extremely short half-life primarily due to rapid uptake by cells as well as deactivation by the circulating enzyme, adenosine deaminase. Half-life is estimated to be between 5 to 10 seconds (Overholt et al., 1988; Somló, 1955; Till, Shinebourne, Rigby, et al., 1989). Due to this short half-life, adenosine will not prevent recurrence of SVT, which is why it is not considered for prophylaxis. Hepatic first-pass metabolism is observed. Adenosine is removed from systemic circulation by cellular uptake of vascular endothelial cells and erythrocytes. It is rapidly metabolized intracellularly by adenosine deaminase to inosine, which is further metabolized to hypoxanthine to uric acid (Möser et al., 1989).

DOSING RECOMMENDATIONS

Adenosine can be administered via IV; if there is no IV access in the hemodynamically unstable infant, the intraosseous (IO) route can be considered. Early studies reported using a starting IV dose ranging from 37 to 50 mcg/kg. Till, Shinebourne, Rigby, and colleagues (1989) reported the range used for effectively restoring normal sinus rhythm in neonates to children was 50 to 250 mcg/kg with a median effective dose of 150 mcg/kg. Dixon and colleagues (2005) in a retrospective chart

TABLE 19.4 Antiarrhythmic Agent Studies

AUTHORS	PURPOSE OF STUDY	STUDY POPULATION	TYPE OF STUDY	RESULTS	NOTEWORTHY CONCLUSIONS
Barton et al. (2015)	To evaluate experience of high-dose (4 mg/kg/day) propranolol in the treatment and prophylaxis of supraventricular arrhythmias.	*N* = 287 Infants <1 year of age who were started on enteral propranolol monotherapy for either reentry SVT or atrial tachycardia over a 10-year period (6/2002–6/2012) from one center Exclusion: Infants with any other documented arrhythmias	Descriptive, retrospective study Limitation: Retrospective nature	Propranolol monotherapy was successful in 67% (*n* = 193) of infants overall. One infant had bradycardia requiring discontinuation of propranolol. Patients who failed therapy as inpatient required either combination therapy or were switched to monotherapy with sotalol, digoxin, amiodarone, or flecainide.	Failed therapy was more common in infants with structural heart defect (31%) or with WPW (20%). Median recurrence as outpatient occurred at 26 days after discharge; only five had occurrence >90 days after discharge.
Capponi et al. (2021)	To describe the experience of a single center with maintenance drug treatment of both re-entry and automatic SVTs in the first year of life.	*N* = 55 *N* = 45/55 reentry SVT[a] *N* = 10/55 automatic tachycardia[b] SVT at onset between the fetal period and the end of the first year of life; placed initially on maintenance therapy with class 1C drugs and beta-blockers, used alone or in combination with additional agents added for unresponsiveness from March 1995 to April 2019	Retrospective, observational Limitations: Small study size and retrospective nature	Flecainide was effective as monotherapy in 51% of infants with reentry tachycardia; better results occurred when given in combination with beta-blockers or digoxin; flecainide was ineffective in only 4.4% of infants. In infants with automatic tachycardias, 30% responded to beta-blocker alone; when combined with flecainide, treatment was 90% effective. Flecainide was associated with significant adverse events in 3.8%, related to accidental overdosages. Beta-blocker therapy was fully tolerated.	The combination of flecainide and beta-blockers was highly effective and well-tolerated as maintenance therapy in infants with reentry of automatic SVTs. However, RCTs are needed to clearly define optimal pharmacotherapy.

Chang et al. (2010)	To compare treatment efficacy and adverse effects of amiodarone versus procainamide therapy in pediatric patients with recurrent SVT.	*N* = 40 episodes of SVT in 37 patients All pediatric patients receiving IV amiodarone or procainamide for treatment of SVT (orthodromic reciprocating tachycardia, intra-arterial reentrant tachycardia, and ectopic atrial tachycardia) from a single center over 25 consecutive months (7/1/2004–8/1/2006) Exclusions: Patients without EKG documentation of SVT, those with documented ventricular arrhythmias, and patients with junctional ectopic tachycardia	Retrospective cohort study Limitation: Small study size and retrospective nature	37 patients with median age of 34 days, 24 had CHD; amiodarone was initial therapy in 26 cases and procainamide in 14 cases; procainamide achieved greater full success in management of recurrent SVT (50%) compared to amiodarone (15%); if full and partial success are combined, procainamide is more successful (71%) compared with amiodarone (34%); 10 patients received the second medication when the first failed; there was no significant difference in adverse events frequency between the two agents; amiodarone adverse events were mainly hypotension and bradycardia; procainamide adverse events were mainly ventricular proarrhythmia and hypotension	Failed therapy was defined as documented recurrence on monotherapy or if therapy needed to be altered to maintain arrhythmia control. This study did not exclude infants with structural heart defects. Monotherapy may be less beneficial to infants with structural heart defects or WPW. Further studies are needed on ideal dose of propranolol, including the efficacy and safety of doses >4 mg/kg/day, as well as the duration of therapy.
Chu et al. (2015)	To understand current practices in SVT management, safety of commonly used medications, and outcomes of hospitalized infants treated for SVT	*N* = 2,848 total *N* = 367 with CHD (16%), and 2,481 without CHD Infants with a diagnosis of SVT who received SVT therapy during the first 120 days of life who were discharged from 348 NICUs managed by Pediatrix Medical Group from 1998–2012	Retrospective, cohort study Limitations: Retrospective nature; limited to hospitalized patients only, did not evaluate SVT recurrence, change in medication regimens, or adverse events in the outpatient population	66% diagnosed with SVT in the first week of life Adenosine was the abortive therapy of choice; overall variation in prescribing choices over this 14-year period; however, amiodarone was the most common therapy used on day 1 of the diagnosis of SVT; for secondary prevention therapies, beta-blockers appeared the last 2 years of the study to replace digoxin; digoxin and beta-blockers were the most common (~65%) multidrug combination; adverse events were seen in 30% of infants on secondary prevention therapy (most common was hypotension in four out of five agents in the study)	Further prospective study needed to compare these agents to develop more specific, effective, and safer guidelines in treatment of pediatric patients with recurrent SVT.

(*continued*)

TABLE 19.4 Antiarrhythmic Agent Studies (*continued*)

AUTHORS	PURPOSE OF STUDY	STUDY POPULATION	TYPE OF STUDY	RESULTS	NOTEWORTHY CONCLUSIONS
Cunningham et al. (2017)	To evaluate the safety and effectiveness of flecainide for treatment of supraventricular or ventricular tachycardia in pediatric patients with no CHD and with CHD or cardiomyopathy	*N* = 175 patients from two pediatric cardiology sites in Canada and the United Kingdom from 1/2000 to 7/2015	Retrospective, cohort study Limitation: Retrospective nature	Treatment duration did not differ between pediatric patients with normal hearts (55 weeks) versus patients with CHD (52 weeks). Flecainide was used as monotherapy in 119 patients; remainder received flecainide in combination with another antiarrhythmic agent. Patients with CHD were not at greater risk for adverse effects compared to patients with normal hearts; fewer than 3% required discontinuation of therapy due to adverse effects, including cardiac dysfunction and proarrhythmia	Flecainide is a safe and effective antiarrhythmic medication in pediatric patients with and without structural cardiac disease. There was no difference in cardiac dysfunction between the two groups that required discontinuation of flecainide therapy; patients with CHD did have QRS widening and prolongation of QTc but this did not result in increased proarrhythmic events. Limitation was small cohort size and only two patients with cardiomyopathy; larger study should be done to validate safety and effectiveness in pediatric patients with CHD and cardiomyopathy.
Dilber et al. (2010)	To report the efficacy and safety[c] of intravenous amiodarone alone or combination with digoxin in neonates and small infants with refractory and life-threatening SVT	*N* = 9, eight with AV reentry[d] and one with atrial flutter All neonates and small infants treated with IV amiodarone alone or in combination with digoxin for life-threatening or resistant tachyarrhythmias between January 2005 and December 2007 Exclusion: Tachyarrhythmia responded to adenosine and controlled with initial digoxin therapy	Retrospective cohort study Limitations: Small study size and retrospective nature	Four patients had recurrence of persistent SVT after adenosine and digoxin therapy requiring addition of amiodarone within 2–4 hours as a third-line therapy; four patients had only temporary conversion of SVT after adenosine and were started initially on amiodarone, two required the addition of digoxin to control the SVT; one patient had atrial flutter with amiodarone initiated and needed to add digoxin for persistence of arrhythmia; amiodarone alone or in combination with digoxin showed complete success in all eight patients with reentrant SVT; only one patient experienced hypotension necessitating inotropic support; two infants had transient rise in TSH that normalized during continuation of treatment	Intravenous amiodarone with or without digoxin is safe and effective in controlling refractory SVT in neonates and infants.

Guerrier et al. (2016)	To describe practice patterns of the management of infants hospitalized with SVT and factors associated with 30-day hospital readmission	*N* = 851 patients; monotherapy: *n* = 234 propranolol, *n* = 128 digoxin, *n* = 85 amiodarone Combination therapy: *n* = 18 propranolol + digoxin, *n* =10 flecainide + digoxin; infants <365 days hospitalized at 43 tertiary care pediatric hospitals from October 2003 to September 2013 with an *ICD-9* code for paroxysmal SVT Exclusions: Infants with atrial or ventricular fibrillation, atrial flutter, primary cardiomyopathy, or nonminor CHD	Retrospective cohort study Limitations: Retrospective nature, risk for inaccurate *ICD-9* coding, underreporting of SVT recurrence on subsequent hospital readmission	Of study population, 86% received monotherapy; propranolol was the most frequently prescribed single-agent antiarrhythmic in high-volume centers; most common multiagent combination was propranolol with digoxin; 5% required hospital readmission for SVT within 30 days of hospital discharge with no significant difference based on antiarrhythmic agent prescribed	Center volume did appear to be a determinant in antiarrhythmic agent choice; this was not associated with difference in patient outcomes. Further quality-improvement projects examining outcome difference and healthcare utilization need to be done. Hospital readmission may be related to intrinsic patient characteristics.
Hornik et al. (2014)	To compare efficacy and safety of digoxin and propranolol for infant SVT prophylaxis	*N* = 457; 342 digoxin, 142 propranolol Infants discharged from 330 NICUs managed by Pediatrix Medical Group from 1998–2012 with SVT treated with digoxin or propranolol in the first 120 days of life Exclusion: Infants discharged prior to completing 2 days of therapy, infants with WPW, atrial flutter, or structural heart defects, or infants on multidrug therapy	Retrospective cohort study Limitations: Retrospective nature	Higher treatment failure (SVT recurrence after 2 days of therapy) in infants on propranolol therapy compared to digoxin (15.4 vs. 6.7/1000 infant-days); hypotension requiring inotropic support more frequent in infants on digoxin therapy compared to propranolol (39.4 vs. 11.1/1000 infant-days)	Use of digoxin declined over time in this study from 100% of infants in 1998 to 48% of infants in 2012 based on provider preference. Study did not provide dosage and intervals administered. Limited to inpatient data. Underestimation of recurrence may have occurred as only need for adenosine or electrical cardioversion were used. Did not have EKG data for type of SVT.

(*continued*)

TABLE 19.4 Antiarrhythmic Agent Studies (*continued*)

AUTHORS	PURPOSE OF STUDY	STUDY POPULATION	TYPE OF STUDY	RESULTS	NOTEWORTHY CONCLUSIONS
Knudson et al. (2011)	To evaluate the safety and ability to control arrhythmia with high-dose sotalol (150 mg/m^2/day) in recurrent neonatal tachycardias that were refractory to first-line pharmacologic therapy	*N* = 78 Infants <2 years of age with SVT who were treated with sotalol after failure of at least one other antiarrhythmic agent from 2001 to 2008 at one children's hospital Median age of SVT diagnosis was 24 days of life; 62% of patients were neonates and 46% of patients had CHD	Retrospective chart review Limitation: Retrospective nature	Seventy inpatients were successfully controlled on sotalol[e]; 53 successfully controlled on sotalol monotherapy, 11 were controlled with sotalol in combination with beta-blocker, four with sotalol in combination with digoxin, and two with sotalol in combination with flecainide; eight patients failed sotalol and required flecainide or amiodarone therapy; no patients experienced proarrhythmia, clinically significant QTc prolongation, worsening cardiac function, or other adverse effects during hospitalization	Further studies are needed to test the hypothesis of higher beginning doses, which allow for more rapid control of tachycardia and decreased length of hospitalization. Future studies should also examine sex-related responses to therapy. Further studies are needed to validate that neonates and infants are less susceptible to the proarrhythmic effects of sotalol.
Kohli (2013)	To evaluate their experience with oral flecainide in acute and medium-term control of SVT in infants not controlled with other first-line antiarrhythmics	*N* = 8 Infants ≤12 months with tachyarrhythmias who did not respond to first-line medications from January 2006 to December 2010 Exclusion: Infants with postsurgical arrhythmias	Prospective study without Randomization and control Limitation: Small study size	All eight infants had termination of their tachyarrhythmia with oral flecainide; 75% of infants had normal sinus rhythm within 24 hours (n = 6), the remaining 25% in less than 3 days; three infants had recurrence of SVT events (1–6 months of age) with resolution occurring with increased dose; 88% of the infants required combination therapy; 88% with propranolol (n = 7) and 33% requiring the addition of digoxin as well (n = 2)	Flecainide is safe. Was found to be useful alone or in combination therapy as second-line management in refractory tachycardia. Limitations: Case series, small number, concern of bias (all infants were hemodynamically stable), and unavailability to monitor drug levels.

Moffett et al. (2015)	To evaluate the efficacy of digoxin and propranolol as first-line enteral therapy for treatment of infants with SVT	*N* = 374; of this number, 199 had CHD Infants <1 year of age hospitalized with a diagnosis of SVT started on either propranolol or digoxin monotherapy from 43 hospitals affiliated with the Child Health Corporation of America from January 2001 to December 2010 Exclusions: Infants receiving any other enteral antiarrhythmic medication in combination with initiation of digoxin or propranolol, who received other IV antiarrhythmic agent (other than adenosine), had a diagnosis of WPW, or death before discharge	Retrospective, cohort study Limitation: Retrospective nature	Digoxin was initial monotherapy in 47.3% of patients, propranolol monotherapy was initial treatment in the remaining 52.7% of patients; median age for initiation was 37 days of life; 45.2% of patients were ≤ 30 days of age; efficacy of treatment was 73.1% for digoxin-treated patients, and 73.5% for propranolol-treated patients	Success was considered as discharge on the initiated enteral monotherapy of digoxin or propranolol without recurrence of SVT; they found both agents may be equally efficacious as monotherapy for infants hospitalized with SVT. Combination of digoxin and propranolol was used in 28% of patients who failed monotherapy. Patients discharged on propranolol monotherapy were more likely to require readmission for SVT; dosing at the higher end of recommended dosing on propranolol may decrease this risk. Limitations included use of *ICD-9* code 427.0, which may include reentrant as well as ectopic focus tachyarrhythmias; inability to assess adverse events associated with either medication; inability to consider variations in practice (broad dosing range, strategies to weight-adjust medications); and effect of other patient comorbidities.

(*continued*)

TABLE 19.4 Antiarrhythmic Agent Studies (*continued*)

AUTHORS	PURPOSE OF STUDY	STUDY POPULATION	TYPE OF STUDY	RESULTS	NOTEWORTHY CONCLUSIONS
Nicastro et al. (2020)	To assess the results and incidence of adverse events of oral propranolol therapy	*N* = 107 Infants <1 year of age with SVT in outpatient clinic from August 2001 to January 2018 receiving oral propranolol 3 mg/kg/day QID for first 3 months followed by 2–5 mg/kg/day TID for 1 year Exclusion: Infants with ectopic atrial tachycardia, atrial flutter without any other associated tachycardia, and infants lost to follow-up	Observational and descriptive Limitations: Adverse event underestimation, masking by other conditions	Median first SVT event was at 190 days; 10 patients had CHD; baseline EKG showed ventricular preexcitation in 25 patients (23.3%); on-treatment recurrent SVT occurred in 33 (30.8%) patients during follow-up period; two patients had severe adverse events requiring discontinuation of propranolol	Therapeutic success in preventing recurrence of SVT may be related to dose used; future randomized studies are needed to determine this dose. Most recurrence events occur in the first month; if initial treatment response is adequate, possibility of later events not as likely.
Price et al. (2002)	To assess the efficacy and safety of flecainide and sotalol combination therapy for the treatment of refractory SVT in children <1 year of age	*N* = 10 Infants <12 months of age treated with combination therapy for a minimum of 72 hours of flecainide and sotalol for SVT after failing at least two antiarrhythmic agents Efficacy, defined as suppression of SVT to no more than rare unsustained events or slowing of SVT to a clinically tolerable rate, occurred in all patients treated with the combination of flecainide and sotalol. This combination may obviate the need for radiofrequency ablation in infants with refractory SVT.	Retrospective review Limitations: Small study size and retrospective nature	Failure rate was reduced from 100% to 0% on combination therapy of flecainide and sotalol; no proarrhythmias occurred	Combination therapy with flecainide and sotalol can safely and effectively control refractory SVT in infants, avoiding the need for radiofrequency ablation.

Sanatani et al. (2012)	To compare digoxin to propranolol prophylactic management with regard to recurrence of SVT requiring medical interventions	N = 61; 27 digoxin, 34 propranolol; infants with SVT (AVRT or AV nodal reentrant tachycardia) presenting from birth to 4 months of age at 14 enrolled centers, from 12/1/2006 through 8/31/2010 Exclusion: Infants with shortening fraction <28% or structural heart disease, infants with WPW, infants with significant comorbidities that could affect medication compliance or tolerance, infants with atrial ectopic tachycardia or junctional reciprocating tachycardia were all excluded	Randomized, double-blind, multicenter study Limitation: Small study size	There was no statistical difference in SVT recurrence after 5 days of therapy in infants on either digoxin or propranolol therapy; both therapies were associated with high initial success rates and no recurrence after 4 months of therapy	Study ended due to inadequate enrollment (target sample size was 220 patients) over almost 4 years. Current practice of treating for 1 year may be too long; further placebo-controlled trials should be done.
Tortoriello et al. (2003)	To determine whether the type of antiarrhythmic therapy required to control SVT, the presence of excitation, or a combination of these factors predict recurrence risk of SVT beyond 1 year	N = 150; n = 116 in group 1[f] (17% with WPW) and n = 34 in group 2 (62% with WPW) Infants who presented with SVT in the first year of life at a single center from January 1984 to December 2000 Exclusions: Infants with permanent form of junctional reciprocating tachycardia, atrial flutter, atrial fibrillation, junctional tachycardia, or atrial ectopic tachycardia	Retrospective Limitation: Retrospective nature, groups were unevenly distributed	Recurrence of SVT occurred in 28% of Group 1; 68% of Group 2; infants with WPW had a 29-fold higher risk of SVT recurrence at >1 year of age compared to infants without preexcitation; infants with WPW who required additional antiarrhythmic agents in addition to digoxin and/or propranolol were at an increased risk for recurrence of SVT	Recurrence of SVT beyond 1 year of age is more likely in patients who require second-line pharmacotherapy and/or those with WPW.

(*continued*)

TABLE 19.4 Antiarrhythmic Agent Studies (*continued*)

AUTHORS	PURPOSE OF STUDY	STUDY POPULATION	TYPE OF STUDY	RESULTS	NOTEWORTHY CONCLUSIONS
Wong et al. (2006)	To assess current cardiologist practice of treating SVT through sending questionnaires	N = 295 (19% return rate); pediatric cardiologists in North America (Canada and the United States)	Survey provided a clinical scenario of a hemodynamically stable infant with SVT refractory to adenosine. Written responses to acute and chronic medical management were elicited. The scenario was modified to include the infant with and without preexcitation. Limitation: Survey response	Surveys were representative of seven provinces in Canada and 40 U.S. states; respondents reported 11 different medications for acute management in the infant without preexcitation; digoxin (42%) and procainamide (21%) were the most common agents used; in the infant with preexcitation, propranolol (34%) and procainamide (23%) were the most common drugs chosen; for chronic management of the infant without preexcitation, respondents reported use of eight different medications with digoxin remaining the most common (52%) followed by propranolol (33%); with known preexcitation, propranolol was the most common chronic antiarrhythmic used (70%)	This survey showed that differences in medication choice were related to presence or absence of preexcitation and whether the respondent had additional electrophysiology training. Limitations include assuming the respondents understood the questions as intended and low response rate. Future randomized, placebo-controlled clinical trials are needed to compare the efficacy of the most commonly prescribed antiarrhythmic agents.

[a]Flecainide was first-line maintenance therapy for reentry SVT; if recurrence of SVT, flecainide was combined with beta-blockers or digoxin.
[b]First-line maintenance therapy for automatic tachycardia was a beta-blocker and if recurrence, combined with flecainide or amiodarone.
[c]Serial outpatient follow-up at 2-week and 3-month intervals for infants receiving digoxin included physical exam, 12-lead EKG, 24-hour Holter monitoring, and serum digoxin level; CXR, liver, and thyroid function tests were done at 3- to 6-month intervals for infants receiving amiodarone.
[d]Seven of the eight patients on admission had congestive heart failure, three had severe cardiovascular collapse, and one died because of significant hemodynamic consequences of the tachyarrhythmias.
[e]Success of inpatient therapy was no tachycardia on telemetry for 48 hours after initiation of sotalol in addition to no signs of tachycardia during remainder of hospitalization. Success during follow-up as outpatient was complete suppression of reentrant SVT or no more than rare, unsustained episodes of focal atrial tachycardia on Holter monitoring; no clinical report of signs or symptoms of tachycardia in outpatient clinic; no ED or hospital admissions for tachycardia. Follow-up was within 1 month for neonates and then every 2 months until 1 year of age with EKG and Holter-monitor testing.
[f]Patients were divided into two groups: Group 1, treatment with digoxin and/or propranolol alone; Group 2, additional agents required (flecainide, sotalol, or amiodarone).
AV, atrioventricular; AVRT, atrioventricular reciprocating tachycardia; CHD, congenital heart defect; CXR, chest x-ray; *ICD-9, International Classification of Diseases*, ninth ed; IV, intravenous; QID, four times a day; SVT, supraventricular tachycardia; TID, three times a day; TSH, thyroid-stimulating hormone; WPW, Wolff-Parkinson-White syndrome.

FIGURE 19.9 Adenosine mechanism of action.

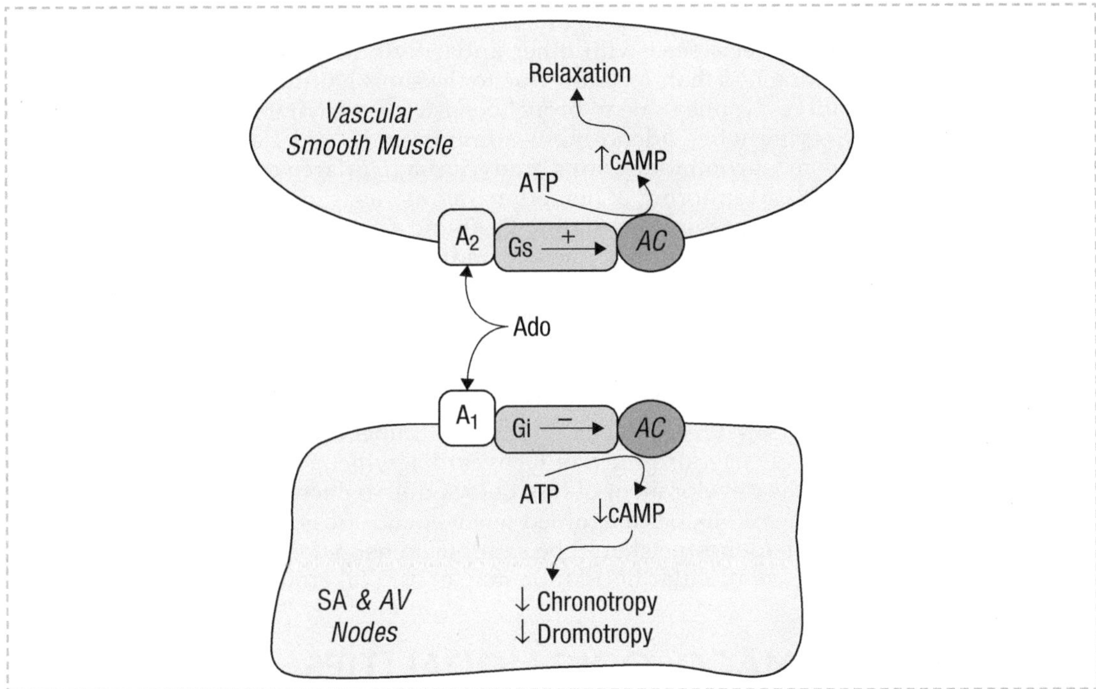

AC, adenylyl cyclase; ATP, adenosine triphosphate; AV, atrioventricular; cAMP, cyclic adenosine monophosphate; Gi, inhibitory G protein receptor; Gs, stimulatory G protein receptor; SA, sinoatrial.

Source: From Klabunde. R. E. (n.d.). *Adenosine*. Image for Cardiovascular Pharmacology Concepts. Retrieved August 18, 2022, from https://www.cvpharmacology.com/antiarrhy/adenosine

review of 23 infants found that a dose of 50 mcg/kg resulted in return to normal sinus rhythm only 9% of the time, a dose of 150 mcg was effective 35% of the time, and a dose of 300 mcg/kg was effective over 90% of the time. The median effective dose in this study was reported to be 200 mcg/kg. Despite these findings, initial recommended starting dosage ranges from 50 to 100 mcg/kg/dose (0.05 to 0.1 mg/kg) over 1 to 2 seconds rapid IV bolus. In cases of refractory SVT, the dosage may be incrementally increased by 50 to 100 mcg/kg/dose every 1 to 2 minutes until termination of SVT occurs or to a maximum of 300 mcg/kg/dose (Berg et al., 2010; Burchum & Rosenthal, 2016; IBM Micromedex Neofax, 2021a; Long, 1998; IBM Micromedex Neofax, 2021a; Taketomo, 2023; Till, Shinebourne, Rigby, et al., 1989). It is imperative to follow with a rapid normal saline (NS) flush to obtain the desired effect of AV blocking before the agent is metabolized by endothelial cells and erythrocytes. For doses less than 600 mcg, it is necessary to dilute the commercially available vial to ensure complete and accurate administration by adding 1 mL (3 mg) adenosine to 2 mL NS for a 1,000 mcg/mL concentration.

For neonates/infants in whom IV access is not available, the IO route has been proposed. Getschman and colleagues (1994) evaluated administration of adenosine via peripheral, central, and IO routes in 30 newly weaned piglets. They found that a higher minimum effective dose was required when adenosine was administered peripherally (158 mcg/kg) in comparison to a dose of 87 mcg/kg when the dose was administered centrally; the minimum effective dose for IO administration was 127 mcg/kg. Small case studies in neonates/infants offered conflicting support of the IO route with three case reports showing the IO route to be effective (Fidanci et al., 2020; Friedman, 1996; Helleman et al., 2017), whereas Goodman and Lu (2012) reported a lack of conversion to normal sinus rhythm despite maximum doses using the IO route in two infants.

Methylxanthines (caffeine, theophylline, aminophylline) block adenosine receptor sites; therefore, larger doses of adenosine are required for infants receiving methylxanthines (Burchum & Rosenthal, 2016; IBM Micromedex Neofax, 2021a; Long, 1998).

CLINICAL-MONITORING PEARLS

The advantages of adenosine as primary treatment are its short half-life and the minimal or absent negative inotropic effects seen with other antiarrhythmic agents. Adverse effects are typically short-lived, lasting less than 1 minute due to the short half-life and may include facial flushing from vasodilation, dyspnea due to bronchoconstriction, irritability, chest pain (which may be evidenced by crying when adenosine is administered), and transient arrhythmias at the time of conversion—most commonly sinus bradycardia (DiMarco et al., 1983; Jezerm et al., 1933; Overholt et al., 1988). Monitoring of hemodynamic status is imperative, including blood pressure, capillary refill, and respiratory status. Profound vasodilation has been reported in some studies after the administration of adenosine, indicating close monitoring of blood pressure for potential hypotension is essential. Other studies have shown the opposite findings with the blood pressure increasing slightly in some cases after administration of adenosine and the return to normal sinus rhythm most likely related to improvement in cardiac output (DiMarco et al., 1983; Greco et al., 1982). Cardiorespiratory and pulse oximeter monitoring are also necessary due to the risk of rare, but possible life-threatening, adverse events such as arrhythmias and apnea (Crosson et al., 1994; Overholt et al., 1988; Till, Shinebourne, Rigby, et al., 1989). The infant must be monitored closely for return of tachycardia, which can be observed up to one-third of the time, and for the development of heart block due to decreased conduction through the AV node. The risk for heart block is magnified when adenosine is given in conjunction with digoxin. Administration of adenosine should be cautious in neonates with WPW syndrome or atrial fibrillation/flutter as ventricular fibrillation may occur (Taketomo, 2023).

CURRENT PHARMACOLOGIC MODALITIES FOR SUPRAVENTRICULAR TACHYCARDIA: LONG-TERM THERAPY

Serial EKGs used to evaluate for appropriate response to pharmacologic management are very important during the initial stages of therapy. Some antiarrhythmic agents may actually produce an arrhythmia that is different from the initially treated arrhythmia or exacerbate the existing arrhythmia; this is referred to as a *proarrhythmia*. Proarrhythmias are more likely to be seen in the early course of treatment. Some antiarrhythmic agents require drug-level monitoring; serum drug levels should be monitored with initiation of therapy, with dosage changes, and if the infant requires other medications that may interact with the antiarrhythmic agent. Steady-state blood concentrations are generally reached after 5 times the drug's half-life. The reader is referred to the sections that follow on first- and second-line pharmacologic agents for long-term management as well as Table 19.4, which summarizes outcomes data from noteworthy studies of antiarrhythmic agents.

PROPHYLACTIC FIRST-LINE PHARMACOLOGIC AGENTS

Digoxin

Digoxin is a cardiac glycoside prepared by extraction from *Digitalis lanata* (Grecian foxglove). It is used in the treatment of heart failure with impaired myocardial contractility in infants with CHDs and in infants with atrial tachycardias or other SVT arrhythmias. Historically, digoxin has been used as first-line therapy for prophylaxis of recurrent SVT despite limited controlled trials (Long, 1998). Success of digoxin for prophylactic therapy ranged from 42% to 65%. The lowest success rate for digoxin-preventing recurrent SVT events was 42% (O'Sullivan et al., 1995); Benson and colleagues (1985) found similar results with only 44% of patients having no recurrence of SVT episodes ($n = 8/18$). Weindling and colleagues (1996) reported digoxin being successful as monotherapy in 62% ($n = 8/13$) of their study patients; Pfammatter and Stocker (1998) found comparable results of success at 65% ($n = 17/26$). Low success rates for maintenance of normal sinus rhythm require either a change in the monotherapy agent or the addition of a second antiarrhythmic agent.

MECHANISM OF ACTION/PHARMACOKINETIC PRINCIPLES

The primary myocardial effects are due to the positive inotropic effect of inhibition of the sodium–potassium pump resulting in an influx of sodium into the cells (Figure 19.10). This influx of sodium influences the sodium–calcium exchanger, leading to an increase in intracellular calcium. Increased intracellular calcium improves myocardial contractility. As a result of the inhibition of the sodium–potassium pump, there is an increase in extracellular potassium. In addition, digoxin slows cardiac conduction through the SA and AV nodes by inhibiting ATPase, resulting in the negative chronotropic actions that decrease the heart rate. Prolongation of the antegrade refractory period in the AV node interrupts the reentrant tachycardia, which includes the AV node as one limb of the reentry circuit. Even though digoxin decreases automaticity in the SA node, automaticity can increase in the Purkinje fibers, resulting in risk for proarrhythmias (Artman et al., 2017; Burchum & Rosenthal, 2016).

The oral bioavailability of digoxin elixir is 75% to 95% and is affected by gastrointestinal motility; peak levels are seen 30 to 90 minutes after oral dosing. The volume of distribution is larger in infants than adults, resulting in a prolonged distribution phase, and the clearance rate is higher in infants in comparison to adults and children. The serum half-life is longer in preterm infants due to slower renal elimination (as long as 60 hours) compared to older infants (approximately 18 hours). Digoxin is primarily excreted unchanged in the urine. Because clearance is related to renal function, the dose must be decreased by 50% in infants with impaired or immature renal function (Alboliras et al., 2018; Artman et al., 2017).

DOSING RECOMMENDATIONS

One of the first studies to evaluate the use of digoxin was a case report of nine infants (all but one was 4 months of age or less, the older infant was 7 months. An initial dose of 0.05 to 0.1 grams of digifoline, a form of digoxin, intramuscularly (IM). Repeated doses of 0.05 to 0.1 grams were given as indicated; total dosing ranged from 0.007 to 0.35 grams per pound given mainly over 1 to 2 days. This dosing was found to promptly restore normal sinus rhythm in most of the cases (Hubbard, 1941). In a study of 32 infants and children with SVT, Klint and colleagues (1972) reported a digitalizing dose of digoxin ranging from 0.033 to 0.066 mg/kg (33 to 66 mcg/kg); one-third of this total dose was given IV or IM with the remaining two-thirds given in two divided doses 4 to 8 hours apart. Successful return to sinus rhythm occurred in 91% ($n = 29/32$) of the patients. Prophylactic dosing was not routinely started unless there was a past history of congestive heart failure. Recurrence was noted and was highest (64%) among patients with WPW; recurrence was treated individually at the time it occurred with digoxin and, if this therapy failed, quinidine (Klint et al., 1972). Lubbers and colleagues (1972) retrospectively evaluated 39 infants younger than 1 year of age at the time of the initial SVT event. Digoxin was the first drug of choice and was administered in a dosage of 0.06 to 0.08 mg/kg (60–80 mcg/kg) in the first 24 hours. Prophylactic dosing of 0.015 to 0.02 mg/kg (15–20 mcg/kg) daily continued after that. In the 28 infants with SVT/WPW who

FIGURE 19.10 Digoxin mechanism of action.

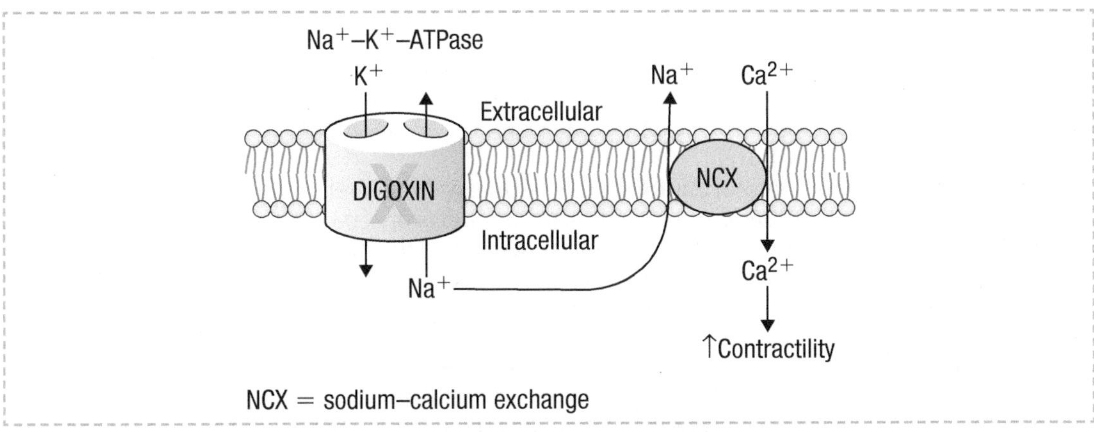

Source: From Artman, M., Mahony, L., Teitel, D. F., & Artman, M. (2017). *Neonatal cardiology*. McGraw-Hill Education.

had the first event prior to the third month of life, 15 had no recurrence and seven had short-lasting events mainly in the first 48 hours after termination of the initial event (Lubbers et al., 1972).

Many of the studies initiated after this that evaluated variations in antiarrhythmic agent selection did not discuss actual dosing used for each of the agents. Sreeram and Wren (1990) described 14 infants receiving digoxin as initial management with doses ranging from 8 to 160 mcg/kg; three of the patients received significant overdoses (375 to 600 mcg), illustrating the concerning risk of miscalculation of digoxin dosing. Strasburger (1991), in a review of the literature, found the total digitalizing dose ranged from 40 to 50 mcg/kg, with maintenance dosing ranging from 10 to 15 mcg/kg/day given in two divided doses or as a single daily dose. O'Sullivan and colleagues (1995), in a retrospective comparison study of digoxin to flecainide, used a prophylactic oral dosing of 8 to 10 mcg/kg/day (dosing interval was not provided), which was effective in 42% of the patients for suppression of SVT. Pfammatter and Stocker (1998), in their retrospective study of 26 newborns (n = 18) and infants (n = 8) with SVT, discussed using an initial IV or oral loading dose given in three to four doses (loading dose was not provided), followed by oral dosing of 0.015 mg/kg/day divided in two doses for patients weighing less than 10 kilograms. Serum drug levels were checked after reaching steady state, approximately 2 to 3 days after initiation of therapy; no difference was noted between those patients who had conversion to sinus rhythm versus those who did not. Srinivasan and Balaji (2019) suggest that if digoxin is used for chronic therapy that dosing should be 8 to 10 mcg/kg/day divided into two doses every 12 hours.

Historically, the loading dose of digoxin is divided into three doses over a 24-hour period due to the large volume of distribution before starting daily maintenance dosing. The total digitalizing dose is lower in the preterm infant (20 mcg/kg) compared to the term infant (30 mcg/kg). Dosing in the infant (>1 month to 2 years) is higher at 40 to 50 mcg/kg (Park & Salamet, 2021). There is a higher incidence of toxic effects in the neonate associated with giving a loading dose; therefore, some providers may employ a different agent while waiting for digoxin to reach steady state (after approximately five doses). Maintenance dosing is approximately 25% to 30% of the total digitalizing dose (Park & Salamet, 2021). Oral dosing is 25% greater than IV dosing, requiring adjustments when changing routes. Many cardiologists still recommend twice-a-day dosing; however, based on pharmacokinetic studies in infants, once-a-day dosing should be considered as it may simplify medication administration after discharge and potentially lead to increased compliance (Artman et al., 2017).

CLINICAL-MONITORING PEARLS

Digoxin has a narrow therapeutic window, making the risk for toxicity high. Neonates with immature renal function or renal failure are especially at risk for digoxin toxicity. Hayes and colleagues (1973) found that toxicity occurred in 16% (n = 5/31) of infants aged 1 week to 11 months who were on maintenance therapy; Levine and Somlyo (1962) reported premature infants being at even higher risk for toxicity, especially within the first 72 hours of dosing. Routine monitoring of serum levels is not done in the neonate due to the presence of endogenous digoxin-like immunoreactive substances, which makes interpretation of the levels more difficult unless the assays are able to exclude this. Lewander and colleagues (1986) found that signs of toxicity were not necessarily proportional to serum digoxin concentrations. Of note, this study looked at acute digoxin accidental or intentional ingestion. If serum drug levels are needed, they should be measured at least 6 hours after a dose or before the administration of the next dose. Therapeutic serum digoxin levels should be between 0.7 to 2 nanograms/mL (IBM Micromedex Neofax, 2021b; Lewander et al., 1986; Ratnasamy et al., 2008; Strasburger, 1991).

Digoxin requires close monitoring for signs of adverse effects related to toxicity. Gastrointestinal symptoms are the most predominant extracardiac effects observed in infants and include feeding intolerance, vomiting, and diarrhea thought to be due to digoxin-mediated increased vagal activity (Runge, 1977). Hyperkalemia can also be seen due to inhibition of the sodium–potassium pump with resultant increased extracellular potassium (Bradberry & Vale, 1995). Central nervous system (CNS) disturbances, such as lethargy or weakness, can be seen in the newborn and infant; in older children and adults, confusion and hallucinations may occur with toxicity. Adverse cardiac effects associated with toxicities may include second- or third-degree heart block with bradycardia, supraventricular and ventricular ectopic beats, and ventricular arrhythmias (Alboliras et al., 2018; IBM Micromedex Neofax, 2021b; Long, 1998). Dosing should be withheld in the infant with a heart rate less than 100 beats per minute or if there is prolongation of the PR interval. Monitoring of renal function, electrolytes, calcium, and magnesium are important as there is increased risk for toxicity in the infant with electrolyte disorders (hypokalemia, hypomagnesemia, hypercalcemia) and renal insufficiency. Medications that predispose the infant to hypokalemia, such as diuretics, and medications that may interfere with digoxin clearance, such as flecainide, amiodarone, or spironolactone, should be used with caution. In cases of life-threatening proarrhythmias, digoxin-specific Fab antibody fragments (DigiFab) should be given (Alboliras et al., 2018; IBM Micromedex Neofax, 2021b; Long, 1998).

Propranolol

Propranolol is a class II antiarrhythmic agent and was the first commercially available beta-adrenergic blocking agent in the United States used in the management of infants with SVT, certain ventricular arrhythmias, congenital long QT syndromes, and hypertrophic cardiomyopathy. Wong and colleagues (2006), in a survey of cardiologists, found that 11 different medications were chosen for acute management and eight medications for long-term prophylaxis. Propranolol was the most common agent chosen by the surveyed cardiologists for acute management of the infant with SVT with preexcitation (34%), as well as for prophylaxis with preexcitation (70%). The success rate for chronic treatment with propranolol ranges from 50% to 90% with no recurrence of SVT (Barton et al., 2015; Begum & Sharker, 2020). Barton and colleagues (2015) reported approximately 70% success in patients with reentrant SVT during initial hospital treatment. Patient follow-up after discharge on propranolol monotherapy showed success rates of almost 88% (n = 167/190) in patients receiving 4 mg/kg/day. In a double-blind, randomized, multicenter study including centers in the United States and Canada, no difference was found between digoxin and propranolol for prophylaxis of SVT, with both agents demonstrating a high initial success rate and no recurrence after 4 months of therapy. The researchers could not conclusively state that this was related to there being no difference between the two agents as the study was underpowered, which may have led to these findings (Sanatani et al., 2012). In a retrospective, large multi-institutional study looking at practice patterns (not on success of therapy), propranolol was the most commonly used agent, followed by digoxin (Seslar et al., 2013).

MECHANISM OF ACTION/PHARMACOKINETIC PRINCIPLES

Propranolol blocks both $beta_1$- and $beta_2$-adrenergic receptor sites, causing the effects seen on the heart and the bronchi, respectively. In infants with SVT, propranolol, due to blocking $beta_1$-adrenergic receptors, affects heart rate, conduction, and myocardial contractility. There is a negative chronotropic effect (suppresses excessive discharge of the SA node) and a negative dromotropic effect on the AV node and accessory pathways, leading to conduction being slowed through the AV node (Nies & Shand, 1975). The blocking of $beta_2$ receptors results in smooth muscle constriction and risk for bronchospasm. Propranolol crosses the blood-brain barrier and can lead to some of the neurologic adverse effects discussed.

Oral bioavailability is 25% to 40% related to extensive first-pass hepatic metabolism (Nies & Shand, 1975). Up to 99% of metabolites are excreted in the urine. Onset of action is rapid with IV dosing (<5 minutes), typically reserved for life-threatening dysrhythmias (Taketomo, 2023). Onset of action for oral dosing is within 1 to 2 hours and peak levels are achieved in approximately 2 hours after oral dosing, with effects lasting 6 to 12 hours. The half-life is probably increased in neonates, and is about 3.5 hours in infants (Taketomo, 2023). Serum half-life is prolonged in infants with liver dysfunction or renal impairment, requiring dosing adjustment to avoid increased risk for adverse effects (Alboliras et al., 2018; Artman et al., 2017; Burchum & Rosenthal, 2016; IBM Micromedex Neofax, 2021c; Severin et al., 2013).

DOSING RECOMMENDATIONS

There are limited data to guide oral dosing of propranolol for SVT, but tertiary references recommend starting at 0.5 to 1 mg/kg for the first dose, then 1 mg/kg/dose every 6 to 8 hours (Barton et al., 2015; Sanatani et al., 2012). IV dosing is much lower at 0.01 to 0.15 mg/kg/dose and should be given via slow push over a 10-minute period. Dosing can be repeated as needed every 6 to 8 hours with a maximum dose of 1 mg/dose (Dalal & Van Hare, 2020; Park & Salamet, 2021).

CLINICAL-MONITORING PEARLS

Propranolol has many contraindications due to effects of beta-adrenergic blocking properties, including hypotension, significant pulmonary disease (history of bronchospasms), second- or third-degree heart block, and bradycardia. Adverse effects related to beta-receptor blockade include decreased myocardial function resulting in hypotension, bradycardia, impaired myocardial contractility, bronchospasms (due to airway smooth muscle constriction from blocking of the beta-2 adrenergic receptors), sleep disturbance (as a result of presence of beta receptors in the brain also being blocked), and risk for hypoglycemia (beta-blockers inhibit hepatic gluconeogenesis and glycogenolysis) especially if oral intake needs to be restricted (Alboliras et al., 2018; Artman et al., 2017; Burchum & Rosenthal, 2016; IBM Micromedex Neofax, 2021c; Severin et al., 2013). If converting from IV to oral or vice versa, use caution as there is a significant difference in dosing. Use with caution with amiodarone as the combination with beta-blockers may enhance the bradycardic effect. Breakthrough recurrent events were seen more commonly within 1 month of discharge and were associated with outgrowing the dose.

SECOND-LINE PHARMACOLOGIC AGENTS

Amiodarone

Amiodarone is an iodinated benzofuran derivative with class III properties; there are potassium channel-blocking effects characterized by prolongation of the action-potential duration and of the refractory period of cardiac cells, resulting in decreased AV conduction and sinus node function (Taketomo, 2023; Weindling et al., 1996). Amiodarone also has sodium channel-blocking effects (class I properties), noncompetitive alpha- and beta-blocking properties (class II properties), and calcium channel-blocking effects (class IV properties; Nattel et al., 1987; Singh, 1983). The combination of these various properties makes amiodarone effective for the broad range of supraventricular and ventricular arrhythmias described in the studies, especially in the patient with impaired cardiac function when other agents may have undesirable negative inotropic effects. Acute administration of amiodarone blocks sodium and calcium channels, resulting in slow upstroke velocity of the cardiac action potential. The effects of sodium channel blockade also include depolarization of the resting membrane potential, causing stronger conduction in the cardiac tissue. Conduction across the AV node is slowed as a result of calcium channel blocking. Long-term maintenance of amiodarone use results mainly in the class III properties of potassium channel blockade, resulting in prolongation of the cardiac action potential and the refractory period (Mujović et al., 2020).

Amiodarone use was first reported in the 1960s, leveraging coronary vasodilation for the treatment of angina in adults (Charlier et al., 1962). Amiodarone was later noted to prolong cardiac action potential, suggesting it may be beneficial for antiarrhythmic effects (Singh & Vaughan Williams, 1970). Rosenbaum and colleagues (1974) found amiodarone successful in controlling the arrhythmias of 11 patients with WPW syndrome. This led to additional clinical trials evaluating the efficacy of amiodarone in patients with ORT and WPW who had failed other antiarrhythmic agents. In 1985, the FDA approved oral amiodarone for treatment of life-threatening ventricular arrhythmias; it was not until 10 years later that IV use was approved by the Parenteral Drug Association. Further clinical trials investigated the role of this agent in treatment of supraventricular tachyarrhythmias (Kopelman & Horowitz, 1989).

There is limited evidence evaluating the safety and efficacy of this agent in the neonatal population, requiring extrapolation from retrospective studies of infants and older children. One of the first studies to evaluate use of amiodarone for treatment of cardiac arrhythmias in infants and older children showed restoration of normal rhythm in 66% of the subjects and clinical improvement in 33% ($n = 135$ with a mean age of 10 years; 8 were less than 1 year of age; Coumel & Fidelle, 1980). Bucknall and colleagues (1986) found similar monotherapy success rates in a study including only a slightly greater number of infants younger than 1 year of age ($n = 11/28$). Shuler and colleagues (1993) evaluated safety and efficacy exclusively in infants younger than 12 months of age. They found variable efficacy in the infants studied (successful in 10 of 17 infants, four with monotherapy and six requiring combination with other antiarrhythmic agent[s]) and the only side effect that was noted was proarrhythmias. In a retrospective study, Burri and colleagues (2003) evaluated the safety and efficacy of IV amiodarone in 23 infants (median age of 8 days). Efficacy for IV amiodarone administration was very good with 19 of 23 infants having the tachycardia terminated; however, it did take a median time of 24 hours to achieve control. It was also observed that there were no severe proarrhythmias. Evaluation of oral dosing indicated that there were no significant proarrhythmias, elevated liver enzymes, or thyroid dysfunction observed (Burri et al., 2003).

The only prospective, randomized, double-blind study in the pediatric population was a dose-response study of the safety and efficacy of amiodarone use in children; the average age was an older child (median of 1.6 years of age). The authors found that overall efficacy and incidence of adverse events was dose related (Saul et al., 2005). Amiodarone was officially supported in the American Heart Association (AHA) Guidelines for Cardiopulmonary Resuscitation and Emergency Care: Pediatric Advanced Life Support algorithms for use in ventricular arrhythmias (AHA, 2000) and later for drug-resistant and countershock-resistant arrhythmia, including SVT (AHA, 2005).

Additional studies evaluating efficacy in neonates and infants demonstrated success rates using amiodarone monotherapy for conversion to normal sinus rhythm as variable, ranging from 33% to 100% (Etheridge et al., 2001; Figa et al., 1994; Perry et al., 1996). Due to the significantly prolonged half-life and risk of significant adverse effects, studies suggest that amiodarone should be reserved for those who have potentially life-threatening arrhythmias for which other antiarrhythmic agents have not been successful (Bucknall et al., 1986; Garson et al., 1984; Kopelman & Horowitz, 1989; McGovern et al., 1983).

MECHANISM OF ACTION/PHARMACOKINETIC PRINCIPLES

Amiodarone acts as previously discussed by several mechanisms as it (a) prolongs repolarization and the duration of the action potential, (b) increases the refractory period in cardiac tissues, and (c) blocks both alpha- and beta-adrenergic receptors as well as calcium channels. These actions result in prolongation of the PR and QT intervals, widening of the T wave, and dampening T wave amplitudes (Rowland & Krikler, 1980; Soult et al., 1995).

Oral bioavailability is approximately 43%. Onset of action is prolonged and considerably variable with oral loading, with effects achieved between 3 days and 3 weeks. Effects can be seen within 30 minutes with an IV loading dose due to faster saturation of the cardiac tissues (Severin et al., 2013). Its duration of effect is between 1 and 3 hours (Latini et al., 1984). Amiodarone is metabolized mainly in the liver with potential for enterohepatic recirculation. Amiodarone is highly lipophilic, meaning that it rapidly distributes from plasma to peripheral tissues; it can accumulate in the liver, spleen, and the lungs (Kopelman & Horowitz, 1989; Latini et al., 1984). Protein binding of amiodarone is approximately 96%; therefore, removal by dialysis is minimal (Latini et al., 1984). Amiodarone follows nonlinear kinetics with a long half-life (6–8 weeks in young patients) and a large volume of distribution (Guccione et al., 1990; Holt et al., 1983). The terminal elimination half-life of desethylamiodarone, the active metabolite, was longer than the parent drug amiodarone after chronic therapy (Holt et al., 1983; Kopelman & Horowitz, 1989). Elimination of amiodarone is slow, so effects, including potential unwanted adverse effects, can be seen for an extended period after discontinuing this agent. Excretion is mainly via the biliary system; less than 1% is excreted as unchanged drug in the urine (Taketomo, 2023).

DOSING RECOMMENDATIONS

Data for oral and IV dosing of amiodarone in neonates/infants are limited. For resistant SVT, an IV loading dose of 5 mg/kg is recommended, followed by continuous IV infusion if arrhythmia is terminated. If the arrhythmia persists, the loading dose can be repeated with total daily dose to not exceed 15 mg/kg/day (Burri et al., 2003; Etheridge et al., 2001; Figa et al., 1994; Haas, 2008; Perry et al., 1996; Soult et al., 1995). Continuous infusion regimens are variable and commonly start at 5 mcg/kg/min with titration to desired response or a maximum of 15 to 25 mcg/kg/min (Burri et al., 2003; Figa et al., 1994; Kovacikova, 2009; Lane et al., 2010; Perry et al., 1996).

As soon as the clinical condition allows, dosing should be switched to the oral route. Bucknall and colleagues (1986) found that higher oral doses were required in the infant younger than 1 year of age, with a mean dose for initial arrhythmia suppression of 15.3 mg/kg/day; dosing was also higher for maintenance, with a mean dose of 8.2 mg/kg/day. They found that when dosage was calculated based instead on surface area (mg/m^2/day), dosage was similar in infants younger than 1 year of age compared to those older than 1 year of age. Etheridge and colleagues (2001), based on a study of 50 neonates/infants (1 to 90 days of age) with SVT, suggested an oral loading dose of 10 to 20 mg/kg/day divided into two doses for 7 to 10 days, with dosage then reduced to 5 to 10 mg/kg/day once daily. The loading dose should always be started at the lowest possible dose capable of terminating the arrhythmia as a higher loading dose is associated with a higher risk of prolonged QT interval. Serum drug concentrations are not helpful due to the long half-life of this agent.

CLINICAL-MONITORING PEARLS

There are many adverse effects associated with the use of amiodarone. Hemodynamic and cardiac status should be closely monitored in patients receiving short-term administration due to risk for hypotension and proarrhythmias. If hypotension occurs during IV amiodarone administration, intravenous volume may be required. The risk for hypotension can be minimized by giving the loading dose over 60 minutes. Long-term administration requires routine monitoring, including liver function (risk for liver toxicity), renal function (risk for toxicity if renal dysfunction present), and thyroid function (risk for hypo- or hyperthyroidism due to high iodine content and inhibition of 5′-deiodinase activity), in addition to pulmonary function tests (risk for pulmonary fibrosis) and ophthalmologic exams (Lane et al., 2010; Long, 1998). Due to the risk of pulmonary toxicity, hepatotoxicity, worsening arrhythmia, or life-threatening arrhythmias, there are black-box warnings for this medication in the United States. Adverse effects typically resolve with discontinuation of the drug. Because of the extremely long half-life, it will take longer to reach steady state; therefore, these adverse effects may not be seen for many months.

In neonates and infants, the literature has discussed risk of cardiac toxicity (worsening of arrhythmia or new onset of significant bradycardia or AV block), gastrointestinal toxicity (poor feeding, emesis, or abnormal liver function tests [LFTs]), neurologic toxicity (lethargy, tremor, developmental delay after start of medication), pulmonary toxicity (tachypnea, hypoxemia, or physical exam abnormal lung findings), dermatologic toxicity (skin discoloration), and thyroid toxicity. The infant should also be monitored for the development of AV block, bradycardia, or other proarrhythmias that can occur due to the β-blocking and calcium channel-blocking effects. Ng and colleagues (2003), in a case report of a 22-day-old, former 42-week gestational-age infant, described the development of a variety of arrhythmias requiring cardiopulmonary resuscitation for a prolonged period after receiving a loading dose of amiodarone for SVT. The dosing followed other researchers' recommended loading dose of 5 mg/kg given over 30 minutes. Ophthalmologic abnormalities, such as optic neuritis, have not been seen in infants (Etheridge et al., 2001). For infants on prolonged therapy, screening of liver and thyroid function should be done every few months to evaluate for potential toxicity. Growth should also be monitored; accelerated bone maturation affecting growth velocity in pediatric patients who develop hyperthyroidism has been described (Ardura et al., 1988). Adverse effects appear to be age dependent and become more frequent with increasing age and duration of treatment; adverse effects are also more common with IV dosing compared to oral dosing (Bucknall et al., 1986; Coumel & Fidelle, 1980; Etheridge et al., 2001).

If amiodarone is used in conjunction with digoxin, the dose of digoxin may need to be lowered as amiodarone increases the level of digoxin. Caution is also warranted when combining amiodarone with another β-blocker due to higher risk for significant bradycardia (Alboliras et al., 2018; Burchum & Rosenthal, 2016; Latini et al., 1984; Long, 1998). Amiodarone should be used with caution in neonates with WPW syndrome or atrial fibrillation/flutter as ventricular fibrillation may occur (Taketomo, 2023). Amiodarone is contraindicated in the infant with AV block, sinus node dysfunction, or sinus bradycardia (Park & Salamet, 2021). The IV formulation may be a vesicant with risk for significant tissue necrosis. If extravasation occurs, stop infusion, gently aspirate extravasated solution through the cannula, and consider hyaluronidase; use of warm compresses and elevation may also be beneficial after these steps. Some preparations contain benzyl alcohol; these solutions should be avoided in the neonate due to risk of a condition described as "gasping syndrome," which consists of metabolic acidosis, respiratory acidosis, gasping respirations, CNS alterations, hypotension, and cardiovascular collapse (Taketomo, 2023).

DRUG SHORTAGE

As of December 2021, there is a current drug shortage of amiodarone for injection (visit ashp.org/drug-shortages for further updates on continued or resolved shortages).

Procainamide

Procainamide is a class 1A agent used for the management of ventricular arrhythmias and SVT. Its metabolite, N-acetylprocainamide (NAPA), has moderate class III actions. The major disadvantages limiting use of this agent are that it must be given via IV and its risk of serious side effects; therefore, it is reserved for cases in which there has been no response to other antiarrhythmic agents.

MECHANISM OF ACTION/PHARMACOKINETIC PRINCIPLES

Procainamide is a sodium channel-blocking agent that acts by decreasing the conduction velocity, decreasing myocardial excitability, and delaying repolarization, which results in increased PR and QT intervals, and widening of the QRS. Myocardial contractility may be depressed by increasing the electrical stimulation threshold of the ventricles and the His-Purkinje system, as well as a result of direct cardiac effects (Taketomo, 2023).

The bioavailability of procainamide is 83% and there is low protein binding (16%). Hepatic metabolism of procainamide results in an active metabolite, NAPA, that is only one-third as potent as the parent compound; this metabolite is excreted renally. Due to hepatic and renal immaturity, the half-life of the parent compound and the active metabolite are longer in neonates than has been reported in older children and adults, requiring adjustments in dosing and dosing interval; half-life in adults is reported to be 2.5 to 5 hours (Taketomo, 2023). However, 67% of the drug is excreted renally as unchanged drug.

DOSING RECOMMENDATIONS

Limited data regarding neonatal dosing are available. Dosing must be titrated to the individual response obtained. Moffett and colleagues (2006), in a retrospective study of 20 neonates, reported a mean loading dose of 9.6 +/- 1.5 mg/kg and a mean continuous infusion rate of 37.56 +/- 13.52 mcg/kg/min. They found that serum concentrations were supratherapeutic in five neonates; four of these were less than 36 weeks' gestation and all had creatinine clearance less than 30 mL/min/1.73 m^2, suggesting that doses should be decreased in preterm infants and those infants with renal impairment (Moffett et al., 2006). Taketomo (2023) suggests an initial IV loading dose of 7 to 10 mg/kg given over 60 minutes followed by a continuous infusion of 20 to 80 mcg/kg/min, whereas Park and Salamet (2021) suggest a lower loading dose of 2 to 6 mg/kg/dose, which can be repeated every 10 to 30 minutes, followed by the maintenance dose. The IO route can be considered in infants in whom IV access cannot be obtained. The onset of action is rapid. IV loading dose should be diluted to a maximum concentration of 20 mg/mL; continuous IV infusion should be diluted to a final concentration of 2 to 4 mg/mL in D_5W.

CLINICAL-MONITORING PEARLS

Adverse effects of procainamide may include feeding intolerance and emesis; with higher serum concentrations, hypotension and arrhythmias may occur (Long, 1998). The FDA black-box warning for potentially fatal blood dyscrasias and drug-induced lupus erythematosus-like syndrome reflect adverse effects in the adult population. A complete blood count (CBC) with differential should be monitored weekly for the first 3 months of treatment and periodically thereafter. Monitoring of EKG and blood pressure (BP) is also recommended. Severe hypotension can occur with rapid administration; to avoid this risk, give the loading dose over 60 minutes in neonates. Procainamide and NAPA serum concentrations should be monitored 6 to 12 hours after start of infusion to avoid toxicity; side effects appear to be plasma-concentration dependent (Bauersfeld et al., 2001). Use caution when administering with other agents, such as amiodarone, that prolong the QT interval. Dosing should be reduced in the neonate with renal dysfunction. Procainamide is commercially available in two different concentrations resulting in risk for under- or overdosing; verify closely the solution provided.

Flecainide

Flecainide is a derivative of procainamide. Flecainide, which received FDA approval in 1984, is effective in restoring normal sinus rhythm in 72% to 90% of patients with AVRT; lower effectiveness was found in patients with WPW. Wren and Campbell (1987) demonstrated either complete suppression of the arrhythmia or control of the ventricular rate in 83% (n = 10/12) of pediatric patients treated with flecainide who had a serious arrhythmia and/or a medically refractory arrhythmia. Zeigler and colleagues (1988) found flecainide successfully controlled SVT in 75% (n = 3/4) of patients with AV node reentry SVTs, but was only 42% effective in patients with accessory connections; their study only focused on pediatric patients and young adults. Perry and colleagues (1989) examined flecainide efficacy and pharmacokinetics in 63 patients with various resistant arrhythmias, of whom 20 were less than 12 months of age. They documented a 60% or greater reduction of arrhythmia burden in 82% of patients with SVT (n = 42/51). In the subgroup with WPW, effectiveness was 69% (n = 11/16); however, proarrhythmias occurred in 31% of subjects (n = 5/16), including one newborn. This contrasts with patients with ORT, in whom flecainide was 78% effective (n = 7/9) with no documented proarrhythmias.

MECHANISM OF ACTION/PHARMACOKINETIC PRINCIPLES

Flecainide is a class 1C antiarrhythmic agent that acts by blocking sodium channels, resulting in decreased conduction velocity (induces anterograde and retrograde conduction block, making this an appealing choice for the patient with WPW) and decreased automaticity (negatively inotropic); it does not have an effect on action potential duration. Flecainide is also effective in prophylactic treatment of AV tachycardia (Till, Shinebourne, Rowland, et al., 1989).

Onset of action is rapid with oral dosing due to relatively fast absorption; bioavailability is nearly 100%. There is a concern of impaired absorption in infants if given concurrently with milk (Perry & Garson, 1992; Russell & Martin, 1989; Severin et al., 2013). Flecainide has a long half-life of 11 to 12 hours in infants younger than 1 year of age and up to 29 hours in the newborn; this longer half-life is most likely reflective of immaturity of hepatic and renal clearance (Taketomo, 2023; Perry et al., 1989). Flecainide is extensively metabolized by hepatic biotransformation and cleared renally as metabolites and unchanged drug (Perry et al., 1989). Peak concentrations are achieved in approximately 3 hours. Flecainide is a little over 40% protein bound.

DOSING RECOMMENDATIONS

There are very limited data regarding neonatal dosing; optimal dosing has not been established. The dose requires individual titration to the desired clinical response in terminating the SVT. Dosing based on body surface area (BSA) compared to weight corresponds better to therapeutic serum levels. Perry and colleagues (1989) used an initial single dose of 25 mg/m^2, followed 24 hours later with 100 mg/m^2/day divided every 12 hours (note that they did initially start with the maintenance dose at 50 mg/m^2/day but found little or no effect so they went to the higher starting dose). If the arrhythmia was not controlled, the dose was titrated upward every five doses to 150 then to 200 mg/m^2/day until effective or a proarrhythmia developed. They also noted that if breakthrough tachycardia occurred prior to the next 12-hour dosing interval, a change of interval to every 8 hours with the same total daily dose was more effective (Perry et al., 1989).

Due to the concern related to dosing based on BSA in neonates, other researchers have suggested dosing based on weight. Wren and Campbell (1987) suggested an oral dose of 3 to 6 mg/kg/day divided every 8 hours and adjusted based on response and/or plasma concentrations. Till, Shinebourne, Rowland and colleagues (1989) found that a dose of 6 mg/kg/day was required to ensure therapeutic serum plasma concentrations. Because neonates may need higher doses, they stressed the importance of monitoring serum levels (Till, Shinebourne, Rowland, et al., 1989). O'Sullivan and colleagues (1995) in a retrospective study utilized flecainide when there was recurrence of SVT in patients treated with digoxin. The dose of oral flecainide ranged from 3.2 to 13.5 mg/kg/day based on plasma levels or ability to control recurrence of SVT. The authors documented a poor correlation between flecainide dose and serum concentration, leading to their recommendations of careful therapeutic drug monitoring. Ferlini and colleagues (2009), in their pilot study of 20 newborns without structural heart disease, initiated oral flecainide 2 mg/kg/day divided into two doses. Flecainide was found to be 85% (n = 17/20) effective in controlling the arrhythmia with a mean dose of 3.35 ± 1.35 mg/kg/day.

Historically, serum levels have been followed closely due to concerns about adverse effects based on adult studies; however, studies in the pediatric population found proarrhythmia occurred in less than 7%, suggesting aggressive therapeutic drug monitoring may not be required in this population unless there is a concern for lack of compliance or signs of toxicity (Price et al., 2002). However, some primary sources disagree on the basis of a poor correlation between serum levels and neonatal dosing based on body weight (O'Sullivan et al., 1995). Importantly, the goal trough range for efficacy remains undefined in the neonatal population, but appears to be lower than the standard for adults (0.2 to 1 mcg/mL). If levels are obtained, they should be drawn after steady state is achieved (more than five doses after starting or changing therapy). Vento and colleagues (2007) demonstrated that hemolysis of the serum drug level may cause a falsely elevated trough level. They hypothesized that since flecainide is a polar substance that can easily diffuse into the cytoplasm of the erythrocyte, plasma levels may only partially reflect the total amount of drug in whole blood. If there are concerns that the specimen is hemolyzed, send a repeat serum drug level before making dosing adjustments (Vento et al., 2007). Use caution in infants with hepatic dysfunction as elimination may be slower; serum concentrations can guide dosing. Milk-based formulas may interfere with absorption; avoid giving medication with feeding and if infant is made nothing by mouth (NPO), the dose will need to be reduced (Russell & Martin, 1989; Thompson, 2012).

CLINICAL-MONITORING PEARLS

Adverse effects include edema, proarrhythmias (black-box warning), and sinus node dysfunction (Alboliras et al., 2018). In neonates or infants with structurally abnormal hearts or those who have impaired ventricular function, the risk for proarrhythmias and even cardiac arrest is more common compared to those with a normal heart (Fish et al., 1991; Perry et al., 1989; Till, Shinebourne, Rowland, et al., 1989). The safety of flecainide in patients with CHD has been revisited more recently. In a retrospective study of 42 children's hospitals, a group of researchers compared flecainide to other antiarrhythmic agents in children with CHD or cardiomyopathy in relation to cardiac arrest or death; they found the incidence was comparable between flecainide and other antiarrhythmic agents (Moffett, Valdes, et al., 2015). Cunningham and colleagues (2017), in a retrospective study that included 20 patients with CHD and two with cardiomyopathy compared to 155 controls with normal hearts, found no difference in the incidence of proarrhythmias and there were no cardiac arrests. Proarrhythmias are more likely to occur during initiation of therapy; therefore, hospitalization during initiation of treatment is recommended (Perry et al., 1989). Monitor BP, pulse, EKG (for increased PR and QRS duration), and liver enzymes. If flecainide is given concurrent with amiodarone, the initial daily dose should be decreased by 20% to 50% as plasma flecainide levels are increased (Perry et al., 1989).

Sotalol

Sotalol has unique properties due to a combination of class II beta-blocking and class III properties. It demonstrates minimal negative inotropic effects and no intrinsic sympathomimetic activity. In patients with WPW, due to the beta-blocking effects, there was slowing of nodal conduction, prolonged AV node refractoriness, and slowing of the SA node. Class III properties were noted with higher doses and showed prolonged refractory periods in the antegrade and retrograde directions of the accessory pathway as well as the ventricular refractory period, leading to increased efficacy in the patient with WPW (Mitchell et al., 1987). Sotalol is highly effective in terminating ARVT in 89% to 95% of patients. In a study of infants younger than 3 months of age, sotalol was effective in the initial treatment of the arrhythmia in 93% (n = 17/18), with two having recurrence related to outgrowing the dose and improper preparation by pharmacy that corrected with increasing the dose and proper preparation, respectively (Tipple & Sandor, 1991). Maragnès and colleagues (1992) reported the highest success of sotalol (89%) was seen in patients with supraventricular reentrant tachycardia with or without preexcitation; their study included 14 infants younger than 3 months who were treated with sotalol alone or in conjunction with digoxin. Pfammatter and colleagues (1995) found complete or partial effectiveness in 93% of children with supraventricular reentrant tachycardia (*n* = 38/41); however, less than one-quarter of the study population was younger than 1 year of age. In a younger population (median age = 2 years), Valdés and colleagues (2018) document acute termination of arrhythmias with IV sotalol in 88% (*n* = 21/24) inclusive of patients with CHD and/or depressed ventricular function; 16 responded with the initial bolus and the remaining five responded to a second bolus.

MECHANISM OF ACTION/PHARMACOKINETIC PRINCIPLES

At higher doses, sotalol functions as a class III antiarrhythmic agent like amiodarone; at lower doses, it also has class II beta-adrenergic blocking properties like propranolol, but due to weaker class II properties, negative inotropic effects are not a concern (Pfammatter et al., 1995). Due to the class III properties, there is a delay in repolarization and a prolongation of the action potential duration, without an associated effect on depolarization. Sotalol is effective in prophylactic treatment of ARVT; however, due to the risk for systemic adverse effects, it has been historically reserved for cases of SVT refractory to other antiarrhythmic agents.

Onset of action is rapid as evaluated by reduction in heart rate (within 5–10 minutes via IV; 1 to 2 hours post dosing when steady state has been achieved with oral therapy; Ho, 1994; Winters, 1993). In adults, oral sotalol is almost completely absorbed (90%–100%; Anttila et al., 1976; Hanyok, 1993). Shi and colleagues (2001), in their study evaluating pharmacokinetic properties in infants and children (including nine neonates ≤1 month and 17 infants >1 month to ≤24 months of age), document similar findings; after a short lag period, sotalol was rapidly absorbed after oral dosing in this younger age group. Two studies in the adult population have shown a modest reduction in bioavailability when sotalol was administered with food, but no studies have evaluated the effect of formula/breast milk feedings on bioavailability. Time to peak serum concentration is 2 to 4 hours after an oral loading dose (Anttila et al., 1976; Hanyok, 1993; Saul, Schaffer, et al., 2001; Winters et al., 1993). The half-life is approximately 10 to 20 hours across all ages in the setting of normal renal function (Anttila et al., 1976; Hanyok, 1993; McDewitt & Shanks, 1977; Saul, Ross, et al., 2001; Shi et al., 2001). Animal studies reflect distribution into a number of tissues, including the heart, liver, and kidney. Due to hydrophilic properties, it poorly distributes to the CNS (Gomoll et al., 1990; Hanyok, 1993). Sotalol is not protein bound (Antilla et al., 1976; Hanyok, 1993). Sotalol is also not metabolized; elimination is primarily by renal excretion with more than 75% of the dose excreted as unchanged drug in urine (Anttila et al., 1976; Hanyok, 1993; Saul, Ross et al., 2001; Saul, Schaffer, et al., 2001; Shi et al., 2001). Due to renal elimination, the dosage must be adjusted with renal dysfunction as clearance will be reduced and the half-life will be markedly prolonged.

DOSING RECOMMENDATIONS

Limited data are available to guide neonatal dosing of sotalol. One of the first case reports of two neonates that developed recurrent SVT resistant to other antiarrhythmic agents found complete control was achieved with oral sotalol dosing of 1.5 to 8 mg/kg/day; there was not detail on initial dosing or increases of dosing to achieve this control (Bowman et al., 1988). Of note, these were premature infants (29 and 36 weeks' gestation) who were delivered secondary to fetal SVT with development of hydrops; caution is needed as the higher dosing may not be required in the neonate without this history. Park and Salamet (2021) suggest a range of 80 to 120 mg/m^2/day divided into three doses for the infant, whereas Maragnès and colleagues (1992) document a higher mean oral dose requirement of 135 mg/m^2/day divided in two doses in their study of 66 patients with 14 patients younger than 3 months of age. Dosing based on BSA was found to reliably correlate with exposure; however, pharmacokinetic studies remain limited, leading to the continued use of body weight for dosing (Saul, Ross, et al., 2001; Shi et al., 2001). Läer and colleagues (2005) suggest an initial oral dose of 2 mg/kg/day divided every 8 hours. Dosing should be gradually increased every 3 days (at steady state) by 1 to 2 mg/kg/day to the desired clinical response with maximum dosing not exceeding 4 mg/kg/day divided every 8 hours (Läer et al., 2005). The 8-hour dosing interval has become standard in modern practice as this interval may be protective in preventing breakthrough arrhythmias (Shi et al., 2001).

Use of IV sotalol was approved by the FDA in 2009 based on data reflecting efficacy and safety in adults. Studies evaluating IV dosing in the pediatric population followed; however, the majority focused on children 2 years of age or older. A case report of two newborns, one with ectopic atrial tachycardia and the other with AVRT, described IV sotalol using the manufacturer-recommended pediatric dose of 30 mg/m^2/dose every 8 hours with an age-related dosage reduction factor to determine the final IV dose, which they administered over 5 hours (Kim et al., 2017). They found the prolonged infusion time produced similar effects to orally administered sotalol; there was transient QTc prolongation after the infusion, highlighting the vital nature of diligent monitoring in clinical practice and further investigation (Kim et al., 2017). Li and colleagues (2017a) used a loading dose of 1 mg/kg over 10 minutes, followed by a maintenance dose of 4.5 mg/kg/day. If the patient remained in normal sinus rhythm, the patient was transitioned to oral dosing. In a post hoc analysis of their cohort, Li and colleagues (2017b) also document close correlation between dosing based on body weight (mg/kg) and body surface area (mg/m^2) in pediatric patients including neonates and infants ($r = 0.977$, $p<0.001$). Valdés and colleagues (2018) used the same loading dose of 1 mg/kg, which was successful in converting to normal sinus rhythm in 88% of their patients after a single dose (67%) or one repeat dose (21%). For maintenance dosing, a median of 120 mg/m^2/day divided two or three times daily and given over 5 hours was required to produce an 83% success rate ($n = 19/23$; Valdés et al., 2018). Borquez and colleagues (2020), in a retrospective study, assessed the use of IV sotalol for acute and maintenance therapy to develop a standardized administration protocol for arrhythmia management in children. For acute therapy ($n = 26$), they used a standardized dose of 30 to 40 mg/m^2 as an initial dose over 15 minutes with no age-related reduction in children younger than 2 years of age. They described mean and median time to conversion in three newborns (median dose 29.82 mg/m^2) and two infants (median dose 37.49 mg/m^2) as 15 minutes. For maintenance IV dosing ($n = 11$), patients required a median dose of 18.2 mg/m^2/dose every 8 hours, infused over 2 hours. Once sinus rhythm was maintained, the patient was transitioned to oral dosing. They found that all of the patients (age range not broken down) with SVT ($n = 9$) converted to sinus rhythm with acute therapy; in addition, the patients maintained sinus rhythm with maintenance therapy. This study was not powered sufficiently to establish a safety profile; however, they did not observe any adverse effects in the study group, suggesting a favorable side effect profile (Borquez et al., 2020).

If QT interval becomes prolonged, decreasing the dose, lengthening the dosing interval, or even discontinuing use of this agent may be required. It is recommended to use lower doses or increased dosing intervals for the infant with renal impairment as half-life will be prolonged. Drug levels are not routinely followed at this time; Läer and colleagues (2005) found an effective sotalol trough serum concentration of 0.4 and 1 mcg/mL was correlated with a 50% and 95% probability, respectively, of the patient converting to sinus rhythm.

CLINICAL-MONITORING PEARLS

Adverse effects include bradycardia, hypotension, proarrhythmias, QTc interval prolongation (as a result of effects on potassium channels) with risk of torsade de pointes, tachycardia, and risk of bronchospasm (Alboliras et al., 2018; Burchum & Rosenthal, 2016). There are conflicting reports on incidence of proarrhythmias, with Pfammatter and colleagues (1995) showing a higher incidence with oral sotalol at 10% compared to other studies. Li and colleagues (2017a) found a lower risk (2%) in their study of intravenous therapy, which excluded patients with decreased cardiac function. Risk for proarrhythmias is most often noted within a few days of starting treatment (Pfammatter et al., 1995). Due to prolonged repolarization, monitor EKG for QTc prolongation, which may be more likely in the neonate (Läer et al., 2005) and more likely with higher blood concentrations associated with a rapid versus slow bolus (Li et al., 2017b). Monitor electrolytes as abnormalities may potentiate toxicity.

MONOTHERAPY VERSUS MULTIDRUG THERAPY

When adenosine is successful in restoring a normal sinus rhythm, propranolol may be prescribed as the first-line prophylactic agent for oral, long-term management. Approximately 33% of infants subject to monotherapy exhibit recurrent episodes of SVT and require multidrug therapy to terminate the arrhythmia (Figure 19.11).

FIGURE 19.11 Management of supraventricular tachycardia.

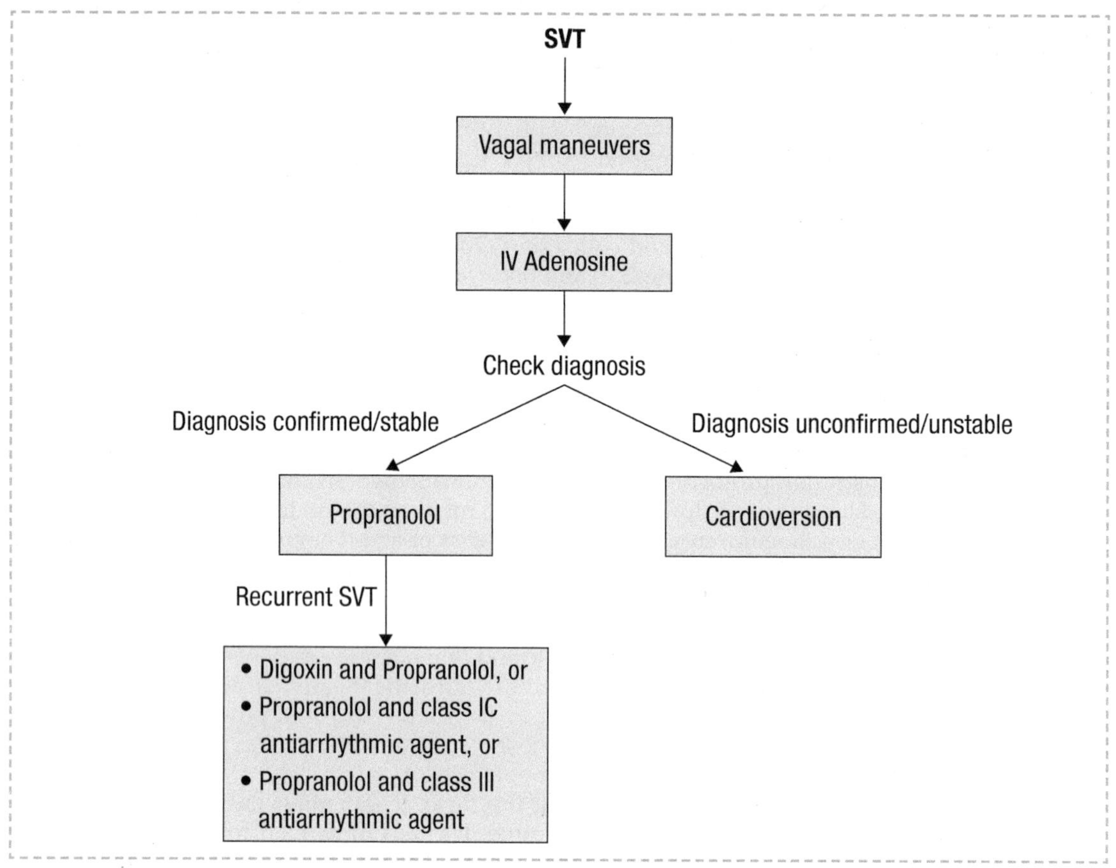

IV, intravenous; SVT, supraventricular tachycardia.

Commonly prescribed multidrug regimens include propranolol and digoxin, or propranolol and another agent, such as sotalol, flecainide, procainamide, or amiodarone (Begum & Sharker, 2020; Knudson et al., 2011; Price et al., 2002; Sanatani et al., 2002; Tavera et al., 2010). Seslar and colleagues (2013), in a retrospective evaluation of multi-institutional children's hospital discharge data of 171 subjects younger than 1 year of age (38% were younger than 30 days of age), found that propranolol was the most common first-line agent used for prophylaxis followed by digoxin; amiodarone, flecainide, and sotalol were also used as prophylactic therapy, but less frequently. Of those infants receiving first-line prophylactic therapy with propranolol or digoxin, 44% required an additional antiarrhythmic agent. Interestingly, they found that 47% of the 171 patients were started on two or more antiarrhythmic agents on the same calendar day. In addition, they observed the pattern that patients who were started on propranolol as first-line prophylactic therapy were combined most frequently with digoxin, followed by amiodarone, sotalol, and then flecainide. The same pattern was found with digoxin; it was most frequently combined with propranolol, followed by amiodarone and then flecainide when combination therapy was required. Use of sotalol in combination with digoxin was not common in this study (Seslar et al., 2013). Selection of the agent should be based on mechanism of action; considering drugs as those that affect the AV node (beta-blockers, digoxin), or that affect both (flecainide), or that affect both (sotalol, amiodarone) is one suggested approach to determine the best agent to initially use (Ratnasamy et al., 2008).

Length of prophylactic therapy for all infants with SVT is variable. Studies have demonstrated that the rate of recurrence drops to less than 50% by 6 to 12 months of age (Garson et al., 1981; Sanatani et al., 2012; Till & Shinebourne, 1991). Newer studies suggest that an infant who remains event free on monotherapy may consider a shorter 4- to 6-month duration of therapy (Aljohani et al., 2021). For the small number of infants who continue to have recurrence of symptomatic SVT, oral prophylactic pharmacologic management is continued until the risk of ablation therapy is lower. Pharmacologic management of the infant with a prior known arrhythmia who presents in congestive heart failure is more complex; these infants may require inotropic support for hypotension, which can provoke arrhythmia recurrence. Use of IV antiarrhythmic agents may also have negative inotropic effects in the infant with heart failure.

PRACTICAL CONSIDERATIONS FOR PRESCRIBERS

SVT is an arrhythmia that typically presents abruptly and requires prompt action by prescribing clinicians. Although adenosine is the customary acute management, there are numerous drugs used for longer term therapy (prophylaxis). Practical considerations that clinicians with prescriptive authority should consider include:

- the efficacy and safety of applicable drugs;
- the relationship between the pharmacokinetic profile of the drug and anticipated developmental changes in the myocardium, ion channels, and the autonomic nervous system in the affected neonate/infant; and
- the state of the science of a particular drug, as most pharmacokinetic data have been extrapolated from adult studies and no expert panel has recommended a specific treatment regimen for neonates and infants, leading to variability among practitioners on selection and dosing of antiarrhythmic agents.

CONCLUSIONS

There are no rigorous, well-controlled clinical trials to evaluate individual antiarrhythmic agents targeting specific arrhythmias in neonates and infants with or without structural heart defects. This leads to variations in clinical practice in choice of agent and dosing regimens, often based on anecdote or institutional and training center biases, not necessarily on evidence. It is prudent of the provider to examine benefits versus risks of pharmacologic management. The best recommendations to date for prophylactic treatment of SVT in neonates and infants is a beta-blocker with the addition of digoxin or procainamide for treatment failures. Regardless of pharmacologic choice, parents will need to be taught how to measure the heart rate in a quiet state, monitor blood sugar if the infant is on a beta-blocker, and perform a vagal maneuver, and should also be trained in cardiopulmonary resuscitation (CPR).

LEARNING TOOLS AND RESOURCES

Advice From the Authors

Amy J. Jnah, DNP, APRN, NNP-BC

This content is complex, and for that reason, will seem intimidating during your first pass. Begin by intently studying normal versus abnormal conduction. Then, move to integrating the mechanism of action of first- and second-line therapies to conduction pathophysiology. This will help discern cause/effect relationships and make recall much faster, particularly during high-stress times!

Jacqui Hoffman, DNP, ARNP, NNP-BC

Arrhythmias can occur in the neonatal period; some are benign, some are related to underlying causes—such as hypoglycemia, fever, and many other etiologies—and will resolve with treating the underlying mechanism, and others are related to disorders of the conduction system and may require pharmacologic management. Neonates with a structurally normal heart can tolerate periods of SVT before becoming hemodynamically unstable; unless this has not been recognized initially, it is rarely a medical emergency. Pharmacologic management is geared to acute termination of the SVT followed by primary and secondary long-term pharmacologic management to prevent reoccurrence in the neonatal/early-infant period. It is easier to understand the broad class of agents to consider for treatment as opposed to memorizing individual agents. As a new neonatal nurse practitioner, I found it helpful to then concentrate on the agents that the cardiologists typically used at this particular agency.

Discussion Prompts

1. You are providing management for a 2-day old, 3.5-kg term infant who presented with poor feeding and pallor. Capillary refill time is 5 to 6 seconds. It is noted that the infant's heart rate is 260 beats per minute. An IV is started and subsequent doses of adenosine are given (100 mcg/kg, 200 mcg/kg, and 300 mcg/kg) with no conversion to normal sinus rhythm. Why do you think that normal sinus rhythm was not restored?
2. You are providing management for a 38-day-old, 1.85-kg, 35.1-week-corrected gestational age (CGA) preterm infant. The infant is on full-volume feeds of mother's own milk with human milk fortifier to 24 kcal/oz with a growth pattern over the past 7 days of 10 grams/day. The infant has been working on nippling, taking 52% to 61% on average, but over the past 3 days the total oral volumes have consistently decreased to only 28% in the past 24 hours. On physical exam this morning, the infant is pale, temperature is 98.8°F/37.1°C, heart rate at rest is 210 beats per minute, respiratory rate is 64 breaths per minute, and blood pressure falls in the 65th percentile for CGA. Why do you think this infant is tachycardic? Do you think this infant requires pharmacologic management?
3. You are doing a neonatology consult in the newborn nursery on a 1-day-old term infant due to heart rate of 270 beats per minute. The infant is active, alert, has been breastfeeding well, and has brisk capillary refill. The postpartum nurse noticed the elevated heart rate during her routine shift vital sign checks. Ice was applied to the face with an abrupt termination of the tachycardia to normal sinus rhythm. The infant was transferred to the NICU for closer monitoring and diagnostic workup, which included a comprehensive metabolic panel, CBC with differential, blood gas with lactate, EKG, echocardiogram, and chest x-ray. The infant had an abrupt onset of tachycardia (heart rate of 252 beats per minute) with a pulse oximeter oxygen saturation unchanged at 98% to 100%. An EKG was performed while ice was applied to the face with heart abruptly back to 110 beats; the EKG showed a slurring of the uptake of the QRS complex. Which pharmacologic first-line agent would most likely be started and why would you choose this?

Mind Map

Acute Management

Medication	Mechanism of Action	Monitoring
Adenosine *not prophylactic-short ½ life	• Binds to A_1 receptors • Stimulates K^+ channels and hyperpolarizes cardiac myocytes slowing conduction of AV node • ↓cAMP blocks Co^+ channels • Shortens action potential duration • ↓Diastolic depolarization	• Hypotension • Dyspnea • Irritability • Chest pain

Second-Line Prophylaxis

Medication	Mechanism of Action	Monitoring
Amiodarone	• Blocks K^+ channels, which prolongs the action potential and refractory period duration • ↑Cardiac tissue conduction by blocking Na^+ channels • Slows conduction across the AV node by blocking Ca^{++} channels • Prolongs P-R + Q-T intervals by blocking α and β receptors	• Hypotension • Arrhythmias • Bradycardia • Feeding intolerance • Tissue necrosis from IV site extravasation • Liver/renal/thyroid functions
Flecainide	• ↓Conduction velocity and myocardial excitability by blocking Na^+ channels	• Edema • Liver function • Proarrhythmias
Procainamide	• ↓Conduction velocity and myocardial excitability by blocking Na^+ channels • Delays repolarization	• Hypertension • Serum levels • Feeding intolerance
Sotalol	• Delayed repolarization • Prolonged action potential duration	• Bradycardia • Hypotension • Proarrhythmias • Bronchospasm • Torsade de pointes tachycardia

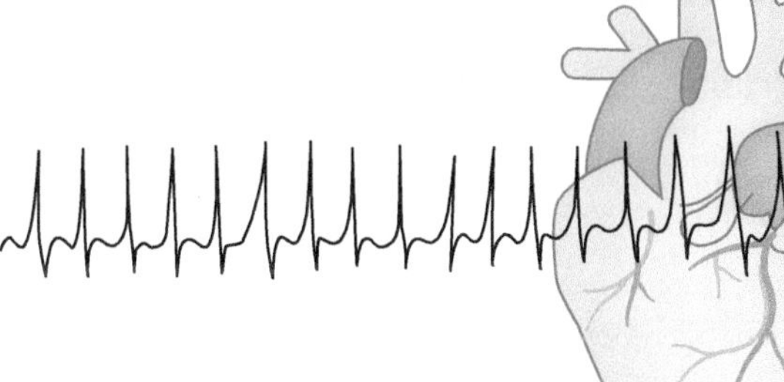

First-Line Prophylaxis

Medication	Mechanism of Action	Monitoring
Digoxin	• ↑Intracellular Ca^{++} to improve myocardial contractility • ↓Extracellular K^+ by inhibiting the Na–K pump • Inhibits ATPase and slows cardiac conduction through AV/SA nodes	• Serum levels for toxicity • Feeding intolerance • Vomiting and diarrhea • Hyperkalemia • Lethargy • Bradycardia
Propranolol	• Blocks β_1 adrenergic receptors to slow heart rate and conduction through AV node	• Hypotension • Bronchospasm • Heart block • Bradycardia • Hypoglycemia

Note: This mind map reflects the design team's interpretation of a portion of one or more concepts addressed in this chapter. Readers should regard the mind maps woven throughout this textbook as examples of multisensory study tools that can be developed to encourage conceptual understanding. Readers are encouraged to develop their own unique mind maps in consultation with academic faculty or clinical preceptors. Design credit: Lindsey Coen, MSN, APRN, NNP-BC, and Samantha Smith, MSN, APRN, NNP.

REFERENCES

References for this chapter are online and available at https://connect.springerpub.com/content/book/978-0-8261-5884-0/part/partIV/toc-part/ch19.

chapter 20

Hypotension and Shock

Jennifer Barnes, Amy J. Jnah, and Patricia L. Dias

LEARNING OBJECTIVES

After completing this chapter, the reader should be able to:

- Define *hypotension* and *shock* and identify the epidemiology of the disease process.
- Explain the physiology of blood pressure (BP) regulation.
- Correlate the pathophysiology of hypotension with the need for pharmacologic treatment.
- Appraise the historical evolution of pharmacologic management of hypotension and shock.
- Evaluate current pharmacologic therapies for treatment of hypotension and shock.

INTRODUCTION

At no other time does the hemodynamic status so drastically and rapidly change as during the transition from fetal to extrauterine life. This transition, in combination with other pertinent disease states, complicates hemodynamic stability. Preterm neonates may experience hypotension due to delayed adaptation to extrauterine life and factors of prematurity such as immature myocardium or secondary to a variety of comorbid states, including but not limited to chorioamnionitis, perinatal asphyxia, hypovolemia, patent ductus arteriosus (PDA), necrotizing enterocolitis, and sepsis. Of those affected by hypotension, approximately 10% to 25% of infants weighing less than 1,500 grams at birth go on to require a vasoactive medication, a relatively static incidence rate (Filippi et al., 2007; Wong et al., 2015). Mortality associated with refractory hypotension is estimated at 31.8% (Ikegami et al., 2010).

The definition of hypotension and the decision to treat are two of the most controversial topics within neonatology. This is in part due to great variability in blood pressure (BP) ranges among neonates. While it is widely known that gestational age, postnatal age including hours from birth, and birth weight factor into BP (Batton et al., 2013), a lack of consensus specific to a definition of hypotension requiring pharmacotherapy persists. Furthermore, there is a dearth of information which correlates which BP values are associated with poor clinical outcomes. In this chapter, we review the definition, pathophysiology, indications for treatment, and pharmacotherapy options for hypotension and shock. In addition, we call attention to seminal and other noteworthy studies that have contributed to the state of the science and helped advance clinical diagnostics and treatment modalities.

DEFINITION OF *HYPOTENSION*

There are two primary methods for measuring BP in a neonate: invasive arterial monitoring and noninvasive monitoring via oscillometric devices. Invasive BP measurement requires umbilical or peripheral arterial access. The pressure transducer in the arterial catheter shows the arterial waveform, which indicates good placement and pressure reliability. Intra-arterial BP monitoring is considered the gold standard BP measurement due to its accuracy and reliability, and because it allows for prompt and frequent BP assessments. Patients with hemodynamic instability should have invasive arterial BP monitoring.

Noninvasive BP monitoring is performed with an oscillometric cuff and monitor. Algorithms within the bedside monitor calculate and display separated systolic, diastolic, and mean arterial blood pressure (MAP) values (Pickering et al., 2005). As the cuff gradually deflates, the maximal amplitude of the pulsation within the artery is considered the MAP. When interpreting the validity of reported values, clinicians must acknowledge that an appropriately sized cuff is important for accurate measurements. The cuff bladder width should be approximately 40% of the arm circumference at the point midway between the olecranon and acromion and thus over the brachial artery. The cuff bladder length should cover 80% to 100% of the circumference of the arm (Batton, 2020). The optimal location of the BP cuff measurement is the right arm because it best reflects the BP of the ascending aorta (Shimokaze et al., 2015).

There is satisfactory literature available that quantifies observed neonatal BP measurements by gestational age, postnatal day of life, and birth weight. Myriad factors affect the postnatal BP, including intrapartum stressors, the rapidly adapting systemic physiology after birth, comorbid conditions linked to preterm birth or critical illness, and variable measurement techniques. Despite this awareness, clinicians are left with an incomplete understanding of how BP values associate with clinical outcomes, such as in cases of impaired cerebral blood flow. As such, there is no generally accepted definition for normotension in the neonatal population.

MAP is most often used to define hyper-, normo-, or hypotensive states in neonates. MAP is calculated as a time-weighted average of systolic blood pressure (SBP) and diastolic blood pressure (DBP) over a cardiac cycle. The most common practice is to define hypotension as MAP lower than the gestational age of the infant (Stranak et al., 2014). This method is likely ubiquitous due to its simplicity and availability. Evidence for this definition is lacking despite its widespread use.

BP dramatically increases over the first hours and week of life; however, comorbid conditions affect BP trends, most significantly within the first hours after birth (Hegyi et al., 1994). Hegyi et al. (1994–1996) investigated SBP and DBP values among preterm infants born between 27 and 36 weeks of gestation and weighing less than 2,000 grams at birth, initially over the first few hours of life followed by trends over the first week of life. Infants were stratified by exposure to maternal hypertension in utero, low Apgar scores at birth, need for mechanical ventilation, and healthy postnatal status. Among infants born preterm, specific to the first 6 hours of postnatal life, SBP and MAP trends did not correlate with gestational age or gender ($p < .05$ Hegyi et al., 1994). However, significant correlations between gestational age and BP ranges were reported across all groups over the first week of life ($p < .05$; Hegyi et al., 1996). Of note, preterm infants who were subject to asphyxia in utero or who received mechanical ventilation manifested with significantly lower SBP and DBP measurements, which subsequently rose over the first week of life, compared with healthy counterparts ($p < .05$). Similarly, the Philadelphia Neonatal Blood Pressure Study Group reported that birth weight and gestational age strongly correlated with SBP on the first day of life for patients admitted to NICUs (Zubrow et al., 1995). BP steadily rose during the first 5 days of life; a more gradual rise in SBP was noted after the first 5 days of life ($p < .05$; Figure 20.1; Zubrow et al., 1995).

An alternative definition for *hypotension* is a noninvasive BP measurement at or below the fifth percentile for gestational and postnatal age (using published percentile references). The most noteworthy study that significantly contributed to this database of percentile references was published by Alonzo et al. (2020). Their work reviewed two billion BP values obtained from over 1,700 neonates and reported moderate correlations between simultaneous noninvasive and invasive BP measurements (Tables 20.1 and 20.2; Alonzo et al., 2020). Readers are encouraged to take time to compare and contrast the invasive and noninvasive MAP values at the fifth percentile as compared with the aforementioned definition for hypotension, which is limited to a MAP that falls below gestational age at birth.

FIGURE 20.1 Systolic and diastolic blood pressure values in the first 5 days of life stratified by gestational age.

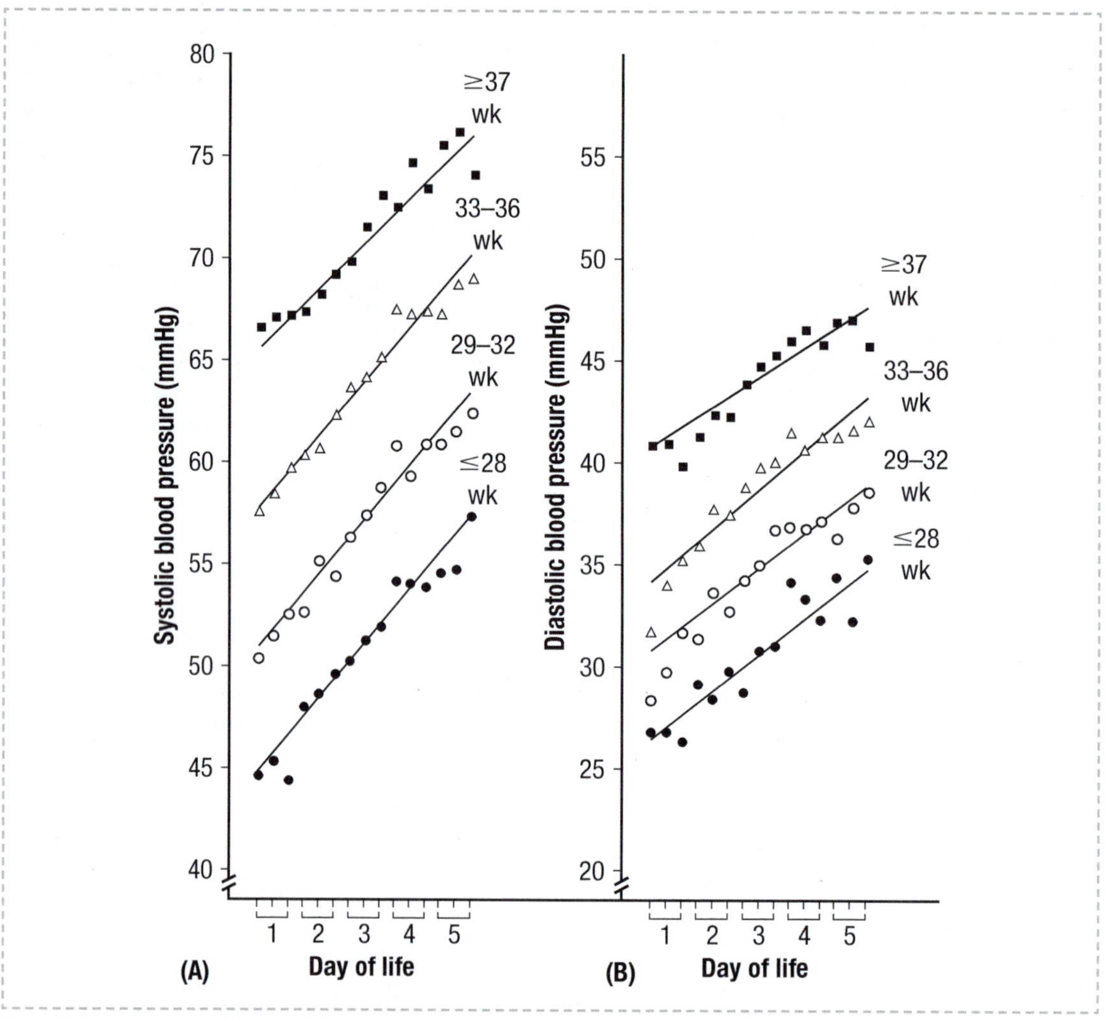

Note: (A) Systolic blood pressure and (B) diastolic blood pressure plotted for the first 5 days of life divided into 8-hour time intervals. Infants were placed into four groups by gestational age: ≤28 weeks (n = 33), 29 to 32 weeks (n = 73), 33 to 36 weeks (n = 100), and ≥37 weeks (n = 110).
Source: From Zubrow, A. B., Hulman, S., Kushner, H., & Falkner, B. (1995). Determinants of blood pressure in infants admitted to neonatal intensive care units: A prospective multicenter study. Philadelphia Neonatal Blood Pressure Study Group. *Journal of Perinatology: Official Journal of the California Perinatal Association, 15*(6), 470–479.

Despite the lack of consensus on hypotensive BP values, BP values are still used as a surrogate marker for underlying pathology in conjunction with clinical findings. A low BP value in conjunction with clinical and/or biochemical markers of tissue ischemia may serve as the best functional definition of hypotensive shock.

PHYSIOLOGY REVIEW: BLOOD PRESSURE REGULATION

As previously discussed, BP is a calculated measurement of the pressure of the circulating blood during a cardiac cycle. Mathematically, MAP is calculated by multiplying left ventricular cardiac output (LVO) by the systemic vascular resistance (SVR). Although APRNs will not be independently calculating MAP, they are responsible for identifying factors that implicate dynamic changes in BP. Adequate BP is necessary to maintain an optimal balance between oxygen delivery to the tissues, cellular health, and later oxygen consumption by those target tissues.

TABLE 20.1 Invasive Mean Arterial Pressure Percentile Reference Table

		DAY OF LIFE						
GESTATIONAL AGE	MAP PERCENTILE	1	2	3	4	5	6	7
23	5th	21	25	25	25	25	26	24
	95th	37	41	47	46	46	43	40
24	5th	22	25	25	26	25	25	25
	95th	38	43	44	46	46	45	44
25	5th	24	27	27	27	27	27	27
	95th	39	43	44	46	47	47	47
26	5th	25	27	27	27	27	27	27
	95th	41	45	49	48	48	52	51
27	5th	25	27	28	28	27	26	28
	95th	43	46	46	51	44	45	45
28	5th	26	30	30	30	31	30	30
	95th	44	46	48	48	50	48	50
29	5th	29	32	32	32	31	31	32
	95th	49	53	54	52	50	51	55
30	5th	29	32	33	33	32	29	31
	95th	50	54	54	54	54	52	52
31	5th	29	31	31	33	33	33	28
	95th	49	55	57	61	57	59	59
32	5th	31	33	35	35	34	30	30
	95th	49	52	54	56	55	52	57
33	5th	31	32	32	33	34	32	34
	95th	51	51	51	53	55	58	52
34	5th	32	34	35	33	34	34	34
	95th	54	55	57	58	69	58	59

Note: Gestational age is shown in weeks.
MAP, mean arterial pressure.
Source: From Alonzo, C. J., Nagraj, V. P., Zschaebitz, J. V., Lake, D. E., Moorman, J. R., & Spaeder, M. C. (2020). Blood pressure ranges via non-invasive and invasive monitoring techniques in premature neonates using high resolution physiologic data. *Journal of Neonatal-Perinatal Medicine, 13*(3), 351–358. https://doi.org/10.3233/NPM-190260.

Cardiac output (CO), which regulates the rate of oxygen delivery to target tissues, is the product of the heart rate (HR) and stroke volume (SV). The HR is contingent on proper autonomic nervous system (ANS) function, as the ANS (made up of the sympathetic and parasympathetic systems) is responsible for stimulating and regulating the rate of cardiac conduction (Figure 20.2). Sympathetic activity is directed to the actin and myosin portions of cardiomyocytes, affecting cardiac contractility. Parasympathetic activity regulates HR in times of stress through the release of acetylcholine, which lowers the HR. Autonomic activity regulates the activity of baroreceptors located at the carotid arteries and aortic arch, which stimulate either vasoconstriction or vasodilation. *Stroke volume* refers to the amount of blood that is ejected from the left ventricle (LV) and is contingent on adequate cardiac preload (force of contraction to eject blood from the ventricles), afterload (force the heart must pump against), and contractility (contractile force of the cardiomyocytes).

The humoral mechanism that contributes to cardiovascular tone and BP is the renin–angiotensin–aldosterone system (RAAS). The RAAS compensatory response is delayed but will sense decreased CO at the afferent arteriole. In response, juxtaglomerular cells located at the afferent arteriole secrete renin, a vasoconstrictive hormone. Renin travels through the circulation and interacts with angiotensinogen to form angiotensin 1. Angiotensin I interacts with the angiotensin converting enzyme (ACE) and changes to its bioactive form, angiotensin II. Angiotensin II thereby stimulates the renal cortex to secrete aldosterone (to encourage sodium and water reabsorption).

TABLE 20.2 Noninvasive Mean Arterial Pressure Percentile Reference Table

GESTATIONAL AGE	MAP PERCENTILE	POSTMENSTRUAL AGE															
		23	24	25	26	27	28	29	30	31	32	33	34	35	36	37	38
23	5th	26	26	27	27	28	30	31	33	33	34	36	38	37	39	42	42
	95th	51	54	51	52	51	55	56	60	59	62	64	66	67	69	69	73
24	5th		26	27	27	28	30	32	33	34	36	37	37	39	41	43	43
	95th		51	50	54	53	57	58	59	60	63	64	64	66	69	72	73
25	5th			26	29	29	31	32	33	33	35	36	38	39	40	41	44
	95th			49	50	53	55	56	58	60	61	62	64	67	68	69	69
26	5th				27	29	31	32	33	35	35	36	36	39	39	41	42
	95th				50	51	57	57	58	61	62	62	64	66	69	71	73
27	5th					29	30	32	33	34	34	35	36	37	39	40	41
	95th					50	55	56	58	60	61	62	64	66	68	72	72
28	5th						29	32	33	34	35	36	36	37	41	40	43
	95th						52	56	58	60	61	62	63	66	68	70	74
29	5th							31	34	35	35	36	37	38	39	41	40
	95th							55	59	61	61	63	64	65	67	68	69
30	5th								32	35	36	37	36	37	37	39	41
	95th								55	61	62	63	63	64	66	66	67
31	5th									33	36	37	37	36	36	38	39
	95th									58	61	64	64	66	66	68	71
32	5th										33	36	38	38	38	37	38
	95th										58	62	63	65	66	66	86
33	5th											34	36	38	39	38	39
	95th											58	63	64	65	66	65
34	5th												35	37	37	37	39
	95th												61	64	64	67	70

Note: Gestational age and postmenstrual age are shown in weeks.
MAP, mean arterial pressure.
Source: From Alonzo, C. J., Nagraj, V. P., Zschaebitz, J. V., Lake, D. E., Moorman, J. R., & Spaeder, M. C. (2020). Blood pressure ranges via non-invasive and invasive monitoring techniques in premature neonates using high resolution physiologic data. *Journal of Neonatal-Perinatal Medicine, 13*(3), 351–358. https://doi.org/10.3233/NPM-190260.

FIGURE 20.2 Neural control of blood pressure (autonomic activity).

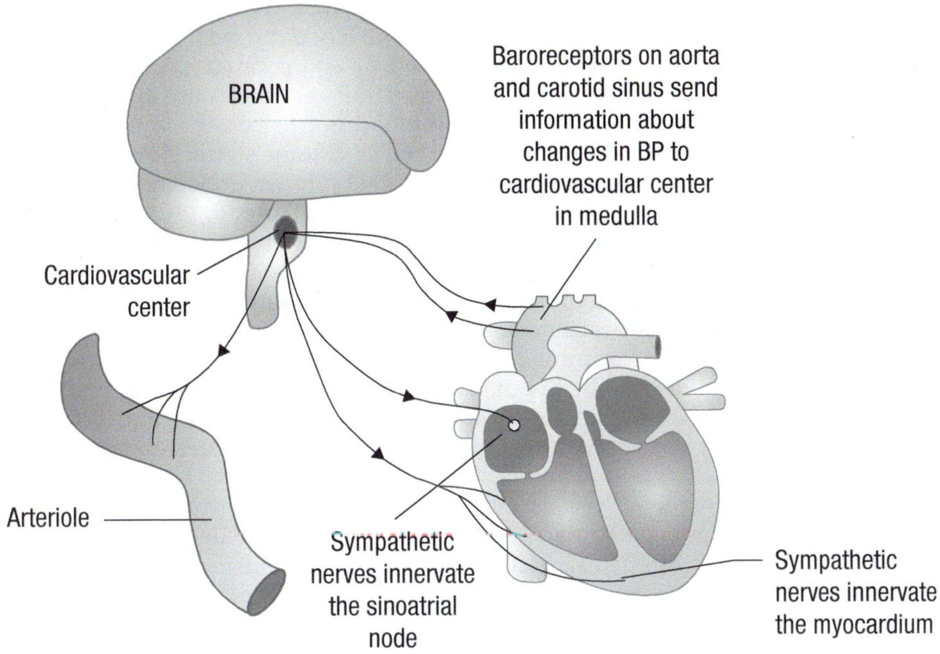

Note: In response to a drop in BP, the autonomic nervous system acts on the baroreceptors to send impulses to the brain, which stimulates the sympathetic nervous system to vasoconstrict or vasodilate to alter blood flow.
BP, blood pressure.
Source: From Shead, S. L. (2015). Pathophysiology of the Cardiovascular System and Neonatal Hypotension. *Neonatal Network. 34*(1):31-9. doi: 10.1891/0730-0832.34.1.31. PMID: 26803043, http://www.academyofneonatalnursing.org/NNT/Cardiac_Pathophysiology.pdf.

At the same time, angiotensin II stimulates the posterior pituitary gland to release stored antidiuretic hormone (ADH; also called *vasopressin*), in an attempt to elicit vasoconstriction and water retention at the distal collecting duct of the nephron. In aggregate, aldosterone and ADH; seek to increase plasma volume.

Chemical mechanisms that impact cardiovascular tone include arterial concentrations of carbon dioxide ($PaCO_2$) and oxygen (PaO_2). For example, a decrease in $PaCO_2$ leads to cerebral vasoconstriction. It is therefore important to tightly regulate acid–base balance during periods of hypotension, as chemical imbalances can exacerbate this pathophysiologic state.

Putting the relevant core concepts together, clinicians should recognize that a decrease in HR, SV, or a combination of both factors, as well as hypoxia or hypocarbia, may reduce CO and BP. Research points to changes in SV as the primary factor that implicates changes in BP and CO among term and preterm infants (de Waal et al., 2017).

PATHOPHYSIOLOGY REVIEW: HYPOTENSION

Hypotension in the neonate is a common symptom of various different pathophysiologic processes. Because BP is the product of CO and SVR, a decrease in one or both parameters will lead to low BP. Determining whether CO or SVR is affected may help to identify the underlying etiology of hypotension in a particular patient. Diagnostic tools such as echocardiography and physical exam can provide additional information on CO and SVR. As previously discussed, most clinicians rely on the MAP to diagnose hypotension, but remember that the MAP is an average of SBP and DBP over a cardiac cycle. Evaluating these two components separately may provide more information on CO and SVR than the MAP alone. For example, consider an infant with a BP of 64/13 mmHg and another infant with a BP of 36/27 mmHg, both have an MAP of 30, but they may be affected by completely different etiologies.

SBP reflects the force of circulating blood exerted on the walls of blood vessels when the heart is contracting. SBP is directly proportional to the SV of the LV. Low SBP suggests a diminished SV and thus a low CO (because CO is the product of SV and HR). A low SV may be attributed broadly to three main factors: low left ventricular preload (not enough blood can get into the LV), high left ventricular afterload (not enough blood can get out of the LV), and poor contractility (not enough LV squeeze). There are many contributing factors that affect SBP and thus cause low CO (Figure 20.3).

DBP, in contrast, reflects the force of circulating blood exerted on the walls of blood vessels when the heart is at rest. It is influenced by SVR as well as volume status. Low DBP suggests low SVR and/or low intravascular volume (from either a total body water deficit or capillary leakage with third spacing). SVR is influenced by the size of the vascular bed, vessel radius, and blood viscosity. Thus, low SVR may be due to an increased number of blood vessels the LV has to fill, vasodilation, or decreased blood viscosity (Figure 20.4).

Combined systolic and diastolic hypotension may be due to multiple etiologies in the same patient, or (more likely) represent continued hemodynamic stress with resulting failure of the entire cardiovascular system. For example, septic shock may initially begin with vasodilation, leading to decreased SVR and diastolic hypotension. This diastolic hypotension can then lead to inadequate end-organ perfusion, which increases lactate production. This metabolic acidosis, in turn, may affect contractility of the myocardium, ultimately leading to decreased CO and systolic hypotension.

Preterm infants are at increased risk of hypotension. In fact, approximately 19% of preterm infants develop hypotension, in particular during the immediate time period after birth (Paradisis et al., 2009). Preterm birth is tightly associated with a delayed transition from fetal to postnatal cardiovascular function. The persistence of fetal circulation, namely at the PDA, results in reduced CO and decreased perfusion to the adrenal glands and nephron. In addition, myocardial function

FIGURE 20.3 Factors leading to low systolic blood pressure and cardiac output.

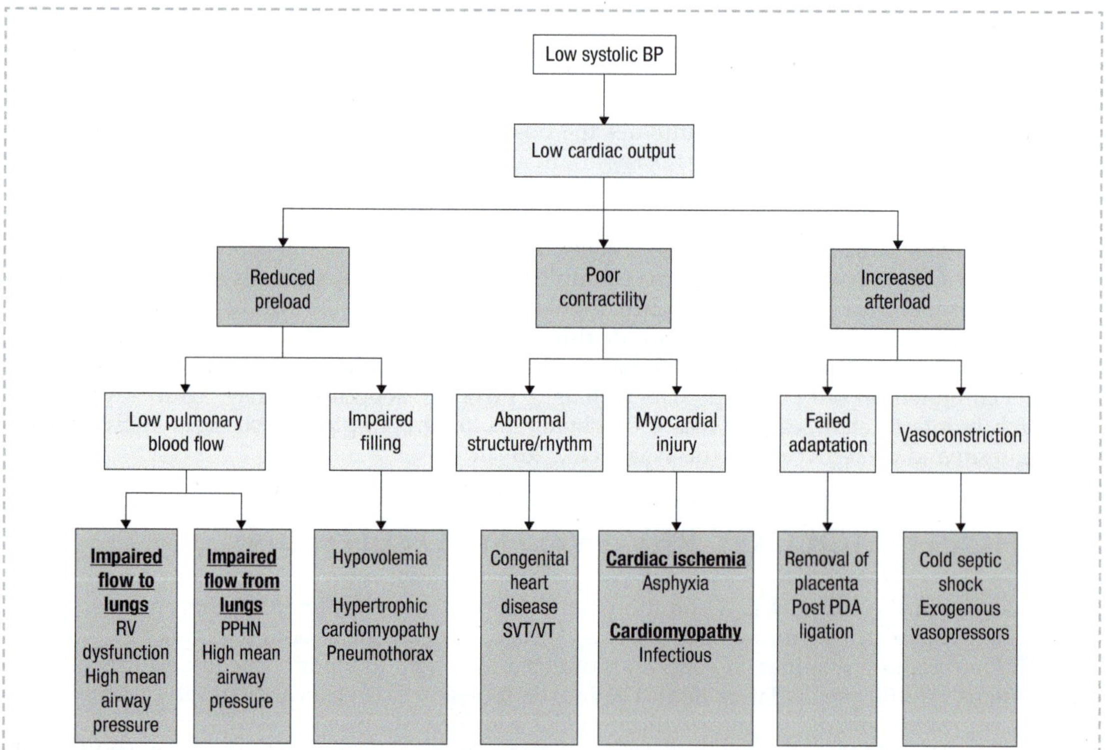

Note: There may be multiple contributing factors leading to an additive effect.

BP, blood pressure; PDA, patent ductus arteriosus; PPHN, persistent pulmonary hypertension; RV, right ventricular; SVT, supraventricular tachycardia; VT, ventricular tachycardia.

Source: Adapted from Giesinger, R. E., & McNamara, P. J. (2016). Hemodynamic instability in the critically ill neonate: An approach to cardiovascular support based on disease pathophysiology. *Seminars in Perinatology, 40*(3), 174–188. https://doi.org/10.1053/j.semperi.2015.12.005.

FIGURE 20.4 Factors leading to low diastolic blood pressure and systemic vascular resistance.

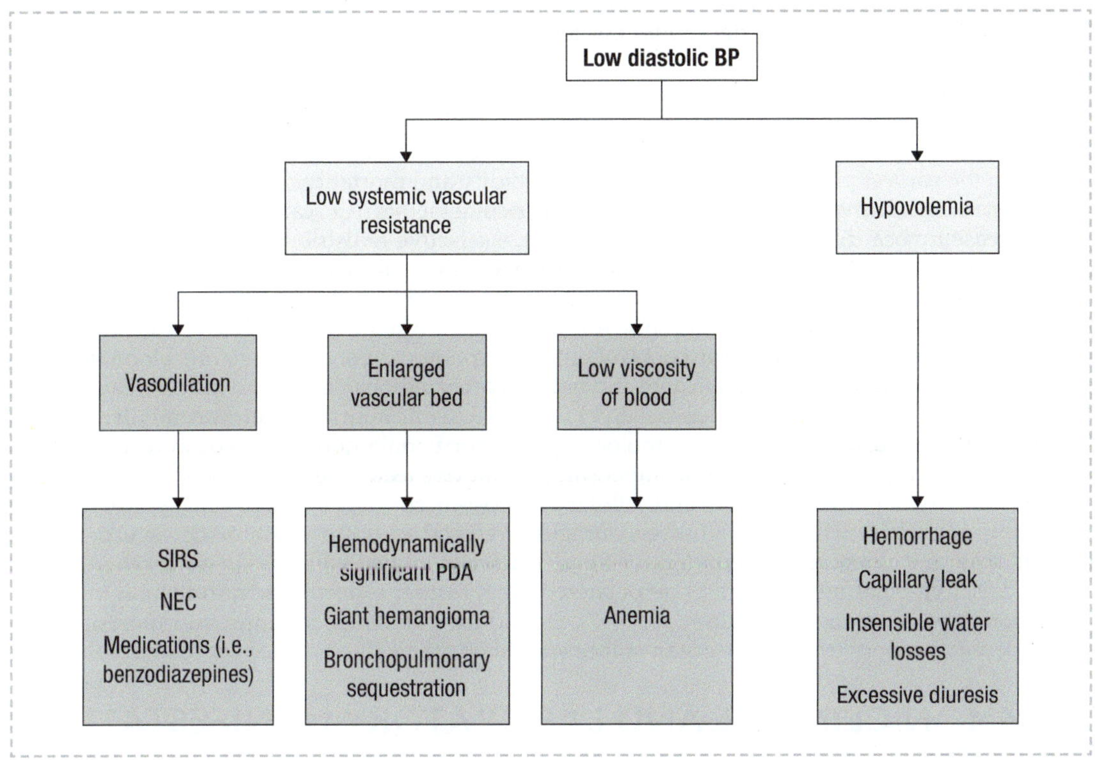

BP, blood pressure; NEC, necrotizing enterocolitis; PDA, patent ductus arteriosus; SIRS, systemic inflammatory response syndrome.
Source: Adapted from Giesinger, R. E., & McNamara, P. J. (2016). Hemodynamic instability in the critically ill neonate: An approach to cardiovascular support based on disease pathophysiology. *Seminars in Perinatology, 40*(3), 174–188. https://doi.org/10.1053/j.semperi.2015.12.005.

(contractility) is immature due to reduced energy stores and mitochondrial activity. In utero, the immature myocardium pumps against the low-resistance placental circulation. At birth, the placenta is removed and thus SVR is abruptly increased. The immature myocardium of a preterm infant may be poorly adapted to overcome this increased afterload, leading to decreased blood flow. Preterm infants may be subject to this state of varied low to low-normal systemic blood flow (SBF) over the first 24 hours of life. This is particularly concerning within the cerebral vasculature, as the reperfusion process is associated with an increased risk of acquired intraventricular hemorrhage (Kluckow & Evans, 2000; Noori et al., 2014).

Vasopressor-resistant hypotension (VRH) develops when hypotensive neonates do not respond to vasopressor or inotrope therapy. More specific, VRH is commonly defined as severe hypotension resulting in inadequate end-organ perfusion despite dopamine and/or dobutamine therapy at doses of 20 mcg/kg/min. Inadequate end-organ perfusion is suspected when oliguria persists for more than 8 hours. This information should assist readers as the chapter progresses and the discussion shifts to currently available pharmacologic management strategies.

PATHOPHYSIOLOGY REVIEW: SHOCK

It is important to note that hypotension in a neonate does not always indicate the presence of shock. *Shock* is defined as a state of cardiovascular compromise that develops when tissues are inadequately supplied with oxygen necessary for cellular and metabolic function. Common etiologies include myocardial dysfunction (*cardiogenic shock*), abnormal distribution of blood volume (*distributive shock*), cardiopulmonary flow restriction (*obstructive shock*), and inadequate blood volume (*hypovolemic shock*). Risk factors for cardiogenic shock include prematurity (immature function), a delayed transition to extrauterine life (poor response to increased left ventricular afterload), or structural heart disease (e.g., ductal-dependent lesion, tachyarrhythmia). Septic shock, a form of distributive shock, is more commonly linked to gram-negative sepsis. Obstructive shock is associated with conditions such as cardiac tamponade and persistent pulmonary hypertension. Hypovolemic shock is less commonly diagnosed in the neonatal population but can be associated with acute blood loss secondary to intrapartum injuries, including fetal–maternal hemorrhage and placental abruption (Singh et al., 2018).

Hypotension, which is commonly used to define shock states in adults, is generally a late finding of shock in neonates. The phases of shock include an initial compensatory phase, uncompensated phase, and a more ominous irreversible phase (Noori et al., 2017). Timely identification of shock, ideally in the earliest phase, is critical to reduce morbidity and mortality risks. The initial compensatory phase of shock involves the release of vasoconstricting factors (e.g., catecholamines, vasopressin) that increase myocardial contractility and HR. Next, a selective redistribution of blood flow to vital organs (e.g., heart, adrenal glands) occurs and urinary output decreases. Although readers may be inclined to assume that the brain will receive preferential blood flow during the early phase of shock, this is not always true. Research has shown that the cerebral cortex is not necessarily considered "vital" in extremely low-birth-weight (ELBW) infants experiencing shock; therefore, blood flow may be preferentially shunted to the brainstem and not the cortex region (Wardle et al., 2000). This puts the ELBW infant at high risk for shock-associated hypoxic ischemic injury and intraventricular bleeding during later reperfusion. Should the pathology persist, hormonal modulation/compensation will be depleted, marking the start of the uncompensated phase of shock. The synthesis of reactive oxygen species (namely, superoxide) surges and cellular apoptosis occurs. An influx of acute-phase reactants including proinflammatory cytokines encourages overproduction of nitric oxide, which induces vasodilation and worsens the hypotensive state. Intracellular potassium leaks out of the cell, and blood vessel vasculature becomes hyperpolarized. This further exacerbates vasodilation through a reduction in vascular tone (Quayle et al., 1997). Should the pathology continue, an irreversible state of shock will develop. Irreversible organ failure and death are likely.

COMMON CLINICAL AND LABORATORY MANIFESTATIONS OF SHOCK

Clinical signs of shock are often nonspecific but very important in determining whether symptomatic hypoperfusion is present. Tachycardia (HR >180 beats per minute) is often an early sign of shock. Decreased peripheral perfusion may be exhibited as pallor, acrocyanosis, cool extremities, and a delayed capillary refill greater than 4 seconds (Miletin et al., 2009). Respiratory complications, such as tachypnea, apnea, and hypoxemia, can also be present. In addition, signs of renal or gastrointestinal dysfunction could represent the compensatory mechanism to maintain adequate perfusion to vital organs (e.g., heart, adrenal glands) at the expense of splanchnic and renal perfusion. Urine output should be monitored and followed closely as a marker of organ perfusion.

Laboratory findings can also help clinicians in the diagnosis of hypotensive shock and decipher the degree of hypoperfusion. The most common biochemical marker of shock is metabolic acidosis, evidenced by elevated serum lactate and decreased serum bicarbonate. Hyperglycemia may also be present due to catecholamine release, except in cases of shock with relative adrenal insufficiency.

DIFFERENTIAL DIAGNOSIS OF HYPOTENSION AND SHOCK

There are numerous etiologies for both hypotension and shock. A discussion of each extends beyond the scope of the chapter; however, Figures 20.3 and 20.4 organize specific causes of neonatal hypotension by their common pathophysiology. Determining the likely etiology of an infant's hypotension allows the clinician to generate an inclusive differential diagnosis and prescribe medications that target the desired physiologic action while avoiding deleterious side effects. As an example, consider again our patient with septic shock. The initial decrease in SVR may be appropriately treated with a medication that causes peripheral vasoconstriction, but if the patient later develops poor cardiac contractility, then afterload reduction may be needed. Specific actions of the commonly used medications for cardiovascular support in the neonate are reviewed in the Current Pharmacological Treatment Modalities section.

HISTORICAL PERSPECTIVE: SEMINAL AND OTHER NOTEWORTHY STUDIES

Hypotension is among the most common problems encountered in the NICU, and yet how to treat neonatal hypotension is fraught with controversy (Evans, 2006; Short et al., 2006). Due to the inherent challenges to conducting randomized controlled trials (RCTs) in this population, there is astonishingly little evidence to guide hemodynamic support of the critically ill neonate (Dempsey & El-Khuffash, 2020; Garvey et al., 2018). Most published trials are underpowered and therefore do not permit clinicians to draw any meaningful conclusions about long-term outcomes. Further, the heterogenous nature of the study populations, inclusion and exclusion criteria, treatments, and outcomes limit the utility of subsequent meta-analyses (Dempsey & El-Khuffash, 2020). As you will discover by reading this section of the chapter, the majority of trials were performed over 20 years ago. Much has changed in the overall management of very premature infants in recent decades, and the state of the science specific to management of hypotension and shock does not completely reflect those changes. Furthermore, prematurity affects the cardiovascular system and receptor maturity, which complicates expected the dose–effect response to various inotropes and vasopressors. Individual and institutional preferences weigh heavily in the choice of drug and the threshold for initiating treatment, leading to significant variation among neonatal clinicians in their approach to infants with low BP (Batton et al., 2013; Rios et al., 2014; Stranak et al., 2014).

The following section serves as a concise overview of the evidence available to guide our choices of the therapeutic agents discussed in the Current Pharmacologic Treatment Modalities for Hypotension and Shock section of this chapter. Table 20.3 is provided to offer readers a more complete look at the relevant RCTs investigating treatments for neonatal hypotension, highlighting those included in various meta-analyses. There are several trends to appreciate when perusing this table. First, most of the trials studied preterm infants, with few studies focusing on term neonates. Second, a number of the studies enrolled infants on the basis of criteria other than hemodynamic status; thus, not all enrolled patients were hypotensive. Third, the majority of patients in these trials were less than 24 hours old, suggesting that delayed transition physiology caused or at least contributed to any cardiovascular instability. Last, there were few appreciable differences in long-term outcomes, likely because of the small numbers of neonates enrolled.

Therefore, despite decades of research, there is still no definitive evidence regarding the impact of treatment for neonatal hypotension, aside from the fact that vasopressors do tend to increase BP (Dempsey & El-Khuffash, 2020; Gupta & Donn, 2014). Dempsey and El Khuffash (2020) offer valuable perspective on the difficulties associated with conducting trials in neonates with hypotension; readers are directed to this excellent review of RCTs conducted in the preterm population for further information.

Preventive Measures

The incidence of hypotension in preterm neonates has decreased in recent years. The most predominant perinatal and postnatal factors leading to this decline include antenatal steroid administration, delayed cord clamping, and a reduction in mechanical ventilation.

Demarini et al. found that very-low-birth-weight infants whose mothers received antenatal steroids had increased BPs during the first 24 hours of life (Demarini et al., 1999). In another study, even incomplete antenatal corticosteroid treatment was associated with a 35% risk reduction in vasopressor requirement when adjusting for gestational age (Elimian et al., 2003). Continued flow in the umbilical vein and arteries at birth through delayed cord clamping may assist with the transition from fetal to neonatal circulation. A recent Cochrane review showed that delayed cord clamping improved infants' MAP in the early hours after birth. Furthermore, a statistically significant reduction in inotropic medications during the first 24 hours of life was also seen with delayed cord clamping (Rabe et al., 2012).

Several studies have shown that mechanical ventilation in preterm infants increases the risk of hypotension due to a negative correlation between increasing mean airway pressures and MAP (Evans & Kluckow, 1996; Kluckow & Evans, 1996; Lakkundi et al., 2014).

In summary, antenatal steroids, delayed cord clamping, and reductions in mechanical ventilation immediately after birth have decreased the frequency of hypotension in the early preterm infant due to improvements in transition to extrauterine life.

TABLE 20.3 Summary of Seminal and Noteworthy Studies Investigating Treatments for Neonatal Hypotension

	AUTHOR, YEAR	POPULATION	INTERVENTIONS	NUMBER	CONCLUSIONS	META-ANALYSES
Volume expansion	Northern Neonatal Nursing Initiative Trial Group, 1996 (The Northern Neonatal Nursing Initiative [NNNI] Trial Group, 1996)	Infants <32 weeks at <2 HOL	FFP versus gelatin-based plasma substitute versus maintenance fluids only	776	Early prophylactic volume expansion had no effect on short-term outcomes (including mortality, P/IVH, PVL, renal impairment, incidence of hypotension, or treatment failure for hypotensive subgroup). A follow-up study showed no difference in risk of severe disability, cerebral palsy, or combined death/severe disability at 2 years of age. (Tin et al., 1996)	Overall conclusions from this Cochrane review (Osborn, 2004): There is insufficient evidence to support volume expansion in very preterm infants, whether hemodynamically stable or with evidence of cardiovascular compromise. Outcomes with meta-analysis: (a) For studies comparing volume expansion with no treatment, there was no difference in mortality (4 studies; Beverley et al., 1985; Gottuso et al., 1976; Lundstrøm et al., 2000; Tin et al., 1996), P/IVH (3 studies; Beverley et al., 1985; Ekblad et al., 1991; Tin et al., 1996), PVL (2 studies; Lundstrøm et al., 2000; Tin et al., 1996), or PDA (2 studies; Beverley et al., 1985; Ekblad et al., 1991). (b) For studies comparing albumin 5% with normal saline in hypotensive infants, there was no difference in mortality, P/IVH, or treatment failure (2 studies; Ekblad et al., 1991; Lynch et al., 2008).
	Beverley et al., 1985	Infants <32 weeks or <1.5 kg at <24 HOL	FFP versus no treatment	73	Prophylactic FFP was associated with a reduction in P/IVH; there was no difference in mortality.	
	Ekblad et al., 1991 and 1992	Infants <35 weeks at <5 HOL	FFP versus no treatment	38	FFP did not significantly influence the pattern of weight change, change in extracellular volume, creatinine clearance, or urinary fractional sodium excretion in the first 5 days of life.	
	Emery et al., 1992	Hypotensive infants <36 weeks at <5 DOL	Albumin 4.5% versus FFP versus control group (5 mL/kg of albumin 20%)	60	Albumin 4.5% and FFP were both associated with a greater increase in MAP compared with the control group. No difference in duration of ventilation was found.	
	Gottuso et al., 1976	Infants <2 kg at <24 HOL	FFP versus no treatment (a third group randomized to exchange transfusion was excluded from the Cochrane review)	59	There was no difference in mortality.	

	Lundstrøm et al., 2000	Normotensive infants <33 weeks at <10 DOL	Albumin 20% versus no treatment (a third group randomized to dopamine was excluded from the Cochrane review)	25	Albumin was associated with a nonsignificant trend toward increased LVO and CBF but had no effect on MAP, PVL, or mortality.	
	Lynch et al., 2008	Hypotensive infants at <4 DOL	Albumin 5% versus normal saline	101	Albumin was associated with a reduction in treatment failure and an increase in MAP.	
	So et al., 1997	Hypotensive infants <35 weeks and <2 kg at <3 HOL	Albumin 5% versus normal saline	63	There was no difference in MAP, treatment failure, CLD, or mortality. Those treated with albumin had more evidence of fluid retention in the first 48 HOL.	
Ino-trope versus volume expan-sion						
	Gill and Weindling, 1993	Hypotensive infants ≤1.5 kg at <24 HOL	Dopamine versus plasma protein fraction (similar to albumin 4.5%)	39	Dopamine was more effective at increasing BP and had a lower rate of treatment failure. Albumin was associated with an increased rate of grade 2–4 P/IVH of borderline statistical significance. There was no difference in mortality, CLD, or ROP. Of note, nearly half of all patients received 20 mL/kg of plasma protein fraction before enrollment for presumed shock.	Overall conclusions from this Cochrane review (Osborn, 2001): There is not enough evidence to determine whether volume expansion or dopamine should be used in preterm infants. Dopamine was superior at increasing blood pressure in hypotensive infants. Neither intervention improved morbidity (P/IVH, CLD, ROP) or mortality. Neither study reported neurodevelopmental outcome.
	Lundstrøm et al., 2000	Normotensive infants <33 DOL	Dopamine versus albumin 20% (a control group receiving no treatment was excluded from the Cochrane review)	24	Dopamine produced a greater percentage increase in MAP compared with volume expansion and no treatment. Both interventions produced similar increases in LVO. Compared with the control group, neither intervention led to a difference in mortality, PVL, or CBF.	

(Continued)

TABLE 20.3 Summary of Seminal and Noteworthy Studies Investigating Treatments for Neonatal Hypotension (*continued*)

	AUTHOR, YEAR	POPULATION	INTERVENTIONS	NUMBER	CONCLUSIONS	META-ANALYSES
Inotrope versus Inotrope						
	Greenough and Emery, 1993	Infants ≤34 weeks with refractory hypotension (s/p volume expansion) at <7 DOL	Dopamine versus dobutamine	40	Dopamine was more effective at increasing BP and had a lower rate of treatment failure.	Overall conclusions from this Cochrane review (Subhedar & Shaw, 2003): No recommendations can be made given the lack of long-term benefit and safety data. Dopamine was more effective in the short-term treatment of hypotensive preterm neonates, although one study showed that dobutamine was more effective at increasing cardiac output (as evidenced by LVO). No study reported data on long-term outcomes. Outcomes with meta-analyses: (a) There was no difference in mortality or PVL (3 studies; Hentschel et al., 1995; Klarr et al., 1994; Rozé et al., 1993), or in grade 3–4 P/IVH (2 studies; Hentschel et al., 1995; Klarr et al., 1994). (b) Dopamine had a lower rate of treatment failure (4 studies Greenough & Emery, 1993; Klarr et al., 1994; Ruelas-Orozco & Vargas-Origel, 2000).
	Rozé et al., 1993	Infants <32 weeks with refractory hypotension (s/p volume expansion)	Dopamine versus dobutamine	20	Dopamine was more effective at increasing/sustaining MAP and trended toward a lower rate of treatment failure; however, dopamine decreased LVO, and dobutamine increased LVO. There was no difference in mortality or PVL.	
	Klarr et al., 1994	Infants ≤34 weeks with RDS and refractory hypotension (s/p volume expansion) at <24 HOL	Dopamine versus dobutamine	63	Dopamine was more effective at increasing BP and trended toward a lower rate of treatment failure. There was no difference in mortality, PVL, or grade 3–4 P/IVH.	
	Hentschel et al., 1995	Infants <37 weeks with refractory hypotension (s/p volume expansion) at <18 DOL	Dopamine versus dobutamine	20	Both interventions were equally effective at increasing MAP and intestinal perfusion (as evidenced by the SMA resistance index). There was no difference in mortality, PVL, or grade 3–4 P/IVH.	
	Ruelas-Orozco and Vargas-Origel, 2000	Infants <37 weeks and ≤1.5kg with refractory hypotension (s/p volume expansion) at <72 HOL	Dopamine versus dobutamine	66	Both interventions were equally effective at increasing MAP. Dopamine trended toward a lower rate of treatment failure.	

	Osborn et al., 2002	Infants <30 weeks with low SVC flow at <12 HOL	Dopamine versus dobutamine (both groups also received normal saline 10 mL/kg)	42	Dobutamine (at the highest dose) produced a greater increase in SVC flow, whereas dopamine resulted in a greater increase in MAP. There was no difference in treatment failure, morbidity (including P/IVH, PVL, NEC, CLD, renal impairment, or ROP), or mortality. A follow-up study showed no difference in cerebral palsy, deafness, or combined death/disability at 3 years of age (Osborn, 2005). Infants treated with dobutamine had a higher developmental quotient, but there was no difference in developmental quotient >2 *SD* below the norm.	Osborn et al., (2002) was the only study eligible for inclusion in a Cochrane review designed to determine the effects of specific inotropes on preterm infants with low SBF. The authors observed that infants receiving dopamine had a greater increase in MAP but little change in SVC flow or RVO. Conversely, infants treated with dobutamine had little change in MAP but a greater increase in SVC flow (a proxy for SBF) at the highest dose (20 mcg/kg/min). Treatment failure was common in both groups (40% of all enrolled neonates did not improve or maintain normal SVC flow). Overall conclusions: Dobutamine was more effective than dopamine at increasing and maintaining SBF, but there was no evidence of any difference in clinical outcomes.
	Filippi et al., 2007	Infants <1.5 kg with refractory hypotension (s/p volume expansion) at <24 HOL	Dopamine versus dobutamine	35	Both interventions increased SBP, but dopamine was more effective. Dopamine was associated with short-term pituitary suppression (as evidenced by reduced serum levels of thyroid-stimulating hormone, total thyroxine, and prolactin), but levels rebounded within 1 day of stopping dopamine. Dobutamine did not alter any hormone levels.	

(*Continued*)

TABLE 20.3 Summary of Seminal and Noteworthy Studies Investigating Treatments for Neonatal Hypotension (*continued*)

	AUTHOR, YEAR	POPULATION	INTERVENTIONS	NUMBER	CONCLUSIONS	META-ANALYSES
	Phillipos et al., 1996	Hypotensive infants at <24 HOL (available data only include infants >1.75 kg)	Dopamine versus epinephrine	20	Both interventions increased mean HR and MAP from baseline (although it was not reported whether there was a difference between the two groups). Dopamine significantly decreased LV stroke volume from baseline, but neither drug had a significant effect on LVO or RVO. There were no data on other clinically important outcomes, including treatment failure, neurodevelopmental impairment, or mortality.	Phillipos et al. (1996) was the only study eligible for inclusion in a Cochrane review (Paradisis & Osborn, 2004) designed to determine the effectiveness and safety of epinephrine in preterm infants with cardiovascular compromise. Note that this study enrolled both term and preterm infants, but the mean GA was 36 weeks. It was also published in abstract form only and had incomplete data on infants <1.75 kg (who were thus excluded from the meta-analysis). Overall conclusions: There is insufficient evidence on the use of epinephrine in preterm infants.
	Pellicer et al., 2005 and Valverde et al., 2006	Hypotensive infants <32 weeks or ≤1.5 kg at <24 HOL	Dopamine versus epinephrine	60	Both interventions increased MAP, HR, cerebral blood volume, and cerebral intravascular oxygenation from baseline (with the only difference between groups being a higher HR change with epinephrine). Dose escalation of either drug did not affect these variables except for a greater HR with higher doses of epinephrine. There was no difference in the rates of treatment failure. Those receiving epinephrine had higher lactate and glucose levels (requiring more insulin therapy). The authors concluded that both low/moderate-dose dopamine and low-dose epinephrine increased cerebral perfusion and MAP in hypotensive LBW infants, but epinephrine was associated with more (transient) adverse effects. A follow-up study (which included 70 normotensive controls) showed no difference in the rates of abnormal neurologic status, developmental delay, or combined death/cerebral palsy/severe NDI at 2–3 years of age. Pellicer et al., 2009	

	Baske et al., 2018	Infants with fluid-resistant septic shock (defined by the presence of low BP and/or other prespecified criteria)	Dopamine versus epinephrine	40	Of the 40 patients, 35 had late-onset neonatal sepsis, and most were hypotensive. Rates of shock reversal, hemodynamic stability during treatment, duration of treatment, lactate clearance, clinical outcomes (including IVH, BPD, NEC, and ROP), and mortality at 28 DOL were similar between groups. Epinephrine was associated with improved hemodynamic stability during treatment in a subgroup analysis of neonates <31 weeks.	
	Rios and Kaiser, 2015	Hypotensive ELBW infants ≤30 weeks at <24 HOL	Dopamine versus vasopressin	20 (+50 normotensive controls)	Both interventions were equally effective at increasing BP. Vasopressin was associated with less tachycardia, fewer doses of surfactant, and lower $PaCO_2$ values. There were no differences in clinically relevant outcomes or mortality.	
Inotrope/lusitrope versus placebo	DiSessa et al., 1981	Normotensive term infants with asphyxia at <24 HOL	Dopamine	14	Low-dose dopamine increased cardiac performance (as measured by echocardiography) and raised SBP in severely asphyxiated newborns. No differences in mortality or long-term neurodevelopmental outcome were found.	DiSessa et al. (1981) was the only study eligible for inclusion in a Cochrane review (Hunt & Osborn, 2002) designed to determine whether dopamine reduces morbidity/mortality in term newborns with perinatal asphyxia. Overall conclusions: There is insufficient evidence to answer this question.
	Cuevas et al., 1991	Infants <37 weeks with RDS at <24 HOL	Low-dose dopamine	49	In a subset of newborns with hypotension, dopamine was effective at normalizing BP. Low-dose dopamine did not significantly improve acid–base balance or clinical outcomes (mortality, CLD, or duration of oxygen therapy).	

(*Continued*)

TABLE 20.3 Summary of Seminal and Noteworthy Studies Investigating Treatments for Neonatal Hypotension (*continued*)

	AUTHOR, YEAR	POPULATION	INTERVENTIONS	NUMBER	CONCLUSIONS	META-ANALYSES
Steroids	Bravo et al., 2015	Infants <31 weeks in low-flow states at <24 HOL	Dobutamine	28	All except two infants achieved/maintained a normal SVC flow; those treated with dobutamine had a higher HR and faster correction of metabolic acidosis. A follow-up study (Bravo et al., 2021) showed no difference in the combined outcome of death or moderate to severe NDI.	
	Paradisis et al., 2009	Infants <30 weeks at <6 HOL	Milrinone	90	Early prophylactic milrinone did not prevent low SBF. There was also no difference in RVO, BP, grade 3–4 P/IVH, or death. Milrinone was associated with a higher HR and slower constriction of the PDA.	
	Dempsey et al., 2021	Hypotensive infants <28 weeks at <72 HOL	Dopamine (both groups also received normal saline 10 mL/kg)	58	The Hypotension In Preterm Infants (HIP) trial terminated early due to significant enrollment issues. Although underpowered, the study did not show any major difference in clinical outcomes, including the primary outcome of survival without CUS abnormality at 36 weeks' PMA.	

	Bourchier and Weston, 1997	Hypotensive infants <1.5 kg at <7 DOL	Dopamine versus hydrocortisone (primary treatment)	40	Both interventions were equally effective at increasing MAP. There were no differences in clinically relevant outcomes (including mortality, IVH, ROP, CLD, NEC, sepsis, symptomatic PDA, or hyperglycemia). Treatment failure was more common in infants treated with hydrocortisone, although this was not statistically significant ($p = .108$) Of note, patients thought to be in shock (requiring immediate inotropic or blood product support) were excluded.	Overall conclusions from this Cochrane review (Ibrahim et al., 2011): There is insufficient evidence to support the routine use of hydrocortisone as primary treatment for hypotension in preterm neonates. Steroids are effective in the treatment of refractory hypotension in preterm neonates, but given the lack of long-term benefit or safety data their use cannot be routinely recommended. Outcomes with meta-analyses (all of which came from 2 trials (Gaissmaier & Pohlandt, 1999; Ng et al., 2006) comparing steroids with placebo for treatment of refractory hypotension): (a) Treatment failure, defined as the persistent need for inotropes, was significantly less in steroid-treated infants. (b) There were no differences in mortality, grade 3–4 IVH, PVL, NEC, or bacterial sepsis.
	Gaissmaier and Pohlandt, 1999	Infants <37 weeks with refractory hypotension (s/p volume expansion and dopamine) at <21 DOL	Dexamethasone versus placebo (both groups were also started on an epinephrine infusion)	1	The duration of epinephrine infusion was shorter in the group who received dexamethasone. There were no differences in clinically relevant outcomes (including mortality, grade 3–4 IVH, PVL, NEC, or bacterial sepsis).	

(*Continued*)

TABLE 20.3 Summary of Seminal and Noteworthy Studies Investigating Treatments for Neonatal Hypotension (*continued*)

	AUTHOR, YEAR	POPULATION	INTERVENTIONS	NUMBER	CONCLUSIONS	META-ANALYSES
	Ng et al., 2006	Infants <32 weeks and <1.5 kg with refractory hypotension (s/p volume expansion and dopamine) at <7 DOL	Hydrocortisone versus placebo	48	More infants in the hydrocortisone group weaned off inotropic support within 72 hours, and the median duration of vasopressor support was halved. Additionally, MAP was consistently higher, less volume expanders and lower cumulative doses of dopamine and dobutamine were required, and treatment failure (defined as a need for a second vasopressor) was less common in those treated with hydrocortisone. There were no differences in clinically relevant outcomes (including mortality, grade 3–4 IVH, PVL, severe ROP, CLD, or NEC). There were also no differences in serious short- and medium-term side effects of steroids (including hyperglycemia, gastric bleeding, GI perforation, or bacterial sepsis).	
	Hochwald et al., 2014	Infants <30 weeks and <1.25 kg with refractory hypotension (s/p volume expansion) at <48 HOL	Hydrocortisone versus placebo (both groups were also started on a dopamine infusion)	22	Those infants treated with hydrocortisone had a higher rate of survival without CLD and a shorter duration of dopamine support. There were no differences in other clinically relevant outcomes (including mortality, grade 3–4 IVH, PVL, CLD, NEC, or bacterial sepsis). Note that the Cochrane review analyzed data from a 2010 abstract (Hochwald et al., 2010) that included 18 of the 22 infants.	
	Kopelman et al., 1999	Infants <28 weeks at <2 HOL	Prophylactic dexamethasone versus placebo	70	Mean BPs were higher in infants who received dexamethasone, but there was no difference in the subsequent use of vasopressors.	

	Efird et al., 2005	Infants <29 weeks and <1 kg at <3 HOL	Prophylactic hydrocortisone versus placebo	34	Infants in the hydrocortisone group required less treatment with vasopressors during the first 2 days of life. There were no differences in clinically relevant outcomes (including mortality, CLD, nosocomial infections, NEC, SIP, IVH, or hyperglycemia).	
	Bonsante et al., 2007	Mechanically ventilated infants ≤30 weeks and <1.5 kg at <48 HOL	Prophylactic hydrocortisone versus placebo	50	Infants in the hydrocortisone group had a higher rate of survival without CLD, higher MAP, decreased incidence of hypotension, and significantly shorter duration of inotropic support. There were no differences in duration of ventilation, PDA, severe ROP, severe IVH, or PVL. There were also no differences in adverse effects of steroids, including GI perforation, NEC, hypertension, hyperglycemia, sepsis, or growth at 36 weeks.	
	Kovacs et al., 2019	Term asphyxiated neonates undergoing therapeutic hypothermia with refractory hypotension (s/p volume expansion)	Hydrocortisone versus placebo (both groups were also started on a dopamine infusion)	35	Infants treated with hydrocortisone were more likely to reach their target MAP, had lower duration of cardiovascular support, and required lower cumulative and peak inotrope dosages. There were no differences in short-term clinical outcomes.	

BP, blood pressure; CBF, cerebral blood flow; CLD, chronic lung disease; CUS, cranial ultrasound; DOL, days of life; ELBW, extremely low birth weight; FFP, fresh frozen plasma; GA, gestational age; GI, gastrointestinal; HOL, hours of life; HR, heart rate; IV, intravenous; IVH, intraventricular hemorrhage; LBW, low birth weight; LV, left ventricle; LVO, left ventricular output; MAP, mean arterial pressure; NDI, neurodevelopmental impairment; NEC, necrotizing enterocolitis; $PaCO_2$, arterial concentration of carbon dioxide; PDA, patent ductus arteriosus; PMA, postmenstrual age; P/IVH, periventricular/intraventricular hemorrhage; PVL, periventricular leukomalacia; RDS, respiratory distress syndrome; ROP, retinopathy of prematurity; RVO, right ventricular output; SBF, systemic blood flow; SBP, systolic blood pressure; SIP, spontaneous intestinal perforation; SMA, superior mesenteric artery; s/p, status post; SVC, superior vena cava.

Volume Expansion

The traditional approach to treating a hypotensive infant included first-line treatment with volume expansion, regardless of the clinical scenario (Dasgupta & Gill, 2003). This approach was prevalent despite awareness that BP measurements in preterm infants correlate poorly with both SBF and blood volume (Barr et al., 1977; Bauer et al., 1993; Kluckow & Evans, 1996, 2000; Osborn et al., 2004). Several observational studies demonstrated risks associated with the use of volume expansion in preterm babies, namely intracranial hemorrhage (ICH) and bronchopulmonary dysplasia (BPD; Goldberg et al., 1980; Van Marter et al., 1990).

Two Cochrane reviews have examined the evidence for use of early volume expansion to prevent morbidity and mortality in very preterm infants (those born ≤32 weeks of gestation or ≤1,500 grams). The first review included RCTs that compared volume expansion with either no treatment or with a different type of volume expansion (Osborn et al., 2004). Eight studies were included, most of which enrolled infants based on gestation or birth weight (and thus included both hypotensive and normotensive babies). Five studies compared volume expansion with no treatment; a meta-analysis of shared outcomes found no difference in mortality, periventricular or intraventricular hemorrhage (P/IVH), periventricular leukomalacia (PVL), or PDA (Osbourne & Evans, 2004). Three of the studies compared different types of volume expansion in hypotensive infants; a meta-analysis of the two studies comparing albumin 5% with normal saline showed no difference in mortality, P/IVH, or treatment failure (Lundstrom et al., 2000; Lynch, 2008; So et al., 1997). Notably, no studies were identified that compared volume expansion with no treatment in infants with cardiovascular compromise. The authors concluded that there is no evidence to support routine volume expansion in hemodynamically stable very preterm infants, and there is insufficient evidence to determine whether volume expansion benefits those infants with cardiovascular compromise (Osbourne & Evans, 2004).

The second Cochrane review included two small studies comparing volume expansion with dopamine in preterm infants (Osborn et al., 2001). Findings showed that dopamine was more likely to increase low BP than volume expansion in hypotensive preterm infants (although many of these patients had already received volume expansion prior to enrollment). Neither intervention, however, reduced morbidity (e.g., IVH, PVL, chronic lung disease, retinopathy of prematurity [ROP], or mortality). Based on these results, the authors gave no recommendation as to whether volume expansion or dopamine should be used to treat preterm infants.

Vasoactive and Inotropic Medications

Dopamine is the most commonly studied inotrope in both preterm and term infants, followed by dobutamine (Garvey et al., 2018; Rios et al., 2014). A Cochrane review compared the efficacy and safety of dopamine versus dobutamine in preterm infants (<37 weeks' gestation) during the first 28 days of life (Subhedar et al., 2003). Five trials with a total of 209 infants were included, all of which enrolled infants who remained hypotensive despite a trial of volume expansion. Infants treated with dopamine were less likely to have persistent hypotension when compared with infants treated with dobutamine. No difference was found in mortality, PVL, or severe P/IVH. One study reported a change in LVO, showing that infants treated with dobutamine had an increase in LVO, whereas infants in the dopamine group surprisingly had a decrease in LVO. It is important to note that none of the included studies examined long-term neurodevelopmental outcome. The authors concluded that dopamine is more effective than dobutamine in the short-term treatment of hypotension, although it may cause a decrease in LVO in some neonates. Because there were no data regarding the long-term benefit and safety of either medication, no firm recommendations were made regarding the treatment of hypotensive preterm neonates.

In one RCT, dopamine versus dobutamine was evaluated in preterm infants with low SBF, rather than hypotension (Osborn et al., 2002). Forty-two infants less than 30 weeks of gestation with low superior vena cava (SVC) flow (as measured by echocardiography) on the first day of life were randomized to either dopamine or dobutamine (after treatment with volume expansion). Results showed that those in the dopamine group had a greater increase in BP but little change in SVC flow or right ventricular output (RVO), whereas neonates treated with dobutamine had a greater increase in SVC flow. Notably, treatment failure was common in both groups. Infants treated with dobutamine had significantly higher scores on developmental assessment at 3 years corrected age (as measured by the Griffiths Mental Development Scales), but there were no differences in other measures of morbidity or mortality. This trial was the only study eligible for inclusion in a Cochrane review with the objective of evaluating the effects of specific inotropes on preterm infants with low SBF (Osborn, Paradisis, et al., 2007).

Another Cochrane review evaluated the impact of dopamine on morbidity and mortality in term infants with perinatal asphyxia (Hunt et al., 2002). Only one study was eligible for inclusion; a total of 14 infants were randomized to either low-dose dopamine or placebo. Unsurprising, those in the dopamine group had higher SBPs, but no difference was found in mortality or neurodevelopmental disability.

Epinephrine is also used in the treatment of neonatal hypotension, often in the setting of pulmonary hypertension (Perkin & Levin, 1982; Zaritsky & Chernow, 1984). A Cochrane review examining the safety and efficacy of epinephrine in preterm infants with cardiovascular compromise identified only one RCT for inclusion (Paradisis & Osborn, 2004). This trial was published in abstract form only and had incomplete data on patients less than 1,750 grams. Thus, the population included in the meta-analysis consisted of 20 babies with a mean gestational age of 36 weeks and birth weights >1,750 grams with hypotension in the first 24 hours of life. Patients were allocated to either dopamine or epinephrine infusions. Clinically important outcomes were not reported, including mortality or treatment failure. Both medications increased HR and BP without having a significant effect on LVO or RVO.

Valverde and colleagues showed that epinephrine dosed 0.125 to 0.5 mcg/kg/min was equally as efficacious as dopamine dosed 2.5 to 10 mcg/kg/min for treating hypotension, with epinephrine producing more chronotropy. However, this study also revealed more adverse side effects with epinephrine, such as hyperglycemia, acidosis requiring bicarbonate, and increased lactate levels (Valverde et al., 2006).

Vasopressin is less frequently used in the NICU, often reserved for infants with refractory hypotension, pulmonary hypertension, or hypotension after cardiac surgery. A Cochrane review was designed to evaluate the effectiveness and safety of vasopressin in neonates with refractory hypotension, but there were no RCTs that met the inclusion criteria (Shivanna et al., 2013). The authors noted that previous case series suggest that vasopressin may increase BP in both extremely preterm and term neonates with catecholamine-resistant shock, but it is unknown whether treatment with vasopressin improves end-organ perfusion, neurodevelopmental outcome, or survival. There are small randomized and observational trials showing that vasopressin is effective in raising BP in extremely preterm infants; however, more studies are needed (Bidegain et al., 2010; Ikegami et al., 2010; Meyer et al., 2006; Rios et al., 2015).

To date, there has been only one RCT that evaluated the use of milrinone in the neonatal population. This trial, which compared early prophylactic milrinone with placebo for the prevention of low SBF in high-risk preterm infants, did not show any significant benefit (Paradisis et al., 2009). Data from a number of case series suggest that milrinone may be useful in certain subpopulations in the NICU, which will be discussed further in the pharmacotherapy section. There is even less evidence regarding the use of norepinephrine in neonates. Although this vasopressor is commonly used as first-line treatment for adult and pediatric vasodilatory shock, it is rarely used in neonates as very few studies (and no RCTs) have been done in this population. However, it is an emerging therapy with a potential role in neonates with septic shock or pulmonary hypertension. The use of norepinephrine in specific subsets of neonatal patients (such as infants with pulmonary hypertension) is reviewed in Chapter 15, "Persistent Pulmonary Hypertension of the Newborn."

Corticosteroids

In preterm infants, relative or absolute adrenal insufficiency is increasingly recognized as a proximate cause of hypotension (Watterberg, 2002). Unlike older patients, preterm infants do not respond to stress with an increase in cortisol concentrations; this may be due to suppression of the hypothalamus–pituitary–adrenal axis or immature endocrine function (reduced enzymes present to convert deoxycortisol to cortisol; Hanna et al., 1997; Huysman et al., 2000; Scott & Watterberg, 1995). In addition, infants treated with dopamine have decreased levels of cortisol, both basal and stimulated (Hochwald et al., 2012; Ng et al., 2004; Scott & Watterberg, 1995). There are fewer data regarding relative adrenal insufficiency in term infants. Studies evaluating specific populations (including patients with congenital diaphragmatic hernia and hypotensive patients with hypoxic ischemic encephalopathy) demonstrated that these term babies also have low cortisol levels (Kamath et al., 2010; Kovacs et al., 2018). Another recent study found that critically ill term infants (requiring vasopressors) had a median basal cortisol of less than 5 mcg/dL, yet a normal stimulated cosyntropin (ACTH) response, suggesting suppression of the feedback loop (Fernandez et al., 2008).

Treatment of neonates with corticosteroids is known to increase their BP (Ng et al., 2006; Watterberg et al., 2004). A Cochrane review investigated the efficacy and safety of corticosteroids for hypotensive preterm infants (<37 weeks' gestation and <28 days' old), either as primary treatment or for refractory hypotension (Ibrahim et al., 2011). Four small RCTs were included with a total of 123 babies. One study evaluated hydrocortisone versus dopamine as primary treatment; persistent hypotension was more common in the group that received hydrocortisone (Bourchier & Weston, 1997). Because this finding was of borderline statistical significance, however, the authors concluded that hydrocortisone may be as effective as dopamine when used as a primary treatment for hypotension. The other three studies evaluated corticosteroid versus placebo as treatment for refractory hypotension (in babies already receiving dopamine or who had been given volume expansion; Ibrahim et al., 2011). Continuing need for inotrope infusion was less common in the babies who received steroids, but there were no other statistically significant effects on any other short- or long-term outcomes. Overall conclusions were that steroids are effective in the treatment of refractory hypotension in preterm infants, but there is insufficient evidence on which to base recommendations given the paucity of data on long-term safety or benefit (see Table 20.3).

CURRENT PHARMACOLOGIC TREATMENT MODALITIES FOR HYPOTENSION AND SHOCK

Treatment for hypotension and distributive shock generally aims to increase BP. After all, BP is the driving force for blood flow; thus, the ultimate goal in treating hypotension is to optimize organ perfusion and clinical outcomes (Heygi et al., 1994). In contrast, cardiogenic shock resolves through augmentation of CO. Pharmacologic agents are often initiated in hypotensive infants or those with compromised CO with evidence of end-organ damage. Management options include volume expansion, vasopressor and inotropic support, and corticosteroids.

Volume Expansion

Volume expansion is frequently used to treat hypotension and shock. However, indiscriminate use of volume expansion should be used with caution, especially in the first several days of life. Hypotension immediately after birth is primarily due to abnormal peripheral vasoregulation and/or myocardial function (Seri, 2001). As mentioned earlier, volume expansion within the first 72 hours of life in very preterm infants did not improve morbidity or mortality (Osborn & Evans, 2004).

In cases of anemia, packed red blood cells may be used. In other instances of hypotension due to documented hypovolemia, an intravenous fluid (IVF) bolus of either normal saline (0.9% NaCl) or lactated Ringer's may be warranted. Isotonic crystalloid solutions are preferred over colloid solutions, such as albumin, or hypotonic solutions, such as 0.45% NaCl, because albumin-containing solutions are associated with increased morbidity risk (Greenough et al., 2002). The volume of IVF bolus should be limited to 10 to 20 mL/kg. Larger volume bolus (>30 mL/kg) in preterm infants has the potential to increase IVH due to rapid fluctuations in cerebral blood flow (Alderliesten et al., 2013). In addition, if a volume bolus is required, give slowly to limit intraluminal pressure changes given the preterm infant's reduced cerebral autoregulatory ability. Even in emergent situations, neonatal resuscitation guidelines recommend a minimum volume bolus duration of 5 to 10 minutes (Aziz et al., 2021).

Vasoactive and Inotropic Medications

Before investigating each common vasoactive drug, it is important to understand the primary difference between a vasopressor and an inotropic drug. *Vasopressors induce vasoconstriction*, which increases the MAP by increasing SVR. In comparison, *inotropes increase cardiac contractility*, which increases perfusion by increasing CO. Both classes of medications aim to better perfuse organs and tissues. Many of the medications discussed have both vasopressor and inotropic effects. Some medications are also lusitropes, which increase the rate of myocardial relaxation. Some medications are also chronotropes, which increase HR. Often the medications will have a dose-dependent effect on receptors and thus produce differing effects at different dosages. These drugs bind to one or more of the following receptors: dopaminergic, beta-adrenergic, and alpha-adrenergic receptors.

D_1 dopaminergic receptors are located at the adrenal cortex, juxtaglomerular cells, renal tubule, and peripheral vascular smooth muscle. D_2 dopaminergic receptors can be found in the central nervous system. Beta-1-adrenergic receptors are predominately located in cardiac muscle and juxtaglomerular cells, whereas alpha-1-adrenergic receptors are found in all peripheral smooth muscle, organs, and glands *except* cardiac muscle and juxtaglomerular cells. Next, alpha-2-adrenergic receptors are found in cardiac presynaptic neurons and vascular postsynaptic neurons. Last, beta-2 adrenergic receptors are found in all peripheral vascular smooth muscle, organs (mainly the lungs), and glands *except* the presynaptic neurons.

Clearly, the stimulation of alpha and beta receptors elicits opposing (but not always proportional) hemodynamic effects. Therefore, it is very important that students and clinicians maintain an understanding of these receptors, their anatomic locus, and the mechanism of action when activated because many of the medications discussed in this section of the chapter bind at more than one receptor and elicit dynamic, dose-dependent vasopressor and inotropic effects.

As with many disease states, clinicians should first optimize nonpharmacologic modalities (e.g., ensure adequate thermoregulation, correct electrolyte imbalances, treat anemia or other underlying causes of hemodynamic instability such as sepsis) before prescribing pharmacotherapies. Should vasoactive or inotropic medications be necessary, readers will discover that these medications must be administered parenterally due to the presence of the intestinal enzyme catechol-O-methyltransferase (COMT), which degrades and inactivates catecholamines. Table 20.4 provides a summary of the vasoactive and inotropic receptors, the mechanism of action, and the clinical effect elicited with administration of the vasoactive and inotropic agonists discussed in this section.

DOPAMINE

Dopamine is the most commonly prescribed and studied medication used in NICUs for treatment of hypotension and shock (Stranak et al., 2014). Dopamine is endogenously produced in the basal ganglia and adrenal medulla, and in times of hemodynamic instability may need to be exogenously supplemented to increase BP and tissue perfusion.

Mechanism of Action/Pharmacokinetic Principles

The mechanism of action of dopamine involves a dose-dependent effect up dopaminergic, beta-1-adrenergic, beta-2-adrenergic and alpha-1-adrenergic receptors (Figure 20.5). This concept is of particular importance because accurate prescribing is critical to elicit the desired response. Low-dose dopamine infusions activate dopaminergic receptors in order to elicit smooth muscle relaxation (via D_1 receptors) as well as to inhibit the release of noradrenaline (via D_2 receptors). Consequently, an increase in renal, mesenteric, and cerebral perfusion occurs. Moderate-dose dopamine infusions activate beta-1-adrenergic receptors, which elicit a positive inotropic and chronotropic effect. Roughly half of the inotropic effect specific to an increase in myocardial contractility is via beta-2-adrenergic receptor stimulation of myocardial norepinephrine release (as norepinephrine increases both HR and myocardial contractility). In addition, approximately 25% of infused dopamine is converted to norepinephrine in the sympathetic nerve endings (Goodall & Alton, 1968). Unfortunately, myocardial norepinephrine stores are quickly depleted, in part because of increased usage and also because norepinephrine stores are reduced in infants compared with children. As a result, dopamine loses some of its inotropic efficacy after 8 to 12 hours in exchange for increased vasopressor efficacy (Seri, 1995). High-dose dopamine infusions further inhibit norepinephrine release and also activate alpha-1-adrenergic receptors located in the peripheral mesenteric and vascular beds. This leads to increased peripheral vascular constriction and SVR, as well as glycogenolysis for the purposes of cellular respiration (adenosine triphosphate [ATP] production). In summary, low-dose dopamine elicits vasodilation and encourages increased renal blood flow. Moderate- and high-dose dopamine lead to a higher ratio of vasopressor to inotropic activity.

TABLE 20.4 Adrenoreceptor Targets for Vasoactive and Inotropic Medications

RECEPTOR	ANATOMIC LOCUS	MECHANISM OF ACTION WHEN STIMULATED	DRUG WITH CARDIAC STIMULATORY EFFECT	DRUG WITH PERIPHERAL VASCULAR STIMULATORY EFFECT
Alpha-1-adrenergic	Cardiomyocytes (myocardium) Peripheral vascular smooth muscle Coronary arteries	Vasoconstriction Glycogenolysis	Dobutamine++ Dopamine++ Epinephrine++ Norepinephrine++	Dobutamine+ Dopamine++++ Epinephrine++++ Norepinephrine++++
Alpha-2-adrenergic	Presynaptic neurons (cardiac) Postsynaptic neurons (Peripheral vascular smooth muscle)	Inhibition of norepinephrine release from presynaptic neurons Inhibition of insulin release from pancreatic beta cells Vasoconstriction via postsynaptic neurons in vasculature	Epinephrine++ Norepinephrine++	Dobutamine+ Epinephrine++++ Norepinephrine++++
Beta-1-adrenergic	Bronchial smooth muscle Cardiomyocytes (myocardium) Peripheral vascular smooth muscle	Bronchoconstriction ↑ Chronotropy ↑ Inotropy ↑ Lusitropy ↑ Dromotropy (rate of conduction across AV node)	Dobutamine++++ Dopamine+++ Epinephrine++++ Norepinephrine++	
Beta-2-adrenergic	Bronchial smooth muscle Peripheral vascular smooth muscle	Vascular and bronchial smooth muscle relaxation Myocardial contraction	Dobutamine++++ Dopamine+++ Epinephrine++++ Norepinephrine++	Dobutamine++ Dopamine++ Epinephrine++++ Norepinephrine+
Dopaminergic-1	Adrenal cortex Juxtaglomerular cells Renal tubules Peripheral vascular smooth muscle	Vascular, renal, and mesenteric smooth muscle relaxation	Dopamine++++	Dopamine++++
Dopaminergic-2	Basal ganglia Presynaptic neurons	Inhibition of noradrenaline release	Dopamine++++	Dopamine++++
Vasopressin-1	Peripheral vascular smooth muscle	Vascular smooth muscle contraction		Vasopressin++++
Vasopressin-2	Peripheral vascular smooth muscle	Vascular smooth muscle relaxation		Vasopressin++++

++++ very high stimulatory effect; +++ high stimulatory effect; ++ moderate stimulatory effect; + low stimulatory effect
AV, atrioventricular.

Sources: From Noori, S., & Seri, I. (2012). Neonatal blood pressure support: The use of inotropes, lusitropes, and other vasopressor agents. *Clinics in Perinatology, 39*(1), 221–238. https://doi.org/10.1016/j.clp.2011.12.010; Phad, N., & de Waal, K. (2020). What inotrope and why? *Clinics in Perinatology*, 47(3), 529–547. https://doi.org/10.1016/j.clp.2020.05.010; Seri, I. (2006). Management of hypotension and low systemic blood flow in the very low birth weight neonate during the first postnatal week. *Journal of Perinatology, 26 Suppl 1*, S8–S13. https://doi.org/10.1038/sj.jp.7211464.

FIGURE 20.5 Dose-dependent effects of dopamine in preterm and term neonates.

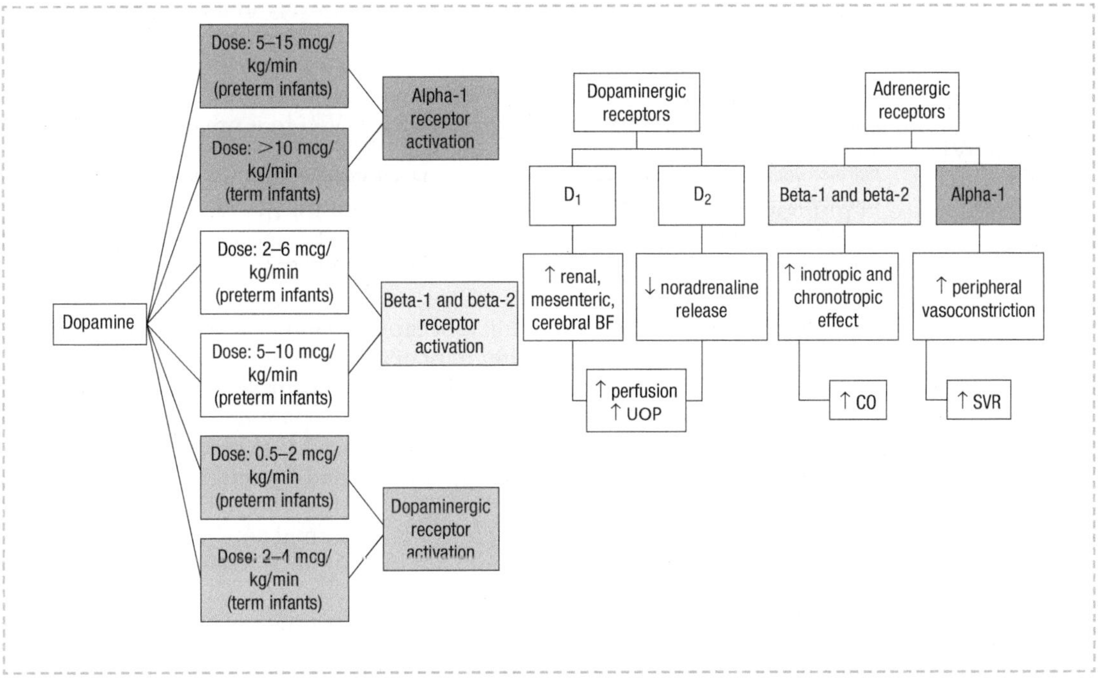

Note: At moderate doses (*light gray*), dopamine stimulates beta-1 receptors in the myocardium (increase heart rate and force of contraction) and beta-2 receptors in the peripheral vasculature (relax vascular smooth muscle and induce peripheral vasodilation) and the myocardium (stimulating norepinephrine release). At high doses (*dark gray*), dopamine stimulates alpha-1 receptors in the myocardium (increase contractility) and peripheral vasculature (increase vasoconstriction).
BF, blood flow; CO, cardiac output; SVR, systemic vascular resistance; UOP, urinary output.
Design credit: Jennifer Barnes and Amy J. Jnah.

The effects of dopamine dosing in preterm infants are extensively debated and are mostly inferred from animal studies and small, underpowered clinical trials. Due to immature adreno-receptor downregulation, preterm neonates may have alpha-adrenergic effects, such as increased BP, even at lower doses. There potentially could even be the paradoxical effect of alpha-adrenergic receptor stimulation prior to beta-adrenergic stimulation in preterm infants (Seri, 1995, 2001; Seri et al., 1993).

Dopamine is administered as an intravenous continuous infusion. The onset of action is generally within 5 minutes. The elimination half-life is 2 minutes in term infants and 4 to 5 minutes in preterm infants (Bhatt-Mehta & Nahata, 1989). Dopamine has demonstrated nonlinear kinetics in children, and at higher doses steady-state concentrations may take longer to achieve (close to 1 hour compared with 10–15 minutes). No pharmacokinetic data specific to the volume of distribution in neonates are available; data in children and adults cannot be extrapolated due to the unique cardiovascular and adrenergic physiology in neonates. Dopamine is metabolized by the liver into mostly inactive metabolites. However, approximately one-quarter of dopamine is metabolized to vasoactive norepinephrine. Dopamine metabolites are eliminated from the body via renal excretion. Clearance of dopamine is prolonged in renal and/or hepatic dysfunction.

Dosing Recommendations

As previously stated, dopaminergic receptors in the renal, mesenteric, and coronary vascular beds are activated at very low dosages (0.5–2 mcg/kg/min among preterm infants and 2–4 mcg/kg/min among term infants; Seri et al., 1993). Moderate dosing is estimated between 2 and 6 mcg/kg/min in preterm infants and 5 to 10 mcg/kg/min in term neonates and infants. High-dose vasopressor activity is reported to occur between 5 and 15 mcg/kg/min in preterm and greater than 10 mcg/kg/min in term neonates and infants (Seri, 1995).

Clinical-Monitoring Pearls

The side effects of dopamine therapy include tachycardia, cardiac arrythmias, worsening vasoconstriction, and suppression of endocrine function. Close monitoring of peripheral perfusion and capillary refill time is necessary, as significant vasoconstriction can lead to peripheral limb necrosis. Dopamine should be given in a central line to prevent extravasation.

Dopamine can also increase pulmonary vascular resistance (PVR) to a greater degree than it increases SVR. Clinicians should carefully consider this risk when prescribing vasoactive medications in patients with persistent pulmonary hypertension of the newborn (PPHN). Alternatively, an increase in pulmonary artery pressure may be beneficial for hypotensive infants with hemodynamically significant PDA with left-to-right shunting. Caution should be used with high doses of dopamine (>10 mcg/kg/min) due to excessive vasoconstriction resulting in decreased CO and cerebral blood flow. Disproportionate vasoconstriction is particularly dangerous in babies who have baseline reduced cardiac contractility, because a failing heart pumping against increased afterload will lead to even lower CO (Soleymani et al., 2010).

Significantly reduced thyroid-stimulating hormone (TSH), T_4, and prolactin levels have been reported in neonates weighing <1,500 grams who have received dopamine (Filippi et al., 2006; Wood et al., 1996). Filippi and colleagues (2007) as well as other scientists discovered that dopamine can suppress anterior pituitary function, which impairs normal thyroid function and gives rise to hypothyroxinemia of prematurity (Soleymani et al., 2010). Therefore, clinicians are encouraged to consider dopamine exposure as a contributing factor to abnormal newborn thyroid screening test results. Of note, effects on the endocrine system are quickly reversible once dopamine is discontinued.

Minimizing fluctuations in BP is optimal, which requires a stable solution of medication, nursing skill during syringe/infusion changeover, and prompt titration of dosage, as needed. Kirupakaran and colleagues (2020) investigated dopamine stability and discovered more rapid degradation after the first hour of compounding with gradual degradation afterward with significant decrease in MAP fluctuations when dopamine infusions were initiated 30 minutes after preparation and dose syringes were changed every 12 hours ($p < .05$, $n = 10$). Given the small sample size and study design, additional research is necessary to generalize these findings. Some institutions use commercially available dopamine infusions for patient-specific syringes, which may also alleviate this issue. However, APRNs should be aware and mindful of these potential MAP fluctuations with daily medication infusion replacements.

Long-term risks are tightly linked to comorbid conditions that develop subsequent to the hypotensive state. Poor organ perfusion increases the risk of IVH, PVL, ROP, and reduced motor and neurocognitive function in childhood.

DOBUTAMINE

Dobutamine is a common inotrope used to treat neonatal hypoperfusion caused by increased PVR and myocardial insufficiency (Martinez et al., 1992). Dobutamine may be preferred in clinical conditions with poor myocardial contractility and normal SVR; however, it increases myocardial oxygen demand. In such instances as perinatal asphyxia or poor transition to extrauterine life, dobutamine's hemodynamic characteristics of increased CO with insignificant or absent vasoconstriction are beneficial.

Mechanism of Action/Pharmacokinetic Principles

Similar to dopamine, the mechanism of action of dobutamine involves a dose-dependent effect on alpha-1- and beta-adrenergic receptors (Figure 20.6). Dobutamine is unique in that its positive and negative isomers have individual receptor affinities. The positive isomer is a beta-adrenergic agonist, whereas the negative isomer is an alpha-1-adrenergic agonist; the effects of the positive isomer exceed the effects of the negative isomer (see Table 20.4). Dobutamine primarily binds to beta-1-adrenergic receptors; the subsequent biochemical response encourages the movement of calcium from the extracellular to intracellular space. This influx of calcium elicits a sympathetic response in the form of increased cardiac contractility, HR, and SV. Although beta-1 activation elicits significant chronotropy in adults, variable and inconsistent changes in HR as well as SVR are reported in neonates and infants. This is likely because beta-2-adrenergic receptors are also activated at the same time and neutralize alpha-1-mediated peripheral vasoconstriction, thus

FIGURE 20.6 Dose-dependent effects of dobutamine in preterm and term neonates.

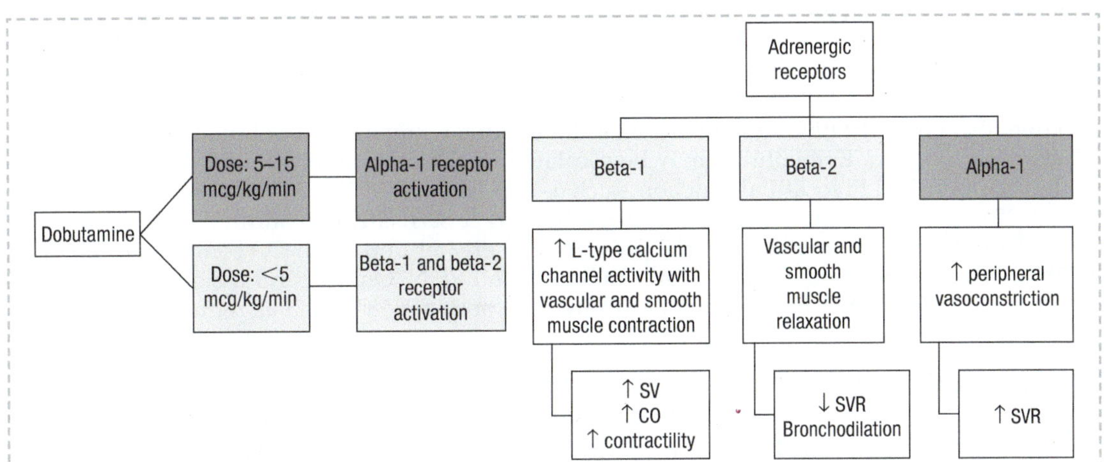

Note: At low doses (*light gray*), dobutamine stimulates beta-1 receptors in the myocardium (increase heart rate and force of contraction) and beta-2 receptors in the peripheral vasculature (relax vascular smooth muscle and neutralizes alpha-1-mediated vasoconstriction). At higher doses (*dark gray*), alpha-1-mediated vasoconstriction is offset by beta-2, eliciting an increase in myocardial contractility and mild peripheral vasodilation. CO, cardiac output; SV, stroke volume; SVR, systemic vascular resistance.
Design credit: Jennifer Barnes and Amy J. Jnah.

decreasing HR and SVR (Giesinger & McNamara, 2016; Mahoney et al., 2015). In fact, several studies reported a 0.6% decrease in SVR with low to moderate dosages and a 10.2% average decrease in SVR with maximum dosages (20 mcg/kg/min; Mahoney et al., 2015).

Similar to dopamine, premature receptor development affects systemic dobutamine dose–response relationships due to delays in beta receptor maturation compared with alpha receptors. Preterm infants may experience enhanced alpha-1-adrenengeic effects at lower doses due to decreased beta receptor sites (Noori & Seri, 2012). Unlike dopamine, dobutamine is not dependent on release of endogenous catecholamines and its inotropic effects last longer (Martinez & Thio, 1992).

Limited pharmacokinetic data specific to neonates and infants are available. Dobutamine is administered as an intravenous continuous infusion. The onset of action is within 1 to 2 minutes. However, time to steady-state concentration varies greatly in neonates from 15 minutes to more than 2 hours (Pellicer et al., 2021). The elimination half-life averages between 2 and 10 minutes in the limited neonatal data available (Pellicer et al., 2021). Dobutamine is quickly metabolized in the liver to inactive metabolites. These inactive metabolites are excreted primarily in the urine with some conjugates excreted in the stool. Clearance of dobutamine is prolonged in renal and/or hepatic dysfunction.

Dosing Recommendations

Dobutamine at low doses (<5 mcg/kg/min) activates beta-1-adrenergic receptors, which leads to increased myocardial contractility with a limited increase in HR. At higher doses (>5 mcg/kg/min), dobutamine will additionally augment CO via an increase in SV. At these doses, there is minimal effect on SVR and thus BP because beta-2 vasodilatation neutralizes alpha-1-mediated vasoconstriction. (Giesinger & McNamara, 2016; Mahoney et al., 2015).

Clinical-Monitoring Pearls

Side effects include increased urinary output, tachycardia, and increased myocardial oxygen demand. Increased urinary output by an average of 2.6 mL/kg/hr has been reported among preterm, oliguric neonates with respiratory distress syndrome (Klarr et al., 1994). Clinicians are encouraged to monitor urinary output as well as serum electrolytes, as imbalances may develop during therapy. Higher doses of dobutamine can lead to tachycardia and increased myocardial oxygen demand, potentially reducing ventricular filling (Noori & Seri, 2012). Other studies have reported that high dosages (10–20 mcg/kg/min) may lower PVR, optimizing right ventricular outflow and reducing ventilation-perfusion mismatching (Osborn, Evans, & Kluckow, 2007; Osborn, Evans, Kluckow, Bowen, et al., 2007).

EPINEPHRINE

Epinephrine is an endogenous catecholamine commonly called *adrenaline* that can also be administered exogenously and has been used to treat hypotension since 1924 (Mahoney et al., 2015). Despite this, there is a significant deficit of well-powered studies to inform its current use in the neonatal population.

Low-dose epinephrine may be used as a therapeutic equivalent to dobutamine, augmenting myocardial function. Epinephrine may be escalated in clinical conditions with low SVR with or without diminished myocardial function, such as sepsis. Epinephrine has also been prescribed to treat hypotension refractory to other inotropes (Noori & Seri, 2012). In addition, epinephrine has a smaller impact on pulmonary arterial pressure and greater impact on CO compared with dopamine, so may be preferred in hypotensive infants with PPHN. On the contrary, epinephrine is not recommended for use in patients with outflow tract obstructions (such as tetralogy of Fallot) or cardiac arrythmias.

Mechanism of Action/Pharmacokinetic Principles

The mechanism of action of epinephrine makes it a potent medication for increasing CO and BP, which can improve cerebral blood flow in hypotensive preterm infants (Figure 20.7; Pellicer et al., 2005). Epinephrine is considered the end product of catecholamine synthesis and exhibits cardiovascular activity by binding to alpha-adrenergic and beta-adrenergic receptors in a dose-dependent fashion. Stimulation of alpha-1-adrenergic receptors leads to increased peripheral vasoconstriction, whereas stimulation of alpha-2-adrenergic receptors increases SVR (postsynaptic) and inhibits norepinephrine release (presynaptic), eliciting coronary vasoconstriction. Stimulation of beta-1-adrenergic receptors induces chronotropy, inotropy, and lusitropy. Beta-2-adrenergic activity leads to increased myocardial contractility and vascular smooth muscle relaxation, but this effect is significantly less in relation to beta-1-activity. As mentioned previously, preterm infants may possess an insufficient or disproportionate number of adrenergic receptors, which can significantly affect drug efficacy and dosing decisions.

Limited data specific to the pharmacokinetics of epinephrine in neonates and infants are available. Similar to the other vasoactive medications described in this chapter, epinephrine is administered via intravenous continuous infusion. Epinephrine is rapid-acting, with an onset of action within 1 to 2 minutes and steady-state concentrations within 10 minutes. The two primary enzymes that metabolize epinephrine are monoamine oxidase (MAO) and COMT (Eisenhofer et al., 2004). As reported by Nakai and Yamada (1983), epinephrine metabolites are rapidly excreted in the urine. Urinary excretion of metabolites increases among neonates with respiratory distress and hypoxemia (Cheek et al., 1963; Mahoney et al., 2012; Schwab et al., 1996). Epinephrine elimination may be extended in renal failure.

Dosing Recommendations

At low doses (0.01–0.1 mcg/kg/min) epinephrine primarily promotes cardiac beta-1 and vascular beta-2 receptors. These effects lead to enhanced myocardial contractility, increased HR and SV (and CO), as well as modest peripheral vasodilatation. At high doses of epinephrine (>0.1 mcg/kg/min), both alpha-1- and alpha-2-adrenergic receptors are stimulated. This results in vasoconstriction (causing increased SVR) as well as increased myocardial contractility. In the neonatal population, epinephrine is generally used as an inotrope and dosed less than 0.1 mcg/kg/min to maximize efficacy while minimizing associated adverse drug reactions, as discussed in the text that follows; alternative agents (dopamine or norepinephrine) are typically preferred as vasopressors.

Clinical-Monitoring Pearls

Side effects include tachycardia, hyperglycemia, hypokalemia, lactic acidosis, and myocardial ischemia (Valverde et al., 2006). Hyperglycemia and lactic acidosis develop secondary to beta-2 activity on the liver and skeletal muscle, which reduces insulin release, increases glycogenolysis, and increases the production of lactate (Noori & Seri, 2012). More recently, G. Lee and colleagues (2021) reported that low-dose epinephrine (<0.05 mcg/kg/min) did not affect blood glucose or lactate levels. Therefore, adverse effects may be dose-related, and lower starting doses may be warranted. Compared with dopamine, epinephrine has been associated with excessive chronotropy, leading to tachycardia. Persistent tachycardia is believed to be the proximate cause of increased myocardial oxygen demand and subsequent ischemia (Zimmerman et al., 2019). Low serum potassium levels

FIGURE 20.7 Dose-dependent effects of epinephrine in preterm and term neonates.

Epinephrine
Dose: >0.1 mcg/kg/min — Alpha-1 and alpha-2 receptor activation
Dose: 0.01–0.1 mcg/kg/min — Beta-1 and beta-2 receptor activation

Adrenergic receptors
Beta-1 — Vascular and smooth muscle contraction — ↑ HR ↑ contractility ↑ lusitropy
Beta-2 — Vascular and smooth muscle relaxation — ↑ coronary art. dilation ↓ SVR Bronchodilation
Alpha-1 — ↑ peripheral vasoconstriction — ↑ SVR
Alpha-2 — Inhibition of norepinephrine release — ↑ SVR Coronary vasoconstriction

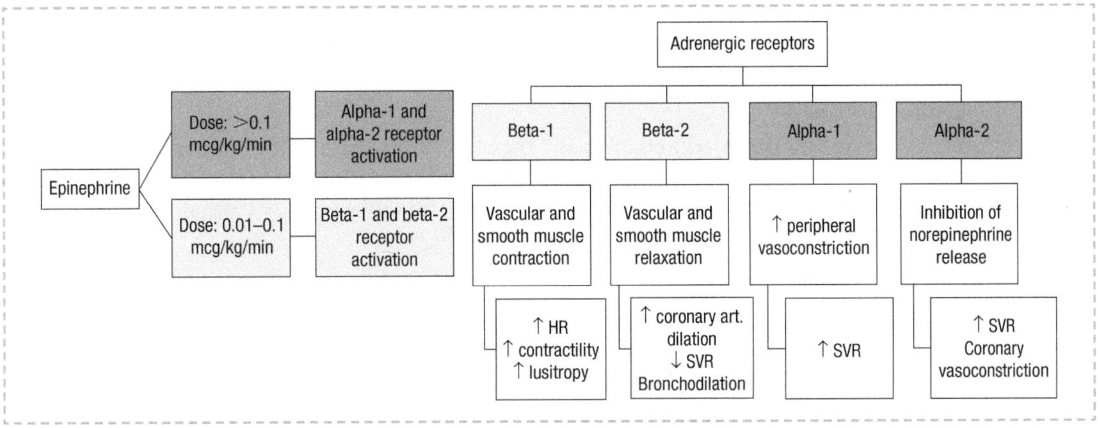

Note: At low doses (*light gray*) epinephrine elicits beta-1 and beta-2 receptors, yielding increased myocardial contractility, increased heart rate, and modest peripheral vasodilatation. At high doses (*dark gray*), alpha-1 and alpha-2 adrenergic receptors are stimulated, yielding increased vasoconstriction, systemic vascular resistance, and myocardial contractility.
HR, heart rate; SVR, systemic vascular resistance.
Design credit: Jennifer Barnes and Amy J. Jnah.

are secondary to an increase in potassium uptake by skeletal muscle cells, especially seen with higher dosage infusions (0.1 mcg/kg/min). Higher dose epinephrine infusions have been reported to reduce serum potassium by 0.8 mEq/L (Brown et al., 1983). Another rare but significant adverse effect of epinephrine and any vasopressor with potent alpha-adrenergic activity is peripheral ischemia and risk of limb necrosis. Epinephrine should be administered in a central line to prevent extravasation.

NOREPINEPHRINE

Norepinephrine is an endogenous catecholamine, also known as *noradrenaline*, with diverse functions as a hormone and neurotransmitter. In the cardiovascular system, norepinephrine has minor positive inotropic effects while producing profound systemic vasoconstriction.

Mechanism of Action/Pharmacokinetic Principles

Norepinephrine produces systemic vasoconstriction through stimulation of both alpha-1 and alpha-2 receptors. The impact on alpha-2 receptors (absent in dopamine) may be responsible for the preferential vasoconstriction of systemic over pulmonary vasculature leveraged in neonates with PPHN (Magnenant et al., 2003). Beta-1 activity is present but minimal compared with dopamine, potentially accounting for decreased arrythmias in adults treated for shock, with increased survival in those with cardiogenic shock (De Backer et al., 2010). As previously discussed, this benefit cannot be directly extrapolated to neonates and careful investigation is required.

Potent systemic vasoconstriction has established norepinephrine as standard of care for adult vasodilatory shock. However, norepinephrine has vasodilatory action in the pulmonary vascular bed of neonates (Magnenant et al., 2003). Consequently, emerging data describe the use of norepinephrine as a vasopressor for septic shock in preterm neonates and hypotension in term neonates with PPHN. In two case series, including 60 preterm neonates with septic shock, norepinephrine normalized BP within 1 hour of initiation; in patients previously requiring other vasopressor infusions, infusions were discontinued within 8 hours; the most frequent adverse effect was tachycardia (Rizk et al., 2018; Rowcliff et al., 2016). In two case series including 29 preterm and term neonates with PPHN exacerbated by systemic hypotension, norepinephrine infusion increased systemic BP while improving oxygenation, LVO, and left pulmonary artery blood flow velocity (Rowcliff et al., 2016; Tourneux et al., 2008). Additional research is clearly required, although these data highlight the potential benefits of norepinephrine compared with traditional vasopressors used in neonatal intensive care.

Limited pharmacokinetic data in neonates and infants are available. Body weight appears to be proportional to norepinephrine clearance and endogenous norepinephrine production (Oualha et al., 2014). In older patients, norepinephrine has a rapid onset of action (1–2 minutes). Norepinephrine metabolism and elimination pathways are identical to epinephrine.

Dosing Recommendations

Norepinephrine is typically initiated at 0.05 to 0.1 mcg/kg/min and titrated in a similar increment to a maximum dose of 2 mcg/kg/min. In neonatal case series, response as determined by normalization of BP occurs at a mean dose of 0.5 mcg/kg/min (Rowcliff et al., 2016) with a typical maximum requirement of 1 mcg/kg/min (Tourneux et al., 2008).

Clinical-Monitoring Pearls

Norepinephrine avoids several adverse effects of epinephrine (lactic acidosis, hyperglycemia) due to minimal beta-2 activity. Excessive vasoconstriction is the major concern, most often evidenced by peripheral ischemia, tachycardia, and/or acidosis (typically occurring at doses greater than or equal to 3.3 mcg/kg/min). Norepinephrine should be administered through a stable central venous catheter due to a high risk of extravasation.

VASOPRESSIN

Vasopressin is an endogenous neuropeptide released from the posterior pituitary gland in order to modulate fluid homeostasis and osmolarity. It stimulates arginine vasopressin (AVP), oxytocin, and purinergic receptors. Vasopressin is considered in the treatment of refractory neonatal hypotension when catecholamines and/or steroid therapies fail to produce a therapeutic response. It may also be considered as first-line treatment for neonatal hypotension that occurs in the setting of increased PVR (as described in the text that follows).

Mechanism of Action/Pharmacokinetic Principles

The mechanism of action of vasopressin involves activation of V_{1a} and V_2 receptors (Figure 20.8). The stimulation of V_{1a} leads to increases in SVR and thus increased arterial BP. Activation of the V_2 receptor conversely causes vasodilation as well as increased water permeability of the kidneys, resulting in increased water reabsorption at the renal collecting duct and an increase in urine osmolarity. V_{1a} predominates at higher doses and thus peripheral vasoconstriction dominates (Dyke & Tobias, 2004).

FIGURE 20.8 Mechanism of action of vasopressin.

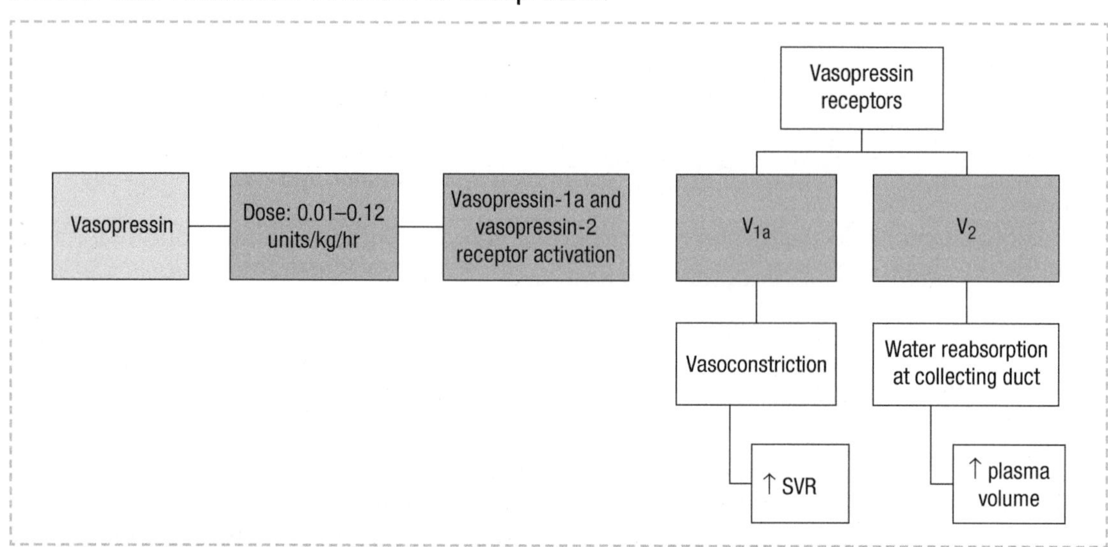

SVR, systemic vascular resistance.
Design credit: Amy J. Jnah.

Vasopressin has marginal chronotropic effects and no clinically relevant effect on CO (Cheung et al., 2012; Meyer et al., 2008). However, vasopressin has been shown to generate direct vasodilation in the pulmonary vascular bed with resulting improvement in oxygenation (Mohamed et al., 2014). This mechanism of action makes vasopressin a potentially optimal agent in patients with PPHN or pulmonary hypertension secondary to congenital heart disease or congenital diaphragmatic hernia (Acker et al., 2014; Lechner et al., 2007; Mohamed et al., 2014; Scheurer et al., 2005).

No pharmacokinetic data in neonates and infants are available. Vasopressin is also given as a continuous intravenous infusion. In children and adults, vasopressin has a quick onset of action, occurring within 15 minutes of infusion initiation. The half-life is approximately 10 to 20 minutes. Vasopressin is metabolized in the liver to inactive conjugates that are predominantly eliminated by the kidneys.

Dosing Recommendations

Vasopressin dosing can be confusing because the neonatal and pediatric literature has described vasopressin in both milliunits/kg/min and units/kg/hr. APRNs need to employ vigilance when comparing dosing from studies with their practice due to conversion calculations. It is advised to be consistent in vasopressin dosing units to prevent errors.

Although there are limited data for vasopressin use in neonates, the studies discussed in this chapter primarily used dosages ranging from 0.01 to 0.12 units/kg/hr. Generally, lower dosing of 0.01 to 0.07 units/kg/hr is recommend for hypotension in PPHN, whereas dosing may go to the higher end of 0.12 units/kg/hr in VRH. Ikegami and colleagues (2010) reported a significant increase in urine output and BP with vasopressin (0.06–0.12 units/kg/hr) administered to neonates with hypotension secondary to septic shock, cardiogenic shock, and adrenal dysfunction ($p < .0001$).

Clinical-Monitoring Pearls

Side effects of vasopressin therapy include decreased urine output, thrombocytopenia, elevated liver enzymes, hyponatremia, and cutaneous ischemia and necrosis (Ikegami et al., 2010; Ruoss et al., 2015). Thrombocytopenia arises due to aggregation of platelets secondary to V_2 receptor activation; the risk increases as dosage increases.

Caution should be used with high doses of vasopressin (>1.2 units/kg/hr) due to a paradoxical increase in pulmonary arterial pressures (Evora et al., 1993). Elevated liver enzymes (total bilirubin and transaminase) are attributed to reduced mesenteric perfusion during therapy (Dünser et al., 2003). Hyponatremia is the most common significant adverse reaction, and close monitoring of electrolytes, fluid balance, and urine output is necessary while on vasopressin. Davalos et al. (2013) showed that, in neonates and infants on vasopressin, a statistically higher incidence of hyponatremia (Na <135 mEq/L) was seen compared with the control group (48% to 17%, $p = .004$).

MILRINONE

Milrinone is a selective type III phosphodiesterase (PDE) inhibitor that elicits inotropic, lusitropic, and vasodilatory effects. This drug is frequently used after congenital cardiac defect corrective surgery to optimize left ventricular filling, preload, contractility, and CO without increasing myocardial oxygen consumption (McNamara et al., 2010; Noori et al., 2007).

Milrinone is not recommended as a first-line therapy for hypoperfusion among preterm neonates (Ruoss et al., 2015). However, among term infants and older preterm infants, the inotropic and lusitropic effects make it an ideal agent to treat low CO in neonates with congenital heart defects after corrective surgery. In addition, milrinone may be used in neonates with PPHN that is refractory to inhaled nitric oxide, as milrinone is known to restore cyclic adenosine monophosphate (cAMP)-mediated pulmonary vasodilation (Chen et al., 2009). However, milrinone is not recommended in neonates with vasoactive-refractory hypotension or neonates with inadequate intravascular volumes.

Mechanism of Action/Pharmacokinetic Principles

Milrinone is a selective type III PDE inhibitor (Figure 20.9). This means that milrinone inhibits PDE III enzymes, which are abundantly located in the myocardial sarcoplasmic reticulum and vascular smooth muscle. Inhibition of PDE III enzymes permits an accumulation of cAMP, and to a lesser extent cyclic guanosine monophosphate (cGMP), inside the cell. As a result, intracellular calcium

FIGURE 20.9 Mechanism of action of milrinone.

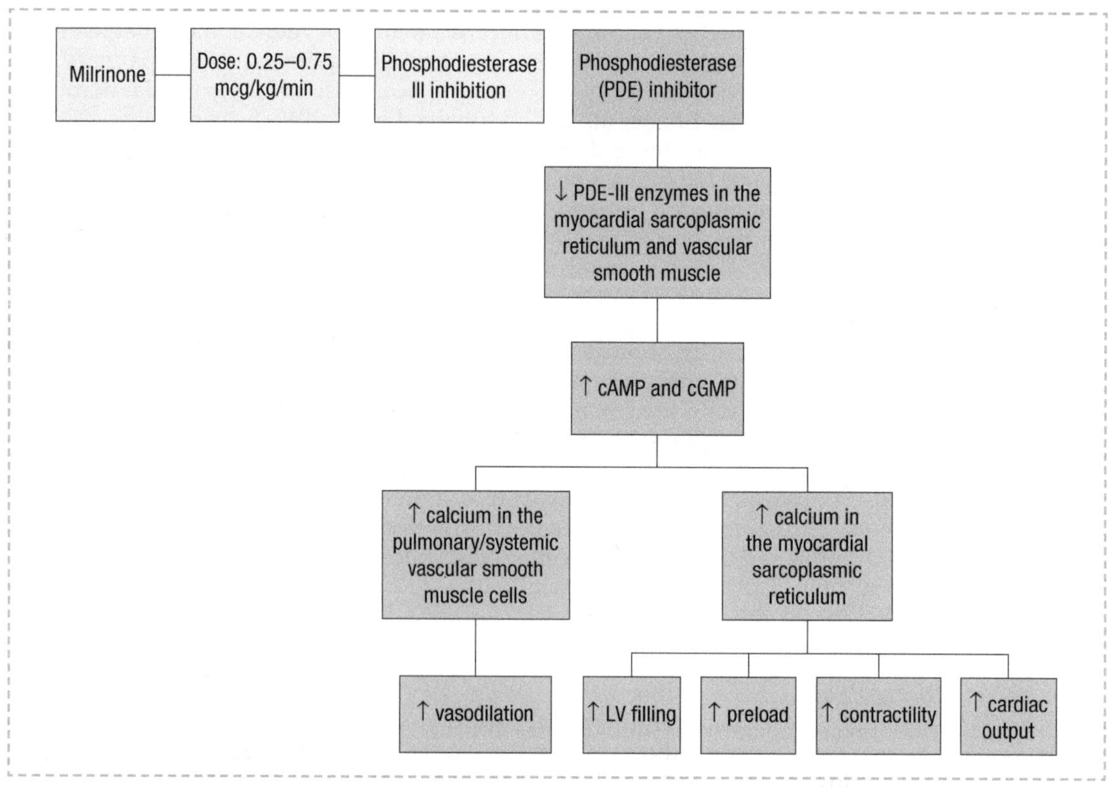

cAMP, cyclic adenosine monophosphate; cGMP, cyclic guanosine monophosphate; LV, left ventricle.
Design credit: Amy J. Jnah.

levels increase, actin and myosin filaments engage, and cardiac systole (contraction) occurs. Calcium also enters smooth muscle cells, and in doing so elicits vasodilation (Ruoss et al., 2015). The net effect of these actions is enhanced left ventricular filling, preload, contractility, and CO, as well as systemic and pulmonary vasodilation (Farrow & Steinhorn, 2011). Of note, animal studies have shown that a specific phosphodiesterase (PDE-IV) is more active for cAMP breakdown in the fetal cardiovascular system and begins to convert to PDE-III at birth. Milrinone has little effect on PDE-IV, which may explain why this drug has little observed efficacy during the first 3 to 7 days of life (Akita et al., 1994; Artman et al., 1988).

Ramamoorthy and colleagues (1998) first investigated the kinetics of milrinone in infants after cardiac surgery. A large volume of distribution was reported, which may require a loading dose to achieve the desired therapeutic effect rapidly. These findings were later confirmed by Hornik et al. (2019). Milrinone is given as an intravenous continuous infusion. The reported half-life is 10 hours in preterm infants and 4 hours in term neonates, which is substantially longer than the half-life of other vasoactive drugs (Paradisis et al., 2007). Milrinone is about 70% protein-bound, resulting in higher active concentrations in neonates and infants with low albumin levels. Most of milrinone is renally eliminated as active drug with only minor liver metabolism. Clearance increases with gestational age and is reported to reach 50% of adult levels between 47 and 68 weeks postmenstrual age (Hornik et al., 2019).

Dosing Recommendations

The dosing range of milrinone as a continuous infusion is typically 0.25 to 0.75 mcg/kg/min (Hansen et al., 2016). Clinicians may initiate therapy with a loading dose (50 mcg/kg/dose) for more rapid therapeutic effects. Loading doses are associated with an increased risk of hypotension (Chang et al., 1995). Loading doses should be given over an hour and extended to over 3 hours in preterm infants to prevent hypotension. Milrinone should not be rapidly titrated, and effects of the medication may be prolonged.

Clinical-Monitoring Pearls

Adverse side effects of milrinone include hypotension, tachycardia, arrythmias, and thrombocytopenia. Milrinone's vasodilation extends from the pulmonary vascular to the peripheral vascular beds, leading to concerns for hypotension. As mentioned previously, hypotension is associated with loading doses but also with the continuous infusion itself. The risk of hypotension is highest with initiation and BPs gradually return to baseline after 24 hours. Neonates with inadequate intravascular volumes and/or aggressive diuresis are also at higher risk of hypotension. Tachycardia has been seen with milrinone therapy. Milrinone may increase HR by 5% to 10% over baseline (McNamara et al., 2013). This tachycardia could have contributed to reports of ventricular arrhythmias resulting from milrinone therapy. Last, thrombocytopenia has been described in children on milrinone. Some studies report much higher incidences of thrombocytopenia, whereas others report rare episodes.

Systemic Corticosteroids

Corticosteroids are commonly prescribed adjunctive medications for neonates with hypotension and shock. Approximately 15% to 30% of hypotensive neonates develop refractory hypotension that is unresponsive to high-dose vasopressor–inotropes (Kumbhat & Noori, 2020). Hydrocortisone is considered the drug of choice for VRH due to its efficacy profile (Higgins et al., 2010; Pellicer 2009). Therefore, we present readers with information specific to hydrocortisone therapy, the most common corticosteroid used to treat hypotension.

HYDROCORTISONE

Hydrocortisone offers balanced mineralocorticoid and glucocorticoid effects, making this drug the optimal corticosteroid for premature and term infants with VRH, asphyxiated newborns, infants recovering from cardiac surgery, and those with septic shock (Kovacs et al., 2019). Recall that cortisol concentrations are inversely related to gestational age and are especially low in infants receiving inotropic support due to adrenergic receptor down regulation (Scott & Watterburg, 1995). Furthermore, premature infants have a limited capacity to increase cortisol production in response to stressful stimuli due to immature adrenal and pituitary signaling systems. This relative adrenal insufficiency has been identified as one cause of refractory hypotension in premature infants (Watterberg, 2002). Thus, hydrocortisone's mineralocorticoid effects are helpful in replacing cortisol directly and thus increasing hemodynamic stability.

Mechanism of Action/Pharmacokinetic Principles

The mechanism of action of hydrocortisone is shown in Figure 20.10. Glucocorticoids increase adrenergic receptor expression, which can cause vasoconstriction and increased CO. The receptor upregulation increases responsiveness to endogenous and exogenous catecholamines (Sasidharan, 1998). There is also an upregulation of angiotensin II receptors and their second-messenger systems, which increases arterial BP. Furthermore, corticosteroids inhibit the production of vasodilatory nitric oxide and prostaglandins (Hausdorff et al., 1990). Within the sympathetic nervous system, hydrocortisone increases the conversion of norepinephrine to epinephrine and inhibits catecholamine metabolism. Hydrocortisone may provide additional positive inotropy by increasing intracellular calcium concentrations (S. R. Lee et al., 2012). Last, corticosteroids may be helpful in reducing capillary leak and are thus especially beneficial in hypovolemic states (Noori et al., 2006).

Hydrocortisone is typically given as intravenous intermittent bolus. Although hydrocortisone is the only medication discussed in this chapter that can be given enterally with an estimated bioavailability of 90%, this route is rarely used in the setting of systemic hypotension. Compared with the continuous infusions discussed earlier, hydrocortisone has a delayed onset of action. Within 2 hours of the initial hydrocortisone dose, significant increases in BP can be seen. Within 6 to 12 hours, after even a single dose of hydrocortisone, a meaningful reduction in vasopressor dosing can be expected (Noori et al., 2006). Vezina and colleagues (2014) report population pharmacokinetics of hydrocortisone in preterm and term neonates. The hydrocortisone half-life is approximately 2.9 hours in term neonates and much longer (approximately 9 hours) in preterm infants less than 35 weeks' postmenstrual age. Hydrocortisone is hepatically metabolized and excreted primarily by the kidneys. Renal clearance increases with advancing gestational age.

FIGURE 20.10 Mechanism of action of hydrocortisone.

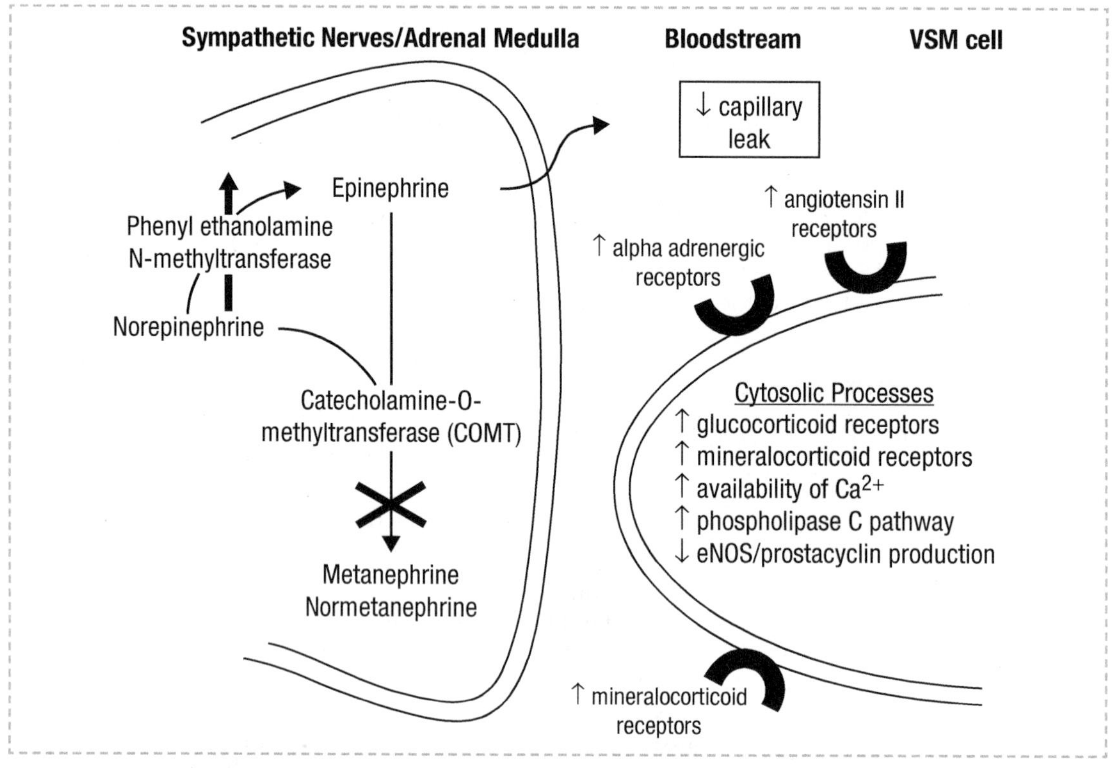

eNOS, endothelial NO synthases; VSM, vascular smooth muscle.

Source: Adapted from Giesinger, R. E., & McNamara, P. J. (2016). Hemodynamic instability in the critically ill neonate: An approach to cardiovascular support based on disease pathophysiology. *Seminars in Perinatology, 40*(3), 174–188. https://doi.org/10.1053/j.semperi.2015.12.005.

Dosing Recommendations (Hypotension-Specific)

Three factors confound dosing decisions: (a) exogenous hydrocortisone mirrors endogenous cortisol levels, (b) bioactive (free) cortisol is not directly measured, and (c) altered metabolic function or decreased cortisol excretion can falsely elevate cortisol values (Kumbhat & Noori, 2020). As such, wide variability in dosing strategies is reported in the available literature. Helbock and colleagues (1993) reported significant increases in BP with an average initial dose of 1.2 mg/kg followed by 1.5 to 6 mg/kg/d maintenance dosing (average 2.3 mg/kg/d). Ng and colleagues in 2006 reported the ability to wean vasopressor/inotropic support after hydrocortisone was administered at 1 mg/kg/d for 5 consecutive days. Seri and colleagues (2001) reported increases in BP and success with vasopressor/inotrope weaning with a dose of 2 to 6 mg/kg/d for up to 3 consecutive days. Finally, Noori and colleagues (2006) reported a significant increase in BP without cardiovascular side effects using an initial hydrocortisone dose of 2 mg/kg/d followed by 1 mg/kg every 12 hours for 2 consecutive days. The most commonly used dosing is 1 mg/kg every 8 hours for hypotension; clinicians are encouraged to titrate to the lowest effective dose after stabilizing BP (Kumbhat & Noori, 2020; Watterberg et al., 2016). When determining the dosing interval for a preterm infant, clinicians should also consider the slower rate of clearance observed in infants less than 35 weeks of gestation. More frequent intervals, such as every 6 hours, may be necessary in post-term neonates.

Clinical-Monitoring Pearls

The use of corticosteroids (including hydrocortisone) can be challenging due to potential adverse effects. Pertinent short-term adverse effects include hyperglycemia, water retention, increased risk of infections (especially fungal), osteopenia, and growth retardation. Gastrointestinal perforation has been reported with concomitant use of nonsteroidal anti-inflammatory drugs, such as indomethacin or ibuprofen, for PDA closure and thus should be avoided (Watterberg et al., 2004). Adrenal insufficiency is another concern with extended corticosteroid courses of 2 weeks or more or multiple repeated steroid exposures (Auron & Raissouni, 2015). Clinicians are encouraged to follow glucose and urine output trends throughout therapy. Given the infectious risk, clinicians should be on high alert for the presence of nonspecific findings that correlate with sepsis.

The use of corticosteroids in neonatology has been controversial due to concerns for neurodevelopmental delays. Early dexamethasone in the first week of life showed an increased incidence of cerebral palsy (Halliday et al., 2003). However, Watterberg et al. (2007) showed that early, low-dose hydrocortisone was not associated with an increase in cerebral palsy. Hydrocortisone-exposed infants even trended toward improved neurodevelopmental scores. However, duration is an important mediator of the association between neurodevelopmental outcomes and corticosteroids. One study showed that hydrocortisone exposure longer than 7 days was associated with reduced motor skill in the first year of life (Patra et al., 2015). With hydrocortisone used to treat hypotension, the duration should be minimized to prevent short- and long-term adverse effects.

CONCLUSIONS

Hypotension is a common pathophysiologic problem encountered in NICUs. Invasive arterial BP monitoring remains the gold standard for diagnosing hypotension and titrating vasopressors and should be pursued if persistently abnormal noninvasive BP measurements are identified. APRNs are expected to generate an appropriate differential diagnosis as a means of identifying the proximate cause for hypotension. Medications used to treat hypotension continue to be prescribed off-label and often in the absence of high quality data (large-scale, multicenter RCTs). Every medication discussed in this chapter can elicit untoward short-term and/or long-term side effects. Therefore, it is crucial that clinicians understand the mechanism of action of vasoactive and inotropic drugs, PDE inhibitors, and corticosteroids to properly prescribe and avoid unnecessary drug exposures. Timely identification and treatment is critical to minimize the risk of long-term injury or irreversible shock and death. APRNs, in particular novice APRNs, are encouraged to pursue a collaborative decision-making approach when prescribing medications for hypotension. This may include collaboration with a pediatric pharmacist and/or specialist, such as a cardiologist, to best match pharmacotherapy with the underlying cause of hypotension/hypoperfusion. This type of synergistic, multidisciplinary approach to managing critically ill neonates helps guarantee the provision of high-quality, timely, and evidence-based care.

LEARNING TOOLS AND RESOURCES

Advice From the Authors

Jennifer Barnes, PharmD, BCPPS

Hypotension and shock in the neonatal population are anxiety-inducing for new and old practitioners alike. I encourage our readers to be thoughtful with selecting the pharmacologic agent and dosing strategy that addresses the underlying cause. It is not a one-size-fits-all approach!

Amy J. Jnah, DNP, APRN, NNP-BC

The approach to managing circulatory insufficiency is anything but simple. Hypotension is regarded as a late symptom of shock, and therefore requires prompt attention and management. Please take pause to study the various drugs covered in this chapter using multisensory strategies (e.g., drawing, concept mapping, study groups) and then test your recall by "teaching back" to a trusted mentor. Mastery is achieved with repetition!

Patricia L. Dias, MD

When approaching a neonatal patient with hypotension, first ask yourself whether treatment is even needed by determining whether shock is present. Next, attempt to determine the etiology of the infant's hypotension by examining the systolic and diastolic components of blood pressure (not just the mean arterial pressure) and using supplemental studies such as an echocardiogram. Finally, select a medication that is tailored for the clinical situation at hand. Managing a hypotensive neonate should truly be an endeavor in personalized medicine.

Discussion Prompts

1. Compare and contrast different methodologies for defining hypotension in the premature infant population.
2. Discuss risk factors in the neonatal population that increase their susceptibility to hypotension and shock.
3. Discuss different receptor targets for vasoactive medications and their effects.
4. Review clinical scenarios in which each vasoactive medication would be preferential and describe why.

Mind Map

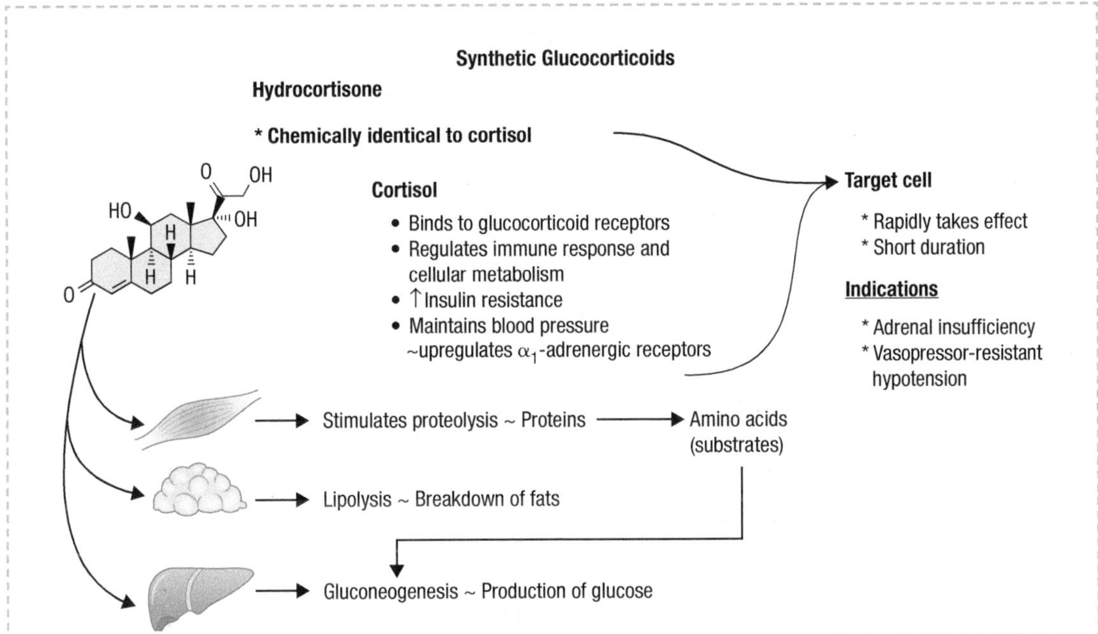

Note: This mind map reflects the design team's interpretation of a portion of one or more concepts addressed in this chapter. Readers should regard the mind maps woven throughout this textbook as examples of multisensory study tools that can be developed to encourage conceptual understanding. Readers are encouraged to develop their own unique mind maps in consultation with academic faculty or clinical preceptors. Design credit: Amy J. Jnah, DNP, APRN, NNP-BC.

REFERENCES

References for this chapter are online and available at https://connect.springerpub.com/content/book/978-0-8261-5884-0/part/partIV/toc-part/ch20.

PART V

Common Gastrointestinal Problems

chapter 21

Human Milk as Medicine

Kelley Baumgartel and Diane L. Spatz

LEARNING OBJECTIVES

After completing this chapter, the reader should be able to:

- Understand the history of human milk as it relates to modern applications.
- Describe critical and protective immune components found in human milk.
- Demonstrate an understanding of the relationship between human milk composition and the developing preterm infant's immune system.
- Identify considerations related to pasteurized donor human milk (PDHM).

INTRODUCTION

The practice of administrating human milk is embedded throughout history; without human milk, our species would not have survived. Human milk exposure during infancy is associated with numerous health benefits. For example, the anti-inflammatory nature of human milk was initially observed by Lucas and Cole (1990), who uncovered its significant protective effect against necrotizing enterocolitis (NEC). This pivotal work led to an entire body of clinical research that examines clinical outcomes as they relate to human milk administration.

Human milk provides a protective extrauterine link between the lactating parent and the critically ill infant. Further, human milk confers protection to critically ill hospitalized infants from disease and mortality by way of highly protective immunofactors. This chapter describes components found in milk that protect against common infant comorbidities. An in-depth understanding of human milk composition variability and the developing neonate is critical for clinicians who work in the NICU. We also identify considerations related to the administration of pasteurized donor human milk (PDHM).

PHYSIOLOGY REVIEW: HUMAN MILK AND THE DEVELOPING IMMUNE SYSTEM

There are 10 times more bacteria in the intestine than there are eukaryotic cells in the body (Walker, 2017), and the milk microbiota is one of the first programmers of infant immunologic, gastrointestinal, and metabolic health (Hunt et al., 2011). Indeed, the immune and gastrointestinal systems develop concurrently (Zhu & Dingess, 2019). Variable colonization patterns are associated with an increased risk for disease in the immediate postnatal period (Butel et al., 2018), with widely noted differences in colonization patterns between formula-fed and breastfed infants (Hunt et al., 2011). Dysbiosis in suboptimal colonization environments may result in susceptibility to infection due to altered immune homeostasis (Wood, 2012).

The preterm infant is at risk for dysbiosis because many receive bovine-based formula, or donor breast milk (which is void of microbiota following pasteurization). In addition, many preterm infants are born via cesarean section, and this delays commensal bacteria colonization (Shao et al., 2019). Adequate colonization with commensal bacteria is important because these bacteria function as a protective "ancillary body organ" (Walker, 2017). However, unlike term infants who are breastfed immediately after birth and discharged soon after delivery, preterm infants often require parenteral nutrition immediately after birth, are fed small volumes of colostrum over the first days of life, are exposed to the unnatural microbiota in the NICU, and may be subject to supplemental preterm formula intake. This increases the risk for dysbiosis (Hartz et al., 2015), which is associated with gastrointestinal and respiratory disease (Jost et al., 2015).

The immediate postnatal window is a critical time in gut barrier establishment and immune modulation via commensal bacteria (Collado, Santaella, et al., 2015). Therefore, immediate feeding of exclusive human milk is strongly encouraged, directly from the lactating parent when possible, during the early postnatal period (Rogier et al., 2014). We refer readers to Chapter 24, "Necrotizing Enterocolitis," for additional discussion of the physiologic development of the gut microbiome.

Innate Immunity

Innate immunity confers protection against infection through induction of natural barriers and inflammatory factors that prevent damage from environmental pathogens (see Chapter 8, "Vaccines and Schedules"). This is highly relevant to NICU clinical practice, as environmental pathogens and multiple invasive medical procedures are common. Innate immunity in preterm infants is limited due to their inability to synthesize protective factors. Preterm infants are born with circulating maternal innate immune factors; however, this protective impact is eliminated once used by the infant.

The neonatal response to infection is compromised, largely due to a significantly limited production of immunoglobulins (Melville & Moss, 2013). As mentioned, many immunoglobulins are maternally transferred in utero after 32 weeks of gestation. The amount of immunoglobulin transfer is positively associated with gestational age, leaving preterm infants at risk due to a deficit of endogenous circulating immunoglobulins when compared to healthy term infants. This is not ideal, as low immunoglobulins lead to pour opsonization and subsequent compromised phagocytosis. This complex process is critical to remove bacteria and infected cells in order to optimize tissue homeostasis and decrease the risk and severity of infection (Rosales & Uribe-Querol, 2017). Phagocytosis is also compromised among preterm infants due to reduced lectin and synthesis of endogenous monocytes and dendritic cells (Melville & Moss, 2013). This may also result in neutropenia, which greatly reduces the infant's ability to fight infection (Correa-Rocha et al., 2012). Recall that neutrophils are the first responders to infection and migrate to the site of infection to kill microorganisms (Jnah & Trembath, 2019). Neutrophils produced by preterm infants are unable to efficiently migrate to the infection site, likely due to a reduction in adhesion molecule expression (Abbas & Lichtman, 2006).

Monocytes are synthesized by bone marrow and differentiate into macrophages, which are highly involved in phagocytosis, bactericidal properties, and antigen presentation (Jnah & Trembath, 2019). Monocytes initiate the inflammatory cascade via cytokine production, pathogenic clearance, and apoptotic cellular removal (de Jong et al., 2017). Preterm monocytes have reduced functionality, another way through which the preterm infant is at risk of infection. The overall ecosystem of human milk is largely anti-inflammatory, which provides preterm infants with additional biologically active proteins to combat disease. For example, toll-like receptors are involved in recognizing pathogens and reduce additional inflammatory responses that would put the infant at greater risk of NEC (Mara et al., 2018).

Adaptive Immunity

Adaptive immunity reflects acquired protection from exposure to vaccines or prior infections. Preterm infants have virtually no adaptive immunity, as they have not had extrauterine exposure to such stimuli prior to birth. Maturation occurs after birth of a healthy term infant, followed by lymphocytic circulatory distribution to peripheral lymphoid organs and spleen. The invasion of pathogens by lymphocytes results in pathogenic and/or tumor cell invasion. B and T cells are differentiated lymphocytes involved in adaptive immunity and continue to differentiate once exposed to an antigen. Following exposure, T and B cells synthesize memory lymphocytes, which work to eliminate the antigen. Preterm infants have a significantly reduced number of circulating lymphocytes, thereby increasing the risk of sepsis and/or death among preterm infants (Jnah & Trembath, 2019).

Passive Immunity

Passive immunity refers to the action of receiving immunologic compounds through either the placenta or human milk (Jnah & Trembath, 2019). As opposed to other immunity types identified previously, this type of immunity is especially relevant to human milk administration. Human milk is the only way through which preterm infants passively receive critical protective milk components, as they are no longer in utero to receive this support via the placenta.

For example, NEC (described earlier as a leading cause of death for preterm infants) is exhibited by increased gastrointestinal permeability. Preterm infants are born with an immature gastrointestinal system, which exhibits poor cellular cohesiveness. The onset of NEC is preceded by the translocation of bacteria across the loose ("leaky") junctions between gastrointestinal epithelial cells. This leakiness between the cells permits the migration of harmful bacteria and other proinflammatory cytokines across the mucosal, submucosal, muscularis, and/or serosal layer of the gut wall. This is accompanied by bacterial proliferation and, possibly, NEC (Remon et al., 2015).

Human milk compounds work to directly oppose such deleterious cycles. For example, human milk oligosaccharides (HMOs) are able to both: (a) compete for binding spots with pathogenic bacteria; and (b) some exhibit prebiotic effects, which promote the growth of commensal bacteria. Immunoglobulin A (IgA) is another example of a critically important compound present in human milk that the infant can ingest and use to further protect an already-compromised gastrointestinal wall. IgA also works to promote a healthy and balanced homeostasis within the gut environment. Together with HMOs, IgA are passively conferred to infants via human milk.

CRITICAL COMPONENTS OF HUMAN MILK

Human milk involves a complex and ever-changing ecosystem. The ability of the lactating parent to produce milk specifically tailored to their infant has been elucidated over the past 25 years. In this section, we provide a high-level overview of some of the most critical components of human milk.

Human milk contains diverse commensal (beneficial) bacteria, which reach the mammary gland through active migration. This is then administered to the infant through the act of direct breastfeeding or nasogastric feeding (Jeurink et al., 2013). This exposure to commensal organisms promotes healthy colonization of the gut with beneficial microbes (Jeurink et al., 2013). The major ingredients found in human milk include oligosaccharides, proteins, enzymes, and immunoglobulins.

Human Milk Oligosaccharides

HMOs and the milk microbiome work synergistically to create an ecologically diverse gastrointestinal microbiome. HMOs constitute nearly 33% of the human milk compositional profile (Diaz et al., 2019), and these carbohydrates are comprised of five monosaccharides (glucose, galactose, N-ethylglucosamine, fucose, and sialic acid) and one disaccharide (lactose).

HMOs participate in modulating the infant immune system and are considered a primary contributor to both the composition and amount of commensal bacteria in breast milk (e.g.,

Bifidobacteria) present in the gut (Moubareck, 2021). Specific immunomodulatory functions of HMOs include inhibition of bacterial adhesion to the gastrointestinal wall, immune signaling, and the induction of immune dendritic cells. HMOs also exhibit a high affinity for certain galectins (Moubareck, 2021), or carbohydrate-bonding proteins linked to proinflammatory diseases (Johannes et al., 2018). When the HMO binds to a specific galectin, it inhibits the ability of the galectin to interact with other cells and elicits a physiologic effect which is often inflammatory in nature.

HMOs are abundant in human milk. When critically ill preterm infants are given colostrum to the cheeks, or when stable preterm or term infants are orally breast- or bottle-fed, HMOs come into direct contact with the respiratory mucosa before descending the esophagus. HMOs that come into contact with the respiratory epithelial cells stimulate the maturation of these cells, improving the immune response to respiratory viruses (e.g., coronavirus, influenza, respiratory syncytial virus). Simultaneously, these HMOs reduce the ability of pathogens to adhere to the respiratory mucosa by acting as decoy receptors.

HMOs that reach the gastrointestinal tract, either by way of swallowing or nasogastric tube, are minimally digested; they reach the large intestine intact and able to encourage the proliferation of commensal bacteria while simultaneously inhibiting bacterial proliferation of pathogenic bacteria. This is particularly beneficial for preterm infants, who are known to have a "leaky" gut, characterized by easily permeable enterocytes at the brush border. Infants who are devoid of adequate HMO intake are at higher risk for acquired comorbid conditions, including gut dysfunction (feeding intolerance), NEC, and diarrhea (Bering, 2018; Morrow et al., 2004).

A small fraction (1%) of HMOs is absorbed through the gut wall and into the systemic circulation, where they bind to cell surface receptors on cells of the immune system and epithelial cells. This modulates the immune response in the gut as well as throughout the body (Triantis, 2018). The remaining 99% of HMOs not absorbed into the circulation continue to the colon, shape the gut microflora in this portion of the large intestine, and are thereby eliminated from the body in the stool (Wiciński et al., 2020).

Bioactive Proteins

Of all bioactive proteins in human milk, lactoferrin is considered the most important. Lactoferrin was discovered as a component of bovine milk in the early 1960s and studied intently over the following decades (Blanc et al., 1963). Years of research elucidated the fact that lactoferrin concentrations are highest in colostrum and slowly decrease across the lactation continuum. Lactoferrin exerts a wide range of anti-infective, anti-inflammatory, antioxidant, immunomodulatory, and prebiotic actions (Albenzio et al., 2016; Ballard & Morrow, 2013). For example, lactoferrin acts as a carrier protein for iron while selectively preventing harmful gut bacteria from interacting with iron. Although most lactoferrin is excreted fully intact in the stool, some is metabolized to lactoferricin, a byproduct that uniquely inhibits the proliferation of some gram-negative bacilli (e.g., *Escherichia coli*) and gram-positive bacilli (e.g., *Staphylococcus*) in the intestinal tract (Brouwer et al., 2011). This is particularly protective for preterm infants. Osteopontin is another human milk protein, typically abundant in colostrum and during early lactation (Jiang & Lönnerdal, 2019). This human milk protein plays an important role in immune function, intestinal maturation, and neurodevelopment (Jiang et al., 2019).

Enzymes

One particular human milk enzyme, superoxide dismutase, found in human milk enhances the antioxidant properties of the milk. This is particularly beneficial for preterm infants who are frequently subjected to oxidative stress after birth, and are unable to neutralize reactive oxygen species. Superoxide dismutase induces vascular relaxation and provides significant antioxidant protection (Lugonja et al., 2013).

Lipase, another critical enzyme found in unpasteurized human milk, was first discovered in the 1950s (Bläckberg et al., 1980). It functions to digest lipids (triacylglycerols) present in unpasteurized human milk. Three types of lipases modulate the digestion of lipids: bile salt-stimulated lipase (BSSL), gastric lipase, and pancreatic lipase. Note that BSSL is inactivated when human milk is pasteurized (e.g., donor human milk), which can reduce lipid digestion and absorption. This supports the use of freshly expressed human milk whenever possible.

Immunoglobulins

Human milk is also a rich source of immunoglobulins, with the most abundant being secretory IgA (Ballard & Morrow, 2013). Like the proteins found in human milk, concentrations of secretory IgA are highest in colostrum. Immunoglobulins protect the mucous membranes and activate phagocytosis (Ballard & Morrow, 2013). The immunoglobulins are ever-changing in human milk in response to the child's environment. For example, during the COVID-19 pandemic, researchers found a robust antibody response in human milk supporting immunologic adaptation to a new environmental pathogen (Fox et al., 2020).

White Blood Cells and Stem Cells

Human milk is also a rich source of white blood cells, stem cells, and immune cells (Hassiotou et al., 2013). Leucocytes in human milk confer active immunity and protect the mammary gland from infection (Hassiotou et al., 2013). Human milk is a rich source of stem cells, which cross the blood–brain barrier and offer neuroprotection. This facilitates myelination in later gestation and improved neurocognitive outcomes (Deoni, 2018; Twigger et al., 2013). Human milk is also an abundant source of cytokines (e.g., interleukins [IL]), which provide both regional and systemic immune support (Ballard & Morrow, 2013). Interleukins (e.g., IL-6) can also cross the blood–brain barrier and augment endogenously produced immune cells, thereby enhancing the immune response (Baumgartel et al., 2016).

Practical Considerations for Clinicians

It is important to understand that human milk is a living, complex, and ever-changing substance. Human milk is always going to be the most potent and beneficial when delivered fresh to the infant. As mentioned in this section, prolonged exposure to a deep freezer and/or pasteurization may completely destroy or reduce the potency of the components of human milk (Table 21.1; Paulaviciene et al., 2020).

HISTORICAL PERSPECTIVES: SEMINAL AND OTHER NOTEWORTHY STUDIES

An ever-increasing number of publications support the accumulating evidence that human milk provides critical protection to neonates, particularly those in the NICU. We call attention to noteworthy studies that have contributed to our current understanding of human milk use in the NICU.

Increased inflammation of the preterm infant gastrointestinal system is associated with NEC and NEC severity. Schanler and colleagues (1999) observed a decreased risk of NEC among preterm infants who received an exclusive human milk-based diet, including fortification (Schanler et al., 1999). This study aimed to describe growth, nutritional status, feeding tolerance, and overall health of preterm infants who receive human milk versus bovine-based milk feedings. This randomized, controlled trial assigned infants into either: (a) early or (b) late feeding initiation. Milk type (human or bovine) was determined by parental choice. A total of 108 infants were included in this study, and those who received an exclusive human milk diet experienced lower rates of NEC compared to infants fed preterm formula (6% vs. 19%, $p \leq .01$). Human milk-fed preterm infants had shorter length of stay and were able to consume more milk than the bovine-based group. This study called attention to the unique properties in human milk which promote the host defense system and gastrointestinal functionality.

It is well established that breastfed preterm infants do not receive adequate protein to allow for optimal growth rates; therefore, fortification is required to promote optimal postnatal growth (Rochow et al., 2021). Sullivan and colleagues (2010) contributed to the state of the

TABLE 21.1 Effects of Freezing and Pasteurization (Heat) on Major Constituents of Human Milk

	ANTIOXIDANTS	COMMENSAL BACTERIA	IMMUNOGLOBULINS			LACTOFERRIN[a]	LEUKOCYTES	LYSOZYME	OSTEOPONTIN	STEM CELLS
			IGA	IGG	IGM					
Major function(s)	Protection from oxidative stress	Formation of the gut microbiota	Host defense at mucosal membranes and gut lumen, intracellular neutralization of viruses, prevention of bacterial translocation	Antimicrobial activity in gut, anti-inflammatory activity, activation of phagocytes, opsonization of gram-negative bacilli	Opsonization of gram-negative bacilli, immune exclusion of antigens, complement activation for pathogen clearance, agglutination	Antimicrobial activity in gut, anti-inflammatory activity, promotion of intestinal maturation, modulation of immune function, opsonization of gram-negative bacilli	Production of antimicrobial proteins and peptides in gut and other tissues, opsonization of bacteria, phagocytosis, protection of mammary glands from infection	Production of antimicrobial cytokines and immunoglobulins in gut, penetrates pathogen membrane and renders bactericidal activity, opsonization of gram-negative and gram-positive bacilli	Immune system regulation, intestinal maturation, myelination	Neuroprotection
Effect of freezing on biologic function(s)	Decreased	**Destroyed**	Decreased	Decreased	Decreased	Decreased	**Destroyed**	Decreased	Decreased	**Destroyed**
Effect of pasteurization on biologic function(s)	Decreased	**Destroyed**	Decreased	Decreased	Decreased	Decreased	**Destroyed**	Decreased	Decreased	**Destroyed**

[a]Lactoferrin is one of the most abundant proteins found in human milk.
IG, immunoglobulin.

Sources: From Ballard, O., & Morrow, A. L. (2013). Human milk composition: Nutrients and bioactive factors. *Pediatric Clinics of North America, 60*, 49–74. https://doi.org/10.1016/j.pcl.2012.10.002; Bollinger, R. R., Everett, M. L., Palestrant, D., Love, S. D., Lin, S. S., & Parker, W. (2003). D. Human secretory immunoglobulin A may contribute to biofilm formation in the gut. *Immunology, 109*(4), 580–587. https://doi.org/10.1046/j.1365-2567.2003.01700.x; Brandtzaeg, P. (2010). The mucosal immune system and its integration with the mammary glands. *Journal of Pediatrics, 156*(2 Suppl.), S8–S15. https://doi.org/10.1016/j.jpeds.2009.11.014; Brouwer, C. P., Rahman, M., & Welling, M. M. (2011). Discovery and development of a synthetic peptide derived from lactoferrin for clinical use. *Peptides, 32*(9), 1953–1963. https://doi.org/10.1016/j.peptides.2011.07.017; Lawrence, R. M., & Pane, C. A. (2007). Human breast milk: Current concepts of immunology and infectious diseases. *Current Problems in Pediatric and Adolescent Health Care, 37*(1), 7–36. https://doi.org/10.1016/j.cppeds.2006.10.002; Lis, J., Orczyk-Pawiłowicz, M., & Kątnik-Prastowska, I. (2013). Proteins of human milk involved in immunologic processes. *Postepy Higieny i Medycyny Doswiadczalnej, 67*, 529–547. https://doi.org/10.5604/17322693.1051648; Liu, B., & Newburg, D. S. (2013). Human milk glycoproteins protect infants against human pathogens. *Breastfeeding Medicine, 8*(4), 354–362. https://doi.org/10.1089/bfm.2013.0016; Paulaviciene, I. J., Liubsys, A., Eidukaite, A., Molyte, A., Tamuliene, L., & Usonis, V. (2020). The effect of prolonged freezing and holder pasteurization on the macronutrient and bioactive protein compositions of human milk. *Breastfeeding Medicine, 15*(9), 583–588. https://doi.org/10.1089/bfm.2020.0219; Trend, S., Strunk, T., Hibbert, J., Kok, C. H., Zhang, G., Doherty, D. A., Richmond, P., Burgner, D., Simmer, K., Davidson, D. J., & Currie, A. J. (2015). Antimicrobial protein and peptide concentrations and activity in human breast milk consumed by preterm infants at risk of late-onset neonatal sepsis. *PLoS One, 10*(2), Article e0117038. https://doi.org/10.1371/journal.pone.0117038

science specific to human milk-based fortification by randomizing extremely preterm infants to receive: (a) human milk-based fortification or (b) bovine-based fortification (Sullivan et al., 2010). This was an international, multicenter study that included 12 NICUs and infants born weighing between 500 and 1,250 grams. In a sample of 207 extremely preterm infants, exclusive human milk diet significantly reduced the rates of NEC and surgical NEC ($p = 0.02$). All cases of surgical NEC were in the bovine-fortification group. As a result, the authors discouraged bovine-based exposure of any kind, and this study provided a template for exclusive human milk-based studies. In other words, this study provided insight into the anti-inflammatory potential of exclusive human milk diets.

Human milk provides anti-inflammatory factors that combat common neonatal morbidities, particularly NEC, as described. Corpeleijn and colleagues (2012) conducted a retrospective multicenter study of very-low-birth-weight infants (<1,500 grams; $n = 349$) who were receiving maternal breast milk (Corpeleijn et al., 2012). The objective of this study was to determine whether the early provision of donor milk instead of preterm formula (when maternal milk is unavailable) reduces the risk of common neonatal complications. Research activities occurred for the first 10 days of life to discern between neonatal outcomes that may be affected by initial diet. This concept is critical, as this milk will prime the infant gut and may serve as a template for subsequent commensal bacteria assemblage (Groer et al., 2014). This study uncovered that early and mostly (>50%) maternal milk feedings are associated with a lower incidence of NEC (relative risk [RR] 0.43, 95% CI: 0.26–0.71). Authors extended the study window to 60 days, which was a critical change in the science and far more generalizable as preterm infants often spend months in the hospital. This change also resulted in more cases (for example, NEC), which increases the power of the study. The authors discuss the matrix of the two milk types (human and bovine) and stress protein fractions between the two milk types are significantly different, with a bovine milk casein fraction that does not match the human milk casein homology. When bovine milk is delivered, systemic inflammation increases and the authors suggest that this exposure exacerbates the infant inflammatory response, thereby increasing the risk of additional complications.

CURRENT HUMAN MILK TREATMENT MODALITIES

With an increasing body of evidence about the benefits of human milk, ethical recommendations surrounding infant nutrition have evolved that reflect the risk of formula feedings (Froh & Spatz, 2014). Research protocols now prohibit the randomization of participants into formula versus human milk groups. This is grounded in the ethical principle of beneficence, as growing evidence clearly indicates that human milk is highly protective, particularly among critically ill infants. The National Health and Medical Research Council (Australia) went so far as to release a recommendation that reflects this pillar of safe research, stating that human milk clinical trials should not threaten the best interest of the infant (Spriggs & Gillam, 2008). Regardless of the research objective, any line of investigation that includes infant nutrition should not interfere with ongoing breastfeeding practices (Franck, 2005).

The protection that human milk affords underdeveloped preterm infants is reflected in a comprehensive body of literature that confirms the protective impact of human milk on neonatal pathology (Altobelli et al., 2020; Nolan et al., 2020; Rocha et al., 2021). We review the protective benefits that human milk offers preterm infants at risk for three of the most common disease processes managed in the NICU and discussed in accompanying chapters in this textbook: bronchopulmonary dysplasia (BPD), NEC, and late-onset sepsis (LOS).

Bronchopulmonary Dysplasia

BPD is one of the most common acquired diseases observed in hospitalized preterm infants (Villamor-Martinez et al., 2019). Those who develop BPD experience a longer length of stay, regardless of gestational age at birth (Kim et al., 2019). The pathogenesis of BPD remains unclear, though some biological processes have been identified that are associated with the onset of BPD. Preterm infant growth and lung development are severely compromised, leaving the infant's respiratory tract vulnerable to pathogens including viruses associated with BPD (Kim et al., 2019). We refer readers to Chapter 16, "Bronchopulmonary Dysplasia," for an expanded discussion of the disease process and pharmacologic management.

Human milk offers protection against oxidative stress, inflammation, and poor postnatal growth, risk factors associated with BPD (Dassios et al., 2021). A significant dose response has been reported in observational studies wherein infants who receive more maternal milk experience a lower risk of developing BPD (Table 21.2; RR 0.84, 95% CI: 0.73–0.96; Miller et al., 2018). However, similar results have not been reported from randomized trials. Therefore, while clearly the most optimal source for enteral nutrition for preterm infants, the relationship between the dose of human milk and risk of BPD remains elusive (Miller et al., 2018). It is possible that the dosage effect of maternal milk, which is reported across observational studies, may be attributed to higher levels of protective factors that are transferred to the infant via human milk, including antioxidants, macronutrients, immunoglobulins, and anti-inflammatory cytokines.

Necrotizing Enterocolitis

NEC is a devastating gastrointestinal complication that affects between 5% and 13% of infants born premature (Ahle et al., 2013; Hackam & Caplan, 2018). As discussed earlier in this chapter, preterm infants who are in the NICU develop a microbiome that reflects their neonatal environment (Brooks et al., 2014). This may introduce dysbiosis, or an imbalance in the gut microbiome, to an anatomically immature and vulnerable gastrointestinal tract. Early provision of human milk encourages the development of a diverse microbiome, which provides a template for subsequent bacterial profiles (Collado, Cernada et al., 2015; Groer et al., 2014; Walker & Iyengar 2015). Further, it is likely that many anti-inflammatory components found in breast milk work in tandem with commensal bacteria to induce an overall anti-inflammatory environment.

A significant reduction in any stage of NEC has been reported with the use of exclusive human milk compared to exclusive preterm formula feedings (Table 21.3; RR: 0.59, 95% CI: 0.39–0.89; Miller et al., 2018). One cohort study investigated the relationship between the dose of exclusive human milk and *severe* NEC; no significant difference was reported (RR: 0.36, 95% CI: 0.06–2.04). Ultimately, Miller and colleagues (2018) concluded that the use of exclusive human milk is associated with a 4.3% risk reduction (2.5–5 per 100 fewer cases of NEC) for any stage of NEC and a 2% risk reduction for severe NEC.

Late-Onset Sepsis

LOS, or sepsis that occurs after 72 hours of life, is a costly and deadly complication in the NICU that affects between 20% and 38% of preterm infants (Tsai et al., 2014). The most significant risk factor associated with the development of LOS is prematurity and/or low birth weight (Shane et al., 2017), as these infants exhibit undeveloped immune systems and are subject to invasive procedures that increase the risk for sepsis. Complications that arise from LOS are also devastating, and include BPD (Stoll et al., 2004), NEC (Tsai et al., 2014), and long-term neurodevelopmental delays (Stoll et al., 2004). A dysbiotic infant gut microbiome compromises the immune response, resulting in a hyperinflamed gastrointestinal environment (Collado, Cernada, et al., 2015).

Human milk combats the proinflammatory impact of systemic sepsis through numerous protective components that mitigate inflammation and increase microbial diversity. Specifically, HMOs in human milk provide a source of nutrition for commensal bacteria, which enhances microbial gut diversity. Other human milk components also favor microbial diversity, including growth factors (Aceti et al., 2017) and immunoglobulins, specifically IgA (Janzon et al., 2019). Lactoferrin, discussed earlier in this chapter, exhibits antimicrobial activity among common pathogens associated with LOS (Trend et al., 2015).

The protective impact of breast milk, as it relates to LOS, was confirmed in a recent meta-analysis, which aimed to examine the impact of various feeding standards on preterm infant health. In this study, human milk dosage was significantly associated with LOS. While modest, the more breast milk the infant receives, the less likely the infant is of developing LOS (RR 1.07, 95% CI: 0.89–1.28; Table 21.4; Miller et al., 2018).

TABLE 21.2 Bronchopulmonary Dysplasia Summary of Findings

COMPARISONS	ANTICIPATED ABSOLUTE EFFECTS[a] (95% CI)		RELATIVE EFFECT (95% CI)	NUMBER OF PARTICIPANTS (STUDIES)	CERTAINTY OF THE EVIDENCE (GRADE)
	RISK WITH PRETERM FORMULA/ PASTEURIZED HUMAN MILK	RISK WITH HUMAN MILK/ UNPASTEURIZED HUMAN MILK			
Bronchopulmonary dysplasia—Exclusive human milk vs. exclusive preterm formula; observational study	Study population		RR: 0.94 (0.26–3.41)	706 (two observational studies)	⊕⊖⊖⊖ VERY LOW [1,2]
	197 per 1,000	185 per 1,000 (51–672)			
Bronchopulmonary dysplasia—Any human milk vs. exclusive preterm formula; observational study	Study population		RR: 1.02 (0.83–1.27)	3,703 (six observational studies)	⊕⊖⊖⊖ VERY LOW [2,3]
	345 per 1,000	352 per 1,000 (286–438)			
Bronchopulmonary dysplasia—Higher vs. lower dose human milk intake; RCT study	Study population		RR: 0.95 (0.73–1.25)	1,075 (four RCTs)	⊕⊕⊖⊖ LOW [2,3]
	263 per 1,000	250 per 1,000 (192–328)			
Bronchopulmonary dysplasia—Higher vs. lower dose human milk intake; observational study	Study population		RR: 0.84 (0.73–0.96)	7,023 (18 observational studies)	⊕⊖⊖⊖ VERY LOW [3]
	305 per 1,000	256 per 1,000 (223–293)			
Bronchopulmonary dysplasia—Unpasteurized vs. pasteurized human milk (MOM or donor); RCT study	Study population		RR: 0.69 (0.43–1.10)	303 (one RCT)	⊕⊕⊖⊖ LOW [4]
	230 per 1,000	159 per 1,000 (99–253)			
Bronchopulmonary dysplasia—Unpasteurized vs. pasteurized human milk (MOM or donor); observational study	Study population		RR: 1.01 (0.72–1.43)	1,644 (five observational studies)	⊕⊖⊖⊖ VERY LOW [2]
	203 per 1,000	205 per 1,000 (146–290)			

Note: GRADE Working Group grades of evidence:
High certainty: We are very confident that the true effect lies close to that of the estimate of the effect.
Moderate certainty: We are moderately confident in the effect estimate: The true effect is likely to be close to the estimate of the effect, but there is a possibility that it is substantially different.
Low certainty: Our confidence in the effect estimate is limited: The true effect may be substantially different from the estimate of the effect.
Very low certainty: We have very little confidence in the effect estimate: The true effect is likely to be substantially different from the estimate of effect.
[1]Substantial heterogeneity, [2]wide CI, [3]moderate heterogeneity; [4]only one study, wide CI.
[a]The risk in the intervention group (and its 95% CI) is based on the assumed risk in the comparison group and the relative effect of the intervention (and its 95% CI).
MOM, mother's own milk; RCT, randomized controlled trial; RR: relative risk.
Source: From Miller, J., Tonkin, E., Damarell, R.A., McPhee, A. J., Suganuma, M., Suganuma, H., Middleton, P. F., Makrides, M., & Collins, C. T. (2013). A systematic review and meta-analysis of human milk feeding and morbidity in very low birth weight infants. *Nutrients, 10*(6), 707. https://doi.org/10.3390/nu10060707

TABLE 21.3 Any Necrotizing Enterocolitis: Summary of Findings

COMPARISONS	ANTICIPATED ABSOLUTE EFFECTS[a] (95% CI)		RELATIVE EFFECT (95% CI)	NUMBER OF PARTICIPANTS (STUDIES)	CERTAINTY OF THE EVIDENCE (GRADE)
	RISK WITH PRETERM FORMULA/ PASTEURIZED HUMAN MILK	RISK WITH HUMAN MILK/ UNPASTEURIZED HUMAN MILK			
Necrotizing enterocolitis—Exclusive human milk vs. exclusive preterm formula; RCT study	Study population 208 per 1,000	35 per 1,000 (4–275)	RR: 0.17 (0.02–1.32)	53 (one RCT)	⊕⊕⊖⊖ LOW [1]
Necrotizing enterocolitis—Exclusive human milk vs. exclusive preterm formula; and observational study	Study population 55 per 1,000	12 per 1,000 (5–30)	RR: 0.22 (0.09–0.54)	993 (three observational studies)	⊕⊕⊕⊖ MODERATE
Necrotizing enterocolitis—Any human milk vs. exclusive preterm formula; observational study	Study population 73 per 1,000	37 per 1,000 (26–56)	RR: 0.51 (0.35–0.76)	3,783 (nine observational studies)	⊕⊕⊕⊖ MODERATE
Necrotizing enterocolitis—Higher vs. lower dose human milk intake; RCT study	Study population 94 per 1,000	51 per 1,000 (26–96)	RR: 0.54 (0.28–1.02)	1,116 (four RCTs)	⊕⊕⊕⊖ MODERATE [2,3]
Necrotizing enterocolitis—Higher vs. lower dose human milk intake; observational study	Study population 80 per 1,000	42 per 1,000 (34–54)	RR: 0.53 (0.42–0.67)	8,778 (22 observational studies)	⊕⊕⊕⊖ MODERATE
Necrotizing enterocolitis—Unpasteurised vs. pasteurized human milk (MoM or donor); RCT study	Study population 59 per 1,000	86 per 1,000 (38–195)	RR: 1.45 (0.64–3.30)	303 (one RCT)	⊕⊕⊖⊖ LOW [4]
Necrotizing enterocolitis —Unpasteurised vs. pasteurised human milk (MOM or donor); observational study	Study population 37 per 1,000	47 per 1,000 (25–90)	RR: 1.28 (0.68–2.43)	1,894 (six observational studies)	⊕⊖⊖⊖ VERY LOW [5]

Note: GRADE Working Group grades of evidence:
High certainty: We are very confident that the true effect lies close to that of the estimate of the effect.
Moderate certainty: We are moderately confident in the effect estimate: The true effect is likely to be close to the estimate of the effect, but there is a possibility that it is substantially different.
Low certainty: Our confidence in the effect estimate is limited: The true effect may be substantially different from the estimate of the effect.
Very low certainty: We have very little confidence in the effect estimate: The true effect is likely to be substantially different from the estimate of effect.
[1]One study, wide CIs, small sample size; [2]Sullivan was not blinded, yet the outcome is objective and unlikely to be biased by this, hence not downgraded; [3]moderate heterogeneity; [4]one study, wide CIs; [5]wide CIs.
[a]The risk in the intervention group (and its 95% CI) is based on the assumed risk in the comparison group and the relative effect of the intervention (and its 95% CI).
MOM, mother's own milk; RCT: randomized controlled trial; RR: relative risk.
Source: Miller, J., Tonkin, E., Damarell, R. A., McPhee, A. J., Suganuma, M., Suganuma, H., Middleton, P. F., Makrides, M., & Collins, C. T. (2018). A systematic review and meta-analysis of human milk feeding and morbidity in very low birth weight infants. *Nutrients, 10*(6), 707. https://doi.org/10.3390/nu10060707

DONOR HUMAN MILK

The American Academy of Pediatrics (AAP) first provided a recommendation on the use of pasteurized donor human milk (PDHM) in 2012 (McGuire, 2012). At that time, they recommended PDHM for very-low-birth-weight infants if the mother's own milk was not available or its use was contraindicated. The first stand-alone position statement by the AAP was published in 2017 (Committee on Nutrition, Section on Breastfeeding, & Committee on Fetus and Newborn, 2017). This AAP position statement focused on the quality and safety of PDHM obtained through the Human Milk Banking Association of North America (HMBANA).

HMBANA oversees all nonprofit milk banks in North America and provides standard guidance for the screening and laboratory evaluation of all donors as well as guidance for Holder pasteurization and postpasteurization culturing of milk. HMBANA milk banks recruit donors from hospitals and the community and all donors undergo a detailed lifestyle and health history screening. The donor must also have paperwork completed by their healthcare clinician to verify that they are in good health. In addition, the infant's healthcare clinician must verify that the infant is healthy and gaining weight (unless the infant is deceased). All HMBANA milk banks in the United States and Canada require serologic testing for HIV, hepatitis B and C, human T-cell lymphotropic virus (HTLV), and syphilis. Once all serologic testing is confirmed to be negative, the milk can be pasteurized. Holder pasteurization heats the milk to 62.5°C (144.5°F) for 30 minutes. Once the milk is pasteurized, one bottle from each batch is sent for bacteriologic screening to ensure there is no growth of pathogens. Once confirmed negative, the milk is ready for distribution to hospitals.

Given the aforementioned screening requirements and pasteurization process, there is a processing fee to purchase milk from an HMBANA milk bank. Research by Spatz and colleagues demonstrated that PDHM from HMBANA is truly cost-effective in the presence of a strong human milk culture and when compared to other common interventions for hospitalized infants such as total parental nutrition (TPN; Spatz et al., 2018). In this study, data was abstracted on 281 infants, some admitted to the NICU while others remained on newborn nursery census requiring hospital treatment (Spatz et al., 2018). The total number of days of PDHM use was calculated, as was the cost of PDHM based on HMBANA PDHM pricing at the time of the research study (Spatz et al., 2018). The average volume of PDHM consumed by infants per day on PDHM was 195 milliliters (range 6–1,335 mL; Spatz et al., 2018). The average cost of PDHM per day on PDHM was $29.19 (range $0.90–$200.23; Spatz et al., 2018). Using the mean cost of PDHM compared to the cost of TPN at the institution at the time of the research, TPN was 44 times as expensive as the cost of PDHM (Spatz et al., 2018). This is significant in that there is strong data to support that when infants are fed an exclusive human milk diet, feeds can be advanced more quickly and the number of days on TPN can be reduced. Thus, if PDHM is administered, both healthcare costs and the risk for acquired diseases can be reduced.

The Academy of Breastfeeding Medicine (Sriraman et al., 2018) recommends the prioritization of PDHM for very-low-birth-weight infants, but also states that donor milk may be important for other populations such as small-for-gestational-age infants, late preterm infants, and infants requiring gastrointestinal surgery. The Academy (Sriraman et al., 2018) further acknowledges the presence of for-profit milk banks and gives strong recommendations against purchasing donor human milk on the internet.

Prolacta Bioscience is a for-profit company based in the United States. Their process of making donor human milk uses the vat pasteurization method. PDHM from Prolacta Bioscience is more expensive than PDHM from HMBANA nonprofit milk banks. Currently, 133/860 of Level 3 and Level 4 NICUs in the United States use PDHM from Prolacta (Prolacta Bioscience, personal communication). In addition to making PDHM, Prolacta Bioscience has 12 formulations of fortifiers made from human milk. These formulations add a variety of nutrients and caloric density to human milk and also include a human milk cream product. There is a large amount of research regarding the benefits of an exclusive human milk diet; however, it is important to note that much of this research has been industry funded (Abrams et al., 2014; Hair et al., 2022).

It is of critical importance to understand that not all donor milk is created equal; the differences come from the method used to process the milk (Spatz & Baumgartel, 2021). Recall that HMBANA (nonprofit) milk banks use the Holder pasteurization method, whereas the Prolacta Bioscience (for-profit) milk bank uses the vat method. In addition to these milk banks, there are other for-profit milk banks (e.g., Medolac, NIC-Q) that produce retort-sterilized milk. *Retorting* is defined as a

TABLE 21.4 Late-Onset Sepsis: Summary of Findings

COMPARISONS	ANTICIPATED ABSOLUTE EFFECTS[a] (95% CI)		RELATIVE EFFECT (95% CI)	NUMBER OF PARTICIPANTS (STUDIES)	CERTAINTY OF THE EVIDENCE (GRADE)
	RISK WITH PRETERM FORMULA/ PASTEURIZED HUMAN MILK	RISK WITH HUMAN MILK/ UNPASTEURIZED HUMAN MILK			
Late-onset sepsis—Exclusive human milk vs. exclusive preterm formula; RCT study	Study population		RR: 0.70 (0.47–1.03)	53 (one RCT)	⊕⊕⊖⊖ LOW [1]
	792 per 1,000	554 per 1,000 (372–815)			
Late-onset sepsis—Exclusive human milk vs. exclusive preterm formula; non-RCT and observational studies	Study population		RR: 0.71 (0.49–1.05)	776 (three observational studies)	⊕⊕⊖⊖ LOW
	174 per 1,000	123 per 1,000 (85–183)			
Late-onset sepsis—Any human milk vs. exclusive preterm formula; observational study	Study population		RR: 0.95 (0.67–1.34)	2,497 (eight observational studies)	⊕⊖⊖⊖ VERY LOW [2 3]
	301 per 1,000	286 per 1,000 (202–404)			
Late-onset sepsis—Higher vs. lower dose human milk intake; RCT study	Study population		RR: 1.07 (0.89–1.28)	1,186 (four RCTs)	⊕⊕⊕⊖ MODERATE [3]
	276 per 1,000	295 per 1,000 (245–353)			
Late-onset sepsis—Higher vs. lower dose human milk intake; observational study	Study population		RR: 0.71 (0.56–0.90)	6,521 (18 observational studies)	⊕⊖⊖⊖ VERY LOW [2]
	230 per 1,000	163 per 1,000 (129–207)			
Late-onset sepsis—Unpasteurized vs. pasteurized human milk (MOM or donor); RCT study	Study population		RR: 0.71 (0.43–1.18)	303 (one RCT)	⊕⊕⊕⊖ MODERATE [4]
	204 per 1,000	145 per 1,000 (88–241)			
Late-onset sepsis—Unpasteurized vs. pasteurized human milk (MOM or donor); observational study	Study population		RR: 1.05 (0.86–1.27)	1,875 (five observational studies)	⊕⊖⊖⊖ VERY LOW [5]
	258 per 1,000	271 per 1,000 (222–328)			

Note: GRADE Working Group grades of evidence:
High certainty: We are very confident that the true effect lies close to that of the estimate of the effect.
Moderate certainty: We are moderately confident in the effect estimate: The true effect is likely to be close to the estimate of the effect, but there is a possibility that it is substantially different.
Low certainty: Our confidence in the effect estimate is limited: The true effect may be substantially different from the estimate of the effect.
Very low certainty: We have very little confidence in the effect estimate: The true effect is likely to be substantially different from the estimate of effect.
[1]Only one study, wide CIs; [2]substantial heterogeneity; [3]wide CI; [4]one study only; [5]moderate heterogeneity.
[a]The risk in the intervention group (and its 95% CI) is based on the assumed risk in the comparison group and the relative effect of the intervention (and its 95% CI).
MOM, mother's own milk; RCT: randomized controlled trial. RR: relative risk.
Source: From Miller, J., Tonkin, E., Damarell, R.A., McPhee, A. J., Suganuma, M., Suganuma, H., Middleton, P. F., Makrides, M., & Collins, C. T. (2018). A systematic review and meta-analysis of human milk feeding and morbidity in very low birth weight infants. *Nutrients, 10*(6), 707. https://doi.org/10.3390/nu10060707

method of heat used to treat low-acid foods prone to microbial spoilage in hermetically sealed containers to extend their shelf life. The goal of retort processing is to obtain commercial sterilization by the application of heat. This process makes it stable at room temperature for up to 3 years. This retort sterilization process destroys many of the beneficial and protective human milk compounds (Spatz & Baumgartel, 2021). Therefore, the authors of this book chapter do not support the use of retort-sterilized milk.

PDHM is useful for parents struggling with a deficient supply of expressed human milk. Use of PDHM permits the continuation of an exclusive human milk diet and the avoidance of infant formula. Among infants born preterm, the most significant benefit of PDHM reported in the research is a reduction in the incidence of comorbid diseases, namely, NEC (Buckle & Taylor, 2017; Cacho et al., 2017; Kantorowska et al., 2016). However, the exclusive use of PDHM is associated with poorer postnatal growth among preterm infants. For this reason, PDHM is often fortified. Although interest in the use of PDHM outside the NICU is expanding it is beyond the scope of this chapter. Of note, PDHM has been used with late preterm infants and certain term infants for supplementation with some HMBANA milk banks to sell PDHM to families in the community; however, the majority of PDHM is earmarked for hospitalized infants. There are significant disparities in access to and use of PDHM in hospitals that serve people of color and low-income families (Baumgartel & Deem, 2019; Spatz, 2021).

It is of paramount importance that both clinicians and parents recognize that PDHM should not be considered a replacement for expressed human milk. All research demonstrates that the best outcomes are achieved with the use of the parent's own milk. This book chapter can serve as a call to action for clinicians to prioritize the use of human milk as a medical intervention.

Hospitals and healthcare personnel should invest time and effort to ensure that all parents make informed feeding choices to provide human milk when their child requires hospitalization at birth. The Spatz 10-step model has been implemented in hospitals throughout the United States and globally with significant increases in human milk feeding at discharge (Spatz, 2004, 2018). The first two steps of the model are informed decision-making and initiation and maintenance of milk supply (Spatz, 2004, 2018). These are the most critical steps for hospital staff to address. Given the tremendous disparities in breastfeeding with lower rates in low-resource families and people of color, it is clear that not all families are given the opportunity to make informed feeding choices. It is of paramount importance that we change the current prenatal care paradigm to help families make informed decisions for the use of human milk and breastfeeding (Spatz, 2021). Research demonstrates that when families participate in group prenatal care and learn the science of human milk and the physiology of lactation, 100% will chose to provide milk for their infant and the majority (87%) will continue through discharge of their infant from the hospital (Froh et al., 2020). With the outcomes of the Spatz 10-step model, the Association of Women's Health, Obstetric and Neonatal Nursing (AWHONN) has adopted this model as the national model for the provision of human milk during parent–infant separation (AWHONN, 2021). The peer-reviewed evidence-based practice guideline provides evidence for each of the 10 steps and step-by-step guidance for clinicians to ensure informed decision-making and the provision of human milk through discharge (AWHONN, 2021).

CONCLUSIONS

In the current practice paradigm, the majority of sick infants are discharged home on formula. This chapter arms clinicians with research and evidence about the components of human milk and how use of human milk is a medical intervention for hospitalized infants. Our goal is that clinicians will use this evidence to empower families to make informed feeding choices for human milk and that hospital administrators invest the necessary resources to support parents in their lactation journeys. It is of paramount important to improve the use of human milk, not just at the initiation of enteral feeds, but throughout the hospital stay. If more infants receive human milk at discharge, breastfeeding continuation rates could increase long term.

LEARNING TOOLS AND RESOURCES

Advice From the Authors

Kelley Baumgartel, PhD, RN

Human milk provides essential protection against many common and devastating neonatal complications. It is critical that healthcare providers understand and implement care that is informed by the abundance of research that supports the practice of human milk administration for vulnerable infants.

Diane L. Spatz, PhD, RN-BC, FAAN

It is essential that clinicians understand that human milk is a critical medical intervention. We all have an important role in ensuring that all families in our care are making informed feeding choices for the use of human milk and provide parents with evidence-based lactation care and interventions to ensure milk supply both short and long term.

Discussion Prompts

1. Human milk is a source of nutrition and immunologic protection, especially for critically ill infants in the NICU. Can you identify three human milk components that provide immunologic protection? How do they exert their functions on the neonate?
2. The administration of PDHM in the NICU is recommended by the AAP when the infant does not have access to maternal milk. How is PDHM different from maternal milk? How might these differences impact clinical outcomes?
3. In clinical research studies, it is unethical to randomize infants into a "formula feeding" group. Can you think of two to three reasons why this research design is unethical?
4. Does your institution ensure that all families are making informed feeding choices? How do families receive information about the science of human milk as a medical intervention?
5. How would you change your institutional culture to increase the provision of parents' own milk versus routine use of PDHM?

Mind Map

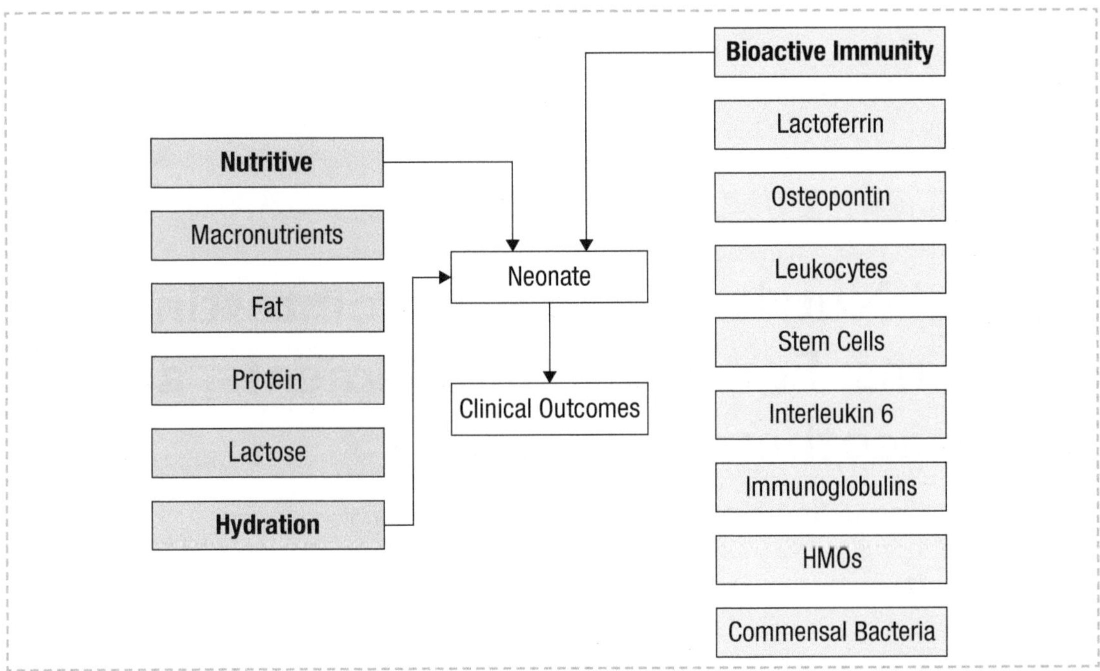

Note: This mind map reflects the design team's interpretation of a portion of one or more concepts addressed in this chapter. Readers should regard the mind maps woven throughout this textbook as examples of multisensory study tools that can be developed to encourage conceptual understanding. Readers are encouraged to develop their own unique mind maps in consultation with academic faculty or clinical preceptors. HMO, human milk oligosaccharide.

REFERENCES

References for this chapter are online and available at https://connect.springerpub.com/content/book/978-0-8261-5884-0/part/partV/toc-part/ch21.

chapter 22

Enteral Nutrition and Gastrointestinal Problems: Formulas, Supplements, and Pharmacotherapeutics

Amy J. Jnah, Carrie Smith, and Stephanie Merlino Barr

LEARNING OBJECTIVES

After completing this chapter, the reader should be able to:

- Explain the physiology of absorption and digestion and the pathophysiology of gastrointestinal (GI) problems.
- Understand the utility of tools used to appraise neonatal and infant growth and development.
- Appraise the historical evolution of scientific inquiries focused on growth and development and early tools used to appraise growth over time.
- Examine term and preterm formulas, fortifiers, and modular additives.
- Evaluate the role of pharmacotherapeutic regimens with respect to pharmacodynamic and pharmacokinetic properties in relation to management/prevention of common GI disorders.

INTRODUCTION

Term infants should regain birth weight by 7 to 10 days after birth and the majority do, whereas preterm infants should regain birth weight within 10 to 14 days after birth and many do not (Koletzko, Wieczorek, et al., 2021; McInerny, 2017). However, problems, including prematurity, metabolic disease, and gastrointestinal (GI) disease, often challenge postnatal growth velocity. Further, the provision of full enteral nutrition is complicated by the risks of feeding intolerance and other more severe GI diseases, such as necrotizing enterocolitis (NEC). These diseases often interrupt or delay enteral feeding advances.

In weight at birth, preterm infants are often appropriate for gestational age (AGA). However, over the first few weeks of life, most preterm infants can tolerate only 38% to 40% of the nutritional intake required to regain birth weight (Harding et al., 2017). Despite multiple changes in nutritional approaches over the weeks and months that follow, many preterm infants fail to reestablish the same rate of growth that would be observed in utero (Brune & Donn, 2018). Rather, most

---

Disclaimer: We seek to be inclusive of all people in our material. We recognize that not all people who give birth and lactate identify as female, and some identify as neither male nor female. Our readers should be aware that the information included in this chapter is intended for all persons, including those who breastfeed, chest feed, or feed with donated expressed human milk.

preterm infants grow parallel to published growth curves and often struggle to maintain adequate growth velocity between 37 and 40 weeks' postconceptual age (PCA; Fenton et al., 2013, 2020). Establishing and sustaining optimal postnatal nutritional intake for preterm infants continues to challenge NICU clinicians and is the subject of ongoing research.

Postnatal growth is generally assessed as size-for-weight gain, which overlooks changes in size-for-length (e.g., head circumference, length) and body composition, all significant factors in overall health outcomes. Johnson et al. (2012) conducted a meta-analysis of former preterm infants' body compositions at birth and at term equivalent age and compared these with a term-born cohort. They found that the former preterm infants had significantly greater total body fat compared with the term-born infants, but they were lighter overall, shorter, and had smaller head circumference (Johnson et al., 2012). Additional studies support the findings of increased adiposity, which may be the primary factor in increased chronic illness in former preterm infants (type 2 diabetes, heart disease, hypertension, and more; Crump et al., 2020; Knop et al., 2018; Uthaya et al., 2005). Thus, although we have made some strides in improving weight gain, ongoing reports of deficits in lean tissue mass and brain growth suggest that additional research is needed to further refine postnatal nutritional management for preterm infants.

In this chapter, we briefly review the core characteristics of the GI tract and the principles of digestion and absorption of enteral nutrients, human milk, formulas, additives, and vitamins available to meet or optimize specific enteral needs. We intentionally emphasize the beneficial relationship among human milk, neurodevelopment, immunologic function, GI health and maturation, and nutrient absorption throughout the chapter. In addition, we examine medications used to treat common GI problems. A fascinating review of the history of the study of human growth and the evolution of commercial formulas is also provided to offer new learners valuable context.

HISTORICAL PERSPECTIVE

Although the concepts and tools discussed in this chapter are commonplace in the current healthcare system, they were missing from use for centuries up to the present time. In fact, few records exist that contextualize the study of human growth over time. We present a concise summary of this remarkably interesting process of scientific inquiry of human growth, based primarily on the work of J. M. Tanner (1981).

The first recorded evidence of human growth data dates all the way back to the sixth century before the common era (BCE). Solon of Athens, a lawyer and poet, recorded the growth of his son in 7-year increments. No attention was paid to the boy's rate of growth or nutritional factors that could have affected his growth, but his statistics mark the beginning of what became centuries of scholarly inquiry and discourse. Tanner (1981) offers a concise interpretation of Solon's writings, as follows:

> A young boy acquires his first ring of teeth as an infant [literally, while unable to speak] and sheds them before he reaches the age of 7 years. When the god brings to an end the next seven-year period, the boy shows the signs of beginning puberty [or: of beginning pubic hair]. In the third hebdomad [seven-year period], the boy enlarges, the chin becomes bearded and the blood of the boy's complexion is lost. In the fourth hebdomad, physical strength is at its peak and is regarded as the criterion of manliness; in the fifth hebdomad a man should take the thought of marriage and seek sons to succeed him. In the sixth hebdomad a man's mind is in all things disciplined by experience and he no longer feels the impulse to uncontrolled behavior. In the seventh he is at his prime in mind and tongue, as also in the eighth, the two together making fourteen years. In the ninth hebdomad, though he still retains some strength, he is too feeble in the mind and speech for his greatest excellence. If a man continues to the end of the tenth hebdomad, he has not encountered death before the due time. (Tanner, 1981, pp. 1–2)

Next, we fast forward to the Renaissance and Reformation. As discussed elsewhere in this book, this period was dominated by medical and artistic inquiries, among others. Numerous drawings of human anatomy were created during this time by noteworthy artists, including Leonardo da Vinci. At some point during this era, physician Jean Fernel (founder of the term *physiology*) began to investigate human physiology or cause/effect relationships. He observed that children grew in stature over time, even in the presence of disease, and concluded (incorrectly) that a "growth faculty" explained this phenomenon. Toward the end of the Renaissance, physician Hippolyt Guarinoni shared his novel cause/effect observation that fatty foods and drink elicit growth and development, and even the onset of menarche. Although also not entirely correct, one might agree that Guarinoni was, thus far, pursuing a line of thought closest to what we know is true in modern society.

Next came more data-driven inquiries. The first individual to focus on anthropometry (and who coined the term) was physician Johann Elsholtz (1623–1688). He sought to measure adult height and did so by inventing a regula (ruler). Next, the book *Anthropometria*, which detailed the proportions of children, was published in 1723 by German painter Johann Bergmüller. He used the geometric principle of proportion to render drawings of children aged 1 to 3, 6, 9, 12, 15, 18, 21, and 24 years. He concluded that, "because growth is often hindered or disturbed, by illness or accident, I have for the most part kept to the average and have presented a neat and well-groomed proportion as the sensible way to represent healthy persons" (Tanner, 1981, p. 50). This book was the impetus for numerous subsequent inquiries and other proportional (but not absolute) drawings of children from infancy through young adulthood. Precision was still lacking.

Next, Herman Boerhaave (1668–1738) shifted attention away from proportion and again toward physiologic cause/effect relationships. His noteworthy observation was that linear growth depended on "elongation of the vessels by the fluid impelled through them." He also concluded that the brunt of human growth occurred in the first year of life and that some children exhibit catch-up growth after illness (Tanner, 1981, p. 69). Although his conclusions were also not entirely correct, as the most rapid period of growth occurs during fetal development, he motivated other scientists to study this phenomenon. The first to correctly identify that the fetus exhibits the most rapid development was Johann Stoller. The first to objectively measure fetuses was George LeClerc (1707–1788), and the first gender-specific growth charts were published in the 18th century by Christian Jampert (Figure 22.1). Readers may find it interesting to compare these charts with the modern gender-specific growth charts used in current NICUs.

Eighteenth-century scientists were interested in documenting long-term growth changes in children. We believe the first report was published in the 18th century by Philibert Montbeillard (1720–1785). Montbeillard used his son as his subject and carefully documented his height and height velocity from birth to age 18. Incidentally, he was also the first to administer a vaccination, the smallpox vaccine, to his son, in 1766 (before he was sadly beheaded by Robespierre). Then, in the United Kingdom, Marine recruits were subject to cohort studies of changes in height.

Additional clinical practice changes occurred during the 19th century. For example, Francois Chaussier, professor of anatomy and physiology, prioritized the assessment of newborn birth weight. He recorded the birth weight for over 7,000 newborns born at a Paris maternity center between 1802 and 1806. These data helped scientists identify the mean birth weight for term or near term (viable) newborns at the time. Next, possibly inspired by the methodology of Bergmüller, Michael Friedlander recorded interval weights for his child, at birth and at 1, 3, 4, 5, 7, 11, and 13 weeks, as well as at 5, 6, and 12 months of age. Notice that interval measurements were

FIGURE 22.1 First gender-specific growth charts.

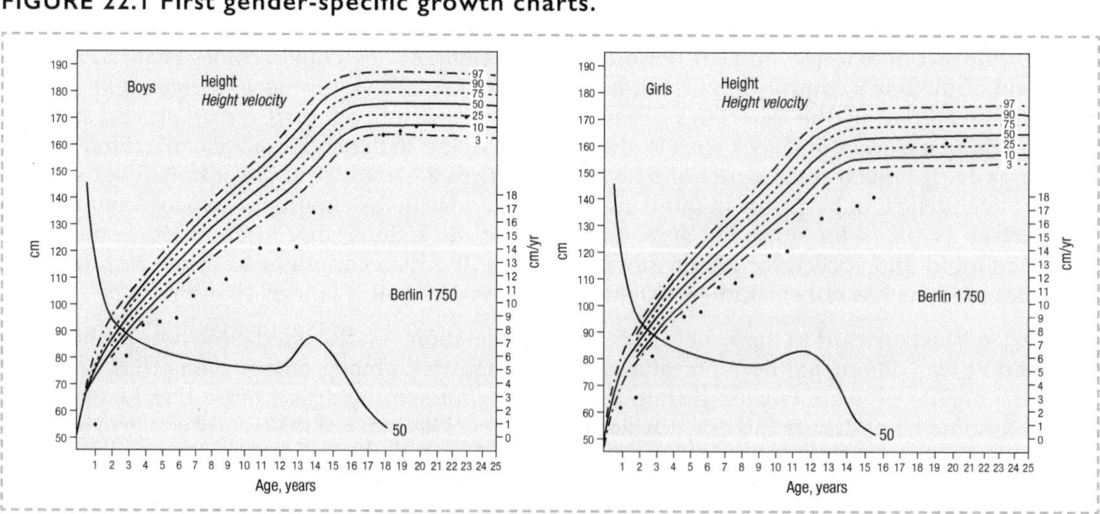

Source: From Tanner, J. M. (1981). *A history of the study of human growth* (pp. 92–93). Cambridge University Press. (Original work published 1920).

more frequent and encompassed a more significant portion of infancy (from birth to 12 months). A closer look at these data indicates that "average" weights observed during the 18th century would be defined as at or near the 10th percentile today!

Adolphe Quetelet (1796–1874) took Bergmüller's line of inquiry and expanded it by recording interval *heights and weights* of males and females from birth to age 25. Then, he began calculating height velocity. None other than *Florence Nightingale* identified the significance of his work and wrote to him on November 8, 1872. She asked for a copy of his book (*Anthropometria*) so that it could be shared with scholars and statesman in the United Kingdom.

Next, Joseph Clarke, an Irish obstetrician who maintained a midwifery practice and dedicated his professional tenure to reducing mortality, introduced the medical profession to taking routine, interval measurements of head circumference beginning at birth. He discovered over the course of his practice that male infants with perceivably larger heads were more difficult to deliver vaginally and mortality risk was higher (50%) in this cohort. In reading his work, we believe it is likely that the high mortality risk was linked to large-for-gestational-age status and shoulder dystocia. Clarke used a varnished piece of linen tape to measure the distance from (a) the most prominent part of the occiput to the frontal sinuses; and (b) one ear, across the anterior fontanelle, and to the opposing ear. The first step of his technique nearly mimics modern-day practice!

By mid- to late 19th century, pediatricians were intent on studying the growth of children over time. Further, pediatricians sought to identify etiologies linked to increases and decreases in weight and the potential relationship with feeding practices. For example, some physicians compared the weights and lengths of breastfed and bottle-fed infants. This led to the realization that growth conferred health. More and more scientists attempted to establish normative growth curves, and these inquiries extended well into the 20th century.

Throughout the 20th century, scientists investigated various aspects of growth and development, namely the relationship between hygiene and growth in learning environments. Other scientists investigated the relationship among growth, heredity, and the environment. The first formulas were created at this point in history, initially concocted at home from pediatrician-created recipes that were focused on providing energy and protein to infants (Schuman, 2003). Families were instructed to use canned milk, corn syrup, and even powdered sugar when mixing the homemade formula (Marriott & Schoenthal, 1929). Next, cases of scurvy increased, and this prompted pediatricians to add orange juice and cod liver to their formula recipes. None of these strategies proved to be entirely safe nor efficacious. Fortunately, commercial formulas were made available in the 1920s; the primary protein source was whey and fat source was milk fat. Later, milk fat was replaced with vegetable oils, still found in some formulas today. Twenty years later, in 1941, the Food and Drug Administration (FDA) put forth formula composition and labeling rules. This helped to standardize and align manufacturing processes with the best nutritional evidence available at the time and curbed the rise in cases of macronutrient and micronutrient deficiencies. Then, in 1967, the American Academy of Pediatrics (AAP) published specific guidelines for the nutritional composition of commercial-based formulas (AAP, 1967). These guidelines (which are occasionally updated) were endorsed by the FDA in 1971 and remain endorsed today. By 1980, the Infant Formula Act was written and passed, which provided even stricter regulatory oversight for commercial-formula manufacturing (Wargo, 2016). As a result of these noteworthy events and actions, systems are in place to protect vulnerable, nonverbal infants from nutritional deficits and infections. History tells us that despite the presence of these strict guidelines, errors occur, and powdered formulas become contaminated (most recently in February 2022). However, thanks to federal oversight, the FDA is quickly able to identify the source, cease production of the specific formula, notify the public and hospital entities, and protect lives.

Currently, 21st-century pediatric dietitians and clinicians continue to research best practices for achieving optimal postnatal growth. We use growth charts to classify a newborn as small-, appropriate-, or large-for-gestational age and assess size-for-age each week that an infant is hospitalized in a NICU. This informs part of the holistic nutritional risk assessment and informs initial nutritional management goals. As infants mature, serial measurements of weight, length, and head circumference are plotted on growth charts integrated within the electronic medical record and are relied upon when evaluating the efficacy and safety of the infant's nutritional regimen.

Given that each hospitalized infant has a nuanced postnatal course, and no consensus has been reached specific to a "gold standard" postnatal feeding regimen, growth charts and body mass index (BMI) charts offer clinicians objective data that can be used when tailoring an enteral feeding regimen. Note that these growth charts (e.g., Fenton, Olsen) are based on fetal-specific growth data, not extrauterine growth trends. Therefore, they cannot identify disproportionate weight gain to length (Olsen et al., 2015). We discuss these current growth charts in the next section of this chapter.

ASSESSMENT OF POSTNATAL GROWTH

Unlike virtually any other aspect of neonatology, the study of human growth actually *began* with infants, backtracked to the fetus, and then moved to the study of growth among school-age children. We have learned many lessons from our predecessors, one being that growth charts are useful tools for assessing postnatal growth across the life span.

Growth Curves

The two growth curves used with preterm (and term) infants, incepted by Fenton (2003) and Olsen et al. (2010), assess size-for-age. These well-tested and validated growth charts are available for use with hospitalized preterm infants born between 22 and 23 weeks of gestation. Each offers clinicians the ability to plot individual head, length, and weight measurements on a graph and compare those measurements with estimated normative age-specific centile markings (e.g., 3%, 10%, 50%, 90%, 97%). Therefore, the Fenton and Olsen growth curves are considered descriptive intrauterine size-for-age curves. These curves exclude the consideration of size-for-length (also referred to as weight-for-length). In contrast, a newer size-for-length tool not yet widely accepted for use in NICUs was incepted in 2021. This tool is titled the INTERGROWTH-21 curve (Villar et al., 2015). The INTERGROWTH-21 permits plotting of measurements as of 27 weeks of gestation, which excludes preterm infants born between 22 and 26 weeks of gestation.

Once a preterm or term infant reaches 42 weeks' postmenstrual age (PMA), clinicians are advised to transition to the World Health Organization (WHO, 2006) growth charts (Taylor & Buck, 2021). We investigate these growth curves in this section of the chapter.

FENTON GENDER-SPECIFIC GROWTH CURVES

The Fenton growth curve was incepted in 2003 and revised in 2013 (Figure 22.2; Fenton & Kim, 2013). Dr. Fenton initially sought to create two gender-specific growth curves which established benchmark indices aligned with expected intrauterine growth rates for preterm males and females.

The 2013 Fenton growth curves were revised to (a) align the curves with WHO metrics published in 2006 (e.g., use of a sample of exclusively breastfed infants whose families were not economically or environmentally constrained, and who did not receive solid food supplementation before 4 months of age); and (b) rescale the x-axis of each chart to reflect PMA rather than completed weeks of gestation (Fenton & Kim, 2013; WHO, 2006). The revised growth curves used data collected from six cross-sectional population-based studies of preterm infants born in the United States, Canada, Germany, Scotland, Italy and Australia, between 23 and 50 weeks' PMA, and published between 1991 and 2007. The sample size was reported to be 34,639 preterm infants <30 weeks of gestation (Fenton et al., 2013).

OLSEN GENDER-SPECIFIC GROWTH CURVES

The Olsen growth curves were incepted in 2010. Dr. Olsen's objective was to update the size-for-length growth curves originally created by Lubchenco and colleagues (1963, 1966). These growth curves, applicable to preterm infants between 22 and 42 weeks' PMA, were developed from a descriptive, cross-sectional population of 257,855 United States born infants born between 1998 and 2006. Preterm infants ≤33 weeks of gestation (N = 16,197) comprised 6.2% of the study population. The two gender-specific preterm growth curves created from these original data remain available for use to NICU clinicians (Olsen et al., 2010).

Olsen Gender-Specific Body Mass Index Curves

The strongest of all available anthropometric indices is the BMI (Taylor & Buck, 2021). BMI is calculated as (weight / length^2). Therefore, in an effort to expand clinician analytical capability and identify disproportionate growth (weight-for-length) in the clinical setting, Olsen et al. (2015)

created gender-specific BMI curves based on data from 254,454 infants born between 1998 and 2006 and between 24 and 41 weeks of gestation.

BMI curves allow clinicians to plot individual size measurements and compare them with centile norms at a given age (size-for-age). However, clinicians must consider potential limitations when using these curves. First, a "normal" (50th percentile) size-for-age-weight at a given gestational age may be disproportionately large (or small) for the infant's length at that same point in time. Second, it is not yet possible to distinguish which body tissues accumulate fat (body composition), nor is it possible to conclude that an increase in BMI confers an increase in body fat in preterm infants (Al-Theyab et al., 2019; Fenton et al., 2020). A particular advantage of the BMI curve is the ability to assess proportionality of growth over time. Ideally, this could reduce the risk of undetected and prolonged suboptimal nutritional intake. Given that a correlation between

FIGURE 22.2 Fenton et al. (2013) gender-specific growth charts.

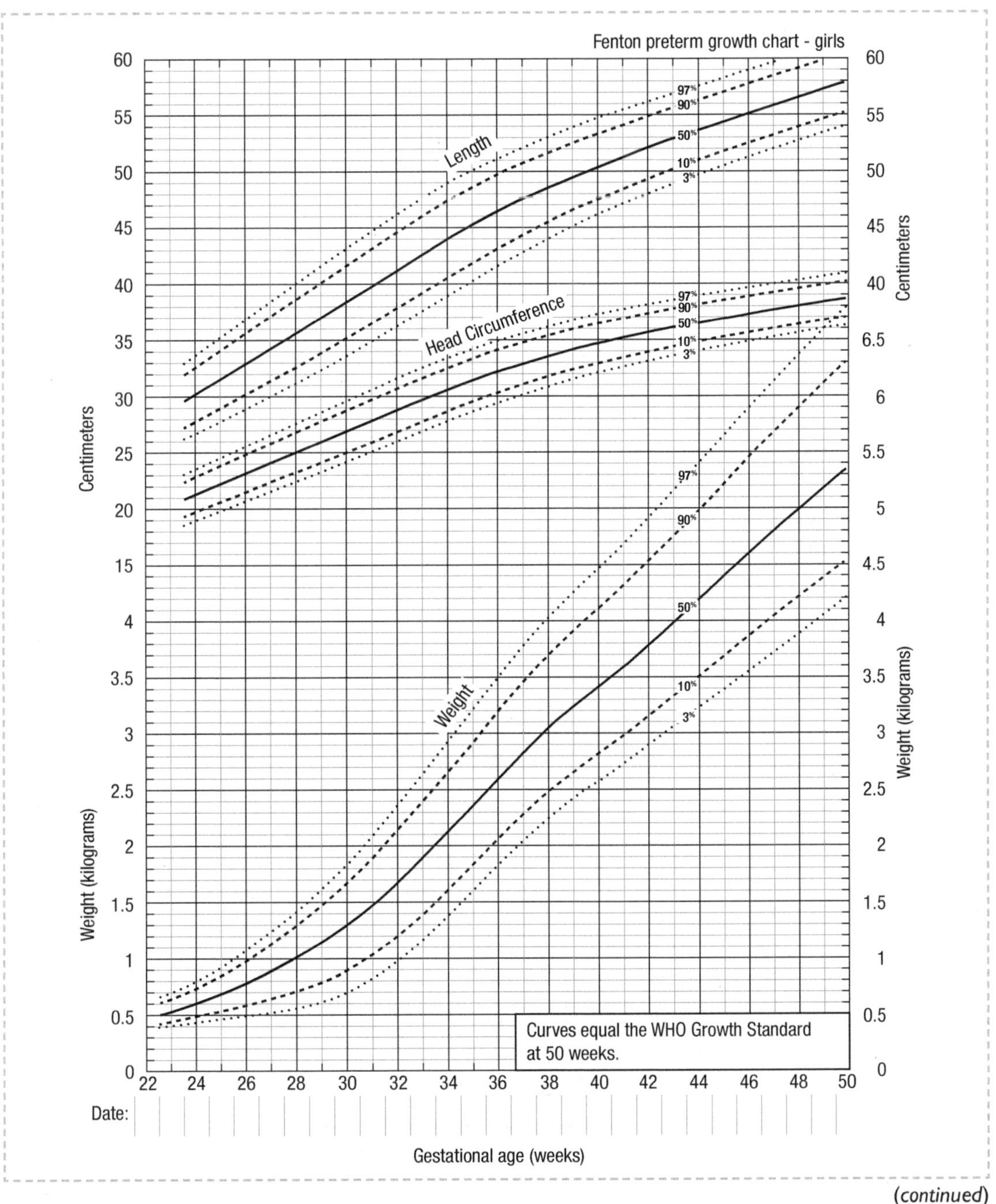

(continued)

FIGURE 22.2 Fenton et al. (2013) gender-specific growth charts. (*continued*)

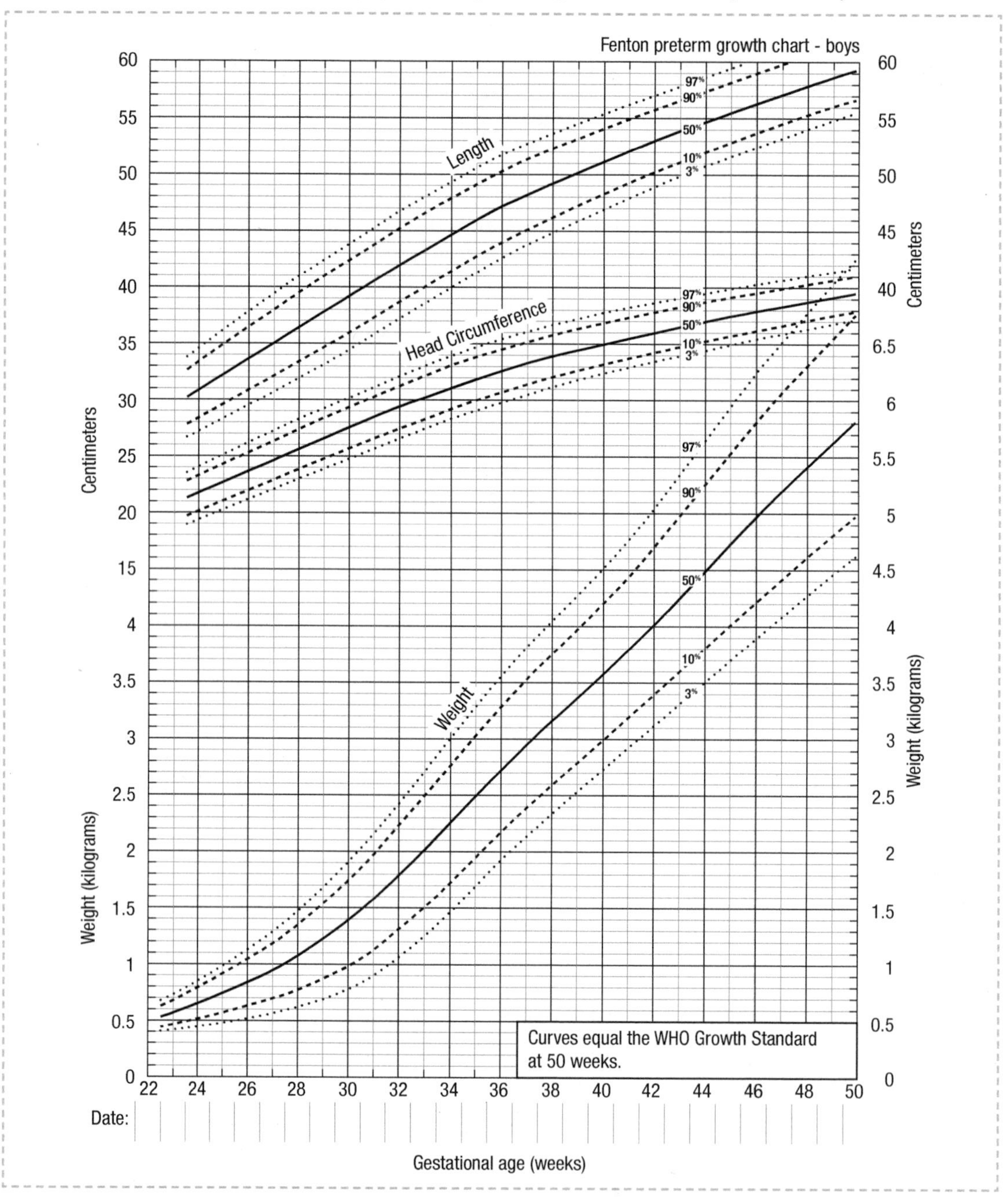

Source: From Fenton, T. R., & Kim, J. H. (2013). A systematic review and meta-analysis to revise the Fenton growth chart for preterm infants. *BMC Pediatrics, 13*, 59. https://doi.org/10.1186/1471-2431-13-59.

preterm birth and latent cardiovascular disease has been reported (Markopoulou et al., 2019; Nakano, 2020; Nuyt et al., 2017), trials that assess the relationship among preterm birth, BMI, and long-term outcomes (e.g., neurodevelopment, obesity, hypertension) are needed.

INTERGROWTH-21 GENDER-SPECIFIC GROWTH CURVES

More recent, in 2015 the INTERGROWTH-21 research team created two growth curves (Figure 22.3). This team used the WHO (2006) framework to study fetal and postnatal growth, health, nutrition, and cognitive development through age 2 and create gender-specific size-for-length growth curves (Villar et al., 2015). These curves were developed from data obtained from two component studies carried out in the United States, United Kingdom, Brazil, Italy, India, Kenya, Oman, and China.

One component study, the Fetal Growth Longitudinal Study (FGLS), recruited a total of 59,137 pregnant women; fetal growth was monitored throughout the duration of these pregnancies (Villar et al., 2014). The other component study, the Newborn Cross-Sectional Study (NCSS), recruited a total of 20,486 pregnant women; all newborns were subject to birth-length measurements.

The curves are indicated for use with newborns older than 27 weeks of gestation at birth. However, only 12 women gave birth to preterm infants less than 33 weeks of gestation. Therefore, until the outcomes of additional research using a larger sample size of preterm infants less than 33 weeks of gestation are disseminated, neonatal experts caution against using this growth chart in the hospital setting and with preterm infants (Fenton et al., 2018).

FIGURE 22.3 INTERGROWTH-21 gender-specific growth charts.

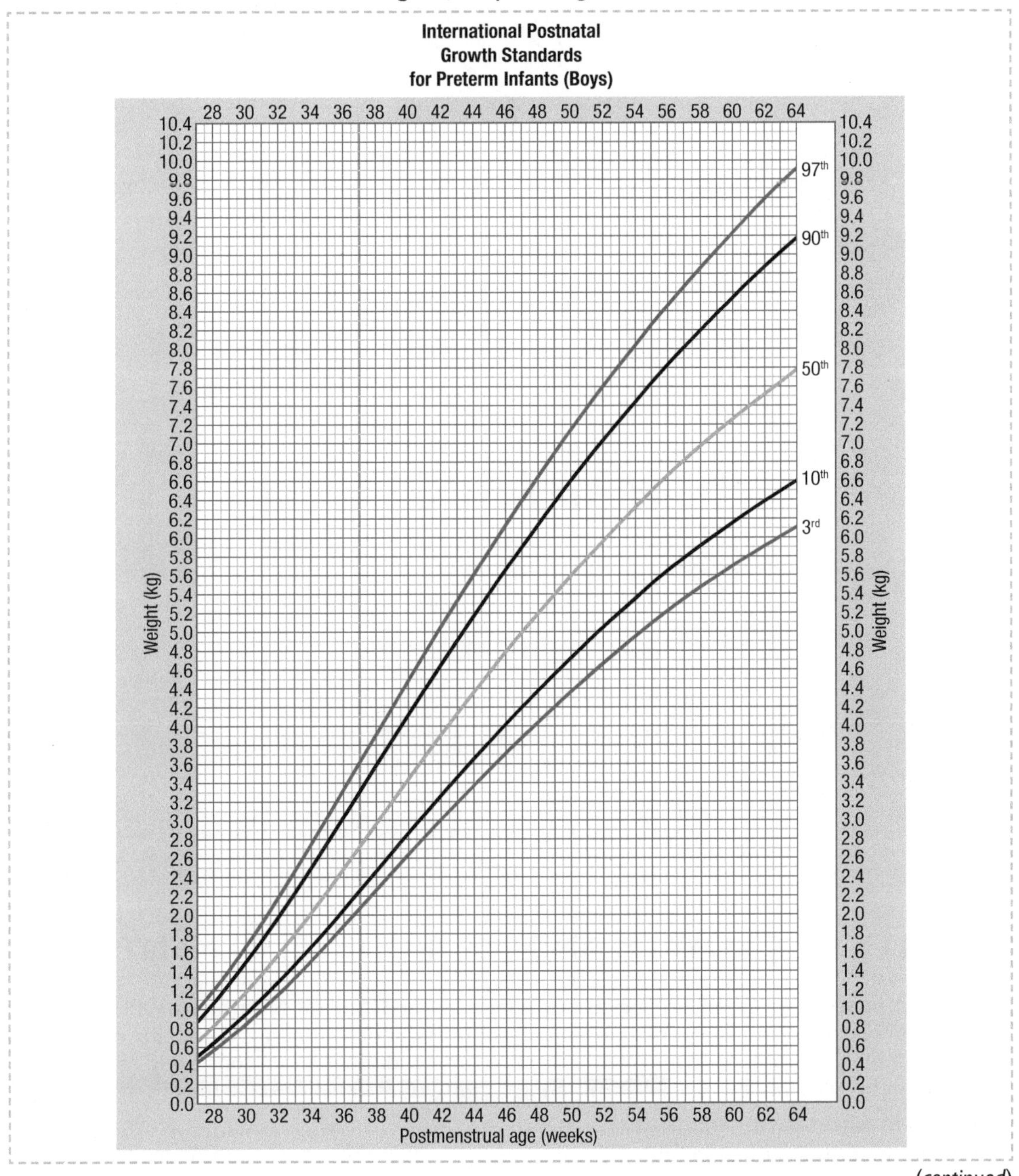

(*continued*)

FIGURE 22.3 INTERGROWTH-21 gender-specific growth charts. (*continued*)

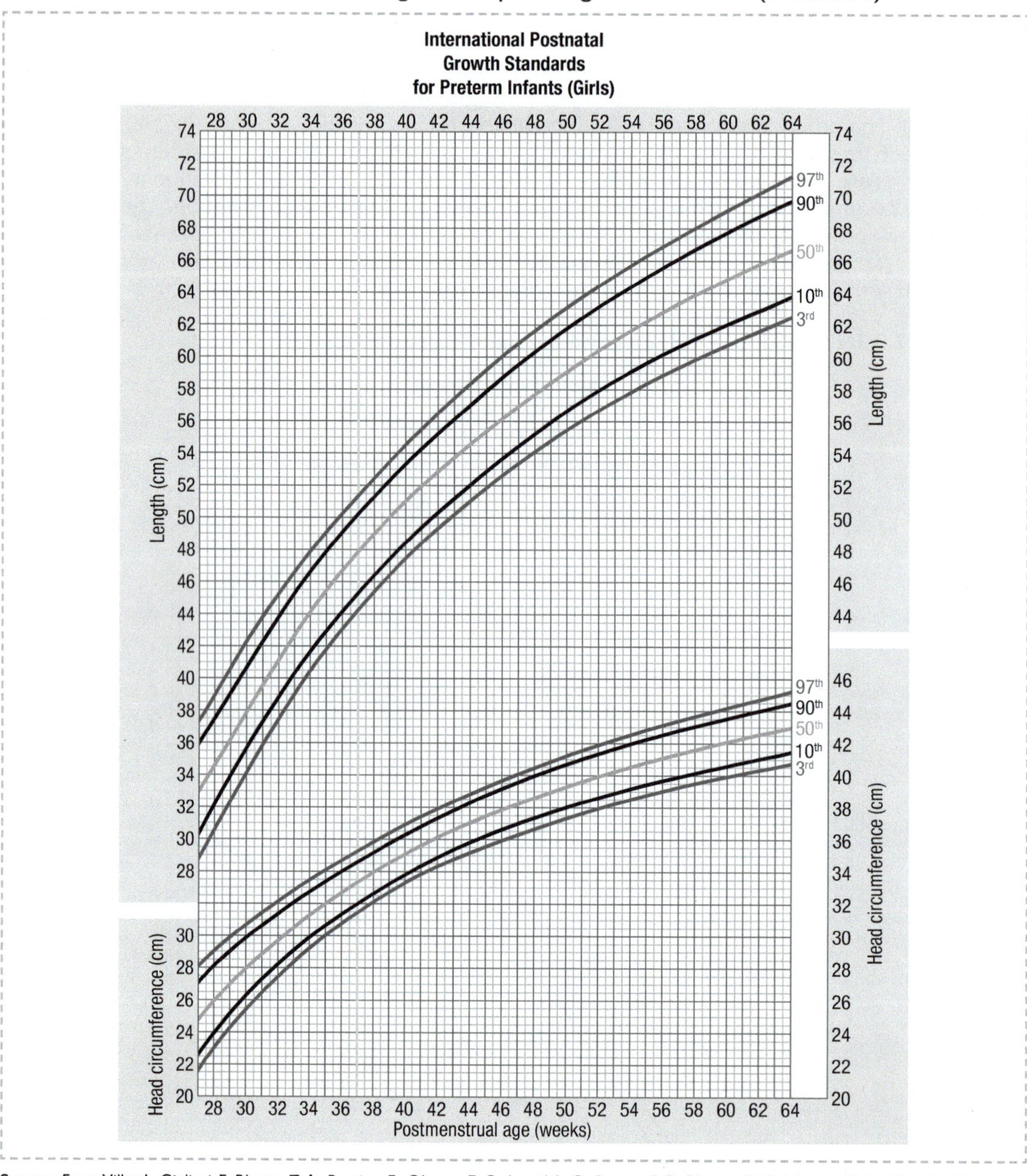

Source: From Villar, J., Giuliani, F., Bhutta, Z. A., Bertino, E., Ohuma, E. O., Ismail, L. C., Barros, F. C., Altman, D. G., Victora, C., Noble, J. A., Gravett, M. G., Purwar, M., Pang, R., Lambert, A., Papageorghiou, A. T., Ochieng, R., Jaffer, Y. A., Kennedy, S. H., & International Fetal and Newborn Growth Consortium for the 21(st) Century. (2015). Postnatal growth standards for preterm infants: The preterm postnatal follow-up study of the INTERGROWTH-21(st) project. *The Lancet Global Health, 3*(11), e681–e691. https://doi.org/10.1016/S2214-109X(15)00163-1.

QUALITY OF GROWTH AND NEURODEVELOPMENT

Two expert panels, the American Society for Parenteral and Enteral Nutrition (ASPEN) and the Academy of Nutrition and Dietetics, published recommendations for assessing quality of growth in preterm infants. Pediatric dietitians refer to these recommendations when consulting on nutritional regimens for hospitalized infants. Three metrics are commonly considered when appraising growth:

- days to regain birth weight
- linear growth velocity
- decline in length-for-age *z*-score

FIGURE 22.4 Interpreting the z-score (sample).

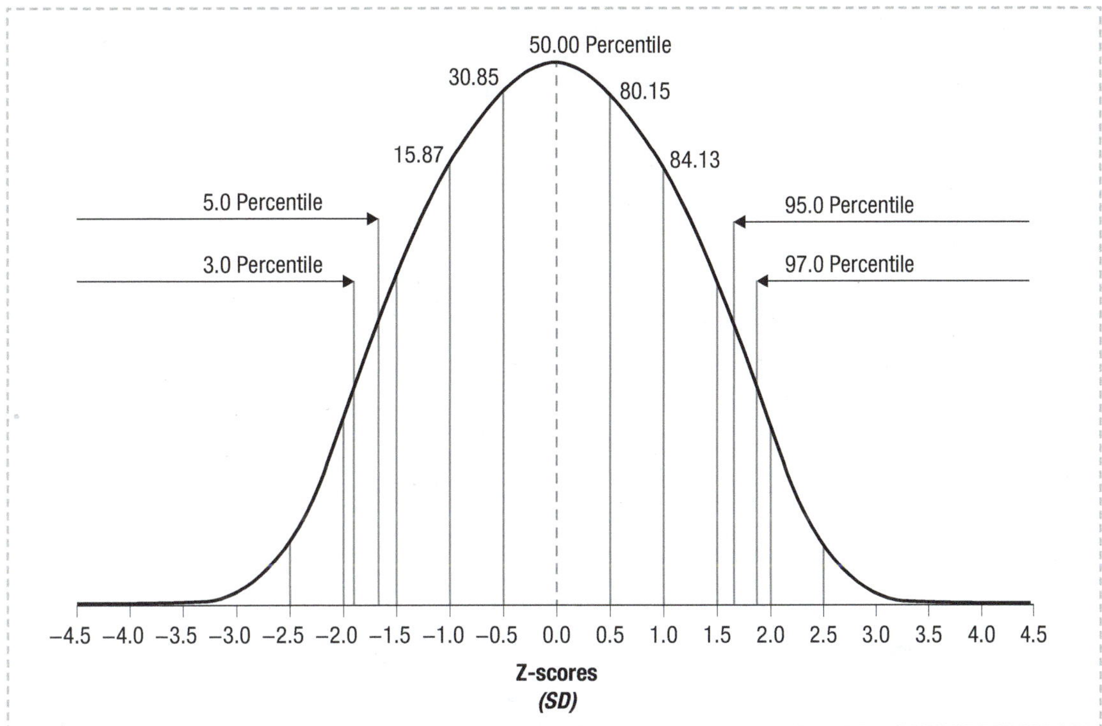

In addition, ASPEN and the Academy of Nutrition and Dietetics encourage clinicians to consider two key metrics when appraising for neonatal malnutrition:

- decline in weight-for-age *z-score*
- weight gain velocity

To clarify, the "*z*-score" is a score that quantifies the distance a growth index is from the mean (Figure 22.4). Specific to the Fenton et al. (2013) and Olsen et al. (2010) growth curves, the *z*-score that corresponds with the mean (50th centile) for growth, length, or head circumference is 0. A weight that plots below the 50th percentile would be assigned a negative *z*-score, whereas a weight that exceeds the 50th percentile corresponds with a positive *z*-score above 0.

Weights that fall below the 50th percentile often receive heightened attention. For many decades, a weight less than 10th percentile at 36 weeks' PMA was defined as *postnatal growth failure* (*PGF*) or *extrauterine growth restriction* (*EUGR*) and associated with an increased risk of poor neurodevelopment. More recent studies published between 1982 and 2018 contradict this historical perspective; weight less than 10th percentile at 36 weeks' PMA is *not unequivocally associated* with poor neurodevelopment (Hack et al., 1982; Shah et al., 2006; Zozaya et al., 2018).

As a result of these new data, Fenton and colleagues (2020) published an opinion paper in favor of retiring the aforementioned diagnoses of PGF and EUGR. Rather, these experts believe that clinicians should focus attention toward appraising postnatal growth over time (Fenton et al., 2020; Fenton, Elrayed, & Alshaikh, 2021). When growth over time and quality of growth are considered during interval nutritional assessments, a holistic and evidence-based approach is offered. In fact, *it is recommended that clinicians appraise the infant's change in z-score over time,* versus change in percentile over time (given that the growth curve centiles appraise growth at that specific gestational age compared with fetal growth at that age). This method offers the best assessment of growth over time. Box 22.1 offers a summary of growth metrics associated with an increased risk for adverse neurodevelopment.

Growth Velocity

Growth velocity is commonly calculated using an exponential or average method, on a weekly (or bi weekly) basis in NICUs (Box 22.2). Growth velocity recommendations for preterm infants, originally established in 1986, targeted a growth velocity of 15 g/kg/d and head and length increase

BOX 22.1 Risk Factors for Poor Neurodevelopment

METRIC
Slow weight gain from birth to discharge
Slow increase in head circumference from birth to discharge
Slow increase in length from birth to discharge
Small size after term

Source: From Fenton, T. R., Al-Wassia, H., Premji, S. S., & Sauve, R. S. (2020). Higher versus lower protein intake in formulated low birth weight infants. *Cochrane Database of Systematic Reviews, 2020*(6), CD003959. https://doi.org/10.1002/14651858.CD003959.pub.

BOX 22.2 Formulas for Calculating Growth Velocity

Exponential Method

$$\frac{1{,}000 \times \ln\,[\text{most recent weight (grams)/weight 5 or 7 days prior (grams)}]}{\text{Duration of time between measurements (days)}}$$

Average Method

$$\frac{[\text{Most recent weight (grams)} - \text{weight on first date (grams)}]/\ \text{mean of weights on most recent and first date}}{\text{Duration of time between measurements (days)}}$$

ln, natural logarithm.

TABLE 22.1 Assessing Growth Velocity

GESTATIONAL AGE	GROWTH VELOCITY	RECOMMENDED GROWTH CURVE
23–36 weeks' PMA	Calculate using serial weights obtained over 5–7 days as grams/kilogram/day.	Fenton et al. (2013) Olsen et al. (2010)
36–42 weeks' PMA	Calculate using serial weights obtained over 5–7 days as average grams/day.	Fenton et al. (2013) Olsen et al. (2010)
>42 weeks' PMA	Calculate daily as grams/day.	WHO (2006)

PMA, postmenstrual age; WHO, World Health Organization.

of 1 cm/wk (Hodges, Johnson, & Merlino-Barr, 2022). New research suggests that the former target of 15 g/kg/d of growth between 23 and 33 weeks' PMA is too low, yet generally appropriate between 34 and 36 weeks' PMA, and too high thereafter (Fenton et al., 2018). Historical head circumference and length targets (1 cm/wk) also did not fit the Fenton and Olsen growth charts after approximately 32 to 33 weeks' PMA.

Currently, *experts recommend a growth velocity target of 15 to 20 g/kg/d for preterm infants between 23 and 36 weeks' PMA and up to 2 kg of weight* (Table 22.1; Fenton et al., 2018; Koletzko, Wieczorek, et al., 2021). This requirement decreases with advancing weight, to 12 to 15 g/kg/d for infants 2 to 3 kg, and 10 to 13 g/kg/d for infants larger than 3 kg (Koletzko, Wieczorek, et al., 2021). The 1 cm/wk head circumference increase remains a reasonable target through approximately 33 weeks' PMA; weekly head growth should slow thereafter in order for normal (and not overly rapid) growth to occur. Likewise, the target of 1 cm/wk length increase is reasonable through 32 weeks' PMA but should increase thereafter in order for infants to demonstrate appropriate growth per the Fenton or Olsen growth curves (Fenton et al., 2018; Kleinman & Greer, 2020). These new data can guide nutritional management decisions after the initial postnatal weight loss period has passed. We refer readers to the superimposed growth calculation figures provided in the Fenton et al. (2018) publication for additional helpful context.

PHYSIOLOGY REVIEW: DIGESTION AND ABSORPTION

Recall that anatomic development of the GI system begins during the fourth week of gestation and is relatively structurally formed by week 20 of gestation (Waskowsky et al., 2019). Noteworthy structural developments that occur during this period include the formation of the intestinal villi and the enteric nervous system. Once the enteric system forms, the fetus begins to swallow and then suck, actions that promote gut motility. Elongation of the GI tract occurs across the final 15 weeks of gestation, commensurate with an increase in gastroesophageal sphincter tone and the number of microvilli and villi lining the endothelial surface of the intestinal tract (Neu & Li, 2002; Parker, 2021). During this time, the fetus swallows as much as 400 mL of amniotic fluid per day, a process thought to aid in physiologic maturation of the GI tract.

Although the GI tract is structurally intact at birth, it is functionally immature. This is particularly true in preterm infants. Therefore, clinicians should understand typical digestive and absorptive processes. Further, clinicians should understand that preterm birth influences digestion and absorption compared with birth at term; enteral nutrition plans need to consider these differences. Digestion begins in the mouth, where salivary enzymes hydrolyze ingested carbohydrates. For infants born prematurely, salivary enzymes do not come into contact with enteral nutrition, as suck–swallow–breathe synchrony only begins to develop around 33 weeks' PMA. Thus, these infants are unable to use salivary amylase or lingual lipase for initial carbohydrate and fat metabolism, respectively.

Once infants are capable of feeding by mouth, the swallowing of enteral nutrition occurs in the following phases: oral (subdivided into oral preparatory and oral transit), pharyngeal, and esophageal. The oral preparatory phase in infants describes the root-to-latch-to-suck sequence. The oral-transit phase describes the propulsion of the bolus of food posteriorly and ends when the bolus leaves the oral cavity. The pharyngeal phase begins with a voluntary swallow, followed by the propulsion of the bolus through the pharynx via a peristaltic wave generated by the tongue base, posterior pharyngeal wall, and opening of the upper esophageal sphincter (UES), also referred to as the *pharyngo-esophageal segment* (*PES*). Coordination of this complicated process is necessary for a safe feed and takes time to develop and mature in the premature infant.

Nutritional components travel from the mouth, through the esophagus, and then enter the stomach. The stomach is a temporary reservoir for nutrition as well as a location for chemical and mechanical digestion. Here, hydrochloric acid is secreted from parietal cells, which activates pepsinogen, converting it to pepsin, and inactivates any ingested bacteria. Pepsin initiates the chemical digestion of ingested proteins, hydrolyzing larger protein molecules into smaller peptide chains. Gastric lipase is also present in the stomach and plays a small role in fat digestion. Other enzymes and hormones are also present within the stomach to help control gastric motility and secretions. Ultimately, a mixture of partially digested food and gastric juices (chyme) travel through the pyloric canal and into the small intestine via gastric emptying.

The small intestine has three parts: the duodenum, the jejunum, and the ileum. In aggregate, this massive system contributes to the final stages of enzymatic digestion and is responsible for nearly all nutrient absorptions in the human body. Although macronutrient digestion and absorption are the focus of this brief review, it is critical to note that vitamin and mineral absorption occurs throughout the small intestine as well. Secretin and cholecystokinin (CKK) are secreted in the duodenum and stimulate the pancreas and the liver to deliver critically necessary digestive enzymes to the duodenum via the pancreatic and common bile ducts. These digestive enzymes include pancreatic proteases, pancreatic amylase, and pancreatic lipase.

Pancreatic proteases (most notably, trypsin, chymotrypsin, and carboxypeptidases) further hydrolyze the peptide chains in the lumen of the small intestine into oligopeptides. Finally, the oligopeptides are hydrolyzed into free amino acids and very small peptides by peptidases on the brush border of the small intestine, readying them for absorption throughout the duodenum and jejunum via sodium-dependent amino acid transporters. Pancreatic amylase breaks down starch (a polysaccharide) into maltose (a disaccharide), maltotriose (a trisaccharide), and alpha-limit dextrins. From there, disaccharides are digested to monosaccharides by brush border hydrolases, including maltase (maltose → glucose + glucose), lactase (lactose → galactose + glucose), and sucrase (sucrose → fructose + glucose). These monosaccharides are then ready for absorption along the intestinal epithelium, which occurs for glucose via active transport using the sodium–glucose cotransporter 1 (SGLT1) transporter, and via facilitated diffusion using the Glut5 transporter for galactose and fructose. Of note, the enzymes used for carbohydrate digestion vary in concentration for preterm infants; pancreatic amylase and lactase activity increases throughout the preterm period.

Fat digestion, partially started with lingual lipase in the mouth and gastric lipase in the stomach, primarily occurs in the small intestine. Bile is created in the liver, stored in the gallbladder, and excreted into the duodenum. Bile emulsifies large triglyceride fat droplets into smaller droplets. Pancreatic lipase then hydrolyzes the emulsified droplets into monoglyceride and free fatty acids. These fat by products form micelles, a temporary structure with a hydrophilic exterior and hydrophobic interior, which are able to transport the fatty acids to the intestinal microvillus for absorption. The majority of fatty acid absorption occurs in the jejunum.

Preterm infants have low levels of pancreatic lipase and bile acids, which can contribute to poor lipid digestion (Koletzko & Lapillonne, 2021). Therefore, medium-chain triglycerides (MCT) are included as a partial fat source in most preterm infant nutrition products as they do not require bile or pancreatic lipase for intestinal absorption (Shah & Limketkai, 2017). In contrast, freshly expressed human milk is naturally designed to promote digestion and absorption in infants because it contains bile salt-stimulated lipase (BSSL). Donor human milk (DHM) loses a substantial amount of BSSL activity due to the denaturing process that occurs during milk processing, which may contribute to the growth challenges that preterm infants face when receiving DHM products.

Once fatty acids enter the epithelial cell, short- and medium-chain fatty acids can be directly absorbed into the bloodstream, whereas long-chain fatty acids reassemble into triglycerides and form chylomicrons with cholesterol and fat-soluble vitamins. Chylomicrons are absorbed into the lymphatic system, travel to the subclavian vein, and exit into the circulation where they travel throughout the body. Triglycerides within the chylomicrons are broken down by lipoprotein lipase into fatty acids and glycerol, which are able to enter cells and undergo beta-oxidation to produce energy, or reform triglycerides for storage.

After the consumed nutrition is digested and absorbed throughout the small intestine, what remains travels to the colon. The ileocecal valve separates the ileum and the colon and is responsible for slowing down intestinal transit to improve absorption and prevent retrograde flow from the large intestine. In infants with short bowel syndrome (SBS), retaining the ileocecal valve is an indicator of likelihood for achieving enteral autonomy (Peters et al., 2022). The large intestine is the final location of digestion in the human body, which includes water and electrolyte reabsorption and secretion, formation and storage of feces, and microbial fermentation. Microbial fermentation is responsible for digesting any remaining carbohydrates (e.g., cellulose) as well, as they synthesize vitamin K and some B vitamins.

In-between feeding cycles, small waves of peristaltic contractions are observed. Gastric hormones, namely motilin and somatostatin, as well as pancreatic polypeptides, modulate this normal physiologic activity. These gentle peristaltic waves, known as *migrating motor complexes* (*MMCs*), expel the remaining food from the stomach and duodenum, encouraging its migration toward the colon.

Although microbial fermentation is a major job in the colon, the development of the gut microbiota is of significant interest in neonatal nutrition at this time. The fetal gut is sterile and only begins to colonize at birth, and is influenced by delivery method, environmental microbes, enteral feed composition, use of probiotics, and antibiotic treatment, among others (Mackie et al., 1999). This microbiota provides host resistance to pathogens in order to resist colonization by invading pathogens (Waskowsky et al., 2019). This is particularly important for preterm infants, as their relative gut immaturity may allow for antigens and pathogens to bypass enzymatic lysis and increase the risk of infection. Intestinal permeability is well documented in premature infants, with utilization of expressed human milk shown to help with gut maturation compared with infant formula in the first weeks of life (Taylor, Basile, Egeling, & Wagner, 2009).

BASIC NUTRIENT NEEDS OF PRETERM INFANTS

Recall that the AAP defines *adequate postnatal nutrition* as that which achieves a postnatal weight gain and rate of growth comparable with what would be observed in a fetus at the same age (Kleinman & Greer, 2020; Shulz & Wagner, 2021). In contrast, the Committee on Nutrition of the

FIGURE 22.5 Schematic depiction of reference nutrient intake for preterm infants.

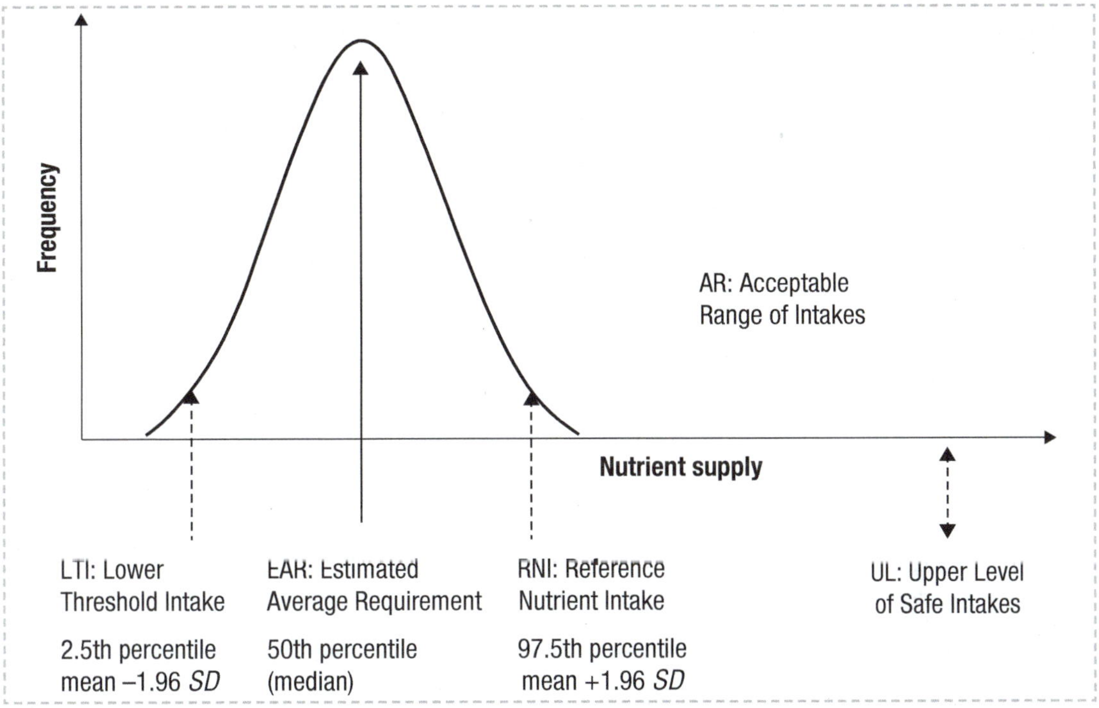

Frequency

AR: Acceptable
Range of Intakes

Nutrient supply

LTI: Lower
Threshold Intake

2.5th percentile
mean −1.96 *SD*

EAR: Estimated
Average Requirement

50th percentile
(median)

RNI: Reference
Nutrient Intake

97.5th percentile
mean +1.96 *SD*

UL: Upper Level
of Safe Intakes

Source: From Koletzko, B., Wieczorek, S., Domellof, M., & Poindexter, B. B. (2021). Defining nutritional needs of preterm infants. In B. Koletzko, F. C. Cheach, M. Domellof, B. B. Poindexter, N. Vain, & J. B. Goudoever (Eds.), *Nutritional care of preterm infants: Scientific basis and practical guidelines* (Vol. 122, pp. 5–11). Karger.

European Society for Paediatric Gastroenterology Hepatology and Nutrition (ESPGHAN) defines *nutritional needs* as the intake required to maintain normal development and health and avoid imposing a nutrient imbalance (Figure 22.5; ESPGHAN, 2010; Koletzko, Wieczorek, et al., 2021).

In order to create the ideal nutritional regimen for a preterm infant, an understanding of benchmark nutritional goals is required. Table 22.2 provides a comprehensive summary of recommendations for daily nutritional intake, per ESPGHAN and the AAP Committee on Nutrition. We offer an expanded discussion of basic water, energy, protein, carbohydrate, and fat needs, as well as a few essential vitamins/minerals, for preterm infants in the next section of this chapter, as these are core considerations for APRNs in the clinical setting.

Water Needs

Recall that the daily total fluid intake represents the recommended daily water intake, which is provided intravenously and/or enterally (human milk and formula comprised approximately 85% water). The recommended daily water (total fluid) goal for neonates less than 1.5 kg at birth is 135 to 200 mL/kg/d (ESPGHAN, 2010; Kleinman & Greer, 2020), a wide range that must be customized to each infant. This requires consideration of applicable comorbidities and risk factors that influence water balance (e.g., mechanical ventilation, immature stratum corneum, sepsis, renal disease). All newborns require a slow advance of total fluid intake to the recommended goal; the initial total fluid goal on admission to a NICU often ranges between 60 and 100 mL/kg/d and is titrated daily, as indicated (Hodges et al., 2022).

Energy Needs

Preterm infants expend significant energy each day while at rest, moving, crying, regulating body temperature, and battling comorbid diseases. Energy expenditures increase sixfold between 22 and 40 weeks of gestation, as the infant matures (Fenton & Kim, 2013). Therefore, adequate exogenous energy must be provided to ensure that energy intake equals that which is excreted in the urine/stool; expended through daily activities/movements; and stored as fat, protein, and glycogen (Huff et al., 2021).

TABLE 22.2 Nutritional Goals for Enterally Fed Preterm Infant Less Than 1,500 Grams

	ESPGHAN (2010)	AAP (2020)	KOLETZKO (2021)
Fluid (mL/kg/d)	135–200	135–200	135–200
Energy (kcal/kg/d)	110–135	110–130	110–130
Carbohydrate (g/100 kcal)	11.6–13.2	11.6–13.2	11–13
Protein (g/kg/d)	4.0–4.5 (<1 kg) 3.5–4.0 (1–1.8 kg)	3.5–4.5	3.5–4.5
Fat (g/kg/d)	4.8–6.6	4.8–6.6	4.55–8.1
Sodium (mg/kg/d)	69–115	69–115	69–115
Potassium (mg/kg/d)	66–132	78–195	78–195
Chloride (mg/kg/d)	105–177	105–177	105–177
Calcium (mg/kg/d)	120–140	120–200	120–122
Magnesium (mg/kg/d)	8–15	8–15	8–15
Phosphorus (mg/kg/d)	60–90	60–140	70–120
Iron (mg/kg/d)	2–3	2–3	1–3
Zinc (mg/kg/d)	1.1–2.0	1.4–2.5	2–3
Copper (mcg/kg/d)	100–132	100–230	120–230
Selenium (mcg/kg/d)	5–10	5–10	7–10
Manganese (mcg/kg/d)	<27.5	1–15	1–15
Fluoride (mcg/kg/d)	1.5–60	1.5–60	–
Iodine (mcg/kg/d)	11–55	10–55	10–55
Chromium (mcg/kg/d)	30–1,230	30–2,250	0.03–2.25
Molybdenum (mcg/kg/d)	0.3–5.0	0.3–5	0.3–5
Thiamin (mcg/kg/d)	140–300	140–300	132–275
Riboflavin (mcg/kg/d)	200–400	200–400	200–430
Niacin (mg/kg/d)	0.38–5.5	1.5–5.0	1.1–5.5
Pantothenic acid (mg/kg/d)	0.33–2.1	0.5–2.1	0.6–2.1
Pyridoxine (mcg/kg/d)	45–300	50–300	66–275
Cobalamin (mcg/kg/d)	0.1–0.77	0.1–0.8	0.12–0.6
Folic acid (mcg/kg/d)	35–100	35–100	22–100
L-ascorbic acid (mg/kg/d)	11–46	20–55	16.5–41
Biotin (mcg/kg/d)	1.7–16.5	1.7–16.5	3.3–15
Vitamin A (mcg/kg/d)	400–1,000	400–1,100	1,332–3,330 (IU)
Vitamin D (IU/d)[a]	800–1,000	400–1,000	400–1,000
Vitamin E (mg/kg/d)	2.2–11	2.2–11	2.2–11
Vitamin K (mg/kg/d)	4.4–28	4.4–28	4.4–28

[a]From feed source plus supplement.

AAP, American Academy of Pediatrics; ESPGHAN, European Society for Paediatric Gastroenterology Hepatology and Nutrition.

Sources: From Agostoni, C., Buonocore, G., Carnielli, V. P., De Curtis, M., Darmaun, D., Decsi, T., Domellöf, M., Embleton, N. D., Fusch, C., Genzel-Boroviczeny, O., Goulet, O., Kalhan, S. C., Kolacek, S., Koletzko, B., Lapillonne, A., Mihatsch, W., Moreno, L., Neu, J., Poindexter, B., … ESPGHAN Committee on Nutrition. (2010). Enteral nutrient supply for preterm infants: Commentary from the European Society for Paediatric Gastroenterology, Hepatology, and Nutrition Committee on Nutrition. *Journal of Pediatric Gastroenterology & Nutrition, 50*(1), 85–91. https://doi.org/10.1097/MPG.0b013e3181adee0; Brion, L. P., Bell, E. F., & Raghuveer, T. S. (2003). Vitamin E supplementation for prevention of morbidity and mortality in preterm infants. *Cochrane Database of Systematic Reviews, 2003*(4), CD003665. https://doi.org/10.1002/14651858.CD003665; Hodges, B. S., Johnson, M., & Merlino-Barr, S. (2022). *Pocket guide to neonatal nutrition* (3rd ed.). Academy of Nutrition and Dietetics. Koletzko, B., Wieczorek, S., Domellof, M., & Poindexter, B. B. (2021). Defining nutritional needs of preterm infants. In B. Koletzko, F. C. Cheach, M. Domellof, B. B. Poindexter, N. Vain, & J. B. Goudoever (Eds.), *Nutritional care of preterm infants: Scientific basis and practical guidelines* (Vol. 122, pp. 5–11). Karger.

Consider that energy excreted through the urine and stool accounts for up to 15 kcal/kg/d of total energy. The average total daily energy expenditure for preterm infants is approximately 65 kcal/kg/d, which is composed of the basal (resting) metabolic rate (40–50 kcal/kg/d); daily activities, including basic body movements, bottle/breast feeding, and in some cases physical or speech therapy (5 kcal/kg/d); and growth (15–74 kcal/kg/d; Huff et al., 2021; Kleinman & Greer, 2020). Energy that is stored as fat, protein, or glycogen accounts for 20 to 30 kcal/kg/d of the total gross intake. Considering these factors, enteral energy intake for preterm infants less than 2 kg averages between 110 and 130 kcal/kg/d; caloric intake needs may increase during growth periods. Nutrition must be customized to each infant, particularly when heat loss increases (e.g., frequent bathing, proximity to air vents, windows), movements are accentuated (e.g., supine vs. prone positioning) or inhibited, and certain medications are prescribed (e.g., caffeine, which increases energy expenditure; Huff et al., 2021). Most preterm infants require enteral fortification, which can be added to human milk feedings (human milk fortifier [HMF]) or preterm formulas. Fortifiers are discussed later in this chapter.

Protein Needs

Adequate intake is essential, beginning immediately after birth, to encourage acceptable protein accretion, lean body mass, and growth over time, and to reduce the risk of retinopathy of prematurity as well as poor neurodevelopment (Huff et al., 2021). Not only is adequate protein intake necessary, but also quality protein intake, as proteins are composed of linked amino acids. Adequate intake of essential amino acids is critical, as the essential amino acids can only be derived from exogenous food sources.

The recommended daily protein intake for preterm infants is 3.5 to 4.5 g/kg/d (ESPGHAN, 2010; Kleinman & Greer, 2020). The total protein intake from enteral nutrition can be calculated using the following process, which is unique to human milk and each type of enteral formula. Clinicians can determine the grams of protein per 100 mL of commercial formula by consulting the nutritional label affixed to the formula. The protein content of preterm human milk is 1.1 g/100 mL and 0.9 g/100 mL in mature term milk (Hodges et al., 2022). The following method can be used to calculate and appraise daily protein intake (g/kg/d):

1. **Identify**: grams of protein per 100 mL.
2. **Identify**: total mL of enteral intake in 24 hours.
3. **Multiply**: protein (g/100 mL) × intake over 24 hours (mL) = protein g/d.
4. **Divide**: protein (g/d) /dosing weight (kg) = protein g/kg/d.

Carbohydrates

Preterm infants cannot endogenously produce the amount of glucose necessary for fatty acid and amino acid synthesis, and brain and cardiovascular growth and function. Glucose needs are inversely proportional to gestational age, primarily because the brain and heart of extremely low-birth-weight infants comprise a significant proportion of total body weight and both these organs have high glucose metabolic rates. Therefore, preterm infants who advance to full enteral feedings need adequate carbohydrate intake for the purposes of energy production, glucose synthesis, and metabolism. Human milk or formula intake at approximately 140 to 160 mL/kg/d provides adequate carbohydrates for glucose production. Clinicians can determine the grams of carbohydrate per 100 mL of commercial formula by consulting the nutritional label affixed to the formula. Every gram of carbohydrate provides approximately 4 kcals (Huff et al., 2021). Glucose intake that exceeds the body's oxidative and glycogen storage capacity may lead to a disproportional increase in fat mass compared with lean body mass; the risk for excess glucose intake is greater when prescribing parenteral nutrition versus enteral intake. The production of fat also stresses the body by increasing energy expenditure, carbon dioxide production, and demand on the respiratory system to expel the volatile gas (by way of increasing minute ventilation).

Fats

Lipids are an essential source of energy for the growing preterm infant. As mentioned in the previous section, preterm infants can synthesize fat from glucose stores; however, this capability is limited. In order to approximate daily intrauterine lipid deposition, which requires intake of 2 g/kg/d in the absence of extrauterine energy expenditure, experts recommend a two- to threefold higher enteral lipid intake of 4.8 to 6.6 g/kg/d (Table 22.2; ESPGHAN, 2010; Kleinman & Greer, 2020; Koletzko & Lapillonne, 2021).

Experts estimate that human milk contains approximately 3.8 g/100 mL of lipids; lipid composition of human milk varies throughout the lactation period. Each gram of lipid yields approximately 9 kcals (Huff et al., 2021; Koletzko & Lapillonne, 2021). Clinicians can determine the grams of lipid per 100 mL of commercial formula by consulting the nutritional label affixed to the formula. The following method can be used to calculate and appraise daily lipid intake (g/kg/d):

1. **Identify**: grams of fat/100 mL.
2. **Identify**: total mL of enteral intake in 24 hours.
3. **Multiply**: fat (g/100 mL) × total intake over 24 hours (mL) = fat g/d.
4. **Divide**: fat (g/d)/weight (kg) = fat g/kg/d.

Vitamins/Minerals

Vitamins and minerals are essential to preterm infant growth and development. Calcium, phosphorus, magnesium, and vitamin D are involved in bone development as well as other metabolic processes. During the third trimester, a fetus sees the highest accretion of calcium and phosphorus; therefore, when an infant is born preterm, they do not have the stores needed for bone development and are at risk of metabolic bone disease (Koletzko, Wieczorek, et al., 2021). Calcium, phosphorus, magnesium, and vitamin D play an important role in respiratory, cardiac, and neurologic function as well. Zinc is needed for optimal growth. Deficiencies may lead to an increased risk for infections (Koletzko, Wieczorek, et al., 2021).

COMMERCIAL FORMULAS

Human milk provides the best nutrition for infants, and clinicians undoubtedly prioritize the provision of human milk except when contraindicated. However, nearly 20% of infants receive formula within the first few days after birth and 31% are consuming formula by 3 months' PMA (Figure 22.6). Infant formula is a life saving tool for infants who need it, with many different types

FIGURE 22.6 Percentage of breastfed children who were supplemented with infant formula, by birth year, National Immunization Survey, United States.

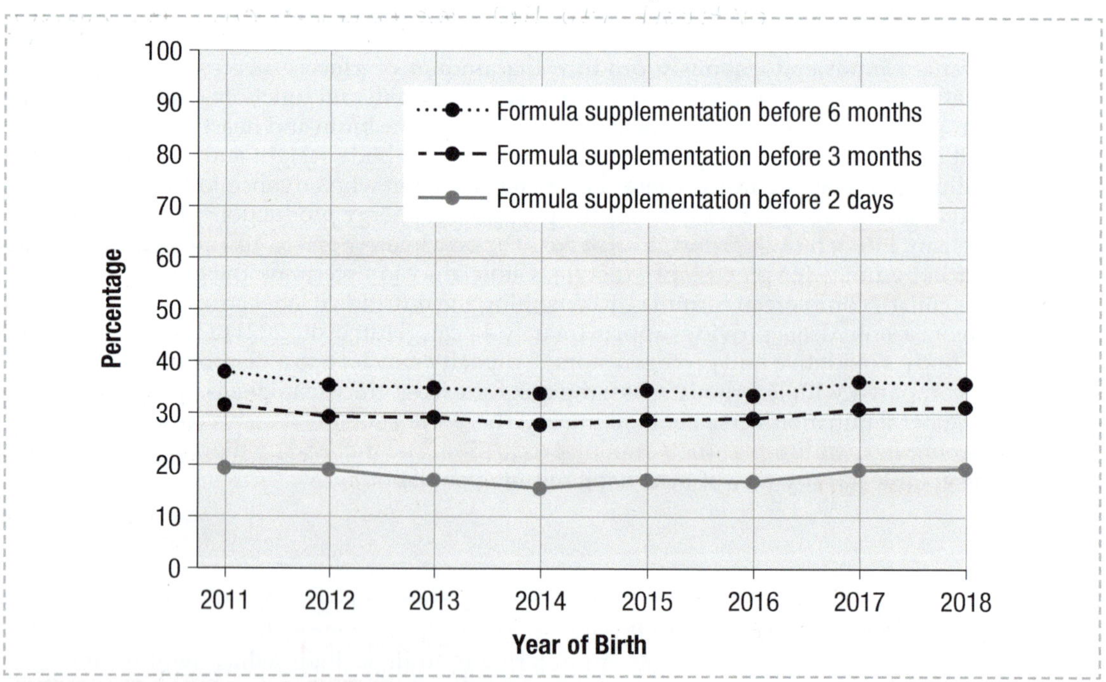

Source: From CDC. *Results: Breastfeeding rates*. https://www.cdc.gov/breastfeeding/data/nis_data/results.html.

of formulas with varying indications on the market. Given the prevalence of formula use in the NICU and newborn nurseries, we present readers with a discussion of core principles specific to the types of commercial formulas.

Infant formulas are available in powdered, ready-to-feed, and concentrated liquid forms. Powdered formulas were the mainstay until the early 21st century, when outbreaks of *Enterobacter* infection were reported and linked to powdered infant formulas. In 2001, van Acker et al. published a report of a 1998 outbreak of *Enterobacter sakazakii* involving 12 cases from one nursery. All infants had received reconstituted powdered formula, which was later found to be the source of the contamination (van Acker et al., 2001). Affected infants presented with NEC; the mortality rate was approximately 16%. Another outbreak of *E. sakazakii* occurred in Tennessee in 2001, when a preterm infant died from *E. sakazakii* meningitis (Bowen & Braden, 2006). Nine other infants tested positive for the bacteria in that same nursery and the bacteria was traced to a can of powered formula, which resulted in a product recall (Centers for Disease Control and Prevention [CDC], 2002). Shortly thereafter, the AAP endorsed CDC and FDA recommendations against the use of powdered formulas in the NICU setting due to the inability to sterilize powders and the concomitant risk of contamination (AAP, 2002; Schulz & Wagner, 2021). The most recent formula recall in February 2022 heavily impacted NICUs due to specific elemental and extensively hydrolyzed protein formulas being recalled (FDA, 2022).

Due to the critical importance of preparing and administering safe feeds to NICU patients, human milk and formula preparation rooms are strongly recommended. Liquid products are the preferred source of formulas and additives due to the risk of infection with powdered products; however, when liquid versions are not available (such as with elemental and metabolic formulas), powder products can be safely provided when appropriate protocols are followed. Units without milk rooms may require bedside RNs to prepare some components of infant feeds (e.g., fortifying human milk); in these circumstances, protocols that include rigorous checks and balances should be in place to reduce the risk of error. It is never best practice to prepare feeds at bedside due to the risk of contamination and error (Academy of Nutrition and Dietetics, Pediatric Nutrition Practice Group, 2019).

Term-Infant Formula

Standard cow's milk protein-based formulas meet the nutritional requirements of healthy term infants, as defined by the Infant Formula Act of 1980. These products are 20 calories per ounce in concentration and are available in a ready-to-feed, powder, and concentrated liquid form, although powdered products are not typically used in hospital settings. The composition of this formula type is summarized in Table 22.3. Although infant formula cannot replace human milk, companies are working to create products that are more similar to human milk in order to provide good alternatives when human milk is unavailable. These formula innovations vary by product and include addition of a milk fat globule membrane and lactoferrin (Chichlowski et al., 2021), supplementation of docosahexaenoic acid (DHA) and arachidonic acid (ARA; Lien et al., 2018), inclusion of human milk oligosaccharides and other prebiotics (Puccio et al., 2017), and addition of probiotics.

Innovations in infant formulas have been shown to be safe and promote infant growth, but there is limited evidence on their impact on other outcomes. For example, since 1966, over 30 randomized trials evaluating DHA and ARA supplementation in formula have been published. A recent Cochrane review explored the benefits (visual acuity, neurodevelopment) of DHA and ARA in term-infant formulas (Jasani et al., 2017). The authors concluded from their meta-analysis that routine supplementation of infant formula with DHA and ARA is not contraindicated, but also does not confer any benefits related to neurodevelopmental and visual acuity outcomes. The quantity of choices and the composition of standard infant formulas are always changing and can be overwhelming to families and providers alike. What is most important to remember is that infant formulas are safe and meet the nutrition requirements of healthy term infants.

Soy Infant Formula

Soy infant formula protein and carbohydrate sources differ from standard cow's milk-based formulas, which can be viewed in Table 22.3. Studies have repeatedly shown that *term infants* fed soy-based

TABLE 22.3 Major Components of Human Milk and Standard Term-Infant Formulas

	TERM HUMAN MILK	COW'S MILK PROTEIN-BASED FORMULA	SOY PROTEIN-BASED FORMULA
Indication for use	Gold standard for enteral feeding in both preterm and term infants	Term infant with human milk unavailable	Galactosemia, hereditary lactase deficiency, vegan preference
Energy (kcal/dL)	65–70	67–68	68
Carbohydrate (g/dL)	Lactose (6.7–7.0) Glucose (<0.01) Human milk oligosaccharides (1.2–1.4)	7.1–7.6 Source: Lactose Corn maltodextrin	7.1–7.6 Source: Corn syrup solids Corn maltodextrin Sucrose
Fat (g/dL)	3.5 Source: Triglyceride (97%–98% total) Cholesterol (0%–0.5% total) Phospholipids (0.6%–0.8% total lipids)	3.4–3.7 Source: Vegetable oils	3.4–3.7 Source: Vegetable oils
Protein (g/dL)	0.9 ± 0.02	1.35–1.4	1.66–1.70 Source: Soy, L-methionine, taurine, L-carnitine
Osmolality (mOsm/kg)	276–300	300–310	170–200
Sodium (mEq/dL)	5–10	0.7–0.8	1.0–1.3
Potassium (mEq/dL)	10–14	1.8–1.9	1.9–2.0
Calcium (mg/dL)	20–25	45–53	70–71
Phosphorus (mg/dL)	12–14	26–29	43–50

Note: Information in this table is provided for teaching purposes and represents the ranges of macronutrients and electrolytes included in term formulas currently on the market. Clinicians should always consult manufacturer information for the most accurate data.

Sources: From Kleinman, R. E., & Greer, F. R. (Eds.). (2020). *Pediatric Nutrition* (8th ed.). American Academy of Pediatrics; Koletzko, B., & Lapillonne, A. (2021). Lipid requirements for preterm infants. In B. Koletzko, F. C. Cheach, M. Domellof, B. B. Poindexter, N. Vain, & J. B. Goudoever (Eds.), *Nutritional care of preterm infants: Scientific basis and practical guidelines* (Vol. 122, pp. 89–102). Karger; Pearson, F., Johnson, M. J., & Leaf, A. A. (2013). Milk osmolality: Does it matter? *Archives of Disease in Childhood: Fetal and Neonatal Edition, 98*(2), F166–F169. https://doi.org/10.1136/adc.2011.300492; https://abbottnutrition.com; https://www.hcp.meadjohnson.com https://medical.gerber.com.

formulas are not deprived of essential nutrients, nor do these infants manifest with immune deficiencies, altered neurodevelopment, thyroid disease, or disorders of sexual differentiation (Bhatia et al., 2008). Soy-based formulas, however, are *not recommended for preterm infants weighing less than 1.8 kg or infants with renal failure* due to an increased risk of aluminum toxicity, metabolic bone disease, and poor growth (Callenbach et al., 1981; Kulkarni et al., 1980). Soy formulas are often used but not typically indicated. Use of soy formula is only recommended in disorders of carbohydrate metabolism (namely, galactosemia and congenital lactase deficiency), if a family has a specific dietary practice (e.g., veganism), and potentially following periods of acute diarrheal disease (Bhatia et al., 2008). Use of soy formula in the setting of cow's milk protein allergy (CMPA) is typically not recommended, as approximately 10% to 14% of infants who have an adverse reaction to cow's milk protein will have a reaction to soybean protein (Klemola et al., 2002; Zeiger et al., 1999).

Tolerance Formulas

Tolerance formulas comprise a varied and growing group of formulas that contain modified carbohydrate and/or protein contents to address symptoms of nonspecific feeding intolerance. Although there are no consistent medical indications for these formulas, they are growing in

TABLE 22.4 Major Components of Nonstandard Term-Infant Formulas

	TOLERANCE FORMULAS	HYPOALLERGENIC FORMULAS	NONALLERGENIC FORMULAS
Indication for use	Symptom management of feeding intolerance (colic, fussiness, gas)	Cow's milk protein allergy, malabsorption	Malabsorption, severe allergy nonresponsive to hypoallergenic formulas
Energy (kcal/dL)	67–68	67–68	67–68
Carbohydrate (g/dL)	7.2–7.4 Source: Corn maltodextrin Corn syrup solids Lactose Human milk oligosaccharides	7.0–7.4 Source: Corn syrup solids Corn maltodextrin Sugar Modified tapioca starch	7.2–7.6 Source: Corn syrup solids Potato starch
Fat (g/dL)	3.4–3.7 Source: Vegetable oils	3.4–3.8 Source: Vegetable oils MCT	3.2–3.4 Source: Vegetable oils MCT
Protein (g/dL)	1.4–1.6 Source: Intact or partially hydrolyzed cow's milk protein	1.8–1.9 Source: Casein hydrolysate Hydrolyzed whey protein isolate	1.8–2.1 Source: Free amino acids
Osmolality (mOsm/kg)	188–220	220–300	300–360
Sodium (mEq/dL)	0.8–1.2	1.1–1.4	1.1–1.3
Potassium (mEq/dL)	1.7–1.8	1.7–1.9	1.6–1.8
Calcium (mg/dL)	49–57	61–64	78–80
Phosphorus (mg/dL)	27–39	35–43	52–56

Note: Information in this table is provided for teaching purposes and represents the customary range of macronutrients and electrolytes included in term formulas currently on the market. Clinicians should always consult manufacturer information for the most accurate data.
MCT, medium-chain triglyceride.
Sources: From https://abbottnutrition.com; https://www.hcp.meadjohnson.com; https://medical.gerber.com.

popularity for at-home use due to their marketing toward infants who are experiencing colic, excessive crying, fussiness, and gas. In a clinical environment, these types of formulas are often used for infants with neonatal opioid withdrawal syndrome (NOWS), although there is limited evidence to support their clinical efficacy (Alsaleem et al., 2020). The utilization of pre- and probiotics, partially hydrolyzed proteins, and differing carbohydrate composition makes this diverse group of formulas difficult to keep track of, although a brief summary can be viewed in Table 22.4.

Hypoallergenic Formulas

Hypoallergenic formulas are characterized predominately by their containing extensively hydrolyzed proteins and varying amounts of MCT (see Table 22.4). The proteins in these types of formulas only contain peptides with a molecular weight of less than 3,000 Da; this differs from tolerance formulas with partially hydrolyzed proteins that have a molecular weight of less than 5,000 Da. Protein hydrolysis often relies on a porcine-derived enzyme for the process, making these products often inappropriate for use with families following a halal or kosher diet. The hydrolysis process also impacts the bioavailability of nitrogen; these products offer higher total protein content to ensure the formula meets the nutritional requirements of a term infant.

The utilization of these hydrolyzed proteins more easily facilitates digestion and absorption while also reducing the risk of allergic reactions. For these reasons, these types of formulas are primarily used for infants with CMPA and malabsorption. Note that these formulas should not be used for preterm infants with the sole goal of improving feed tolerance as related to prematurity.

Similarly, these products should not be used with the intention of preventing NEC as there is no evidence of such benefit (Ng et al., 2019).

Nonallergenic Formulas

Nonallergenic formulas, also referred to as *elemental formulas*, are peptide-free and contain a mixture of essential and nonessential amino acids. Elemental formulas are only available in powdered form and thus require a formula/milk room to be safely prepared. These formulas are indicated for infants with malabsorption (e.g., as with short gut syndrome) and milk protein allergy nonresponsive to utilization of a hypoallergenic formulas. Both hypoallergenic and nonallergenic formulas are hyperosmolar. Rapid administration of hyperosmolar formulas increases the risk of GI cramping and osmotic diarrhea and dehydration. Clinicians must be mindful of this risk when initiating and progressing enteral feeds.

Preterm-Infant Formulas

Preterm infants have higher total nutrition requirements due to exponential growth requirements, being in a catabolic state due to critical illness, and accumulation of nutrient deficits in the setting of minimal nutrient stores. Preterm infants miss the opportunity for in utero accretion of nutrients, which occurs during the third trimester. It is the current standard of care to provide nutrient-dense formula to meet these elevated needs. Protein is whey-predominant and also fortified, which meets the ESPGHAN (2010) and the AAP (2020) recommended goal of 3.5 to 4.5 g/kg/d of enteral protein intake (Table 22.5). Fat is provided as predominantly MCTs, which are easier to digest. Vitamins, electrolytes, and minerals are added in higher levels to preterm formulas to offset the lack of third-trimester intrauterine transfer.

Preterm-infant formulas are typically used at a 24 kcal/oz concentration but are also available in 20 and 30 kcal/oz ready-to-feed concentrations. Preterm infants may require customized fortification to meet nutritional needs, particularly those who exhibit poor growth velocity and a concurrent need for fluid restriction (e.g., cases of bronchopulmonary dysplasia [BPD]). Concentrating preterm formulas to 26 kcal/oz, 27 kcal/oz, and 28 kcal/oz can be prepared using the ready-to-feed, 24-calorie-per-ounce and 30-calorie-per-ounce concentrations and manufacturer ratio mixing volumes.

Preterm-infant formulas may be used following NICU discharge up until an infant reaches a weight of 3.6 kg; the weight limit exists to prevent excessive nutrient intake as total daily volume increases. Although preterm-infant formulas are not always readily available commercially, the Women, Infants, and Children Supplemental Nutrition Program (WIC) does cover preterm-infant formulas in many states. Formula companies also have programs to ship preterm-infant formula to patient homes free of charge. When preterm-infant formulas are no longer nutritionally appropriate, a transition to preterm discharge formula is indicated (see Table 22.5).

Preterm discharge formulas generally offer approximately 72 to 74 kcal/100 mL of energy intake and 1.8 to 1.9 g/100 mL of protein intake. Utilizing preterm discharge formula that has energy, protein, and nutrient enrichment is beneficial to growth outcomes and may be beneficial for neurodevelopmental outcomes. This is particularly true for the smallest infants (born <1,250 grams), with longer times of use of this product being indicated for infants born at a smaller birth weight/earlier gestational age (Kleinman & Greer, 2020; Teller et al., 2016). These products may be used up to 12 months corrected age. Primary care pediatricians and nurse practitioners must closely monitor growth velocity and total daily protein load in infants consuming more than 24 kcal/oz formulas.

HUMAN MILK

Human milk from the lactating parent is the gold standard for infant feeding and is the most important medication that is administered in the NICU. Preterm infants especially benefit from utilization of the parent's own human milk, which has been associated with decreased risk of NEC, BPD, late-onset sepsis, and retinopathy of prematurity (Altobelli et al., 2020; Hair et al., 2016; A. L. Patel et al., 2017; Raghuveer & Zackula, 2020). Human milk also contains unique nutritive and non nutritive factors that contribute to its improved digestion and tolerance compared with infant formulas. Chapter 21, "Human Milk as Medicine," provides further discussion on this complex and vital substance.

Although we have published estimates of human milk composition (see Tables 22.3 and 22.5), human milk is a dynamic substance that can greatly vary among lactating individuals, within a single person's lactation journey, and even within a single milk expression. When calculating intakes of human milk fed infants in the NICU, it is critical to remember that these are estimated rather than actual values. For healthy, term infants, the variations within human milk are not important; for preterm infants, lower-than-average energy or protein milk may result in poor growth.

TABLE 22.5 Major Components of Preterm Formula and Preterm Human Milk

	PRETERM HUMAN MILK	PASTEURIZED DONOR MILK	PRETERM FORMULA	PRETERM DISCHARGE FORMULA
Indication for use	Gold standard for preterm infants	High-risk infants when expressed human milk is unavailable with priority to infants born <1,500 grams	<1.8 kg at birth	<37 weeks' GA at birth, or <1.8 kg at birth, now >3.6 kg
Energy (kcal/dL)	67	43–86	80	74–75
Carbohydrate (g/dL)	7.3	7–7.3	8.2–8.8 Source: Corn syrup solids Lactose	7.6–7.7 Source: Corn syrup solids Lactose
Fat (g/dL)	3.5	1.7–7.4	4.1–4.3 Source: Vegetable oils MCT	3.9–4.1 Source: Vegetable oils MCT
Protein (g/dL)	1.62	0.8–2.2	2.4–2.7 Source: Whey protein concentrate	2.1 Source: Whey protein concentrate
Osmolality (mOsm/kg)	290	Not available	300–320	230–310
Sodium (mEq/dL)	1.2	0.4 ± 0.1	1.5–2.5	1–1.2
Potassium (mEq/dL)	1.3	1± 0.1	2–2.6	2–2.7
Calcium (mg/dL)	25	23.7 ± 5.3	134–144	79–89
Phosphorus (mg/dL)	14.5	13.2 ± 3.2	73–80	47–48

Note: Nutritional composition of human milk from individuals is qualitatively and quantitatively variable; composition of donor human milk greatly varies among the types of products available on today's market. Information in this table is provided for teaching purposes and represents the customary range of macronutrients and electrolytes included in preterm-infant formulas. This information is not brand-specific. Clinicians should always consult manufacturer information for the most accurate data.
GA, gestational age; MCT, medium-chain triglyceride.

Sources: From Committee on Nutrition, Section on Breastfeeding, & Committee on Fetus and Newborn. (2017). Donor human milk for the high-risk infant: Preparation, safety, and usage options in the United States. *Pediatrics, 139*(1), e20163440. https://doi.org/10.1542/peds.2016-3440; Kleinman, R. E., & Greer, F. R. (Eds.). (2020). *Pediatric Nutrition* (8th ed.). American Academy of Pediatrics; Koletzko, B., Cheah, F. C., Domellöf, M., van Goudoever, J. B., Poindexter, B. B., & Vain, N. (2021). Scientific basis and practical application of nutritional care for preterm infants. *World Review of Nutrition and Dietetics, 122*, XIII–XIV. https://doi.org/10.1159/000514773; Perrin, M. T., Belfort, M. B., Hagadorn, J. I., McGrath, J. M., Taylor, S. N., Tosi, L. M., & Brownell, E. A. (2020). The nutritional composition and energy content of donor human milk: A systematic review. *Advances in Nutrition, 11*(4), 960–970. https://doi.org/10.1093/advances/nmaa014; https://abbottnutrition.com/; https://www.hcp.meadjohnson.com.

Donor Human Milk

DHM is an important tool for for prevention of NEC in very low-birth weight infants. The AAP specifically recommends use of DHM for high-risk infants when expressed human milk is unavailable, with priority given to infants born less than 1,500 grams (Committee on Nutrition, Section on Breastfeeding, & Committee on Fetus and Newborn, 2017). Similar to expressed human milk, DHM does not meet the nutritional needs of growing preterm infants. Further, the nutritional composition of DHM can vary widely (see Table 22.5).

Clinicians should recognize that, although the composition of freshly expressed maternal milk is well documented, the composition of DHM can be widely variable. Factors that contribute to this variability include the stage of lactation of the donor, DHM bank practices (e.g., mixing and pooling of donated samples, transferring of milk between containers prior to distribution), method of DHM processing, and length of DHM storage. Experts have demonstrated that these factors influence the true composition of the donated milk. An outstanding visual depiction of these factors was created by Perrin and associates (2020) and is provided in Figure 22.7.

Availability of nutritional information (energy, macronutrient) depends on the source of the DHM. The availability of a human milk analyzer approved by the FDA for clinical use (MIRIS Human Milk Analyzer, MIRIS AB, Uppsala, Sweden) has improved the feasibility of DHM banks in providing energy and macronutrient information. The micronutrient composition of DHM is not easily tested nor commonly available from commercial and nonprofit DHM banks. The potential for unknown DHM nutritional composition can impede the ability of clinicians to appraise the extent of fortification required to promote optimal postnatal growth and development.

As discussed in Chapter 21, "Human Milk as Medicine," DHM is subject to processing via Holder pasteurization, vat pasteurization, or retort sterilization. Although necessary, these

FIGURE 22.7 Factors that affect the nutrient profile of donor human milk.

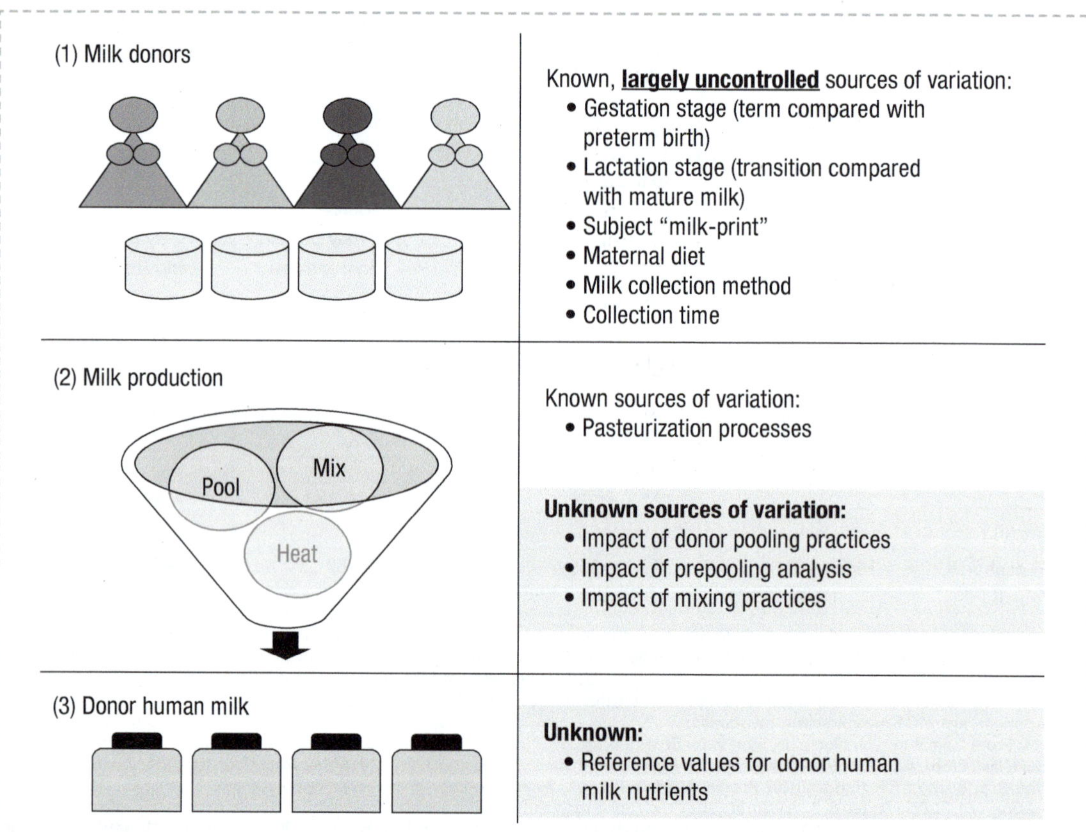

Source: From Perrin, M. T., Belfort, M. B., Hagadorn, J. I., McGrath, J. M., Taylor, S. N., Tosi, L. M., & Brownell, E. A. (2020). The nutritional composition and energy content of donor human milk: A systematic review. *Advances in Nutrition, 11*(4), 960–970. https://doi.org/10.1093/advances/nmaa014.

processes degrade or demolish the bioactive components found in human milk. For example, following Holder pasteurization, BSSL is abolished (Neu, 2019); immune protective proteins like immunoglobulin A (IgA) and lactoferrin are decimated by retort sterilization (Meredith-Dennis et al., 2018). Cacho et al. (2017) introduced a promising strategy to reintroduce commensal bacteria to human milk fed to preterm infants, which involves adding freshly expressed maternal milk to DHM. This strategy may facilitate the establishment of a healthy gut microbiota and resist pathogenic invasion. More research is needed before this strategy can be adopted into hospital-based feeding protocols in U.S. NICUs.

Human Milk Fortifiers

After reviewing Tables 22.4 and 22.6, readers should recognize that human milk, donor or freshly expressed, cannot solely provide a growing preterm infant with adequate nutritional intake to meet the recommended postnatal growth velocity. Preterm human milk alone provides far less than the estimated requirements of a preterm infant; even if higher volumes are used to meet an infant's estimated energy requirements, human milk cannot meet a preterm infant's protein or micronutrient requirements (see Table 22.6). This should not confer inferiority to preterm formulas, as human milk unequivocally reduces the risk of GI disease in preterm infants and is associated with improved neurocognitive development. Rather, the use of human milk should be complemented with the use of HMFs, which provide the additional and necessary nutrient intake to optimize postnatal growth velocity, linear growth, and head growth (Abrams et al., 2013; Kuschel & Harding, 2014).

Currently, two types of HMF are available for use in the hospital setting: human milk-based liquid fortifier and bovine-based fortifiers. When HMF is added to human milk, it is referred to as fully *fortified milk*. This fully fortified human milk (as shown in Table 22.6 as *HMF 1:25* or *Prolact+4*) is nutritionally adequate to optimize postnatal growth velocity among preterm infants. In situations where HMF supply is limited, expressed breast milk may be fortified using preterm-infant formula.

BOVINE-BASED LIQUID FORTIFIERS

Recall that the AAP recommends that preterm infants, especially those born less than 2,000 grams, receive HMF (Abrams et al., 2013). The most commonly used HMFs in NICUs are bovine-based. Initially prepared as acidified and nonacidified preparations, clinicians quickly learned that the use of the acidified HMF preparations was associated with reduced growth and acquired metabolic acidosis; its use was discontinued (Cibulskis & Armbrecht, 2015; Darrow et al., 2020; Lainwala et al., 2017). Currently, nonacidified and hydrolyzed bovine-based HMF (B-HMF) products are available and recommended for use in NICUs (Schulz & Wager, 2021).

HUMAN MILK-BASED LIQUID FORTIFIERS

As discussed in Chapter 24, "Necrotizing Enterocolitis," exposure to infant formula is a modifiable risk factor for NEC. Therefore, clinicians hypothesize that exclusive use of human milk-derived nutrition reduces the risk of NEC in high-risk neonates. This includes the use of freshly expressed

TABLE 22.6 Intake for a 1-kg Infant at ~120 kcal/kg/d

NUTRIENT	ESTIMATED NEEDS	HUMAN MILK (PT)	HMF 1:25	HM: PT HP 1:1	HM: PT 30 1:1	PROLACT+4
Volume (mL/kg)	135–200	180	150	165	145	145
Protein (g/kg)	3.5–4.5	2.5	4.3	3.1	3.1	3.6
Calcium (mg/kg)	120–200	44	182	130	148	179
Potassium (mg/kg)	60–140	23	102	72	82	96
Zinc (mcg/kg)	1,400–2,500	612	1,992	1,206	1,332	2,160

HM, human milk; HMF, human milk fortifier; PT HP, preterm 24 kcal/oz high protein infant formula; PT 30, preterm 30 kcal/oz infant formula.
Sources: From https://abbottnutrition.com; https://www.prolacta.com.

human milk and donor milk, as well as HMF. In 2006, in order to support the use of exclusive human milk throughout the birth hospitalization, the first DHM-based HMF (DHM-HMF) was manufactured. Manufacturing and distribution expanded thereafter and continues at present. Although the FDA does not regulate DHM banks, it does regulate the manufacturing and distribution of DHM-generated HMF. These regulations are outlined in the Infant Formula Act of 1980 as well as the Code of Federal Regulations (21 CFR 107.50; Steele et al., 2019).

"WHAT DO I PRESCRIBE?" COMPARING HUMAN VERSUS BOVINE-BASED FORTIFIERS

There is a substantial amount of research available for clinicians to review that is specific to the utilization of DHM-based fortifiers (DHM-HMF), although much of it is industry-funded. For example, Sullivan and colleagues (2010) reported the outcomes of a randomized trial involving DHM-HMF and B-HMF. The incidence of combined mortality and death was substantially lower among infants fed DHM-HMF compared with B-HMF, and all cases of surgical NEC were observed in infants who received B-HMF (Sullivan et al., 2010). Although the difference in NEC rates was impressive, generalization of these findings was limited by the study design. Despite the availability of DHM on the unit, the B-HMF group received preterm-infant formula if no maternally expressed human milk was available, whereas the DHM-HMF group received DHM if no maternally expressed human milk was available.

Cristofalo and colleagues (2013) reported the outcomes of a small randomized multicenter trial that concluded the use of DHM-HMF (vs. B-HMF) was associated with reduced days of parenteral nutrition (27 vs. 36 days, $p = .04$) and incidence of NEC (3% vs. 21%, $p = .08$). This study was limited by the small sample size ($N = 53$) and a higher-than-average rate of NEC among infants fed B-HMF, substantially above typical NICU NEC rates. Five years later, O'Connor and colleagues (2018) published the outcomes of a small, blinded randomized trial. Their results contrasted with previous studies; no significant difference in feeding intolerance or mortality and morbidity was identified ($p = .07$). Although this study was not industry-funded, it was not powered to determine the impact of fortification method on NEC occurrence.

Common factors that impact the ability of clinicians to prescribe DHM-HMF versus B-HMF include supply-chain limitations and the enormous cost of DHM-HMF. For reference, Prolact+2 HMF costs approximately $6.25 per mL. Therefore, the associated cost for a 1-kg infant receiving maternally expressed human milk fortified with Prolact+2 HMF exceeds $180 per day. In contrast, B-HMF costs approximately $1.30 per packet. The cost to feed the same 1-kg infant with maternally expressed human milk fortified with B-HMF is $7.80 per day (Ganapathy et al., 2012). Although there is potential for cost savings with the prevention of a single case of NEC, further evaluation of HM-HMF from nonindustry-funded research is required to better understand the potential benefits of its use in the NICU population.

Modular Additives

Modular additives are incomplete dietary supplements that contain fat, protein, and/or carbohydrates. Individual macronutrient modulars are used to meet the unique nutrient requirements of infants that formula and human milk alone cannot meet. Combination modulars are useful for increasing total energy content within a feed (e.g., increasing a formula to 28 kcal/oz).

Additional fats may be indicated for infants requiring extra energy in a small volume. These products are commonly used for infants with fluid restrictions that limit their total nutrient intake, often seen with BPD or congenital heart defects. One common method for adding fat calories to a nutritional regimen is through the inclusion of MCT oil. Generally speaking, 1 mL of MCT oil provides 4.5 to 7.7 calories; clinicians should consult the product label to confirm energy offerings. Most clinicians begin therapy by providing an additional 10 kcal/kg of MCT oil and assess for tolerance and response; however, dosing decisions should be tailored to each patient and in consultation with the NICU dietitian. Clinicians and bedside staff should be educated that MCT oil can adhere to and deteriorate plastics (feeding tubes) over time and thus should be administered as a bolus medication prior to the provision of the scheduled feeding. In comparison, for infants feeding orally, emulsified MCT products may be easily mixed with feeds for oral administration.

Additional protein may be required to optimize protein intake goals in preterm infants. Protein modulars are often used for individualized fortification among infants with inadequate protein intake due to low total protein content in human milk despite standard fortification. Extensively hydrolyzed liquid protein (e.g., LiquiProtein®) is approved for use in infants and associated with excellent weight gain and tolerance (Kim et al., 2015). Two other protein modulars, powdered intact protein and amino acid-based protein, are occasionally used off-label in the NICU.

Although persistent hypoglycemia is typically treated with a pharmacologic agent (e.g., diazoxide) or titration of the glucose infusion rate, enteral carbohydrate supplementation may be needed. This scenario typically results from congenital hyperinsulinism or being an infant of a diabetic mother (IDM). Utilization of higher carbohydrate-containing formulas and/or concentrating formulas may be a useful approach to dietary hypoglycemia management. Clinicians should recognize that maltodextrin-based carbohydrate modulars (e.g., SolCarb®) are not customarily recommended in preterm infants due to the risk of maldigestion, hyperosmotic load, and NEC (Buddington et al., 2018; Singh et al., 2020; Thymann et al., 2009). In addition, cornstarch is not appropriate for use in preterm or term infants due to diminished pancreatic amylase activity.

NUTRITIONAL IMPLICATIONS OF DISEASE STATES

In addition to special formula and supplementation requirements related to preterm birth, genetic or metabolic disorders and certain developmental and GI problems of the neonate contribute to special enteral needs. We will identify nutrition considerations related to disease states commonly seen in the NICU. Details on pharmacologic agents are provided later in the chapter.

Bronchopulmonary Dysplasia

Chapter 16, "Bronchopulmonary Dysplasia," reviews enteral nutrition-related strategies for infants with BPD. Clinicians must recognize that adequate nutrient intake is vital to prevent, treat, and grow and develop in the setting of acquired respiratory diseases. Dietary regimens must be customized to the needs of the infant and often differ from the routine feeding regimens of healthy counterparts. For example, infants with BPD demonstrate higher energy needs secondary to energy demands imposed by the disease process (Bauer et al., 2021). Hypercaloric feedings in the setting of fluid restriction are often prescribed (Hodges et al., 2022). Electrolyte replacement is common, as diuretic therapy is often pursued in the setting of pulmonary congestion. Later, particularly among infants who require tracheostomy and demonstrate reduced work of breathing and energy losses over time, feeding regimens may need to be adjusted (e.g., discontinuation of hypercaloric feedings).

Chylothorax

Chylothorax may develop during fetal development or after a traumatic event, such as cardiac surgery (Tutor, 2014). Fat droplets and lymph (chyle) accumulate in the pleural space, via the thoracic duct. Although early treatment customarily involves parenteral nutrition, once enteral feedings are resumed, use of a formula high in MCTs is necessary. MCTs bypass lymphatic drainage and are transported directly to the portal circulation for absorption (Jackson & Jnah, 2021; Schild et al., 2013). This reduces the formation of chylomicrons and lymphatic flow within the thoracic duct. Alternatively, newer data suggest that the use of skimmed human milk may be a suitable regimen for affected infants (Höck et al., 2021).

Cow's Milk Protein Allergy

CMPA is one of the most common allergies in infants and young children. CMPA may present with immunoglobulin E (IgE)- and non-IgE-mediated symptoms, including bloody stools, diarrhea, emesis, eczema, and failure to thrive/weight loss. Scoring tools have been created to help improve accuracy in diagnosing infants with CMPA, which is often a diagnosis of exclusion, as there is no singular marker used to make a diagnosis (Salvatore et al., 2019).

The recommended nutritional regimen for an infant with CMPA involves the initial use of an extensively hydrolyzed protein formula. If symptoms persist with the use of the extensively hydrolyzed formula, clinicians often prescribe an amino acid-based formula (Vandenplas et al., 2007). For infants receiving human milk, dietitians may counsel lactating mothers to undergo a strict elimination diet. This requires close oversight from a dietitian to ensure both appropriate elimination of all cow's milk protein-containing food items and appropriate inclusion of necessary nutrients in the setting of a restrictive diet.

Gastroesophageal Reflux Disease

Gastroesophageal reflux (*GER*) is defined as *retrograde* movement of gastric contents into the distal esophagus (Gulati & Jadcherla, 2019). Decreased lower esophageal segment pressure and delayed gastric emptying may contribute to GER (Neu & Li, 2002). Manifestations may be *gastrointestinal* (e.g., emesis, abdominal distension), *cardiorespiratory* (e.g., apnea, tachypnea or periodic breathing, bradycardia or tachycardia), *somatosensory* (e.g., crying, grimacing, arching of lower back), or *aerodigestive* (uncoordinated sucking and swallowing, coughing, choking, or sneezing; Gulati & Jadcherla, 2019). Nonpharmacologic treatments include reduced feeding volumes, modified positioning during and in-between feedings (left lateral positioning), and in some cases use of thickeners. In symptomatic gastroesophageal reflux disease (GERD), pharmacologic treatment often includes judicious use of histamine-2 (H2) receptor antagonists and/or proton pump inhibitors (PPIs) to decrease or suppress acid production and prokinetics to enhance gastric emptying (Tighe et al., 2014). If a protein allergy is thought to be triggering GER, changing to a protein hydrolysate or elemental formula may be appropriate (Tighe et al., 2014).

Gastroparesis (Dysmotility/Hypomotility)

As previously discussed, motor function is immature in preterm infants, particularly those born less than 34 weeks of gestation, yet improves with advancing postnatal age. Reduced gastroduodenal motor function, which is observed in some preterm infants who are approaching or have reached full enteral feeding volumes, precipitates varying degrees of GI dysmotility. Dysmotility is associated with delayed gastric emptying and slower transit times. Common manifestations include increased prefeed gastric residuals and abdominal distension. During fasting states, MMC activity is either absent or reduced, which hinders the clearing of the stomach and duodenum and forward movement of residual content. Clinicians should consider dysmotility as part of the differential diagnosis in infants who present with findings as described earlier. To improve GI motility, prokinetic drugs (e.g., erythromycin) may be prescribed in these situations (Lam & Ng, 2011).

Inherited Metabolic Disorders

Inherited metabolic disorders require specialized lifelong enteral management in order to prevent nutritional deficiencies, neurodevelopmental impairment, and death. Many of these disorders are detected on newborn screening done in the first days of life. In this section, we review a few of the more common inherited metabolic disorders.

CYSTIC FIBROSIS

Cystic fibrosis (CF) is an autosomal recessive genetic disorder caused by a mutation at the CF *transmembrane conductance regulator (CTFR)* gene. Under normal circumstances, the *CTFR* gene, located on chromosome 7, encodes a protein in epithelial cells which regulates electrolyte (chloride) and water transport across cell membranes. When functional, the *CTFR* gene facilitates the production of a thin, easily cleared mucus that coats major passageways (e.g., conducting airways, pancreas, GI tract). Mutations in the *CFTR* gene impair the flow of chloride ions and water across cell membranes (Waskowsky et al., 2019), leading to the formation of an unusually thick and sticky mucus; meconium ileus is a common GI finding that develops as a consequence of this gene mutation.

All infants with CF, who may be breastfed or bottle-fed, require close monitoring of pancreatic function because an insufficient release of digestive enzymes can precipitate weight loss and failure to thrive. Affected infants require fat-soluble vitamin and pancreatic enzyme supplementation (e.g., Creon®, Pancreaze®, Zenpep®) and close monitoring of caloric intake. The dose of the selected enzyme supplement is titrated based on the fat content of the prescribed nutritional regimen, as the primary mechanism of action is to assist in the breakdown of ingested fats and proteins (Larson-Nath et al., 2020). Use of a multidisciplinary approach to the care of the affected infant, which includes a pediatric pulmonology team and a pediatric dietitian, is essential to optimize treatment and outcomes.

PHENYLKETONURIA

Phenylketonuria (PKU) is a genetic disorder involving a mutation in the *PAH* gene, the gene responsible for synthesizing phenylalanine hydroxylase. Affected neonates cannot enzymatically convert phenylalanine to tyrosine, a necessary precursor for dopamine synthesis. This leads to abnormally high levels of phenylalanine, or hyperphenylalaninemia. Sustained hyperphenylalaninemia is linked to developmental delays and neurobehavioral problems.

Infants with PKU require a specialized phenylalanine-free formula (Kleinman & Greer, 2020) and careful dietary monitoring to support normal growth and neurodevelopment (Williams et al., 2008). Breastfeeding is challenging but possible in infants with PKU; a combination of human milk and phenylalanine-free formula that maintains a safe serum phenylalanine level in the infant can be determined by the metabolic team via sequential blood testing (Banta-Wright et al., 2012). Supplementation with phenylalanine-free amino acids usually begins during infancy to provide sufficient protein intake for normal growth (Williams et al., 2008).

GALACTOSEMIA

Galactosemia involves a group of genetic disorders in which a gene mutation leads to a deficiency in one of the three enzymes responsible for processing galactose. Classic galactosemia, the most common and severe type, is caused by a deficiency of the galactose-1-phosphate uridyl transferase (GALT) enzyme (Waskowsky et al., 2019). The deficiency of the GALT enzyme prevents the metabolism of galactose and leads to a buildup of galactose 1-phosphate if proper dietary management is not achieved (Haskovic et al., 2020). Associated comorbidities include failure to thrive, cognitive impairment, and developmental delays.

Lactose, a disaccharide formed from glucose and galactose, is the primary carbohydrate found in human milk and cow's milk. Thus, galactosemia is one of the few absolute contraindications to human milk feeding. Infants with galactosemia require soy formula as it is lactose-free.

Ready-to-feed and concentrated liquid soy formulas manufactured in the United States use carrageenan, a natural gum emulsifier, as a thickener and stabilizing agent; carrageenan is roughly 27% bound galactose, by weight (Acosta, 2001; Kulkarni & Shaw, 2016). The significance of the galactose in carrageenan in regard to individuals with galactosemia has not been fully determined. One report from 1970 found that carrageenan is unlikely to release free galactose for absorption in the GI tract, and thus is likely safe to include in the diet for individuals with galactosemia (Bott et al., 1970). This report noted that, in cases of gastroenteritis, bacterial degradation may have the potential to hydrolyze glycosidic linkages of carrageen and release free galactose; avoidance of carrageenan should be considered in these instances. Utilization of a powdered soy infant formula is recommended as it is a lactose- and galactose-free product. For infants with galactosemia born less than 1,800 grams or with renal failure, soy formulas are not considered appropriate due to its elevated aluminum content with potential for toxicity and increased risk of metabolic bone disease (Bhatia et al., 2008). In this instance, amino acid-based formulas are most typically used in conjunction with calcium and phosphorus supplementation to improve bone mineralization.

Lactose Intolerance

Lactose intolerance is critically different from galactosemia (an inherited metabolic disorder) and CMPA (an immunologic reaction to one or more cow's milk protein). Lactose intolerance results from the maldigestion of lactose due to a deficiency of lactase, an enzyme in the brush border of the small intestine that hydrolyzes D-lactose to form D-galactose and D-glucose, which are absorbed into the bloodstream. Lactose intolerance, although common in adults globally, is very rare in children under the age of 5 and is not typically of clinical concern in infancy. Clinicians should recognize that preterm infants are born with lower lactase enzyme activity, but lactase activity is quickly stimulated with the introduction of enteral feeds after birth (Shulman et al., 1998). Following acute gastroenteritis or other intestinal mucosa injury, a temporary lactose intolerance (known as secondary lactase deficiency) may occur but should not be confused with a lactose intolerance.

Necrotizing Enterocolitis

NEC is a devastating intestinal disease with high risk of morbidity and mortality. Chapter 24, "Necrotizing Enterocolitis," reviews enteral nutrition-related strategies critical for NEC prevention, including the utilization of human milk for enteral nutrition, standardized feeding guidelines, and probiotics. Infants are made nothing by mouth (NPO) when concerns for NEC arise and when the confirmatory diagnosis is rendered. Enteral feeds are typically resumed once hemodynamic and respiratory stability is established, the empirical antibiotic course is completed, electrolyte homeostasis is restored, and the abdominal examination is reassuring. Expressed human milk is the preferred feeding modality following NEC diagnosis, although DHM, extensively hydrolyzed protein formulas, or elemental formulas may be used if unavailable (Christian et al., 2018).

Neonatal Abstinence Syndrome/Neonatal Opioid Withdrawal Syndrome

Infants with NOWS frequently have GI symptoms, including loose stools and reflux, related to withdrawal. Mother's own milk, when appropriate, remains the best nutrition for this population and has consistently been linked to a lower requirement for pharmacotherapy and shorter length of hospital stay (Holmes et al., 2017). Recent data indicate that only 20% of infants with NOWS are exclusively breastfed beyond 1 month of life and 8.3% beyond 6 months of life, indicating that this population likely requires greater lactation support to meet breastfeeding goals (Hicks et al., 2018). Although low-lactose formulas are commonly used in this population, there is no evidence to suggest that this practice lessens duration of pharmacologic treatment or reduces length of hospital stay (Alsaleem et al., 2020; Pandey et al., 2021). Due to their hypermetabolic state, infants with NOWS often require a hypercaloric formula to meet their elevated energy requirements and to support growth (Hudak et al., 2012). See Chapter 9, "Neonatal Abstinence Syndrome," for further discussion on this topic.

Short Bowel Syndrome

SBS is the most common long-term morbidity associated with surgical NEC. In other cases, congenital malformations are the proximate cause of SBS. As a result, SBS is not always preventable. Among affected infants, parenteral nutrition is required postsurgery and followed by a slow transition to enteral nutrition. Enteral feedings are typically initiated at trophic volumes and cautiously advanced, as tolerated. Titration of feeding volumes is common, and many infants demonstrate tolerance and more optimal absorption with the provision of continuous (vs. bolus) feedings. In some cases, postpyloric feedings may be necessary to avoid recurrent intolerances and/or malabsorption.

Human milk is the preferred feeding source for infants with SBS; however, if human milk is not available, an extensively hydrolyzed or elemental formula may be prescribed to optimize absorption. Clinicians most closely monitor stool and ostomy output during the initiation and advancement of enteral feeding. Fluid and electrolyte replacement may be necessary, as well as titration of the total fluid volume/caloric density.

Stress Gastritis

Stress-induced gastritis may cause erosion of the GI mucosa and lead to GI bleeding in critically ill infants. Bleeding can be superficial or involve hemorrhage requiring blood transfusion. Infants (>1 month of age) with stress-induced gastritis may require treatment with H2-receptor antagonists (e.g., famotidine) or PPIs (e.g., omeprazole, lansoprazole, pantoprazole), which act to reduce or suppress acid production.

CURRENT PHARMACOLOGIC TREATMENT MODALITIES FOR SPECIAL ENTERAL NUTRITION AND COMMON GASTROINTESTINAL PROBLEMS

Histamine-2 Receptor Antagonists

H2-receptor antagonists (blockers) are a commonly prescribed class of medication in NICUs in preterm infants less than 1,500 grams to improve GER by suppressing gastric acid production despite limited evidence, safety concerns, and side effects (Santos et al., 2019). However, due to concerns for increased risk of developing hospital-acquired infections (Bianconi et al., 2007) and NEC in preterm neonates from chronic acid suppression, a more judicious use in this population has been warranted (Terrin et al., 2012).

Given the absence of clear safety and efficacy data, *these agents should not be utilized in clinical practice for treatment of GER.* Additional studies are needed to examine and identify optimal regimens and durations of treatment for pathologic GERD. Likewise, additional information is required prior to routine prophylaxis regimens for GI erosions from common therapies or medications similar to that in older children and adults (Mills et al., 2020).

MECHANISM OF ACTION/PHARMACOKINETIC PRINCIPLES

H2-receptor antagonists reduce gastric acid secretion and act by competitive reversible binding of histamine H2 receptors located on the basolateral (antiluminal) surface of gastric parietal cell. This class of medications acts as competitive antagonists interfering with pathways of gastric acid production and secretion and reduces both volume and acidity. H2-receptor antagonists suppress basal and meal-stimulated acid secretion in a dose-dependent manner (Nugent et al., 2022). They are particularly effective in blocking nocturnal acid secretion since it is largely dependent on histamine. H2-receptor antagonists have little to no effect on histamine type 1 receptors, which are blocked by antihistamines used to treat allergic reactions and seasonal allergies. There are four available medications in this class and the initial H2-receptor antagonist approved for use in the United States was cimetidine (1977), which was followed by ranitidine (1983), famotidine (1986), and nizatidine (1988). Cimetidine and nizatidine have limited/absent data in neonates and are generally not used. Ranitidine was recently withdrawn from the market in the United States.

Famotidine has a thiazole ring and is 10 to 15 times more potent than ranitidine and 40 to 60 times more potent than cimetidine (Sewing, 1988). Famotidine undergoes hepatic metabolism to famotidine S-oxide and 30% to 35% of the drug is eliminated in this form. About 65% to 70% of the total administered dose of famotidine undergoes renal elimination as unchanged drug. Famotidine has low protein binding (15%–20%) and bioavailability (40%–45%) and a time to peak concentration of 1 to 3 hours after oral administration (Buck, 1998; Wenning et al., 2005).

DOSING RECOMMENDATIONS

Famotidine is dosed at 0.5 to 1 mg/kg/dose by mouth once daily for GERD or 0.25 to 0.5 mg/kg/dose intravenously once daily for stress ulcer prophylaxis (Taketomo, 2023). Doses of H2-receptor antagonists should be adjusted in acute renal failure (Gladziwa & Klotz, 1993).

CLINICAL-MONITORING PEARLS

The administration of H2-receptor antagonists in neonates has been associated with an increased risk of NEC (Terrin et al., 2011), increased risk of late-onset sepsis (Bianconi et al., 2007), and independent risk for *Candida parapsilosis* (Saiman et al., 2001). Chronic gastric-acid suppression is associated with healthcare- and community-associated *Clostridium difficile* infection in children (Khanna & Pardi, 2012). In addition, there is an increased risk of acute gastroenteritis and community-acquired pneumonia (Canani et al., 2006). Neonates requiring therapy should be monitored carefully for the development of these conditions, and the duration of therapy should be limited to the minimum necessary.

Acute clinical monitoring should include a complete blood cell count, liver enzymes, heart rate, blood urea nitrogen, and serum creatinine (Kuusela, 1998). Transient and reversible effects on liver function have been reported (Glade et al., 1980).

Proton Pump Inhibitors

PPIs represent the most highly prescribed medication class in the adult population for acid suppression therapy (Rababa & Rababa'h, 2021). PPIs provide superior acid suppression, ulcer healing, and pain relief when compared with H2-receptor antagonists. Acid suppression therapy is widely prescribed as well in the neonatal population, despite a lack of scientific data to support the routine use for suspected GER and GERD in infants less than 1 year old. Optimal dosing, duration, and potential long-term toxicity profiles of PPIs have not yet been fully elucidated (Illueca et al., 2014). This significant knowledge gap has resulted in many variations at practice sites across the country in terms of agents used, doses, and duration of treatment. The AAP has targeted an initiative to decrease the frequency of use of antireflux therapies since they are among the most commonly prescribed drugs in neonatal intensive care (Angelidou et al., 2017).

The long-term use of these agents for chronic suppression of acid is not without side effects. Potential adverse effects associated with widespread H2-receptor antagonist utilization (NEC, infection) can likely be extrapolated to PPIs. Infant use of PPIs alone or together with H2-receptor antagonists is associated with an increased risk of childhood fracture, which appears amplified by days of use and earlier initiation of acid suppression therapies. The decision to initiate therapy should be weighed carefully against possible fracture risk. Other long-term side effects include electrolyte disturbances, GI and respiratory tract infections, vitamin B_{12} deficiency, hypochlorhydria, and rebound hyperacidity after discontinuation (Buck, 2019).

MECHANISM OF ACTION/PHARMACOKINETIC PRINCIPLES

PPIs undergo acidic activation within the parietal cell of the GI tract to be ionized to form covalent disulfide bonds with cysteines of the H^+–K^+-adenosine triphosphatase (H^+–K^+-ATPase) pump. PPIs inhibit the function of the proton pump responsible for the terminal step in gastric acid secretion (Vanderhoff & Tabhoub, 2002). PPIs are rapidly absorbed with variable bioavailability impacted by the timing of administration with respect to meals. This class of drug is highly protein-bound, and extensively metabolized by the liver via cytochrome-P450 isoenzymes, principally CYP2C19 and CYP3A4. Metabolites are excreted in the urine and bile.

DOSING RECOMMENDATIONS

PPIs are administered orally generally once daily and up to twice daily. Oral absorption is decreased with the administration of food; administration in adults occurs 30 minutes prior to meals; however, the clinical impact of this approach has not been validated in neonates. Pantoprazole is the only medication in this class with an intravenous formulation. This class of medication represents a large variation in practice among NICUs in terms of dosing and duration of treatment. Reported dose ranges are 0.7 to 3.3 mg/kg/d divided once to twice daily, 0.5 to 1.5 mg/kg/d and up to 3 mg/kg/d divided once to twice daily, and 2.5 mg daily for omeprazole, lansoprazole, and pantoprazole, respectively (Romano et al., 2011). There are no dose adjustments required for renal impairment. The area under the curve (AUC) and half-life are increased in patients with mild to moderate hepatic impairment (Child–Pugh class A or B); AUC is increased sixfold and half-life increased fivefold in compensated/decompensated cirrhosis (A. S. Patel et al., 2003; Tolia & Boyer, 2008).

CLINICAL-MONITORING PEARLS

PPIs are indicated for use in pediatric patients for peptic ulcer disease, eradication of *Helicobacter pylori* infections, GERD, stress ulcer prophylaxis, treatment and prevention of nonsteroidal anti-inflammatory drug (NSAID) gastroduodenal ulcers, and Zollinger–Ellison syndrome. Cautious use in neonates is recommended due to a paucity of data. When initiated, use the lowest effective doses for the shortest effective duration. The long-term effects of chronic acid suppression are unknown (Romano, 2011). Routine use is not recommended in preterm neonates (Eichenwald et al., 2018) due to lack of clinical efficacy data and the potential for adverse effects, such as heart valve thickening observed in animal models and an increased risk of childhood fracture, which is amplified by days of use and early initiation of acid suppressive therapy (Malchodi et al., 2019).

Acute clinical monitoring should include evaluation of the serum complete blood count, electrolytes, alkaline phosphatase, blood urea nitrogen, and serum creatinine. Vitamin B_{12} levels should be evaluated with chronic use. In addition, an increased index of suspicion for respiratory infections, fungal infections, and NEC is warranted given the association between acid suppressive therapy and these morbidities (Illueca et al., 2014).

Prokinetic Agents

Prokinetic agents activate motilin receptors on smooth muscle and cholinergic nerves and enhance gastric (antral) contractility. This improves function by enhancing gastric emptying and reducing the risk of reflux into the esophagus. GI dysmotility is a common condition that affects premature infants and delays the time to full enteral feeding volume and thereby increases the risks associated with prolonged parenteral nutrition. Published studies regarding the efficacy of prokinetic agents have been conflicting and systematic reviews or guideline statements have not supported the routine use of prokinetics for GERD (Gieruszczak-Białek et al., 2015; Rosen et al., 2018; Van der Pol et al., 2011).

ERYTHROMYCIN

Erythromycin, discovered in 1952, is a broad-spectrum macrolide antibiotic produced by a strain of *Saccharopolyspora erythraea* (formerly *Streptomyces erythraeus*) containing a 14-membered lactone ring with 10 asymmetric centers and two sugars: L-cladinose and D-desoamine. A meta-analysis of 10 randomized controlled trials reported no improvement in feeding tolerance and demonstrated no benefit of erythromycin use as a prokinetic agent in preterm neonates. The authors concluded that the conflicting results of individual randomized controlled trials were attributable to varying gestational and postnatal ages, differences in dose and route of administration of erythromycin, and in variability in GI motor responses in the presence of different feeding conditions, which included intermittent and continuous feeding (Patole et al., 2005). As erythromycin represents the only prokinetic without a prohibitive adverse effect profile in neonates, it may be trialed in a small subset of patients with clinically significant, intractable GI hypomotility.

Mechanism of Action/Pharmacokinetic Principles

Erythromycin is a motilin agonist and potent stimulant of small bowel motor activity and directly stimulates smooth muscle cells by a calcium-mediated event, thereby increasing GI motility and improving gastric emptying (Hawkyard & Koerner, 2007). Erythromycin has poor oral absorption (18%–45%), which is variable based on salt or base form. Protein binding is 73% to 81%. It is metabolized by the liver via CYP3A4 by demethylation and has a half-life of 2 hours. Erythromycin also inhibits CYP3A4, resulting in multiple drug–drug interactions, which require careful evaluation during prescription.

Dose Recommendations

Published studies regarding the efficacy of erythromycin for this indication are limited and dosing regimens have varied with limited reported efficacy (Chicella et al., 2005). Dosing regimens reported are 1.5 to 2.5 mg/kg/dose PO every 6 hours, 5 mg/kg/dose PO every 6 hours, and 10 to 12.5 mg/kg/dose PO every 6 to 8 hours for low-dose, intermediate-dose, and high-dose regimens, respectively. Variable efficacy in trials does not correlate with dose, so clinicians may trial low-dose therapy, escalate dosing if indicated, and withdraw therapy in patients without clear efficacy from high-dose therapy. There are no dose adjustments required for renal impairment and no dose adjustments required for hepatic impairment.

Clinical-Monitoring Pearls

Clinical monitoring during administration includes blood pressure, heart rate, liver enzymes, blood urea nitrogen, serum creatinine, and electrocardiography to evaluate QTc interval. Neonates initiated on erythromycin therapy who are less than 14 days old experience a 10-fold increase in risk of hypertrophic pyloric stenosis. Rare but life-threatening side effects include QTc prolongation, ventricular arrhythmias, and torsade de pointes. QT-prolonging class IA, IB, and III may enhance the QT-prolonging effects of erythromycin (Patole et al., 2005).

Antiflatulents

SIMETHICONE

Simethicone has a long history of use in infants after FDA approval in 1952 (Voepel-Lewis et al., 1998). A randomized, double-blind, placebo-controlled trial evaluated infants with colic in three general pediatric practices in distant geographic regions. There were no statistically detectable differences in symptoms and simethicone was no more effective than placebo in the treatment of colic (Metcalf et al., 1994). In fact, no randomized trials have demonstrated any effect from simethicone on symptoms of colic or GI discomfort (Lucassen et al., 1998). It is important to note that simethicone is not systemically absorbed and also lacks any appreciable side effects. Therefore, simethicone has historically been and will remain the most widely utilized placebo in newborn medicine.

Mechanism of Action/Pharmacokinetic Principles

Simethicone is an orally administered antifoaming agent, a silicone-based surfactant, and is used to relieve painful pressure caused by excess gas in the stomach and intestines. It contains a mixture of polydimethylsiloxane and hydrated silica gel. Simethicone decreases the surface tension of the GI gas bubbles, thereby reducing gas for patients with recurrent flatulence. Simethicone exerts its action locally in the GI tract and is not systemically absorbed into the bloodstream and as such has a favorable safety profile in infants. Simethicone is orally administered and is excreted in the feces.

Dosing Recommendations

Simethicone is administered for gas pain or discomfort at a dose of 20 mg by mouth four times a day as needed, with a maximum of 12 doses in 24 hours. There are no dose adjustments required for renal or hepatic impairment.

Clinical-Monitoring Pearls

Simethicone is physiologically inert and is not systemically absorbed. However, inactive ingredients may include sodium benzoate/benzoic acid, which has been linked to neonatal gasping syndrome, and products may also contain artificial dyes or artificial flavors.

Oral Vitamin/Mineral Supplements

MULTIVITAMINS

Multivitamin supplements are recommended in infants less than 2.5 kg and who are receiving less than 300 kcal/d. Clinicians must consider the estimated vitamin content contained within the feeding regimen when determining the necessary daily dosage of water-soluble vitamin supplementation. Water-soluble vitamins provide a source of vitamins A, C, D, E, B1, B2, B3, and B6.

In most circumstances involving enteral feedings with human milk, preterm infants require orally administered liquid multivitamin supplementation dosed between 0.5 and 1 mL daily (e.g., Poly-Vi-Sol®). When dosing Poly-Vi-Sol with Iron® for infants who are less than 2.5 kg, a reduced dosage of 0.5 mL daily is recommended to avoid iron overload.

D-Vi-Sol® (Vitamin D Cholecalciferol)

Vitamin D cholecalciferol (D_3) contains 400 international units (IU), which is equal to 10 mcg, per 1 mL volume. Supplementation of oral vitamin D is recommended for all infants (breast- and formula-fed) and should begin shortly after birth. The current recommended daily vitamin D intake for fully enterally fed preterm infants is 400 to 1,000 IU/d (Kleinman & Greer, 2020). Supplementation should continue until infants are weaned from breast milk and are consuming the recommended daily dosage from enteral feedings.

DEKA®

Some infants will require a specialized supplement that delivers fat-soluble vitamins in a water-soluble formulation. This vitamin, DEKA®, is typically reserved for infants with a history of cholestasis with direct hyperbilirubinemia or malabsorption. DEKA therapy is initiated when an infant is tolerating adequate enteral feeding volume. Supplement 1 mL by mouth daily.

Iron

Preterm infants (<37 weeks of gestation) who are fed human milk should receive a supplement of elemental iron at 2 mg/kg/d starting at 1 month of age and extending through 12 months of age. This can be provided as medicinal iron or in iron-fortified complementary foods. Preterm infants fed a standard preterm- or standard term-infant formula will receive approximately 1.8 to 2.7 mg/kg/d of iron, assuming a formula intake of 150 mL/kg/d. Despite the use of iron-containing formulas, 14% of preterm infants develop iron deficiency between 4 and 8 months of age. Some formula-fed preterm infants may need additional oral iron supplementation for treatment of anemia of prematurity of 2 to 6 mg/kg/d of elemental iron. Exceptions to this iron supplementation practice in preterm infants would be infants who received multiple transfusions during hospitalization, who might not need any iron supplementation. Consider waiting for a period of 2 weeks post-transfusion prior to initiation of any oral iron supplementation (Rao & Georgieff, 2009). Orders for oral iron supplementation should be based on desired elemental iron per day.

CONCLUSIONS

Management of infants with special enteral nutrition needs due to prematurity, GI problems, or genetic or metabolic disorders may involve a range of evidence-based best-practice interventions. Best treatment options often include a combination of interventions, including conservative non-pharmacologic management, caloric and/or vitamin supplementation, or ultimately the use of pharmacologic agents. APRNs are encouraged to appraise disease severity when evaluating the need for special formulas and/or nutritional supplementation. This judicious approach can facilitate optimal growth and development and minimize the onset of adverse effects.

Ideally, clinicians will benefit from use of a growth chart that resists skewing in the face of various enteral feeding regimens (Villar et al., 2014). This type of pragmatic tool meets the needs of all NICUs in the United States and beyond, and is likely of use to researchers studying the safety and efficacy of standardized enteral feeding regimens. This may also facilitate standardization of growth assessments, per PMA, including the method used to report growth velocity (g/kg/d vs. g/d). In the meantime, the Fenton et al. (2013), Olsen et al. (2010), and Olsen et al. BMI-for-age (2015) growth charts offer clinicians an excellent means to record, trend, and analyze growth over time. Concurrent use of multiple tools (e.g., size-for-age *and* BMI-for-age growth charts) is recommended to provide optimal data that can be used to customize nutritional regimens for preterm infants.

LEARNING TOOLS AND RESOURCES

Advice From the Authors

Amy J. Jnah, DNP, APRN, NNP-BC

Prescribing a nutritional regimen is just as important as prescribing therapeutic agents for other disease processes. Be sure to stay aware of the state of the science, explain risks and benefits to parents, and regularly seek perspective from NICU dietitians before ordering a nutritional regimen. If you work at a smaller NICU, make time to confer with your collaborating neonatologist with the intent to learn something new, that you can share with others!

Carrie Smith, MS, RD, CSP, LD

Look at every moment in life as a learning opportunity. Utilize your resources. Once you think you know something, seek out additional information to keep learning and building on that foundation. Although there are guidelines and evidence-based practices, remember that each patient (infant, child, adolescent, adult) is unique and is a human. They should be treated with the respect that comes from that.

Stephanie Merlino Barr, MS, RDN, LD

The NICU relies on multidisciplinary collaboration to ensure optimal outcomes of our incredibly fragile patients. Learning how to care for these patients should similarly be a multidisciplinary effort. Talk with your NICU dietitians to help learn about enteral nutrition management and administration in the NICU! In addition, remembering all the different formula types can be daunting. Taste testing is an effective and memorable approach I use with all my trainees in the NICU; once you taste an extensively hydrolyzed protein formula, you won't forget it.

Discussion Prompts

1. Consider a situation in which a preterm infant is being fed maternal milk fortified with a human milk fortifier to 26 kcal/oz. The infant reaches full enteral feeding volumes and is tolerating the nutritional regimen. However, the serum phosphorus level steadily rises above the reference range. An intervention is warranted to normalize the serum phosphorus level. Discuss the differential diagnosis and treatment options, citing appropriate evidence to support your decision.
2. Discuss the pros and cons associated with each type of formula available for use with term newborns. Then, consider the newborn with NOWS. Which type of term formula is preferred for an infant suffering withdrawal and why? How do energy requirements differ between a newborn with NOWS and a healthy term counterpart?
3. Consider the growth charts that you use to appraise postnatal growth. Next, consider the following question: Could the exclusive use of size-for-age growth charts (which do not consider BMI) increase the risk for persistently elevated BMI levels in infancy and confer inadvertent increased risk for latent disease?

Mind Map

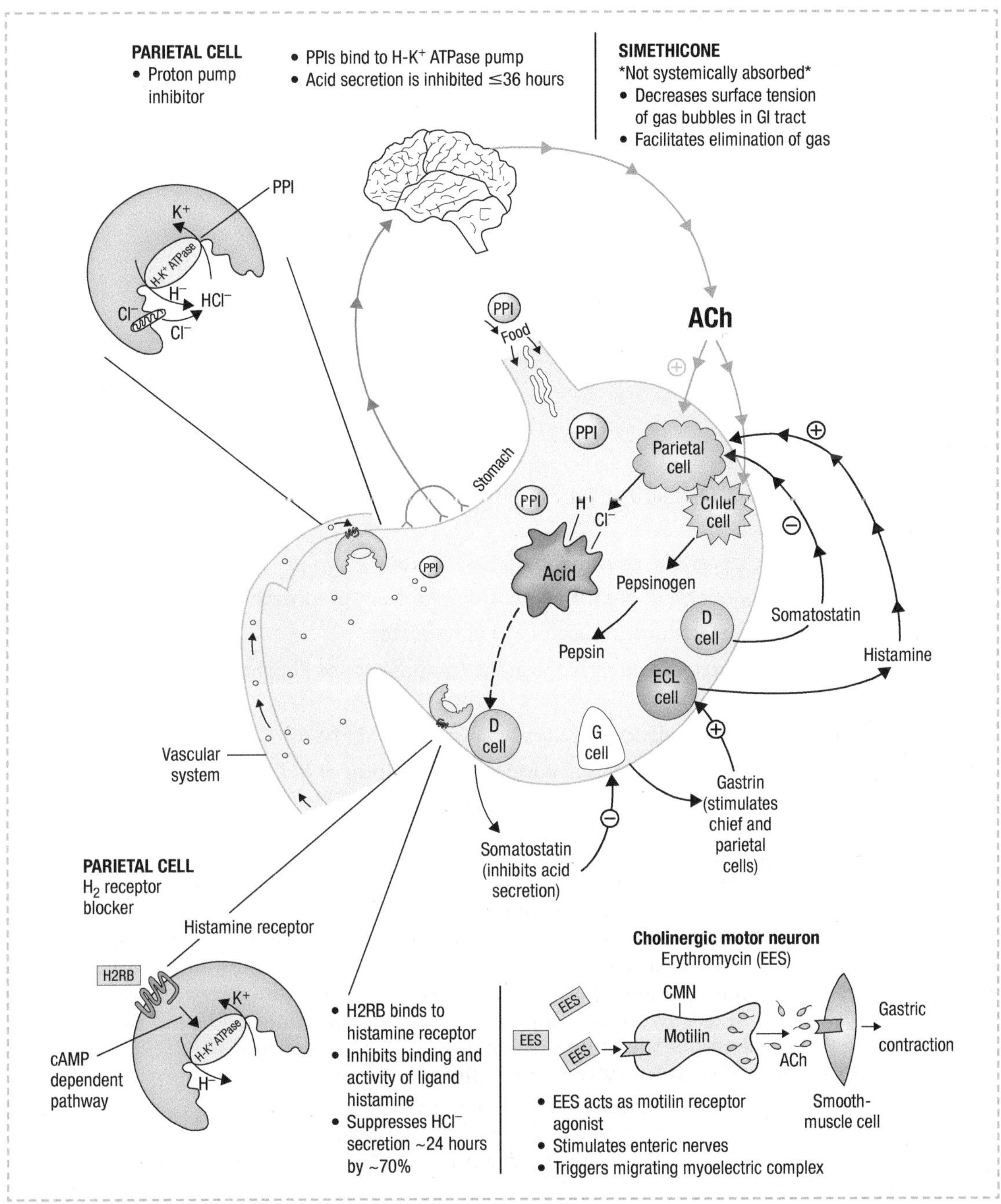

Note: This mind map reflects the design team's interpretation of a portion of one or more concepts addressed in this chapter. Readers should regard the mind maps woven throughout this textbook as examples of multisensory study tools that can be developed to encourage conceptual understanding. Readers are encouraged to develop their own unique mind maps in consultation with academic faculty or clinical preceptors.
ACh, acetylcholine; cAMP, cyclic adenosine monophosphate; ECL, enterochromaffin-like; GI, gastrointestinal; H2, histamine2; H2RB, histamine2 receptor blocker; PPI, proton pump inhibitor.
Design credit: Lara Golden, PhD, MSN, RN, and Sarah Willis, MSN, APRN, NNP-BC, East Carolina University Neonatal Nurse Practitioner Program.

REFERENCES

References for this chapter are online and available at https://connect.springerpub.com/content/book/978-0-8261-5884-0/part/partV/toc-part/ch22.

chapter 23

Parenteral Nutrition

Amy J. Jnah, Tracy Rickard, Elizabeth Sharpe, and Van Tran

LEARNING OBJECTIVES

After completing this chapter, the reader should be able to:

- Explore the historical contributions made in the development of parenteral nutrition (PN).
- Identify appropriate indications for use of PN in neonates.
- Describe the macronutrient and micronutrient components of PN and its role in nutritional support.
- Discuss current recommendations in the administration of PN.
- Review relevant monitoring strategies during administration of PN.

INTRODUCTION

Parenteral nutrition (PN), also known as *hyperalimentation*, has been used in neonates for decades with the goal of achieving adequate nutrition for extrauterine growth and development (ElHassan & Kaiser, 2011). Early nutritional initiation as well as optimal dosing of nutrients have been found to be relevant factors for neurocognitive development (Schneider & Garcia-Rodenas, 2017). PN can be prepared as a two-in-one solution, composed of amino acids and carbohydrates with intravenous (IV) fat emulsions prepared separately, or a three-in-one solution, which offers the two-in-one (amino acids, carbohydrates) and lipids in one solution.

The goal of PN is to provide adequate energy for optimal growth and to prevent the development of malnutrition, refeeding syndrome (RS), and an essential-fatty-acid deficiency (EFAD; Gargasz, 2012). PN often serves as the sole or primary source of nutritional support for neonates weighing less than 1,500 grams at birth, whose gastrointestinal tracts are too anatomically and physiologically immature to tolerate full enteral feeds immediately after birth. As the neonate transitions to extrauterine life and stabilizes, a gradual increase in enteral feedings is typically accompanied by weaning PN (ElHassan & Kaiser, 2011). In other circumstances (e.g., postoperative scenarios), PN may temporarily nourish a neonate until the gastrointestinal tract resumes adequate motility and enteral nutrition can be resumed.

APRNs order PN almost daily in Level III to V NICUs across the United States. Although this is customarily executed in collaboration with a neonatologist and pediatric pharmacist, it is essential that APRNs identify the macronutrients and micronutrients that comprise PN; the role of each component in promoting health and development; and then disease states that warrant the inclusion, supplementation, or removal of certain components. Despite significant advances in neonatal care, as many as 50% of preterm infants weighing between 500 and 1,500 grams at birth do not demonstrate adequate postnatal growth and 25% are affected by severe growth failure (Kleinman & Greer, 2020). Therefore, this chapter reviews all components that must be considered when initiating and continuing PN in the NICU.

HISTORICAL PERSPECTIVE: SEMINAL AND OTHER NOTEWORTHY STUDIES

It has been said that we ride on the shoulders of our predecessors. This section of the chapter examines seminal and noteworthy scientific discoveries made over the past several hundred years, which informed the current PN recipe used in NICUs today. Early events that led up to the inception of PN are summarized in Table 23.1.

The evolution of IV nutrition began more than 350 years ago, around 1616, with William Harvey. A physician and avid hunter, Harvey took interest in understanding why valves in the veins worked in only one direction. He opted to experiment with deer carcasses, and in doing so he discovered that the heart propelled blood in one direction. He once said:

TABLE 23.1 Early Contributors to the Development of Parenteral Nutrition

YEAR	HISTORIC EVENT	INVESTIGATOR
1616	Discovery of the phenomena of blood circulation within the body	Harvey
1626	Seminal report of blood circulation	Harvey
1658	Seminal report of IV injections using animal models (dogs)	Wren
1832	Seminal investigation of IV water and sodium repletion among premorbid patients with cholera	Latta
1843–1859	IV sugar, milk, and egg infusions used in animal models (leads to the discovery of glycogen)	Bernard
1896	Seminal report of IV glucose infusion in adults	Beidl/Krauts
1923	Sterility is identified as necessary to avoid infiltration of pyrogens into IV solutions	Siebert
1924	Seminal report of IV "drip" infusion in adults	Matas
1935	Seminal report of IV oil emulsion in adults	Holt
1938	Identification of the essential amino acids	Rose
1940	Seminal report of IV amino acid infusion in adults	Stohl/Blackfan/Dennis
1945	Polyethylene intravenous catheters adopted for use in humans (in the absence of sterile technique) First fat emulsion prepared using soy phospholipids	Zimmerman Stare
1961	First large-scale soybean oil emulsion experiment conducted in 422 patients	Schuberth/Wretlind
1965–1966	Seminal report of long-term PN in animal models (beagle puppies) associated with adequate growth and development	Dudrick/Wilmore/Vars/Rhoads
1967	Seminal report of adequate growth in neonates subjected to 44 days of exclusive PN secondary to small-bowel atresia	Wilmore/Dudrick

IV, intravenous; PN, parenteral nutrition.

Sources: From Dudrick, S. J., & Malkan, A. D. (2013). The history, principles, and practice of parenteral nutrition in preterm neonates. In S. Patole (Ed.), *Nutrition for the preterm neonate: A clinical perspective* (pp. 193–213). Springer Publishing Company; Dudrick, S. J., Wilmore, D. W., Vars, H. M., & Rhoads, J. E. (1968). Long-term total parenteral nutrition with growth, development, and positive nitrogen balance. *Nutrition Reviews, 39*(7), 278–281. https://doi.org/10.1111/j.1753-4887.1981.tb06788.x; Matas, R. (1924). The continued intravenous "drip": With remarks on the value of continued gastric drainage and irrigation by nasal intubation with a gastroduodenal tube (jutte) in surgical practice. *Annals of Surgery, 79*(5), 643–661. https://doi.org/10.1097/00000658-192405000-00001; Millam, D. (1996). The history of intravenous therapy. *Journal of Intravenous Nursing, 19*(1), 5–14; Mundi, M. S., Martindale, R. G., & Hurt, R. T. (2017). Emergence of mixed-oil fat emulsions for use in parenteral nutrition. *Journal of Parenteral and Enteral Nutrition, 41*(1 Suppl.), 3S–13S. https://doi.org/10.1177/0148607117742595; Silverman, M. E. (2007). De motu cordis the lumleian lecture of 1616: An imagined playlet concerning the discovery of the circulation of the blood by William Harvey. *Journal of the Royal Society of Medicine, 100*(4), 199–204. https://www.ncbi.nlm.nih.gov/pmc/articles/PMC1847732; Wilmore, D. W., & Dudrick, S. J. (1968). Growth and development of an infant receiving all nutrients exclusively by vein. *The Journal of the American Medical Association, 203*(10), 860–864. https://doi.org/10.1001/jama.1968.03140100042009; Zimmermann, B. (1945). Intravenous tubing for parenteral therapy. *Science, 101*(2631), 567–568. https://doi.org/10.1126/science.101.2631.567

> the valves in the veins of so many parts of the body, were so plac'd that they gave free passage to the blood towards the heart, but oppos'd the passage of the venal blood the contrary way... that, since the blood could not well, because of the interposing valves, be sent by the veins to the limbs; it should be sent through the arteries and return through the veins, whose valves did not oppose its course that way. (Boyle, 1688, pp. 157–158)

Harvey's novel discovery provided physicians, scientists, and others with a better understanding of the function of valves in veins and the concept that blood flowed in a set direction. Now, experts were stimulated to investigate the effects associated with the injection of substances into veins. Christopher Wren, a 24-year-old budding architect with a distinct interest in medicine, was one of the first to learn of Harvey's findings. A curious individual by nature, Wren invented a syringe and injected ale, wine, and opium into the veins of dogs (Gibson, 1970). His rather unconventional (and unethical) experiments led to the conclusion that intravenously administered alcohol elicited the same inebriating effect as orally consumed alcohol. He wrote:

> The most considerable experiment I have made of late is this: I injected wine and ale into the mass of blood in a living dog, by a vein, in good quantities, till he became extremely drunk; but soon after voided it by urine. It will be too long to tell you the effects of opium, scammony, and other things which I have tried in this way. I am in further pursuit of the experiment, which I take to be of great concernment, and what will give great light to the theory and practice of physic. (Gibson, 1970, p. 334)

The first to infuse a relatively safe solution (saline) into a patient was Thomas Latta, a Scottish physician (MacGillivray, 2006). His discovery coincided with the cholera epidemic of 1832. Latta identified that patients with cholera-induced diarrhea developed severe dehydration, or "black blood," along with a water and salt deficiency (Hyman et al., 1971). He used IV saline infusions to replenish the fluid and electrolytes and restore the "arterial qualities" of the blood. In 1843, Claude Bernard, a prominent French physiologist, investigated the basic biochemical nature of nutrient substances, namely, glucose. He infused various sugar solutions into animals in an attempt to discover the origin of sugar isolated in the liver. In 1859, he was credited with illustrating the importance of glucose as an energy source essential to maintaining normal metabolism (Dudrick & Palesty, 2011). The use of glucose and electrolyte-containing fluids gained widespread acceptance in the 1880s secondary to successful outcomes linked to fluid resuscitation in hypovolemic pregnant women suffering an antepartum hemorrhage (Srinivasa & Hill, 2012).

Next, in 1896, Drs. Arthur Beidl and Rudely Krauts discovered that the rate at which IV nutrients were infused may provoke complex (and toxic) responses among patients with a normal metabolism as well as pathologic disease states (Vinnars & Wilmore, 2003). In response, Woodyatt and colleagues (1915) introduced the concept of regulating the rate of glucose-containing fluids. The research team proposed that the body's ability to tolerate and utilize supplemental glucose was dependent on the dose and rate of the glucose infusion (Woodyatt et al., 1915). This established the notion of the dose-response relationship. As Dr. Woodyatt wrote:

> ...the power of the body to utilize glucose must depend on the rate at which the tissues are able to abstract glucose from the blood by their combined powers to burn it, to reduce it into fat or to polymerize it into glycogen. (Woodyatt et al., 1915, p. 2067)

However, the interrelationship among IV access, substrates, microbiology, and pyrogens had yet to be elucidated. This changed in 1909, when IV salvarsan injections were adopted for use in patients with syphilis. Nearly every patient developed a severe fever after the infusion was complete. By 1923, Florence Siebert discerned that microbial contamination of the IV fluids, with or without evidence of aseptic technique used during preparation of the fluid or administration of the antimicrobial agent, encouraged the accumulation of pyrogens and onset of hospital-acquired infection. Clearly, asepsis had to be a priority if IV infusions were to continue in the hospital setting.

By the turn of the 20th century, physicians accepted that crystalloid IV fluids could be used to treat transient pathophysiologic conditions but could not satisfy the long-term nutritional needs of critically ill patients. Therefore, physician researchers shifted their focus toward identifying all essential nutrients necessary for growth and development. This led to the creation of oil emulsions (1935) and the identification of the essential amino acids in 1938 (Dudrick, 2003). Shortly thereafter, Robert Elman discovered that amino acids, essential macronutrients, could be safely added to IV solutions in the form of protein hydrolysate (Elman, 1940). Around this same time, Stanley Dudrick, a surgical resident at the University of Pennsylvania, was tasked with identifying the nutritional needs (macronutrients and micronutrients) of animals (dogs), and created a concentrated PN solution that contained all the necessary nutrients, and aseptically administered the nutrient solution (Dudrick, 2005). Dudrick offered an eloquent reflection of his early steps in a recent publication:

> The compatibility of the individual components of the intravenous nutrient regimen had to be determined, assured, and maintained under a number of variable situations, including a wide range of ambient temperature changes, exposure to light, time from formulation to infusion, instability during transportation, duration of shelf life, etc. The risk of infection had to be eliminated or minimized to an acceptable level. As the former was probably impossible, in view of the fact that a foreign body had to be passed through the skin into the bloodstream and remain in place for prolonged periods of time, the latter was essential. Pharmaceutical and medical technology companies had to be convinced to develop, produce, and market the nutrient components and apparatus for safe formulation and administration of TPN within a reasonably affordable cost. Procedures and tests had to be established to assess and monitor the safety and efficacy of a TPN program. Continuous infusion of the solution at a constant rate throughout each 24 h period had to be maintained in order to ensure the administration of the maximally utilizable dosages of each of the nutrients in the mixture for the support of cellular metabolism. This concept was quite different from the usual infusion practices at that time. Furthermore, it was essential to overcome decades of written and verbal expressions by prominent physicians and scientists that long-term total parenteral nutrition was either impossible, improbable, impractical, unaffordable, or folly. Plausible fundamental evidence to the contrary had to be generated if skepticism and prejudices were to be neutralized or overcome, and if widespread clinical acceptance was eventually to occur. Accordingly, efforts were directed toward designing experiments in the laboratory to explore and verify the efficacy and safety of TPN with the ultimate goal of applying clinically to patients, the basic knowledge, skills and techniques acquired, developed and mastered in animals. (Dudrick & Malkan, 2013, pp. 196–197)

The inclusion of amino acids and fat emulsions in IV solutions marked the genesis of PN. Historically, all IV fluids were administered peripherally; however, the osmolarity of this more complex PN solution was sixfold greater than historic solutions. Therefore, catheters capable of infusing the hyperosmolar fluid were necessary. The first flexible polyethylene catheters were introduced by Zimmerman (1945). This was followed by commercial development of glass containers and tubing that could tolerate the osmolarity of PN without producing precipitates.

Neonatal nurses may find the initial procedure used to prepare a PN infusion particularly intriguing. First, the parenteral solution was poured into an open glass flask and a plug of gauze was used to cover the neck of the flask. The glass flasks were often wrapped in hot water bottles to "prevent shock" (cold stress). Then, infusion tubing was connected to the patient. Next, a rubber stopper was attached to the neck of the flask. A glass tube was inserted through the stopper and used as a conduit between the fluid in the flask and rubber IV tubing. When the nurse was ready to begin the drip infusion, a metal screw clamp was carefully loosened and the flow rate was set (Dudrick & Palesty, 2011). Infusions took a few hours, and the nurse was expected to remain continuously at the bedside to observe the patient.

Now that equipment was available to administer the PN and the nutrient needs of animals (beagle puppies) were determined, Wilmore and Dudrick (1968) focused on concentrating the PN nutrient solution for each puppy. Ultimately, the osmolarity of the PN solutions ranged between 1,800 to 2,400 mOsm/L. The external jugular vein was used for central catheter insertion, with tip placement confirmed within the superior vena cava. Puppies received PN for 72 to 256 consecutive days and each demonstrated adequate weight gain, anabolism, and a positive nitrogen balance (Nakayama, 2017). This novel success paved the way for decades of subsequent research and enhancement of PN for use in adults, children, and infants.

Seminal Use of Parenteral Nutrition in an Infant

The very first infant who received PN was a term female born in 1967 serendipitously close to Dudrick's laboratory in Pennsylvania. Dudrick had just finished his "beagle" research when he learned of the infant, who required a significant intestinal resection and anastomosis of the duodenum to the terminal ileum secondary to a severe small-bowel atresia. Over the course of 19 postoperative days, the infant had lost over 20% of her birth weight (2.3 kg at birth to 1.8 kg). Dudrick described the infant as "catabolic, hypometabolic, and moribund" (Dudrick & Malkan, 2013, p. 199). With parental consent, a central venous catheter (CVC) was inserted into the external jugular vein and PN was initiated using the "beagle formula." After 45 consecutive days of treatment, the infant weighed 3.4 kg. The infant's length increased by 5.5 cm and her head circumference increased by 6.5 cm.

GOALS AND INDICATIONS FOR PARENTERAL NUTRITION

The minimum acceptable standards for the provision of PN, as developed by Dudrick and Malkan (2013), call on pharmacists and neonatal clinicians to:

- Anticipate, avoid, and correct nutritional and metabolic imbalances, derangements, or adverse reactions.
- Concentrate the nutrient substrate components (up to 5 to 6 times isotonicity) in order to remain within acceptable total fluid limitations for the patient.
- Demonstrate the absence of adverse interactions or precipitation.
- Demonstrate and maintain the practicality, efficacy, and safety of long-term continuous central venous access and infusion of hypertonic nutrient solution.
- Maintain meticulous asepsis and antisepsis throughout the entire continuum of solution preparation, admixture, and infusion.

Common indications for the use of PN include intestinal insults (e.g., surgery), intestinal inflammation (e.g., necrotizing enterocolitis [NEC]), intestinal obstruction (e.g., imperforated anus, ileus, atresia), intestinal malabsorption, intestinal immaturity, intestinal dysmotility, and extraintestinal disorders resulting in malnutrition (Kleinman & Greer, 2020). Novice clinicians should consider the following guiding questions when considering the use of PN (Gargasz, 2012):

1. What is the indication for use of PN in the patient?
2. What venous access is available for use?
3. What are the patient's current dietary needs?
4. Is the patient at risk for RS?

ROUTES OF ADMINISTRATION

PN can be administered by way of peripheral venous catheters and CVCs. Peripheral administration may be indicated when short-term PN (less than 2 weeks) is anticipated and the osmolarity of the PN solution remains less than 900 mOsm/L (Table 23.2; Boullata et al., 2014); however, many clinicians permit an osmolarity between 900 and 1,250 mOsm/L for peripheral PN when short-term

TABLE 23.2 Recommendations for Maximum Osmolarity in Peripheral Parenteral Nutrition Solutions

ORGANIZATION	MAXIMUM RECOMMENDED OSMOLARITY
AAP	900 mOsm/L
ASPEN	900 mOsm/L
ESPEN	850 mOsm/L
INS	900 mOsm/L

Note: Many hospitals permit higher peripheral PN osmolarity considering stability and site of access.

AAP, American Academy of Pediatrics; ASPEN, American Society for Parenteral and Enteral Nutrition; ESPEN, European Society for Parenteral and Enteral Nutrition; INS, Infusion Nurses Society; PN, parenteral nutrition.

Sources: From Boullata, J. I., Gilbert, K., Sacks, G., Labossiere, R. J., Crill, C., Goday, P., Kumpf, V. J., Mattox, T. W., Plogsted, S., Holcombe, B., & American Society for Parenteral and Enteral Nutrition. (2014). A.S.P.E.N. clinical guidelines: Parenteral nutrition ordering, order review, compounding, labeling, and dispensing. *Journal of Parenteral and Enteral Nutrition, 38*(3), 334–377. https://doi.org/10.1177/0148607114521833; Gorski, L., Hadaway, L., Hagle, M., Broadhurst, D., Clare, S., Kleidon, T., Meyer, B., Nickel, B., Rowley, S., Sharpe, E., & Alexander, M. (2021). Infusion therapy standards of practice, 8th edition. *Journal of Infusion Nursing, 44*(1S), S1–S224. https://doi.org/10.1097/NAN.0000000000000396; Kleinman, R. E., & Greer, F. R. (Eds.). (2020). *Pediatric nutrition* (8th ed.). American Academy of Pediatrics; Pittiruti, M., Hamilton, H., Biffi, R., MacFie, J., Pertkiewicz, M., & ESPEN. (2009). ESPEN guidelines on parenteral nutrition: Central venous catheters (access, care, diagnosis and therapy of complications). *Clinical Nutrition, 28*(4), 365–377. https://doi.org/10.1016/j.clnu.2009.03.015

PN needs are anticipated in order to avoid risks associated with CVC insertion and maintenance. Clinicians must appraise the integrity and locus (e.g., scalp vs. larger antecubital vein) of the peripheral IV catheter when determining whether peripheral access is safe for the parenteral infusion. Conversely, central venous access is recommended when long-term PN therapy (>14 days) is indicated and/or an osmolarity greater than 900 mOsm/L is required (ElHassan & Kaiser, 2011; Kleinman & Greer, 2020). Among hospitalized infants, peripherally inserted central catheters (PICCs) and tunneled CVCs (e.g., broviac) are used for administration of prolonged PN (Kolaček et al., 2018).

FLUID AND ENERGY REQUIREMENTS

Water is a major component of the human body and an essential carrier for nutrients and metabolites (Jochum et al., 2018; Joosten et al., 2018). Early in gestational development, water accounts for 94% of fetal body composition. This decreases incrementally as the fetus matures. By 24 weeks of gestation, water accounts for 90% of body composition, decreasing to 75% at term, and 50% by adulthood (Jochum et al., 2018; Joosten et al., 2018).

The ultimate goal when prescribing a total daily fluid requirement is to provide enough fluid to maintain homeostasis (avoid dehydration and overhydration), euglycemia, and acid-base balance (Kleinman & Greer, 2020). Fluid intake recommendations offered by leading consensus groups consider body composition and postnatal factors (e.g., skin immaturity, use of mechanical ventilation) that can increase water loss (Table 23.3). Among neonates less than 1,500 grams at birth, the use of 90% humidity paired with maintenance of a thermal-neutral isolette air temperature can reduce postnatal water loss by 30% (Jochum et al., 2018). Among neonates who require mechanical ventilation, the use of heated and humidified air mitigates insensible losses through the respiratory tract. Once clinicians estimate insensible losses and determine the neonate's total daily fluid requirement, the total volume of PN, fat emulsion (IV lipid emulsion [ILE]), and enteral feeding volume (as applicable) can be calculated. It is also important to consider the total fluid volume of medication infusions, which include standard umbilical arterial catheter maintenance fluids, as a part of the total daily fluid requirement, in particular among neonates weighing less than 1,000 grams at birth. A summary of conditions commonly associated with the need for higher or lower daily total fluid intake is provided in Table 23.4.

Energy requirements loosely coincide 1:1 with water requirements (1 mL water per 1 kcal); however, energy intake is always individualized to meet basal metabolic requirements and growth needs for infants (Jochum et al., 2018). The basal metabolic requirement for exclusively

TABLE 23.3 Recommended Daily Fluid Intake (mL/kg/d)

ESPGHAN	DAY 1 (BIRTH)	DAY 2	DAY 3	DAY 4	DAY 5
Term	40–60	50–70	60–80	60–100	100–140
Preterm (>1,500 g)	60–80	80–100	100–120	120–140	140–160
Preterm (1,000–1,500 g)	70–90	90–110	110–130	130–150	160–180
Preterm (<1,000 g)	80–100	100–120	120–140	140–160	160–180
AAP	**DAY 1 (BIRTH)**	**DAY 2**	**DAY 3**	**DAY 4**	**DAY 5**
Term					100–150
Preterm (≥1,000 g)	60–80	80–100	100–120	120–140	140–160
Preterm (<1,000 g)	80–100	*	*	*	140–160

*The AAP does not specify precise titration parameters for daily fluid intake for preterm infants weighing less than 1,000 grams at birth beyond the date of birth. Rather, the recommendation is to titrate daily total fluid intake based on urine output and insensible water losses.
AAP, American Academy of Pediatrics; ESPGHAN, European Society for Paediatric Gastroenterology Hepatology and Nutrition.
Sources: From Jochum, F., Moltu, S. J., Senterre, T., Nomayo, A., Goulet, O., Iacobelli, S., Braegger, C., Bronsky, J., Cai, W., Campoy, C., Carnielli, V., Darmaun, D., Decsi, T., Domellöf, M., Embleton, N., Fewtrell, M., Fidler Mis, N., Franz, A., Goulet, O., … ESPGHAN/ESPEN/ESPR/CSPEN Working Group on Pediatric Parenteral Nutrition. (2018). ESPGHAN/ESPEN/ESPR/CSPEN guidelines on pediatric parenteral nutrition: Fluid and electrolytes. *Clinical Nutrition, 37*(6), 2344–2353. https://doi.org/10.1016/j.clnu.2018.06.948; Kleinman, R. E., & Greer, F. R. (Eds.). (2020). *Pediatric nutrition* (8th ed.). American Academy of Pediatrics.

TABLE 23.4 Conditions That Commonly Require Adjusted Daily Total Fluid Intake

CHANGE FROM RECOMMENDED DAILY FLUID INTAKE	COMMON COMORBID CONDITIONS
Increased total fluid goal	• Abdominal wall defects • Exposure to ambient air (use of radiant warmer) • High-output renal failure • Preterm birth <28 weeks of gestation
Decreased total fluid goal	• Humidification with use of double-wall isolette • Large patent ductus arteriosus with retrograde flow • Oliguric renal failure • Whole body cooling

parenterally fed infants is 40 to 60 kcal/kg/d and approximately 3 to 4.5 calories are required to gain 1 gram of weight. As readers will learn in the upcoming section of this chapter, macronutrients provide varied caloric yield and must be optimized for infants to achieve the desired weight gain of 15 to 20 grams/kg/d (Table 23.5; Kleinman & Greer, 2020). Optimization of energy requirements is particularly important with certain comorbid conditions (e.g., bronchopulmonary dysplasia [BPD]), as these diseases are associated with increased energy use. Affected infants may require additional calories (often while fluid restricted) for adequate growth.

COMPONENTS OF PARENTERAL NUTRITION

Because the intestines serve as an important site of metabolism, parenterally fed neonates are at risk for nutritional deficiencies. Therefore, PN should be composed of macronutrients and micronutrients in specific proportions in order to maintain growth and prevent malnutrition, deficiencies, and toxicities. Macronutrients are composed of protein, carbohydrates, and lipids, whereas micronutrients include electrolytes, trace elements, and vitamins.

Presently, nutritional intake recommendations have been constructed by specific organizations, including the American Academy of Pediatrics (AAP), the American Society for Parenteral and Enteral Nutrition (ASPEN), and the European Society for Paediatric Gastroenterology Hepatology and Nutrition (ESPGHAN). Generally, amino acids, dextrose, and lipids should make up 10% to 15%, 45% to 60%, and 25% to 40% of a patient's caloric needs, respectively (Kleinman & Greer, 2020). We review each component in this section of the chapter.

Macronutrients

PROTEIN

Proteins are major constituents of all cells in the human body and are composed of a specific number and sequence of amino acids. The protein source in PN is amino acids, which supply the body with essential amounts of nitrogen necessary to maintain lean body mass and support neurotransmission, tissue turnover, and repair (Gargasz, 2012; Vlaardingerbroek et al., 2011). Amino acids are categorized into three groups: essential, nonessential, and semi-essential. Essential amino acids are necessary for normal physiologic function and not endogenously synthesized; therefore, it is essential that these amino acids be included in the daily nutritional regimen (Vlaardingerbroek et al., 2011). These essential amino acids include histidine, isoleucine, leucine, lysine, methionine, phenylalanine, threonine, tryptophan, and valine (van Goudoever et al., 2018). Commercially prepared pediatric formulations of amino acids used with neonates and infants supply these indispensable amino acids, as well as nonessential amino acids (Table 23.6; Plogsted et al., 2016).

Parenterally administered amino acids are 100% bioavailable; therefore, the parenteral daily requirement is lower compared to enteral diets. Each gram of amino acid yields 4 kcal of energy.

PN protein intake should exceed 1.2 grams/kg/d in order to account for daily protein breakdown and urinary protein output, and promote a positive nitrogen balance (Kleinman & Greer, 2020;

TABLE 23.5 Recommended Daily Energy Requirements With Parenteral Nutrition

	ASPEN		AAP		ESPGHAN	
Energy requirements	Preterm (PMA <34 weeks 0/7)	85–111 kcal/kg/d	<1,000 g	105–115 kcal/kg/d	Preterm	90–120 kcal/kg/d
	Late Preterm (PMA 34 weeks 0/7 to 36 weeks 6/7)	100–110 kcal/kg/d	1,000–1,500 g	90–100 kcal/kg/d	Term	90–100 kcal/kg/d
			0–3 months	(89 × weight [kg] − 100) + 175 kcal	0–7 months	75–90 kcal/kg/d
	Term (PMA ≥ 37 weeks 0/7)	90–108 kcal/kg/d	4–6 months	(89 × weight [kg] − 100) + 56 kcal	7–12 months	75–90 kcal/kg/d

Note: Recommendations apply to clinically stable, growing, preterm infants. Caloric needs of infants receiving exclusive PN are approximately 10% to 15% lower compared to enteral feeding needs.
AAP, American Academy of Pediatrics; ASPEN, American Society for Parenteral and Enteral Nutrition; ESPGHAN, European Society for Paediatric Gastroenterology Hepatology and Nutrition; PMA, postmenstrual age.
Sources: From the American Society for Parenteral and Enteral Nutrition. (2019). *ASPEN recommendations on appropriate dosing for parenteral nutrition for neonatal and pediatric patients.* https://nutritotal.com.br/pro/wp-content/uploads/sites/3/2019/04/PN-DosingASPEN.pdf; Joosten, K., Embleton, N., Yan, W., Senterre, T., Braegger, C., Bronsky, J., Cai, W., Campoy, C., Carnielli, V., Darmaun, D., Decsi, T., Domellöf, M., Embleton, N., Fewtrell, M., Fidler Mis, N., Franz, A., Goulet, O., Hartman, C., Hill, S., … ESPGHAN/ESPEN/ESPR/CSPEN Working Group on Pediatric Parenteral Nutrition. (2018). ESPGHAN/ESPEN/ESPR/CSPEN guidelines on pediatric parenteral nutrition: Energy. *Clinical Nutrition, 37*(6), 2309–2314. https://doi.org/10.1016/j.clnu.2018.06.944; Kleinman, R. E., & Greer, F. R. (Eds.). (2020). *Pediatric nutrition* (8th ed.). American Academy of Pediatrics.

TABLE 23.6 Composition of the Three Commercially Available Pediatric Mixed Amino Acid Solutions

	AMINOSYN-PF	PREMASOL (6%, 10%)	TROPHAMINE (6%, 10%)
Essential amino acids	Histidine[a] Isoleucine Leucine Lysine[a] Methionine[a] Phenylalanine Threonine Tryptophan Tyrosine Valine	Histidine[a] Isoleucine Leucine Lysine[a] Methionine[a] Phenylalanine Threonine Tryptophan Tyrosine Valine	Histidine[a] Isoleucine Leucine Lysine[a] Methionine[a] Phenylalanine Threonine Tryptophan Tyrosine Valine
Nonessential amino acids	Alanine Arginine[a] Aspartic acid[b] Glutamic acid[b] Glycine Proline Serine Taurine	Alanine Arginine[a] Aspartic acid[b] Glutamic acid[b] Glycine Proline Serine Taurine	Alanine Arginine[a] Aspartic acid[b] Glutamic acid[b] Glycine Proline Serine Taurine

Note: Amino acid solutions are contraindicated for use in infants with suspected and confirmed inborn errors of *amino acid* metabolism (e.g., maple syrup urine disease, isovoleric acidemia). Measured amounts of each individual amino acid vary per commercial formulation.
[a]Indicates cationic amino acid (positive charge).
[b]Indicates anionic amino acid (negative charge).

Osborn et al., 2018; van Goudoever et al., 2018). Currently, most clinicians prescribe 1.5 to 3 grams/kg/d of amino acid on admission or within the first day of life and advance by 0.5 to 1 gram/kg/d toward a maximum of 4 grams/kg/day (Table 23.7).

Certain comorbid conditions require adjustments to amino acid intake. For example, neonates with renal failure may require a reduced protein load of 0.8 to 2 grams/kg/d due to reduced

TABLE 23.7 Recommendations for Daily Protein Intake

	ASPEN		AAP		ESPGHAN	
Protein (gram/kg/d)	Preterm	Initiation: 1–3 Advance by: N/A Goal: 3–4 (max 3–4)	Preterm <1,000 grams	Initiation: 2–3 Goal: 3.5–4 (max 4)	Preterm	Initiation: 1.5 Advance by: 1/d Goal: 2.5–3.5 (max 3.5)
	Term	Initiation: 2.5–3 Advance by: N/A Goal: 2.5–3 (max 3–4)	Preterm >1,000 grams	Initiation: 2–3 Goal: 3–3.8 (max 4)	Term	Initiation: 2.5–3 Advance by: N/A Goal: 2.5–3 (max 3)

AAP, American Academy of Pediatrics; ASPEN, American Society for Parenteral and Enteral Nutrition; ESPEN, European Society for Parenteral and Enteral Nutrition; N/A, not available.

Sources: From the American Society for Parenteral and Enteral Nutrition. (2019). *ASPEN recommendations on appropriate dosing for parenteral nutrition for neonatal and pediatric patients*. https://nutritotal.com.br/pro/wp-content/uploads/sites/3/2019/04/PN-DosingASPEN.pdf; Kleinman, R. E., & Greer, F. R. (Eds.). (2020). *Pediatric nutrition* (8th ed.). American Academy of Pediatrics; van Goudoever, J. B., Carnielli, V., Darmaun, D., Sainz de Pipaon, M., Braegger, C., Bronsky, J., Cai, W., Campoy, C., Carnielli, V., Darmaun, D., Decsi, T., Domellöf, M., Embleton, N., Fewtrell, M., Fidler Mis, N., Franz, A., Goulet, O., Hartman, C., Hill, S., ... ESPGHAN/ESPEN/ESPR/CSPEN Working Group on Pediatric Parenteral Nutrition. (2018). ESPGHAN/ESPEN/ESPR/CSPEN guidelines on pediatric parenteral nutrition: Amino acids. *Clinical Nutrition, 37*(6), 2315–2323. https://doi.org/10.1016/j.clnu.2018.06.945

urinary protein excretion. Neonates with gastrointestinal diseases (e.g., NEC) may require a higher protein load of 3 to 4 grams/kg/d to offset gastrointestinal losses (Carlson & Kavars, 2016; Gargasz, 2012).

The provision of amino acids is not without complications. Short-term adverse effects are usually observed in infants with renal disease (and who receive a standard amino acid dose) or those who receive an excessive amino acid dosage. One particular short-term adverse effect, which has fallen subject to debate over the years, is metabolic acidosis (MA). The mechanism by which MA develops is worthy of consideration. Synthetically produced "essential" amino acids are stratified as cationic or anionic amino acids, based on the charge associated with the amino acid. Positively charged (cationic) amino acids include arginine, histidine, lysine, methionine, and cysteine; hydrogen (H+) ions are produced as these amino acids are metabolized. Negatively charged amino acids include aspartic acid and glutamic acid; H+ ions are consumed as these amino acids are metabolized. Therefore, an imbalance/excess of cationic acids may precipitate a cation gap and MA. This may be further exacerbated by an excessive chloride load in PN, in particular among preterm infants. However, given that commercially prepared PN solutions offer a mix of positively and negatively charged amino acids, and amino acids are used for protein synthesis and energy, the onset of MA is more likely secondary to urinary losses or a pathologic disease process than a consequence of parenteral protein load.

Amino acids that are not used to synthesize new protein are subject to hepatic metabolism and renal excretion. Amino acid metabolism yields the production of ammonia molecules, which are hepatically transformed into urea and renally excreted (Weiner et al., 2015). Early PN use is not associated with an increased risk for elevated urea or ammonia levels, despite their role in nitrogen excretion. Therefore, routine surveillance of either indice is not indicated for the purpose of analyzing amino acid tolerance during PN therapy. Rather, clinical conditions that alter water homeostasis or renal function (e.g., acute kidney injury) can reduce nitrogen excretion, causing blood urea and ammonia buildup.

Protein cannot be the sole energy source for growing infants. Rather, calories from nitrogen energy sources (amino acids) must be blended with calories from nonnitrogen energy sources (carbohydrates & lipids). The recommended ratio for optimal growth is 20 to 30 kcals of carbohydrate/lipid energy for every 1 gram of amino acid during the neonatal period and 40 kcals of carbohydrate/lipid energy for every 1 gram of amino acids during infancy (National Institute for Health and Care Excellence [NICE], 2020; van Goudoever et al., 2018). Insufficient nonnitrogen energy (<20 kcal per 1 gram of amino acids) may lead to oxidation of amino acids, increased blood urea levels, and poor growth. In contrast, an excess of nonnitrogen energy (>30 kcals per 1 gram of amino acids) could increase fat deposition and the risk for latent chronic disease (e.g., hypertriglyceridemia, diabetes) in adulthood (NICE, 2020).

CARBOHYDRATES (DEXTROSE)

Glucose is the primary source for energy metabolism during fetal development and postnatal life. Adequate circulating glucose is necessary for optimal metabolic function, particularly in the brain and heart. Dextrose is the type of sugar provided in PN, yielding 3.4 kcal of energy per gram (Gargasz, 2012). In comparison, the sugar in enteral food sources includes corn syrup, modified corn starch, fructose, sucrose, maltodextrin, or lactose (human milk).

When initiating neonatal PN, carbohydrate delivery should consider the glucose infusion rate (GIR). The GIR reflects the amount of dextrose (glucose) in milligrams infused per kilogram of body weight, per minute (mg/kg/min). The following equation is used to calculate the GIR:

$$\text{GIR (mg/kg/min)} = \text{infusion rate (mL/hr)} \times \text{dextrose concentration (g/dL)} \times 1{,}000\ \text{(mg/g)}/(\text{weight [kg]} \times 60\ [\text{min/hr}] \times 100\ [\text{mL/dL}]).$$

The customary initial GIR for preterm and term infants ranges between 4 and 8 mg/kg/min (Table 23.8), because this rate accounts for the higher glucose utilization rate in infants compared to adults (Thornton et al., 2015). Clinicians are expected to appraise the prenatal and delivery history to identify risk factors for poor glycemic control. In addition, postnatal factors (e.g., late preterm gestation, small for gestational age, sepsis) may inform the initial ordered GIR. Circumstances that preclude the administration of fat emulsions (e.g., fungemia, hypertriglyceridemia) may require a compensatory increase in the GIR.

Clinicians should gradually and cautiously increase the GIR, typically by no more than 1 to 3 mg/kg/min daily (lower end of range in preterm infants <1,500 grams), toward a maximum of 10 to 14 mg/kg/min, as tolerated (ASPEN, 2019; Kleinman & Greer, 2020; Lapillonne et al., 2018; Mesotten et al., 2018; van Goudoever et al., 2018). The upper rate of GIR represents the maximum glucose oxidative capacity for energy production and glycogen deposition; exceeding the recommended maximum GIR could lead to increased carbon dioxide production and exacerbation of lung disease, particularly in preterm infants (ElHassan & Kaiser, 2011).

Accurate and regular blood glucose monitoring, through arterial or capillary glucose sampling, is recommended to avoid prolonged states of hypo- or hyperglycemia. The definition of hypoglycemia is unclear, as no consensus has been established to date. The AAP defines *refractory hypoglycemia* as less than 40 mg/dL in the first 4 hours of life or less than 45 mg/dL between 4 and 24 hours of life; no recommendations beyond the first 24 hours of life are published. The Pediatric Endocrine Society suggests that altered neurogenic responses may be observed with plasma glucose levels less than 50 mg/dL in the first 48 hours of life and less than 60 mg/dL thereafter (Thornton et al., 2015). Clinicians should consider these expert opinions when determining the threshold for titration of the GIR.

TABLE 23.8 Recommendations for Daily Carbohydrate Intake

	ASPEN		AAP		ESPGHAN	
Carbohydrates (mg/kg/min)	Preterm	Initiation: 6–8 Advance by: 1–2/d Goal: 10–14 (max 14–18)	Preterm <1,000 grams	Initiation: 5–7 Goal: 11.3–16.2	Preterm	Initiation: 4–8 Advance stepwise over the next 2–3 days Goal: 10–12 (max 12)
	Term	Initiation: 6–8 Advance by: 1–2/d Goal: 10–14 (max 14–18)	Preterm >1,000–1,500 grams	Initiation: 5–7 Goal: 9.7–16.7	Term	Initiation: 2.5–5 Advance stepwise over the next 2–3 days Goal: 10–12 (max 12)

AAP, American Academy of Pediatrics; ASPEN, American Society for Parenteral and Enteral Nutrition; ESPEN, European Society for Parenteral and Enteral Nutrition.

Sources: From the American Society for Parenteral and Enteral Nutrition. (2019). *ASPEN recommendations on appropriate dosing for parenteral nutrition for neonatal and pediatric patients*. https://nutritotal.com.br/pro/wp-content/uploads/sites/3/2019/04/PN-DosingASPEN.pdf; Kleinman, R. E., & Greer, F. R. (Eds.). (2020). *Pediatric nutrition* (8th ed.). American Academy of Pediatrics; Mesotten, D., Joosten, K., van Kempen, A., Verbruggen, S., Braegger, C., Bronsky, J., Cai, W., Campoy, C., Carnielli, V., Darmaun, D., Decsi, T., Domellöf, M., Embleton, N., Fewtrell, M., Fidler Mis, N., Franz, A., Goulet, O., Hartman, C., Hill, S., … ESPGHAN/ESPEN/ESPR/CSPEN Working Group on Pediatric Parenteral Nutrition. (2018). ESPGHAN/ESPEN/ESPR/CSPEN guidelines on pediatric parenteral nutrition: Carbohydrates. *Clinical Nutrition, 37*(6), 2337–2343. https://doi.org/10.1016/j.clnu.2018.06.947

On the opposite end of the spectrum, hyperglycemia (plasma glucose >150 mg/dL) has been associated with increased morbidity (Ramel & Rao, 2020). Clinicians should avoid reducing the GIR below the basal metabolic rate when treating hyperglycemia, as this will deprive infants of necessary caloric intake for effective growth and development (Mitanchez, 2007). Other adjuvant therapies include optimizing parenteral amino acid intake or enteral feedings, as this increases endogenous insulin secretion. Reducing or stopping fat emulsions can reduce glucose levels, as well as correct a low phosphorus level. If adjuvant therapies and/or titration of the GIR to the lowest (basal) rate is unsuccessful, low-dose insulin therapy is the preferred treatment for hyperglycemia (Mesotten et al., 2018). Clinicians must recognize that although an exogenous insulin infusion is effective, this therapy increases cellular glucose uptake, which can elicit a severe and acute state of hypoglycemia. Interval surveillance of plasma glucose levels (at least hourly) is indicated throughout insulin therapy.

LIPIDS

ILEs offer a concentrated source of energy and essential fatty acids: 9 kcal of energy per 1 gram (Cober et al., 2021; Gargasz, 2012; Lapillonne et al., 2018). ILEs are composed of a lipid source (comprised of fatty acids) and an emulsifier (Table 23.9). The emulsifier, which consists of egg yolk-derived phospholipids, envelopes the lipid globules in order to maintain the solubility of the emulsion (Lapillonne et al., 2018). The 20% concentration is prescribed to infants because it contains the ideal ratio of lipid and emulsifier and is prepared in a much lower volume than the 10% ILE concentration (Lapillonne et al., 2018). This iso-osmolar 20% concentration offers the most efficient triglyceride clearance, which is particularly advantageous with preterm neonates.

Pure soybean oil-based ILEs have been widely used in neonatal units in the United States for decades. The composition of soybean oil-based ILEs is unique in that they contain high concentrations of essential fatty acids, lack appreciable amounts of long-chain polyunsaturated fatty acids (PUFAs), and contain low amounts of vitamin E (Lapillonne et al., 2018). Vitamin E is the most important lipophilic antioxidant as it prevents the oxidation (premature breakdown) of essential

TABLE 23.9 Composition of Pediatric Intralipid Emulsions

TYPE	LIPID SOURCES (%)	FATTY ACIDS	FDA APPROVAL (YEAR)
Intralipid	100% soybean oil	Linoleic Linolenic Oleic Palmitic Stearic	1996
Soy-oil and mixed-oil lipid emulsions (SMOFlipid)	30% soybean 30% MCT 25% olive oil 15% fish oil	Caprylic Capric Docosahexaenoic Eicosapentaenoic Linoleic Linolenic Palmitic Stearic	2016
Fish-oil lipid emulsions (Omegaven)	100% fish oil	Arachidonic Docosahexaenoic Eicosapentaenoic Myristic Oleic Palmitic Palmitoleic	2018

MCT, medium chain triglyceride.

Sources: From Food and Drug Administration. (1996). *Intralipid 20%*. https://www.accessdata.fda.gov/drugsatfda_docs/label/2007/017643s072,018449s039lbl.pdf; Food and Drug Administration. (2016). *SMOFlipid*. https://www.accessdata.fda.gov/drugsatfda_docs/label/2016/207648lbl.pdf; Food and Drug Administration. (2018). *Omegaven*. https://www.accessdata.fda.gov/drugsatfda_docs/label/2018/0210589s000lbledt.pdf

fatty acids (Raederstorff et al., 2015). Given that PUFAs are uniquely found in high concentrations in the brain and retina, an adequate level of vitamin E is critical to promote normal brain and ocular development and function.

The newer ILEs include SMOFlipid and Omegaven. Compared to Intralipid, both formulations offer increased proportions of anti-inflammatory omega-3 fatty acids (n-6 and n-3 long-chain fatty acids) and vitamin E. The substitution of SMOFlipid for Intralipid is a reasonable approach to limit exposure to soybean oil-based ILE. However, clinicians must ensure delivery of the minimum dose of essential fatty acids when utilizing this unique formulation. Omegaven, pure fish-oil ILE, is approved with a dose limitation of 1 gram/kg/d. This dose restriction may limit the aggregate intake of essential fatty acids over time, which could impede optimal brain and ocular development. Therefore, long-term use is usually restricted to infants with pathologic jaundice (cholestasis). We refer readers to Chapter 25, "Hyperbilirubinemia," for additional discussion of ILE and use in cases of cholestasis.

In addition to optimizing central nervous system development and retinal growth and function, ILEs also assist in the delivery of lipid-soluble vitamins (e.g., vitamins A, D, E, K), decrease carbon dioxide production (as compared to carbohydrates), and contribute to positive net nitrogen balance (Gargasz, 2012; Kleinman & Greer, 2020; Lapillonne et al., 2018). As previously mentioned, lipids contribute to the glucose load. Therefore, the inclusion of ILE usually reduces the GIR necessary to maintain euglycemia (Lapillonne et al., 2018). Finally, ILE can offset the high osmolarity of an amino acid-glucose solution when infused simultaneously into the same vein, which can spare peripheral veins (Kleinman & Greer, 2020).

ILE is typically initiated within the first 2 days of life. In fact, early initiation encourages a positive nitrogen balance, lower plasma urea concentrations, and enhanced albumin synthesis (Table 23.10). However, careful monitoring of triglyceride and glucose concentrations may be warranted (Lapillonne et al., 2018). The omission of ILEs is discouraged, as this can also lead to the development of an EFAD. In order to prevent EFAD, ESPGHAN recommends the inclusion of a minimum of 0.25 gram/kg/d of *soy-based lipids* in preterm infant diets and 0.1 gram/kg/d in term infant diets (Lapillonne et al., 2018). In contrast, the AAP recommends a minimum of 0.5 to 1 gram/kg/d of soybean oil-based ILE (Kleinman & Greer, 2020). Therefore, most U.S.-based neonatal clinicians order a minimum of 0.5 gram/kg/d of soy-based ILE; exceptions apply to infants with cholestasis. Refer to the Complications section in the following text for an expanded discussion of EFAD.

Neonatal clinicians have remained conscious of the potential risk of light exposure during administration of PN. Light exposure can encourage the synthesis of peroxides (by-products of lipid peroxidation), which can induce oxidative damage (Baird, 2001; Cober et al., 2021). Among preterm infants, the most notable acquired disease associated with oxidative stress and damage is BPD. Prior to the 21st century, it was common to find PN bags, syringes, and tubing shielded from light. More recently, shielding has fallen out of favor. Sherlock and Chessex (2009) investigated the incidence of "shielding" PN in Canadian NICUs. They found that nearly 50% of Level III neonatal units offered partial

TABLE 23.10 Recommendations for Daily Intralipid Emulsion Intake

	ASPEN		AAP		ESPGHAN	
Intralipid emulsions (gram/kg/d)	Preterm	Initiation: 0.5–1 Daily advance: 0.5–1 Goal: 3 Max infusion rate 0.15 gram/kg/hr	Preterm	Initiation: 0.5–3 Daily advance: N/A Goal: N/A Max infusion rate 3–4 grams/kg/d	Preterm	Initiation: N/A Daily advance: N/A Goal: N/A Max infusion rate 4 grams/kg/d

AAP, American Academy of Pediatrics; ASPEN, American Society for Parenteral and Enteral Nutrition; ESPEN, European Society for Parenteral and Enteral Nutrition; N/A, not available.

Sources: From the American Society for Parenteral and Enteral Nutrition. (2019). *ASPEN recommendations on appropriate dosing for parenteral nutrition for neonatal and pediatric patients.* https://nutritotal.com.br/pro/wp-content/uploads/sites/3/2019/04/PN-DosingASPEN.pdf; Kleinman, R. E., & Greer, F. R. (Eds.). (2020). *Pediatric nutrition* (8th ed.). American Academy of Pediatrics; Lapillonne, A., Fidler Mis, N., Goulet, O., van den Akker, C. H. P., Wu, J., Koletzko, B., Braegger, C., Bronsky, J., Cai, W., Campoy, C., Carnielli, V., Darmaun, D., Decsi, T., Domellöf, M., Embleton, N., Fewtrell, M., Fidler Mis, N., Franz, A., Goulet, O., … ESPGHAN/ESPEN/ESPR/CSPEN Working Group on Pediatric Parenteral Nutrition. (2018). ESPGHAN/ESPEN/ESPR/CSPEN guidelines on pediatric parenteral nutrition: Lipids. *Clinical Nutrition, 37*(6), 2324–2336. https://doi.org/10.1016/j.clnu.2018.06.946

shielding (light protection to PN bag only, lipids exposed to light) and no units offered complete shielding (Sherlock & Chessex, 2009). Currently, ASPEN recommends complete PN light protection beginning as soon as possible during the PN compounding process and continued until the entire PN and/or ILE admixture or infusion is complete (Cober et al., 2021; Robinson et al., 2021). Y-site compatibility with medications should be verified prior to initiation of administration to ensure compatibility of infusions.

Micronutrients

ELECTROLYTES AND MINERALS

Electrolytes and minerals must be supplied in PN and tailored specifically to each patient. Precise dose requirements are not known; therefore, we offer readers a summary of recommendations from expert panels in Table 23.11. Metabolic complications can result from deficiencies and excess amounts of electrolytes and minerals. Therefore, routine monitoring is warranted to prevent development of these metabolic complications (see monitoring section for more detailed information).

Electrolytes are added to PN as ions (e.g., mEq, mmol) or salts. Careful attention to ordering units is required to reduce the risk for error. Monovalent anions and cations include sodium (Na), potassium (K), chloride (Cl), acetate, calcium (Ca), and magnesium (Mg); whereas phosphorous presents as phosphate (PO_4; McNamara & Gray, 2017). Since ions cannot exist alone, they will always bind to another ion in the environment to be electrically neutral, forming a salt before separating and rebinding to other ions in solution (McNamara & Gray, 2017). That being said, in order to balance a solution, clinicians must determine the amount of Na and K required. Next, clinicians determine the amount of PO_4 that is necessary for bone mineralization and growth. PO_4 is bound to either ion as sodium phosphate or potassium phosphate. The remaining unbound Na and K can be paired with acetate or Cl (e.g., sodium acetate, sodium chloride, potassium acetate,

TABLE 23.11 Daily Micronutrient Recommendations

ELECTROLYTES	ASPEN		AAP		ESPGHAN	
Sodium (mEq/kg)	Preterm	2–5	Preterm	2–4	Preterm	2–5
	Term		Term		Term	2–3
Potassium (mEq/kg)	Preterm	2–4	Preterm	2–4	Preterm	1–5
	Term		Term		Term	1–3
Calcium (mEq/kg)	Preterm	2–4	Preterm	0.45–4	Preterm	1.6–4 (up to 7)
	Term	0.5–4	Term		Term	1.5–3
Phosphate (mmol/kg)	Preterm	1–2	Preterm	0.5–2	Preterm	1–3.5
	Term	0.5–2	Term		Term	0.7–1.3
Magnesium (mEq/kg)	Preterm	0.3–0.5	Preterm	0.25–1	Preterm	0.2–0.5
	Term		Term		Term	0.2–0.3
Acetate (mEq/kg)	Preterm	As needed to maintain acid–base balance	Preterm	N/A	Preterm	N/A
	Term		Term		Term	
Chloride (mEq/kg)	Preterm		Preterm	2–4	Preterm	1–5
	Term		Term		Term	1–3

AAP, American Academy of Pediatrics; ASPEN, American Society for Parenteral and Enteral Nutrition; ESPEN, European Society for Parenteral and Enteral Nutrition; N/A, not available.

Sources: From the American Society for Parenteral and Enteral Nutrition. (2019). *ASPEN recommendations on appropriate dosing for parenteral nutrition for neonatal and pediatric patients*. https://nutritotal.com.br/pro/wp-content/uploads/sites/3/2019/04/PN-DosingASPEN.pdf; Jochum, F., Moltu, S. J., Senterre, T., Nomayo, A., Goulet, O., Iacobelli, S., Braegger, C., Bronsky, J., Cai, W., Campoy, C., Carnielli, V., Darmaun, D., Decsi, T., Domellöf, M., Embleton, N., Fewtrell, M., Fidler Mis, N., Franz, A., Goulet, O., … ESPGHAN/ESPEN/ESPR/CSPEN Working Group on Pediatric Parenteral Nutrition. (2018). ESPGHAN/ESPEN/ESPR/CSPEN guidelines on pediatric parenteral nutrition: Fluid and electrolytes. *Clinical Nutrition, 37*(6), 2344–2353. https://doi.org/10.1016/j.clnu.2018.06.948; Kleinman, R. E., & Greer, F. R. (Eds.). (2020). *Pediatric nutrition* (8th ed.). American Academy of Pediatrics; Mihatsch, W., Fewtrell, M., Goulet, O., Molgaard, C., Picaud, J.-C., Senterre, T., & ESPGHAN/ESPEN/ESPR/CSPEN Working Group on Pediatric Parenteral Nutrition. (2018). ESPGHAN/ESPEN/ESPR/CSPEN guidelines on pediatric parenteral nutrition: Calcium, phosphorus and magnesium. *Clinical Nutrition*, 37(6 Pt B), 2360–2365. https://doi.org/10.1016/j.clnu.2018.06.950

or potassium chloride). Note that changes in ions (e.g., increasing acetate) will require changes to their salt formulation (e.g., changing sodium chloride to sodium acetate or increasing sodium acetate or potassium acetate) as ions do not exist by themselves.

In parenterally fed infants, the ratio of Ca mEq to PO_4 mmol intake should be 2:1, respectively. The goal for standard PO_4 intake is 39 to 67 mg/kg/d and the target calcium intake is 60 to 80 mg/kg/d; these targets are associated with acceptable plasma ion levels (Kleinman & Greer, 2020). However, clinicians should prioritize the provision of sufficient Ca and PO_4 in PN for bone and tissue accretion more so than targeting therapy to achieve specific plasma concentrations, as this reduces the risk for acquired metabolic bone disease (osteopenia of prematurity). This goal is often challenged by PN solubility curves, given the volume limits of neonatal PN. One particularly helpful strategy used to reduce the pH of PN and permit additional inclusion of Ca and PO_4 is to include cysteine in the PN. Cysteine lowers the pH of PN, leaving room for additional Ca and PO_4. Clinicians should also be prepared to identify infants at risk for hypophosphatemia, as additional supplementation may be necessary soon after birth. Preterm infants who suffered intrauterine growth restriction incur increased risk for severe hypophosphatemia. This can lead to muscle weakness, respiratory failure, cardiac dysfunction, and death (Mihatsch et al., 2018).

Customarily, a maximum of 0.5 mEq/kg/d of Mg is included in PN, as hypermagnesemia is associated with increased risk for hypotonia, bradycardia, decreased gastrointestinal motility, and death (Das et al., 2015). Infants prenatally exposed to maternal Mg therapy (e.g., preeclampsia, tocolysis) are most likely to present with elevated plasma Mg levels in the first few days of life (Mihatsch et al., 2018). Further, Mg excretion may be stalled during the initial transitional period after birth. Therefore, clinicians usually avoid the inclusion of Mg over the first few days of life, until glomerular filtration normalizes, and the blood Mg concentration is verified.

TRACE ELEMENTS

Routine administration of trace elements is considered standard of care to prevent deficiencies. Trace elements are commercially available as separate ingredients or in multiple-trace-element solutions (e.g., Multrys, Multitrace-4 Neo) for use in PN. However, the compositions of commercial pediatric trace element solutions vary widely, which complicates experts' ability to render dosing recommendations (Zemrani et al., 2018). Additional challenges include interchanging products due to shortages or clinical status for which specific trace elements should be omitted (e.g., cholestasis or renal impairment).

Essential nutrients, or trace elements, include zinc, copper, manganese, and selenium. These components must be supplied in PN to prevent deficiencies and optimize growth, especially in premature infants. Guidelines from expert panels are presented in Table 23.12 and each component is discussed in further detail in the following text.

Zinc is involved in the metabolism of proteins, carbohydrates, lipids, and nucleic acids (Domellöf et al., 2018). In addition, zinc is also essential for tissue accretion. Zinc deficiencies have been reported to include failure to thrive, growth retardation, alopecia, diarrhea, dermatitis (commonly perianal), ocular changes, rash (crusted, erythematous, involving face, extremities, and anogenital areas), nail hypoplasia or dysplasia, and increased risk of infections (Domellöf et al., 2018; ElHassan & Kaiser, 2011). The recommended daily dose of zinc is 400 to 500 mcg/kg/d in premature infants, 250 mcg/kg/d in term infants up to 3 months of age, and 100 to 250 mcg/kg/d for infants 3 to 12 months of age (ASPEN, 2019; Domellöf et al., 2018). In patients who are receiving PN long term or those with high gastrointestinal fluid output (e.g., ileostomy), periodic monitoring is recommended as these patients are likely to have significantly higher zinc losses (Domellöf et al., 2018). Zinc toxicity is associated with depressed phagocytic and bacterial leukocytic activity and pancreatitis (ElHassan & Kaiser, 2011).

Copper is a functional component for several enzymes and can be found in high content in gastrointestinal fluids (Domellöf et al., 2018). Copper deficiency, a risk for those on long-term PN, has been associated with pancytopenia, osteoporosis, anemia, depigmentation of hair and skin, neutropenia, poor weight gain, hypotonia, and ataxia later in life (Domellöf et al., 2018; ElHassan & Kaiser, 2011). The recommended daily dose for copper ranges between 20 and 40 mcg/kg for term and preterm infants (ASPEN, 2019; Domellöf et al., 2018). *Copper is excreted through bile and should be decreased or excluded from PN in patients with cholestasis.* Copper toxicity is associated with hepatic cirrhosis.

TABLE 23.12 Daily Trace Element Recommendations

TRACE ELEMENT	ASPEN		AAP		ESPGHAN	
Zinc (mcg/kg)	Preterm	400	Infants	Varies by product Multitrace-4 Neonatal: 0.2 mL/kg Multrys: 0.3 mL/kg (max 1 mL)	Preterm	400–500
	Term and Infants (3–10 kg)	250			Term (to 3 months)	250
					Infants (3–12 months)	100
Copper (mcg/kg)	Preterm	20			Preterm	40
	Term	20			Term	20
Manganese (mcg/kg)	Preterm	1			Preterm	1
	Term				Term	
Chromium (mcg/kg)	Preterm	0.05–0.3			Preterm	0.2
	Term	0.2			Term	
Selenium (mcg/kg)	Preterm	2	Preterm	2	Preterm	7
	Term		Term		Term	2–3

AAP, American Academy of Pediatrics; ASPEN, American Society for Parenteral and Enteral Nutrition; ESPEN, European Society for Parenteral and Enteral Nutrition.

Sources: From the American Society for Parenteral and Enteral Nutrition. (2019). *ASPEN recommendations on appropriate dosing for parenteral nutrition for neonatal and pediatric patients.* https://nutritotal.com.br/pro/wp-content/uploads/sites/3/2019/04/PN-DosingASPEN.pdf; Domellof, M., Szitanyi, P., Simchowitz, V., Franz, A., Mimouni, F., & ESPGHAN/ESPEN/ESPR/CSPEN Working Group on Pediatric Parenteral Nutrition. (2018) ESPGHAN/ESPEN/ESPR/CSPEN guidelines on pediatric parenteral nutrition: Iron and trace minerals. *Clinical Nutrition*, 37(6 Pt B), 2354–2359. https://doi.org/10.1016/j.clnu.2018.06.949; Kleinman, R. E., & Greer, F. R. (Eds.). (2020). *Pediatric nutrition* (8th ed.). American Academy of Pediatrics.

Manganese plays a role in enzyme activation (e.g., superoxide dismutase), carbohydrate metabolism, and normal bone structure (ElHassan & Kaiser, 2011). Manganese deficiency is associated with nausea, vomiting, dermatitis, hair depigmentation, and growth retardation. The daily dose should not exceed 1 mcg/kg/d. *Manganese is also excreted through bile and should be excluded from PN in patients with cholestasis.* Toxicity is associated with basal ganglia damage, neurotoxicity, and cholestasis.

Chromium is required for carbohydrate and lipid metabolism and is a regulator of insulin action (ElHassan & Kaiser, 2011). Chromium deficiency is not reported in the neonatal population and the risk for inclusion in PN usually outweighs the benefit. Despite purposeful exclusion from a PN recipe, contaminates in PN lead to a daily chromium intake of 0.2 to 0.3 mcg/kg/d (max 5 mcg/kg/d) among term and preterm infants. *Chromium should be excluded from PN in patients with renal disease.* Chromium toxicity is associated with chronic renal failure and an interference with iron metabolism and storage (Domellöf et al., 2018; ElHassan & Kaiser, 2011).

Selenium acts as an antioxidant, representing a component of glutathione peroxidase used in thyroid metabolism (Domellöf et al., 2018; ElHassan & Kaiser, 2011). Deficiencies have been associated with erythrocyte macrocytosis, depigmentation, and muscle weakness. The recommended dose of selenium is 2 to 7 mcg/kg/d in preterm infants and 2 to 3 mcg/kg/d in term infants (ASPEN, 2019; Domellöf et al., 2018). *Selenium should be excluded from PN in patients with renal disease.* No reports of selenium toxicity in neonates have been published; however, selenium toxicity in adults is associated with hair and nail loss, skin rash, teeth discoloration, paresthesia, and paralysis (Domellöf et al., 2018).

CARNITINE

Carnitine, an amino acid synthesized in the liver, modulates the transport of long-chain PUFAs across mitochondrial membranes and into the mitochondrial matrix, where enzymes necessary for fatty acid oxidation (metabolism) reside. Infants cannot synthesize adequate carnitine from fatty acids (e.g., lysine, methionine) or store carnitine; however, human milk and infant formulas provide infants with necessary carnitine, and it can be added to PN. Clinicians may notice that carnitine is not automatically included in PN formulations, but rather can be added during the ordering process. Although it is clear that carnitine levels are low in nonsupplemented parenterally fed infants, likely due to demand associated with postnatal growth and development, it remains unclear whether carnitine supplementation is necessary. One meta-analysis has been published to date, which reviewed data from all randomized trials ($n = 6$) that included carnitine supplementation. The authors concluded that insufficient evidence exists to support routine carnitine supplementation in PN (Cairns & Stalker, 2000). An updated meta-analysis showed no benefit of carnitine supplementation on lipid tolerance, ketogenesis, or weight gain in infants requiring PN (Mirtallo, 2010).

Despite the conclusion from Cairns and Stalker (2000), the AAP recommends that preterm and term infants subjected to prolonged (>4 weeks) PN receive between 2.4 and 10 mg/kg/d of carnitine supplementation (ElHassan & Kaiser, 2011; Lapillonne et al., 2018). We see this as a recommendation that thoughtfully considers risk:benefit and is therefore protective by design versus preventative. Earlier supplementation is indicated in cases of renal or hepatic impairment.

Vitamins

Due to poor stores, preterm infants are especially at high risk for vitamin deficiencies, which can lead to system-wide poor growth and development (Bronsky et al., 2018; ElHassan & Kaiser, 2011). The optimal time to initiate vitamin supplementation remains unknown, although many clinicians begin within the first few days of birth and continue on a daily basis through discharge to home (ElHassan & Kaiser, 2011). Recommended vitamin intake levels are presented in Table 23.13. When prescribing parenteral multivitamin (MVI), the recommended dose is 2 mL/kg to a maximum of 5 mL, which accounts for a portion of a reconstituted single-dose (5 mL) MVI vial in infants less than 2.5 kg (Kleinman & Greer, 2020). Parenteral MVI supplementation is usually discontinued once enteral feedings are tolerated, at approximately 120 mL/kg/d (Kleinman & Greer, 2020).

Because there is a concern for free radical formation secondary to light exposure (similar to our discussion of ILEs), clinicians may opt to shield PN preparations that contain MVIs. This will decrease the formation of hydrogen peroxide by at least 50% (ElHassan & Kaiser, 2011). Last, clinicians should be aware that commercially prepared vitamin formulations offer the recommended dose of vitamins A, D, E, and K, but exceed the recommended dose of vitamin B_{12}. There have been no reports of B_{12} toxicity to date.

Heparin

Heparin is added to IV solutions, including PN, to prevent thrombotic catheter occlusion and increase intended completion of therapy (Shah & Shah, 2008). Heparin is a naturally occurring glycosaminoglycan carbohydrate found in the mast cells in the body that enhances catheter patency by suppressing clot formation (Burcham & Rosenthal, 2019). Heparin is preferentially included in IV solutions that infuse through a central venous or arterial catheter. However, Isemann and colleagues (2012) demonstrated that heparin could be omitted from continuous infusions when short term without compromising catheter usability (Isemann et al., 2012).

MECHANISM OF ACTION/PHARMACOKINETIC PRINCIPLES

The mechanism of action of heparin involves enhancing the activity of antithrombin in order to elicit the inactivation of two coagulation factors: thrombin and factor Xa. Heparin has a more rapid clearance in neonates with an increased volume of distribution and a short half-life between 35 and 42 minutes in neonates younger than 36 weeks (Taketomo, 2023).

DOSING RECOMMENDATIONS

For neonates with central venous access devices, the prophylactic recommendation to maintain patency with unfractionated heparin continuous infusion is 0.5 units/kg/hour (Gorski et al., 2021; Monagle et al., 2012). In two randomized controlled trials of neonates with PICCs, 0.5 units/kg/hour was effective in prolonging duration of catheter usability without increasing adverse effects (Shah et al., 2007; Uslu et al., 2010). Further, no increase in risk for heparin-induced thrombocytopenia or hemorrhage has been identified with the inclusion of 0.5 units/kg/hour of heparin (Monagle et al., 2012). Some neonatal units prefer to include heparin in the PN admixture. Continuous infusion of heparin at 1.5 units/kg/hour was equally effective as heparin of 0.5 units/mL at sustaining catheter patency (Barekatain et al., 2018).

TABLE 23.13 Daily Vitamin Recommendations

	ASPEN	AAP	ESPGHAN	
Vitamin A (IU/kg)	Using pediatric multivitamins[a] Weight <1 kg: 1.5 mL Weight 1–3 kg: 3.25 mL Weight >3 kg: 5 mL OR Weight <2.5 kg: 2 mL/kg Weight ≥2.5 kg: 5 mL	Using pediatric multivitamins[a] Weight <2.5 kg: 2 mL/kg Weight ≥2.5 kg: 5 mL	Preterm	700–1,500
			Term to 12 months	150–300
Vitamin D (IU)			Preterm	200–100
			Term to 12 months	400
Vitamin E (IU/kg)			Preterm	2.8–3.5
			Term to 12 months	
Vitamin K (mcg/kg)			Preterm	10
			Term to 12 months	
Thiamine (mg/kg)			Preterm	0.35–0.5
			Term to 12 months	
Riboflavin (mg/kg)			Preterm	0.15–0.2
			Term to 12 months	
Pyridoxine (mg/kg)			Preterm	0.15–0.2
			Term to 12 months	
Niacin (mg/kg)			Preterm	4–6.8
			Term to 12 months	
Vitamin B_{12} (mcg/kg)			Preterm	0.3
			Term to 12 months	
Pantothenic acid (mg/kg)			Preterm	2.5
			Term to 12 months	
Biotin (mcg/kg)			Preterm	5–8
			Term to 12 months	
Folic acid (mcg/kg)			Preterm	56
			Term to 12 months	

[a]Pediatric multivitamins include infuvite pediatric (Baxter) and MVI pediatric (Hospira).

AAP, American Academy of Pediatrics; ASPEN, American Society for Parenteral and Enteral Nutrition; ESPEN, European Society for Parenteral and Enteral Nutrition.

Sources: From the American Society for Parenteral and Enteral Nutrition. (2019). *ASPEN recommendations on appropriate dosing for parenteral nutrition for neonatal and pediatric patients.* https://nutritotal.com.br/pro/wp-content/uploads/sites/3/2019/04/PN-DosingASPEN.pdf; Bronsky, J., Campoy, C., Braegger, C., Braegger, C., Bronsky, J., Cai, W., Campoy, C., Carnielli, V., Darmaun, D., Decsi, T., Domellöf, M., Embleton, N., Fewtrell, M., Fidler Mis, N., Franz, A., Goulet, O., Hartman, C., Hill, S., Hojsak, I., … ESPGHAN/ESPEN/ESPR/CSPEN Working Group on Pediatric Parenteral Nutrition. (2018). ESPGHAN/ESPEN/ESPR/CSPEN guidelines on pediatric parenteral nutrition: Vitamins. *Clinical Nutrition, 37*(6), 2366–2378. https://doi.org/10.1016/j.clnu.2018.06.951; Kleinman, R. E., & Greer, F. R. (Eds.). (2020). *Pediatric nutrition* (8th ed.). American Academy of Pediatrics.

COMPLICATIONS

Complications may arise from PN administration that include central line-associated infections, metabolic disturbances, or even mechanical complications (e.g., pneumothorax, air embolus, thrombotic events; Hartman et al., 2018; Kleinman & Greer, 2020). Long-term noncentral line PN-associated complications in neonates include hepatobiliary complications and metabolic bone disease (Hartman et al., 2018). These complications and recommendations for management are discussed in further detail in the text that follows including recommendations for management.

Electrolyte and Metabolic Abnormalities

As briefly mentioned earlier, electrolyte and metabolic abnormalities can occur if there are deficiencies or ions are given in excess. After ruling out underlying causes of metabolic and electrolyte disorders (e.g., renal tubular acidosis, dehydration, medication induced, etc.), inspect the patient's PN closely to determine whether the PN solution may be the cause. If the PN solution is not the cause, then consider it a "pharmacotherapy" to assist in supplementation of these electrolytes and minerals. Table 23.14 offers a sample laboratory monitoring schedule for infants who are receiving PN.

TABLE 23.14 Suggested Laboratory Monitoring Schedule During Parenteral Nutrition Therapy

LAB INDICES	INITIAL MONITORING (PENDING ATTAINMENT OF TOTAL INTAKE GOAL)	MAINTENANCE MONITORING
Sodium, potassium, chloride (serum)	Daily	Twice weekly
Carbon dioxide (serum)	Daily	Twice weekly
Urea nitrogen, creatinine (serum)	Daily	Twice weekly
Glucose (serum)	Daily until goal GIR is achieved As needed with clinical instability	Twice weekly
Phosphorus (serum)	Daily until total kcal intake at goal As needed with clinical instability	Twice weekly
Calcium (serum)	Daily until intake at goal or any period of metabolic instability	Twice weekly
Magnesium (serum)	Daily until normalized after birth As needed with clinical instability	Twice weekly
Triglyceride (serum)	Daily until lipid intake at goal As needed with clinical instability	Twice weekly
Liver function (serum)	Weekly	Every other week

GIR, glucose infusion rate.

Essential Fatty Acid Deficiency

Fat is an essential part of the diet as it serves multiple functions, including formation of cell membranes. In the setting of inadequate or absent linoleic acid (LNA), oleic acid is metabolized to mead acid (also known as *eicosatrienoic acid* [*triene*]) and production of arachidonic acid (also known as *eicosatetraenoic acid* [*tetraene*]) is reduced. An elevated triene:tetraene ratio is suggestive of EFAD, with a ratio greater than 0.2 confirming a diagnosis of EFAD (Hamilton et al., 2006; Sardesai, 1992).

Impaired fat intake, digestion, absorption, and/or metabolism can increase the risk of EFAD. Patients with these risk factors need to be monitored closely for evidence of EFAD. Clinical symptoms of EFAD include dry/scaly scalp, hair loss, hair depigmentation, poor wound healing, growth restriction, and increased susceptibility to infection. It is important to note these nonspecific signs overlap with other deficiencies, which therefore need to be ruled out. Additional laboratory evidence of EFAD includes elevated liver function tests, hyperlipidemia, thrombocytopenia, and altered platelet aggregation.

Once EFAD has been identified, the cause of EFAD must be determined. Recalculation of the fat content in the PN solution should be done to determine the amount of LNA provided. The minimum amount of soybean oil may be increased in order to treat preexisting EFAD. Unfortunately, there is no dosing guidelines for how much ILE should be administered. Gradual incremental increases of the percentage of calories from LNA should be provided for a defined period of time (e.g., 2 to 4 weeks) followed by another triene:tetraene ratio. As patients with EFAD may also be at risk for carnitine deficiency, PN-dependent patients should be evaluated and supplemented as appropriate. For patients who are not able to receive ILE (e.g., severe hypertriglyceridemia, severe cholestasis, or shortage of ILEs), topical oils may be considered. However, limited evidence indicates this method may not be effective (Friedman, 1976; Solanki et al., 2005).

Parenteral Nutrition-Associated Liver Disease

Infants subject to long-term PN incur increased risk for pathologic jaundice (cholestasis) and parenteral nutrition-associated liver disease (PNALD), also known as *intestinal failure-associated liver disease* (*IFALD*) or PN-induced cholestasis (Gargasz, 2012; Wales et al., 2014). We refer readers to Chapter 25, "Hyperbilirubinemia," for an expanded discussion of cholestasis and treatment recommendations.

The risk for PNALD is higher in preterm infants secondary to hepatic immaturity and the increased likelihood for a longer duration of PN exposure. Hepatic immaturity manifests with reduced enzymatic activity, bile salt uptake, and excretion. As patients with intestinal failure are typically unable to feed, lack of enteral feeding impairs the enterohepatic circulation and bile acid secretion/absorption, leading to mucosal atrophy and increasing the risk of bacterial translocation.

Refeeding Syndrome

As discussed throughout this chapter, preterm infants are born prior to the third trimester of pregnancy, when the majority of macronutrient and micronutrient stores accumulate. Many are exposed to poor nutrient transfer in utero and subject to intrauterine growth restriction. Therefore, at birth, clinicians prioritize the timely and efficient provision of PN to replete protein, fat, and glycogen stores. However, some preterm infants whose anthropometric indices indicate poor intrauterine growth, and who are subject to amino acid and glucose infusion after this period of nutritional deprivation, can manifest with significant electrolyte disturbances. These infants are diagnosed with RS.

RS involves a pathologic response to the provision of amino acids, glucose, and vitamins/nutrients after a period of fasting. This most often occurs within the first 5 days after preterm birth following a prolonged period of insufficient placental nutrient uptake (Figure 23.1). Recall

FIGURE 23.1 Pathogenesis of refeeding syndrome.

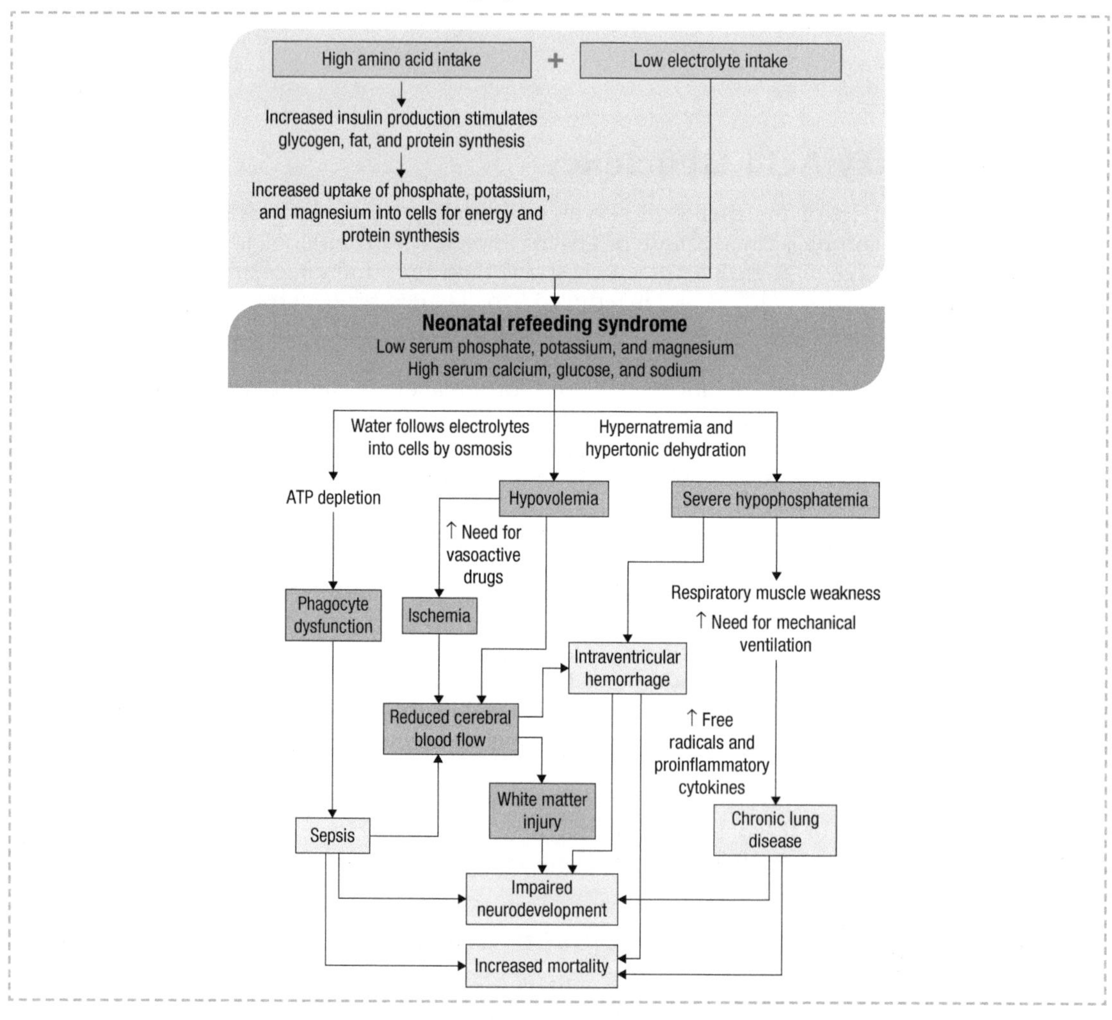

ATP, adenosine triphosphate.
Source: From Cormack, B. E., Jiang, Y., Harding, J. E., Crowther, C. A., Bloomfield, F. H., & ProVIDe Trial Group. (2021). Neonatal refeeding syndrome and clinical outcome in extremely low-birth-weight babies: Secondary cohort analysis from the ProVIDe trial. *Journal of Parenteral and Enteral Nutrition, 45*(1), 65–78. https://doi.org/10.1002/jpen.1934

that total water intake (total fluid intake) is low in the first 1 to 2 days after birth. This induces a transient state of hypovolemia (compared to intrauterine fluid intake) and may induce hypertonic dehydration and hypernatremia. The introduction of glucose and amino acids activates insulin synthesis and secretion. Cellular phosphate uptake increases to produce energy and proteins necessary for postnatal growth. Increased osteoclast activity occurs, which liberates available calcium from the bone and into the plasma, inducing a state of hypercalcemia (Cormack et al., 2021). Then, within 5 days of refeeding, as nutrient supplementation increases in PN, the following electrolyte disturbances develop:

- hypercalcemia,
- hyperglycemia,
- hypernatremia,
- hypokalemia,
- hypomagnesemia,
- hypophosphatemia

Some of these electrolyte disturbances (e.g., hypophosphatemia) increase the risk for brain injury (e.g., intraventricular hemorrhage [IVH]). Hypophosphatemia is known to cause thrombocytopenia and prolonged coagulation times, making this cause/effect relationship understandable. In addition, low protein and albumin levels are associated with IVH (Cormack et al., 2021). Although more research is indicated to fully understand the risks of RS, it is certainly necessary for clinicians to maintain awareness of this pathologic state and closely monitor biochemical indices to prevent the onset of extreme shifts (hyper- or hypo-availability of ions).

CONCLUSIONS

Poor nutrition and growth are associated with negative outcomes, including neurocognitive developmental delays. By recognizing limitations in nutritional absorption and digestion, the nutritional requirements of preterm and term infants can be optimized by APRNs, who play a crucial role in identifying, prescribing, and monitoring PN in critically ill neonates. National nutritional and pediatric organizations such as ASPEN (ASPEN, 2019; Cober et al., 2021), AAP (Kleinman & Greer, 2020), and ESPGHAN (Bronsky et al., 2018; Domellof et al., 2018; Hartman et al., 2018; Jochum et al., 2018; Joosten et al., 2018; Kolacek et al., 2018; Lapillonne et al., 2018; Mesotten et al., 2018; Mihatsch et al., 2018; van Goudoever et al., 2018) have published recommendations for usual dosing ranges of macronutrients and micronutrients making up PN solutions for infants as well as monitoring parameters to avoid development of any adverse effects.

LEARNING TOOLS AND RESOURCES

Advice From the Authors

Amy J. Jnah, DNP, APRN, NNP-BC

Pace yourself. Ordering total parenteral nutrition (TPN) is always intimidating to NNP students and new graduate NNPs. I suggest you begin by studying the macronutrients and dosages recommended by expert panels. Then, do the same with micronutrients. Last and probably even more important, discuss your customized TPN plan with your colleagues, including the pediatric pharmacist. I assure you, this dialogue will prove invaluable over time as you become familiar with strategies used to maintain acid/base balance and homeostasis despite the presence of comorbid conditions.

Tracy Rickard, MSN, APRN, NNP-BC

Don't ever lose a desire to learn. We are never too old, too proud, or too experienced to learn new things. Always, always know why you are giving a patient a medication and what it does to the patient!

Elizabeth Sharpe, DNP, APRN, NNP-BC, VA-BC, FAANP, FAAN

Exquisite knowledge of parenteral nutrition and its administration will form an essential cornerstone for your day-to-day patient management. Knowing chemical characteristics will enable you to match intravenous therapies with appropriate vascular access devices and prevent harm due to complications. Take the time to learn something new every day!

Van Tran, PharmD, BCPS, BCPPS, MBA

I've always loved the quote, "If you're not willing to learn, no one can help you. If you're determined to learn, no one can stop you" (Zig Ziglar). Sometimes, it can be overwhelming, but remember, even the greatest of the great started where you are right now. So, take one concept at a time, learn and teach each other (because it truly does help retain and apply the information), and love what you do.

Discussion Prompts

1. Compare and contrast the parameters (e.g., osmolarity, dextrose concentration, potassium concentration) for peripheral and central parenteral nutrition.
2. Discuss the risks, inclusive of short- and long-term complications, and benefits of parenteral nutrition.
3. What parenteral nutrition components would you consider decreasing or removing in patients with organ dysfunction (e.g., renal impairment, hepatic impairment)?
4. Compare and contrast the components of various lipid emulsions. Are there limitations to each lipid emulsion? What considerations need to take place with lipid administration?

Mind Map

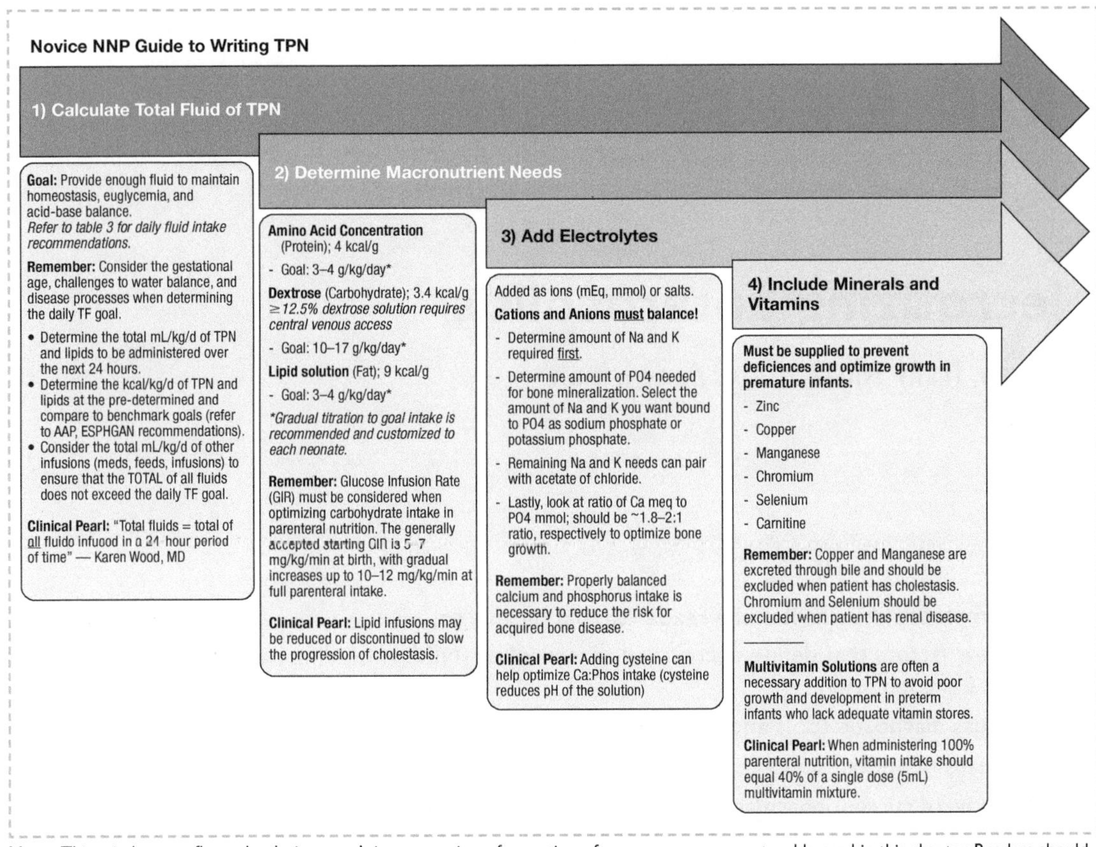

Note: This mind map reflects the design team's interpretation of a portion of one or more concepts addressed in this chapter. Readers should regard the mind maps woven throughout this textbook as examples of multisensory study tools that can be developed to encourage conceptual understanding. Readers are encouraged to develop their own unique mind maps in consultation with academic faculty or clinical preceptors.
AAP, American Academy of Pediatrics; NNP, neonatal nurse practitioner; TF, ; TPN, total parenteral nutrition.
Design credit: Meredith McSwain, MSN, APRN, NNP-BC, and Lauren Lucas, MSN, APRN, NNP-BC, East Carolina University Neonatal Nurse Practitioner Program.

REFERENCES

References for this chapter are online and available at https://connect.springerpub.com/content/book/978-0-8261-5884-0/part/partV/toc-part/ch23.

chapter 24

Necrotizing Enterocolitis

Van Tran, Tracy Rickard, and Amy J. Jnah

LEARNING OBJECTIVES

After completing this chapter, the reader should be able to:

- Review factors that define necrotizing enterocolitis (NEC), including pathophysiology and clinical presentation.
- Discuss diagnostic tools and indicators confirming NEC.
- Evaluate nonpharmacologic options for prevention of NEC in neonatal patients.
- Investigate current pharmacologic treatment recommendations for NEC.
- Examine opportunities for further research of NEC in the neonatal population.

INTRODUCTION

Necrotizing enterocolitis (NEC) is a life-threatening acute inflammatory disease of the bowel with clinically significant complications that uniquely affect neonates (Bazacliu & Neu, 2019; de Waard et al., 2019; Juhl et al., 2019; Neu & Walker, 2011; Rich & Dolgin, 2017). The incidence of NEC has increased proportionally over the years due to a concurrent increase in survival among infants born prematurely (Ahle et al., 2013; Hackam & Caplan, 2018). NEC is reported in 5% to 13% of very-low-birth-weight (VLBW) preterm infants born in the United States and Canada, nearly double the incidence of 1% to 7.5% reported in the mid-1970s (Duchon et al., 2021; Horbar et al., 2017; Marseglia et al., 2015). Morbidity is as high as 30%, particularly among infants requiring surgery; infants with NEC also incur increased risk of bronchopulmonary dysplasia (BPD) and long-term neurodevelopmental delay (Neu & Walker, 2011).

Most cases of NEC occur in infants less than 32 weeks' gestation with a birth weight of less than 1,500 grams (Horbar et al., 2017; Wertheimer et al., 2019). The onset of NEC is inversely related to gestational age in that the earlier the gestational age at birth, the later the postnatal age at which NEC develops. For example, for infants born at less than 30 weeks' gestation, the average age at onset is 20.2 days. For infants born at 31 to 33 weeks' gestation, the average age at onset is 13.8 days, and for infants born after 36 weeks the onset is 5.4 days (Wertheimer et al., 2019). Gordon and associates (2014) reported that among preterm infants, the peak onset for most cases of NEC is between 29 and 32 weeks' postmenstrual age (PMA). Clearly, the onset of symptoms varies by gestational age and among studies.

The two most significant risk factors for NEC are prematurity and birth weight less than 1,500 grams; these risks are considered unmodifiable for clinicians staffing NICUs. The one *modifiable* risk factor is preterm formula use, and because of this clinicians are consistently reminded to prescribe human milk or donor breast milk in lieu of formula, whenever possible (Rose & Patel, 2018). The American Academy of Pediatrics Committee on Nutrition (Daniels, 2017) issued a policy statement to this effect, recommending the use of donor milk for preterm infants weighing less than 1,500 grams at birth. One other significant risk is prolonged antibiotic exposure and its effect on the intestinal microbiota of the gut, to include delayed commensal colonization and reduced diversity of the gut microflora (Li et al., 2020; Raba et al., 2021). Alternatively, new data suggest that preterm infants weighing ≤1,500 grams at birth and who receive early empiric broad-spectrum antibiotics within the first 3 postnatal days incur a lower risk of later development of NEC (Bell stage ≥II; odds ratio [OR]: 0.25; 95% confidence interval [CI]: 0.12–0.47; $p < .0001$; Li et al., 2020). Judicious prescribing practices are necessary. Other factors associated with an increased and decreased risk of NEC, which neonatal clinicians must be aware of and that are reported from randomized controlled trials (RCTs), are summarized in Table 24.1.

From an economic standpoint, the annual burden of NEC is estimated between $500 million and $1 billion (Bazacliu & Neu, 2019; Neu & Walker, 2011). Approximately one-third to one-half of affected infants will require surgical intervention, which significantly contributes to this economic burden (Rich & Dolgin, 2017). Short-term morbidities include poor postnatal growth, increased BPD, patent ductus arteriosus (PDA), retinopathy of prematurity (ROP), and gastrointestinal (GI) issues (Bazacliu & Neu, 2019). Long-term morbidities include a 24.8% to 59.3% risk of neurodevelopmental delay, failure to thrive, and GI complications such as strictures, adhesions, cholestasis, and short bowel syndrome with or without intestinal failure (IF; Bazacliu & Neu, 2019; Flahive et al., 2020). Mortality risk is estimated at 23.5% among infants diagnosed with Bell stage ≥II (Jones & Hall, 2020). Even more ominous is the 50.9% postsurgical mortality risk among infants weighing less than 1,000 grams at birth and who develop advanced NEC (Fullerton et al., 2016; Hull et al., 2014).

This chapter provides a brief overview of the pathophysiology and epidemiology of NEC and its risk factors, clinical presentation, laboratory evaluation, diagnosis, as well as treatment and prevention recommendations. Common pathogenic organisms and opportunities for antibiotic stewardship are also described.

TABLE 24.1 Commonly Proposed Risks for Necrotizing Enterocolitis

PRENATAL PERIOD	INTRAPARTUM PERIOD	POSTNATAL PERIOD
↓ Antenatal steroid exposure	~ Intrapartum antibiotics	~ Anemia and PRBC transfusion
~ Maternal hypertension[a]		↓ Arginine
↓ Progesterone use		↑ Birth weight <1,500 grams
~ Tocolytics		↓ Breast milk/donor milk
↑ Congenital heart disease[a]		~ Empiric antibiotics
		↓ Erythropoietin
		↓ Fluid restriction
		↑ Glycerin suppository
		↓ Oral lactoferrin
		↓ Parenteral arginine
		↑ Prematurity
		↑ Preterm formula
		~ PDA
		↓ Probiotic supplementation
		~ Surfactant
		~ Umbilical catheter

Note: ↑ increased risk, ↓ decreased risk, ~ mixed results.

[a]Congenital heart diseases, which encourage diastolic flow reversal, include left-sided obstructive lesions, total anomalous pulmonary venous return, truncus arteriosus, and Ebstein anomaly.

PDA, patent ductus arteriosus; PRBC, packed red blood cell.

Sources: From Kelleher, S. T., McMahon, C. J., & James, A. (2021). Necrotizing enterocolitis in children with congenital heart disease: A literature review. *Pediatric Cardiology, 42*(8), 1688–1699. https://doi.org/10.1007/s00246-021-02691-1; Moss, 2008; Patel, A. L., Panagos, P. G., & Silvestri, J. M. (2017). Reducing incidence of necrotizing enterocolitis. *Clinics in Perinatology, 44*(3), 683–700. https://doi.org/10.1016/j.clp.2017.05.004; Rose, A. T., & Patel, R. M. (2018). A critical analysis of risk factors for necrotizing enterocolitis. *Seminars in Fetal & Neonatal Medicine, 23*(6), 374–379. https://doi.org/10.1016/j.siny.2018.07.005.

PHYSIOLOGY REVIEW: THE GUT MICROBIOME

Before we progress to a discussion of the pathophysiology of NEC, it is pertinent to review the physiologic establishment of the gut microbiome. Although once disputed, we now are aware that early colonization of the fetal GI tract begins within the womb. The mechanism by which this occurs involves the migration of oral bacteria from the pregnant mother into maternal circulation and then to the placenta, fetal membranes, and umbilical vein (Kim & Claud, 2019). Studies have confirmed the presence of maternal oral flora in meconium and amniotic fluid (Jiménez et al., 2008).

Postnatal changes to the gut microbiome occur in a well-choreographed and orderly manner. Three species of bacteria colonize within the gut in a sequential order true for all newborns. These three species present over the first 3 weeks of life after birth and begin with gram-positive species (e.g., staphylococci, streptococci, enterococci), followed by gram-negative rods or Gammaproteobacteria (e.g., *Escherichia coli*), and last Clostridia species. The length of time required for each species to colonize and the time between transitional changes is believed to be influenced by gestational age at birth, method of delivery, postnatal feeding practices, and duration of antibiotic exposure. La Rosa and colleagues (2014) reported that preterm infants' stool samples contained more Gammaproteobacteria compared with their term counterparts at the same PMA. Additional research is needed to fully understand the relationship between gestational age and gut maturation. Specific to method of birth, the GI tract of neonates delivered vaginally include flora contained within the maternal vaginal canal (e.g., *Lactobacillus*), whereas neonates born by Cesarean section manifest with gut flora consistent with the mother's skin (e.g., *Staphylococcus, E. coli*).

Feeding practices influence colonization within the gut microbiome and maturation of host defenses within this region of the body. Newborns who are breastfed tend to accumulate *Bifidobacterium* at a greater proportion compared with other bacterial species. This is beneficial to the newborn, as *Bifidobacterium* facilitates maturation of innate and adaptive immune responses (Palmeira & Carneiro-Sampaio, 2016). As discussed in Chapter 21, "Human Milk as Medicine," human milk contains fats, proteins, and carbohydrates, namely oligosaccharides. The absorption of oligosaccharides is enhanced in the presence of *Bifidobacterium*, a probiotic that increases significantly among human-milk-fed babies. *Bifidobacterium* found in the colon produce lacto-N-biosidase, an enzyme with a particular affinity for oligosaccharides. This enhances macronutrient absorption. In contrast, Stark and Lee (1982) analyzed the GI tract of formula-fed babies and found that *Bifidobacterium* species were lower and anaerobic species (e.g., *Clostridium*) higher than human-milk-fed counterparts. Over time, as the maternal milk supply wanes, *Bifidobacterium* species decline, whereas *Bacteroides* and *Firmicutes* bacterial loads increase, a normal part of the maturational process.

Eventually, by the end of the first year of life, the GI microbiome transitions to a symbiotic environment full of approximately 10^{14} bacterial cells of varied species working in harmony to offer necessary host defenses and digestive assistance (Round & Mazmanian, 2009). Viral or bacterial infections and prolonged use of antibiotics often disrupt this delicate balance, thrusting the GI system into dysbiosis, which limits host defenses, digestion, and nutrient absorption.

PATHOPHYSIOLOGY REVIEW

The gut microbiome undergoes dynamic changes after birth. Among neonates born preterm, in particular those born weighing less than 1,500 grams, birth followed by a NICU admission abruptly alters gut maturation. It is likely that periods of dysbiosis, which occur when there is an increased proportion of pathogenic to commensal bacteria, increase the susceptibility of the intestinal mucosa to injury (Duchon et al., 2021; Kim & Claud, 2019; Rich & Dolgin, 2017). Other factors that increase the risk of NEC among preterm infants include immunologic factors (decreased secretory immunoglobulin A [IgA] and lymphocytes, and immature innate immunity), luminal factors (reduced hydrogen ion production and enzyme activity, decreased peristalsis), and barrier immaturity (thinner mucosal layer and junctions between epithelial cells; Chandran et al., 2021).

Common pathogens found within NICUs include *Enterococcus faecium, Staphylococcus aureus,* Enterobacteriaceae species (e.g., *E. coli, Klebsiella pneumoniae*), *Acinetobacter baumannii, Pseudomonas aeruginosa,* and *Enterobacter* species. Similar pathogens have been isolated from peritoneal fluid and blood culture samples taken from infants with NEC (Brook, 2008). The most common pathogens reported in cases of NEC include Gammaproteobacteria (e.g., *E. coli*, *K. pneumoniae*), *Clostridium*, enteric pathogens (*Salmonella*, Coxsackie B2 virus, coronavirus, rotavirus), and *Bacteroides fragilis*. Multimicrobial contamination of the peritoneal cavity has been reported in up to 50% of affected infants, and of these patients nearly 25% manifested with mixed aerobic–anaerobic peritoneal flora (Bell et al., 1980).

The multifactorial pathogenesis that occurs and leads to mild, moderate, or severe disease remains to be elucidated. Three factors have been proposed to contribute to the pathogenesis of this disease and these are (a) GI dysbiosis between pathogenic and commensal bacteria, (b) injury to the intestinal lining, and (c) activation of the innate immune response with uncontrolled inflammation (Wertheimer et al., 2019). First, disruption of a homeostatic intestinal bacterial load by invading pathogens (e.g., gram-positive anaerobic bacteria or gram-negative bacteria) induces a state of dysbiosis. Next, pathogenic bacteria translocate across the intestinal epithelia. Lastly the innate immune response is activated. Neal and colleagues (2006) studied the relationship between gram-negative bacterial invasion and NEC. They found that lipopolysaccharides on the wall of gram-negative bacteria activate toll-like receptors (TLRs) on the wall of the intestinal mucosa (Hackam & Caplan, 2018). This elicits the innate immune response. TLR-4 phagocytizes the bacteria. Other TLRs activate signaling pathways, which encourage the infiltration of proinflammatory cytokines (e.g., tumor necrosis factor, interleukins, procalcitonin, and C-reactive protein). The consequential inflammatory response tends to be abundant in cases of NEC.

Few histopathologic studies of tissue sections of the alimentary tract have identified varied depths of necrosis, inflammation, bacterial overgrowth, and pneumatosis at the mucosa, submucosa, and muscularis layers, and the serosa. Remon and colleagues (2015) evaluated the tissue samples of 33 infants with NEC and reported findings that help elucidate the relationship between the migration of proinflammatory cells and bacteria and disease severity. They identified a median depth of necrosis to the muscularis layer; strong correlations between the depth and the extent of necrosis were observed ($r = 0.807$, $p < 0.001$). Proinflammatory cells, primarily macrophages and neutrophils, were identified in 81.8% of tissue samples. The depth of invasion of these infiltrates extended across all layers and correlated with the depth of bacterial invasion ($r = 0.372$, $p = .03$) and disease severity. Bacterial populations were primarily mixed (cocci and bacilli) and found within all layers of the GI tract: mucosa (9.1%), submucosa (18.2%), muscularis (30.3%), and serosa (3%). Fungal species were present in 6% of all cases and corresponded with severe necrosis. Pneumatosis was identified in 42.2% of all tissue samples. Although these statistics should not be generalized as they reflect the outcomes of one study, the basic principle that pathogens and inflammatory mediators can penetrate each layer of the wall of the alimentary tract is important. The depth of penetration and the surface area involved often correspond with advancing disease severity.

Clinical Manifestations of Necrotizing Enterocolitis

The clinical presentation of NEC is often nonspecific and variable (Table 24.2). The most commonly reported GI signs of NEC include an "acute abdomen," which is customarily defined as new-onset abdominal distension, bilious aspirate or emesis, and hematochezia in the absence of a rectal

TABLE 24.2 Common Manifestations of Necrotizing Enterocolitis

Gastrointestinal manifestations	Abdominal distension Abdominal tenderness/guarding Absent bowel sounds Gastric aspirate (bilious, bloody) Ileus (reduced peristalsis) Occult positive stool
Sepsis manifestations	Apnea and bradycardia Coagulopathy Metabolic acidosis Shock Temperature instability

fissure (Knell et al., 2019). Infants may present with "sepsis like" features, including temperature instability, lethargy, pallor, apnea, and bradycardia (Jnah & Trembath, 2019). The progression of symptoms may be slow or involve a rapid onset with fulminant progression; mortality risk is high in these situations (Wertheimer et al., 2019). We encourage readers to refer to *Fetal and Neonatal Physiology for the Advanced Practice Nurse* (Jnah & Trembath, 2019) for an expanded discussion of manifestations, which includes helpful radiographic images.

Evaluation

Customary evaluation indices include radiographic studies, abdominal ultrasound, and hematologic and metabolic studies. Common radiographic findings include a gasless abdomen, dilated loops of bowel, portal venous (hepatobiliary) gas, pneumatosis intestinalis, or pneumoperitoneum (Bell et al., 1978; Berrington & Embleton, 2021; Knell et al., 2019). Abdominal ultrasound is emerging as an adjunct to radiographic studies, offering reduced radiation exposure and a more granular assessment of the bowel wall, perfusion, gut motility, or abnormal findings such as peritoneal fluid (Lazow et al., 2021). Studies are currently underway to determine whether ultrasonography can aid decision-making specific to the need for surgical intervention. Hematologic and metabolic findings often include thrombocytopenia, neutropenia, elevated C-reactive protein level, metabolic acidosis, electrolyte abnormalities, and coagulopathies (D'Angelo et al., 2018). A sepsis evaluation is customary; however, positive blood culture results are not consistently reported among infants with NEC. Stoll and colleagues (2002) reported that 21% of infants with NEC had at least one positive blood culture (late-onset sepsis). Bizzaro and associates (2014) reported a substantially higher incidence (44%) of NEC-associated bloodstream infections among a population of exclusively VLBW infants. The majority of positive blood cultures contained gram-negative Enterobacteriaceae (Bizzarro et al., 2014).

Staging

In an effort to enable uniform staging stratification of infants, Dr. Martin Bell proposed the original clinical criteria used to stage NEC cases (Bell et al., 1978). Three stages were outlined, enhancing the ability to recognize, diagnose, and treat each cohort of patients. As our understanding of NEC has evolved, staging was updated to include three major stages with substages, to better appraise and communicate the severity of the disease process (Table 24.3).

HISTORICAL PERSPECTIVE: SEMINAL AND OTHER NOTEWORTHY PHARMACOLOGY-SPECIFIC STUDIES

Readers have likely noticed that this section is customarily dedicated to a retrospective look at the evolution of pharmacotherapies used to treat the disease process of interest. For example, Chapter 10, "Apnea of Prematurity," discusses the Caffeine for Apnea of Prematurity (CAP) trial and Chapter 25, "Hyperbilirubinemia," discusses the evolution of pharmacotherapies used to treat both pathologic and physiologic hyperbilirubinemia. In those cases, the etiology and pathogenesis of the disease process are well understood. NEC, however, may develop from the infiltration of a number of pathogens into the gut lumen, and blood culture results may remain negative despite the presence of clinical illness. Our review of the literature revealed six historical studies that specifically investigated the relationship between antimicrobial therapy and NEC.

The earliest studies of antimicrobial therapy for NEC were published in the 1970s and reported the outcomes associated with a combination of intravenous (IV) and oral antibiotics. The first report was published by Bell et al. (1973), who sought to share the outcomes associated with their hospital-specific treatment regimen. Infants diagnosed with NEC were given IV penicillin and kanamycin or gentamicin, plus oral kanamycin or gentamicin at a dosage of two to three times the IV dose ($N = 14$). The authors reported that no infants subject to antimicrobial therapy developed an intestinal perforation. Bell and colleagues (1978) reported the outcomes associated with combination antimicrobial therapy ($N = 48$). This team of researchers initially prescribed a combination

TABLE 24.3. Modified Bell's Staging Criteria for Necrotizing Enterocolitis

STAGE	CLASSIFICATION	SYSTEMIC SIGNS	INTESTINAL SIGNS	RADIOLOGIC SIGNS	TREATMENT
IA	Suspected NEC	Temperature instability, apnea, bradycardia, lethargy	Elevated pre-gavage residuals, mild abdominal distension, emesis, guaiac-positive stool	Normal or intestinal dilation, mild ileus	NPO, antibiotics × 3 days pending culture
IB			Same as IA, *plus* bright red blood from rectum		
IIA	Definite NEC (mildly ill)		Same as IB, *plus* absent bowel sounds, +/- abdominal distension	Intestinal dilation, ileus, pneumatosis intestinalis	NPO, antibiotics × 7-10 days if exam is normal in 24-48 hours
IIB	Definite NEC (moderately ill)	Same as above, *plus* mild metabolic acidosis, mild thrombocytopenia	Same as IB, *plus* absent bowel sounds, *definite* abdominal distension, +/- abdominal cellulitis or right lower quadrant mass	Same as IIA, *plus* portal vein gas, +/- ascites	NPO, antibiotics × 14 days, sodium bicarbonate for acidosis
IIIA	Advanced NEC (severely ill, bowel intact)	Same as IIB, *plus* hypotension, bradycardia, severe apnea, combined respiratory andmetabolic acidosis, disseminated intravascular coagulation, neutropenia	Same as IIB, *plus* signs of generalized peritonitis, marked tenderness, and distension of abdomen	Same as IIB, *plus* definite ascites	Same as IIB, *plus* 200+ mL/kg fluids, inotropic agents, ventilation therapy, paracentesis
IIIB	Advanced NEC (severely ill, bowel perforation)			Same as IIB, *plus* pneumoperitoneum	Same as IIIA, *plus* surgical intervention

NEC, necrotizing enterocolitis; NPO, nothing by mouth.
Source: From Walsh, M. C. & Kliegman, R. M. (1986). Necrotizing enterocolitis: Treatment based on staging criteria. *Pediatric Clinics of North America, 33*(1), 179-201. https://doi.org/10.1016/s0031-3955(16)34975-6

of a semisynthetic penicillin (most often, ampicillin) plus an aminoglycoside (kanamycin) over a span of 6 days. Then, partway through the study period, the team changed the antimicrobial study protocol to a combination of IV gentamicin and clindamycin plus oral gentamicin for a total of 3 to 5 days of therapy. All neonates with stage I NEC survived, and 85% of those with stage II/III disease survived. Blood culture samples from four of the neonates who died yielded Gammaproteobacteria (*E. coli, Klebsiella*). Complications included intestinal strictures requiring operative intervention; one stricture-related death was reported. Bell and colleagues (1979) investigated the changes in gastric flora in a subset of preterm infants from the previous study with a mean birth weight of 1,660 grams, before and after administration of triple therapy involving IV gentamicin and clindamycin plus oral gentamicin. Pretreatment intestinal microflora included gram-negative organisms (*Klebsiella, E. coli, Enterobacter*, and *Citrobacter)* and gram-positive organisms (*S. epidermidis, S. aureus*, and *Streptococcus* species). After therapy, a significant reduction in both gram-positive and gram-negative species were reported ($p < .02$). This study helped elucidate the pathogens that may play a role in the development of NEC, which helped inform prescribing decisions.

The early 1980s marked a shift in research toward comparing outcomes of exclusive IV combination therapy versus combination IV and oral therapy. Hansen and colleagues (1980) published an RCT comparing IV ampicillin and gentamicin (A/G) with IV ampicillin and gentamicin with oral gentamicin for a total of 4 days of therapy. This particular study randomized infants who were greater than 1,500 grams at birth and with an average gestational age of 34.7 to 35.6 weeks, significantly above the customary risk threshold for NEC. The study reported comparable clinical outcomes between groups, although the methodology (randomization/blinding protocol) was poorly defined and the study was underpowered to detect a difference in mortality; therefore, it was not relied on in the clinical setting.

As of mid-1980s, oral antimicrobial use ceased. Physicians exclusively treated NEC with IV therapy, although one particular regimen was never agreed upon. Schiefele and colleagues (1987) investigated the use of a (longer) 7- to 10-day course of IV A/G versus vancomycin and ceftriaxone (V/C) among 90 infants with NEC. Reductions in gut flora (specifically, staphylococci and coliforms; $p < .001$), surgical need ($p = .04$), and mortality rate ($p < .048$) were detected among infants treated with V/C. These data elucidated the relationship between broad-spectrum treatment and reduced morbidity and mortality rates. However, the single-center nature of this study and the lack of replication have resulted in limited uptake of this broad-spectrum regimen (V/C) in clinical practice as standard of care. Next, Faix and associates (1988) added to the evidence by publishing a randomized trial comparing IV A/G with triple therapy of ampicillin, gentamicin, and clindamycin (A/G/C). The researchers further extended the duration of antimicrobial therapy, compared with prior studies, to 10 to 14 days. The incidences of intestinal perforation and death were similar between groups; however, the inclusion of clindamycin was associated with intestinal strictures (A/G group 1/18 vs. A/G/C 6/15, $p = .022$) and therefore the trial was ended prematurely. Note that a more recent retrospective, case–control study ($N = 2{,}780$) published by Autmizguine and colleagues (2015) confirmed the association of anaerobic therapy with an increased risk of intestinal strictures (OR: 1.73, 95% CI: 1.11–2.72). It is important to note that mortality was less common among infants with surgical NEC treated with an antimicrobial regimen including anaerobic coverage (OR: 0.71, 95% CI: 0.52–0.95).

One systematic review, published in 2012, examined the efficacy of antibiotic treatment regimens for NEC, specific to surgical need and mortality (Shah & Sinn, 2012). This review considered two studies, Hansen et al. (1980) and Faix et al. (1988), as no other studies met the criteria for meta-analyses. No statistically significant differences in death or bowel perforation were identified. As a result, the authors could not recommend one particular antibiotic treatment regimen. However, the authors did caution against the use of clindamycin secondary to the development of intestinal strictures.

CURRENT PHARMACOLOGIC TREATMENT MODALITIES USED TO PREVENT NECROTIZING ENTEROCOLITIS

Before we discuss current pharmacotherapies prescribed to treat NEC, it is prudent to discuss current preventive strategies. Prolonged antimicrobial use can erode the microbiome by reducing gut *Bifidobacterium*, a risk factor of NEC (Penders et al., 2006). Therefore, judicious use of antimicrobial agents is essential. Further, use of enteral feeding protocols that incrementally increase the osmolality of nutritional substances, use of human milk, and use of probiotics may reduce the risk of NEC. Chandran and colleagues (2021) reported that providing colostrum to the cheeks shortly after birth, prescribing human milk using a standardized feeding protocol (SFP) to optimize the osmolality of milk using dilution guidelines, using probiotics, and avoiding histamine type-2 receptor antagonists (H2RAs) and long-term broad-spectrum antibiotic use were associated with zero cases of NEC over a 1-year period at a single center. We explore these preventive strategies in this section of the chapter.

Early Colostrum, Human Milk, and Standardized Feeding Protocols

Early exposure to maternal colostrum is associated with immune maturation and reduction in risk of NEC. Recall that secretory IgA levels are reduced in preterm infants, increasing the risk of a deficient immune response in the face of pathogenic infiltration. Early human milk (colostrum) is saturated with secretory IgA (Garofalo, 2010; Rodriguez et al., 2009), which is then transferred to the preterm infant when colostrum is swabbed into the mouth in the first days of life. This offers valuable protection to the vulnerable neonate. Lee and colleagues (2015) reported the outcomes of an RCT that explored the efficacy of early colostrum use on the immune system. This team reported reduced incidences of clinical sepsis (50% vs. 92%, $p = .003$) and duration of antibiotic exposure (6 vs. 9 days, $p = .014$). No difference in the incidence of NEC was observed; however, the aforementioned benefits are encouraging, as antibiotic exposure is associated with an increased risk of NEC.

Experts have reported for decades that variable feeding practices increase the risk of NEC among preterm infants (Uauy et al., 1991). The use of SFPs is known to reduce total central-line days and the duration of parenteral nutrition, two risk factors for sepsis in hospitalized neonates (Kung et al., 2016; Rozé et al., 2017). A recently published systematic review by Jasani and Patole (2017) investigated the efficacy of SFPs in reducing the incidence of NEC among infants weighing less than 2,500 grams at birth and less than 37 weeks' gestation. Their meta-analysis of the data showed that SFPs significantly reduced the risk of NEC (relative risk [RR]: 0.26, 95% CI: 0.19–0.35, $p < .00001$).

The use of human milk as the sole source of enteral nutrition is strongly associated with a reduced incidence of NEC. We refer readers to Chapter 21, "Human Milk as Medicine," for an expanded discussion.

Low-Osmolality Feedings

Osmolality is defined as the number of particles of a solute per kilogram of solvent (Ernst et al., 1983; Latheef et al., 2021). Substances that have a high osmolality are associated with GI intolerances in preterm babies, as the increase in solute can negatively affect the gut mucosa (Ellis et al., 2019; Kreins et al., 2018). Animal studies (rat models) have shown that the continuous administration of hyperosmolar substances into the GI tract induces irreversible damage to the intestinal wall. This, in turn, encourages the accumulation of excess pathogenic bacteria and translocation of microorganisms into the abdominal cavity (Latheef et al., 2021). Given the predisposition of the preterm gut to injury, clinicians seek to minimize the administration of high-osmolality (>450 mOsm/kg) substances until feeding tolerance is established (Barness et al., 1976).

Consider that the fetal gut is exposed to amniotic fluid with an osmolality of approximately 275 mOsm/kg and normally tolerates this osmolality without issue (Latheef et al., 2021). Preterm birth abruptly removes the presence of amniotic fluid, and the gut is quickly exposed to enteral nutrition. Unfortified breast milk has an average osmolality of 300 mOsm/kg, whereas preterm formula has an average osmolality of 268.5 to 315.3 mOsm/kg (Latheef et al., 2021; Pereira-da-Silva et al., 2008). The addition of substances, including higher caloric-density formulas, human milk fortifiers, or nutritional supplements, increases the osmolality of the milk. For example, the osmolality of ferrous sulfate, potassium phosphate, and standard multivitamins is 714 mOsm/kg, 1,470 mOsm/kg, and greater than 2,000 mOsm/kg, respectively. This exceeds the 450 mOsm/kg threshold recommended by the American Academy of Pediatrics (Shah & Sinn, 2021). Therefore, slow enteral feeding advances and incremental introduction of fortification or nutritional supplements are indicated.

Some studies have shown that mixing oral medications with enteral feedings increases osmolality and risk of NEC (Atakent et al., 1984; Book et al., 1975; Mutz & Obladen, 1985; Shah & Sinn, 2021). In contrast, other studies did not find a significant difference in the incidence of NEC following administration of hyperosmolar feeds and/or medications (Latheef et al., 2021; Kim et al., 2015; Rigo et al., 2017; Singh et al., 2017). Further studies in larger cohorts are needed to better understand the osmolality threshold associated with NEC, stratified by gestational age or birth weight and day of life (Latheef et al., 2021). With such conflicting data, avoidance of enteral medications may be a reasonable consideration until adequate enteral feeding volume is achieved.

Probiotics

Probiotics are live microorganisms that can be beneficial when used in appropriate amounts; they promote gut health by limiting pathogen growth, promoting enterocyte differentiation, downregulating intestinal inflammation, and improving mucosal barrier integrity (Razak et al., 2021). The most commonly prescribed and investigated probiotics include *Bifidobacterium, Lactobacillus, Saccharomyces*, and *Streptococcus* species.

A 2020 Cochrane review of 56 RCTs that included 10,812 preterm infants showed infants who received probiotics had a lower risk of NEC (16 trials with low risk of bias including 4,597 infants, RR: 0.70, 95% CI: 0.55–0.89) among other outcomes, including reduced mortality risk (McGuire et al., 2020). However, the authors importantly noted that all studies yielded evidence of either low or moderate certainty; therefore, higher quality trials are still necessary to generalize these findings. Similarly, a 2021 meta-analysis of 30 high-quality nonrandomized studies including 77,018 infants showed reduced NEC, reduced mortality, and reduced late-onset sepsis (Deshmukh & Patole, 2021). The number needed to treat (NNT) to prevent one case of NEC ≥ stage II, late-onset sepsis, and all-cause mortality by routine probiotic supplementation was 39, 68, and 77, respectively. Despite these results, the certainty of evidence was downgraded to low quality due to limitations in study designs or the nonrandomized nature of the trials.

Although these results may favor the use of probiotics, uncertainty lingers and limits use in clinical practice (Barbian et al., 2019; Razak et al., 2021). For example, unlike pharmaceutical products, currently available probiotics are not regulated by the U.S. Food and Drug Administration (FDA) to ensure safety and efficacy (Razak et al., 2021). In addition, probiotics are considered dietary supplements and manufacturers do not guarantee the amount of bacteria or the purity of bacterial strains (Barbian et al., 2019). Importantly, there are concerns for possible systemic sepsis with the organisms present in the probiotic preparations. Supplementation with *Lactobacillus rhamnosus* GG specifically has been associated with the development of sepsis (Dani et al., 2016).

As the number of infants who need to receive supplementation to prevent a case of NEC (NNT) would be relatively high, it is reasonable to avoid the use of probiotics when the incidence or risk of NEC is low. Many clinicians remain reluctant to use probiotics until higher quality evidence is available, or probiotic manufacturing and distribution are regulated (Razak et al., 2021). Given the lack of FDA-regulated pharmaceutical-grade products in the United States, conflicting data on safety and efficacy, and potential for harm in a highly vulnerable population, current evidence does not support the routine, universal administration of probiotics to preterm infants, especially those with a birth weight of less than 1,000 grams (Poindexter & COFN, 2021). Clinicians who choose to utilize probiotics in their practice should do so with a local guideline specifying patient criteria, the exact product to be used, the prophylaxis regimen, efforts to prevent contamination, and methods of monitoring for adverse events to ensure consistent supplementation practices (Razak et al., 2021). Another potential supplementation that may optimize the preterm intestinal microbiome composition is prebiotics, nondigestible products promoting the growth of desirable commensal bacteria (Duchon et al., 2021). However, prebiotic supplementation has not been shown to reduce NEC incidence in preterm infants and is not recommended until further evidence becomes available (Duchon et al., 2021).

Avoidance of Histamine-2 Receptor Antagonists and Proton Pump Inhibitor Medications

Medications suppressing gastric acid, including H2RAs and proton pump inhibitors (PPI), have been prescribed for treatment of gastroesophageal reflux disease (GERD) and stress ulcer prophylaxis in the neonatal population (Slaughter et al., 2016). However, H2RAs and PPIs are believed to alter the intestinal microbiome by inhibiting the synthesis of gastric acids, raising gastric pH levels, and decreasing immune responses (Chandran et al., 2021). The net effect is a relative increase of bacterial species that can transfer across the mucosal layer and into the deeper layers of the intestinal wall. For these reasons, use of H2RA and PPI is associated with an increased risk of NEC (Duchon et al., 2021; N. Singh et al., 2016). Well-powered randomized trials are needed to examine the comparative effectiveness as well as the safety of these medications for use in neonatal patients. In the meantime and in the absence of a compelling indication (e.g., documented ulceration), it is reasonable to avoid the administration of antacid medications to preterm infants.

EARLY SUPPORTIVE CARE FOR NECROTIZING ENTEROCOLITIS

Early medical management of NEC involves supportive care, including bowel rest, gastric decompression, and provision of parenteral nutrition (Knell et al., 2019). Bowel (GI) rest is essential to facilitate resolution of the intestinal inflammatory process. Gastric decompression can be provided by placing an orogastric (OG) or nasogastric (NG) tube to drain any fluid or air from the stomach, therefore allowing the bowel to rest (Duchon et al., 2021; Rich & Dolgin, 2017). Obtaining central venous access, often with a peripherally inserted central catheter (PICC), is advantageous for administration of prolonged IV nutrition (e.g., parenteral nutrition) and any necessary continuous infusions such as IV vasopressors (Rich & Dolgin, 2017).

If clinically necessary, fluid resuscitation, correction of any hematologic or metabolic issues, as well as cardiac and/or respiratory support may be needed (Knell et al., 2019). Sepsis guidelines for pediatrics recommend crystalloid, rather than albumin, for the initial resuscitation of pediatric patients with septic shock or other sepsis-associated organ dysfunction (Weis et al., 2020). In the setting of symptomatic thrombocytopenia, anemia, and coagulopathy, transfusions of platelets, packed red blood cells, and fresh frozen plasma may be required, respectively (Rich & Dolgin, 2017).

Given the abdominal disease and distension that manifests secondary to NEC, most affected infants have limited pulmonary reserve and require respiratory support; this is particularly true in infants with BPD (Rich & Dolgin, 2017). Data suggest that these interventions in conjunction with use of broad-spectrum antibiotics are associated with a 60% to 80% recovery rate in patients with stage I or II NEC without the need for surgery (Berman & Moss, 2011; Knell et al., 2019).

CURRENT PHARMACOLOGIC TREATMENT MODALITIES FOR NECROTIZING ENTEROCOLITIS

Given the epidemiologic data discussed throughout this chapter, a combination of antimicrobial therapy that treats gram-positive (e.g., ampicillin, vancomycin) and gram-negative (e.g., gentamicin, ceftazidime) bacteria is indicated to treat infants with medical NEC (Duchon et al., 2021; Rich & Dolgin, 2017). The Infectious Diseases Society of America (IDSA) recommends one of three regimens for intra-abdominal infections: (a) ampicillin, gentamicin, and metronidazole; (b) ampicillin, cefotaxime/ceftazidime, and metronidazole; or (c) meropenem. However, there is no standard combination of empiric antimicrobial agents and no standard duration of treatment for NEC, specifically.

Although there is no standard combination of empiric antimicrobial agents used for NEC, ampicillin and gentamicin provide adequate coverage for stage I/II NEC. The addition of metronidazole (or substitution of meropenem or piperacillin-tazobactam with or without an aminoglycoside) is common with cases of stage III NEC. Although the aforementioned regimen (beta-lactam with or without an aminoglycoside) generally provides adequate coverage against gram-positive and gram-negative organisms, anaerobic coverage may be added in situations where a clinical response is not observed. Metronidazole, clindamycin, piperacillin-tazobactam, or meropenem offers adjunctive anaerobic coverage. Clinicians should take note that the evidence is weak for the addition of anaerobic coverage; however, clinicians continue to use anaerobic agents with preference to metronidazole over piperacillin-tazobactam, especially with cases of surgical NEC (Donà et al., 2023). Recall that previous studies have suggested there is a risk of late stricture formation from routine inclusion of anaerobic coverage in the treatment of medical NEC without necrosis or perforation (Faix et al., 1988).

Taking into consideration that concomitant bacteremia is present in up to one-third of patients with NEC (Bell et al., 1980), the choice of empiric antimicrobials should be targeted to cover organisms associated with previous infections or per region/facility-specific antibiograms (refer to Chapter 28, "Neonatal Sepsis and Meningitis"; Duchon et al., 2021). Antifungals are typically not used in cases of NEC except in instances of positive fungal cultures or in patients who are clinically worsening (Rich & Dolgin, 2017). Vancomycin may be indicated in those colonized with methicillin-resistant *S. aureus* (MRSA) or coagulase-negative staphylococci (CoNS), or if the rates of hospital-associated MRSA are concerning (Duchon et al., 2021). If MRSA or ampicillin-resistant *Enterococcus* infections are suspected, the combination regimen may be altered to vancomycin plus aminoglycoside for stage I/II NEC, with the addition of metronidazole for stage III NEC. A systematic review in 2020 (two RCTs, three observational studies including a total of 3,161 patients) did not show any antibiotics to be superior to ampicillin and gentamicin in decreasing mortality and preventing clinical deterioration (Donà et al., 2023). Although used quite frequently nationwide, the safety and efficacy of the combinations of antibiotics mentioned previously in infants with complicated intra-abdominal infections have not been established.

To fill this informational gap of antibiotic combinations, the Safety of Clindamycin, Ampicillin, Metronidazole, and Piperacillin-tazobactam (SCAMP) trial was conducted in premature infants ≤33 weeks' gestation (N = 180) with complicated intra-abdominal infections to evaluate the safety and efficacy of these antibiotic regimens when received for 10 days or less (Smith et al., 2021). The most common diagnosis in the study group was NEC (59%). Patients were exposed to either ampicillin, gentamicin, and metronidazole (group 1); ampicillin, gentamicin, and clindamycin (group 2); or piperacillin-tazobactam and gentamicin (group 3). Other/adjunctive gram-positive antibiotics (e.g., vancomycin) were prescribed at the discretion of the medical team. The authors concluded that no antibiotic regimen for intra-abdominal infections showed superiority specific to safety or mortality.

Mechanism of Action/Core Pharmacokinetic Principles

Beta-lactam antibiotics encompass penicillins, carbapenems, and cephalosporins. Commonly prescribed beta-lactam antibiotics include ampicillin and ceftazidime. In cases of multidrug-resistant Enterobacteriaceae, meropenem may be considered. Beta-lactam antibiotics disrupt bacterial cell wall synthesis. The specific mechanism that leads to this effect is best studied as a stepwise sequence of events. First, the drug molecules bind to one or more penicillin-binding proteins (PBPs). This blocks peptidoglycan units on bacterial cells from reproducing and cross-linking. As a result, bacterial cells cannot form a cell wall (Kohanski et al., 2010). A concurrent increase in autolysins, enzymes that enhance peptidoglycan turnover in favor of formation of newer peptidoglycans, occurs. This rather uncontrolled upregulation of autolysin synthesis increases bacterial cell disruption and ultimately cell death.

Ampicillin offers time-dependent pharmacodynamic activity against susceptible gram-positive and gram-negative bacteria. Ampicillin does not resist destruction by penicillinase, an extracellular enzyme that inactivates the antibiotic around it. From a pharmacokinetic standpoint, the half-life decreases as PMA increases (Rivera-Chaparro et al., 2017). Tremoulet and colleagues (2014) reported a half-life of 3.2 to 5 hours among preterm infants younger than 7 days and 2.4 to 4 hours among preterm infants ≥8 and ≤28 days of life. There are no dosage adjustments for renal impairment provided in the manufacturer's labeling; however, dosing adjustments should be considered in patients with severe impairment (Taketomo, 2023). Ampicillin is excreted largely unchanged in the urine and clearance increases with advancing gestational age, by approximately 56% in neonates greater than 34 weeks' gestation compared with those ≤34 weeks (Tremoulet et al., 2014). Generally, ampicillin is well tolerated by most patients without adverse reactions.

Piperacillin, a semisynthetic beta-lactam derived from ampicillin, is customarily prescribed in combination with tazobactam (a beta-lactamase inhibitor), yielding *piperacillin-tazobactam*. Tazobactam is paired with piperacillin for synergy against some resistant organisms as it prevents the breakdown of piperacillin by inhibiting beta-lactamase. This allows the effect of piperacillin (inhibition of bacterial cell wall synthesis). Similar to ampicillin, this drug offers time-dependent pharmacodynamic activity against gram-positive, gram-negative, and anaerobic bacteria (Rivera-Chaparro et al., 2017). This drug is FDA-approved for use in infants older than 2 months of age but not in preterm infants (Federal Drug Administration, 2007). Piperacillin-tazobactam is primarily eliminated by glomerular filtration and tubular secretion. Elimination is slow among infants compared with children and adults and clearance increases with advancing postnatal age. Although evidence is limited, this drug appears to be relatively well tolerated among preterm infants.

Aminoglycosides, namely *gentamicin*, exhibit concentration-dependent activity against gram-negative bacteria. Gentamicin is *not* effective at killing anaerobic bacteria because it requires oxygen-dependent active transport to penetrate the bacterial wall. The mechanism of action is best understood as a stepwise sequence of events. Drug molecules use oxygen-dependent active transport pathways to penetrate the bacterial wall. Next, gentamicin molecules bind to 16S RNA units in bacteria, which inhibits further bacterial protein synthesis (O'Sullivan et al., 2020). The clinical response to gentamicin is associated with the ratio of the peak concentration over the minimum inhibitory concentration (MIC) of the bacteria. Ototoxicity and nephrotoxicity have been reported, especially in those with higher than recommended trough concentrations, as well as in those who receive concomitant ototoxic and/or nephrotoxic medications. Infants with renal insufficiency are at increased risk of toxicity as gentamicin is excreted mainly unchanged in the urine; therefore, doses need to be adjusted accordingly, or gentamicin should be avoided, if renal dysfunction is severe. In these cases, a beta-lactam antibiotic with similar spectrum of activity (e.g., ceftazidime) may be substituted.

Clindamycin, first produced in 1966, is a lincosamide antibiotic. This drug is used in the treatment of gram-positive cocci (e.g., *Streptococcus*) as well as both gram-positive and gram-negative anaerobic bacteria (e.g., *Bacteroides, Clostridium*). The mechanism of action involves initial binding of drug molecules to the 50S RNA unit in bacteria. Similar to the mechanism of gentamicin, this process of binding inhibits transpeptidation, which prevents bacterial synthesis (elongation) and decreases the ability of the bacteria to adhere to other cells and tissues (Rivera-Chaparro et al., 2017). Ultimately, the bacteria are destroyed and phagocytized. Clindamycin is considered bacteriostatic, although it can be bactericidal against some strains of staphylococci, streptococci, and anaerobes. Like metronidazole, it is often used in neonates for suspected or confirmed anaerobic infections. No dose adjustments are necessary in patients with renal or hepatic impairment, although caution is warranted if used in those with severe hepatic impairment (Taketomo, 2023). Some preparations of IV clindamycin contain benzyl alcohol, and these should be avoided in neonates. Clindamycin utilization for stage III NEC has decreased significantly due to the emergence of resistant *Bacteroides* species.

Metronidazole, first produced in the 1950s for treatment of vaginal trichomoniasis, is a concentration-dependent nitroimidazole antibiotic used in the treatment of gram-negative anaerobic (e.g., *Bacteroides*) and protozoal infections (Rivera-Chapparro et al., 2017). Metronidazole has largely replaced clindamycin as the preferred anaerobic coverage for patients with stage III NEC. The mechanism of action begins when drug molecules enter the cell through passive diffusion. Next, the nitro side chain of the drug molecule undergoes chemical changes to produce a toxic nitro radical. This activates the drug and creates a concentration gradient favoring additional drug uptake within the bacteria. Finally, DNA destabilization develops, followed by apoptosis (Nagel & Aronoff, 2020). Metronidazole has excellent bioavailability; more than 90% of the drug is absorbed after enteral administration, although this route of administration is not relevant in the treatment of NEC. This drug is hepatically metabolized; therefore, dose adjustments are not necessary in infants with renal insufficiency.

Dosing Recommendations

Pharmacokinetic studies regarding antimicrobial agents in preterm neonates are rapidly emerging. Clinicians should refer to perpetually updated, evidence-based electronic tertiary references for the most recent dosing recommendations. Doses of beta-lactam and aminoglycoside antibiotics should be adjusted based on renal insufficiency; serum creatinine is a useful surrogate of renal perfusion and drug clearance. In addition to those with renal impairment, consideration should be taken in patients with underlying physiologic factors and those who may have altered drug dispositions due to critical illness (Rivera-Chaparro et al., 2017).

Clinical-Monitoring Pearls

Customary lab monitoring includes surveillance of blood urea nitrogen (BUN) and creatinine levels. Renal function should be monitored regularly in patients on ampicillin, gentamicin, or vancomycin (Rivera-Chaparro et al., 2017). Specific to gentamicin (a concentration-dependent antibiotic), high doses are administered with long intervals between doses in order to achieve the desired therapeutic effect and allow enough time for clearance to avoid nephrotoxicity (Neeli et al., 2021). This explains why trough levels (drawn prior to a dose; goal <1 mcg/mL) are essential to evaluate for toxicity and prevent further accumulation, and peak levels (drawn after a dose) are essential to evaluate for drug efficacy.

Adjustments in antimicrobial therapy should be made based on blood culture results and sensitivity data. Given advancements in real-time polymerase chain reaction (PCR) for cultures, clinicians should be familiar with the scope of this technology in their institution and the potential impact on timely de-escalation of therapy. In terms of duration of antimicrobial use, the time frame ranges from 7 to 14 days for medically managed NEC but may be longer in more complex cases of NEC requiring surgical intervention (Duchon et al., 2021).

Discharge planning should always include a hearing screening test. Many factors increase the risk of acquired hearing loss, including preterm birth, exposure to sounds exceeding 45 dB, and exposure to aminoglycosides. A recent Cochrane review estimated that infants exposed to one dose of an aminoglycoside per day, for an extended time, incur a 1.4% risk of ototoxicity ($n = 3/214$ infants; Rao et al., 2016). Excess accumulation of gentamicin is believed to elicit uptake at the renal and cochlear hair cells, and induce mitochondrial stress and apoptosis, leading to renal injury and/or hearing loss (Smits et al., 2017). Given that acquired hearing loss is more common compared with congenital hearing loss, clinicians are encouraged to consider mitigating risks as much as possible through careful therapeutic drug monitoring.

CONCLUSIONS

The exact causes of NEC in infants remain one of the most complex mysteries in neonatology and are likely multifactorial. As it has remained for decades, the medical management of NEC remains limited to supportive care and preventive measures. With no clear evidence-based consensus on antimicrobial regimens for treatment of NEC, expert consensus remains that initial antimicrobials of choice should cover the most commonly isolated pathogens. Prevention remains essential in decreasing the incidence of NEC with judicious antimicrobial stewardship, avoidance of highly osmolar agents, and optimal feeding approaches.

LEARNING TOOLS AND RESOURCES

Advice From the Authors

Van Tran, PharmD, BCPS, BCPPS, MBA

I've always loved the quote "If you're not willing to learn, no one can help you. If you're determined to learn, no one can stop you" (Zig Ziglar). Sometimes, it can be overwhelming, but remember, even the greatest of the great started where you are right now. So, take one concept at a time, learn and teach each other (because it truly does help retain and apply the information), and love what you do.

Tracy Rickard, MSN, APRN, NNP-BC

Don't ever lose a desire to learn. We are never too old, too proud, or too experienced to learn new things. Always, always know why you are giving a patient a medication and what it does to the patient!

Amy J. Jnah, DNP, APRN, NNP-BC

NEC can be such a devastating disease process. Your best ammunition is to know the pathogenesis of the disease, risk factors, and proactively appraise each patient, every shift, for NEC risk. Empower your colleagues at the bedside by teaching them about the disease, manifestations, and pharmacologic regimens. In doing so, you strengthen the team and provide excellent care to vulnerable babies!

Discussion Prompts

1. The patient you are managing is suspected of having NEC. Create a checklist of (supportive care and medical management) tasks to ensure the management of this patient is complete.
2. In addition to early supportive care, antibiotics continue to play a crucial role in the management of NEC. Create an antibiotic plan for your patient in each stage of the Bell criteria.
    a. Which antibiotic(s) or combination of antibiotics would you consider for your patient? Which organisms would you want coverage against? Create at least three different combinations. This allows for various practices and problem-solving, especially in times of drug shortages.
    b. Would your regimens vary for intact bowel versus perforated or necrotizing/ischemic NEC?
    c. How would the duration of antibiotics vary depending on the staging of NEC?
    d. If your patient has renal insufficiency, are there antibiotics you would avoid or renally adjust or monitor closely?
3. Discuss the pros and cons of probiotic use in the NICU with your pediatric pharmacist and dietitian. Then, compare your findings with the results from current studies. What new perspective can be gained from this type of scholarly inquiry?

Mind Map

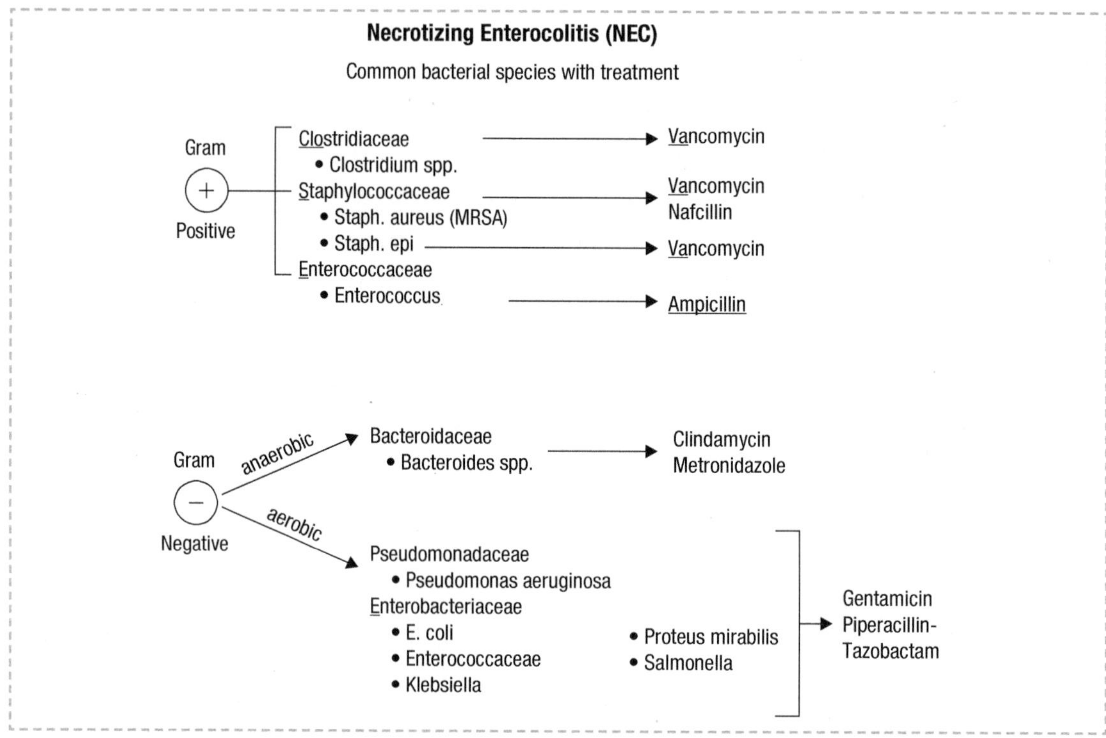

Note: This mind map reflects the design team's interpretation of a portion of one or more concepts addressed in this chapter. Readers should regard the mind maps woven throughout this textbook as examples of multisensory study tools that can be developed to encourage conceptual understanding. Readers are encouraged to develop their own unique mind maps in consultation with academic faculty or clinical preceptors.
MRSA, methicillin-resistant *Staphylococcus aureus*.
Design credit: Meredith McSwain, MSN, APRN, NNP-BC, East Carolina University College of Nursing, Neonatal Nurse Practitioner Program.

REFERENCES

References for this chapter are online and available at https://connect.springerpub.com/content/book/978-0-8261-5884-0/part/partV/toc-part/ch24.

PART VI

Common Hematopoietic and Endocrine Problems

chapter 25

Hyperbilirubinemia

Amy J. Jnah and Keliana O'Mara

LEARNING OBJECTIVES

After completing this chapter, the reader should be able to:

- Define *hyperbilirubinemia* and identify the epidemiology of its disease process.
- Enumerate the most common risk factors for indirect and direct hyperbilirubinemia.
- Explain the physiology of bilirubin metabolism.
- Correlate the pathophysiology of indirect and direct hyperbilirubinemia with the need for pharmacologic treatment.
- Appraise the historical evolution of pharmacologic management for hyperbilirubinemia.
- Evaluate the role of pharmacotherapeutic regimens with respect to pharmacodynamic and pharmacokinetic properties in relation to management/prevention of hyperbilirubinemia.

INTRODUCTION

Icterus has been observed in newborns for nearly two centuries. The earliest report of neonatal jaundice dates back to 1724, when both physicians and nurses reported cases of otherwise healthy newborns whose skin developed a yellow hue within the first few days of life (Lauer & Spector, 2011). Many of these infants developed severe hyperbilirubinemia, manifested with signs of encephalopathy, and died. Consequently, mortality risk throughout the 18th and 19th centuries was disturbingly high.

Fortunately, a novel discovery was made by Sister J. Ward, a charge nurse assigned to the premature unit at Rochford General Hospital in Essex, England, in the mid-1900s. Sister Ward was known for taking her preterm patients out onto a hospital terrace for fresh air and sunshine. Sister Ward would strip the neonates down to a diaper and let them enjoy the sun and fresh air. Not surprising, several neonates were icteric at the time and Sister Ward astutely observed that the icteric skin paled when exposed to sunlight. This single observation was the catalyst for decades of research into hyperbilirubinemia and undoubtedly saved the lives of countless preterm (and term) infants. As Drs. Dobbs and Cremer (Sister Ward's attending physicians) wrote in an editorial, her discovery prompted other questions, which led to the novel discovery that sunlight (more specifically, blue light) degraded bilirubin. We encourage you to pause and read the entirety of the Dobbs and Cremer (1975) article to obtain valuable historical perspective.

It is now widely accepted that up to 50% of full-term and 80% of preterm newborns manifest with physiologic hyperbilirubinemia after birth (Bhutani et al., 2013; Woodgate & Jardine, 2015). Given the prevalence of icterus, neonatal APRNs must remain aware of the state of the science.

Deviations from the standard of care are associated with increased risk for both short- and long-term injury, including but not limited to bilirubin-induced neurotoxicity and kernicterus, two devastating, yet *preventable*, morbidities that significantly damage the basal ganglia (Kemper et al., 2022; Maisels et al., 2012). Although the incidence of bilirubin-induced neurologic dysfunction (BIND) and kernicterus has decreased over the years, the incidence is not zero. Experts must continue to teach and reteach the basics of bilirubin metabolism and the pathogenesis of indirect and direct hyperbilirubinemia. All clinicians should maintain awareness of prophylactic and definitive pharmacotherapeutic strategies that are informed by well-powered studies.

This chapter has been carefully crafted to provide readers with a timely refresher of basic physiology specific to bilirubin metabolism. From there, we discuss the pathogenesis of both unconjugated and conjugated hyperbilirubinemia. To aid readers' ability to execute proper diagnostic reasoning in the clinical setting, common causes for unconjugated and conjugated hyperbilirubinemia are identified to aid readers' ability to execute proper diagnostic reasoning in the clinical setting. Next, we take a step back and identify seminal and other noteworthy studies that informed pharmacologic treatment of hyperbilirubinemia. Last, we present the current state of the science specific to pharmacologic treatment of unconjugated and conjugated hyperbilirubinemia. Readers are encouraged to consult the formulary in Chapter 31 as needed for additional information on pharmacotherapeutics discussed in this chapter. Learning tools and resources, provided at the end of this chapter, are offered to stimulate additional scholarly conversation both in the classroom and clinical settings, as well as encourage active learning habits for those preparing for clinical rotations or a board certification examination.

PHYSIOLOGY REVIEW: BILIRUBIN METABOLISM

Within the reticuloendothelial system, red blood cells (RBC) are broken into globin, heme, and eventually bilirubin and other by-products. This process begins with macrophages, which ingest RBCs and initiate heme catabolism. Globin and heme dissociate from one another. Globin is degraded and recycled, whereas heme is dissociated into iron (Fe2+), carbon monoxide (a catalyst), and porphyrin. Iron is preserved within the circulation. Porphyrin is further oxidized to biliverdin, and subsequently reduced to bilirubin—that bright yellow molecule that neonatal clinicians are all too familiar with. Bilirubin is not water soluble, and, as such, requires albumin for transport to the liver. Once bound to albumin, bilirubin enters the liver and detaches from albumin. Next, the enzyme uridine diphosphate glucanosyltransferase (UDP1A1) interacts with bilirubin and catalyzes the binding of bilirubin with glucuronic acid. The newly conjugated bilirubin is excreted into the biliary system, and then the intestinal tract. Normally, enzymes within the intestinal tract interact with the majority (98%) of conjugated bilirubin, converting it (by way of oxidation) to stercobilin. Stercobilin is excreted in the stool. A smaller portion (2%) of conjugated bilirubin is converted to urobilinogen, absorbed back into the bloodstream, converted (by way of oxidation) to urobilin, and excreted in the urine.

PATHOPHYSIOLOGY OF UNCONJUGATED HYPERBILIRUBINEMIA

Factors that customarily contribute to hyperbilirubinemia (Table 25.1) derange the physiologic process described in the prior section of this chapter. When a contributing factor is considered neurotoxic, a rapid and toxic accumulation of unconjugated bilirubin can develop, cross the blood-brain barrier, and threaten the infant's long-term neurologic and physical well-being.

Newborns have increased bilirubin production due to higher RBC volume per kilogram than adults, as well as a shorter RBC life span (Watson, 2009). The shorter life span of hemoglobin increases RBC catabolism and the rate of release of bilirubin into the plasma (Watson, 2009). Examples of conditions that predispose newborns to increased bilirubin production include hemolytic jaundice, polycythemia, and extravascular blood accumulation from birth trauma (Table 25.2). Most experts agree that hemolytic diseases of the newborn (e.g., ABO incompatibility, Rh isoimmunization, and glucose-6-phosphate dehydrogenase [G6PD] deficiency) pose the greatest neurotoxic threat to the newborn. A brief review of the pathophysiology of these diseases is provided.

TABLE 25.1 Contributing (Risk) Factors for Hyperbilirubinemia in Newborns

NEUROTOXIC RISK FACTORS	RISKS FOR DEVELOPING SIGNIFICANT HYPERBILIRUBINEMIA

• Albumin <3.0 g/dL
• Gestational age <38 weeks
• Hemolytic diseases of the newborn
  ◦ Rh factor incompatibility
  ◦ ABO incompatibility
  ◦ G6PD deficiency
  ◦ RBC membrane defects (e.g., hereditary spherocytosis)
• Sepsis
• Clinical instability
	• Bruising (e.g., cephalohematoma)
	• Family history (parent or sibling) of phototherapy or exchange transfusion
	• Genetic ancestry associated with risk for enzymopathy or other inherited RBC disorder (e.g., G6PD, hereditary spherocytosis)
	• Gestational age <40 weeks (risk is inversely proportional to degree of prematurity)
	• Icterus documented within the first 24 hours of life
	• Infant of a diabetic mother
	• Phototherapy required prior to discharge from birth hospitalization
	• Rate of rise (TcB or TsB) >0.3 mg/dL/hr within first 24 hours of life
	• Rate of rise (TcB or TsB) >0.2 mg/dL/hr after 24 hours of life
	• Suboptimal intake hyperbilirubinemia
	• TcB or TsB result near phototherapy threshold prior to discharge from birth hospitalization
	• Trisomy 21

Note: It is imperative that clinicians carefully review the maternal/family history to identify risk factors for the development of severe hyperbilirubinemia. In addition, a full analysis of all bilirubin test results is indicated, which includes (a) determining the phototherapy threshold for the infant based on assigned neurotoxicity risk stratification, (b) plotting the test result on the hour-specific nomogram for risk stratification and assigning the appropriate risk category, (c) identifying the threshold for exchange transfusion, and (d) ensuring that follow-up bilirubin testing aligns with standards of practice recommended by the American Academy of Pediatrics.

DAT, direct antiglobulin test; G6PD, glucose-6-phosphate dehydrogenase; RBC, red blood cell; TcB, transcutaneous bilirubin; TsB, total serum bilirubin.

Source: From Kemper, A. R., Newman, T. B., Slaughter, J. L., Maisels, M. J., Watchko, J. F., Downs, S. M., Grout, R. W., Bundy, D. G., Stark, A. R., Bogen, D. L., Holmes, A. V., Feldman-Winter, L. B., Bhutani, V. K., Brown, S. R., Maradiaga Panayotti, G. M., Okechukwu, K., Rappo, P. D., & Russell, T. L. (2022). Clinical practice guideline revision: Management of hyperbilirubinemia in the newborn infant 35 or more weeks of gestation. *Pediatrics, 150*(3), Article e2022058859. https://doi.org/10.1542/peds.2022-058859

TABLE 25.2 Common Etiologies for Pathologic Unconjugated Hyperbilirubinemia

HEMOLYTIC CAUSES	NONHEMOLYTIC CAUSES	IMPAIRED CONJUGATION

• Immune-mediated hemolysis
  ◦ Rh incompatibility
  ◦ ABO incompatibility
• RBC enzyme defects
  ◦ G6PD deficiency
• RBC membrane defects
  ◦ Hereditary spherocytosis
• Hemoglobinopathies
  ◦ Thalassemia
  ◦ Sickle cell disease
	• Extravascular blood accumulation
	  ◦ Birth trauma (cephalohematoma, subgaleal hematoma)
	• Polycythemia
	• Enterohepatic recirculation
		• Physiologic transition to extrauterine life as enzyme levels increase
		• UDP-glucanosyltransferase enzyme deficiencies (Crigler-Najjar syndrome, Gilbert syndrome)
		• Congenital hyperthyroidism
		• Breast milk jaundice

G6PD, glucose-6-phosphate dehydrogenase; RBC, red blood cell; UDP, uridine diphosphate.

Isoimmune Hemolytic Diseases

Blood type (ABO) incompatibility and Rhesus (Rh) incompatibility are the two most common causes for antibody-mediated hemolysis. It is estimated that 25% of mother/infant dyads are ABO incompatible (Pan et al., 2021). Less than 1% of affected infants undergo exchange transfusion (ET; Bhutani et al., 2013). Timely diagnosis and targeted initiation of appropriate pharmacotherapies, namely intensive phototherapy, are necessary to continue to avoid the need for ET.

ABO Incompatibility

The term *incompatible* suggests conflict or mismatch. Therefore, ABO incompatibility involves a conflict/mismatch between the mother's and fetus/newborn's blood type. Since individuals with type O blood carry both anti-A and anti-B antibodies, the infant of a mother with type O blood is considered at increased risk for ABO incompatibility, postnatal hemolysis, hyperbilirubinemia, and mild anemia. To facilitate early identification of this blood type incompatibility, cord blood sampling is performed to determine the newborn's blood type. Targeted pharmacotherapy, discussed in detail later in this chapter, customarily involves the use of phototherapy to facilitate rapid extrahepatic removal of excess unconjugated bilirubin deposited in the tissues and, in rare cases, ET, to reduce circulating maternal anti-A or anti-B antibodies. In some cases when total serum bilirubin levels are rising at a rate of greater than 0.2 mg/dL per hour despite intensive phototherapy, or measured levels are within 2 to 3 mg/dL of the threshold for ET, intravenous immune globulin (IVIg) may be prescribed (Hansen & Watchko, 2019).

Rh Disease

Rh hemolytic disease, a consequence of alloimmunization, is now rarely reported because of postpartum administration of Rho(D) immune globulin (RhoGAM) to Rh-negative mothers. With Rh hemolytic disease, antigenic fetal blood group factors are passed from the father to the fetus. These antigenic factors pass through the umbilical vein and enter the maternal circulation, usually secondary to a fetal–maternal hemorrhage, and elicit an immune response in the mother. Maternal immunoglobulin G (IgG) antibodies, referred to as *anti-Rh antibodies*, are produced after the exposure to the Rh-positive fetal blood, enter the fetal circulation, and elicit hemolysis. Increased production of fetal erythroblasts during pregnancy can lead to erythroblastosis fetalis, which is fatal if untreated. Most cases involve the D antigen, which explains the use of anti-D IgG during pregnancy. RhoGAM has successfully reduced the incidence of alloimmunization from 13% to 16% to 0.13 to 0.2% (de Haas et al., 2014).

Targeted pharmacotherapies may include fetal blood transfusions (to reduce or totally suppress fetal erythropoiesis), postnatal phototherapy, intravenous immunoglobulin (IVIg), and ET. Phototherapy facilitates bilirubin excretion, IVIg is thought to decrease the rate of hemolysis by blocking Fc receptor sites within the reticuloendothelial system, and ET removes unconjugated bilirubin and maternal anti-Rh antibodies, which decreases the rate of hemolysis.

Glucose-6-Phosphate Dehydrogenase Deficiency

The enzyme G6PD was first discovered in 1932 by scientists Walter Christian and Otto Warburg. From there, scientists identified the G6PD enzyme on all human cells, including RBCs. An X-linked recessive disorder that more frequently affects males, G6PD deficiency involves reduced levels of this antioxidant enzyme. The G6PD enzyme is a critical component of the pentose phosphate pathway, a pathway that produces nicotinamide adenine dinucleotide phosphate (NADPH). NADPH protects RBCs from oxidative damage (and hemolysis). Therefore, a deficiency leaves RBCs vulnerable to oxidative damage, lysis, and acute hemolysis.

There are currently 186 known G6PD mutations; the A- and Mediterranean mutations are most common (Minucci et al., 2012). Disease prevalence varies, but generally speaking, infants of East and Southeast Asian descent are up to 29% likely to carry the G6PD gene mutation. The prevalence of malaria in Southeast Asia explains the high prevalence of G6PD-deficient individuals in this geographic region, given the potential protection against life-threatening disease in affected individuals (Flatz et al., 1963; Iwai et al., 2001; Nuchprayoon et al., 2002). Infants of Sub-Saharan African, Mediterranean, Middle Eastern, and Arabian descent are also considered at increased risk for this disease (Kemper et al., 2022). More specifically, African American males incur a 13% risk for G6PD, whereas African American females incur a 4% risk for the disease (Kemper et al., 2022).

It is important to recognize that confirmatory diagnosis of G6PD deficiency requires selective allele–allele testing, which can take several days to report. Therefore, neonatal APRNs must thoroughly review the maternal history and the newborn's clinical presentation to quickly identify the at-risk infant. For example, newborns who require phototherapy during the birth hospitalization, formula-fed infants with hyperbilirubinemia (an atypical presentation), or infants who manifest with late-onset hyperbilirubinemia should be considered at risk for G6PD deficiency (Kemper et al., 2022). In many cases, acute infection (e.g., urinary tract infection) can trigger rapid hemolysis and severe hyperbilirubinemia, which can develop during the birth hospitalization in an infant requiring intermediate or intensive care, or after discharge in a late preterm or term newborn discharged within the first 24 to 72 hours after birth. Targeted pharmacotherapies discussed later in this chapter include phototherapy, IVIg, and ET.

PATHOPHYSIOLOGY OF CONJUGATED HYPERBILIRUBINEMIA

Conjugated hyperbilirubinemia, or cholestatic liver disease, manifests as decreased canalicular bile flow (Watson, 2009). Biliary atresia is the most common extrahepatic cause for cholestasis and affects approximately one per 1,2000 live births (Zagory et al., 2015). Bile is unable to flow from the liver, through the biliary tree, and into the intestinal tract due to a blockage (atresia) of bile flow within the biliary tree. Progressively worsening sclerosis within these extrahepatic bile ducts creates the obstructive state. In cases that involve both intra- and extrahepatic occlusion of bile ducts, concomitant congenital cytomegalovirus is often suspected. Other etiologies, including prolonged use of parenteral nutrition, sepsis, congenital malformations that affect the biliary system, and idiopathic neonatal hepatitis, are summarized in Table 25.3 (Niemi, 2020; Suchy, 2004; Watson, 2009).

Occasionally, cholestasis is considered a transient, "physiologic" state because infants born prematurely present with immature hepatic enzyme function, which matures over time. Among infants with pathologic cholestasis, the pathogenesis involves failed bilirubin excretion and a consequential accumulation of bile acids and cholesterol within the blood and extrahepatic tissues (Watson, 2009). Because conjugated bilirubin is inadequately delivered to the gastrointestinal tract, a deficiency of bile salts is observed. This inhibits the absorption of essential fats and fat-soluble vitamins (A, D, E, K). Affected infants initially manifest with jaundice, dark-colored urine, and acholic stools. Prolonged disease states include the development of fat-soluble vitamin deficiencies and poor growth velocity. Severe cases are associated with liver fibrosis and cirrhosis, portal hypertension, and ascites. We discuss the use of targeted vitamin pharmacotherapies later in this chapter.

HISTORICAL PERSPECTIVE: SEMINAL AND OTHER NOTEWORTHY STUDIES

Several pivotal studies helped shape our ability to identify, diagnose, and initiate evidence-guided pharmacotherapies for infants with hyperbilirubinemia. Identifying these landmark studies offers unique insight into the genesis of scientific inquiries into hyperbilirubinemia and the evolution of the state of the science. Some therapies, namely phototherapy and ET, remain in use today. Other prospects, including probiotic supplementation and tin metalloporphyrin, did not significantly reduce the duration of phototherapy or effectively modulate bilirubin production. Neither therapy is recommended for use in the United States.

TABLE 25.3 Common Etiologies for Pathologic Conjugated Hyperbilirubinemia

INTRAHEPATIC ETIOLOGIES	EXTRAHEPATIC ETIOLOGIES

• Genetic disorders
  ◦ Alagille syndrome
• Metabolic and endocrine disorders
  ◦ Galactosemia
  ◦ Hypopituitarism
  ◦ Hypothyroidism
  ◦ Tyrosinemia
• Neonatal lupus
• Prolonged parenteral nutrition
• Short gut syndrome
• Viral or bacterial infection
  ◦ Cytomegalovirus
  ◦ Herpes simplex virus
  ◦ HIV
	• Biliary atresia
	• Choledochal cysts
	• Cystic fibrosis
	• Gallstones
	• Mucus plugging

Sources: From Pace, E. J., Brown, C. M., & DeGeorge, K. C. (2019). Neonatal hyperbilirubinemia: An evidence-based approach. *The Journal of Family Practice, 68*(1), E4–E11. https://www.mdedge.com/familymedicine/article/193251/pediatrics/neonatal-hyperbilirubinemia-evidence-based-approach; Suchy, F. J. (2004). Neonatal cholestasis. *Pediatrics in Review, 25*(11), 388–396. https://doi.org/10.1542/pir.25-11-388; Watson, R. L. (2009). Hyperbilirubinemia. *Critical Care Nursing Clinics of North America, 21*(1), 97–120. https://doi.org/10.1016/j.ccell.2008.11.001

Exchange Transfusion

The safety of ET is well documented in the literature. One of the first (if not the very first) report of mortality secondary to severe hyperbilirubinemia dates back to the 18th century. In a letter to Dr. Hans Sloane, physician to King George II, Dr. W. H. Cheselden makes a plea for help for a newborn:

> At the request of a patient of mine, I give you the following short account. The case of the gentlewoman has been very extraordinary. She has had the misfortune to lose three fine boys who came into the world with very healthful symptoms for the first 2 days and then the strongest signs of icterus appeared, the epidermis being all over tinctured alike, which bad symptoms provide most certainly mortal in a few days … I hope that you'll be so good as to put this lady into a more successful method, which I do assure you will give a great deal of satisfaction to. (Smith, 2023)

Dr. Cheselden's letter illuminates the helplessness and desperation felt by physicians forced to practice medicine in the absence of adequate evidence. In this example, Dr. Cheselden knew a pathologic process was responsible for the infant's mortality but did not have current evidence or resources to investigate the phenomenon. For the next 200 years, and in the absence of research, numerous other physicians struggled to make sense of the pathogenesis of severe Rh isoimmunization and hemolytic disease of the newborn (HDN).

Finally, in 1924 came the ET, the first major breakthrough in the treatment of severe hyperbilirubinemia. The first neonatal ET was performed in Toronto, Canada, on December 18, 1924. Dr. Alfred Hart, a physician overseeing the care of an infant with (undiagnosed) Rhesus factor positive (Rh+) isoimmune disease, reported the need for a "drastic" intervention capable of removing an "unknown toxin circulating in the blood." He wrote the following:

> The baby was a perfectly healthy, fine specimen of male child weighing between 8 and 9 lb. The family history, however, was so remarkable that one was prepared for trouble. As the father informed me, they had had six boys born previously, all apparently as healthy and strong at birth as this baby. They all, however, had developed jaundice within the first 24 hours, and the condition had become progressively worse until death occurred in from 3 to 11 days. (Hart, 1924, as cited in Dunn, 1993, p. 95)

Dr. Hart concluded that an "exsanguination transfusion" was a necessary life-saving procedure. His technique modeled that of Dr. Bruce Robertson, the physician credited with inventing this procedure during his service with the Canadian Army during WWI (1914–1918). Dr. Hart began by withdrawing approximately 100 to 250 mL of blood from the superior sagittal sinus of the affected newborn. Then, he performed a cutdown procedure at the ankle and transfused approximately 335 mL, donated by the infant's father, into the left saphenous vein. While this primitive technique increased survival rates, cases of kernicterus and associated intellectual disability persisted because an insufficient quantity of Rh-positive (D) cells was removed prior to the ET. Scientists and clinicians did not yet recognize that removal of Rh-positive (D) cells slows hemolysis and helps prevent migration of indirect bilirubin across the blood-brain barrier.

This changed in 1945, when Dr. Harry Wallerstein performed an ET on a newborn with erythroblastosis fetalis, whose mother had an Rh antibody titer on record of 1:1,024 (Pochedly, 1970). Wallerstein began by infusing isotonic sodium chloride by way of a peripheral intravenous catheter. Next, he inserted a 19-gauge needle into the anterior fontanelle and withdrew approximately 50 to 60 mL of blood. Then, Wallerstein transfused Rh-negative blood through the peripheral catheter and continued this procedure until the volume of blood transfused exceeded that which was withdrawn (by approximately 75–100 mL).

In the years that followed, Wallerstein's method was aborted due to the significant risks associated with puncturing at the anterior fontanelle. Rather, scientists investigated alternative procedural techniques. Wiener and Wexler (1946) used the saphenous vein to inject donor blood and radial artery for the removal of blood. Both access points were established using a cutdown procedure. Blood that was removed was poured into medicine glasses and measured. Next, in 1951, L. K. Diamond and colleagues introduced use of the umbilical vessels. The first procedure involved the use of needles; one needle was inserted into an umbilical vessel and used to withdraw blood while a second needle was inserted into a different vessel and used to transfuse blood. Given the complexity of this method, needles were replaced with rubber catheters. Then, the rubber catheters were replaced by the use of one polyethylene catheter. Blood was withdrawn and then transfused using that same catheter (Pochedly, 1970).

In 1967, Mammen published a retrospective review of 27 ETs and concluded that the following factors were essential to a successful ET: (a) O negative cross-matched blood, (b) transparent umbilical catheter to facilitate identification of air bubbles, (c) stepwise removal of small aliquots of neonatal blood followed by the administration of comparable aliquot of donated blood, and (d) monitoring of serum calcium levels throughout the procedure.

The next novel discovery was made as scientists focused on the stepwise removal of neonatal blood and administration of donated blood: one double volume exchange transfusion (DVET) cleared approximately 90% of neonatal RBCs and reduced unconjugated bilirubin levels by 50% (Mammen, 1967). Finally, the medical and nursing community had a quantifiable outcome measure.

Scientists then directed attention to infectious, immunologic, and other risks associated with ET. Grajwer and colleagues (1976) investigated the use of fresh whole blood (<5 days old) versus frozen erythrocytes diluted in plasma. Freeze-preserved erythrocytes offered increased shelf-life, preservation of 2,3-diphosphoglycerate (DPG) levels, rare blood type availability, and inventory control. Given that freeze-preserved red cells had to be thawed and washed, all leukocytes, platelets, antigens, and antibodies were also removed during this process (Grajwer et al., 1976). Disadvantages included increased costs and the risk for bacterial contamination during thawing, cleansing, and preparation (Grajwer et al., 1976). Barnard and colleagues (1977) analyzed fresh blood, 4-day-old stored blood, and reconstituted blood from 4-day-old packed cells and fresh frozen plasma. Their results introduced the use of dacron wool microfilters, which removed microaggregates from donated, prepared blood. In 1984, Setzer and colleagues investigated the relationship between ET and hyperkalemia. The team reported a significant decrease in mean plasma potassium concentrations after washing red cells (18.6 ± 8.8 mEq/L vs. 1.6 ± 0.7 mEq/L, respectively).

By 1987, the American Association of Blood Banks (AABB) published standards that required hospital blood banks to prepare plasma-reduced whole blood or packed red blood cells reconstituted with plasma, with or without the addition of citrate phosphate dextrose for anticoagulation. The blood had to be fresh (<7 days preferred), leukocyte-depleted, with a hematocrit between 45% to 60%, negative for viruses, including HIV, hepatitis B virus and cytomegalovirus, and preferably irradiated to prevent graft-versus-host disease (Holland & Schmidt, 1987). These developments were promising, given the significant risks associated with ET.

Around the same time that the AABB published standards for the ET, research was accumulating specific to phototherapy as a first-line therapy. Brown and colleagues (1985) investigated the efficacy of phototherapy as a first-line therapy for hyperbilirubinemia compared to ET. Among infants less than 2,000 grams at birth, 4.8% of infants who received phototherapy went on to require an ET, whereas 23.9% of infants who did not receive phototherapy required an ET (p <.001). Phototherapy seemed to significantly decrease the need for ET among infants with birth weight of 2,000 to 2,499 grams (4.3% vs. 25.4%, p =.001). Among term infants with hemolytic disease, early initiation of phototherapy was believed to optimize the efficacy of ET.

In 2004, the American Academy of Pediatrics (AAP) outlined other significant risks with ET, including death (3/1,000 procedures), apnea, bradycardia, cyanosis, vasospasm, thrombosis, necrotizing enterocolitis (NEC), hypoxic–ischemic encephalopathy, and AIDS (AAP, 2004). In 2006, Nasseri and colleagues investigated the use of IVIg in infants with ABO and Rh isoimmunization; combination use of IVIg with phototherapy was associated with decreases in unconjugated bilirubin levels, further marginalizing the use of ET. Chitty and colleagues (2013) associated ET with an increased need for endotracheal intubation and mechanical ventilation, two procedures that also impose risks on ill neonates. Zwiers and colleagues (2018) reported adverse effects, including thrombocytopenia, hypocalcemia, hypokalemia, pulmonary hemorrhage, sepsis, NEC, intraventricular hemorrhage, and seizures (Zwiers et al., 2018). The risk for severe adverse effects ranged from 3% to 10%; less severe adverse effects are linked to as many as 74% of ETs (Zwiers et al., 2018). Generally, over the past 50 years, mortality risk linked to ET has ranged between 0.53% and 4.7% (Badiee, 2007; Boggs & Westphal, 1960; Guaran et al., 1992; Jackson, 1997; Keenan et al., 1985; Panagopoulos et al., 1969; Patra et al., 2004).

More recently, Wolf and colleagues (2020) published results of a retrospective multicenter cohort study that characterized the prevalence of ET among 1,247,425 infants born between 1997 and 2016. The incidence of ET decreased from 0.3% to 0.05%over the 9-year study period, whereas the incidence of phototherapy and IVIg therapy increased. ET-associated mortality risk was greatest among infants 29 weeks of gestation or younger compared to term infants (adjusted odds ratio [OR]: 20.08, 95% confidence interval [CI]: 7.32 - 55.07]).

In summary, nearly 100 years have elapsed since the first ET was performed on a newborn with hemolytic disease. Thanks to a century of research, we are now well aware of the risks and benefits associated with ET and have outstanding quality-control processes in place to provide high-quality blood products to neonates. Neonatal clinicians should make every attempt to discuss those risks, benefits, and prognostics with the family, before initiating what is often an urgent, time-sensitive, and "life and limb" pharmacotherapy.

Phototherapy

Leave it to a nurse (Sister J. Ward) to exhibit the extraordinary deductive reasoning necessary to stimulate scientific inquiry and save countless lives! The story of phototherapy as a therapy for icterus began in the summer of 1956, as alluded to earlier in this chapter. Nurse Ward anecdotally reported the novel observation that skin of premature infants exposed to sunlight became paler compared to areas covered by a diaper (Hansen et al., 2020). This observation prompted the physician team of Drs. R. J. Cremer, P. W. Perryman, and D. H. Richards to investigate (albeit without the rigor we are accustomed to at present) the influence of (*sun*)light on unconjugated bilirubin. Naked preterm infants were placed into direct *sun*light, eyes covered with plastic shields, for approximately 20 consecutive minutes. Postintervention total bilirubin measurements were lower than pretherapy measurements. Further, a dose–response relationship was identified and reported as follows: "the longer the exposure time, the greater the fall in serum bilirubin" (Hansen et al., 2020, p. 1096). This discovery led to the invention of the first inpatient (indoor) *photon* light (phototherapy) device, an adjustable hemicylindrical stainless steel apparatus affixed with eight blue fluorescent 40-watt tubes which emitted 420 to 480 mμ (Figure 25.1). The height of the apparatus was adjusted solely to maintain euthermia among treated neonates and not (yet) to maintain a certain irradiance.

Thanks to this research, nearly one thousand icteric infants born in the United Kingdom were treated with phototherapy between 1958 and 1967; no adverse effects were reported. American pediatricians were certainly aware of UK successes, but clinical equipoise in the United States slowed the adoption of phototherapy for nearly another decade. According to Dr. Maisels, who wrote about his lived experience during this very time frame, hundreds of ETs were performed during his pediatric residency (early 1960s) with no discussion of phototherapy (Maisels, 2001).

In 1968, results of the first randomized controlled trial (RCT) using phototherapy in the United States confirmed the efficacy of phototherapy as a therapy for hyperbilirubinemia of prematurity (Lucey et al., 1968). Further, this research paved the way for modifications to the phototherapy apparatus, to include ten 20-watt bulbs (Figure 25.2). Finally, in the words of Dr. Maisels, "phototherapy had arrived" (p. S93)! Numerous studies followed, which confirmed the efficacy of the blue-green phototherapy light spectrum. By 1985, Brown and colleagues discovered that early (prophylactic) phototherapy (initiated at 24 ± 12 hours of life) effectively prevented hyperbilirubinemia among infants less than 2,000 grams at birth (p <.001). Decades of additional research followed, which confirmed these findings, firmly establishing phototherapy as the first-line standard of practice for prophylaxis and treatment of indirect hyperbilirubinemia (Ahlfors et al., 2007; Bender et al., 2007; Morris et al., 2008; Oh et al., 2010).

Exogenous Albumin Therapy

Recall that adequate circulating albumin levels are necessary to optimize bilirubin binding and transport to the liver for conjugation and later excretion. This begged the question: Could exogenous albumin dosing expedite resolution of the disease process? Early studies favored adjunctive exogenous albumin therapy. Tsau and colleagues (1972) and Brodersen and Hansen (1977) reported that 1 g/kg of exogenous albumin dosing adequately increased albumin reserve and, thus, provided additional binding sites for unconjugated bilirubin. Hosono and colleagues (2001) reported similar outcomes and illuminated a mathematic relationship between albumin and unconjugated bilirubin: 1 g of albumin could bind with 8.3 mg/dL of unconjugated bilirubin. In other words, a neonate with a serum albumin concentration of 3.0 mg/dL could bind approximately 24.9 mg/dL

FIGURE 25.1 First phototherapy chamber used in the United States.

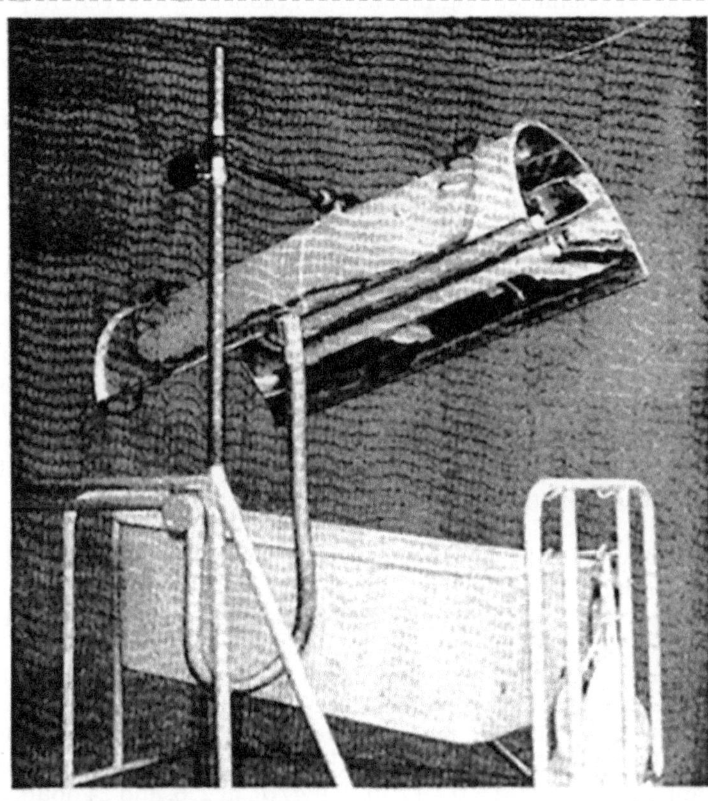

Source: From Cremer, R. J., Perryman, P. W., & Richards, D. H. (1958). Influence of light on the hyperbilirubinaemia of infants. *The Lancet, 1*(7030), 1094–1097. https://doi.org/10.1016/s0140-6736(58)91849-x

FIGURE 25.2 Second phototherapy light chamber used in the United States.

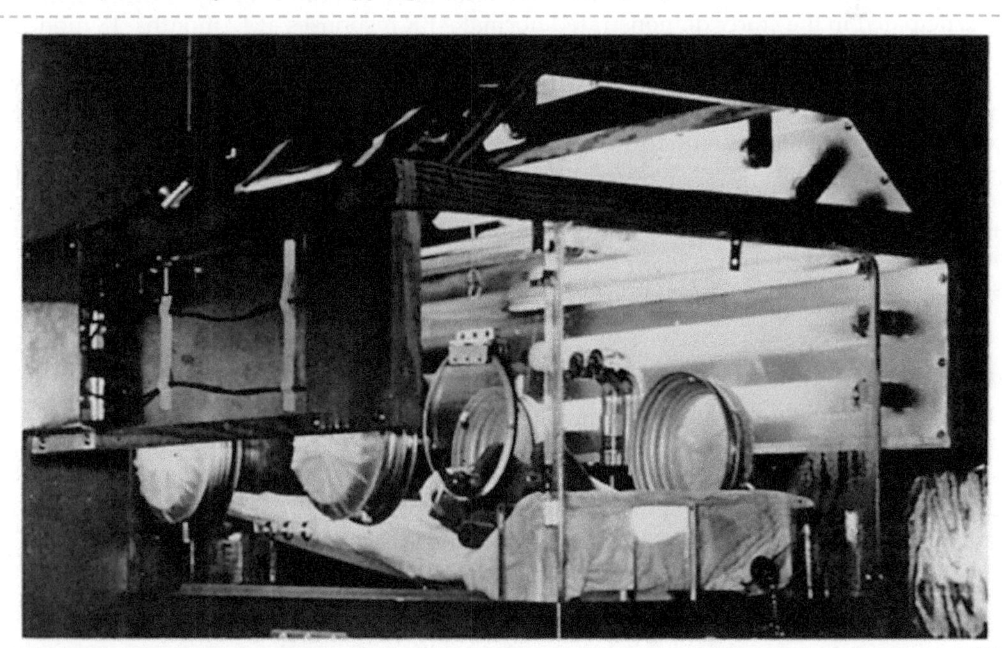

Source: From Lucey, J., Ferriero, M., & Hewitt, J. (1968). Prevention of hyperbilirubinemia of prematurity by phototherapy. *Pediatrics, 41*(6), 1047–1054. https://doi.org/10.1542/peds.41.6.1047

of bilirubin. As a result of these and other studies, numerous neonatology groups subscribed to the provision of exogenous albumin among infants with moderate to severe hyperbilirubinemia. In fact, this author (Dr. Jnah) recalls drawing up and administering albumin to icteric neonates while serving as a commissioned U.S. Navy Nurse Corps Officer at Naval Medical Center Portsmouth, Virginia (1994–1996).

Around the same time that these albumin-binding studies were underway, other scientists began investigating combination therapies, including (a) albumin administration with phototherapy and (b) albumin administration with ET. Theoretically, scientists believed that ET would increase bilirubin binding capacity because plasma albumin in adult (donor) blood has a greater binding capability compared to neonatal albumin (Cepeda & Shankaran, 1985). Therefore, researchers questioned the efficacy of a "loading dose" of albumin to be administered prior to an ET. In a case series of three patients, Ruys and Van Gelderen (1962) observed a temporary increase in blood volume when albumin was administered prior to an ET, increasing the risk for overload syndrome. Researchers suggested that risks may exceed any possible benefits (Ruys & Van Gelderen, 1962). Additional conflicting data were reported over the years; some studies reported that bilirubin levels decreased more slowly in infants who received combination therapy versus phototherapy only, whereas other studies reported opposing conclusions (Cepeda & Shankaran, 1985; Chan et al., 1971; Porto et al., 1969). Finally, in 1985, the landmark National Institute of Child Health and Human Development (NICHD) phototherapy study offered much needed clarity. To eliminate methodologic variabilities observed in prior studies, the NICHD team used the two laboratory testing methods (1-[4-hydroxyazobenzene] benzoic acid [HBABA] dye binding and sephadex G-25 gel column chromatography) singularly reported in other trials. Therefore, each blood specimen was subject to both testing methods and researchers were able to conclude that combination therapy did not significantly affect bilirubin-albumin binding.

In 2001, Hosono and colleagues (2001) published results of data collected between 1988 and 1998, which in part reaffirmed findings from the 1985 NICHD phototherapy study. The team also investigated outcomes of combination therapy. Interestingly, infants who received phototherapy in combination with albumin presented with higher serum bilirubin levels compared to infants who received phototherapy only ($M = 0.4 +/-0.19$ mg/dL at 2, 6, and 24 hours postalbumin treatment; $p < .01$); albumin therapy seemed to liberate additional bilirubin formerly sequestered to the tissues and facilitated its transport to the liver. Then, the research team went on to follow the infants for 2 additional years to assess auditory brainstem response (ABR) test results. Hosono and colleagues (2002) reported a significant decrease in the incidence of abnormal ABR test results in infants who received both phototherapy and albumin at 6 months of age; however, all infants who participated in the study demonstrated normal ABR responses at 12 months, 18 months, and 2 years of age (Hosono et al., 2002).

More recently, Magai and colleagues (2019) reported no difference in serum bilirubin levels in infants who received combination phototherapy and albumin therapy versus those who received phototherapy and fluid resuscitation (Magai et al., 2019). There were also no significant differences in need for ET, repeat phototherapy, death, and discharge. Developmental outcomes among infants randomized to either arm of the study were similar at 12 months of age (Magai et al., 2019). As a result of these seminal studies and other case reports, albumin supplementation *was not recommended* by the AAP (2004) and albumin supplementation was not included as a part of the revised AAP (Kemper et al., 2022) clinical practice guideline.

Intravenous Immune Globulin

Our historic look at IVIg is focused on the use of this drug in infants with isoimmune hemolytic diseases. Recall from our earlier physiology discussion that macrophages mediate the destruction of red cells. Drugs that can reduce the rate of hemolysis slow the rate of rise of unconjugated bilirubin in the plasma, giving more time for intensive phototherapy to exert a therapeutic effect. IVIg is thought to reduce the rate of hemolysis by blocking Fc-receptors on macrophages.

Nearly 60 years ago, Rewald and Suringar (1965) published one of the first case reports of six fetal deaths linked to Rh incompatibility. Three years later, Rewald and Lora (1968) reported the use of high-dose IVIg to the same women during their subsequent pregnancies. Five out of the six women went on to deliver healthy newborns. These and other reports of successful IVIg administration in pregnant women prompted neonatal clinicians to adopt IVIg use (in the absence of high-quality outcomes data) in newborns with isoimmune hemolytic disease and worsening hyperbilirubinemia refractory to aggressive phototherapy.

Two decades later, Sato and colleagues (1991) and Rübo and colleagues (1992) reported seminal results of IVIg administration to neonates with isoimmune hemolytic disease; IVIg significantly slowed the rate of rise of serum unconjugated bilirubin and, more specifically, did so for a span of 24 to 48 hours. Sato and colleagues (1991) administered IVIg (1 g/kg) over 6 to 8 hours with concurrent administration of double phototherapy. Rübo and colleagues (1992) designed an RCT: Infants randomized to the intervention arm were treated with 10 mL/kg of IVIg administered over 2 hours. Researchers noted a significant difference in the need for ETs between the control group and interventional group (69% ET rate in control group vs. 12.5% ET rate in the intervention group, $p = .003$).

The first Cochrane review was published by Alcock and Liley (2002). The authors considered the results of three of the seven RCTs or quasi-RCTs in circulation at the time. Although the rate of ET decreased in infants treated with IVIg (typical relative risk [RR]: 0.28, 95% CI: 0.17–0.47; typical risk difference [RD]: −0.37, 95% CI: −0.49 to −0.26; number needed to treat [NNT] 2.7), study quality was poor and generalizability limited. Contrary to clinical practice at the time, the authors did not recommend IVIg use.

Gottstein and Cooke (2003) published the second Cochrane review of IVIg use in neonates with isoimmune hemolytic disease. Like the Soto and colleagues (1991) and Rübo and colleagues (1992) studies, the authors concluded that IVIg slowed the rate of rise of serum unconjugated bilirubin levels, reducing the need for ET and even shortening the total number of hours of phototherapy. No adverse effects were reported. Further, the authors calculated the NNT to be quite low, at 2.7 (95% CI: 2.0–3.8). The authors concluded that a delay in the widespread adoption of IVIg (0.5–1 g/kg) in combination with phototherapy for the treatment of isoimmune hemolytic disease was arguably unethical (Gottstein & Cooke, 2003).

Two years later, in 2004, the AAP critically appraised the evidence in 75 publications and published the first clinical practice guidelines for managing hyperbilirubinemia in infants at 35 or more weeks of gestation (AAP Subcommittee on Hyperbilirubinemia, 2004). More specifically, IVIg (0.5–1 g/kg over 2 hours, and every 12 hours, as needed) was recommended for infants with isoimmune hemolytic disease whose serum unconjugated bilirubin levels were increasing despite the use of intensive phototherapy (blue–green light spectrum, 430–490 nm, irradiance of at least 30 watts per microW/cm^2 per nm, over maximum body surface area).

PHARMACOTHERAPIES THAT DISPLACE BILIRUBIN

Although numerous research teams focused on studying treatment regimens for hyperbilirubinemia, other teams sought to better understand whether pharmacotherapies could displace bilirubin from albumin binding sites. In 1961, Nyhan linked sulfonamide antibiotics with bilirubin displacement from albumin binding sites and kernicterus in premature neonates (Nyhan, 1961). In 1988, Wadsworth and Suh expanded on Nyhan's work by exploring plasma protein binding and bilirubin displacement in 52 antibiotics. Variable levels (high, intermediate, low) of bilirubin displacement were reported with the administration of oxacillin, cefotaxime, ceftriaxone, gentamicin, and clindamycin, antibiotics commonly administered to septic or potentially septic neonates (Table 25.4; Wadsworth & Suh, 1988). Most of the sulfonamides, with the exception of sulfamethoxine, demonstrated high levels of bilirubin displacement (Wadsworth & Suh, 1988). In fact, one particular antibiotic, ceftriaxone, significantly and critically displaced bilirubin from albumin. This discovery led to a 2007 combined Food and Drug Administration (FDA) and Roche Laboratories advisory statement cautioning providers against prescribing ceftriaxone in newborns. Antibiotics demonstrating an intermediate level of bilirubin displacement included nafcillin, cefoxitin, imipenem, vancomycin, cephalexin, and erythromycin (Wadsworth & Suh, 1988). Last, cefazolin, amoxicillin, cefuroxime, penicillin G, amikacin, and aminoglycosides displaced bilirubin at low levels (Wadsworth & Suh, 1988). Between 1982 and 2017, additional studies linked drugs, including ibuprofen and diuretics (i.e., bumetanide, furosemide), to bilirubin displacement (Ahlfors & Wennberg, 2004; Cooper-Peel et al., 1996; Mitra & Rennie, 2017). These landmark discoveries help frame current clinical decision-making and prescriptive practices, most notably among jaundiced newborn infants.

TABLE 25.4 Antibiotics Known to Displace Bilirubin From Albumin

HIGH RISK	INTERMEDIATE RISK	LOW RISK
Sulfonamides	Nafcillin	Cefazolin
Ceftriaxone	Cefoxitin	Amoxicillin
	Imipenem	Cefuroxime
	Vancomycin	Penicillin G
	Cephalexin	Amikacin
	Erythromycin	Aminoglycosides

Sources: From Ahlfors, C. E., & Wennberg, R. P. (2004). Bilirubin-albumin binding and neonatal jaundice. *Seminars in Perinatology, 28*(5), 334–339. https://doi.org/10.1053/j.semperi.2004.09.002; Cooper-Peel, C., Brodersen, R., & Robertson, A. (1996). Does ibuprofen affect bilirubin-albumin binding in newborn infant serum?. *Pharmacology & Toxicology, 79*(6), 297–299. https://doi.org/10.1111/j.1600-0773.1996.tb00012.x; Mitra, S., & Rennie, J. (2017). Neonatal jaundice: Aetiology, diagnosis and treatment. *British Journal of Hospital Medicine, 78*(12), 699–704. https://doi.org/10.12968/hmed.2017.78.12.699; Nyhan, W. L. (1961). Toxicity of drugs in the neonatal period. *The Journal of Pediatrics, 59*(1), 1–20. https://doi.org/10.1016/S0022-3476(61)80204-7; Wadsworth, S. J., & Suh, B. (1988). In vitro displacement of bilirubin by antibiotics and 2-hydroxybenzoylglycine in newborns. *Antimicrobial Agents and Chemotherapy, 32*(10), 1571–1575. https://doi.org/10.1128/AAC.32.10.1571

CURRENT PHARMACOLOGIC TREATMENT MODALITIES FOR UNCONJUGATED HYPERBILIRUBINEMIA

From an economic lens, hospital costs average $21,556 for infants who require treatment for hemolytic disease compared to $12,986 for infants who do not (Yu et al., 2019). More broadly, therapies for hemolytic hyperbilirubinemia cost approximately $271.9 million per year in comparison to the $177 million in costs for newborns without hyperbilirubinemia (Yu et al., 2019).

Pharmacologic management of unconjugated hyperbilirubinemia is often prescribed in partnership with phototherapy. Therapeutic goals are aimed at decreasing serum bilirubin levels and preventing the development of bilirubin-associated neurodevelopmental sequelae. In addition, management should avoid unintended harms, including inducing maternal anxiety, decreased breastfeeding, and unnecessary treatment or costs (Kemper et al., 2022). Current recommendations specific to these common pharmacotherapeutic regimens are discussed in this section of the chapter.

Phototherapy

Phototherapy remains the first-line therapy for the management of elevated bilirubin, a rapid rise in indirect bilirubin (>0.2 mg/dL per hour), or for newborns who absolutely need a timely initiation of phototherapy (Hansen et al., 2020). Phototherapy is a biomolecular process that ushers toxic bilirubin molecules to elimination pathways without the need for hepatic conjugation. In most circumstances, properly administered intensive phototherapy (≥30 microW/cm^2 at wavelength 475 nm) can prevent bilirubin-induced neurologic disorder (BIND) and kernicterus; however, a lack of ethically designed scientific trials has made it difficult to quantify this relationship.

MECHANISM OF ACTION/PHARMACOKINETIC PRINCIPLES

Phototherapy should be considered a drug. Similar to drug molecules, a dose of photons of energy is prescribed and emitted from a phototherapy device. This induces photochemical reactions that occur within seconds as the blue–green light diffuses into the epidermis, dermis, and small proportion of subdermal skin layers (Figure 25.3). Next, unbound bilirubin molecules absorb the blue-light therapy. At the proper dose, an irradiance of 30 to 45 microW/cm^2 in the blue–green light wavelength (460 to 490 nm), configurational isomers, structural isomers (lumirubin), and oxidation products are formed (Maisels & McDonagh, 2008). These low molecular weight and water-soluble isomers and oxidation by-products bypass hepatic conjugation and are excreted into the bile or urine (AAP, 2004).

FIGURE 25.3 Mechanism of action of phototherapy.

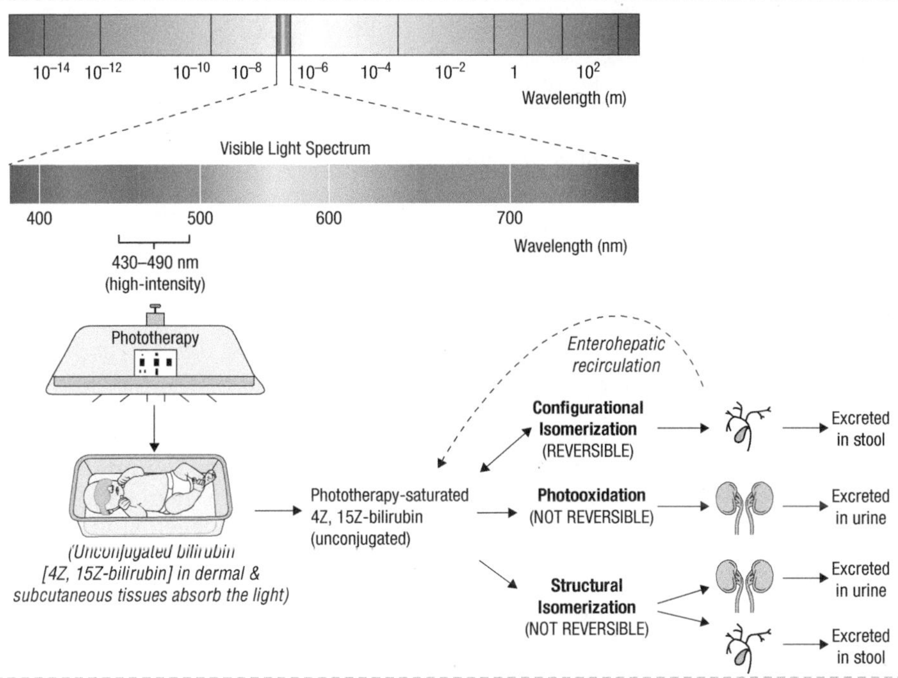

Note: Readers are encouraged to shade the light spectrum between 430 and 460 blue and shade the light spectrum 460 and 490 blue–green. Refer to the ebook content for a colored version of this figure.
Source: Design credit: Amy J. Jnah. Created with Biorender.com

DOSING RECOMMENDATIONS

The delivered dose of phototherapy depends on the physical and photobiologic characteristics of the device, which include emission spectral data and irradiance, as well as body surface area exposure. Dosing is altered by increasing/decreasing the number of phototherapy sources, changing the distance between the baby and the light source, and increasing or decreasing the exposed body surface area.

Various types of phototherapy delivery devices are available, including light-emitting diodes (LEDs), fluorescent light, halogen light, and halogen fiberoptic pads/blankets. More recent blue-spectrum LEDs have been widely adopted for use in neonatal units in the United States, as these lights are less obtrusive compared to older models that used fluorescent bulbs, can be integrated into isolette design, and can be easily adjusted (irradiance) by nursing staff.

It is important to note that phototherapy converts toxic bilirubin to water-soluble bilirubin, which is not neurotoxic. Studies have shown that the transformation of bilirubin to the water-soluble form is significantly evident within approximately 15 to 60 minutes of the onset of phototherapy and a 20% decrease in circulating unconjugated bilirubin can be observed within 2 hours of the onset of therapy (AAP, 2004; Balasundaram & Bhutani, 2016; Bhutani et al., 2011). Therefore, the timely identification of moderate, severe, extreme, and hazardous hyperbilirubinemia is as critical as the prompt and proper initiation of phototherapy (Table 25.5; Bhutani et al., 2004).

CLINICAL-MONITORING PEARLS

Side effects of phototherapy include impaired neonatal temperature control, insensible water loss, and retinal damage if undergoing prolonged direct exposure to the light sources. If used in neonates with cholestatic jaundice, exposure to phototherapy can result in "bronze baby syndrome," a benign skin reaction. Additional skin reactions include purpuric and bullous rashes. Phototherapy may also prolong patent ductus arteriosus patency and change mesenteric blood flow in low-birth-weight premature infants. Albeit rare, exposure to phototherapy also increases the risk for childhood-onset epilepsy (Kemper et al., 2022).

TABLE 25.5 Standard Definitions for Neonatal Hyperbilirubinemia

TYPE OF HYPERBILIRUBINEMIA	DEFINITION (INDIRECT BILIRUBIN MEASUREMENT AT >72 HOURS OF LIFE)	PERCENTILE
Mild	<14 mg/dL	<40th
Moderate	>17 to ≤ 20 mg/dL	>95th
Severe	>20 to ≤ 25 mg/dL	>98th
Extreme	>25 to ≤ 30 mg/dL	>99.9th
Hazardous	>30 mg/dL	>99.99th

Source: From Balasundaram, M., & Bhutani, V. K. (2016). *Severe hyperbilirubinemia (SHP Toolkit)*. https://www.cpqcc.org/sites/default/files/pdf/toolkit/Severe%20Hyperbilirubinemia%20Prevention%20Toolkit_rev%2010.2016%20v2.pdf

Intravenous Immune Globulin

IVIg is a blood product extrapolated from pooled plasma composed primarily (98%) of IgG antibodies (Figure 25.4; Navarro et al., 2010). IVIg is known to play a role in immunomodulation in various disease states (e.g., neonatal autoimmune thrombocytopenia, hemochromatosis, neutropenia, and Kawasaki disease). More commonly, high-dose IVIg has been studied as a pharmacotherapeutic agent among neonates with unconjugated hyperbilirubinemia secondary to ABO isoimmunization or rhesus disease (RhD; Miqdad et al., 2004; Rübo & Wahn, 1991; Santos et al., 2013; Smits-Wintiens et al., 2011; Tanyer et al., 2001; Zwiers et al., 2018). The use of IVIg with each of the aforementioned disease states (among neonates and infants) is off label.

MECHANISM OF ACTION/PHARMACOKINETIC PRINCIPLES

Recall that maternal–fetal antibody/antigen interactions require transplacental transfer of maternal antibodies into the fetal circulation. Pregnant females with type A and B blood groups produce immunoglobulin M (IgM), a large immunoglobulin that cannot cross the placenta. On the contrary, type-O mothers produce IgG antibodies, which can cross the placenta. Maternal anti-A or anti-B antibodies can therefore induce fetal hemolysis when the fetal blood type is type A or type B. In these situations, maternal isoantibody interacts with fetal antigens (on the RBC); this is the stimulus for the activation of hemolysis. In addition, alloimmunization, particularly involving the Rh blood group system and D antigen, can elicit hemolysis.

Although the exact mechanism by which IVIg reduces hemolysis remains elusive, evidence suggests IVIg occupies the reticuloendothelial cell surface (Fc) antibody receptors and prevents the aforementioned antigen/antibody interaction. The effect is decreased uptake of antibody-coated RBCs and decreased heme catabolism. Given that off-label use of IVIg in neonates is directed at treating antigen/antibody interactions and excess heme catabolism in neonates with severe hyperbilirubinemia, this proposed mechanism of action seems reasonable.

DOSING RECOMMENDATIONS

Recent clinical data used to inform current prescribing practices are somewhat limited and conflicting. A meta-analysis by Cortey and colleagues (2014) describes its use in neonates with ABO incompatibility and found that IVIg 0.5 to 1.5 g/kg/dose (up to three doses) in conjunction with phototherapy was associated with decreased need for ET (RR = 0.27, p <.00001, NNT = 5) compared to no IVIg. Concomitant IVIg was also associated with a shorter duration of phototherapy by 0.84 days, without notable adverse effects.

At least one study has evaluated the use of IVIg as prophylaxis for ET in neonates with RhD (Smits-Wintjens et al., 2011). Infants (n = 80) received IVIg 0.75 g/kg (n = 41) or placebo as 5% dextrose (n = 39). There was no difference in need for ET between the IVIg and placebo groups (17% vs. 15%, p = 0.99). In addition, there were no differences in number of ETs (4.7 vs. 5.1, p = .34) or maximum bilirubin level (14.8 vs. 14.1 mg/dL, p = .52) for those that received IVIg.

Zwiers and colleagues (2018) published the second Cochrane review focused on IVIg use among infants with isoimmune hemolytic diseases. The authors considered data published in nine RCTs or quasi-RCTs, all involving the provision of IVIg to infants with Rh and ABO incompatibility.

FIGURE 25.4 Chemical structure of immunoglobulin G.

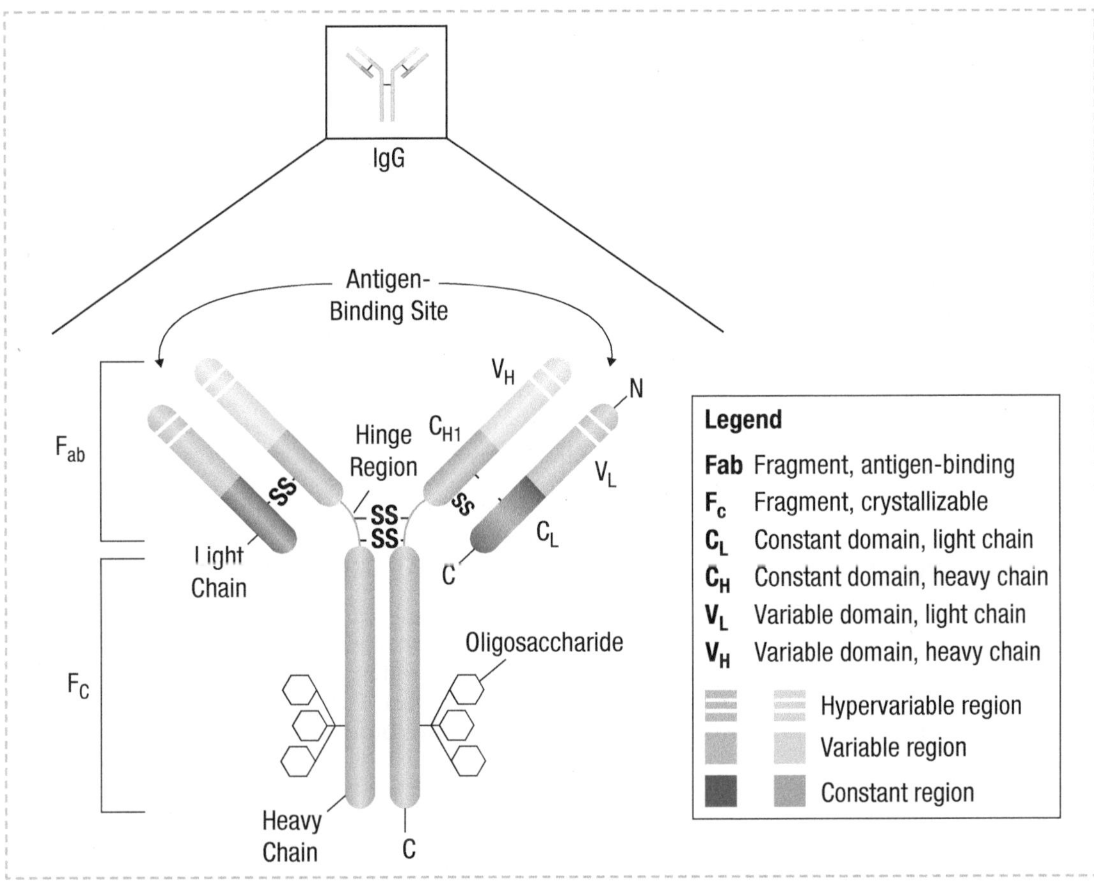

Note: The immunoglobulin G antibody is composed of two protein chains that form a "Y" shape. The top portions of the "Y" shape are known as *light chains* and the bottom are known as *heavy chains*. Each chain consists of a variable and constant region. Antigens bind to immunoglobulin at the variable region, or the *fragment of antigen-binding* (*Fab*) region. Constant regions, in particular on the heavy chain of the immunoglobulin, crystallize and form a *fragment crystallizable* (*Fc*) region. These Fc regions on the immunoglobulin are capable of binding with Fc receptors on other cells, such as reticuloendothelial cells, and trigger immune-mediated hemolysis. Intravenous immunoglobulin blocks Fc receptor sites and prevents antigen/antibody reactions and subsequent hemolysis of red blood cells within the reticuloendothelial system.

Similar to results from the 2002 Cochrane review, Zwier and colleagues (2018) reported a decrease in the rate of ET in infants treated with IVIg (typical RR: 0.28, 95% CI: 0.17–0.47; typical RD: −0.37, 95% CI: −0.49 to −0.26; NNT = 2.7). However, study quality was poor; only two of the nine studies were double-blinded, and as a result, Zwiers and colleagues (2018) did not recommend routine use of IVIg. Their conclusion was met with swift criticism from some members of the scientific community. Hansen and Watchko (2019) agreed that IVIg should not be routinely prescribed but offered strong support for the use of IVIg as recommended by the AAP Subcommittee on Hyperbilirubinemia (Kemper et al., 2022). IVIg use for prophylaxis is discouraged.

> KAS 21: Intravenous immune globulin (IVIG; 0.5 to 1 g/kg) over 2 hours may be provided to infants with isoimmune hemolytic disease (ie, positive DAT) whose TSB reaches or exceeds escalation of care threshold. The dose can be repeated in 12 hours. (Aggregate Evidence Quality Grade C, Option). (Kemper et al., 2022, p. 13)

Neonatal APRNs must recognize that the administration of IVIg risks fluid overload as well as hyperosmolar-induced fluid shifts. The customary osmolarity of IVIg is greater than 1,000 mOsm/L compared to plasma osmolarity less than 300 mOsm/L. Some studies have illuminated a potential relationship between IVIg administration and an increased risk for thromboemboli and NEC secondary to hyperviscosity-induced intestinal ischemia (Figueras-Aloy et al., 2010; Kemper et al., 2022; Marshall et al., 1993; Merlob et al., 1990; Navarro et al., 2009). In addition, IVIg solutions that include stabilizers, such as sucrose, can impair renal function.

CLINICAL-MONITORING PEARLS

Overall, it appears that IVIg is relatively safe in infants with isoimmune hemolytic diseases and may decrease the duration of phototherapy and need for ET. Further clinical trials are needed to determine whether the efficacy differences seen in previous studies are related to the underlying etiology, dosing/timing of IVIg, or from other patient-related factors that have not thus far been elucidated. Only two studies have been published that include an assessment of long-term outcomes. Both studies reported favorable results in that no cases of cerebral palsy, deafness, or kernicterus were identified among infants treated with IVIg (Miqdad et al., 2004; Santos et al., 2013). More research is needed to better illuminate long-term risks and benefits. It appears, based on the existing evidence and AAP (Kemper et al., 2022) guidance, that use of IVIg for severe unconjugated hyperbilirubinemia will not fall out of favor in the near future.

Exchange Transfusion

ET is utilized in neonates with persistently elevated unconjugated bilirubin despite treatment with phototherapy and adequate hydration and in those newborns with anemia secondary to in utero hemolysis (Murki & Kumar, 2011).

MECHANISM OF ACTION/PHARMACOKINETIC PRINCIPLES

The mechanism of action of the ETs involves the direct removal of circulating antibody-coated RBCs and products of hemolysis. Unlike many therapies, the mechanism of action is quite basic; however, the steps involved in determining the dose and duration of therapy, as well as mechanical steps involved in administering this therapy, are complex. For these reasons, we digress to discuss these issues, as errors are directly associated with morbidity and mortality risk.

DOSING RECOMMENDATIONS

ET requires removal of the infant's blood in incremental steps while concurrently replenishing the baby with fresh donor RBCs. To complete the transfusion, the clinician must calculate the estimated blood volume for the patient. Premature infants have an estimated volume of 95 mL/kg (example: 57 mL in a 0.6-kg baby) and term infants have an estimated volume of 85 mL/kg (example: 255 mL in a 3-kg baby). A single ET requires 85 to 95 mL/kg of donor blood (Murki & Kumar, 2011). A DVET requires 170 to 190 mL/kg of donor blood (Murki & Kumar, 2011). When performed properly, total bilirubin levels decrease during and immediately after ET. The most recent Cochrane review specific to ET versus DVET reported that a single volume exchange lowers indirect bilirubin levels by a mean of 1.47 mg/dL (SD ± 24) as compared to 1.62 mg/dL (SD ± 47) with DVET (Thayyil & Milligan, 2006).

There are various techniques that may be utilized to perform an ET, which include use of a single umbilical venous catheter, a single umbilical venous and umbilical artery catheter, or a catheter placed in a peripheral artery (usually radial) and/or a large peripheral vein (Murki & Kumar, 2011). In the single umbilical catheter pull–push technique, the catheter is ideally placed in the inferior vena cava below its junction with the right atrium. The umbilical venous catheter should be connected to two three-way or one four-way stopcock. The four stopcock channels should connect to the following catheters (prefilled with normal saline to prevent air cavitation): umbilical catheter, the catheter draining the withdrawn blood, donor blood, and a saline syringe. To prevent air embolism, the catheters and connections should never be left open to prevent air embolism. Aliquots of donor blood (term infants: 5%–8% total blood volume at 5 mL/kg/min, preterm: 5 mL/kg of blood volume) are exchanged with the infant's blood until the total target exchange volume has been completed. The infant should be made nothing by mouth (NPO) prior to the procedure and continuous cardiorespiratory monitoring should be completed during the procedure. Accurate counts of total blood volume infused and removed should be closely monitored during the procedure. The double-catheter pull–push technique follows a similar procedure but allows the removal of blood through the umbilical artery while simultaneously infusing donor blood through the umbilical vein.

If umbilical vessels are not available for use, the peripheral route may be considered. Removal and replacement of blood can happen simultaneously with two large-bore peripheral catheters.

A 24-gauge catheter should be inserted into the peripheral artery (radial or posterior tibial) and adequacy of collateral circulation should be confirmed before proceeding. The catheter is then connected to a syringe with a three-way stopcock. Another catheter is then inserted into a peripheral vein of another limb and connected to a three-way stopcock. Two people are required to complete this procedure, with one removing blood and one transfusing blood via each catheter (5–10 mL/min). To prevent occlusion, the person utilizing the arterial catheter may need to intermittently flush with heparinized saline. Technical challenges include difficulty maintaining the placement of the peripheral arterial catheter, limb ischemia from rapid removal of blood, and catheter occlusions secondary to negative suction applied during blood removal.

CLINICAL-MONITORING PEARLS

Potential adverse effects include vascular injuries, cardiovascular complications, hematologic laboratory disturbances (e.g., hypocalcemia, hypomagnesemia, hyperkalemia, thrombocytopenia, hyperglycemia), and infection (Murki & Kumar, 2011; Patra et al., 2004; Thayyil & Milligan, 2006). Hypocalcemia and hypomagnesemia manifest when citrate anticoagulants are present in donor blood. Hyperkalemia and thrombocytopenia may occur when using older blood (>5 days) because it contains higher potassium and lower platelets. Cold donor blood may contain excess glucose molecules and elicit rebound hypoglycemia. Interval hematologic monitoring can help identify neonates at risk for lab derangements. Infants receiving medications that require specific blood concentrations for their action, such as antibiotics, may need to be redosed after the ET is complete. The ET is a technically complex procedure; following procedures to maintain procedural competency is critical.

CURRENT PHARMACOLOGIC TREATMENT MODALITIES FOR CONJUGATED HYPERBILIRUBINEMIA

Recall that true liver disease, or *cholestasis*, is defined as an increased serum conjugated bilirubin level (>2 mg/dL) that manifests as a result of decreased bilirubin excretion into the biliary system (Fawaz et al., 2017). However, a direct serum bilirubin level that is increasing or greater than 1 mg/dL is abnormal and should raise the index of suspicion for cholestasis (Kemper et al., 2022). The risk for developing cholestasis is estimated at up to 70% among infants born preterm, and of these infants, 50% who manifest with cholestasis are less than 1 kg at birth (Niccum et al., 2019). The classic triad of clinical indices that suggest cholestasis include prolonged jaundice, persistent and/or worsening direct hyperbilirubinemia, and acholic stool. The more common causes for neonatal/infant cholestasis include intestinal failure-associated liver disease (IFALD), obstructive disorders (e.g., biliary atresia), congenital viral infections (STORCH), bile acid synthesis disorders (e.g., Alagille syndrome), and disorders identified on most state newborn screening tests (e.g., cystic fibrosis, hypothyroidism, galactosemia, tyrosinemia, alpha-1 antitrypsin deficiency; Harpavat et al., 2011, 2016, 2018; Kemper et al., 2022). Readers are referred to Chapter 23, "Parenteral Nutrition," for a discussion of IFALD.

Common manifestations of cholestasis include increased metabolic demand, poor absorption of fat, and impaired macronutrient (namely, protein and carbohydrates) metabolism. Although a detailed discussion of the diagnostic workup is beyond the scope of this textbook, the customary diagnostic pathway includes analysis of the serum glucose level; liver function, including indirect and direct bilirubin, gammaglutamyltransferase (GGT), and prothrombin time/international normalized ratio (INR), as well as a hepatic ultrasound to evaluate for obstructive or vascular abnormalities. Mortality risk among infants with IFALD is estimated at up to 30%, although this statistic is confounded by other morbidity risks (Colby et al., 2007).

Pharmacologic management of cholestasis is focused on treating the proximate cause for abnormal hepatobiliary function and improving liver function, postnatal growth, visual and neurodevelopment, and platelet and immune function. Cholestatic infants often require additional caloric intake to offset metabolic demands, upward of 125% of the recommended daily allowance, and a daily protein intake of 3.5 to 4 g/kg/d for preterm and 2.5 to 3 g/kg/d for term infants (American Society for Parenteral and Enteral Nutrition [ASPEN], 2019; Kleinman et al., 2020; Lapillonne et al., 2018; Mesotten et al., 2018; van Goudoever et al., 2018). In addition, vitamin supplementation is indicated and customarily extends for several months beyond the resolution of symptoms. Supportive therapies include fat-soluble vitamin (A, D, E, K) supplementation, medium-chain triglyceride (MCT) supplements, adequate caloric intake, and, in some cases, ursodeoxycholic acid therapy. Infants who require aqueous parenteral nutrition may benefit from the titration of choline, carnitine, and N-acetylcysteine; studies are underway to test the efficacy of these micronutrients in restoring biliary flow among infants with cholestasis.

Here we present a discussion of current pharmacotherapies used in the treatment of cholestatic jaundice. We begin with a discussion of intravenous lipid emulsions (ILEs), a therapy with known benefits (e.g., reduced mortality and optimized postnatal growth) and risks (e.g., IFALD and sepsis).

Intravenous Lipid Emulsion

Fatty acids are an essential part of the daily nutritional regimen for neonates and infants (see Chapter 23, "Parenteral Nutrition"). Preterm infants are particularly vulnerable to fatty acid deficiencies, as fetal acquisition of maternally donated long-chain polyunsaturated fatty acids (PUFA) occurs in the third trimester of pregnancy. ILEs are prescribed to preterm infants in order to provide a source of calories and omega-3 and omega-6 fatty acids, precursors required for functional maturation of platelets, development of the immune response, and neurocognitive and visual development (Cober et al., 2021; Tomsits et al., 2010).

Three types of lipid emulsions are available in the United States: Intralipid, SMOFLipid, and Omegaven (Table 25.6). Intralipid is composed of 100% soybean oil (major constituent being omega-6 PUFA). Use of this lipid emulsion began in the 1970s; FDA approval was issued in 1996. SMOFLipid is a mixed oil-based ILE composed of 30% soybean oil, 30% medium-chain triglycerides, 25% olive oil, and 15% fish oil. It is not FDA approved for use in pediatric patients but is used in preterm infants considered at risk for IFALD, formerly known as *parenteral nutrition-associated liver disease* (*PNALD*), or those with confirmed IFALD. Omegaven, the only FDA-approved ILE for use in preterm infants with IFALD, consists of 100% fish oil (Cober et al., 2021). This lipid emulsion earned FDA approval in 2018; however, a black-box warning has been issued for preterm infants, specific to the risk for death in preterm infants secondary to poor clearance, increased plasma fatty acid accumulation, and the potential for sequestering of intravascular fat deposits in the lungs (Fresenius Kabi, 2020).

TABLE 25.6 Composition of Oils in SMOF Lipid Emulsion and Reported Benefits

INGREDIENT	BENEFITS
Soybean oil *(30% less than Intralipid)*	Avoids excessive LA intake, reducing the risk for proinflammatory effects (inflammation, oxidative stress, lipid peroxidation) linked to high PUFA intake
Medium-chain triglycerides *(30% more than Intralipid)*	Direct hepatic uptake and production of energy Carnitine free Does not accumulate in the hepatic system Less susceptible to lipid peroxidation
Olive oil *(25% more than Intralipid)*	Enhances vitamin E intake, which prevents lipid peroxidation-induced cell damage
Fish oil *(15% more than Intralipid)*	Anti-inflammatory properties Enhances phospholipid production

Note: Carnitine is customarily removed from aqueous parenteral nutrition when cholestasis is suspected or confirmed; therefore, a carnitine-free LE is desirable. Although fish oil administration is associated with clinical advantages, and accounts for the smallest ingredient in SMOF, clinicians should recognize that this fatty acid is comprised of two PUFAs susceptible to lipid peroxidation (degradation).

LA, linoleic acid; LE, lipid emulsion; PUFA, polyunsaturated fatty acid, SMOF, soybean oil, medium-chain triglycerides, olive oil, fish oil.

Sources: From Tomsits, E., Pataki, M., Tolgyesi, A., Fekete, G., Rischak, K., & Szollar, L. (2010). Safety and efficacy of a lipid emulsion containing a mixture of soybean oil, medium-chain triglycerides, olive oil, and fish oil: A randomised, double-blind clinical trial in premature infants requiring parenteral nutrition. *Journal of Pediatric Gastroenterology & Nutrition, 51*, 514–521. https://doi.org/10.1097/MPG.0b013e3181de210c; Torgalkar, R., Dave, S., Shah, J., Ostad, N., Kotsopoulos, K., Unger, S., & Shah, P. S. (2019). Multi-component lipid emulsion vs soy-based lipid emulsion for very low birth weight preterm neonates: A pre-post comparative study. *Journal of Perinatology, 39*(8), 1118–1124. https://doi.org/10.1038/s41372-019-0425-7

SOY OIL- AND MIXED OIL-BASED LIPID EMULSIONS

The earliest double-blind RCT investigating the safety, tolerability, and efficacy of SMOF ILE compared to Intralipid ILE in preterm infants was conducted by Rayyan and colleagues (2012). Their results suggested that SMOF could be safely administered to preterm infants up to a maximum dose of 3.5 g/kg/d. Gura and colleagues (2008) reported infants treated with SMOF ILE were 4.8 times more likely to recover from cholestasis compared to infants treated with Intralipid. Tomsits and colleagues (2010) conducted a similar trial involving 60 preterm infants (≤34 weeks of gestation) randomized to receive SMOF or Intralipid infusions, which were initiated at a dose of 0.5 g/kg/d and advanced by 0.5 g/kg/d to a maximum dose of 2 g/kg/d. Enteral feedings complemented parenteral nutrition, as tolerated. Triglyceride levels were monitored throughout the study, as preterm infants have reduced fat and muscle mass as well as decreased lipoprotein lipase (LPL) enzyme levels. LPL hydrolyzes triglycerides, which releases the fatty acids and permits delivery to target tissues. Triglyceride levels were similar between groups within the first week of life (<1 mmol/L). Plasma γ-glutamyl transferase (GGT) levels increased from baseline in both the study and control groups (69.1–154.4 IU/L, p = .01) but were not significantly different between groups. More recently, Rayyan and associates (2012) investigated the use of SMOF versus Intralipid in preterm infants (≤34 weeks of gestation). Triglyceride levels were not significantly different between groups; however, direct bilirubin levels were significantly different. Preterm infants treated with SMOF infusions manifested with significantly lower direct bilirubin levels (0.73 mg/dL baseline vs. 0.6 mg/dL) compared to infants who received Intralipid (0.47 mg/dL baseline vs. 0.75 mg/dL) after 8 days of therapy (p = .036). Given that IFALD is diagnosed after approximately 14 to 30 consecutive days of parenteral nutrition, the duration of this study may limit the quality of the results. Other studies also reported a statistically significant reversal of cholestasis (direct bilirubin <2 mg/dL) with SMOF ILE. Vayalthrikkovil and colleagues (2017), in a systematic review inclusive of four RCTs and two observational studies, reported that SMOF ILE reduced the incidence of cholestasis compared to Intralipid (RCTs, n = 386, RR: 0.40, 95% CI: 0.22–0.76, NNT = 11; observational studies, n = 421, RR: 0.1, 95% CI: 0.02–0.60, NNT = 17).

In 2016, I. Diamond and colleagues investigated SMOF in infants. The authors reported that SMOF use was significantly associated with a reduction in conjugated bilirubin levels when compared to traditional Intralipid use (27% vs. 69%, p = .04). More recently, Casson and colleagues (2020) conducted a retrospective analysis of infants who received either SMOF or Intralipid. The authors reported that infants who received full aqueous parenteral nutrition with SMOF were less likely to meet diagnostic criteria for cholestasis (conjugated bilirubin >2 mg/dL) compared to infants who received full aqueous parenteral nutrition and Intralipids (78% vs. 92%, p = .057). No significant difference in the primary outcomes of cholestasis was observed among infants who received combined enteral, aqueous parenteral nutrition, and either Intralipid or SMOF infusions (91% vs. 76%, p = .18).

Additional adequately powered RCTs are needed to further evaluate short- and long-term effects of SMOF use in preterm infants. One particular short-term effect of ILE, as reported by multiple research teams, is the potential for sepsis in preterm infants. Freeman and colleagues (1990) reported a 56% increase in sepsis diagnoses among preterm infants receiving ILE. In contrast, multiple other studies reported no increased risk for sepsis (Brine & Judith, 2004; Gilbertson et al., 1991; Hammerman & Aramburo, 1988; Toce & Keenan, 1995). Long-term effects worthy of additional investigation include the incidence of visual impairment (retinopathy of prematurity [ROP]) and osteopenia of prematurity among infants treated with SMOF compared to other ILE. Torgalkar and colleagues (2019) published the largest investigation of long-term outcomes linked to SMOF versus Intralipid therapy among infants younger than 32 weeks or less than 1,500 grams at birth and who received at least 7 days of ILE. Dosing was initiated at 1 g/kg/d and increased by 1 g/kg/d to a maximum dose of 3 to 3.5 g/kg/d. No significant difference in the incidence of ROP, bronchopulmonary dysplasia (BPD), or NEC was observed. As a result of these and other studies, many NICUs have adopted SMOF ILE for use in preterm infants.

FISH-OIL BASED LIPID EMULSIONS

Fish-oil ILE, namely, Omegaven®, is FDA approved for use in preterm neonates with cholestatic jaundice. This lipid emulsion is composed entirely of fish oils; supplemental vitamin E is added to the composition of the product. Prophylactic use has not been shown to prevent the development of IFALD in preterm infants. Gura and colleagues (2006) published the first report of successful fish-oil ILE use (dose = 1 g/kg/d) in two infants with IFALD; disease resolution was reported after 60 days of pharmacotherapy. Lam and colleagues (2014) published the first double-blind RCT comparing the use of soy-oil and fish-oil ILE in infants with IFALD. Both groups of infants were advanced on enteral feeds during the interventional period. Infants receiving fish-oil ILE demonstrated a slower rate of increase (per week) in conjugated bilirubin levels compared to infants receiving soy-based ILE (0.0067 mg/dL vs. 0.1527 mg/dL, respectively, $p = .03$). Further, infants who received fish-oil ILE exhibited faster disease resolution, defined as decreasing conjugated bilirubin levels, once advanced to full enteral feeds ($r = -.31$, $p = .002$). On the basis of these data, Omegaven may be used in infants with severe cholestasis. However, additional studies are indicated to appraise long-term growth and hematologic (platelet) function among preterm infants provided exclusively fish-oil based ILE (Guthrie & Burrin, 2021).

MECHANISM OF ACTION/PHARMACOKINETIC PRINCIPLES OF LIPID EMULSIONS

Enterally ingested lipids are absorbed by chylomicrons in the gut, transported to the lymphatics, general circulation, and then transported to target tissues and the liver. Infants intractable to enteral nutrition require ILE, which are administered directly into the general circulation. The composition of ILE mimics a chylomicron, which facilitates efficient transport of lipid to the tissues and liver. Reduced clearance is reported among preterm and small-for-gestational-age infants (Fresenius Kabi, 2016).

DOSING RECOMMENDATIONS (INTRALIPID AND SMOFLIPID)

A dosing range of 0.5 to 3.5 g/kg/d of Intralipid is recommended to avoid the onset of an essential fatty acid deficiency (EFAD) and promote growth (Cober et al., 2021; Kleinman & Greer, 2020; Martindale & Klek, 2020). These recommendations align with an absolute minimum dose of 0.25 g/kg/d (preterm infants) to 0.1 g/kg/d (term infants) of linoleic PUFA (Koletzko et al., 2005). Therefore, among infants diagnosed with ILFAD, a reduction in the Intralipid dose to 1 g/kg may be indicated.

SMOFLipid does not deliver the same proportion of linoleic PUFA as Intralipid. The recommendation from the international summit "Lipids in Parenteral Nutrition" (Calder et al., 2020) specific to fish-oil containing ILEs (SMOF) in neonates, which contain the minimum amount of linoleic PUFA at the lowest recommended dose, is 1 g/kg/d (on day 1 of life), followed by 2 g/kg/d (day 2 of life) and 3 g/kg/d (day 3 and beyond; Martindale & Klek, 2020). The maximum dose for infants and children, per the consensus statement, is 3 g/kg/d (Martindale & Klek, 2020). Dose reduction of SMOFLipid has been associated with EFAD and should be avoided (Cary et al., 2019).

DOSING RECOMMENDATIONS (OMEGAVEN)

A dose of 1.0 to 1.5 g/kg/d is reported in the literature in order to avoid the onset of an EFAD. A dose of 1.0 g/kg/d effectively maintains fatty acid levels (de Meijer et al., 2010) and one case report reported reversal of an EFAD with the administration of 1.5 g/kg/d (Riedy et al., 2017).

CLINICAL-MONITORING PEARLS

Although generally considered safe, caution should be applied when administering ILEs given the risk for hypertriglyceridemia, inflammation, oxidative stress, and infection. Common clinical chemistry parameters are summarized in Box 25.1 and discussed in Chapter 23, "Parenteral Nutrition." Close monitoring for deviations in physiologic homeostasis that may suggest sepsis, while avoiding unnecessary antibiotic use, is indicated.

Vitamin A, D, E, and K Supplementation

Cholestasis can lead to fat malabsorption secondary to decreased secretion of bile salts. Oral fat-soluble vitamin absorption is dependent on intestinal bile acid solubilization, so a deficiency can arise in patients with cholestatic liver disease (serum direct bilirubin >2 mg/dL). In fact, Sokol

BOX 25.1 Chemistry Parameters Monitored With Lipid Emulsion Therapy

Basic metabolic panel
Phosphate
Liver function panel
Complete blood count
Triglyceride
Total cholesterol
HDL cholesterol
LDL cholesterol
Glucose

Note: Screening of a complete blood count may be reserved for circumstances involving an inadvertent rapid infusion of a lipid emulsion, which raises suspicion for fat overload. This may predispose the infant to decreased platelet adhesion and bleeding. No clinically significant bleeding has been reported, to date, due to incorrect programming of an infusion pump.
HDL, high-density lipoprotein; LDL, low-density lipoprotein.
Source: Cober, M. P., Gura, K. M., Mirtallo, J. M., Ayers, P., Boullata, J., Anderson, C. R., Plogsted, S., & ASPEN Parenteral Nutrition Safety Committee. (2021). ASPEN lipid injectable emulsion safety recommendations part 2: Neonate and pediatric considerations. *Nutrition in Clinical Practice, 36*(6), 1106–1125. https://doi.org/10.1002/ncp.10778

and colleagues (1983) published novel findings linking decreased bile acid concentrations with vitamin E deficiency, tocopherol depletion, spinocerebellar degeneration, and peripheral neuropathy. Supplementation is necessary to prevent a deficient state of vitamins A, D, E, and K, but has also been found to be relatively ineffective in the setting of severe cholestasis. Although parenteral vitamin supplementation has been reported as successful, the need for daily intramuscular injections, associated pain, and parental concerns for home administration preclude its use.

MECHANISM OF ACTION/PHARMACOKINETIC PRINCIPLES

In the presence of bile and pancreatic enzymes, fat-soluble vitamins are emulsified and absorbed into the cytoplasm of micelles, or clusters of lipids. Micelles transport the fat-soluble vitamins to the intestinal microvilli and bile salts are then recycled. Once absorbed across the intestinal epithelium and into intestinal enterocytes, fat-soluble vitamins are engulfed by chylomicrons, which transport the vitamins to the lymphatic vessels, and then to the bloodstream. Chylomicrons remain bound to fat-soluble vitamins until metabolized by lipoprotein lipase. It is at this time that the fat-soluble vitamins are released from the blood to the tissues (Reddy & Jialal, 2020). Clearly, bile salts are essential for successful absorption of fat-soluble vitamins; a deficit of intestinal bile salts will stunt the absorption of these vitamins irrespective of the dose of enteral supplementation. This is the challenge clinicians face when trying to prevent or treat vitamin deficiencies in cholestatic infants.

Vitamin E is a more general term used to reference tocopherol and tocotrienol molecules. These molecules are antioxidants that prevent lipid peroxidation and EFAD. A natural, water-soluble isomer of vitamin E, or d-α-tocopheryl polyethylene glycol 1,000 succinate (TPGS), has shown to be effective at increasing vitamin E levels in infants with cholestasis. TPGS can form micelles in the absence of bile and pancreatic enzymes and be absorbed directly into the intestinal enterocyte. A multicenter trial that included infants as young as 6 months of age evaluated the efficacy and safety of TPGS and reported that enteral TPGS supplementation induced an increase in vitamin E levels after 6 months of treatment (p <.05; Heseker et al., 1993). No adverse effects were reported across the duration of the study period.

DOSING RECOMMENDATIONS

A study evaluating fat-soluble vitamin status in infants with biliary atresia receiving oral liquid supplementation (n = 92) found that deficiency is common, and vitamin levels are inversely proportional to serum total bilirubin levels (Shneider et al., 2012). Those infants with a total bilirubin of 2 mg/dL or more were more likely to have biochemical fat-soluble vitamin deficiency despite oral supplementation. Therefore, infants with cholestatic liver disease should receive vitamin supplementation at the following doses: vitamin A 5,000 to 25,000 IU/d, vitamin D 400 to 1,200 IU/d, vitamin E TPGS (micellar form) 25 IU/d, and vitamin K 7.5 mg/wk divided into three 2.5-mg daily doses (Balistreri et al., 2014).

One small pediatric study evaluated dosing of oral multivitamin (MVI) with additional AquADEK compared to a conventional oral or intramuscular MVI injection in pediatric patients with a variety of underlying etiologies for chronic cholestasis (Shen et al., 2012). A total of 23 patients were evaluated. The median age was 6.8 years (range: 0.3–18) and weight was 16.6 kg (range: 5.6–53.1 kg). The baseline median direct bilirubin was 3.7 mg/dL (range: 0.1–23.9 mg/dL). Twelve of the 23 patients transitioned to 3 months of oral MVI with AquADEK, but two patients were returned to the conventional treatment group within a month after dropping out secondary to taste aversion. There were no statistically significant differences in baseline characteristics or vitamin deficiency outcomes between groups. Overall rates of vitamin K deficiency were low, and there was a trend toward improved vitamin D deficiency in the MVI with the AquADEK group (60% vs. 100%, $p = 0.09$).

ADEK and AquADEK were more recently replaced with alternative fat-soluble ADEK enteral vitamin supplement that offers a miscible form of vitamin E. This product, DEKA Essential Liquid (Callion Pharm, Jonesboro, TN), was developed in consultation with the Childhood Liver Disease Research Network (CHiLDReN) and is reported to enhance vitamin E supplementation by maximizing vitamin E TPGS. The recommended dose is 25 IU/d; use is off label in infants and children.

Although data in cholestatic neonates are lacking, some recommendations for enteral supplementation in preterm neonates may help guide initial supplementation goals (Table 25.7; Agostoni et al., 2010). This may be achieved using a variety of methods, including oral supplementation of individual vitamins, combination oral products (MVI with ADEK), DEKA Essential Liquid with TPGS, and injectable vitamin preparations.

CLINICAL-MONITORING PEARLS

It is recommended that fat-soluble vitamin levels are measured in neonates with cholestasis and supplemented if required (Mouzaki et al., 2019). Routine clinical monitoring priorities include interval measurements of serum 25-hydroxyvitamin D, triglyceride, and serum direct bilirubin. Less often, the prothrombin time/INR may be measured. While there is an inversely proportional relationship between the INR and vitamin K level (elevated INR suggests vitamin K deficiency), the INR is not a reliable marker for vitamin K deficiency in infants (Shneider et al., 2012).

Signs and symptoms of deficiency may be difficult to determine in the neonatal patient (Agostoni et al., 2010). Vitamin A deficiency may be associated with vision impairment, so ophthalmology follow-up should be considered. Vitamin D deficiency may manifest as osteopenia and rickets. Further workup should include consideration of measurement of serum parathyroid hormone, calcium, and phosphate levels. Vitamin E deficiency can present as neurologic symptoms that may not be reversible with supplementation. Presence of RBC acanthocytosis on peripheral blood smear may also be indicative of vitamin E deficiency. Last, vitamin K deficiency is classically associated with disturbances in the clotting cascade, but it may also impair bone mineralization even in the presence of normal INR.

Medium-Chain Triglycerides

Maldigestion and malabsorption associated with impaired bile acid function can lead to impaired nutritional status in infants with cholestasis (Kriegermeier & Green, 2020; Mouzaki et al., 2019; Suchy, 2004). Depending on the severity of liver disease, infant formulas enriched with MCTs may be utilized.

MECHANISM OF ACTION/PHARMACOKINETIC PRINCIPLES

MCT-based saturated fats passively diffuse through intestinal enterocytes because they do not require carnitine transport (Guthrie & Burrin, 2021). This may allow for enhanced nutritional impact since traditional fat preparations may have decreased intestinal absorption. Absorption is

TABLE 25.7 Fat-Soluble Vitamins

FAT-SOLUBLE VITAMIN	ENTERAL DOSING RANGE	CONCENTRATION IN MVI WITH ADEK (PER 0.5 ML)	CONCENTRATION IN DEKA ESSENTIAL LIQUID (PER 0.5 ML)	SERUM REFERENCE RANGE
A	400–1,000 mcg/kg/d	375 mcg	375 mcg	300–800 mcg/mL
D	800–1,000 IU/d	1,000 IU	1,000 IU	25(OH) vitamin D: >50 mnol/L
E	2.2–11 mg/kg/d	25 mg	25 mg (miscible form)	1–2 mg/dL
K	4.4–28 mg/kg/d	1,000 mcg	1,000 mcg	No specific laboratory test International normalized ratio is not an accurate representation of total vitamin K status Undercarboxylated serum vitamin K-dependent proteins may be used as biomarkers of vitamin K deficiency

MVI, multivitamin.

Source: From Agostoni, C., Buoncore G., Carinelli, V. P., De Curtis, M., Darmaun, D., Desci, T., Domellof, M., Embleton, N. D., Fusch, C., Genzel-Boroviczeny, O., Goulet, O., Kalhan S. C., Kolacek, S., Koletzko, B., Lapillonne, A., Mihatsch, W., Moreno, L., Neu, J., . . . Ziegler, E. E. (2010). Enteral nutrient supply for preterm infants: Commentary from the European Society for Paediatric Gastroenterology, Hepatology, and Nutrition Committee on Nutrition. *Journal of Pediatric Hastroenterology and Nutrition, 50*(1), 85–91. https://doi.org/10.1097/MPG.0b013e3181adaee0

facilitated because MCTs do not require bile acids or lipase for digestion (Taketomo, 2023). These MCT-based fats also suppress hepatic TLR4 signaling, a pathway that initiates the innate immune response and association inflammation. The benefits associated with this anti-inflammatory property require further investigation. No kinetic data specific to absorption, distribution, metabolism, and excretion in infants is available in the literature.

DOSING RECOMMENDATIONS

Dosing customarily begins at 1 to 2 g/kg/d (1–2 mL/kg/d) and may be advanced to meet the nutritional needs of the neonate (Taketomo, 2023). The daily dose is customarily divided into three to four smaller doses and mixed with enteral feedings.

CLINICAL-MONITORING PEARLS

Caution must be applied if providing long-term nutrition (>4–6 weeks) high in MCTs, as EFAD can occur in the absence of adequate long-chain fatty acid intake (Mouzaki et al., 2019). Fat-soluble vitamin deficiency often occurs in conjunction with EFAD and should be evaluated if infants present with symptoms of deficiency for either of these. Increased fat intake may be necessary if the infant has evidence of excessive fecal fat loss. Supplementation should be individualized to the patient. Options include vegetable/canola oil, coconut oil (unsaturated fat), MCT oil, Liquigen (emulsified MCT oil), and microlipid. MCT oil or Liquigen are generally preferred in liver disease because they do not require bile acid or pancreatic enzymes to break down (Suchy, 2004). Clinicians are encouraged to monitor growth velocity and anthropometric indices throughout therapy as well as the color, consistency, and frequency of stool output.

Ursodeoxycholic Acid

Recall that both bile acids and intestinal lipase enzymes are necessary for the digestion of fats. Bile acids emulsify fats and activate lipases, which break down fats into free fatty acids and glycerol, facilitating absorption and transport to the liver and other body tissues. Gastric lipolysis is of particular importance, as it is responsible for 25% to 60% of total fat digestion (Hamosh, 2006). Preterm infants are vulnerable to poor fat absorption as both lipase activity and the presence of bile salts are abnormally low compared to term counterparts. The development of parenteral nutrition associated cholestasis (PNAC) exacerbates this issue and may require pharmacotherapeutic intervention to augment existing bile salt concentrations and reverse cholestasis.

Ursodeoxycholic acid, otherwise known as *ursodiol*, is a hydrophilic natural bile acid used to treat confirmed ILFAD. Although not approved by the FDA for use in neonates or infants, ursodiol has been prescribed off-label for decades. The utility of prophylactic use to enhance fat absorption in preterm infants remains under investigation.

MECHANISM OF ACTION/PHARMACOKINETIC PRINCIPLES

Ursodeoxycholic acid is a hydrophilic bile acid with three major mechanisms of action: (a) protects cholangiocytes from biliary acid toxicity, (b) increases bile acid secretion, and (c) protects hepatocytes from apoptosis. The protection of cholangiocytes promotes choleresis (flow of bile) through increased chloride and bicarbonate secretion from cholangiocytes. Protection of hepatocytes occurs by way of mitochondrial membrane stabilization and displacement of cytotoxic bile acids, which also decreases inflammation by reducing immunoglobulin and cytokine production (Lewis et al., 2018; Suchy, 2004). These actions improve biliary function and bile flow.

Gordi and colleagues (2014) published the very first pharmacokinetic study specific to ursodiol; this report was largely underpowered; therefore, additional data are necessary to generalize these findings. The authors reported that ursodiol exhibited linear pharmacokinetics. This refers to zero-order kinetics; the rate of drug elimination is constant regardless of the plasma concentration.

DOSING RECOMMENDATIONS

Ursodiol dosing is 10 to 30 mg/kg/d in divided doses (typically every 8 hours) and is only available in an enteral formulation (Taketomo, 2023). Diarrhea is the most common side effect and may limit its utility in infants with underlying cholestasis etiologies such as intestinal failure/short bowel syndrome.

The efficacy of ursodiol versus phenobarbital in the treatment of cholestasis has been a focus of attention of late, as phenobarbital use has been prescribed in the past as a therapy for cholestatic jaundice. Lewis and colleagues (2018) retrospectively compared direct bilirubin levels following treatment with ursodiol versus phenobarbital in neonates with cholestatic jaundice (n = 68). The median ursodiol dose was 27 mg/kg/d compared to a median phenobarbital dose of 4.48 mg/kg/d. After a 17-day course of therapy, a significantly decreased direct bilirubin level was observed among infants treated with ursodiol compared to phenobarbital (4.98 vs. 7.84 mg/dL, respectively, p = 0.02). When adjusting for pertinent demographics, such as baseline direct bilirubin, intrauterine growth restriction, and limited lipid infusions, ursodiol was significantly superior to phenobarbital for lowering of direct bilirubin (3.65 vs. 7.89, p <.01).

CLINICAL-MONITORING PEARLS

Despite a lack of robust data, ursodiol appears to be a reasonable treatment option for neonatal cholestasis in infants who tolerate enteral medications, particularly in those with parenteral nutrition as their likely underlying etiology. Routine surveillance of GGT levels, the earliest and most sensitive marker of cholestasis, and direct bilirubin levels is indicated. Most clinicians stop therapy when the direct bilirubin level is less than 2 mg/dL.

Phenobarbital

Recall the prior discussion of findings reported by Lewis and colleagues (2018). Their study was the first focused on comparing the efficacy of phenobarbital versus ursodiol in the treatment of cholestasis in neonates. Phenobarbital has been historically prescribed to cholestatic infants unable to tolerate sufficient enteral feeding volumes to warrant oral medication administration (e.g., ursodiol). Like many pharmacotherapeutic regimens, the use of phenobarbital for cholestatic jaundice is off-label and prescribed in the absence of quality data. In fact, while investigating phenobarbital use for neurologic disease, Gleghorn and colleagues (1986) followed direct bilirubin levels and found that 66% of all neonates went on to develop cholestasis despite receiving phenobarbital (5 mg/kg/d) compared to 33% of neonates who were not exposed to phenobarbital and developed cholestasis.

MECHANISM OF ACTION/PHARMACOKINETIC PRINCIPLES

Specific to cholestatic disease, the mechanism of action of phenobarbital involves the induction of microsomal liver enzymes and control of hepatocellular metabolism via action at the constitutive androstane receptors. The effect is an increase in enzyme and bile acid secretion and bile acid flow (Gleghorn et al., 1986; Suchy, 2004). Subsequently, the concentration of circulating bile acids decreases. Phenobarbital is primarily metabolized by hepatic cytochrome P450 enzymes (CYP2C9, CYP2C19, and CYP2E1). Drug half-life is longest in preterm infants (141 hours) and the volume of distribution of the drug is two-fold that of adults (Pacifici, 2016). However, given that phenobarbital induces hepatic enzymes that can, in turn, metabolize the drug, drug half-life decreases with prolonged therapy. Metabolites are renally excreted. Clearance matures with advancing weight (increases by 36.7% for every 1 kg in weight gain) and advancing postnatal age (increases by 5.3% per postnatal day of life; Völler et al., 2017).

DOSING RECOMMENDATIONS

Phenobarbital dosing for neonatal cholestasis is typically 3 to 5 mg/kg/d and can be given enterally or intravenously (Taketomo, 2023). Sedation is the most notable side effect, but potential for neuronal apoptosis and developmental delays, as seen in animal models, may limit its place in clinical practice. In the retrospective study by Gleghorn and colleagues (1986), briefly discussed earlier, of 31 infants born less than 1,500 grams who received more than 14 days of exclusive parenteral nutrition, patients who received concurrent intravenous phenobarbital 5 mg/kg/d ($n = 10$) were compared against those who did not ($n = 21$). Total parenteral nutrition (TPN)-associated cholestasis was defined as a serum total bilirubin greater than 3 mg/dL at more than 3 weeks of life. Infants with neurologic conditions, such as seizures, possible seizures, or seizure prophylaxis following intraventricular hemorrhage, generally received phenobarbital for those comorbid conditions, not specifically for TPN-induced cholestasis. The authors concluded that use of phenobarbital was not effective in preventing TPN-associated cholestasis.

CLINICAL-MONITORING PEARLS

Given its relative lack of efficacy and potential for neurotoxicity, phenobarbital should be evaluated judiciously prior to use for cholestasis. Clinicians should consider the risks and benefits associated with phenobarbital use and consider delaying pharmacotherapy until the infant is capable of tolerating oral ursodiol dosing. Routine surveillance of direct bilirubin levels during phenobarbital therapy, prompt discontinuation of dosing upon resolution of cholestasis (direct bilirubin level <2 mg/dL), and long-term neurocognitive assessments are indicated.

CONCLUSIONS

Jaundice is one of the most common problems identified in neonatal intensive care that is linked to diagnostic workups. Indirect hyperbilirubinemia, when left untreated, risks severe and irreversible neurotoxicity. The mainstays of pharmacotherapy have been and still include phototherapy and, in rare circumstances, ET. The efficacy of prophylactic or adjunctive IVIg therapy remains poorly understood; additional research is needed to better understand the mechanism of action and long-term risks and benefits.

Direct hyperbilirubinemia is less frequently diagnosed when compared to its counterpart (indirect hyperbilirubinemia). When left untreated, cholestatic liver disease is associated with significant morbidity and mortality risks. Fortunately, routine liver function testing, in particular among at-risk neonates, is commonplace in U.S. NICUs. Nutritional therapy is of primary importance and should be optimized to facilitate adequate macronutrient and vitamin absorption. The mainstay of pharmacotherapy has been ursodeoxycholic acid, a drug that promotes choleresis in cases of cholestasis excluding parenteral nutrition-induced disease. However, the clinical response to treatment can be insufficient. Emerging molecular diagnostics may allow for customized pharmacotherapies, including the administration of farnesoid X receptor (FXR) agonists, a drug class currently under investigation in animal models.

LEARNING TOOLS AND RESOURCES

Advice From the Authors

Amy J. Jnah, DNP, APRN, NNP-BC

Hyperbilirubinemia, either physiologic or pathologic, is one of the most common conditions you will diagnose as a neonatal nurse practitioner. A systems approach to diagnosing and treating this condition is essential to protect newborns from bilirubin neurotoxicity or, in cases of cholestatic disease, vitamin deficiency. I suggest you draw out complex concepts because this encourages active learning. Then, fact check your work with a trusted mentor, and pay it forward if a peer voices a similar struggle!

Keliana O'Mara, PharmD, BCPPS

Medications and treatment modalities often change with time as new literature and drugs are developed. If you train yourself to understand the basic pathophysiology and pharmacology associated with the disease states, it better prepares you to keep up with new therapies as they emerge.

Discussion Prompts

1. Phototherapy decreases bilirubin values in most circumstances and prevents kernicterus, but a paucity of data limits our ability to fully understand this relationship. What factors likely contribute to the lack of ethically designed scientific trials focused on quantifying this important relationship?
2. Discuss the risks and benefits of IVIg as an adjunctive pharmacotherapy to phototherapy among infants with isoimmune hemolytic diseases. Then, compare the data with your institution's policy and procedure.
3. Compare and contrast the mechanism of action of ursodeoxycholic acid and phenobarbital as it pertains to the restoration of bile flow in infants with cholestasis.

Mind Map

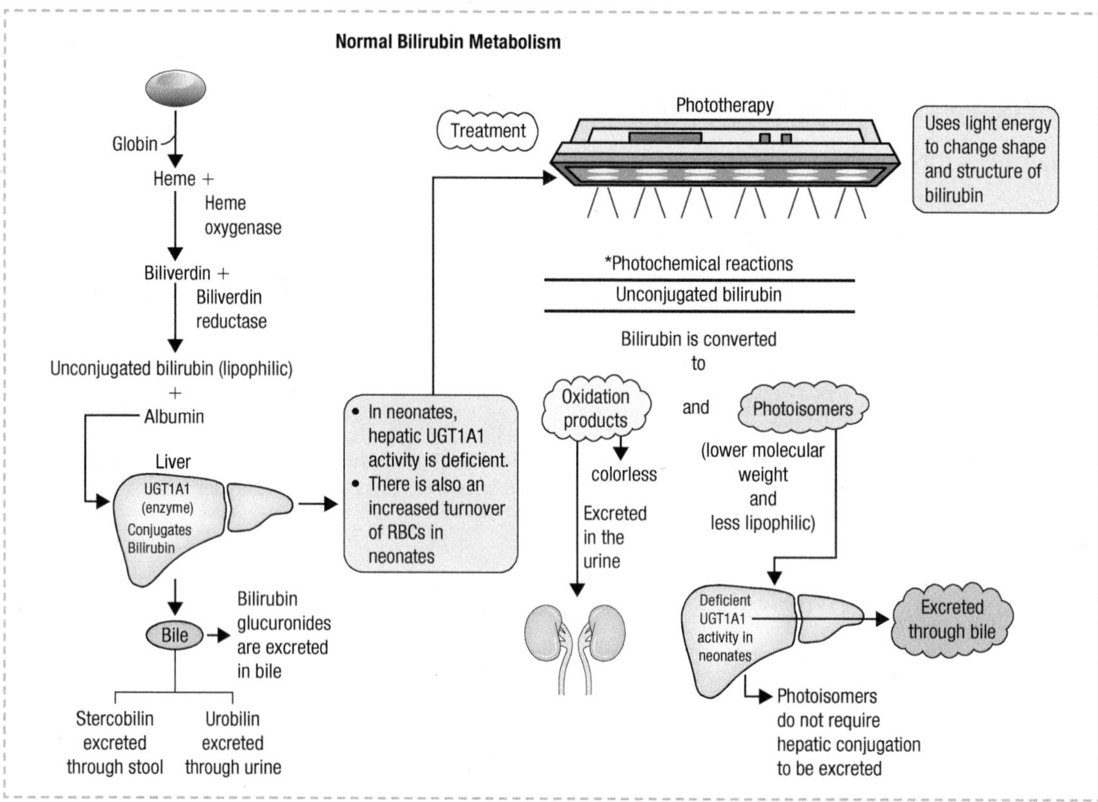

Note: This mind map reflects the design team's interpretation of a portion of one or more concepts addressed in this chapter. Readers should regard the mind maps woven throughout this textbook as examples of multisensory study tools that can be developed to encourage conceptual understanding. Readers are encouraged to develop their own unique mind maps in consultation with academic faculty or clinical.
RBC, red blood cell.
Source: Design credit: Jordan Lewis, MSN, and Rebecca Judy, MSN, East Carolina Neonatal Nurse Practitioner Program.

REFERENCES

References for this chapter are online and available at https://connect.springerpub.com/content/book/978-0-8261-5884-0/part/partVI/toc-part/ch25.

chapter 26

Osteopenia of Prematurity

Valarie A. Artigas, Mary Whalen, and Mehran Nesari Asdigha

LEARNING OBJECTIVES

After completing this chapter, the reader should be able to:

- Define *osteopenia of prematurity* (*OoP*) and identify the epidemiology of the disease process.
- Enumerate the most common risk factors for OoP.
- Explain the physiology of fetal bone accretion.
- Correlate the pathophysiology of OoP with the need for pharmacologic treatment.
- Appraise the historical evolution of pharmacologic management of OoP.
- Evaluate current pharmacologic therapies for treatment of OoP.

INTRODUCTION

With the advancement and acceptance of the importance of the nutritional sciences, healthcare clinicians are able to recognize and prevent diseases that are caused by nutritional deficiencies. Despite these advancements, metabolic bone disease in at-risk premature infants is a common, and potentially serious, comorbid condition in preterm, low-birth-weight, and chronically ill or medically fragile infants and children (Rustico et al., 2014). Metabolic bone disease may also be referred to as *osteopenia of prematurity (OoP)* or *osteopathy*, and may lead to rickets of prematurity if untreated. Given the lack of consensus among neonatal and pediatric clinicians in regard to terminology, definitions, screening, and treatment, the quantifiable incidence of metabolic bone disease remains elusive; however, it has been approximated that between 23% and 60% of preterm infants with a birth weight between 1,000 and 1,500 grams will be affected by some degree of metabolic bone disease (Rayannavar & Calabria, 2020; Sabroske et al., 2020).

Given the prevalence and significant comorbidity in preterm infants, routine evaluation is imperative to prevent, recognize, and treat this form of osteopathy. This routine evaluation should include examination of bone mineralization in an at-risk group of infants, including those born before 30 weeks' gestation, of low birth weight, receiving prolonged parenteral nutrition, lacking of basic turning and positioning due to the severity of illness, and exposed to common drugs in the NICU, such as diuretics, caffeine, and corticosteroids, which are considered osteolytic (Rayannavar & Calabria, 2020). However, the best approach is the prevention of this symptomatic disease.

Although consensus exists among neonatal providers regarding the risk factors leading to this osteopathic condition, the lack of normative data and clinical trials leads to variation in screening practices among neonatologists (Rayannavar & Calabria, 2020). Consensus of screening for metabolic bone health did not exist until 2013 when the American Academy of Pediatrics' (AAP) Committee on

Nutrition (CON) released their report focusing on mineral and hormonal balances and their effects regarding bone disease in preterm infants (Abrams, 2013). If metabolic bone disease is not recognized and treated, these affected infants may experience rickets and other long-term consequences, which include smaller/shorter stature as well as osteopenia during their young adult years.

Although the authors recognize the diversity of given terminology, their intent is to use the term *OoP* for the present-day discussion within the chapter. OoP is used for infants demonstrating evidence of compromised bone mineralization without radiographic changes. The term *rickets* will be reserved for the chronic disorder of calcium and mineral dysfunction, which is characterized by radiologic evidence of bone demineralization and elevated serum alkaline phosphatase (ALP) levels (Koo et al., 1982).

This chapter presents a step back in time and history to identify the seminal work and research from the centuries-old scientists and physicians who have shaped our understanding of bone disease among newborns and children. This chapter has been thoughtfully constructed to provide readers with a timely refresher of basic physiology and pathophysiology specific to OoP. From there, we discuss how to identify preterm infants at risk of developing OoP as it relates to the common causes of this metabolic bone condition. We review fetal and postnatal bone homeostasis, as well as describe the mechanisms required for the accretion of nutrients. Discussion ensues regarding therapies common to the neonate's care that are considered osteolytic in nature (methylxanthines, loop diuretics, and glucocorticoids).

The robust discussion offered within this chapter will prepare readers to prescribe evidence-based diagnostic practices, as well as identify therapeutic interventions in both the inpatient and post-discharge clinical care setting for these fragile neonates. Last, we present the current state of the science specific to screening for and the pharmacologic treatment of OoP. Readers are encouraged to consult the Appendix, "Formulary," as needed, for additional information on pharmacotherapeutics discussed in this chapter. Learning tools and resources, provided at the end of the chapter, are offered to stimulate additional scholarly conversation both in the classroom and clinical settings, as well as to encourage active learning practices for those preparing to take the board certification examination.

HISTORICAL PERSPECTIVE: SEMINAL AND OTHER NOTEWORTHY STUDIES

Although nutritional deficiencies have been recorded since ancient times, most physicians believed that disease processes occurred due to the lack of cleanliness or through the mysticism of ancient gods. The Greek physician Soranus, who practiced in Rome, reported deformation of the bones in infants as early as the first and second centuries CE. He attributed these deformities to be the result of failure of Roman mothers to properly nurture and clean their children, but did not directly implicate poor diet in the condition (Hess, 1929). As noted by Soranus as well as other first- and second-century physicians, this condition came to be known as *rickets*. Although early descriptions of these "rachitic" children are documented, it was not until the mid-17th century that a true interpretation and evidence were presented. Medical historians credit Cambridge physician Francis Glisson for his work in the identification and treatment of rickets as a specific disease process. Glisson's work resulted from direct observation in both the clinical and postmortem setting (Rajakumar, 2003). Glisson emphasized the importance of acknowledging rickets as a disease of not just the bones but also the systemic implications contributing to the mortality rates of children (Gibbs, 1994). Despite the early documentation of rickets, there would be no new advances in the medical communities concerning the condition until the 20th century. At the turn of the 20th century, rickets became an endemic condition among underprivileged infants whose families resided in the northern cities of the United States and Europe, especially England. Childhood rickets was the most common cause of all deformities. Affected children (Figure 26.1) demonstrated clinical manifestations of macrocephaly in relation to their very thin arms and bowed, thin legs, which limited their ability to move and walk normally (Gibbs, 1994).

During the 19th century and through the work of such healthcare clinicians as Florence Nightingale, the founder of modern nursing, and Hugh Owen Thomas, a physician treating "crippled" rachitic children, many improvements were made in the overall health of children. Growing knowledge about the importance of cleanliness, fresh air, UV lights, and nutritious meals promoted wellness and cured illness. The early 20th century was witness to the expansion of knowledge regarding the nutritional sciences, especially in treating rickets in infants and children. Understanding the pathophysiology of rickets, advances in biochemical and radiologic testing, clarification surrounding the antirachitic effects of ingesting cod liver oil (Figure 26.2), the importance of skin exposure to UV light (sunlight), and improvements in sanitary living conditions were in

FIGURE 26.1 Children affected by rickets.

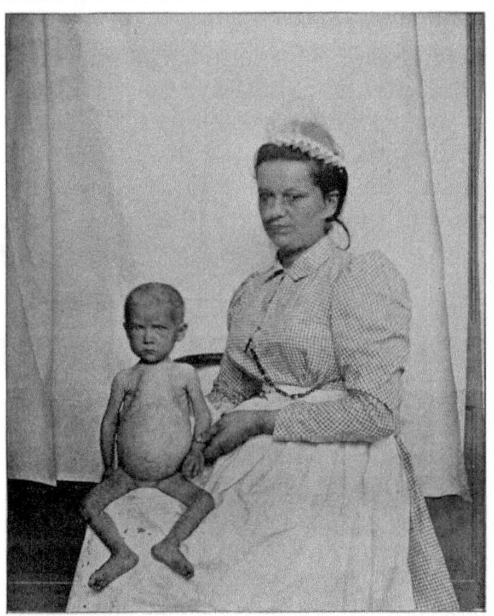

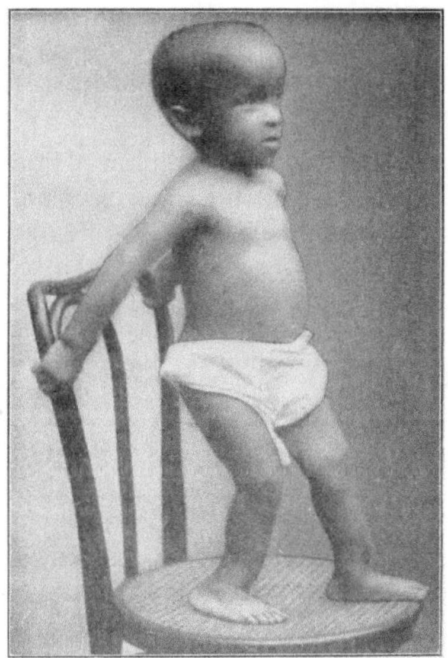

Source: From The Reading Room/Alamy Stock Photo. Image ID: 2AN5RG8.

FIGURE 26.2 Nurse administering cod liver oil to children at school (1910).

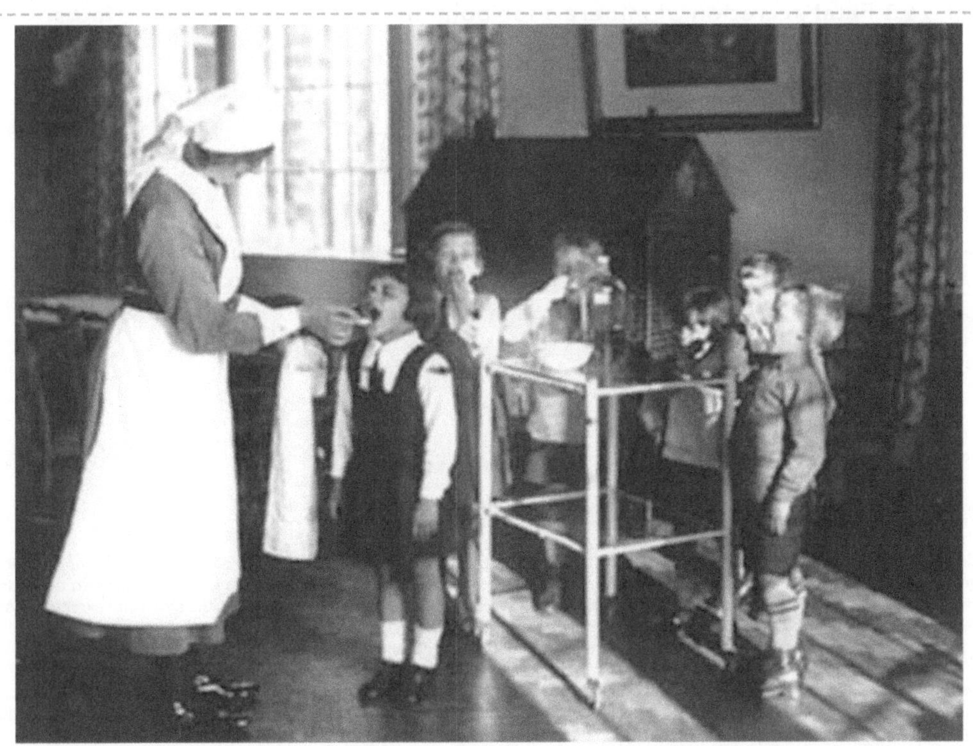

Source: From Hernigou, P., Auregan, J. C., & Dubory, A. (2019). Vitamin D: Part II; cod liver oil, ultraviolet radiation, and eradication of rickets. *International Orthopaedics, 43*(3), 735–749. https://doi.org/10.1007/s00264-019-04288-z.

combination paramount in eradicating rickets in this underserved population of infants and children (Hess, 1929). Cod liver oil had been used for centuries to relieve joint pain and treat rickets in children. Every 5 mL of cod liver oil provides 90% of the daily requirement for vitamin A and 113% of the requirement for vitamin D (Rajakumar, 2003; Raman, 2017).

An English physician, Edward Mellanby, identified the role that diet played in the development of rickets, postulating that sufficient intake of vitamin A, calcium, and phosphorus possessed "antirachitic" properties; across the pond, Elmer McCollum, a nutritional biochemist whose work included biological analysis of the contents of foods, discovered the vitamins contained in certain foods (McCollum, 1957). Clinical studies performed by Dr. Harriette Chick and colleagues in the 1920s and 1930s confirmed the preventive and therapeutic value of cod liver oil and sunlight to prevent rickets in infants (Weick, 1967). The seasonal variation in the incidence of rickets, the role of skin pigmentation in exacerbation of rickets during the winter months, the role of diet, and the appreciation that human milk was not an adequate source of vitamin D were now understood (Rajakumar, 2003). The eventual public health prevention strategy to fortify milk with vitamin D led to the eradication of rickets in the United States among term newborns (Weick, 1967).

PHYSIOLOGY REVIEW: FETAL SKELETAL DEVELOPMENT

The placenta plays a pivotal role in fetal skeletal development as calcium is actively transported transplacentally with a maternal to fetal calcium gradient of 1:4 (Moreira et al., 2015) In addition, activation of vitamin D to 1,25-dihydroxycholecalciferol (1,25[OH]$_2$D) also occurs in the placenta, which is an essential element of transplacental phosphate transfer (Faienza et al., 2019). Calcium and phosphorus readily cross the placenta to the fetus via active transport, and as such are stored by the developing fetus, as shown in Figure 26.3 (Perino, 2020).

The fetus experiences a "hypercalcemic" state, which is necessary for proper skeletal development, during which calcium and phosphorus promote the formation of bone. Vitamins A, C, and D, as well as hormones including thyroid hormone, growth hormone, and parathyroid

FIGURE 26.3 Fetal accretion of minerals for bone health in the developing fetus.

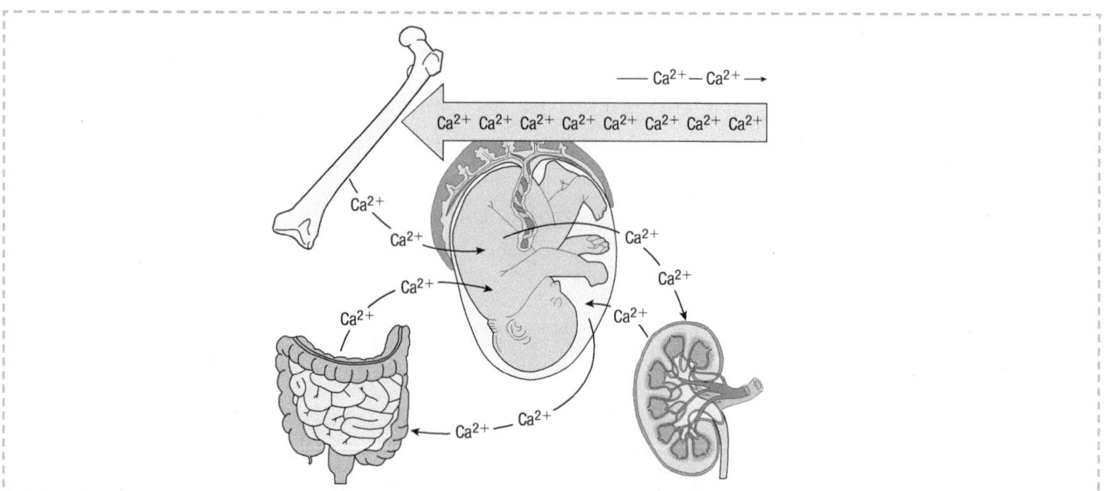

Note: Circulation of minerals within the fetal-placental unit. Calcium is represented here, but these statements apply to phosphorus (phosphate) and magnesium as well. At the *top right*, the main flux of mineral comes across the placenta and through the fetal circulation into the bone; however, some mineral returns to the maternal circulation (back flux). On the *bottom right*, the fetal kidneys filter the blood and excrete minerals into the urine, which in turn makes up much of the volume of amniotic fluid. On the *bottom left*, amniotic fluid is swallowed, and its mineral content can be absorbed by the fetal intestines, thereby restoring it to the circulation. The renal-amniotic-intestinal loop is likely a minor component for fetal mineral homeostasis. At the *top left*, although the net flux of mineral is into the bone, some minerals are reabsorbed from the developing skeleton to reenter the fetal circulation. If placental delivery of minerals is deficient, fetal secondary hyperparathyroidism ensues, which causes more substantial resorption of mineral from the fetal skeleton, reduced skeletal mineral content, and possible fractures occurring in utero or during the birthing process.

Source: From Kovacs, C. S. (2014). Bone development and mineral homeostasis in the fetus and neonate: Roles of the calciotropic and phosphotropic hormones. *Physiological Reviews, 94*(4), 1143–1218. https://doi.org/10.1152/physrev.00014.2014.

hormone (PTH), also have a role in influencing bone growth in utero (Gomella, 2020). Calcium and phosphorus are deposited into an organic matrix called the *osteoid*. Osteoblasts, which are bone-forming cells, work to create or model bone. They cover the surface of the spongiosa as well as make new layers of bone matrix. Osteoblasts have PTH receptors, which can increase the production of osteoclasts. Osteoclasts are the remodelers of bone—they break down and resorb bone (Rigo et al., 2007). Infants born prematurely cannot achieve optimal bone mineralization compared with full-term infants. In addition, poor mineral intake and absorption after a preterm birth result in a hypomineralization process; in other words, the new bone growth has decreased bone density.

Neonatal Bone Homeostasis

All newborns experience a hypocalcemic state shortly after birth. Calcium levels reach a nadir at 24 to 48 hours postdelivery related to the reversal of fetal physiologic mechanisms. After delivery, the hypocalcemic state occurs due to separation from maternal and placental circulation, and conditions become less favorable for mineralization, especially in preterm infants whose calcium and phosphorus stores are incomplete (Moreira et al., 2015; Rayannavar & Calabria, 2020). With removal of the placenta and low enteral intake in the first 24 hours, there is a precipitous drop in serum calcium, which leads to a hypocalcemic state. This leads to the release of PTH, which is blunted during the first 24 to 48 hours. Calcium levels quickly return to normal by 48 hours of life due to PTH, which stimulates release of calcium from the bone, renal reabsorption of calcium, and excretion of phosphorus. Mobilization of calcium, phosphorus, and even magnesium shares important functions in maintaining mineral homeostasis.

Renal function also plays a pivotal role in the regulation of these minerals to prevent excess urinary losses. In order to maintain homeostasis of these minerals in serum for cell function, these physiologic mechanisms may promote loss of bone integrity. Therefore, infants born prematurely with an already compromised skeletal system will mobilize minerals into the blood and consequently lose more bone strength in response to triggers to maintain homeostasis, as with acidosis commonly seen in preterm infants. To maintain homeostasis within acidotic conditions, the bone releases sodium bicarbonate, calcium carbonate, and dicalcium phosphate into the bloodstream, risking the already compromised strength and formation of bones (Moreira et al., 2015).

Noteworthy to the neonatal clinician is an understanding of the physiologic mechanisms responsible for bone homeostasis. Serum calcium homeostasis is maintained and controlled primarily by the relationship among PTH, calcitonin, and vitamin D. This reciprocal relationship exhibits their effects on the gastrointestinal (GI) tract, kidneys, and bones. The movement of calcium from the GI tract and bone determines the serum calcium concentration, establishing calcium homeostasis. This negative feedback system begins at birth with loss of the placenta. Calcium levels fall, stimulating PTH secretion. PTH stimulates receptors in the renal tubule and osteoblast. The receptors on the osteoblast in turn stimulate the osteoclasts to begin bone resorption, releasing calcium and phosphorus to the circulation and promoting reabsorption of calcium and excretion of phosphorus via the renal tubule, leading to increased serum calcium. In addition, PTH stimulates the kidney to release calcitriol. This stimulates proteins in the intestine to bind calcium and phosphorus increasing intestinal absorption. As serum concentrations of calcium normalize, PTH decreases and the thyroid secretes calcitonin. This stimulates osteoblasts to absorb calcium and phosphorus, decreasing intestinal and renal reabsorption of these minerals, as represented in Figure 26.4 (Chacham et al., 2020; Perino, 2020; Rayannavar & Calabria, 2020). The serum concentration of phosphate is primarily regulated by way of the kidney with tubular reabsorption of phosphate. The kidney also appears to be a primary site for maintaining normal serum magnesium levels. Normal calcium values over the first few days of life are summarized in Table 26.1.

ANTENATAL AND NEONATAL RISK FACTORS FOR OSTEOPENIA OF PREMATURITY

There are a number of both antenatal and neonatal (postnatal) risk factors summarized in Boxes 26.1 and 26.2 that are associated with OoP, although the main pathogenic mechanism is represented by the reduced placental transfer of calcium and phosphate related to preterm birth (Faienza et al., 2019). In addition, suboptimal maternal vascular supply of nutrients leads to poor growth

FIGURE 26.4 Calcium homeostasis.

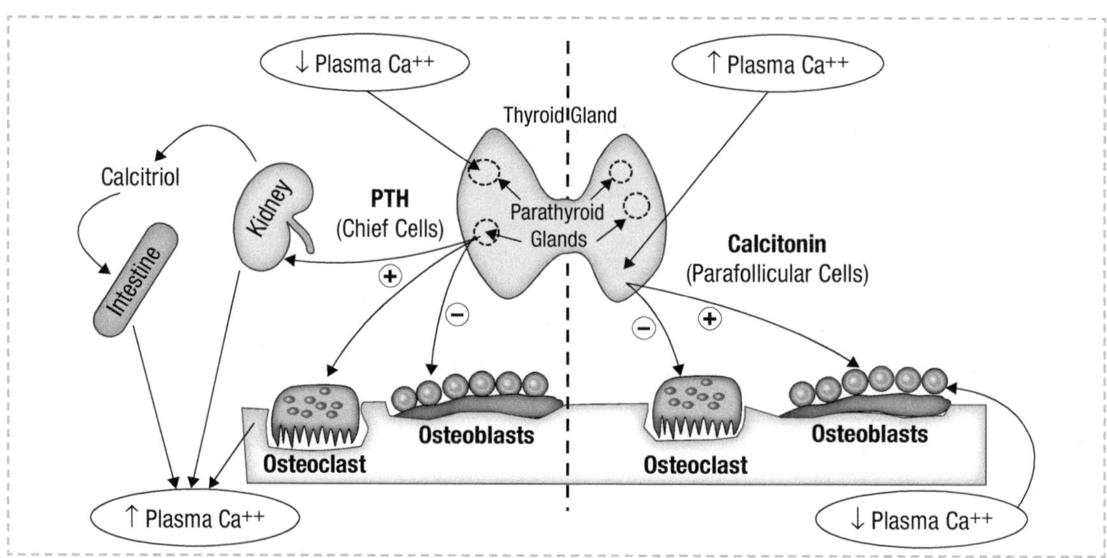

Note: When blood calcium levels drop, the parathyroid gland responds by releasing PTH. Conversely, high blood calcium levels stimulate the thyroid gland to release calcitonin to decrease calcium levels.
PTH, parathyroid hormone.
Source: From Perino, J. M. (2020). Calcium levels in the neonate. *Neonatal Network, 39*(1), 35–39. http://doi.org/10.1891/0703-0832.39.1.35. Image courtesy of Dr. W. Diehl-Jones.

TABLE 26.1 Newborn Calcium Values in the First 48 Hours of Life

	AGE	NORMAL VALUES SERUM CONCENTRATION (mg/dL)
Calcium, total	Cord blood	9–11.5
	Newborn 3–24 hours	9–10.6
	Newborn 24–48 hours	7–12
	4–7 days	9–10.9
Calcium, ionized, whole blood	Cord blood	5–6
	Newborn 3–24 hours	4.3–5.1
	Newborn 24–48 hours	4–4.7
	≥2 days	4.8–4.92

Source: Adapted from Taketomo, C. K. (Ed.). (2023). Pediatric & neonatal dosage handbook: An extensive resource for clinicians treating pediatric and neonatal patients (29th ed.). Lexicomp/Wolters Kluwer.

of the developing fetus. Several maternal conditions may obstruct maternal vascular flow to the fetus, including hypertension, diabetes, anemia, smoking, or use of cocaine (Abrams, 2017; Chacham et al., 2020; Moreira et al., 2015).

Having lost the last trimester of accelerated calcium and phosphorus absorption and bone growth puts the preterm infant at greatest risk. This is further compromised by the dysmature digestive functions of the preterm infant and limited amount of calcium and phosphorus in human milk and full-term formulas, which leads to inadequate absorption of nutrients needed for bone health and growth. This is exacerbated by impaired calcium and phosphorus absorption frequently identified in infants with necrotizing enterocolitis (NEC) and short bowel syndrome.

Other common neonatal morbidities that may impair bone remodeling by reducing osteoblast proliferation, activating osteoclast activity, and/or decreasing calcium absorption include sepsis, acidosis, and cholestatic jaundice. Chronic acidosis has been implicated in the pathogenesis of enhanced bone resorption and osteopenia, resulting in a loss of bone mineral content. The postulated mechanism for bone involvement includes acidosis-mediated exaggerated osteoclastic bone resorption. Other contributory factors include abnormal renal handling of phosphate,

BOX 26.1 Antenatal Risk Factors For Osteopenia of Prematurity

Chorioamnionitis
Genetic polymorphisms (vitamin D receptors, placental hormones: estrogens and collagen alpha-1)
Male gender fetus
Maternal malnutrition
Maternal use of tobacco
Maternal vitamin D deficiency
Placental insufficiency
Preeclampsia

Sources: Adapted from Abrams, S. A. (2017). Osteopenia (metabolic bone disease) of Prematurity. In E. C. Eichenwald, A. R. Hansen, C. Martin, & A. R. Stark (Eds). *Cloherty and Stark's manual of neonatal care* (8th ed., pp. 853–857) Wolters Kluwer; Chacham, S., Pasi, R., Chegondi, M., Ahmad, N., & Mohanty, S. B. (2020). Metabolic bone disease in premature neonates: An unmet challenge. *Journal of Clinical Research in Pediatric Endocrinology, 12*(4), 332. https://doi.org/10.4274/jcrpe.galenos.2019.2019.0091; Faienza, M. F., D'Amato, E., Natale, M. P., Grano, M., Chiarito, M., Brunetti, G., & D'Amato, G. (2019). Metabolic bone disease of prematurity: Diagnosis and management. *Frontiers in Pediatrics, 7*, 143. https://doi.org/10.3389/fped.2019.00143

BOX 26.2 Neonatal Risk Factors for Osteopenia of Prematurity

Extreme prematurity and VLBW, lack of movement, critically ill with sedation, lack of repositioning and support of proper body alignment care
Prolonged need for parenteral nutrition, unfortified human-milk feedings
Inadequate supply versus intake of calcium, phosphorus, and vitamin D
Chronic conditions/sequelae such as BPD, PVL/IVH, and NEC with short bowel/malabsorption/dumping phenomena
Hepatic (cholestatic jaundice) and renal (osteodystrophy) dysfunction
Medications (loop diuretics, caffeine, and glucocorticoids) that alter bone formation/compromise bone mineralization and osteolytic medications

BPD, bronchopulmonary dysplasia; IVH, intraventricular hemorrhage; NEC, necrotizng enterocolitis; PVL, periventricular leukomalacia; VLBW, very low birth weight.
Sources: Adapted from Abrams, S. A. (2017). Osteopenia (metabolic bone Disease) of Prematurity. In E. C. Eichenwald, A. R. Hansen, C. Martin, & A. R. Stark (Eds)., Cloherty and Stark's manual of neonatal care. 8th ed. (pp. 853–857). Philadelphia: Wolters Kluwer; Chacham, S., Pasi, R., Chegondi, M., Ahmad, N., & Mohanty, S. B. (2020). Metabolic bone disease in premature neonates: An unmet challenge. *Journal of Clinical Research in Pediatric Endocrinology, 12*(4), 332. https://doi.org/10.4274/jcrpe.galenos.2019.2019.0091; Faienza, M. F., D'Amato, E., Natale, M. P., Grano, M., Chiarito, M., Brunetti, G., & D'Amato, G. (2019). Metabolic bone disease of prematurity: Diagnosis and management. *Frontiers in Pediatrics, 7*, 143. https://doi.org/10.3389/fped.2019.00143; Moreira, A., Jacob, R., Lavender, L., & Escaname, E. (2015). Metabolic bone disease of prematurity. *NeoReviews, 16*(11), e631–e641. https://doi.org/10.1542/neo.16-11-e631

leading to hypophosphatemia in proximal renal tubular acidosis (RTA), and impaired vitamin D metabolism and action (Karpen, 2018). Other medical conditions that require the use of osteolytic medications (diuretics, glucocorticoids, and methylxanthines), such as bronchopulmonary dysplasia (BPD) and congestive heart failure (CHF), promote bone demineralization in the already-compromised infant (Faienza et al., 2019). Further in the chapter, we discuss osteolytic medications as a causative risk for OoP.

OSTEOPENIA OF PREMATURITY

OoP is a multifaceted postnatal bone disease commonly detected in very-low-birth-weight (VLBW; <1,500 grams) newborns, with a greater incidence in those preterm infants exhibiting extremely low-birth-weight (ELBW; <1,000 grams). The prevalence of OoP is difficult to discern related to the varying recommendations that exist in regard to the diagnosis, management, and treatment of osteopenia or metabolic bone disease (Faienza et al., 2019). OoP is characterized by biochemical and radiologic findings related to bone demineralization. Of note, OoP occurs due to intake and/or absorption of calcium and phosphorus inadequate to meet the normal bone growth demands. This results in varying degrees of hypomineralization of the skeleton when compared with fetal accretion rates. Rickets, however, presents with the radiologic features of a "washed out" appearance of the metaphysis of the long bone with or without evidence of fractures (Avila-Alvarez et al., 2020).

Clinicians should be aware that radiographic bone changes, such as fraying/cupping of the metaphyses and fractures, are only evident after 20% to 40% of bone loss has occurred in the affected infant, and oftentimes these changes are noted incidentally on the radiograph (Rayannavar & Calabria, 2020). Bone mineralization occurs in two phases. In phase 1, the osteoblasts are responsible for forming the osteoid (organic bone matrix). In phase 2, the accumulated minerals, primarily calcium and phosphorus, embed themselves within the bone matrix.

Pathophysiology of Osteopenia of Prematurity

Bone health is preserved within a tightly controlled balance of calcium and phosphorus. For infants who have lost the last trimester of mineral accretion as well as those with poor enteral absorption, it is important to employ preventive measures through fortified parenteral and enteral nutrition, vitamin supplementation, and routine monitoring to prevent bone demineralization and assess risk for OoP. Moreover, when inadequate mineral levels are recognized, additional supplementation of those and supporting elements should be provided to promote bone formation.

The incidence of rickets (confirmatory bony changes/fractures) is inversely proportional to gestational age (GA); currently 10% to 20% of those with a birth weight of less than 1,000 grams will develop this complication. Although the risk has decreased since the employment of fortified human milk and formulas and preventive vitamin D supplementation, risk, which is multifactorial, remains high as a complication of prematurity, feeding intolerance, and medication administration (Abrams & CON, 2013; Kelly et al., 2014; Mutlu et al., 2023; Perino, 2020). The body employs multiple mechanisms and feedback systems in an effort to maintain normal serum levels of calcium and phosphorus. As previously mentioned, these include secretion of PTH and calcitonin, intestinal absorption of calcium and phosphorus, renal absorption of calcium and excretion of phosphorus, and bone resorption and formation (Chacham et al., 2020).

One such feedback system occurs via the parathyroid gland. When serum calcium levels are low, PTH is secreted from the parathyroid gland to increase serum calcium. This causes the osteoclasts to release calcium into the bloodstream. In turn, phosphate excretion is increased via the kidney at the level of the distal tubule. PTH also stimulates the renal and intestinal absorption of calcium. As levels normalize, the mobilization of calcium from the bone decreases, as does renal and intestinal absorption. In turn, when calcium levels are increased, the parathyroid gland secretes calcitonin, which encourages bone osteoblasts to absorb calcium, stimulating bone formation, as shown in Figure 26.4.

In response to hypophosphatemia, calcitriol is released, stimulating phosphorus absorption by way of the intestine and osteoclast activity in the bone. However, this also stimulates the release of calcium from the bone, much like PTH, as well as reabsorption of calcium through the intestine and kidney. With osteoclast (bone resorption) activity, ultimately bone mass will decrease if adequate supplementation is not provided. In addition, in response to hypophosphatemia, the 1-α-hydroxylase enzyme is activated, leading to increased $1,25(OH)_2D$ levels, independent of PTH, supporting intestinal reabsorption of calcium and phosphorus. If $1,25(OH)_2D$ levels are low, additional vitamin D supplementation is needed to support adequate absorption of calcium and phosphorus in support of bone health (Auron & Alon, 2018; Chilakapati et al., 2019). When calcium and phosphorus levels normalize, 1-α-hydroxylase works to degrade calcitriol to the less active form, decreasing absorption of these minerals (Olmos-Ortiz et al., 2015).

In severe cases of hypophosphatemia, phosphorus levels will be low and calcium levels will be normal to high. This is due to mechanisms working to increase phosphorus levels, which also mobilize calcium. Given what is happening physiologically, it is important to recognize that phosphorus as well as calcium supplementation must be provided to prevent further loss of bone calcium, despite normal calcium levels. Furthermore, providing calcium increases ionized calcium (iCa) levels, thereby decreasing PTH secretion and thus decreasing phosphorus renal losses, both processes necessary to increase serum phosphorus, decrease bone reabsorption, and promote bone formation (Auron & Alon, 2018; Chinoy et al., 2019, 2021). These processes identify biochemical markers helpful in screening bone health.

PHARMACOTHERAPIES WITH OSTEOLYTIC PROPERTIES

Diuretics

Premature infants who develop breathing problems related to immaturity, such as apnea of prematurity or BPD, may require diuretics to facilitate gas exchange (Orth & O'Mara, 2018). Although clinical trials have yet to show that long-term use of diuretics prevents or lessens BPD, they are often used to treat preterm infants with concerns for chronic lung disease (McPherson, 2019). Diuretics work via the kidneys to reduce sodium reabsorption, thereby influencing the volume of water reabsorbed into circulation.

By increasing urine output, diuretics are able to reduce preload stress on both the lungs and heart. Pulmonary edema has been linked to reduced gas exchange in the alveoli, so it is critical for babies with respiratory conditions to avoid volume overload to help reduce the need for oxygen or mechanical ventilation. However, diuretics also lead to electrolyte imbalances, which include calcium and phosphorus renal losses and metabolic alkalosis, further contributing to calcium loses (by increased calcium binding to protein decreasing bio-availability) and increasing risk for bone demineralization, as well as reduction in growth velocity (Davies, 2015; McPherson, 2019; Orth & O'Mara, 2018; Perino, 2020).

By far, the diuretic class that carries the largest risk of bone demineralization in preterm neonates is loop diuretics (Chinoy, 2019). Loop diuretics, such as furosemide, block calcium reabsorption by blocking the Na/K/2Cl cotransporter at the loop of Henle and calcium paracellular excretion, further contributing to calcium and magnesium losses (Auron & Alon, 2018). Thiazide diuretics are associated with osteomalacia (soft bones) in neonates but through a different mechanism. Thiazide diuretics, such as chlorothiazide, increase calcium reabsorption and phosphorus loss via the distal and proximal convoluted tubules (Liamis et al., 2010; Orth & O'Mara, 2018). Rarely contributing to hypercalcemia, thiazide diuretics promote renal clearance of phosphate, leading to hypophosphatemia, which stimulates bone resorption in an attempt to reestablish normal serum phosphate levels (Auron & Alon, 2018; Orth & O'Mara, 2018).

Glucocorticoids

Corticosteroids are routinely used to treat severe BPD as they have demonstrated efficacy in reducing the duration of ventilation dependency of these infants (Cummings, 2022). Corticosteroids, especially glucocorticoids, have suppressive effects on bone formation and growth and have been demonstrated to reduce gut absorption of calcium, as well as increase urinary excretion of calcium (Canalis, 1996). The lack of calcium impacts bone homeostasis as low serum calcium promotes osteoclast maturation and subsequent bone demineralization. Prolonged courses of high-dose glucocorticoids, often dexamethasone, have been identified as a risk factor for the development of OoP and should be used at the lowest effective dose for the shortest duration possible (Ukarapong et al., 2017). Although a threshold dose per day has not yet been determined in neonates, an earlier study showed that neonatal exposure as tapering high-dose dexamethasone (cumulative dose 6–8 mg) was associated with significantly shorter stature and reduced bone mass later in life (Wang et al., 2007).

Caffeine

In the NICU, caffeine is the most prescribed agent to treat apnea of prematurity due to its wide therapeutic index and ability to be dosed once daily (Abdel-Hady et al., 2015; Ali et al., 2018). Caffeine works in the treatment of neonatal apnea of prematurity by stimulating the respiratory center in the medulla, as well as increases the body's peripheral sensitivity to carbon dioxide, enhances diaphragmatic contractility to aid with the mechanical process of breathing, and increases skeletal muscle tone, minute ventilation, metabolic rate, and oxygen consumption (Abdel-Hady et al., 2015). Caffeine enhances bone resorption by promoting osteoclast differentiation and by inhibition of tubular reabsorption of calcium in the kidneys, which also contributes to increased urine output (Abdel-Hady et al., 2015).

In the neonatal population, a randomized controlled trial evaluated the rate of calcium excretion in the urine in preterm infants treated with either theophylline or caffeine (methylxanthines) compared with controls (Zenardo et al., 1995). The investigators found babies treated with methylxanthines had a higher rate of urinary calcium excretion 10 to 15 times that of controls, further supporting the urinary calcium excretion hypothesis (Zenardo et al., 1995). Although daily doses of caffeine may not necessarily be linked to increased risk of osteopenia, a retrospective study led by Ali and colleagues discovered an association between higher cumulative doses of caffeine and increased risk of OoP (Ali et al., 2018). The study included 109 VLBW infants with GA less than 31 weeks and both biochemical markers of bone demineralization as well as radiographs were used to diagnose osteopenia. The authors accounted for potential covariables which could confound study outcomes, including diuretic/vitamin D/corticosteroid use, GA, and weight. The authors still concluded even with those adjustments that for every 5-mg/kg increase in cumulative caffeine dose, the infant was 1.10 times more likely to develop osteopenia (95% CI: 1.05–1.15). In addition, the probability of osteopenia increased as the duration of caffeine therapy was extended ($p = .02$).

Clinicians should be mindful of the impact any of these medications may have on the population of infants already at risk for osteopenia. Combining these medications to treat disease further increases the risk for OoP. Optimal nutrition (including calcium/phosphate/vitamin D) is critical, and growth should be monitored and maximized to reduce the risk of developing osteopenia.

PREVENTION AND SCREENING OF OSTEOPENIA OF PREMATURITY

OoP is an evasive disease that does not present with signs and/or symptoms until significant bone loss has occurred. Although guidelines for screening do exist (Abrams et al., 2013; American Society for Parenteral and Enteral Nutrition [ASPEN], 2013), a survey by Kelly and colleagues in 2014 demonstrated that even though experts agree that routine screening for this disease in preterm and sick neonates is necessary, which tests used to screen, when to screen, and when to provide treatment are inconsistent among neonatologists (Chinoy et al., 2021; Kelly et al., 2014; Rayannavar & Calabria, 2020).

OoP requires monitoring of several biochemical markers, as well as radiologic and ultrasonographic investigation, when OoP is suspected. The principal approach is prevention of this disease through meticulous screening of all preterm infants at risk of developing OoP, particularly those ≤2,000 grams and ≤32 weeks' gestation, infants who have been on long-term parenteral nutrition, those who do not tolerate fortification, as well as infants requiring fortified human milk and formulas (Abrams & CON, 2013). Most often, calcium, phosphorus, and ALP are used to monitor bone health for those at risk, beginning by 4 weeks of age and biweekly thereafter until fortification can be discontinued (Abrams et al., 2013; ASPEN, 2013). However, more recent evidence supports the use of PTH in identifying early disease.

A study conducted by Chinoy and colleagues published in 2021 highlights the delicate balance between calcium and phosphorus and the importance of the provider recognizing how these elements work in tandem to promote bone health. To determine the role of hyperparathyroidism screening in infants with OoP, the authors conducted a survey study to examine the practices used to screen and treat OoP among neonatologists and endocrinologists in the United Kingdom. The authors found that fewer neonatologist respondents use PTH levels to determine OoP risk compared with endocrinologists ($p < .001$). PTH is as sensitive and more specific for OoP than ALP, and additionally beneficial when monitoring response to treatment (Moreira et al., 2014).

Furthermore, neonatologists most often reported treating infants with phosphate supplements alone without calcium for hypophosphatemia in addition to either a multivitamin for vitamin D or vitamin D supplements. The consequence of not providing calcium supplementation when calcium levels appear normal in combination with low phosphorus levels is that both calcium and phosphorus will be leached from the bone in an effort to normalize serum phosphorus levels. This then leads to hyperparathyroidism secondary to an imbalance in the ratio of serum calcium to phosphorus, as well as bone reabsorption (mobilizes calcium and phosphorus from the bone), inhibiting bone formation (Chilakapati et al., 2019; Chinoy et al., 2021).

When using ALP as a screening tool, it is important to also consider other factors or physiologic properties that may affect ALP levels. First, PTH increases in response to low calcium levels. ALP levels will then increase in response to elevated PTH. However, ALP will also increase in response to liver disease, decreasing the specificity of this marker for bone disease until late in the disease (Newsome et al., 2018). With elevated ALP, bone-specific ALP and osteocalcin levels can be obtained to help determine elevation of this enzyme from the bone or liver, although preterm normative levels do not exist (Abrams & CON, 2013). Gamma-glutamyl transferase (GGT) can also be used to differentiate the source of elevated ALP, as it is not found in bone, but abundant in liver. If GGT is elevated, indicating liver disease, it is more likely that the liver is the cause of elevated ALP (Newsome et al., 2018).

Since PTH increases first, it is a more sensitive marker (71% vs. 26%) of movement of calcium from the bone compared with ALP and elevates before hypophosphatemia develops. Elevated PTH (>180 pg/dL) combined with low phosphorus increases the sensitivity to 100% and specificity to 94% for OoP (Moreira et al., 2013). Although hypophosphatemia, in addition to elevated ALP, increases the sensitivity as a marker of OoP, this occurs late in the disease (Auron & Alon, 2018; Chinoy et al., 2021; Rayannavar & Calabria 2020). These findings highlight the importance that PTH levels can have for OoP screening. The authors recommend screening PTH levels in addition to ALP, calcium, and phosphorus as part of monitoring for OoP to begin at 3 to 4 weeks of life and biweekly for low-birth-weight infants and those less than 32 weeks' gestation (Chinoy et al., 2019).

Last, isolated hypophosphatemia may be present. Screening the tubular reabsorption of phosphorus (TRP) is helpful to determine the cause and what to supplement. TRP will be high in an attempt to conserve phosphorus, whereas PTH will be low/normal. This indicates a need for phosphorus supplementation most likely due to low intake or poor phosphate intestinal absorption. If TRP is low, this favors phosphorus renal excretion as seen with increased PTH, which encourages phosphorus excretion, indicating the need to supplement both calcium and phosphorus for hypophosphatemia (Rayannavar & Calabria 2020).

Radiographic studies are indicated when fracture is suspected on physical examination or when lab results are concerning for OoP, which is ALP greater than 900 IU/L or greater than 500 IU/L and trending up with normal GGT, in combination with hypophosphatemia. The most valuable radiographs are those of the wrist and knee (Abrams & CON, 2013; Chinoy et al., 2019, 2021). Table 26.2 summarizes several biomarkers used to test for OoP with normative value ranges.

CURRENT NONPHARMACOLOGIC TREATMENT MODALITY FOR OSTEOPENIA OF PREMATURITY: MOBILIZATION

Immobilization inhibits osteoblast activity and bone remodeling. This can occur in infants with induced immobility receiving sedative medications or muscle weakness as with hypoxic-ischemic encephalopathy (HIE) and hypophosphatemia (Avila-Alverez et al, 2020). A systematic review of literature showed that physical activity, including a protocol of passive range of motion (ROM) and joint compression performed 5 to 15 minutes daily for 4 to 8 weeks, can improve bone mineralization in preterm infants, as demonstrated through quantitative ultrasound (QUS) and biochemical markers of bone turnover. Current evidence suggests that therapeutic positioning against flexible boundaries is the safest means of promoting active bone loading for preterm and chronically ill infants. Future studies should explore a holistic, developmental care model and use of positioning aids that allow for movement against flexible resistance while continuing to incorporate an interdisciplinary approach. In addition, larger sample sizes and longitudinal studies are needed to determine long-term outcomes of physical activity on fracture reduction and bone health in preterm infants (Schulzke et al., 2014; Stalnaker & Poskey, 2016). Table 26.3 provides a summary of the key points of discussion for infants at risk of OoP.

TABLE 26.2 Common Biomarkers Used for Screening in Osteopenia of Prematurity

BIOMARKERS	NORMAL VALUE RANGES	ASSOCIATED RISK
ALP Bone turnover marker	**Term:** 90–540 IU/L **Preterm:** Values peak at 400–800 IU/L in VLBW 4–6 weeks, then decrease if OoP is not present and infant is receiving supplementation with fortification. **Key point:** ALP increases physiologically over the first 3 weeks of life and then peaks by 6–12 weeks. ALP is a poor indicator of OoP as a stand-alone marker unless serum phosphorus levels are also low.	Can be affected by hepatic dysfunction particularly cholestasis. Screen GGT to help interpret ALP. • Greater than 500 IU/L and trending up suggests impaired bone homeostasis. • Greater than 700 IU/L reflects bone demineralization despite absence of clinical signs. • Greater than 900 IU/L without hepatic dysfunction, less than 32 weeks' GA, and low phosphorus levels <4.6 mg/dL (1.8 mmol/L), should consider radiograph evaluation; these values have a diagnostic sensitivity of 100% and a diagnostic specificity of 70%. • Greater than 1,200 IU/L is associated with short stature in childhood.
Total calcium (bound + unbound)	**Term:** 8.5–10.2 mg/dL (2.1–2.6 mmol/L) **Preterm:** 7–9 mg/dL (1.8–2.6 mmol/L) **Key point:** Alone, not a reliable screening marker. Infants with bone loss may still have normal serum calcium levels.	40% of total calcium is bound to albumin and unavailable for cell function. • Calcium value falls 0.8 mg/dL (0.2 mmol/L) for every 1 g/dL decrease in albumin. • Calcium values may also be affected by phosphate depletion.
Ionized calcium (available)	4.4–5.3 mg/dL (1.1–1.35 mmol/L)	Affected by pH, increased availability with low pH. (A change of 0.1 pH unit may alter ionized calcium by 10% without altering total calcium concentration.)
PTH	1.6–9.3 pmol/L (15.1–87.7 pg/mL)	Increases first with low calcium; elevated PTH (>180 pg/dL) combined with low phosphorus increases the sensitivity to 100% and specificity to 94% for OoP.
Phosphate	5.0–8.8 mg/dL (1.25–2.2 mmol/L) **Key point:** Hypophosphatemia is the EARLIEST marker of impaired mineral homeostasis.	Less than 4.6 mg/dL (<1.1 mmol/L) at 3 weeks of age. Oral phosphorus supplementation binds with ionized calcium, further decreasing ionized calcium levels leading to further PTH secretion.

GTT	Mean range (IU/L) at 3–7 days of life 22–25 weeks: 76.6 ± 58.1 26–29 weeks: 147.4 ± 123.4 30–36 weeks: 175.5 ± 95.00 37–39 weeks: 144.8 ± 90.4 40–42 weeks. 116.8 ± 73.3	
Serum 25(OH)D levels	Sufficiency: 20–100 ng/mL (50–250 nmol/L) Insufficiency: 15–20 ng/mL (37.5–50 nmol/L)) Deficiency: <15 ng/mL (<37.5 nmol/L) Severe deficiency: ≤5 ng/mL (≤12.5 nmol/L) Intoxication: ≥150 ng/mL (375 nmol/L)	1,25(OH)$_2$D should not be used for monitoring vitamin D concentration, not representative of vitamin D exposure; very unstable.
Long bone radiographs of wrist and knee	Radiographic changes usually evident after 20%–40% mineral loss has occurred; recognition of fractures usually an incidental finding	Obtain radiographs for VLBW infants whose ALP levels are >900 IU/L when measured 1 week apart for two consecutive measurements.
Urine calcium: Urine creatinine (spot urine)	<3.8 mmol/mmol (1.3 mg/mg)	It is not reliable in detecting OoP; affected by preterm kidney. Use of loop diuretics/methylxanthines may affect levels.
QUS DEXA scan (considered the gold standard for assessing bone mineralization and fragility) SOS US	Used in research settings and not widely available; used to determine mineral content SOS: measures bone density, predicting bone turnover	QUS can be done at bedside. DEXA scans cannot be done at bedside, radiation exposure; guidelines for children are lacking. SOS has no radiation, has reference ranges for term and preterm infants, and not widely available.
TRP	85%–95% when serum phosphorous level is <5.5 mg/dL Key point: Obtain serum phosphorous and creatinine at the same time of urine.	↑ with phosphorus depletion, poor intake, or absorption.

1,25(OH)$_2$D, 1,25-dihydroxycholecalciferol; ALP, alanine phosphatase; DEXA, dual x-ray absorptiometry; GA, gestational age; GGT, gamma-glutamyl transferease; OoP, osteopenia of prematurity; PTH, parathyroid hormone; QUS, quantitative ultrasound; SOS, speed of sound; TRP, tubular reabsorption of phosphate; US, ultrasound; VLBW, very low birth weight.

Sources: Adapted from Abrams, S. A., Committee on Nutrition (2013). Calcium and vitamin D requirements of enterally fed preterm infants. *Pediatrics, 131*(5), e1676–e1683. https://doi.org/10.1542/peds.2013-0420; Auron, A., & Alon, U. S. (2018). Hypercalcemia: A consultant's approach. *Pediatric Nephrology, 33*(9), 1475–1488. https://doi.org/10.1007/s00467-017-3788-z; Chacham, S., Pasi, R., Chegondi, M., Ahmad, N., & Mohanty, S. B. (2020). Metabolic bone disease in premature neonates: An unmet challenge. *Journal of Clinical Research in Pediatric Endocrinology, 12*(4), 332. https://doi.org/ 0.4274/jcrpe.galenos.2019.2019.0091; Chinoy, A., Mughal, M. Z., & Padidela, R. (2019). Metabolic bone disease of prematurity: Causes, recognition, prevention, treatment and long-term consequences. *Archives of Disease in Childhood Fetal and Neonatal Edition, 104*(5), F560–F566. https://doi.org/10.1136/archdischild-2018-316330; Davies, J. H. (2015). Approach to the child with hypercalcaemia. *Endocrine Development, 28*, 101–118. https://doi.org/10.1159/000380998; Perino, J. M. (2020). Calcium levels in the neonate. *Neonatal Network, 39*(1), 35–39. http://doi.org/10.1891/0703-0832.39.1.35; Zhou, P., & Markowitz, M. (2009). Hypocalcemia in infants and children. Pediatrics in review, *30*(5), 190–192. https://doi.org/10.1542/pir.30-5-190; and Rayannavar, A., & Calabria, A. C. (2020). Screening for metabolic bone disease of prematurity. Seminars in fetal and neonatal medicine, *25*(1), 101086. https://doi.org/10.1016/j.siny.2020.101086.

TABLE 26.3 Pharmacotherapeutic Osteopenia of Prematurity Risk

DISEASE	PREVENTION/TREATMENT STRATEGIES	COMPETING EFFECTS THAT CONTRIBUTE TO OoP
BPD	• Loop diuretics • Thiazide diuretic • Glucocorticoids (steroids)	• Loop diuretics enhance calcium renal losses with long-term use. • There is risk of bone calcium/phosphorus demineralization with thiazide diuretics. These should be reserved for infants demonstrating pulmonary edema, avoiding chronic administration. • Steroids promote osteoclast maturation inhibiting bone formation, decrease gut absorption of calcium/phosphorous, plus increase renal excretion of calcium.
Diseases preventing adequate enteral nutrition: short-gut syndrome, NEC, diseases requiring fluid restriction, slow advancement, and intolerance to enteral nutrition	• Parenteral nutrition	• Limited calcium/phosphorous administration unable to meet physiologic demand due to compatibility within the solution. Adequate protein is required to support calcium and phosphorus solubility in parenteral nutrition. As solutions become concentrated, intake of these elements becomes limited. Decreased concentrations when not administered centrally, due to risk of IV infiltration and alterations in the skin's integrity. • As a contaminant, aluminum content in parenteral nutrition varies, accumulation interferes with other minerals interfering with bone formation. • Increased renal calcium losses occur. • In NEC, disrupted microbiome and gut atrophy inhibit secretion of intestinal enzymes, limiting calcium/phosphorous absorption.
Apnea of prematurity	• Caffeine	• Caffeine increases osteoclast activity and renal losses of calcium. This increases with longer duration of use.
Seizures and cholestasis	• Anticonvulsants	• Use of phenytoin/phenobarbital promotes increased hepatic metabolism (CYP450), which leads to decreased vitamin D availability, which directly affects calcium levels.
HIE	• Calcium	• Hypoxia interferes with magnesium, allowing cellular influx of calcium and low serum calcium levels. Therapeutic hypothermia will increase levels. Close monitoring is needed. • Immobilization occurs with sedative medications. • Hypophosphatemia decreases osteoblast activity.

Malabsorption	• Addition of fat-soluble vitamins A, D, E, and K	• Causes poor gut calcium and phosphorus absorption with limited vitamin D availability.
Hyperbilirubinemia	• Phototherapy	• Encourages calcium bone osteoclast absorption.
GERD GI surgeries GI anomalies or disease	• Proton pump inhibitors: omeprazole • H_2 antagonists: famotidine, ranitidine	• Inhibit intestinal absorption of calcium.
Osteopenia	• Calcium and phosphate supplementation	• If administered together, causes precipitation without absorption. • Phosphorus should not be administered with formula as it will inhibit calcium absorption. • Calcium administered simultaneously with phosphorus will bind with phosphorus in feeding, inhibiting absorption. Calcium should be administered separately from feeding and phosphorus administration.

BPD, bronchopulmonary dysplasia; GERD, gastroesophageal reflux disease; GI, gastrointestinal; HIE, hypoxic-ischemic encephalopathy; IV, intravenous; NEC, necrotizing enterocolitis; OoP, osteopenia of prematurity.

Sources: Adapted from Abrams, S. A., Committee on Nutrition (2013). Calcium and vitamin D requirements of enterally fed preterm infants. *Pediatrics, 131*(5), e1676–e1683. https://doi.org/10.1542/peds.2013-0420; ASPEN. (2013). Clinical guidelines: Nutritional support of neonatal patients at risk for metabolic bone disease. *Journal of Parenteral and Enteral Nutrition, 37*(5), 570–598. https://doi.org/10.1177/0148607113487216; Avila-Alvarez, A., Urisarri, A., Fuentes-Carballal, J., Mandiá, N., Sucasas-Alonso, A., & Couce, M. L. (2020). Metabolic bone disease of prematurity: Risk factors and associated short-term outcomes. *Nutrients, 12*(12), 3786. https://doi.org/10.3390/nu12123786; Perino, J. M. (2020). Calcium levels in the neonate. *Neonatal Network, 39*(1), 35–39. http://doi.org/10.1891/0703-0832.39.1.35; Chinoy, A., Mughal, M. Z., & Padidela, R. (2019). Metabolic bone disease of prematurity: Causes, recognition, prevention, treatment and long-term consequences. *Archives of Disease in Childhood-Fetal and Neonatal Edition, 104*(5), F560–F566. https://doi.org/10.1136/archdischild-2018-316330; McPherson, C. (2019). Pharmacotherapy for the prevention of bronchopulmonary sysplasia: Can anything compete with caffeine and corticosteroids? *Neonatal Network, 38*(4), 242–249. https://doi.org/10.1891/0730-0832.38.4.242; Mutlu, M., Aktürk-Acar, F., Kader, S., Aslan, Y., & Karagüzel, G. (2023). Risk factors and clinical characteristics of metabolic bone disease of prematurity. *American Journal of Perinatology, 40*(5), 519-524. https://doi.org/10.1055/s-0041-1729559; Sabroske, E. M., Payne, D. H., Stine, C. N., Kathen, C. M., Sollohub, H. M., Kohlleppel, K. L., Lorbieski, P. L., Carney, J. E., Motta, C. L., Pierce, M. R., & Ahmad, K. A. (2020). Effect on metabolic bone disease markers in the neonatal intensive care unit with implementation of a practice guideline. *Journal of Perinatology, 40*(8), 1267–1272. https://doi.org/10.1038/s41372-020-0693-2

CURRENT PHARMACOLOGIC TREATMENT MODALITIES FOR OSTEOPENIA OF PREMATURITY

As neonatal clinicians, our goal should always be to focus on primary prevention. Despite the best evidence-based neonatal nutritional advancements, there remain those infants who require pharmacologic therapies to address their OoP. Recommendations for prescribing calcium, phosphorus, and vitamin D vary greatly across the world. One treatment plan that has gained a global consensus among neonatal providers is that premature infants be fed fortified human milk or a preterm formula to optimize bone mineralization. In addition, neonatal providers should be conscious to limit the chronic use of diuretics and methylxanthines, which will reduce mineral stores and glucocorticoids, which will enhance bone resorption.

Nutritional Supplementation

The last trimester is when 80% of calcium and phosphorus accretion occurs, putting the preterm infant less than 27 weeks' gestation at greatest risk (Chinoy et al., 2021). During this period, absorption rates increase to provide calcium 100 to 130 mg/kg/d and phosphorus 60 to 70 mg/kg/d (Mutlu et al., 2023). Therefore, for this population, it is imperative that supplementation of these minerals be provided to avoid the bone demineralization seen with OoP. The recommendation for prevention of OoP in preterm infants is to provide adequate calcium of 120 to 220 mg/kg/d and phosphorous of 60 to 140 mg/kg/d to maintain a calcium to phosphorus ratio of 2:1 (Abrams et al., 2013; Chacham et al., 2020; Chinoy et al., 2019). Vitamin D supplementation is recommended for all infants (Abrams et al., 2013). Providing mothers who are breastfeeding with vitamin D supplementation of 600 IU/d has also been shown to have a preventive effect (Chacham et al., 2020).

Although human milk is the gold standard to support neonatal nutrition, it is very low in calcium and phosphorus and unable to meet the needs of the preterm infant's growth. Since fortifying human milk with calcium, phosphorus, and other elements has become widespread, OoP has decreased. This advent has left those infants who receive competing medications and those with complications that leave the neonate vulnerable to long-term parenteral nutrition, poor enteral intake, and immobilization to be most vulnerable to OoP (Chacham et al., 2020; Chinoy et al., 2021). It is recommended that preterm infants receive human milk with fortification or preterm formulas up to 34 weeks' postmenstrual age or until their weight exceeds 1,800 to 2,000 grams before transitioning off supplementation (Abrams et al., 2013).

Additional supplementation of calcium, phosphorus, and/or vitamin D would be driven by screening results (Figure 26.5). As previously described, there is a balance between calcium and phosphorus that requires the evaluation of more than one lab test to determine treatment. With elevated PTH greater than 180 pg/dL and iCa less than 4.5 mg/dL, the infant requires calcium supplementation. Calcium carbonate oral suspension is the preferred oral supplementation. Absorption occurs in the small intestine and is dependent on calcitriol and vitamin D. Calcium primarily distributes in the form of hydroxyapatite crystal in the skeleton (99%) and is protein-bound to albumin (40%). Calcium does not undergo direct metabolism and is excreted in feces (75%) and urine.

When phosphorus levels are less than 4.6 mg/dL, phosphorus should be supplemented as well (Chacham et al., 2020; Faienza et al., 2019; Moreira et al., 2015). Only when TRP is increased greater than 85%, indicating renal absorption of phosphorus with hypophosphatemia and normal calcium levels, should phosphorus be supplemented alone. Phosphorus can be supplemented with either potassium phosphate (Neutra-Phos-K) or sodium and potassium phosphate (Phos-Nak or Neutra-Phos). Phosphorus salt absorbs well from the upper GI tract and enters cells through active transport from extracellular fluid found in the skeleton in combination with calcium. Of the serum phosphate, 85% is free and ultra-filterable and only 15% is protein-bound. Like calcium, phosphorus does not undergo direct metabolism and is excreted in the urine, with more than 80% of the dose resorbable by the kidneys. Additional vitamin D supplementation should be provided if levels of 25(OH)D are less than 20 IU/dL. The algorithm for prevention, screening, and treatment of OoP provides a systematic approach to management (see Figure 26.5).

FIGURE 26.5 Algorithm for prevention, screening, and treatment of osteopenia of prematurity.

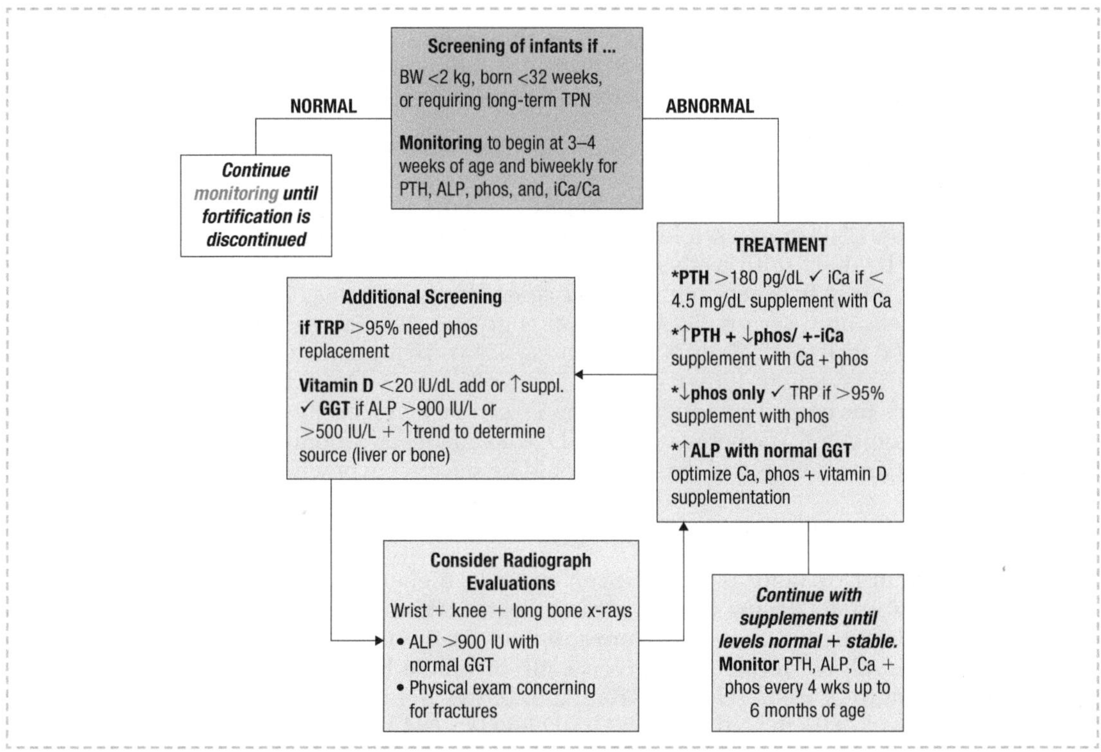

ALP, alkaline phosphatase; BW, birth weight; Ca, calcium; GGT, gamma-glutamyl transferase; iCa, ionized calcium; IU, international units; phos, phosphorus; PTH, parathyroid hormone; TPN, total parenteral nutrition; TRP, tubular reabsorption of phosphate.

Vitamin D: Pharmacokinetic Principles

Vitamin D is a fat-soluble vitamin available in two forms. Vitamin D_3, or cholecalciferol, produced endogenously in skin with sunlight exposure, can also be consumed via animal-based foods. Vitamin D_2, or ergocalciferol, is plant-based and produced synthetically from ergosterol found in plants. Both forms are provitamins that must be activated by 25-hydroxylase in the liver to form 25(OH)D (calcidiol) and then by 1-α-hydroxylase in the kidney to produce the active metabolite $1,25(OH)_2D$ (calcitriol; Auron & Alon, 2018; Olmos-Ortiz e al., 2015). Structurally, the two forms differ by one side chain; vitamin D_2 has an additional methyl chain (Figure 26.6; Kane, 2015). Vitamin D works by stimulating intestinal absorption of calcium and phosphorus,

FIGURE 26.6 Two forms of vitamin D (D_2 and D_3).

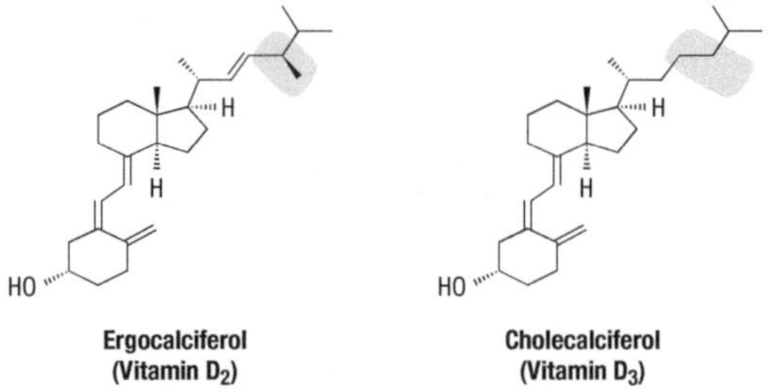

Ergocalciferol (Vitamin D_2)

Cholecalciferol (Vitamin D_3)

Source: From Kane, S. P. (2015, July 19). *It's time to say "goodbye" to vitamin D2 (ergocalciferol)*. https://www.ClinCalc.com.

promoting renal reabsorption of filtered calcium, and by mobilizing calcium from bone to blood. Onset of action for both vitamin D_2 and D_3, defined as rise in serum 25(OH)D, appears to be the same (Armas et al., 2004). In addition, although the rise of serum 25(OH)D was similar between vitamin D_2 and D_3, the potency of vitamin D_3 is three times greater than vitamin D_2, achieving higher levels of 25(OH)D (Tripkovic et al., 2012). Excretion of either vitamin D_2 or vitamin D_3 is via bile (feces) with minimal renal elimination.

DOSING RECOMMENDATIONS

The AAP recommends 200 IU daily for premature neonates less than 1,500 grams and 400 IU for infants greater than 1,500 grams if tolerating full enteral nutrition. For term neonates, the recommendation is 400 IU daily until feeds are between 800 and 1,000 mL/d with vitamin D-fortified formula (Abrams, 2013). In severe symptomatic cases, doses as high as 2,000 IU have been recommended for 6 weeks until serum 25(OH)D level is greater than 20 ng/mL, followed by a maintenance dose of 400 to 1000 IU daily (Golden et al., 2014). Treatment should include calcium and phosphorus supplementation. Either vitamin D_3 or vitamin D_2 should be administered using a syringe to measure the correct quantity. Vitamin D_3 can be given orally as a liquid formulation of 10 mcg/mL (400 units/mL), whereas vitamin D_2 is available as an oral 8,000 -unit/mL solution. Formulations that are alcohol- and dye-free should be selected in newborns.

CLINICAL-MONITORING PEARLS

The risk of vitamin D toxicity is rare but can occur in higher doses. Toxicity is more likely to occur from inappropriate dosing during home administration of vitamin D by parents. Two case reports identify breastfed infants who were supplemented with vitamin D (Bilbao, 2017). In the first case, a 3.5-month-old female was given 1 mL of Whole Foods over-the-counter vitamin D daily with a strength of 2,000 IU/mL. After 2.5 months, the infant presented to the ED with a serum calcium level of 21 mg/dL and 25(OH)D level of 644 ng/mL. In the second case report, a 2.5-month-old male was given 1 mL of Hi-Po Emulsi-D3 daily, which has a strength of 2,000 IU per drop. This medication is a prescription-only formulation and was initially prescribed by a chiropractor for adult use. After receiving 20,000 IU daily (10 drops) for 1.5 weeks, the infant was admitted to the ED with a serum calcium of 15 mg/dL and 25(OH)D level of 680 ng/mL. Signs and symptoms of vitamin D toxicity include poor feeding, constipation, lethargy, polyuria, failure to thrive, emesis, and diarrhea. These case reports demonstrate the importance of patient counseling upon discharge to prevent inappropriate dosing and toxicity. Notable drug–drug interactions include bile acid sequestrants like cholestyramine, which impairs the absorption of vitamin D; thus, administration time should be separated by several hours (Robien et al., 2013). Multivitamins may already contain adequate daily vitamin D doses and combining it with other vitamin D formulations is considered duplicative therapy and should not be recommended. Vitamin D levels do not need to be evaluated routinely in healthy preterm infants (Abrams, 2020). For infants at higher risk for deficiency, routine 25(OH)D levels should be performed every 3 months until stable (Jain et al., 2010).

Calcitriol: Pharmacokinetic Principles

Calcitriol is a vitamin D analog and is the active form of vitamin D ($1,25[OH]_2D$). It is recommended in neonates with symptomatic acute hypocalcemia requiring active vitamin D to boost calcium absorption. It is also recommended in infants with deficiency of hydroxylase enzymes, unable to convert vitamin D to its active form. Calcitriol binds to vitamin D receptors in the gut, parathyroid gland, kidneys, and bone to increase serum calcium. These binding processes stimulate intestinal absorption and transport of calcium from the gut into circulation, promote renal tubular reabsorption of calcium, and mobilize calcium from the bone back to circulation. Calcitriol is rapidly absorbed in the small intestine, with a quick onset of 4 hours and a duration between 3 and 5 days. Calcitriol is highly protein-bound (99%) and is metabolized hepatically via CYP3A4; enterohepatic recycling and biliary excretion also occur. Unabsorbed calcitriol is primarily excreted via feces, whereas absorbed calcitriol is eliminated unchanged via urine. Calcitriol should not be used in the setting of renal dysfunction, particularly in preterm infants.

DOSING RECOMMENDATIONS

In a study conducted by Lin et al., oral calcitriol was dosed at 0.1 mcg daily in neonates with early-onset hypocalcemia, which resulted in a significant increase in serum calcium after 5 days compared with the placebo group. In another well-documented study by Miller et al. (2012), a 0.05 mcg/kg/d dose of oral calcitriol was used. This dose was reported to cause rebound hypercalcemia and was decreased to 0.02 mcg/kg/d. With a slow titration back to 0.05 mcg/kg/d, a second hypercalcemic episode occurred; finally, the calcitriol dose was maintained at 0.03 mcg/kg/d. Amaral et al. (2010) reported using intravenous (IV) calcitriol at 0.25 mcg daily with a switch to per os (PO) calcitriol for maintenance. Overall a recommendation of 0.02 to 0.06 mcg/kg/d is well documented (Jain et al., 2010; Vuralli, 2019).

CLINICAL-MONITORING PEARLS

Adequate calcium intake is necessary to achieve the therapeutic effect of calcitriol; dietary modifications of phosphate and magnesium may also be required (Vuralli, 2019). If hypomagnesemia is the cause, magnesium levels must be corrected first. Similarly, if there is excess phosphate, dietary phosphorus may need to be restricted during therapy. It is important to note that calcitriol does not replace vitamin D stores in the body; thus, it must be administered with either vitamin D_3 or D_2 to replenish stores (Misra et al., 2008). Calcitriol's adverse reaction profile is similar to vitamin D_3 and D_2, which is the risk of hypercalcemia and vitamin D toxicity from prolonged use. One case report of a 24-week-old infant found polyuria as a sign of hypercalcemia (Rodd et al., 1999). A second case report from the same study found dehydration, failure to thrive, and excess calcium excretion as clinical signs of hypercalcemia. Calcitriol is not suggested for use in the setting of renal dysfunction due to the consequences of hypercalcemia. In a recent review by Lavinia Negrea (2019), dose-dependent consequences of calcitriol use can be exaggerated in renal impairment. Negrea notes hypercalcemia and hyperphosphatemia with possible risk for vascular calcifications and development of adynamic bone disease. Notable drug–drug interactions include bile acid sequestrants like cholestyramine, which impair the absorption of vitamin D, and as such may impair the intestinal absorption of calcitriol; thus, administration time should be separated by several hours (Robien et al., 2013). Multivitamins may already contain adequate daily vitamin D doses; thus, combinations should be avoided. During the treatment of hypocalcemia, calcitriol therapy should be monitored by checking serum calcium and phosphorous levels weekly following initiation and during dosage adjustments, then periodically during therapy (Jain et al., 2010). 25(OH)D levels should be obtained 1 month following initiation and repeated at 3-month intervals until normal.

CONCLUSIONS

Preterm and chronically ill infants are at risk of developing OoP. Despite the recommendations released by the AAP in 2013, there remains variation in practice related to screening, prevention, and treatment of OoP among neonatal clinicians. This lack of consensus inhibits the description and quantification of the prevalence of OoP among high-risk infants. Given the medical advancements in both the neonatal and technological sciences, there has been a significant decrease in this disease. However, variation in practice remains, highlighting the importance of identifying evidence-based practices and guidelines. Knowledge gaps remain, validating the need for continued research that will generate best practices for screening and treatment of these fragile infants. For the neonatal population, noninvasive diagnostic tools that limit radiation exposure and healthcare costs should also be explored and made readily available.

Prevention is paramount in decreasing the incidence of OoP. The optimization of total parenteral nutrition and the success of early achievement of full enteral feedings are important goals for the prevention and management of OoP (Faienza et al., 2019). Adequate supplementation to support bone growth is important to prevent significant bone loss and rickets. Long-term risk exists if OoP is inadequately treated or not treated at all. Sequelae for the affected infant/toddler include poor linear growth, leading to short stature and osteopathy in the teenage and young-adult years. As our infants prepare for discharge, it is important to educate the family regarding ongoing nutritional needs, including the benefits of intermediate formulas for the preterm infant and vitamin D supplementation. Postdischarge nutritional supplementation will often be driven by growth parameters. Infants requiring postdischarge use of calcium and/or phosphorus or those on calcitriol should have biomarkers monitored as previously discussed (Faienza et al., 2019; Rustico et al., 2014). A basic understanding of the physiology involved in adequate bone health and development provides neonatal clinicians and nurses with strategies for instruction to parents and pediatric outpatient clinicians.

LEARNING TOOLS AND RESOURCES

Advice From the Authors

Valarie A. Artigas, DNP, APRN, NNP-BC

Osteopenia of prematurity is all about bodybuilding! It is our sincerest wish that you enjoyed this chapter. Our professional journey as nurses lends itself to caring for a diverse set of patients and parents. We learn so much from each parent we touch with our knowledge and compassion for their little one who has been entrusted to us to heal. We are privileged to share in their journeys of endless love, hope, and sorrow for those babies whose sunrise in this world may only be for a fleeting moment in time. Remember to be a lifelong learner, know your style of learning for academic success, and understand that you will forever be transforming your role as an APRN and leader. Create your path of success to caring for those little ones who challenge us to critically think and who amaze us every day with their resilience to live. They are counting on us!!

Mary Whalen, DNP, APRN, NNP-BC

While osteopenia has decreased significantly in the neonatal population with preventative measures, this complication still exists and is greatest for our most fragile infants. As clinicians, neonatal nurse practitioners are well positioned to identify best evidence to educate other NNPs and our interdisciplinary colleagues on the prevention, identification, and treatment of this disease. Engaging in research and quality initiatives to further the science and evidence is well within the grasp of the NNP and should be encouraged and supported by our health organizations. As NNPs we can and will make a difference in the outcomes and health of the population we serve.

Mehran Nesari Asdigha, PharmD

The importance of adequate vitamin D status during pregnancy and early infancy has become increasingly acknowledged in recent years; nevertheless, osteopenia of prematurity remains common among extremely low-birth-weight premature infants. There is a need to reexamine our understanding of both nonpharmacologic as well as pharmacologic treatment options, particularly in our most fragile infants. My hope is that this chapter brings you the knowledge, awareness, and mindful tools for prevention, detection, and treatment of this disease.

Discussion Prompts

1. Preterm infants less than 32 weeks' gestation and with a birth weight less than 2,000 grams are at increased risk of developing OoP. Discuss the antenatal and neonatal factors that predispose preterm infants to disruption of normal bone and mineral homeostasis.
2. Describe the importance of and strategies for screening the at-risk infant for OoP.
3. Identify evidence-based interventions for the prevention and treatment of OoP.
4. Recognize the effects of osteolytic medication use in the NICU that promote bone demineralization.
5. One of the most commonly used drugs in the preterm infant is caffeine. Describe the benefits of caffeine in this population and the associated risk for OoP.
6. List the physiologic effects PTH secretion has for serum calcium and the effects secretion of this hormone can have for bone health.
7. Describe the advantages and disadvantages of the screening tools available to monitor bone health. Include the importance of identifying the source of elevated ALP in determining treatment.
8. Identify the neonates at risk for OoP. Which of these infants is at greatest risk for this complication and why?

Mind Map

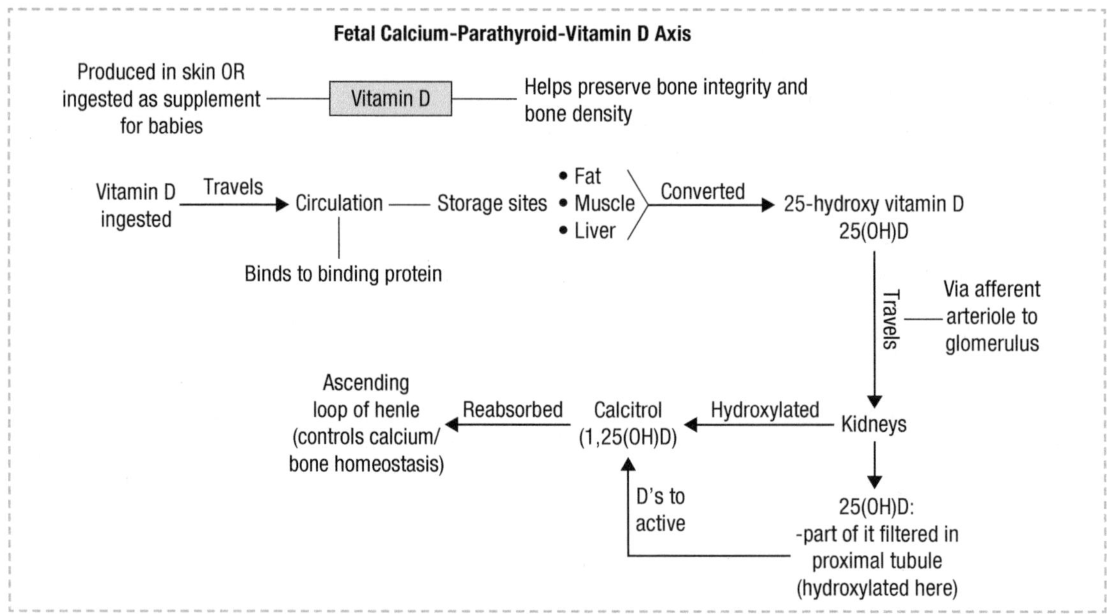

Note: This mind map reflects one neonatal APRN's interpretation of a portion of one or more concepts addressed in this chapter. Readers should regard the mind maps woven throughout this textbook as examples of multisensory study tools that can be developed to encourage conceptual understanding. Readers are encouraged to develop their own unique mind maps in consultation with academic faculty or clinical instructors.
Design credit: Valarie A. Artigas, DNP, APRN, NNP-BC and Mary Whalen, DNP, APRN, NNP-BC

REFERENCES

References for this chapter are online and available at https://connect.springerpub.com/content/book/978-0-8261-5884-0/part/partVI/toc-part/ch26.

PART VII

Common Infectious Disease Problems

chapter 27

Congenital Viral Infections

Christopher McPherson

LEARNING OBJECTIVES

After completing this chapter, the reader should be able to:

- Name the commonly acquired congenital viral infections and identify the epidemiology of the disease process.
- Explain the physiology of viral replication and the body's natural defense system.
- Correlate the pathophysiology of a congenitally acquired viral infection with the need for pharmacologic treatment.
- Appraise the historical evolution of pharmacologic management for congenital viral infections.
- Evaluate the role of pharmacotherapeutic regimens with respect to pharmacodynamic and pharmacokinetic properties in relation to management of congenital viral infections.

INTRODUCTION

Congenital viral infections have the potential to profoundly impact neonatal and childhood outcomes, ranging in presentation from dramatic neonatal shock to asymptomatic infection with significant deficits detected in childhood. A common acronym applied to congenital infections, inclusive of major viral pathogens, is TORCH. **T**oxoplasmosis is caused by the protozoan parasite *Toxoplasma gondii*, presenting with the classic triad of chorioretinitis, cerebral calcifications, and hydrocephalus. **O**ther typically refers to syphilis, caused by the spirochete *Treponema pallidum*, but may also capture viral infections, including parvovirus, varicella zoster, and Zika virus. **R**ubella is a virus typically presenting as a classic "blueberry muffin" rash and is associated with multiple neonatal anomalies. **C**ytomegalovirus (CMV) is the most common intrauterine infection and the leading cause of nongenetic deafness and learning disability; it is the secondary focus of this chapter. **H** captures a diverse array of neonatal exposures, including hepatitis B, HIV, and, most common, herpes simplex virus (HSV). Historically, congenital HSV has been a devastating neonatal infection, although dramatic advances in pharmacotherapy have recently improved outcomes; HSV is the primary focus of this chapter. Prompt recognition of the hallmark symptoms of neonatal congenital infections followed by appropriate diagnostic testing facilitates optimal treatment, giving these high-risk neonates the best possible outcome.

PHYSIOLOGY REVIEW: VIRAL REPLICATION

Viruses enter the body through several routes, including the respiratory tract, gastrointestinal (GI) tract, and genital tract. Neonatal infection occurs when the fetus becomes the target organ of a pathogen via the placenta (transplacental transmission), when a maternally acquired virus contacts mucosal barriers of the neonate during delivery (vertical transmission), or after birth from contact with infected individuals (horizontal transmission). DNA viruses are the focus of this chapter, and replication involves attachment to a host cell; fusion to the plasma membrane; capsid transport of viral DNA to the cellular nucleus; transcription of viral DNA into mRNA in the case of lytic infections; translation of mRNA into proteins, including viral DNA polymerase; and utilization of these proteins for viral DNA duplication. To fully understand the mechanisms of action discussed throughout this chapter, the reader should be familiar with the process of DNA replication described in Chapter 4, "Neonatal Pharmacogenomics and Pharmacogenetics." After viral replication, the viral copies can spread locally to adjacent cells via extracellular (most common) or intracellular pathways (herpes virus). Intracellular spread is uniquely protected by the lack of antibodies within cellular membranes. Infection occurs if cells in a target organ support attachment, replication, and release of a virus. In many cases, the site of infection is the primary target organ, including respiratory tract infections like influenza and rhinovirus, and GI tract infections like rotavirus. In other cases, viruses may spread to multiple organs within the body through the blood or peripheral nerves; for example, HSV displays high neurovirulence with virions traveling along axons from the point of entry to the nuclei of sensory neurons where viral replication occurs (J. G. Stevens & Cook, 1971).

The body defends against viral replication and spread via multiple mechanisms. Viral entry activates the innate immune system. Viral proteins and nucleic acids are recognized as invaders via cellular proteins called *pattern recognition receptors*. Upon recognition of RNA signatures of virus, these receptors initiate the synthesis of cytokines. Cytokines function locally by binding cell surface receptors, producing innate antiviral activity in neighboring cells and an inflammatory response. The inflammatory response facilitates elimination of some viruses by increasing blood flow and capillary permeability at the site of infection to allow influx of phagocytic cells attracted by cytokines (neutrophils, for example). Sentinel cells are an additional component of the innate response, including dendritic cells, which detect infection and amplify the cytokine response. If the innate immune system fails to eradicate a virus, the adaptive immune system responds. Antibodies may prevent infection by recognizing an invading virus to neutralize, agglutinate, or destroy the virus via phagocytosis or the complement system. After infection, cells display fragments of viral peptides via class I major histocompatibility complex proteins (MHC class I). Circulating cytotoxic T cells utilize receptors to recognize viral peptides and release cytotoxic factors to kill the infected cell. Some viruses inhibit MHC molecules from displaying their peptides. Cells infected by these viruses are invisible to T cells, but susceptible to natural killer cells that eliminate cells displaying abnormal MHC molecules. A component of both the innate and adaptive immune system, circulating interferons are small proteins produced and released by infected cells. Interferons signal viral presence to nearby cells to upregulate MHC class I molecule display. Interferons also directly interfere with replication of viruses through activation of intracellular inhibitors of protein synthesis. Failure of the innate and adaptive immune response to eradicate or attenuate viral infection results in the consequences of disease described in subsequent sections of this chapter.

PATHOPHYSIOLOGY OF CONGENITAL VIRAL INFECTIONS

The fetus and neonate are uniquely susceptible to viral infection because innate and adaptive immune defenses are immature, and placental transfer of maternal immunity is partial. Congenital viral infections, especially those occurring in the first trimester, may cause maldeveloped organs due to the undifferentiated nature of many fetal cells at this stage; Rubella, CMV, and Zika virus are all well-known causes of microcephaly, for example. Viral transmission near birth or during delivery may cause significant subclinical (CMV), localized (HSV of the skin, eyes, and mouth), and disseminated disease (disseminated, symptomatic CMV or HSV). The following text briefly describes the specific pathophysiology of the most common and/or consequential congenital viral infections (with the notable exception of HIV, which is discussed in Chapter 7, "Common Medications Prescribed in the Newborn Nursery").

Cytomegalovirus

CMV is the most common intrauterine infection, impacting 0.5% to 2% of all newborns. Although acutely asymptomatic in most cases, CMV is the leading cause of nongenetic deafness and learning disability. CMV is transmitted through bodily fluids, including saliva, urine, blood, and breast milk. The incidence of congenital CMV in a population reflects the rate of maternal seropositivity, with dramatic differences across populations (Lantos et al., 2015). For example, the rate of seropositivity in White women in the United States is approximately 40%, rising with age, and approaching 70% beyond 60 years of age. In Black women, 60% population seropositivity occurs by age 10 with rates escalating to 70% to 80% through childbearing years. The risk of transmission in women with latent disease is 0.5% to 2% (Fowler et al., 2003). Given the ubiquitous nature of this virus in the general population, seroconversion during pregnancy is relatively common at 2.3% (Hyde et al., 2010). This poses a much higher risk to the fetus, with transmission rates of 40% to 50% from primary maternal infection (Picone et al., 2013).

The pathogenesis of CMV infection involves either intrauterine (transplacental) transmission, intrapartum (vertical) transmission, or postnatal (horizontal) transmission during breastfeeding. The exact mechanisms that facilitate transplacental transmission remain unknown (Pass & Arav-Boger, 2018). Transplacental infection occurs when infected cells migrate to the placenta, invade the trophoblast layer, and transfer into the fetal endothelial capillaries (located at the chorionic villi; Gabrielli et al., 2001). Intrapartum transmission involves direct contact between infectious cells and the fetal mucosa, and viral cells thereby migrate to the vascular endothelium. The vascular endothelium is targeted because this location favors rapid viral replication. Approximately 16 hours after the virus is transmitted to the fetus, rapid viral DNA replication begins (Emery et al., 2002). Infected cells can then disseminate to the epithelium of various organs, including the inner ear, brain, lungs, kidneys, and biliary tree (Griffiths, 2000). As alluded to earlier in this section, innate and adaptive immune responses in neonates are insufficient to contain viral replication. Therefore, replication persists and may lead to organ maldevelopment (e.g., microcephaly, chorioretinis) or dysfunction (e.g., pathologic jaundice).

Herpes Simplex Virus

Disseminated HSV infection represents a potentially devastating condition that is associated with extremely high morbidity and mortality. Infection in adults may be orolabial (HSV-1) or genital (HSV-1 or HSV-2). The seroprevalence of HSV-2 is approximately 16% in the United States, although only 8% to 15% of seropositive women shed virus at the time of delivery (American College of Obstetricians and Gynecologists [ACOG] Committee on Practice Bulletins, 2007; Bradley et al., 2014). It is important to note that less than 2% of infants exposed in this manner will develop neonatal infection (Brown et al., 1997). In fact, the highest risk to the neonate is posed by primary genital HSV infection (odds ratio [OR]: 33.1, 95% confidence interval [CI]: 6.5–168, $p < .001$), which is asymptomatic in the mother approximately two-thirds of the time (Brown et al., 1997, 2003). Maternal antibody status, duration of membrane rupture, mode of delivery, and integrity of the neonatal skin barrier also influence perinatal transmission rates. Prenatal and postnatal acquisition of HSV is less common, accounting for only 15% of neonatal cases. Overall, the estimated rate of occurrence of neonatal HSV is between 13 and 60 cases per 100,000 live births (Baldwin & Whitley, 1989).

The pathogenesis of HSV infection involves penetration of viral cells through mucosal surfaces with subsequent viral replication. Neonatal HSV infections are classified by organ involvement: (a) disease localized to the skin, eyes, and/or mouth is known as *skin, eyes, and mouth (SEM)* disease; (b) disease infecting the brain with or without skin, eyes, or mouth involvement is central nervous system (CNS) disease; and (c) disease involving multiple organs, including the brain, lungs, liver, or adrenal glands with or without the skin, eyes, and/or mouth, is disseminated disease. Skin lesions may present with any of these disease subtypes. Therefore, we begin by discussing the pathogenesis of HSV skin and mucosal lesions.

Once within the mucosa, HSV cells replicate, enter cutaneous neurons, and travel along those peripheral neurons until they reach the ends of the sensory ganglia. At this point, infectious viral cells are synthesized. These infectious cells subsequently migrate backward and to the initial site of inoculation, where they undergo additional replication (Whitley & Roizman, 2001). This process of replication damages the epithelium. Cellular debris and inflammatory mediators accumulate, yielding the appearance of a vesicle (Stanberry et al., 1982). As more and more inflammatory mediators aggregate at the site of inoculation, the vesicle takes on the appearance of a pus-filled lesion.

Recall that dorsal ganglia contain numerous sensory nerve endings (from peripheral tissues such as the skin) that extend through that dorsal nerve root and into the CNS. When HSV cells travel along neurons, reach the ends of peripheral sensory ganglia, and penetrate past this point and into the dorsal (posterior) root region and beyond, generalized infection manifests. Among fetuses and neonates, innate and adaptive immune responses are often unable to contain viral replication. Therefore, replication persists and may lead to disseminated migration of infectious cells into numerous organ systems, including the CNS.

CLINICAL MANIFESTATIONS AND DIAGNOSIS

Cytomegalovirus

Clinical symptoms of congenital CMV infection occur in 10% to 15% of infected neonates, signifying that more than 85% of infected neonates are asymptomatic at birth. Common presenting symptoms include microcephaly, direct hyperbilirubinemia and jaundice, hepatosplenomegaly, lethargy, and petechial rash. Radiology and ophthalmologic examinations reveal periventricular calcifications, chorioretinitis, and bone abnormalities or abnormal dentition, including hypocalcified enamel. Common laboratory findings include thrombocytopenia, anemia, elevated transaminases, and elevated conjugated bilirubin levels. The developmental hallmark of CMV is sensorineural hearing loss presenting at any point from birth to 4 years of age, which occurs in 50% to 90% of symptomatic patients and 10% to 15% of asymptomatic patients (Madden et al., 2005; Pass, 2005). Of all infants with hearing loss detected during the birth hospitalization, approximately 20% of cases are linked to congenital CMV (Kimberlin et al., 2021).

Congenital CMV infection may be detected by culture or PCR of neonatal urine or saliva. Early testing in suspected cases is vital to avoid confusion with postnatally acquired disease. Brain imaging and serial hearing evaluation are also indicated in symptomatic infants. Currently, population screening for asymptomatic disease is not standard of care, although studies examining the feasibility and appropriateness of this approach are emerging (Nagel et al., 2020; Shlonsky et al., 2021).

Herpes Simplex Virus

Neonatal HSV SEM disease accounts for approximately 45% of cases, CNS disease accounts for approximately 30% of cases, and disseminated disease accounts for approximately 25% of cases (Kimberlin, 2007). Neonates with perinatally acquired SEM or disseminated disease experience symptoms at a mean age of 6 days, whereas CNS disease presents at a mean of 12 days of age (Kimberlin, Lin, Jacobs, Powell, Frenkel, et al., 2001). Localized disease often progresses to disseminated disease in the absence of antiviral therapy (Whitley et al., 1980). Morbidity and mortality are progressively higher with disseminated disease, compared to CNS, and compared to SEM disease (far left columns of Figure 27.1).

The timing of HSV acquisition influences presentation of postnatal disease. Congenital HSV is present at birth and presents with some combination of topical (scarring, lesions, altered pigmentation, aplasia cutis, erythematous macular exanthema), ophthalmologic (microphthalmia, retinal dysplasia, optic atrophy, chorioretinitis), and/or CNS abnormalities (microcephaly, encephalomalacia, hydranencephaly, intracranial calcifications; Florman et al., 1973). Skin vesicles are the most common presenting symptom of neonatal HSV (83% of patients with SEM disease, 63% of patients with CNS disease, and 58% of patients with disseminated disease). Neonates with SEM disease may also present with conjunctivitis, lethargy, and/or fever. The hallmarks of neonatal CNS disease are seizures, irritability, tremors, poor feeding, and/or bulging fontanelle. Disseminated disease also generally presents as encephalitis, with subsequent organ system involvement detected clinically (e.g., pneumonitis) or biochemically (e.g., coagulopathy, hepatic dysfunction).

When postnatal symptoms raise the index of suspicion for neonatal HSV, five tests should be pursued to confirm or rule out the disease process (Kimberlin et al., 2021). A single swab specimen of skin vesicles and another swab specimen of surface mucosa (conjunctivae, mouth, nasopharynx, and anus) should be obtained for HSV culture or HSV DNA polymerase chain reaction (PCR)

FIGURE 27.1 Survival (panel 1) and disability-free survival (panel 2) in neonates with congenital herpes simplex virus enrolled in randomized controlled trials of vidarabine and acyclovir.

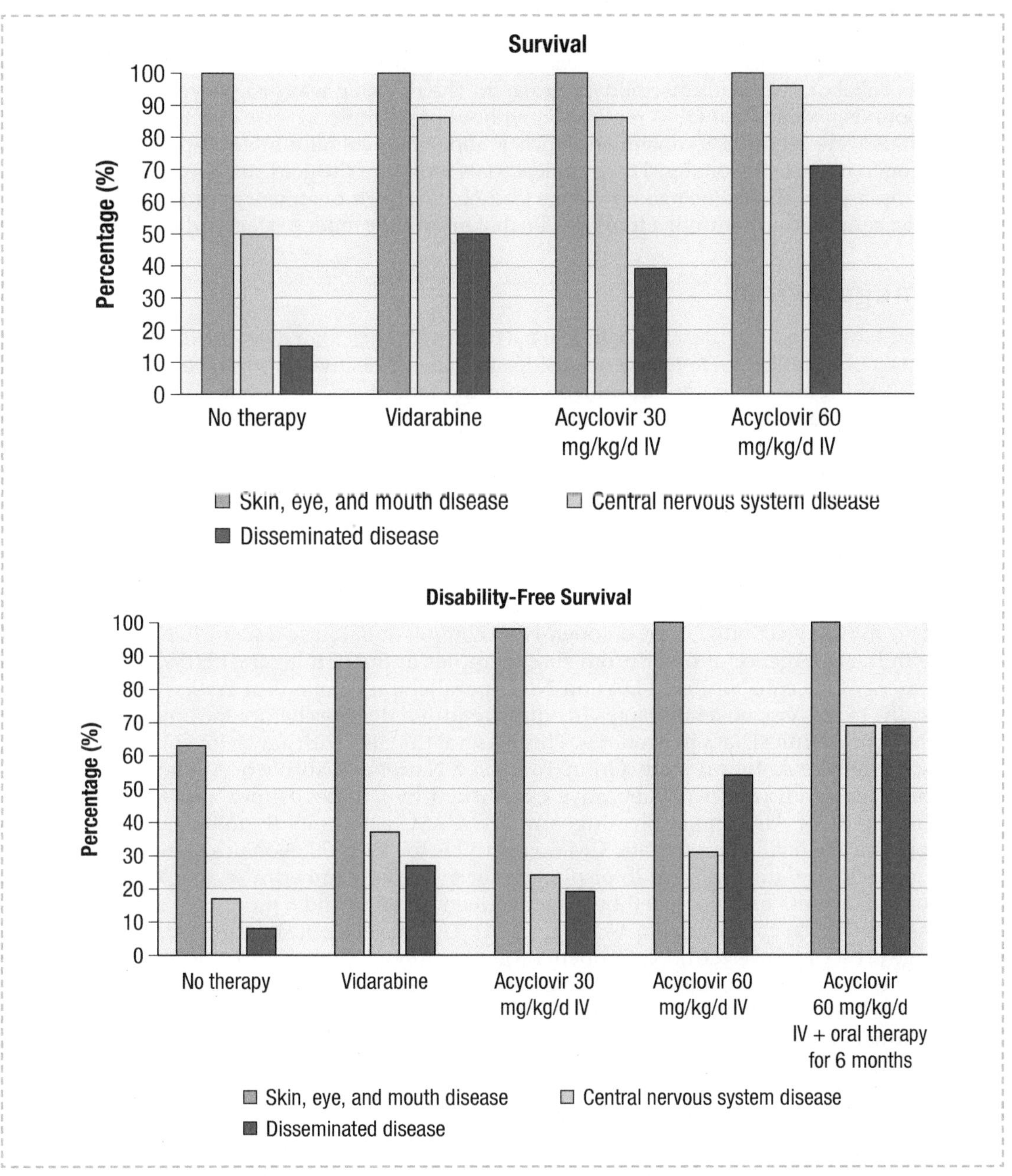

Note: No therapy represents placebo controls in the initial trial of vidarabine for 10 days. Subsequently, acyclovir 30 mg/kg/d for 10 days was compared to vidarabine, acyclovir 60 mg/kg/d for 21 days was compared to historic controls, and 6 months of combined intravenous and oral acyclovir was compared to acyclovir 60 mg/kg/d for 21 days.
IV, intravenous.

assay. Whole blood should be evaluated for alanine aminotransferase (ALT) and analyzed for the presence of virus via HSV DNA PCR assay (Kimberlin et al., 1996). In addition, cerebrospinal fluid (CSF) should be obtained and sent for HSV DNA PCR. Intravenous (IV; parenteral) acyclovir therapy, which is discussed in more detail later in this chapter, should be initiated pending culture and/or PCR results. Neonates with CNS or disseminated disease should receive repeat CSF studies before completion of IV antiviral therapy. Neonates with confirmed infection should undergo ophthalmologic examination and neuroimaging.

HISTORICAL PERSPECTIVE: SEMINAL AND OTHER NOTEWORTHY STUDIES

The approach to neonates diagnosed with congenital viral infection has been dramatically altered by decades of collaborative, multidisciplinary research. The first step was drug development, identifying compounds toxic to viral DNA replication without prohibitive adverse effects in the host. Next, clinical trials were required to document efficacy and safety, initially in adult patients with rapid progression to impacted neonates. These clinical trials represent the gold standard for relatively rare neonatal diseases, with advancing knowledge leading to refined treatment approaches evaluated in multicenter randomized controlled trials (RCTs) that inform the modern standard of clinical practice.

Cytomegalovirus

Congenital CMV was first described in 1904. The drug ganciclovir was developed in the early 1980s as part of the effort to develop nucleoside analogues selective for viral, not host, DNA (Martin et al., 1983). Ganciclovir rapidly moved from the laboratory to human use in May 1984 for the compassionate treatment of a 29-year-old female with CMV pneumonia after bone marrow transplantation, a universally fatal diagnosis at the time (Buhles, 2011). After successful use in this case, ganciclovir compassionate use rapidly expanded to patients with CMV retinitis secondary to AIDS, resulting in publication of the first cohort study regarding ganciclovir in 1986 (Collaborative DHPG Treatment Study Group, 1986). Historically, the U.S. Food and Drug Administration (FDA) requires randomized placebo-controlled trials for approval of novel therapeutic agents. However, the devastating nature of CMV retinitis and clear efficacy of ganciclovir made this traditional approach unacceptable to scientists and AIDS activists. This activism led to the FDA approval of ganciclovir for CMV retinitis based on open-label compassionate-use data in 1989. This approval, along with the emergence of other promising therapies in the fight against HIV/AIDS, led to the development of the collaborative FDA and NIH "parallel track policy" in 1990.

Typically, in this era, novel therapies in adults required decades before the emergence of pharmacokinetic and clinical data in neonates. This was not the case with ganciclovir, due to the efforts of the Collaborative Antiviral Study Group (CASG), a National Institute of Allergy and Infectious Diseases-funded multicenter collaborative established by Charles Alford and Richard Whitley of the University of Alabama at Birmingham. The CASG acted rapidly to determine the role of ganciclovir for neonatal symptomatic CMV. From 1991 to 1999, 100 neonates were randomized to receive ganciclovir 6 mg/kg IV q12h or placebo for 6 weeks (Kimberlin et al., 2003). None of the ganciclovir recipients had worsened hearing between baseline and 6 months of age compared to nearly half of the placebo group (0% vs. 41%, $p < .01$). The rate of stable hearing was also higher at 1 year of age (21% vs. 68%, $p < .01$). Neutropenia was a common adverse effect, occurring in roughly two out of every three patients who received the study drug. Two other concerning issues were noted in this trial—maintaining IV access for 6 weeks was challenging, and viral loads returned to pretreatment levels rapidly after discontinuation of active therapy. These issues were addressed in two subsequent trials. In 2008, investigators documented the pharmacokinetic equivalence of valganciclovir (the oral prodrug of ganciclovir) 16 mg/kg given orally every 12 hours with treatment dosing of IV ganciclovir (Kimberlin et al., 2008). Pharmacokinetic study to guide dosing facilitated a CASG trial of 6 weeks of valganciclovir therapy versus a prolonged 6-month course, published in 2015 (Kimberlin et al., 2015). Although sensorineural hearing was similar at 6 months between groups, improvement or normalcy was more likely at 12 months (73% vs. 57%, $p = .01$) and 24 months (77% vs. 64%, $p = .04$) in the prolonged therapy group. The prolonged therapy group also had superior neurodevelopmental scores at 24 months, specifically in the domains of language and receptive communication. It is important to note that the incidence of neutropenia was not different between study groups and was lower than the initial trial of ganciclovir (21% in the prolonged treatment group). This series of trials represents a giant leap forward for neonates with symptomatic congenital CMV. Unfortunately, 85% to 90% of infants with congenital CMV are asymptomatic at birth. Neonates with asymptomatic disease have a much lower risk of complications, but still experience a 10% to 15% incidence of sensorineural hearing loss, a 2.5% incidence of chorioretinitis, and a nearly 4% incidence of IQ less than 70. The prevalence of congenital CMV in populations with low socioeconomic status makes optimization of the approach to asymptomatic congenital CMV a public health imperative.

Herpes Simplex Virus

HSV infection was first reported in neonates in the 1930s (Batignani, 1934; Hass, 1935). In the absence of pharmacotherapy, mortality from CNS or disseminated HSV is common in both neonates and adults (approximately 70%; Olson et al., 1967). In this setting, high-risk/high-reward clinical trials were conducted as novel agents were identified as active against HSV. The first generation of antiviral agents arose from efforts to develop chemotherapy in the fight against cancer. The first antiviral agent (idoxuridine) was synthesized in the late 1950s. Idoxuridine, a nucleoside analogue, mimics the nucleic acid base thymidine (see Figures 4.3 and 4.4 of Chapter 4, "Neonatal Pharmacogenomics and Pharmacogenetics"). However, incorporation into viral DNA during replication blocks base pairing, due to the iodine atom in idoxuridine halting viral DNA synthesis. In response to widespread case reports of open-label use of idoxuridine for HSV in the 1970s, a clinical trial randomized adult patients with HSV encephalitis to idoxuridine or placebo (Boston Interhospital Virus Study Group & NIAID-Sponsored Cooperative Antiviral Clinical Study, 1975). Of nine patients randomized to active therapy, seven died and one was neurologically devastated. In addition, six of eight patients who completed 14 days of therapy experienced hematologic toxicity, including severe neutropenia, anemia, and thrombocytopenia. Note that this generation of agents identified to halt DNA replication in rapidly proliferating cancer cells effectively targeted and destroyed cancer, viral, and host cells.

The quest for more selective antiviral agents led to the examination of naturally occurring biologic compounds. The Caribbean sponge *Cryptobenthic crypta* has intrinsic antiviral activity. Isolation of the arabinosyl nucleoside in the 1960s led to the synthesis of two chemotherapeutic agents with activity against HSV, cytarabine and vidarabine. Cytarabine and vidarabine mimic the nucleic acid bases cytosine and adenine, respectively (again, please refer to Figures 4.3 and 4.4 of Chapter 4, "Neonatal Pharmacogenomics and Pharmacogenetics"). After incorporation into viral DNA, these compounds inhibit DNA polymerase, resulting in decreased DNA synthesis. Unfortunately, cytarabine was not clinically effective and produced prohibitive toxicity in an RCT of 39 adults with disseminated HSV (D. A. Stevens et al., 1973). Cytarabine remains in clinical use today for the treatment of leukemia and lymphoma rather than HSV. However, in 1977, vidarabine became the first systemic agent approved by the FDA for the treatment of HSV. Vidarabine also became the first agent examined systematically for the treatment of neonatal HSV by the CASG. A controlled trial randomized 56 newborns with SEM disease ($N = 13$), CNS disease ($N = 16$), or disseminated disease ($N = 27$) to vidarabine or placebo (Whitley et al., 1983). No patients with SEM infection died (Figure 27.1); however, only one patient (25%) in the treatment group developed mild chorioretinitis at 2 years of age, compared to three (38%) in the control group who developed severe chorioretinitis and/or neurologic deficits during the first year of life. Mortality was significantly reduced in neonates with CNS or disseminated disease randomized to vidarabine (38% vs. 74%, $p = .014$). However, only 14% of treated neonates avoided severe disability at 1 year of age (absence of spasticity, microcephaly, seizures, blindness; compared to 8% of the placebo group). No evidence of acute toxicity was identified. Increasing the dose of vidarabine did not improve clinical effect (Whitley et al., 1983).

The dramatic improvement in mortality from antiviral therapy was encouraging. However, the desire to further decrease mortality and simultaneously decrease morbidity led to continued research. Acyclovir was synthesized in the mid-1970s through modification of the sugar moiety of the nucleoside base of vidarabine (Laport et al., 2009). Unlike the relatively nonspecific vidarabine, acyclovir is selective for herpes viruses, including HSV, CMV, and varicella zoster. Hence, acyclovir is far more efficient and less toxic than previous antiviral agents. In addition, acyclovir (maximum concentration 7 mg/mL) is substantially more soluble than vidarabine (maximum concentration 0.7 mg/mL), facilitating intermittent infusion of acyclovir over 1 hour as compared to 12 hours for vidarabine infusion. Acyclovir was patented in 1974 and approved for human use by the FDA in 1982. Even before formal approval, the CASG began a trial to examine acyclovir for neonatal HSV.

The initial clinical trial for neonatal HSV enrolled 202 neonates from 27 centers and randomized to acyclovir or vidarabine, both dosed at 30 mg/kg/d for 10 days (acyclovir was given as 10 mg/kg/dose over 1 hour every 8 hours; the total dose of vidarabine was given over 12 hours once daily; Whitley et al., 1991). No patients with SEM disease died; 88% of the vidarabine group and 98% of the acyclovir group were developing normally at 1 year of age ($p > .05$; see Figure 27.1). Mortality was equivalent between groups for babies with CNS disease (14% in both groups); 37%

treated with vidarabine and 24% treated with acyclovir were developing normally at 1 year of age ($p > .05$). Mortality was much higher in patients with disseminated disease but not different between groups (50% for vidarabine vs. 61% for acyclovir, $p > .05$); normal development at 1 year of age was rare (27% for vidarabine vs. 19% for acyclovir, $p > .05$). Serious toxicity was not observed with either therapy. The authors hypothesized that earlier initiation of therapy likely accounted for superior outcomes in all groups compared to previous trials. Despite acyclovir's lack of therapeutic superiority in this trial, it supplanted vidarabine as the standard of care for neonatal HSV, given the relative ease of acyclovir administration. However, the emergence of DNA PCR as a diagnostic tool led to consideration of modification of acyclovir therapy. In a retrospective study, several CSF samples tested positive for HSV DNA after completion of 10 days of antiviral therapy, including neonates originally classified with only SEM disease (Kimberlin et al., 1996). This finding led investigators to consider alteration of both the dose and duration of IV acyclovir therapy.

The next trial by the CASG examined both interventions, comparing 79 neonates who received acyclovir 45 mg/kg/d for 21 d ($N = 13$) and 60 mg/kg/d for 21 d ($N = 66$) to historic controls from the previous trial (Kimberlin, Lin, Jacobs, Powell, Corey, et al., 2001). Survival rates remained high and were similar between high-dose acyclovir and historic controls for neonates with SEM or CNS disease (see Figure 27.1). However, the survival rate for neonates with disseminated HSV disease treated with high-dose acyclovir was significantly higher than historic controls (69% vs. 39%; OR: 3.3, 95% CI: 1.4–7.9). In addition, across all disease categories, neonates treated with high-dose acyclovir trended toward a higher likelihood of normal development at 12 months of age compared to historic controls (adjusted OR: 6.6, 95% CI: 0.8–113.6, $p = .051$). This trend was largely driven by neonates treated with high-dose acyclovir for disseminated disease (54% normal at 12 months compared to 19% of historic controls, $p > .13$). The most common adverse effect in neonates treated with high-dose therapy was myelosuppression, with 13% experiencing anemia, 19% neutropenia, and 15% thrombocytopenia. Nephrotoxicity was not common with high-dose acyclovir (6%, exclusively patients with disseminated disease), suggesting this adverse effect may be less prevalent in neonates compared to older populations (Rao et al., 2015). Subsequent retrospective assessment of 89 infants treated with high-dose acyclovir suggests an even lower rate of nephrotoxicity (2%; Ericson et al., 2017). Given the manageable nature of acyclovir toxicity in neonates, investigators considered whether further prolongation of the treatment course would improve outcomes in childhood.

After acute IV therapy, inert HSV implants in sensory ganglia and periodically reactivates as localized disease (Kimberlin & Rouse, 2004). Suppressive therapy has been documented to prevent these localized recurrences in adults with orolabial or genital HSV infections (Douglas et al., 1984; Spruance et al., 1988). Soon after acyclovir became available, investigators noted recurrence of disease in neonates with CNS disease that could be blunted with prolonged oral acyclovir therapy (Gutman et al., 1986). In the CASG trial comparing acyclovir and vidarabine, the investigators noted an association between adverse neurologic outcome and three or more recurrences of vesicles after completion of therapy in infants with SEM disease (79% normal development at 1 year of age compared to 100% with two or fewer recurrences, $p = .04$; Whitley et al., 1991). In response, the CASG launched a phase I/II trial (safety and dose finding) of suppressive oral acyclovir for 6 months (300 mg/m^2/dose either twice or three times daily) in 26 infants (Kimberlin et al., 1996). Three-times-daily therapy was largely effective at preventing recurrence of lesions (81% vs. 54% of historic controls). Neutropenia remained the most common adverse effect (46%).

In 2011, the CASG's 21-center, phase-III trial of prolonged oral acyclovir therapy was published (Kimberlin et al., 2011). This trial randomized 74 neonates with HSV (45 with CNS disease and 29 with SEM disease) to oral acyclovir 300 mg/m^2/dose three times daily or placebo for 6 months. In the overall cohort, oral therapy prolonged the time to two cutaneous recurrences by 2.5 months ($p = .009$). Assessment of 28 infants with CNS disease at 1 year of age revealed significantly higher Bayley mental development scores in the treatment group (88 vs. 68, $p = .046$). Among infants assigned to long-term suppressive therapy, 69% had normal neurologic outcomes and 6% had only mild impairment. This compares favorably to 33% with normal outcomes and 8% with mild impairment in the placebo group. There was no significant difference in the incidence of neutropenia between groups (23% vs. 6%, $p = .09$); however, the strong trend highlights the importance of continued monitoring for this adverse effect in clinical practice. High-dose IV acyclovir for 14 to 21 days followed by 6 months of oral suppressive therapy represents the current standard of care for neonatal HSV.

CURRENT PHARMACOLOGIC TREATMENT MODALITIES FOR CONGENITAL VIRAL INFECTIONS

Available RCTs inform current treatment recommendations. The definitive source for current standard of care is the Report of the American Academy of Pediatrics' Committee on Infectious Diseases, known as the *Red Book* (Kimberlin et al., 2021). The following sections focus on pharmacotherapy and monitoring, directly reflecting guidance from the most recent edition of this report. Despite clear guidance in this essential tertiary reference, a local collaborative approach remains vital, including consultation with a pediatric infectious diseases specialist for guidance on infection prevention during the hospital stay and longitudinal monitoring and support after discharge. Additional vital team members include lactation specialists to support safe pumping and breastfeeding in the absence of lesions on the breasts. Engagement of other multidisciplinary team members may be required based on the clinical presentation and morbidities of specific neonates.

Cytomegalovirus

As previously described, ganciclovir or valganciclovir is indicated for symptomatic congenital CMV disease.

GANCICLOVIR/VALGANCICLOVIR

Mechanism of Action/Pharmacokinetic Principles

Like vidarabine and acyclovir, ganciclovir and valganciclovir mimic the nucleic acid base adenine. After incorporation into viral DNA, these compounds inhibit DNA polymerase, resulting in decreased DNA synthesis. However, ganciclovir is highly selective for the herpes virus CMV due to a single carboxyl side chain, which facilitates phosphorylation by a protein kinase encoded by the CMV gene *UL97*.

Ganciclovir has a relatively short half-life in neonates of 2.4 hours with renal elimination of unchanged drug. Although ganciclovir has enteral bioavailability of 5% to 10%, valganciclovir is 50% to 60% bioavailable through the addition of an L-valyl ester, which is cleaved in the intestines and liver during enteral absorption.

Dosing Recommendations

Neonates with confirmed infection should be treated with oral valganciclovir 16 mg/kg/dose orally every 12 hours for 6 months; if the neonate cannot tolerate enteral medications, ganciclovir 6 mg/kg/dose IV every 12 hours may be utilized as a portion of the total course. At minimum, the dose should be adjusted monthly for weight gain.

Clinical-Monitoring Pearls

Absolute neutrophil counts should be monitored weekly for 6 weeks, then at 8 weeks, then monthly for the duration of therapy if they are stable. Neutropenia below 500 cells/mm^3 may be treated with granulocyte colony-stimulating factor, generally daily for up to 3 days. Serum ALT concentration should be measured monthly during treatment. Progression of disease should be evaluated with serial audiologic assessments through childhood.

At present, antiviral pharmacotherapy is not recommended for neonates with asymptomatic or mild symptomatic disease outside of a study protocol (including omission of therapy in those with isolated sensorineural hearing loss). Preterm infants with symptomatic disease were also not included in the trial of long-term valganciclovir therapy and may receive a shorter course (2–4 weeks) of IV ganciclovir with close follow-up and consultation with infectious disease specialists.

Herpes Simplex Virus

Experts agree that antiviral therapy to cover HSV should not be added to the standard antimicrobial cocktail used to rule out early-onset or late-onset sepsis in neonates. Guidelines exist detailing indications for antiviral therapy in asymptomatic neonates born to women with active genital herpes lesions (Kimberlin et al., 2013). However, the majority of neonatal HSV occurs after birth to asymptomatic women. Commonly, antiviral therapy is added for seizures after birth, even though

CNS or disseminated HSV present with seizures in the second or third week of neonatal life. Clinicians must be familiar with the classic symptoms and timing of congenital HSV to appropriately select patients likely to benefit from antiviral therapy.

ACYCLOVIR

Mechanism of Action/Pharmacokinetic Principles

Recall that acyclovir mimics the nucleic acid base adenine and inhibits DNA polymerase, resulting in decreased DNA synthesis. Also, acyclovir is selective for herpes viruses, including HSV, CMV, and varicella zoster, compared to less specific historic treatments like vidarabine. Specifically, acyclovir has high affinity for a form of the enzyme thymidine kinase encoded by herpes viruses, which catalyzes the first step toward conversion of acyclovir to acyclovir triphosphate, a nucleoside analogue that competitively inhibits viral DNA polymerase by acting as an analog to deoxyguanosine triphosphate (dGTP; Elion, 1982).

Acyclovir has a half-life of approximately 4 hours in neonates with normal renal function. Oral dosing results in substantially lower exposure due to the poor absorption of acyclovir in the GI tract.

Dosing Recommendations

Neonates should receive acyclovir 20 mg/kg intravenously every 8 hours for 21 days for proven disseminated or CNS HSV or 14 days for proven SEM disease, followed by 300 mg/m^2/dose three times daily for a minimum of 6 months (Kimberlin et al., 2021). In patients with disseminated or CNS disease, IV therapy should be prolonged by at least 1 week if CSF studies are still positive at the end of the initial treatment course. Consultation with a pediatric infectious diseases specialist is recommended in these cases if it has not already occurred earlier in the clinical course.

Clinical-Monitoring Pearls

Complete blood count with differential, with specific attention to absolute neutrophil count, must be monitored at least twice weekly during the IV course (Kimberlin, Lin, Jacobs, Powell, Corey, et al., 2001). Generally, granulocyte colony-stimulating factor should be administered for persistent absolute neutrophil counts below 500 cells per mm^3. In infants with stable neutrophil counts, monitoring should occur at 2 and 4 weeks after initiation of long-term oral therapy and monthly thereafter (Kimberlin et al., 2021).

Other TORCH Infections

Additional congenital infections captured by the TORCH pneumonic occur in neonates and warrant rapid recognition. Toxoplasmosis may present with significant clinical illness but is typically detected with specific testing, including dilated eye examination (revealing chorioretinitis) and CNS imaging (documenting cerebral calcifications and hydrocephalus). Visual or hearing impairment and severe developmental delay are common, but not apparent until later in life. Diagnosis is confirmed by postnatal serologic testing for Toxoplasma immunoglobulin G (IgG), IgM, and IgA and PCR of CSF, urine, and whole blood. Toxoplasmosis is treated with 3 to 12 months of pyrimethamine, sulfadiazine, and folinic acid (shorter and longer durations are the minimum for asymptomatic and symptomatic infection, respectively). The dosing regimen is relatively complex, and readers should reference an updated tertiary dosing reference and/or the American Academy of Pediatrics *Red Book* (Kimberlin et al., 2021). Monitoring parameters for these agents include complete blood counts with differential to evaluate for neutropenia weekly for 4 weeks, then every 2 weeks for 2 to 3 months, then every 3 to 4 weeks for the duration of therapy. Ongoing evaluation of the disease process should include ophthalmologic evaluations every 3 to 6 months for the first 3 years of life and long-term neurodevelopmental follow-up. Toxoplasmosis treatment should always occur under the supervision of a pediatric infectious diseases specialist. Discharge planning should begin as soon as diagnosis is confirmed, given the vital nature of follow-up evaluations and the unique challenge of the need for prior insurance authorization and limited outpatient pharmacy availability for these uncommon medications.

The approach to "other" infections varies from definitive treatment to supportive care. Chapter 7, "Common Medications Prescribed in the Newborn Nursery," describes congenital syphilis treatment in detail. Neonates whose mothers had varicella in the immediate peripartum period should be treated with varicella zoster immune globulin intramuscularly as soon as possible within 10 days of exposure. The dose is 62.5 units for neonates weighing less than or equal to 2 kg and 125 units for neonates over 2 kg. The most common adverse effect is injection-site reactions. Care for "other" viruses, specifically parvovirus and Zika virus, is exclusively supportive to address immediate symptoms in the neonate.

Congenital rubella may present as growth restriction, interstitial pneumonia, radiolucent bone disease, hepatosplenomegaly, thrombocytopenia, and/or the classic "blueberry muffin" rash. Congenital anomalies of the eyes (cataracts, pigmentary retinopathy, microphthalmos, glaucoma) and heart (patent ductus arteriosus, peripheral pulmonary artery stenosis) have also been associated with disease, and long-term auditory and neurologic impacts (including autism) are common. Diagnosis is confirmed by the detection of rubella-specific IgM antibody. Treatment is exclusively supportive.

CONCLUSIONS

Congenital infections can have devastating short-term or long-term impacts on the neonate. Prompt identification of disease and early initiation of indicated therapy dramatically improves outcome. For common viral infections specifically, the outcomes of neonates exposed to CMV, HSV, and HIV have been dramatically altered by collaborative trials identifying and evaluating novel agents and optimizing their dose and duration. Treatment of CMV, an infrequent cause of mortality but a common cause of hearing loss, has dramatically improved outcomes for symptomatic neonates. However, the optimal approach to treat the large population of neonates with asymptomatic disease remains unclear. Survival in neonates with disseminated HSV has increased from 15% to 70% with standard IV acyclovir. Survival without developmental disability has increased from less than 10% to 70% with the addition of prolonged oral therapy. Collaborative trials hold the promise of identifying treatments for other viral infections with no direct pharmacotherapeutic options (parvovirus, Zika virus, rubella). Knowledge of historic trials and involvement in future trials offer the clinician scientist a unique opportunity to optimize direct patient care as well as the care of generations of neonates in the future. We hope that this chapter has provided readers with a clear understanding of the pathophysiology, history, diagnosis, and treatment of CMV and HSV infections. Chapter 7, "Common Medications Prescribed in the Newborn Nursery," describes prophylaxis for exposure to the other *Hs*, hepatitis B and HIV.

LEARNING TOOLS AND RESOURCES

Advice From the Author

Christopher McPherson, PharmD, BCPPS

I have trouble remembering isolated facts or numbers, but I can easily remember a good story. The evolution of neonatal HSV therapy is a great story. Examining the trials chronologically helps me link the pieces of this story together and allows me to understand the decisions made in initial trials and how they informed the next trial. Knowing the story and walking with these scientists as they made breakthroughs and learned from mistakes, it's much easier to remember the nuts and bolts of clinical practice like dosing and monitoring parameters. I strongly recommend this approach for all neonatal pharmacotherapies.

Discussion Prompts

1. Collaborative, multicenter RCTs have revolutionized the care of neonates with symptomatic CMV and congenital HSV. Does your institution participate in multicenter RCTs in neonates? What challenges exist at a participating center or what barriers prevent participation in these trials?
2. Asymptomatic congenital CMV represents a leading cause of sensorineural hearing loss. Explore new and ongoing research on the screening and treatment of asymptomatic congenital CMV and discuss next steps.
3. In the interest of brevity, the specific dosing approach for congenital toxoplasmosis was not included in this chapter. Utilizing the *Red Book*, identify the standard dosing algorithm for pyrimethamine, sulfadiazine, and folinic acid. Does the electronic ordering system at your hospital provide this dosing to prescribers?

Mind Map

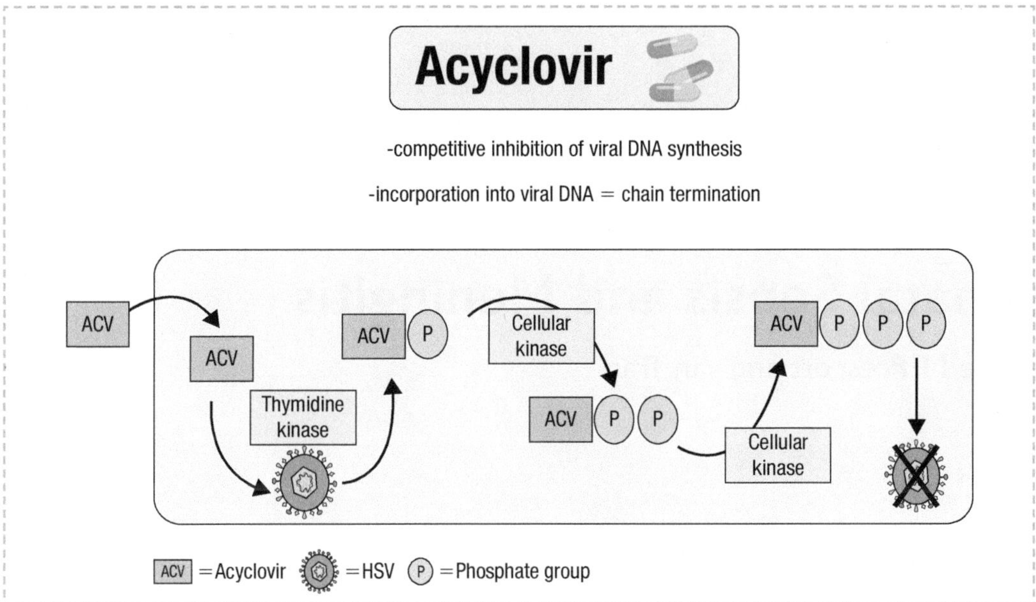

Note: This mind map reflects the design team's interpretation of a portion of one or more concepts addressed in this chapter. Readers should regard the mind maps woven throughout this textbook as examples of multisensory study tools that can be developed to encourage conceptual understanding. Readers are encouraged to develop their own unique mind maps in consultation with academic faculty or clinical preceptors. HSV, herpes simplex virus.

Design credit: Laura Cline, MSN, APRN, NNP-BC, and Hannah Hardesty, MSN, APRN, NNP-BC, East Carolina University Neonatal Nurse Practitioner Program.

REFERENCES

References for this chapter are online and available at https://connect.springerpub.com/content/book/978-0-8261-5884-0/part/partVII/toc-part/ch27.

chapter 28

Neonatal Sepsis and Meningitis

Stephanie M. Prescott and Van Tran

LEARNING OBJECTIVES

After completing this chapter, the reader should be able to:

- Examine the seminal studies that shaped the state of science specific to neonatal sepsis.
- Describe the physiology of the neonatal immune system.
- Enumerate the most common causes of sepsis in the neonatal period.
- Explain the pathophysiology of neonatal early-onset sepsis (EOS) and late-onset sepsis (LOS).
- Explain the pathophysiology of meningitis.
- Investigate current pharmacotherapeutic regimens for infants with neonatal sepsis and meningitis.

INTRODUCTION

Neonatal sepsis and meningitis, previously known as *childbed fever* or *puerperal septicemia,* have long been major contributors to maternal and neonatal morbidity and mortality over the years. By definition, sepsis involves a bacterial, viral, or fungal infection that imposes significant morbidity and mortality risk to preterm and term infants. This chapter focuses on bacterial and fungal infections.

Sepsis and meningitis are categorized as early onset or late onset, based on the hour or day of life in which one or more pathogens are isolated from blood (sepsis) or cerebrospinal fluid (CSF; meningitis). This is further subdivided for preterm and term infants (Table 28.1). EOS involves vertical transmission of a pathogen, from the mother to the fetus, most often during the birth process. Risk factors are summarized in Table 28.2.

EOS most often involves the vertical transmission of organisms residing in the maternal genitourinary tract by way of (a) hematogenous transplacental intra-amniotic infection, (b) ascending vaginal infection through ruptured membranes, or (c) fetal contact with the vaginal canal during descent through the vaginal canal in the intrapartum period (Walker et al., 2019). In contrast, LOS most often involves the horizontal transmission of a pathogen from the hospital environment, community, or caregiver to the infant (Glaser et al., 2021). As it is nearly impossible to clinically distinguish bacteremia from meningitis, clinicians rely on the laboratory analysis of CSF to confirm the diagnosis and guide treatment (Bentlin & de Souza Rugolo, 2010).

The most common organisms responsible for neonatal EOS include *Streptococcus agalactiae* (also known as group B *Streptococcus* [GBS]), *Escherichia coli, Staphylococcus aureus, Haemophilus influenzae,* Candida spp., and *Listeria monocytogenes.* GBS is a gram-positive, facultative anaerobic coccus (round bacteria) that tends to form chains (Shabayek & Spellerberg, 2018). In comparison, *E. coli*

TABLE 28.1 Early- and Late-Onset Sepsis and Meningitis in Neonates

TYPE OF INFECTION	TIMING OF PATHOGEN IDENTIFICATION IN PRETERM NEONATES	TIMING OF PATHOGEN IDENTIFICATION IN TERM NEONATES
Early-onset sepsis or meningitis	Pathogen detected in blood or CSF ≤**72 hours** of birth	Pathogen detected in blood or CSF ≤**7 days** after birth
Late-onset sepsis or meningitis	Pathogen detected in blood or CSF >**72 hours** after birth	Pathogen detected in blood or CSF >**7 days** after birth

CSF, cerebrospinal fluid.
Source: From Mukhopadhyay, S., & Puopolo, K. M. (2012). Risk assessment in neonatal early onset sepsis. *Seminars in Perinatology*, *36*(6), 408–415. https://doi.org/10.1053/j.semperi.2012.06.002.

TABLE 28.2 Risk Factors for Early-Onset Sepsis in Newborns

MATERNAL RISK FACTORS	INFANT RISK FACTORS	SOCIAL RISK FACTORS
• Chorioamnionitis • Frequent digital examinations • GBS bacteriuria • Internal fetal monitoring device • Maternal fever • Meconium-stained amniotic fluid • Premature rupture of membranes • Previous infant with GBS infection • Procedures during pregnancy, e.g., cervical cerclage, amniocentesis • Prolonged rupture or labor • Vaginal colonization with GBS	• Apgar score ≤6 at 5 minutes • Black race • Congenital anomalies • Fetal distress • Fetal tachycardia • Instrument-assisted delivery • Intravenous access • Intubation • Low birth weight • Male sex • Prematurity	• Low socioeconomic status • Poor/late prenatal care • Poor maternal nutrition • Substance abuse

GBS, group B *Streptococcus*.
Sources: From Mukhopadhyay, S., & Puopolo, K. M. (2012). Risk assessment in neonatal early onset sepsis. *Seminars in Perinatology*, *36*(6), 408–415. https://doi.org/10.1053/j.semperi.2012.06.002; Puopolo, K. M., Benitz, W. E., Zaoutis, T. E., Committee On Fetus and Newborn, & Committee On Infectious Diseases. (2018a). Management of neonates born at ≤34 6/7 weeks' gestation with suspected or proven early-onset bacterial sepsis. *Pediatrics*, *142*(6), e20182896. https://doi.org/10.1542/peds.2018-2896; Puopolo, K. M., Benitz, W. E., Zaoutis, T. E., Committee On Fetus and Newborn, & Committee On Infectious Diseases. (2018b). Management of neonates born at ≥35 0/7 weeks' gestation with suspected or proven early-onset bacterial sepsis. *Pediatrics*, *142*(6), e20182894. https://doi.org/10.1542/peds.2018-2894; Puopolo et al., 2019; Simonsen, K. A., Anderson-Berry, A. L., Delair, S. F., & Davies, H. D. (2014). Early-onset neonatal sepsis. *Clinical Microbiology Reviews*, *27*(1), 21–47. https://doi.org/10.1128/CMR.00031-13.

are rod-shaped, gram-negative, facultative anaerobic bacteria (Conway et al., 2004; Tenaillon et al., 2010). GBS remains the most common cause of EOS in term newborns, whereas *E. coli* is the most common cause of EOS in preterm newborns (Pantell et al., 2021). Preterm newborns are particularly vulnerable to EOS; the rate of EOS is 30 times higher in preterm newborns less than 28 weeks of gestation and 11 times higher in those between 29 and 33 weeks of gestation at birth compared with term newborns (Singh & Yu, 2019).

The reduced incidence of GBS EOS and the consequential increased incidence of gram-negative EOS (*E. coli*) in newborns are attributed to the widespread implementation of the 1996 Centers for Disease Control and Prevention (CDC) consensus guidelines for intrapartum GBS antibiotic prophylaxis (IAP). In 1996, the incidence of EOS was approximately 3 to 4 cases per 1,000 live births and nearly all cases involved GBS infection. In the years that followed, the incidence of EOS declined to 0.8 per 1,000 live births (Schrag et al., 2016). More recently, the incidence of EOS was estimated to be 0.5 cases per 1,000 infants born at term (≥37 weeks of gestation), 1 per 1,000 infants born between 34 and 36 weeks of gestation, 6 cases per 1,000 infants born between 29 and 34 weeks of gestation, 20 cases per 1,000 infants born between 25 and 28 weeks of gestation, and 32 cases per 1,000 infants born between 22 and 24 weeks of gestation (Schrag et al., 2016; Weston et al., 2011). The mortality risk is estimated to be 1.6% for neonates ≥37 weeks of gestation at birth,

30% between 25 and 28 weeks of gestation, and 50% for infants between 22 and 24 weeks of gestation (Stoll et al., 2020). Infants with very low birth weight (VLBW) account for the majority (75%) of deaths from EOS (Stoll et al., 2020).

Although IAP in high-risk pregnant women has been remarkably successful, it has not reduced the incidence of LOS, including GBS LOS (Puopolo et al., 2018b; Toyofuku et al., 2017). The incidence of LOS is estimated at 10% to 30% in VLBW infants (Greenberg et al., 2017; Horbar et al., 2017). GBS LOS is associated with a high risk of meningitis (up to 57.7%) and postinfectious neurologic sequelae (e.g., hydrocephalus, empyema, encephalomalacia). *Pseudomonas* accounts for up to 25% of gram-negative LOS-associated mortality (Tsai, Chu, et al., 2014). The overall incidence of LOS meningitis is 0.3 per 1,000 live births, which is likely underreported, because less than 50% of preterm neonates with LOS are stable enough to receive a lumbar puncture, or receive it after antibiotic administration has begun (Bundy & Noor, 2021). The risk of neurodevelopmental impairment (NDI) increases as the number of LOS episodes increases. Based on the results of a recent cohort study, three or more LOS episodes are associated with a 42% risk of NDI (Mukhopadhyay & Puopolo, 2012). Overall mortality risk in VLBW infants is 15% with a positive blood culture and 9% for VLBW infants with a negative blood culture ($p < .001$; Hornik, Fort, et al., 2012). Mortality risk is 11%, 21%, and 29% among infants with gram-positive, gram-negative, and fungal infections, respectively (Hornik, Fort, et al., 2012).

Fungemia is the third leading cause of LOS in VLBW infants (Lovero et al., 2016). *Candida* spp. are responsible for 3% of EOS and 11% of LOS, primarily in VLBW infants (Benjamin et al., 2006; Wynn & Wong, 2017). Of all extremely low-birth-weight (ELBW) infants (<1,000 grams), 4% to 8% acquire fungal bloodstream infections and 30% of affected infants die (Lovero et al., 2016). Long-term neurodevelopmental complications, cerebral palsy, blindness, and hearing deficits are reported among survivors (Benjamin et al., 2006).

The high morbidity and mortality burden of neonatal sepsis and meningitis highlights the importance of clear understanding of the physiology of neonatal immunity, the pathophysiology and risk factors for the disease, and the optimal targeted and timely treatment. This chapter provides a brief overview of the physiology of fetal and neonatal immune development and the blood–brain barrier (BBB); the pathophysiology of neonatal sepsis, meningitis, and vertical transfer; the risk factors, clinical presentation, laboratory evaluation, and treatment recommendations for EOS and LOS; common pathogenic organisms; and opportunities for antibiotic stewardship.

HISTORICAL PERSPECTIVE: SEMINAL AND OTHER NOTEWORTHY STUDIES

Ancient Greek and Hindi texts indicated that cleanliness was necessary for midwives to protect neonatal health. If this advice was followed worldwide through modern times, many lives could perhaps have been spared. However, as bacteria was an unknown concept at the time, causes of early sudden fever and death in postpartum women and their infants were attributed to many, often bizarre, causes. These theorized causes included unbalanced humors, obstructed lochia, rising too soon after childbirth, milk circulating in the blood, hard labor, miasma, extreme fear of childbirth, and extreme joy for the expectant birth. Treatment included bleeding, applying cupping glasses to the groin and hips, opening veins of the knees and thighs, using aromatics to induce sweat, applying leeches to hemorrhoids, as well as using purgatives and laxatives (Peckham, 1935). It was not until the early 1800s, when women began delivering at "lying in" hospitals, that the epidemic nature of the disease was recognized. Women were then isolated, and their linen burned in addition to the aforementioned "treatments." Finally, in the mid-1800s, the dual nature of postpartum sepsis was observed and obstetrical cleanliness was again recommended. Shortly after, in 1887, GBS was identified.

> The occurrence of childbed fever among the newborn can be explained in two ways. [It] may be caused by factors operating on the mother during intrauterine life of the fetus, and the mother can then impart the disease on the infant. Alternatively, the cause may affect the infant itself after birth, in which case the mother may or may not be affected. Thus, the infant dies, not because the disease has been imparted, as in the first case, but rather because childbed fever originates in the infant itself. (Semmelweis, 1861/1983)

By 1935, the most common causative organism in EOS, hemolytic *Streptococcus*, had been identified, but treatments such as isolation, vitamin enrichment, serum from patients with scarlet fever, quinine, disulfamine, iodine, mercury, and arsenic remained largely ineffective and often dangerous (Lindsay, 1935). Although British surgeon Joseph Lister's antiseptic methods had been disseminated in the late 1800s, it took more than 30 years for antiseptic techniques to be widely accepted in the United States (Herr, 2007). In the early 20th century, 6 to 9 per 1,000 women died of pregnancy complications and 10% to 30% of infants died within the first year (CDC, 1999). Fortunately, antiseptic techniques and penicillin were adopted into practice in the 1940s; these strategies reduced neonatal mortality by 40% (CDC, 1999). By the 1970s, clinical trials informed clinicians that GBS EOS could be largely prevented with the use of properly timed intrapartum antimicrobial prophylaxis; ampicillin and an aminoglycoside were recommended for use in at-risk neonates in the 1970s as well. By 1996, the CDC recommended routine intrapartum GBS prophylaxis with at-risk pregnancies. Widespread adoption of these guidelines resulted in a decrease in mortality from 55% in 1970, to 5% in 2004, and to 0.15% in 2017 among neonates with invasive GBS disease (Dermer et al., 2004; Kamal et al., 2019). In 2002, the CDC recommended that obstetric providers screen all pregnant women for GBS between 35 and 37 weeks of gestation. In 2010, the CDC clarified the definition of adequate IAP and published an algorithm to help neonatal clinicians determine whether routine care, 48-hour observation, a limited laboratory evaluation, or full evaluation with antimicrobial therapy were indicated (Verani et al., 2010). This unintentionally led to a significant increase in painful procedures and antibiotic exposures among otherwise well-appearing term newborns.

As of 2017, nearly 67% of infant deaths in the United States occurred during the neonatal period (Singh & Yu, 2019). Note that GBS remained the leading cause of sepsis in term neonates; however, *E. coli* emerged as the leading cause of EOS-related mortality in preterm neonates, particularly those subject to premature rupture of membranes (Puopolo et al., 2017).

Next, a computer-based predictive EOS calculator emerged, created by Puopolo and colleagues (2011), to help clinicians distinguish between late preterm and term infants who require immediate treatment, and those who may safely be observed before treatment is initiated. This calculator considered the highest maternal antepartum temperature, duration of rupture of membranes, GBS status, use of intrapartum antibiotic therapy, and gestational age to estimate the risk of EOS. Neonatal clinicians observed the infant after birth, and based on the clinical presentation classified the infant as well appearing, equivocal, or clinically unwell. This classification informed whether clinical observation only, observation and laboratory evaluation, or empirical pharmacologic therapy were indicated (Escobar et al., 2014).

In 2018, the CDC appointed the American College of Obstetricians and Gynecologists (ACOG) and American Academy of Pediatrics (AAP), and the American Society for Microbiology (ASM) as stewards for GBS prophylaxis in pregnant women and newborns, and laboratory practices for the detection and identification of GBS, respectively. Within 1 year of this change ACOG (2019) published updated guidelines that retired the CDC 2010 guidance. Most notable, this new guidance shifted prenatal GBS screening to 36 0/7 to 37 6/7 weeks to ensure accuracy in results through 41 weeks of pregnancy, recommended antibiotics for IAP to prevent GBS infection (ampicillin, penicillin G), and recommended allergy testing for women who self-report a penicillin allergy. Cefazolin was recommended for use in women with a penicillin allergy at low risk for anaphylaxis and clindamycin for women considered at high risk for anaphylaxis. One month later, in July 2019, the AAP endorsed ACOG's guidance and recommended that clinicians use one of three possible methods to appraise EOS risk in newborns ≥35 weeks of gestation: (a) categorical risk assessment, (b) EOS calculator, or (c) risk assessment based on the newborn's clinical condition. The most recent updates to the ASM (2021) guidelines were published on July 23, 2021.

Some wrong turns have been made along the way, such as the use of chloramphenicol (see Chapter 1, "Pediatric Drug Regulation in the United States"), a promising antibiotic that led to "gray baby syndrome," hyperbilirubinemia, kernicterus, shock, and death (Cummings et al., 2021). Successes, though, namely the use of IAP in high-risk women and the EOS calculator in late preterm and term newborns, have drastically reduced the burden of EOS surveillance and treatment worldwide. Antibiotic stewardship efforts continue to prioritize use of the minimum effective antibiotic regimen for cases of suspected and confirmed EOS and LOS. There is much work to be done, including pharmacokinetic studies of antimicrobial agents prescribed to neonates.

PHYSIOLOGY REVIEW: NEONATAL IMMUNE DEVELOPMENT AND RESPONSES

Embryonic hematopoiesis begins in the aorta at 3 to 6 weeks' postconception, moves to the liver, then transitions to the bone marrow, the site of adult hematopoiesis, by 24 weeks of gestation (Zhang et al., 2017). Progenitor immune cells are present in fetal tissues, liver, bone marrow, thymus and blood, and exhibit both pro- and anti-inflammatory capabilities (De Kleer et al., 2014). The fetus must achieve a balance between tolerance and activation when faced with a constant stream of foreign proteins and cells throughout gestation via the placenta. The neonate must then tolerate massive microbial exposure at delivery after residing in a sterile or nearly sterile uterine environment.

Immunogenic tolerance of the fetus and neonate is mitigated by transplacental immunoglobulin transfer and breast milk-derived, pathogen-specific antibodies (Albrecht & Arck, 2020). Immunoglobulin G (IgG), the most abundant antibody in maternal circulation and the only immunoglobulin capable of traversing the placenta, binds and neutralizes toxins, opsonizes pathogen surfaces, and initiates immune pathways to protect the fetus from pathogens recognized by the maternal immune system. This provides the fetus with passive immunity during gestation and during the first few months of life (Albrecht & Arck, 2020; Jnah & Trembath, 2019; Vidarsson et al., 2014). Fetal IgG concentrations increase during the second half of pregnancy, which leaves very preterm neonates (and ELBW neonates) devoid of adequate IgG for immune defenses (Wynn & Wong, 2017). As previously mentioned, the rate of LOS is 3 to 10 times higher in preterm infants, and poor IgG transfer is one reason for the increased risk of sepsis in these vulnerable preterm infants (Shane et al., 2017).

After birth, innate immune defenses are primarily modulated by neutrophils, monocytes, macrophages, dendritic cells, T cells and B cells. Normally, these cells sense bacterial signatures and elicit potent proinflammatory and antimicrobial activity. However, neonates are affixed with a reduced neutrophil count compared with older infants and children, which inhibits phagocytic activity (Glaser et al., 2021). Monocyte and macrophage counts and function are also reduced, which hinders proinflammatory and antigen-presenting responses. Reduced dendritic cell function hinders activation of the adaptive immune response (Figure 28.1; Danis et al., 2008; Zhang et al., 2017). Further, given that acquired immunity requires pathogenic exposures and the formation of memory T and B cells, the naïve state exhibited by newborns accustomed to a sterile environment means that weeks and months are required before an efficient response is observed. Thus, cellular responses are uniquely programmed toward tolerance of foreign antigens, and, in the case of premature infants, intolerance of lifesaving measures that generate oxygen radicals, such as supplemental oxygen administration, during the first several days of life.

The neonatal immune system is best supported with the provision of freshly expressed human milk. This unpasteurized human milk contains not only maternal IgG, but also immunoglobulin M (IgM), immunoglobulin A (IgA), and other immune-modulatory compounds, including cytokines, chemokines, and antibacterial proteins and peptides (Edwards et al., 2021; M'Rabet et al., 2008). These immunogenic compounds provide short-term protection against pathogens while the infant's quiescent immune system matures in the face of commensal microbial colonization. Preterm infants benefit most from the provision of fresh human milk; however, they are more likely to experience short- or long-term feeding intolerances and interruptions in human milk feedings. In addition, preterm infants are more likely to receive pasteurized human milk, which is devoid of immunoglobulins (Demers-Mathieu et al., 2019). These factors contribute to the increased risk of LOS in the preterm population. We refer readers to Chapter 6, "Postpartum Pharmacology," and Chapter 21, "Human Milk as Medicine," for additional helpful information specific to human milk.

Commensal microbes also play a role in infant immune programing (Jnah & Trembath, 2019). Maternal gastrointestinal, vaginal, mammary, salivary, and skin microbes colonize the newborn (Dunn et al., 2017; Gomez de Agüero et al., 2016; Makino, 2018). Early microbial colonization disruptions as a result of Cesarean delivery, feeding intolerances, formula feeding, and antibiotic administration have been shown to have lasting consequences to later health, including allergy, obesity, and inflammatory bowel conditions (Arboleya et al., 2018; Butel et al., 2018; Mueller et al., 2015; Nash et al., 2017; Turta & Rautava, 2016; Yasmin et al., 2017).

FIGURE 28.1 Innate versus adaptive immunity.

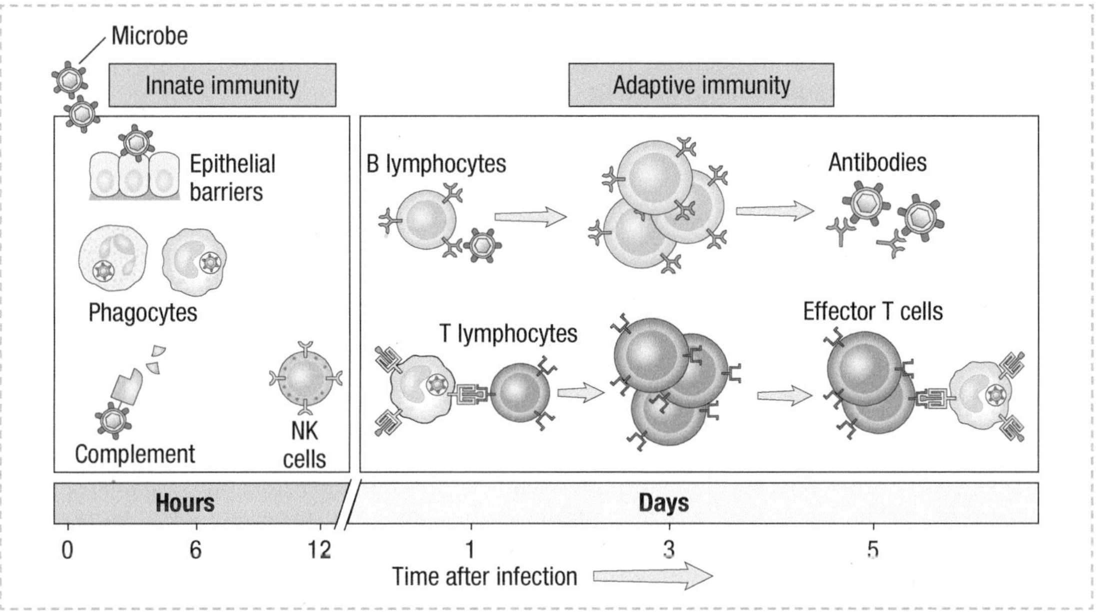

Microbe
Innate immunity
Adaptive immunity
Epithelial barriers
Phagocytes
Complement
NK cells
B lymphocytes
Antibodies
T lymphocytes
Effector T cells
Hours
Days
0 6 12 1 3 5
Time after infection

NK, natural killer.
Source: From Abbas, A. K., Lichtman, A. H., & Pillai, S. (2010). *Basic immunology updated edition: Functions and disorders of the immune system.* Elsevier Health Sciences.

Immune defenses also depend on intact and mature skin (the largest organ) and ample vernix. The outermost layer of the skin (stratum corneum) and the vernix matures in the third trimester. Therefore, neonates born preterm present with limited innate defenses. This compromises the ability to withstand bacterial invasion over the first 8 to 12 weeks of life (Evans & Rutter, 1986; Jnah & Trembath, 2019; Visscher et al., 2005). Over the first few months of life, massive surface colonization by commensal bacteria occurs, which strengthens the skin barrier and innate immune responses.

PATHOPHYSIOLOGY REVIEW: BACTEREMIA, MENINGITIS, AND FUNGEMIA

Bacteremia

Vascular endothelial cells become activated in response to bacterial constituents, leading to the production and release of adhesion molecules, cytokines, and chemokines for the purpose of attracting immune cells and containment of the pathogen (Sampah & Hackam, 2020). Vasoactive substances are released from the activated immune cells, including prostaglandin, nitric oxide, histamine, and platelet-activating factor (Marom et al., 2004; Sellin et al., 2018). This cascade of responses to bacterial substances may lead to endothelial cell apoptosis, loss of vascular tone, and capillary leak, thereby contributing to acute respiratory distress syndrome and pulmonary hypertension seen in conjunction with sepsis even when originating in extrapulmonary localized tissues. Systemic activation of vascular endothelial cells may lead to systemic inflammatory response syndrome (SIRS) in which systemic overproduction of cytokines leads to loss of vascular tone, hypovolemia, disseminated intravascular coagulation (DIC), shock, and death (Chang, 2019).

Meningitis

The BBB is an anatomic and functional barrier of endothelial cells present in the capillaries of the brain that limits communication between the central nervous system (CNS) and the bloodstream (Kadry et al., 2020). Bacteria that infiltrate the bloodstream may penetrate the BBB in the fetus or neonate, causing inflammation of the meninges. Mechanisms by which bacteria cross the BBB in neonates are poorly understood, but are believed to be multifactorial and bacterial concentration-dependent (Huang et al., 2000). Symptoms of neonatal meningitis are often nonspecific and so must be suspected in cases of neonatal bacteremia due to immature neonatal immune function, especially in preterm infants (Bundy & Noor, 2021).

Fungemia

Systemic fungal infections are three to four times more deadly than systemic infections with gram-positive bacteria and carry about the same risk of mortality as systemic gram-negative bacterial infections. Of the fungal species, *Candida* spp. are most frequently associated with neonatal sepsis (Ershad et al., 2019). Fungemia, as with other instances of LOS, is associated with central-line use, mechanical ventilation, prolonged antibiotic exposure, prolonged parenteral nutrition (PN), long-term hospitalization, prematurity, and low birth weight (Lovero et al., 2016). Fungal infection of the skin and/or mucous membranes, such as dermatitis, oral thrush, and congenital candidiasis, may spread to the blood and other organs via breaks in epithelial barriers from premature skin and invasive procedures or catheters. Invasive fungal dermatitis occurs in ELBW infants, causing extensive erosion of the skin, and often leads to disseminated infection. *Candida* spp. can be cultured from skin, blood, CSF, gastric aspirate, tracheal aspirate, urine, and stool. More sites of fungal colonization lead to greater risk of invasive fungal infection (Manzoni et al., 2007). Invasive disseminated candidiasis is associated with spontaneous intestinal perforation in ELBW infants, distinct from necrotizing enterocolitis (NEC), with up to 33% of affected neonates having positive blood, peritoneal fluid, CSF, or urine cultures with histopathologic evidence of fungal infection at the site of intestinal perforation (Bendel, 2005).

Candida is a normal part of the human gastrointestinal and vaginal microbiota. The most common method of acquiring fungal bloodstream infections is via damaged mucosa or epithelium in the gut or premature skin (Mora Carpio & Climaco, 2021). PN and intravenous (IV) lipid emulsions increase biofilm production in candidiasis, thereby increasing virulence (Mora Carpio & Climaco, 2021). Prolonged antibiotic exposure confers a selective advantage to fungus as intestinal bacteria killed by targeted antibiotics normally function to stimulate the mucosa to secrete antifungal peptides (McCarty & Pappas, 2016). *Candida* spp. are able to adhere to tissue and plastic surfaces and form biofilms that then secrete antifungal resistance molecules, making it difficult to eradicate established fungal infections (McCarty & Pappas, 2016). The neonatal immune tolerance profile prevents optimal opsonization and killing of disseminated fungal infections and contributes to the refractory response of antifungals in this population.

EARLY-ONSET SEPSIS: MICROBIOLOGY, MANIFESTATIONS, AND DIAGNOSTICS

Clinical Manifestations

Infants with EOS present with symptoms that vary depending on gestational age, severity of infection, and the invading pathogenic organism. Decreased gestational age is a strong predictor of EOS as nearly two-thirds of preterm infants are delivered after preterm labor, prolonged rupture of membranes, use of instrumentation during pregnancy, frequent maternal exam, and maternal infection (Goldenberg et al., 2008; Puopolo et al., 2018a).

Clinical manifestations of EOS in preterm infants include apnea, bradycardia, and cyanosis. In comparison, signs of EOS in late preterm and term infants include tachypnea, tachycardia, temperature instability, and/or a need for supplemental oxygen, noninvasive or invasive respiratory support (Puopolo et al., 2019; Simonsen et al., 2014).

Diagnostics

The gold standard for the diagnosis of EOS is a positive blood culture; however, the prevalence of low-colony-count sepsis in neonates complicates the interpretation of negative cultures, and in some cases the positive result is due to type 1 error (contamination; Hornik, Benjamin, et al., 2012; Kellogg et al., 1997). Therefore, clinicians must ensure optimal blood volume and phlebotomy technique to detect pathogens even at low colony counts (Cantey & Sanchez, 2011). Most antibiotic therapies may be discontinued when culture results have been negative for 36 to 48 hours, except for cases where there is evidence of site-specific infection (Puopolo et al., 2018a). Other diagnostic tests include a complete blood count with differential, which yields a low positive predictive value for sepsis but helps clinicians appraise red blood cell indices.

When meningitis is suspected or a positive blood culture is reported, CSF sampling is indicated (Swanson, 2015). Ideally, the CSF sample should be obtained before antimicrobial therapy is started, as the medications selected are those with optimal CNS penetration. CSF studies help determine the dose and duration of antibiotic therapy necessary to adequately treat the infection (Aleem & Greenberg, 2019; Puopolo et al., 2018b).

Current Pharmacologic Treatment Modalities for Early-Onset Sepsis

Bacterial resistance resulting from widespread antibiotic use has become an important problem in recent times requiring strict antibiotic stewardship to avoid unnecessary or prolonged antibiotic use. This provides opportunity for the growth and selection of resistant organisms. Unnecessary investigation and treatment with antibiotics results in maternal–infant separation, prolonged hospital stay, breastfeeding difficulties, increased hospital costs, and risks of chronic diseases associated with early antibiotic exposure, such as asthma, allergy, autoimmune disease, and obesity (Deshmukh et al., 2021; Risnes et al., 2011; Saari et al., 2015; Sobko et al., 2010).

Various randomized controlled trials (RCTs) have evaluated different regimens for EOS (Hammerberg et al., 1989; Metsvaht et al., 2010; Miall-Allen et al., 1988; Snelling et al., 1983; Tewari & Jain, 2014). A recent 2021 Cochrane review including five RCTs (Korang, Gordon et al., 2021), with 865 cumulative infants, did not find any difference among regimens when assessing death from all causes, serious adverse events, respiratory support, circulatory support, nephrotoxicity, neurologic developmental impairment, ototoxicity, or NEC. However, all these trials were at high risk of bias and had very low certainty of evidence. Due to scarce data, it cannot be concluded that one regimen is superior to another.

As antibiotics have become one of the most used therapeutics in the NICU, risk versus benefit must be considered, especially when continuing empirical antibiotics in the absence of a culture-confirmed infection (Puopolo et al., 2018a). The routine empirical use of broad-spectrum antibiotic agents is neither recommended nor justified and may promote bacterial antibiotic resistance, alteration of gut colonization, increased risk of *Candida* colonization and subsequent invasive candidiasis, and increased risk of death, NEC, and LOS (Puopolo et al., 2018a; Tzialla et al., 2012). Antimicrobial resistance patterns of bacterial isolates commonly detected in the local NICU or community settings should guide choice of empirical antimicrobial therapy in newborns who are critically ill until culture results are available (Puopolo et al., 2018a; Shane et al., 2017). For more complex cases (e.g. meningitis, other site-specific infections, resistant/atypical organisms), consultation with pediatric infectious diseases specialists should be considered (Puopolo et al., 2018a).

Given the prevalence of GBS and *E. coli, the initial antibiotic regimen for suspected EOS should target both gram-positive and gram-negative organisms*. Therefore, combination therapy, including a beta-lactam (ampicillin) and an aminoglycoside (gentamicin) or cephalosporin (cefotaxime, ceftazidime), is indicated (Shane et al., 2017). This combination provides effective coverage against GBS, *E. coli,* most other streptococcal and enterococcal species, and *L. monocytogenes*, as well as offers synergistic bacterial killing (Puopolo et al., 2018a; Sivanandan et al., 2011).

BETA-LACTAM (AMPICILLIN)

Recall that gram-negative bacteria are surrounded by a thin peptidoglycan cell wall with an outer membrane containing lipopolysaccharides, whereas gram-positive bacteria lack the outer membrane but are surrounded by much thicker layers of peptidoglycan. Knowing bacterial cellular composition is essential in understanding how antibiotics inhibit cellular processes to contribute to cell death. Ampicillin offers bactericidal activity against gram-positive and gram-negative aerobic and anaerobic bacteria by binding to penicillin-binding proteins (PBPs) in order to inhibit cell wall synthesis (Kapoor et al., 2017).

Mechanism of Action/Pharmacokinetic Principles

The mechanism of action of beta-lactam antibiotics (as well as penicillins, carbapenems, and cephalosporins) involves binding to one or more of the PBPs. This prevents cross-linking of peptidoglycan units and inhibits the final transpeptidation step of peptidoglycan synthesis within bacterial cell walls (Kohanski et al., 2010). The decrease in peptidoglycan synthesis and increase in autolysins lead to cell lysis, and ultimately bacterial cell death (Kapoor et al., 2017).

Ampicillin is administered via IV, making the drug 100% bioavailable. Protein binding in neonates is low (10%), lipophilicity is high, and ampicillin exhibits a relatively stable volume of distribution among preterm and term neonates (Padari et al., 2021). CNS penetration is poor (3%–5%) in the absence of meningitis and increases to approximately 40% with inflamed meninges, which explains the increased dosing requirement for meningitis compared with sepsis. Ampicillin is excreted largely unchanged in the urine, with the half-life decreasing as postmenstrual age (PMA) increases for infants with postnatal age of less than 28 days (Rivera-Chaparro et al., 2017).

Dosing Recommendations

Active pharmacokinetic study informs the dosing and duration of ampicillin for EOS, LOS, and meningitis. Dose and/or interval vary by PMA, postnatal age, and indication. Current AAP (2021a) *Red Book* recommendations reflect a robust pharmacokinetic study (Tremoulet et al., 2014); however, data continue to emerge (Padari, 2021). Clinicians must refer to updated tertiary references or guidelines for the most recent, evidence-based recommendations. The following is the current standard IV dosing regimen that can be used with cases of EOS based on gestational age and postnatal age:

- **≤34 weeks and <7 days of life**: 50 mg/kg/dose every 12 hours
- **>34 weeks of gestation and ≤28 days of life**: 50 mg/kg/dose every 8 hours

The standard duration of treatment for uncomplicated GBS bacteremia is 10 days and for *Listeria* bacteremia is 14 days. If meningitis is caused by a penicillin-susceptible organism, increasing the dose of ampicillin may be considered to achieve adequate CNS penetration and the duration of therapy may be extended to a minimum of 14 to 21 days (Taketomo, 2023).

Clinical-Monitoring Pearls

Generally, ampicillin administration is well tolerated and without adverse reactions. However, Hornik and colleagues (2016) report an increased risk for neonatal seizures with exposure to high-dose ampicillin (>50 mg/kg/dose). These data highlight the importance of optimal dose and duration selection based on the pathogen and site of infection. Renal function should be monitored throughout therapy; dosage adjustments may be indicated with renal insufficiency (Rivera-Chaparro et al., 2017).

AMINOGLYCOSIDE (GENTAMICIN)

Ampicillin is customarily paired with gentamicin (or a cephalosporin) to treat suspected EOS. Gentamicin is one of the most commonly used antibiotics in the neonatal period. Although two-thirds of *E. coli* EOS isolates being resistant to ampicillin, the majority remain sensitive to gentamicin (Stoll et al., 2020).

Mechanism of Action/Pharmacokinetic Principles

Aminoglycosides exhibit concentration-dependent killing with postantibiotic effect by inhibiting bacterial cell protein synthesis. This is accomplished by binding to the 30S ribosomal subunit of the bacterial cell, which induces translational errors and destroys the cell membrane.

Gentamicin, like other antimicrobial agents, is administered intravenously and is 100% bioavailable. Low protein binding is observed and volume of distribution is inversely proportional to PMA. Pathologic conditions that may further increase the volume of distribution include edema, ascites, and fluid overload. Wide variability in elimination half-life also exists (approximately 3–11.5 hours among neonates <7 days of life), with half-life also inversely associated with gestational and postnatal age. Gentamicin is excreted, primarily unchanged, in the urine (Taketomo, 2023).

Dosing Recommendations

As with ampicillin, it is vital to consult updated tertiary dosing references regarding gentamicin dosing. The following is the current approach for neonates in the first 1 to 2 weeks of life from Le and Bradley (2018) as well as from the AAP (2021a) based on gestational age and day of life:

- **<30 weeks and ≤14 days of life**: 5 mg/kg/dose every 48 hours
- **30 to 34 weeks and ≤10 days of life**: 5 mg/kg/dose every 36 hours
- **≥35 weeks and ≤7 days of life**: 4 mg/kg/dose every 24 hours

Note the higher weight-based dose in more premature neonates, reflective of increased volume of distribution in this population. Also note the longer interval in this population, reflective of greater immaturity of renal clearance.

Clinical-Monitoring Pearls

Monitoring of gentamicin peak and trough levels and renal function, as well as urine output, is warranted given that the drug is renally excreted. Peak levels impact efficacy for this concentration-dependent killer; goal levels for optimal bactericidal activity should be 10 times the minimum inhibitory concentration (MIC) of the target organism, or 8 to 12 mcg/mL in most settings (Touw et al., 2009). Toxicity risk is linked to insufficient drug clearance, which occurs if renal function is impaired (e.g., abnormally elevated serum creatinine, oliguria <1 mL/kg/hr). Trough levels are drawn prior to administration of a scheduled dose. Clinicians should ensure that bedside staff understand the necessity of properly timing blood sampling for the trough level and the need to hold the ordered dose of gentamicin until the trough result is reported and interpreted. The goal trough level is <1 mg/L (Touw et al., 2009). Ototoxicity and nephrotoxicity have been reported, especially in those with higher-than-recommended troughs as well as in those who receive concomitant ototoxic and/or nephrotoxic medications.

Multiple therapeutic drug monitoring strategies exist for aminoglycosides (peak and trough vs. trough only vs. random levels with pharmacokinetic extrapolation). The timing of therapeutic drug monitoring should ideally occur in consultation with a clinical pharmacist and the existing laboratory schedule of the infant should be considered. Generally, therapeutic drug monitoring should occur as soon as possible after the medical team decides to extend treatment beyond 36 to 48 hours.

THIRD-GENERATION CEPHALOSPORIN (CEFOTAXIME, CEFTAZIDIME)

In cases of renal insufficiency or concerns for meningitis, ampicillin may be paired with a third-generation cephalosporin, namely cefotaxime or ceftazidime. Cephalosporins are categorized into five different classes according to their spectrum of activity, ranging from gram-positive organisms to resistant gram-negative organisms with newer generations (i.e., going from first generation to second, etc.; Table 28.3; Rivera-Chaparro et al. 2017). Cefotaxime and ceftazidime, both third-generation cephalosporins, are commonly prescribed in place of gentamicin for treatment of suspected EOS, when renal function is impaired, or when gram-negative meningitis is suspected. Third- and fourth-generation cephalosporins are reserved for patients with impaired renal function, as the risk of additive gentamicin toxicity is unacceptable in this setting, and for suspected gram-negative meningitis, as these agents exhibit optimal CNS penetration (Shane et al., 2017). However, they should not replace gentamicin as empirical EOS therapy in the absence of these indications (see Clinical Monitoring Pearls section).

Mechanism of Action/Pharmacokinetic Principles

Third-generation cephalosporins exhibit a similar mechanism of action to ampicillin, as cephalosporins are also beta-lactam antibiotics. Cephalosporins exhibit bactericidal activity by binding to PBPs on the membrane of the bacterial cell wall. PBPs are necessary to maintain cell wall integrity (rigidity). The binding of a beta-lactam antibiotic to the PBP weakens the bacterial cell wall, induces lysis, and inhibits further bacterial cell wall synthesis.

Cefotaxime and ceftazidime are administered via IV and are 100% bioavailable. The volume of distribution is high as third-generation cephalosporins widely distribute to tissues (including the lungs and CNS). CNS penetration is optimized when the meninges are inflamed (Taketomo, 2023). Cefotaxime is hepatically metabolized and renally excreted. Approximately 60% of the drug is excreted unchanged and the remainder is excreted as metabolites (Taketomo, 2023).

TABLE 28.3 Common Cephalosporins Prescribed to Neonates, By Generation

GENERATION	EFFICACY	DRUG PRESCRIBED TO NEONATES
First generation	Effective against most gram-positive bacteria and modest activity against gram-negative bacteria	Cefazolin Cephalexin
Second generation	Effective against most gram-positive bacteria with increased bactericidal activity against gram-negative bacteria (compared with first generation)	Cefoxitin
Third generation	Variable efficacy against gram-positive bacteria (cefotaxime > ceftazidime) with increased efficacy against gram-negative bacteria (compared with second-generation drugs); increased BBB penetration compared with earlier generations	Cefotaxime Ceftazidime Ceftriaxone
Fourth generation	Effective against gram-positive and gram-negative bacteria (e.g., Enterobacteriaceae, *Pseudomonas*)	Cefepime
Fifth generation	Effective against most gram-positive bacteria (including MRSA, VISA, and VRSA) and susceptible gram-negative bacteria (no activity against *Acinetobacter* and limited activity against *Pseudomonas*)	Ceftaroline

BBB, blood–brain barrier; MRSA, methicillin-resistant *Staphylococcus aureus*; VISA, vancomycin-intermediate *Staphylococcus aureus*; VRSA, vancomycin-resistant *Staphylococcus aureus*.
Source: From Bui, T., & Preuss, C.V. (2021). Cephalosporins. In *StatPearls*. StatPearls Publishing. https://www.statpearls.com/.

Dosing Recommendations

For the purpose of treating EOS, the AAP (2021a) recommends cefotaxime and ceftazidime dosing of 50 mg/kg/dose every 12 hours. With a high index of suspicion for meningitis, the dosing interval should be decreased to every 8 hours for infants ≥32 weeks gestational age (Chen et al., 2018; Kafetzis et al., 1982; Leroux et al., 2016). More frequent dosing is also indicated when these agents are used for LOS, as renal function matures with advancing PMA; in the setting of severe renal dysfunction, dose/interval adjustment may also be required; please refer to updated tertiary references for dosing tables based on available pharmacokinetic data.

Clinical-Monitoring Pearls

Cephalosporins are generally well tolerated. Clinicians typically monitor renal function throughout therapy, as the majority of the drug is renally excreted. Prolonged therapy warrants monitoring for myelosuppression, a rare complication of extended courses of beta-lactam antibiotics. The primary concern regarding widespread utilization of third-generation cephalosporins in neonates is subsequent fungal infections and colonization with resistant organisms. Numerous retrospective studies have associated third-generation cephalosporin exposure in preterm neonates with increased risk of fungal infections and death (Aliaga et al., 2014; Clark et al., 2006; Cotten et al., 2006). A landmark RCT documents frequent colonization with resistant gram-negative bacilli after treatment with cefotaxime, a rare occurrence in neonates randomized to empirical aminoglycoside (de Man et al., 2000). These long-term adverse effects highlight the importance of judicious utilization of cephalosporins despite the advantages of these agents over aminoglycosides (minimal toxicity, lack of therapeutic drug monitoring, and better penetration of lungs/CSF).

LATE-ONSET SEPSIS: MICROBIOLOGY, MANIFESTATIONS, AND DIAGNOSTICS

Although most cases of EOS are antenatally acquired, LOS is acquired postnatally from the hospital or community and presents after 72 hours in preterm infants and from 7 to 28 days in term infants (Ershad et al., 2019; Tsai, Hsu, et al., 2014). Risk factors associated with LOS in the NICU include the need for invasive procedures and indwelling catheters (e.g., percutaneous, peripheral, central venous lines), prolonged PN, endotracheal intubation, prolonged hospitalization, underlying respiratory/cardiovascular diseases, failure of early enteral feeding with breast milk, and formula feeding (El Manouni El Hassani et al., 2019; Tsai, Hsu, et al., 2019). Gram-positive organisms are the most common pathogens in LOS, although gram-negative, fungal, and viral causes have been reported (Table 28.4).

Clinical Presentation

There is great variation in clinical characteristics between different types of gram-negative and gram-positive organisms (Tsai, Hsu, et al., 2014). Neonates with LOS may be febrile or hypothermic, but may also remain well appearing or exhibit nonspecific signs and symptoms such as irritability, poor feeding, vomiting, diarrhea, abdominal distension, hyper- or hypoglycemia, tachypnea, jaundice, somnolence, decreased perfusion, or general malaise (Ershad et al., 2019; Pantell et al., 2021; Tsai, Hsu, et al., 2014). Conversely, infants may present with serious symptoms such as seizures, hypotonia, decreased consciousness, abnormal reflexes, cyanosis, apnea, respiratory distress, tachycardia, or bradycardia (Ershad et al., 2019). Petechia, mottling, and rash may also be present (Bundy & Noor, 2021; Tsai, Hsu, et al., 2014).

Diagnostics

Customary diagnostic tests include blood culture, complete blood count with differential, urine culture, and lumbar puncture. Recall that blood culture is the gold standard test for diagnosing bacteremia; attention to adequate blood volume and sterile technique is vital; blood cultures should be obtained from multiple sites (e.g., peripherally inserted central catheter [PICC] and and peripheral venipuncture), when feasible (Hornik, Benjamin, et al., 2012). White blood count (WBC), absolute neutrophil count (ANC), immature to total neutrophil ratio (I:T), and platelet count yield only moderate sensitivity and specificity (Box 28.1), which decreases with advancing gestational age (Hornik, Benjamin, et al., 2012). Neutrophil to lymphocyte ratio (NLR) and inflammatory markers, such as C-reactive protein (CRP) and procalcitonin (PCT), have recently been proposed as more accurate predictors of LOS in symptomatic infants (Goldberg et al., 2020). Serial measures must be used, however, due to the delay in inflammatory marker production in both the liver and the thyroid. PCT is both more responsive to bacteria and more rapidly detectable, making this marker superior to CRP when available (Adib et al., 2012). However, both markers have excellent negative predictive value, but poor positive predictive value (i.e., normal results rule out infection; abnormal results do not reliably indicate the presence of infection).

Lumbar puncture is recommended for all infants >72 hours of age with suspected LOS as bacteremia is not always present in the setting of CSF culture-positive meningitis (Aleem & Greenberg, 2019; Stoll et al., 2004). Urinalysis should be performed on all infants with LOS. There is no single laboratory evaluation shown to be both sensitive and specific enough to reliably predict LOS in

TABLE 28.4 Common Organisms Identified in Infants With Late-Onset Sepsis

GRAM-POSITIVE (61%)	GRAM-NEGATIVE (26%)	FUNGAL (11%)	VIRAL (2%)
• Coagulase-negative *Staphylococcus* • *Staphylococcus aureus* • *Streptococcus agalactiae* (GBS) • *Listeria monocytogenes*	• *Escherichia coli* • *Enterobacter* spp. • *Klebsiella* spp. • *Pseudomonas* spp. • *Serratia* spp.	• *Candida albicans* • *Candida parapsilosis*	• Herpes simplex virus • Enterovirus

GBS, group B *Streptococcus*.

Sources: From Boghossian, N. S., Page, G. P., Bell, E. F., Stoll, B. J., Murray, J. C., Cotten, C. M., Shankaran, S., Walsh, M. C., Laptook, A. R., Newman, N. S., Hale, E. C., McDonald, S. A., Das, A., Higgins, R. D., & Eunice Kennedy Shriver National Institute of Child Health and Human Development Neonatal Research Network. (2013). Late-onset sepsis in very low birth weight infants from singleton and multiple-gestation births. *Journal of Pediatrics, 162*(6), 1120–4, 1124.e1. https://doi.org/10.1016/j.jpeds.2012.11.089; Shane, A. L., Sánchez, P. J., & Stoll, B. J. (2017). Neonatal sepsis. *The Lancet, 390*(10104), 1770–1780. https://doi.org/10.1016/S0140-6736(17)31002-4; Wynn, J. L., & Wong, H. R. (2017). Pathophysiology of neonatal sepsis. In R. A. Polin, S. H. Abman, D. H. Rowitch, W. E. Benitz, & W. W. Fox (Eds.), *Fetal and neonatal physiology* (pp. 1536–1552.e10). Elsevier. https://doi.org/10.1016/B978-0-323-35214-7.00152-9).

BOX 28.1 Sensitivity and Specificity

Remember, *sensitivity* is the measure of a test's ability to correctly identify persons with a disease, whereas *specificity* refers to a test's ability to identify persons who do not have the disease. Greater than 90% on either of these measures represents a strong result.

this population; therefore, clinicians must rely on clinical evaluation, physiologic monitoring, and imperfect laboratory measures in combination to assist with real-time decision-making (Goldberg et al., 2020). Studies are underway to investigate genomic diagnostic methods (Pantell et al., 2021).

Current Pharmacologic Treatment Modalities for Late-Onset Sepsis

A recent 2021 Cochrane review of five RCTs (N = 580 infants) compared various antimicrobial regimens for LOS (Korang, Greisen, et al., 2021). The authors did not find any difference among regimens in all-cause mortality, serious adverse events, circulatory support, nephrotoxicity, neurologic developmental impairment, or NEC. However, the included trials yielded low certainty of evidence. Therefore, due to a paucity of quality data, no antimicrobial regimen is considered superior to another for the empirical treatment of suspected LOS.

The antibiotic regimen for suspected LOS should target both gram-positive and gram-negative organisms inclusive of known environmental pathogens (staphylococcal and gram-negative bacteria; Pammi & Weisman, 2015; Sivanandan et al., 2011). The presence of coagulase-negative *Staphylococcus* (CoNS) as the most frequently isolated LOS pathogen and methicillin-resistant *Staphylococcus aureus* (MRSA) as one of the more devastating complicates selection of gram-positive coverage. Empirical vancomycin is required to cover both organisms; however, national efforts target a reduction in vancomycin utilization to reduce alarming rates of enterococcal and staphylococcal resistance (Iosifidis et al., 2013). In addition, as with broad-spectrum gram-negative antimicrobials, vancomycin exposure increases the risk of subsequent resistant gram-negative infection in neonates (Smith et al., 2010; Somily et al., 2014). To avoid empirical vancomycin utilization for LOS, clinicians must first recognize that CoNS bacteremia generally produces mild clinical symptoms. In fact, delaying definitive therapy for CoNS does not impact morbidity or mortality rates in affected neonates (Ericson et al., 2015). Second, neonatal units should consider screening for colonization with MRSA (Giuffrè et al., 2013). Recall that MRSA accounts for approximately 3% of neonatal LOS, whereas methicillin-sensitive *Staphylococcus aureus* (MSSA) accounts for approximately 6% (Shane et al., 2012). Delaying definitive coverage for MRSA bacteremia dramatically worsens clinical outcome (Thaden et al., 2015); however, vancomycin is inferior to oxacillin/nafcillin for treatment of MSSA (higher mortality; Kim et al., 2008). Therefore, colonization status of an individual infant may guide optimal empirical treatment selection. In cases of clinical LOS, defined as illness subject to antimicrobial therapy in the absence of a culture-identified organism, in the absence of MRSA colonization or a history of MRSA infection, an acceptable regimen would include a beta-lactam antibiotic (ampicillin or nafcillin/oxacillin) and an aminoglycoside (gentamicin) or cephalosporin for more optimal CNS penetration (cefotaxime, ceftazidime; Sivanandan et al., 2011). Readers should refer to Table 28.5 for alternative antimicrobial regimens based on additional clinical details.

BETA-LACTAMS (NAFCILLIN/OXACILLIN)

Mechanism of Action/Pharmacokinetic Principles

Nafcillin and oxacillin are narrow-spectrum beta-lactam penicillinase-resistant (antistaphylococcal) antibiotics that bind to PBP. This interferes with bacterial cell wall synthesis of susceptible bacteria, including methicillin-sensitive *Staphylococcus* spp.

The volume of distribution of nafcillin/oxacillin is low in neonates compared with children and adults, and increases with advancing postnatal age, resulting in higher weight-based doses in children compared with neonates. Nafcillin/oxacillin are highly protein-bound. Most drug undergoes hepatic metabolism prior to excretion in the urine; a small percentage is excreted unchanged. The

TABLE 28.5 Commonly Prescribed Antimicrobial Regimens for Late-Onset Sepsis

INDICATION FOR TREATMENT	COMBINATION THERAPY	ANTIMICROBIAL AGENT(S)
Suspected LOS (no history/risk of MRSA)	Beta-lactam + Aminoglycoside	Nafcillin/oxacillin
		Gentamicin
Suspected LOS (history/risk of MRSA)	Glycopeptide + Aminoglycoside	Vancomycin
		Gentamicin
Suspected LOS with cardiorespiratory collapse or no response to beta-lactam + aminoglycoside regimen	Glycopeptide + Third-generation cephalosporin	Vancomycin
		Cefotaxime or ceftazidime
Suspected LOS with concern for gastrointestinal involvement (NEC)	Beta-lactam + Aminoglycoside	Ampicillin
		Gentamicin
Adjunctive anaerobic coverage	Penicillin/beta-lactamase inhibitor or Nitroimidazole antibiotic or Lincosamide antibiotic	Piperacillin/tazobactam
		Metronidazole
		Clindamycin

LOS, late-onset sepsis; MRSA, methicillin-resistant *Staphylococcus aureus*; NEC, necrotizing enterocolitis.

elimination half-life is approximately 2 to 6 hours in neonates younger than 7 days of life (Taketomo, 2023). Hepatic metabolism and renal elimination mature with advancing PMA, resulting in more frequent dosing in older subjects.

Dosing Recommendations

For the purpose of treating LOS in neonates ≤28 days of life, the AAP (2021a) recommends IV dosing based on gestational age and day of life:

- **≤34 weeks and >7 days of life**: 25 mg/kg/dose every 8 hours
- **>34 weeks and >7 days of life**: 25 mg/kg/dose every 6 hours

For the purpose of treating LOS in infants older than 28 days of life, the AAP (2021a) recommends IV (or intramuscular) dosing of 100 to 200 mg/kg/d divided into four to six doses. Regardless of postnatal age, 50 mg/kg/dose should be utilized for suspected or proven meningitis. Given that nafcillin is hepatically metabolized and renally eliminated, infants with hepatic or renal dysfunction may require a wider interval between doses to ensure adequate excretion and avoid toxicity. Pharmacokinetic studies of nafcillin/oxacillin in the neonatal population are sparse; readers should utilize tertiary references for updated recommendations that may emerge from future studies.

Clinical-Monitoring Pearls

The most common adverse effect associated with nafcillin is phlebitis at the injection site. Therefore, some neonatal units restrict nafcillin to patients with central venous access. Oxacillin produces a lower rate of phlebitis, but higher risk of transaminitis, making this agent appropriate for peripheral administration but requiring periodic monitoring of hepatic enzymes. As with other beta-lactams, myelosuppression may occur from prolonged therapy.

GLYCOPEPTIDE ANTIBIOTIC (VANCOMYCIN)

Mechanism of Action/Pharmacokinetic Principles

Vancomycin is a tricyclic glycopeptide antibiotic that weakens bacterial cell walls by blocking glycopeptide polymerization. This enables leakage of intracellular contents and ultimately induces bacterial cell death (Patel et al., 2021).

An increased volume of distribution of vancomycin is observed in neonates and infants, which decreases with advancing age; however, overall exposure determines the therapeutic effect for this time-dependent killer, so weight-based dosing is relatively homogenous across populations, whereas the dosing interval is highly variable. Vancomycin is protein-bound and is not subject to hepatic metabolism. Renal clearance, by way of glomerular filtration, is reported (Taketomo, 2023). As postnatal glomerular filtration correlates with gestational age and postnatal age, longer dosing intervals are required to achieve goal trough concentrations in more immature patients.

Dosing Recommendations

A common dosing regimen for this medication has been difficult to establish due to the variable pharmacokinetics that occur with physiologic changes in the neonate during development (Rivera-Chaparro et al., 2017). For the purpose of treating LOS in neonates ≤28 days of life, the AAP (2021a) recommends an IV loading dose of vancomycin (20 mg/kg) followed by maintenance dosing customized to gestational age and renal function. This approach relies on serum creatinine, a marker that may reflect maternal values in the first week of life and may fluctuate significantly in acute illness after that. For the purpose of treating LOS in infants greater than 28 days of life, the AAP (2021a) recommends an IV dose of 45 to 60 mg/kg/d divided into three to four doses. These general recommendations highlight the need for continued attention to emerging studies of vancomycin pharmacokinetics that inform optimal dosing.

Clinical-Monitoring Pearls

Vancomycin use is associated with risk of nephrotoxicity and ototoxicity, as well as phlebitis. These risks increase with concomitant aminoglycoside use. Given that vancomycin is excreted primarily via glomerular filtration, and nephrotoxicity is a potential adverse effect, renal function should be monitored throughout therapy (Taketomo, 2023). In addition, clinicians should monitor drug levels and adjust therapy accordingly to ensure that the optimal exposure of an organism to the antibiotic as measured by the area under the curve (AUC) and the minimum concentration of an antibiotic needed to inhibit the growth of an organism MIC is achieved and toxicity is avoided. The most recent guidelines of the Infectious Diseases Society of America state that an AUC/MIC between 400 and 600 mg/hr/L is ideal for treatment of invasive MRSA infections (Rybak et al., 2020). Due to practical limitations in calculating the AUC/MIC in hospitalized infants, trough levels guide prescribing practices. Although the correlation between trough levels and AUC/MIC remains an area of active study in neonates, generally accepted trough targets include 5 to 15 mcg/mL for CoNS infection, 7 to 11 mcg/mL for MRSA bacteremia, and 15 to 20 mcg/mL for meningitis. It is important to note that consultation with pediatric infectious diseases specialists is advisable for the latter indications, as newer therapies (e.g., ceftaroline) may be preferred.

PENICILLIN/BETA-LACTAMASE INHIBITOR (PIPERACILLIN/TAZOBACTAM)

Mechanism of Action/Pharmacokinetic Principles

Piperacillin, a semisynthetic beta-lactam derived from ampicillin, is used in combination with tazobactam, a beta-lactamase inhibitor (Rivera-Chaparro et al., 2017). Piperacillin-tazobactam provides broad-spectrum coverage against gram-positive, gram-negative, and anaerobic bacteria. The mechanism of action is elicited by piperacillin, which binds with PBPs, and in doing so inhibits bacterial cell wall synthesis. Tazobactam binds to beta-lactamases, which protects the integrity of piperacillin. Poor CNS penetration of tazobactam is reported, making this a suboptimal drug for use with cases of meningitis.

A low volume of distribution is reported in infants (0.37 ± 0.1 L/kg; Taketomo, 2023), as this drug exhibits low lipophilicity and volume of distribution loosely reflects total body water content. This principle informs higher weight-based doses in more immature infants. The elimination half-life in neonates is approximately 1.7 to 9 hours, and this decreases to a more stable elimination half-life of 1.4 ± 0.5 hours in infancy. Piperacillin is primarily excreted in the urine as unchanged drug, and to a lesser extent in the stool. Tazobactam is solely eliminated in the urine, mainly in the form of unchanged drug molecules (Taketomo, 2023). Therefore, dosing interval reflects the maturity of renal function, with more frequent dosing required in more mature subjects.

Dosing Recommendations

For the purpose of treating LOS in neonates ≤28 days of life, the AAP (2021a) recommends dosing based on PMA:

- **≤30 weeks**: 100 mg/kg/dose every 8 hours
- **>30 weeks**: 80 mg/kg/dose every 6 hours

It is important to note that this dosing recommendation is based on recent and robust pharmacokinetic study, although emerging evidence may inform further optimization. For the purpose of treating LOS in infants older than 28 days of life, the AAP (2021a) recommends an IV dose of 240 to 300 mg/kg/d divided into three to four doses.

Clinical-Monitoring Pearls

Piperacillin-tazobactam use is associated with limited adverse effects, including leukopenia, neutropenia, and hypokalemia. Given that this drug is primarily eliminated by glomerular filtration and tubular secretion, renal function should be monitored during therapy. Dosage adjustments may be indicated in infants with renal impairment. In addition, administration with concomitant nephrotoxins (i.e., vancomycin) significantly increases the risk of renal toxicity.

NITROIMIDAZOLE ANTIBIOTIC (METRONIDAZOLE)

Mechanism of Action/Pharmacokinetic Principles

Metronidazole is a concentration-dependent nitroimidazole antibiotic effective against anaerobic and protozoal infections. Metronidazole enters the bacterial cell (or protozoa) through passive diffusion and migrates to the DNA helix. The drug molecules destabilize and break the DNA, which inhibits protein synthesis and leads to bacterial (or protozoal) cell death.

Metronidazole is primarily administered IV in cases of LOS, which is associated with 100% bioavailability. Hepatic metabolism is reported and drug metabolites are excreted in the urine.

Dosing Recommendations

Metronidazole is initiated with an IV loading dose of 15 mg/kg (AAP, 2021a). For the purpose of treating LOS in neonates ≤28 days of life, the AAP (2021a) recommends IV dosing based on gestational age:

- **<34 weeks**: 7.5 mg/kg/dose every 12 hours
- **34 to 40 weeks**: 7.5 mg/kg/dose every 8 hours
- **>40 weeks:** 10 mg/kg/dose every 8 hours

This approach is informed by recent pharmacokinetic studies, including prospective validation, although ongoing investigation may inform future modifications. For the purpose of treating LOS in infants older than 28 days of life, the AAP (2021a) recommends an IV dose of 22.5 to 40 mg/kg/d divided into three to four doses.

Clinical-Monitoring Pearls

Adverse effects include GI disturbances and neutropenia. Prolonged therapy warrants monitoring of complete blood count with differential.

LINCOSAMIDE ANTIBIOTIC (CLINDAMYCIN)

Mechanism of Action/Pharmacokinetic Principles

Clindamycin, a lincosamide antibiotic, inhibits protein synthesis by binding to the 50S subunit of susceptible bacterial ribosomes close to the peptidyl transferase center (Rivera-Chaparro et al., 2017). Clindamycin distributes widely into body fluids and tissues, with the exception of minimal passage into the CSF. Clindamycin is metabolized by CYP3A4, with excretion predominantly in the feces.

Dosing Recommendations

For the purpose of treating LOS in neonates ≤28 days of life, the AAP (2021a) recommends IV dosing based on gestational age:

- **≤32 weeks:** 5 mg/kg/dose every 8 hours
- **33 to 40 weeks**: 7 mg/kg/dose every 8 hours
- **>40 weeks**: 9 mg/kg/dose every 8 hours

Recent pharmacokinetic studies, including prospective validation, form the basis for these recommendations, although emerging evidence may modify this approach. For the purpose of treating LOS in infants older than 28 days of life, the AAP (2021a) recommends an IV dose of 20 to 40 mg/kg/d divided into three to four doses.

Clinical-Monitoring Pearls

Adverse effects associated with clindamycin therapy include phlebitis during IV administration and colitis during prolonged therapy. The primary limitation of clindamycin in neonatal intensive care is growing resistance among *Bacteroides* strains. Neonatal units should ensure adequate sensitivity among organisms empirically targeted by clindamycin and consider alternative therapies in the setting of unacceptable resistance.

FUNGEMIA

A national surveillance study conducted in Great Britain in 2006 revealed that more than 90% of cases of neonatal fungal sepsis were due to *Candida* species, a third of infected infants had previously diagnosed surface colonization, and a third had previously received either oral or IV antifungal prophylaxis (Clerihew et al., 2006). Candidemia was found to have a significantly higher rate of infectious complications (30.8%), persistent bloodstream infection (19.2%), and sepsis-attributable mortality (23.1%; Tsai, Hsu, et al., 2014).

Clinical Evaluation

Early presentation of fungemia is difficult to distinguish from bacterial sepsis but progresses to DIC, coagulopathy, leukopenia, thrombocytopenia, anemia, and metabolic acidosis significantly more often than the more common gram-positive bacterial infections and leads to the highest incidence of septic shock and death compared with other pathogenic organisms (Clerihew et al., 2006; Tsai, Hsu, et al., 2014). Congenital candidiasis can be distinguished from erythema toxicum or miliaria because fungal lesions will be present on the palms and soles of the feet (Pammi, 2021). Disseminated fungal infection presents with lethargy, feeding intolerance, cardiac instability, apnea, respiratory distress, and hyperbilirubinemia, much like bacterial sepsis, but the hallmark of fungemia is persistent hyperglycemia and thrombocytopenia (Mokhtar et al., 2014; Pammi, 2021).

Laboratory Evaluation

Persistent hyperglycemia and thrombocytopenia are common with neutropenia associated with overwhelming disease (Bendel, 2005). Platelet-consuming fungal balls may form on the ends of catheters, in the urinary tract, on heart valves, and/or in the eyes, brain, liver, and kidneys. Therefore, suspected fungemia evaluation must include cultures of the blood, CSF, and urine; dilated eye exam; echocardiography; and sonograms of the liver, spleen, kidneys, head, and catheter tips to rule out vegetation or clots (Barton et al., 2014; Noyola et al., 2001; Pammi, 2021).

Current Pharmacologic Treatment Modalities for Fungemia

Invasive fungal infection should be elevated in the differential diagnosis in infants who have central vascular access, an endotracheal tube, thrombocytopenia (platelets <100 K/mm^3), exposure to broad-spectrum cephalosporins or carbapenem, and gestational age less than 28 weeks (Sivanandan et. al., 2011). Although these risk factors are not diagnostic or exclusive to fungal infections, they should raise the index of suspicion for a possible fungal infection. Amphotericin B and fluconazole are the antifungal drugs of choice for treatment of *Candida* spp. (Lovero et al., 2016). The common *Candida* spp. (e.g., *C. albicans, C. parapsilosis,* and *C. glabrata*) all remain sensitive to amphotericin B (Lovero et al., 2016). However, up to 50% of *C. glabrata* are intrinsically resistant to fluconazole, so the agent of choice is dependent on exhibited resistance to fluconazole and the prevalence of specific species in the local environment (Bendel, 2005; Lovero et al., 2016). We present the state of science specific to amphotericin B and fluconazole in this section of the chapter, such that readers can compare the pharmacokinetic profile and dosing regimens and recognize essential clinical-monitoring priorities.

AMPHOTERICIN B

There are two formulations of amphotericin B: deoxycholate (conventional) and lipid formulations (e.g., liposomal, lipid complex; Greenberg & Benjamin, 2014). Amphotericin B deoxycholate, or conventional, is most commonly used in the treatment of systemic *Candida* infections in neonates and infants. Lipid-associated amphotericin preparations appear to be safe and effective in neonates but not superior to conventional formulations, especially in the urinary tract as a result of poor penetration (Bendel, 2005; Taketomo, 2023).

Mechanism of Action/Pharmacokinetic Principles

Amphotericin B is a polyene that binds to ergosterol, a compound that resides on the cell membranes of fungi, and thus alters cell membrane permeability, causing leakage of cell components and subsequent cell death (Taketomo, 2023). Amphotericin B also stimulates phagocytes in the neonatal immune system, which assists with fungal clearance (Noor & Preuss, 2021).

Amphotericin is administered IV, which yields 100% bioavailability. Amphotericin has a long half-life in infants and older patients, supporting once-daily dosing. The metabolism and elimination of amphotericin are poorly understood, involving minor renal and biliary excretion. The role of metabolism or other elimination pathways has not been quantified, although hepatic and/or renal dysfunction do not appear to impact serum concentrations.

Lipid preparations of amphotericin B produce significantly lower rates of nephrotoxicity and infusion reactions in adults (Loo et al., 2013). Lipid preparations of amphotericin B bind preferentially to high-density lipoprotein (HDL) compared with low-density lipoprotein (LDL); renal cells exhibit lower HDL receptor expression. This property of lipid preparations also increases uptake by the mononuclear phagocyte system, preferentially distributing drug to the liver, spleen, lung, and bone marrow (over the kidneys). In addition, lipid preparations of amphotericin B are intrinsically more selective than conventional preparations for fungal versus mammalian cell membranes, a property that does not impact efficacy but clearly may play a role in the stark difference in toxicity profile. It is important to note that nephrotoxicity is not a frequent adverse effect of conventional amphotericin B in neonates (Turkova et al., 2011). Given the frequent involvement of multiple organ systems in neonatal fungemia, conventional amphotericin B is preferred to ensure adequate renal penetration. However, specific clinical circumstances may alter this standard approach.

Dosing Recommendations

The AAP (2021b) recommends customized dosing regimens based on the specific formulation of amphotericin to be used. The recommended IV dose of amphotericin B deoxycholate is 1 mg/kg/d, which should be administered over 2 to 4 hours. The recommended IV dose of amphotericin B lipid complex (Abelcet) is 3 to 5 mg/kg/d, which should be infused over 2 hours. Amphotericin B liposomal (Ambisome) is dosed at 3 to 7 mg/kg/d and infused over 2 hours.

Clinical-Monitoring Pearls

Urine output should be monitored carefully during amphotericin therapy. Renal function (e.g., serum creatinine and blood urea nitrogen [BUN]) should be monitored at least every other day when therapy is initiated/titrated and at least weekly thereafter (Taketomo, 2023). Serum electrolytes should be monitored during therapy, as amphotericin B can accumulate in the tissues and cause hypokalemia and hypomagnesemia, particularly with prolonged use (Noor & Preuss, 2021). Liver function, coagulation indices, and complete blood count should be monitored frequently during therapy (Noor & Preuss, 2021).

Bedside clinicians must recognize that amphotericin B is only compatible with dextrose. As such, PN may need to be infused over a 22-hour period to allow an infusion window for amphotericin B, particularly if IV access is limited.

FLUCONAZOLE

Fluconazole prophylaxis may be protective in a specific subset of high-risk preterm neonates (Weimer et al., 2022) but also contributes to the emergence of azole resistance, as many *Candida* species are currently resistant to fluconazole (AAP, 2021b). Before initiating prophylactic therapy, clinicians may consider pursuing a multidisciplinary discussion, including neonatologists, pharmacists, and pediatric infectious diseases providers. Unit-specific epidemiology is helpful when considering fungemia prophylaxis. If the If the candidemia incidence is low, clinicians may consider saving fluconazole for treatment of confirmed documented infections (Lovero et al., 2016).

Mechanism of Action/Pharmacokinetic Principles

Fluconazole is an azole antifungal agent that interferes with fungal cytochrome P450 enzyme activity, decreasing ergosterol synthesis, a critical part of the fungal cell wall membrane, and inhibiting cell membrane formation (Govindarajan et al., 2021). Fluconazole penetrates the CSF, eyes, peritoneal fluids, skin, sputum, and urine (Taketomo, 2023).

Fluconazole is primarily excreted (80%) unchanged into the urine, making it an excellent choice for fungemia involving the urinary tract (Taketomo, 2023). A small proportion of the drug is hepatically cleared.

Dosing Recommendations

If fluconazole is used, administration of a loading dose (25 mg/kg) can help facilitate faster achievement of target therapeutic AUC and was found to be safe in a small cohort of infants (Greenberg et al., 2014). In cases of systemic candidiasis, the AAP (2021b) recommends an IV dose of 12 mg/kg/d.

Clinical-Monitoring Pearls

Routine surveillance of renal and hepatic function, as well as serum electrolytes, is indicated throughout fluconazole therapy. Monitoring of renal function is indicated because fluconazole is renally excreted. Note that, despite the fact that minimal hepatic metabolism is reported, a risk of hepatotoxicity is reported and is unrelated to the duration or dose of exposure. Additional adverse effects include prolonged QTc interval.

CONCLUSIONS

Understanding of normal and abnormal microbial colonization and pathogenicity; the mechanisms of microbial structure, ecology, and function; and the means with which to reduce or eradicate pathogens has decreased the incidence of sepsis in the neonate since the days when childbed fever struck women and their infants in seemingly random patterns. Neonates are nearly sterile at delivery when they enter the world of microbes. Their immune systems are designed to tolerate the massive microbial colonization that must take place to ensure a fully functioning metabolism, immune system, and neurodevelopment. Premature infants, deprived of the maternal antibodies and immune modifications that occur during the last trimester in preparation for birth and possibly compromised from the circumstances that led to preterm delivery, are particularly vulnerable to invasion from opportunistic or pathogenic organisms. Disrupted epithelial and mucosal barriers, suppressed innate and adaptive immune function, inability to consume protective breast milk, invasive procedures, prolonged exposure to antibiotics and PN, altered initial microbial colonization from Cesarean delivery, and prolonged hospital stays all contribute to increased risk of EOS and LOS in this population. The nonspecific nature of presenting symptoms and the inadequacy of laboratory testing make diagnosis and treatment especially difficult. Practitioners must be aware of the common microbes that inhabit their environment and the therapies that target them while simultaneously practicing antimicrobial stewardship to reduce resistance. Utmost care should be exercised to prevent contamination of indwelling catheters and tubes. Handwashing is one of the easiest and most effective strategies used to protect neonates from infection. Critical thinking and clinical observation are the first steps to preventing, recognizing, assessing, and diagnosing neonatal EOS and LOS.

Although the EOS calculator has remained effective at reducing inappropriate antibiotic use, unnecessary laboratory tests, and shortening hospitalization, its use is limited to infants older than 34 weeks of gestation (Deshmukh et al., 2021). Many preterm infants present with nonspecific symptoms of EOS (e.g., respiratory distress, hypotension), when other factors associated with premature birth present, and prophylactic antibiotic treatment is employed to reduce morbidity and mortality risks from EOS (Puopolo et al., 2018a; Singh & Yu, 2019). Although the duration of antibiotic exposure for suspected sepsis has decreased (e.g., 36 hours vs. 48 hours), no objective tools are available to further discriminate symptoms of sepsis and refine prescribing practices. Ideally, this will change over the years and additional tools will be introduced for use among the preterm population.

LEARNING TOOLS AND RESOURCES

Advice From the Authors

Stephanie M. Prescott, PhD, MSN, APRN, NNP-BC

Nurses are the frontline caregivers who are always the first to recognize when something is wrong with their patients. Be guardians who battle unclean hands, monitor sterility during procedures, be critical observers that recognize danger signals early. Advocate for neonates by understanding environmental pathogens and how to reduce them, limiting exposure to unnecessary therapies, and promoting immune-supporting activities like breastfeeding.

Van Tran, PharmD, BCPS, BCPPS, MBA

I've always loved this quote from Zig Ziglar: "If you're not willing to learn, no one can help you. If you're determined to learn, no one can stop you." All this information can be overwhelming, but remember, even the greatest of the great started where you are right now. So, take one concept at a time, learn and teach each other (because it truly does help retain and apply the information), and love what you do.

Discussion Prompts

1. Describe the risk factors for early-onset sepsis and distinguish those that are modifiable from those that are fixed.
2. Utilize the EOS risk calculator in several newborn term babies in your unit. Does your care match the calculator's recommendation?
3. Examine the recommended regimens in Table 28.5 and describe the differences in microbial coverage between the various indications for treatment.

Mind Map

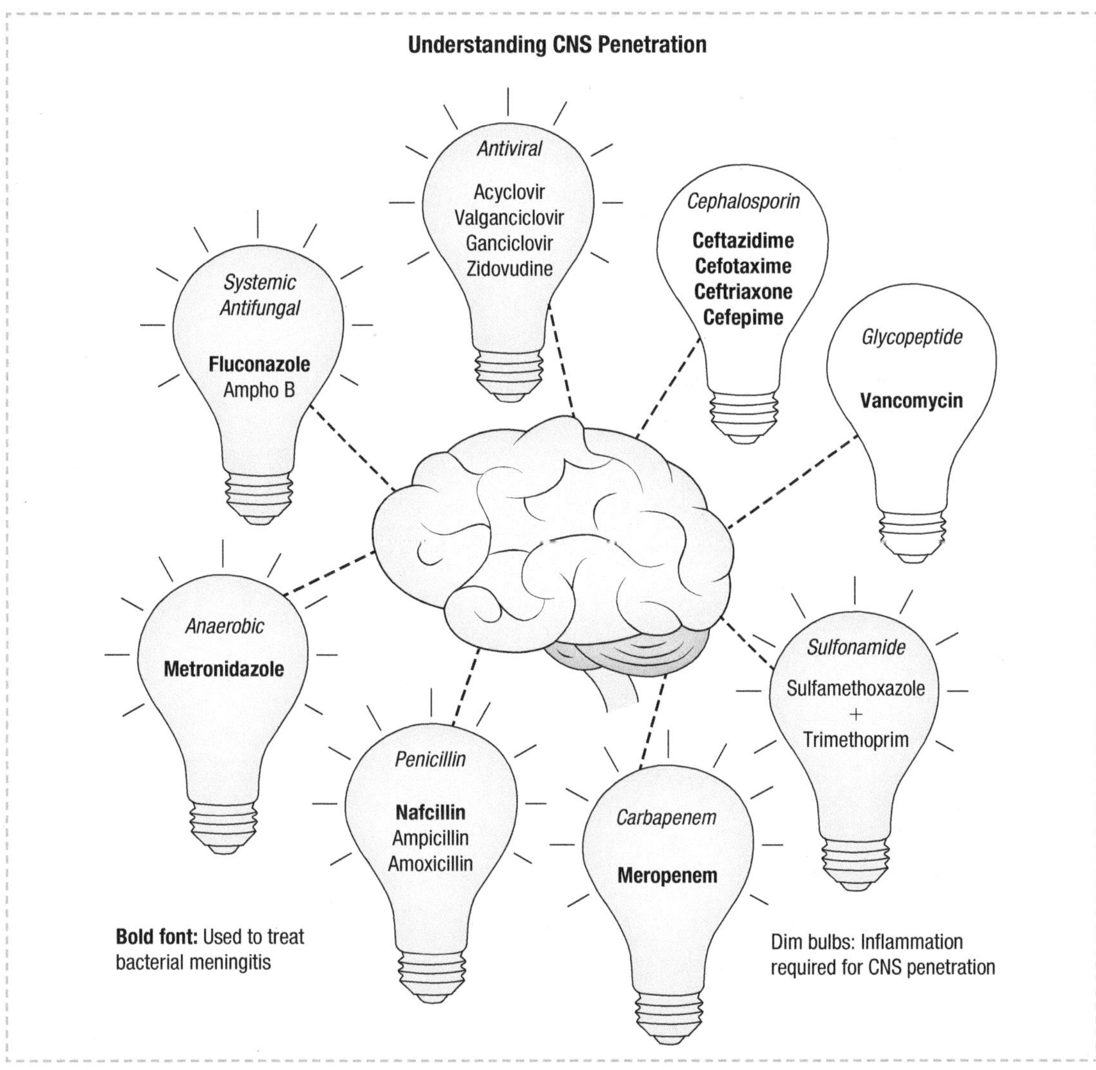

Note: This mind map reflects the design team's interpretation of a portion of one or more concepts addressed in this chapter. Readers should regard the mind maps woven throughout this textbook as examples of multisensory study tools that can be developed to encourage conceptual understanding. Readers are encouraged to develop their own unique mind maps in consultation with academic faculty or clinical preceptors.
CNS, central nervous system.
Design credit: Jessica Mazzei, MSN, APRN, NNP, RNC-NIC, East Carolina University Neonatal Nurse Practitioner Program.

REFERENCES

References for this chapter are online and available at https://connect.springerpub.com/content/book/978-0-8261-5884-0/part/partVII/toc-part/ch28.

PART VIII

Common Ocular Problems

chapter 29

Retinopathy of Prematurity

Debbie Fraser and William Diehl-Jones

LEARNING OBJECTIVES

After completing this chapter, the reader should be able to:

- Define *retinopathy of prematurity* (*ROP*).
- Outline the pathophysiology of ROP.
- Describe the process for screening and diagnosis of ROP.
- Identify strategies to prevent ROP.
- Discuss the current treatments for ROP.

INTRODUCTION

Retinopathy of prematurity (ROP), first described by physician Theodore Terry (1942) as retrolental fibroplasia (RLF) or a "fibroblastic overgrowth," was responsible for an epidemic of blindness in the 1940s and 1950s. A seminal randomized study of oxygen therapy, published by Kinsey in 1956, demonstrated that RLF was more likely to occur in infants receiving unrestricted oxygen (>50%) rather than only enough oxygen to prevent hypoxia. Findings from this study, and other novel studies discussed later in this chapter, led to restrictions in the use of oxygen to a maximum concentration of 40%. This limitation ultimately decreased the incidence of blindness in premature infants but increased morbidity and mortality specific to cerebral palsy and lung disease (Cross, 1973; Fleck & McIntosh, 2008). In addition, as survival rates for low-birth-weight infants in the 1970s and 1980s increased concurrent with increased use of mechanical ventilation and other invasive lifesaving therapies, a resurgence of ROP was observed (Fleck & McIntosh, 2008).

By the mid-1990s there was a significant improvement in the rates of ROP, especially in developed countries. This was attributed to standardized screening and treatment protocols along with significant efforts to better control the oxygen saturation levels in low-birth-weight infants (Almė et al., 2008; Chow et al., 2003). In comparison, a third epidemic of ROP emerged throughout middle-income countries such as areas in Latin America and South Asia. This was attributed to increased survival rates of premature newborns in the absence of consistent practices around ROP screening and treatment in these countries (Gilbert et al., 2019). Today, rates of ROP are still rising in developing areas, such as parts of Africa and in India. Therefore, public health efforts continue.

It is now widely understood that ROP is an eye disease that targets the developing vasculature of the retina in premature infants. Severe disease can progress to retinal detachment resulting in blindness in the affected eye (Fierson et al., 2018). Occurring almost exclusively in infants born at less than 32 weeks of gestation, it is currently estimated that 50% to 57% of infants born at less than 1,250 grams in the United States have some degree of ROP. Of those, 90% will have mild disease requiring no treatment, whereas 1,100 to 1,500 infants, or 8% to 9%, require treatment, and 400 to 600, or 1% to 2% of infants, will be declared legally blind (National Eye Institute, 2019).

The history of diseases, such as ROP, teaches us valuable lessons about the potential iatrogenic harms of seemingly innocent treatments such as administering oxygen. Further, a review of current therapies, such as anti-vascular endothelial growth factor (anti-VEGF) therapy, suggests the need for a cautious approach to systemic therapies in neonates who are still in a rapid phase of growth and development. This chapter reviews the history, incidence, and risk factors for development, pathophysiology, and the screening and diagnosis of ROP. Strategies to prevent ROP are outlined followed by an in-depth review of the surgical and pharmacologic treatment of this disease.

PHYSIOLOGY REVIEW: RETINAL VASCULARIZATION

Before we begin to investigate the pathophysiology of ROP, as well as prevention, screening, and treatment modalities, it is prudent to review the core components of normal retinal vascularization. The first phase of retinal vascularization begins at 15 to 16 weeks' gestation with the formation of spindle cells at the head of the optic nerve. These spindle cells develop into primitive vascular tubules and move along the pathway of future major retinal blood vessels to the optic disc. Spindle cells disappear by 21 weeks' gestation. The second phase of retinal vascularization is marked by angiogenesis, or the formation of new vessels. During week 17 to 18 of gestation, networks of capillaries form from the major radial vessels on the nasal side of the retina along the leading edge of the peripheral retina (Fleck & McIntosh, 2008). Vessel development is complete when it reaches the temporal ora serrata at approximately 40 to 44 weeks' gestation (Dogra et al., 2017). The process of angiogenesis is driven by the relative level of hypoxia that exists in the intrauterine environment. Hypoxia results in increased levels of vascular endothelial growth factor (VEGF), which is secreted by retinal astrocytes and Müller cells. A second substance, insulin-like growth factor (IGF-1), also plays a role in stimulating angiogenesis. The role of IGF-1 in retinal development is less clear but it has been demonstrated that retinal vessels develop more slowly in the absence of IGF-1 (Smith, 2003). In utero, IGF-1 is supplied by the placenta and amniotic fluid and levels decline after birth until endogenous production in the liver takes over. Following preterm birth, levels of IGF-1 fall and may remain low for some time, resulting in the accumulation of VEGF and, ultimately, more severe ROP (Lin & Binenbaum, 2019).

PATHOPHYSIOLOGY OF RETINOPATHY OF PREMATURITY

ROP is a two-phase process beginning with exposure to a hyperoxic environment during the period of retinal vasoproliferation (Eldweik & Mantagos, 2016; Hellström & Hård, 2019). In infants born before retinal vascularization is complete, hyperoxia suppresses VEGF synthesis and secretion (Eldweik & Mantagos, 2016). Hyperoxia and VEGF suppression, combined with factors, including undernutrition, low levels of IGF-1, respiratory distress, and sepsis, cause a reduction in retinal vessel growth and regression of existing blood vessels (Hellström & Hård, 2019). As the retina continues to grow, the nonvascularized area of the retina becomes hypoxic, leading to the second phase of ROP.

The second phase of ROP begins between 32 and 34 weeks' postmenstrual age as a critical level of tissue hypoxia is reached, which, in turn, stimulates the release of VEGF. VEGF secretion leads to an angiogenic response and new vessel growth (neovascularization). Upregulation of IGF-1 contributes to the development of new blood vessel growth by enhancing the effect of VEGF on angiogenesis. As a result of increased VEGF secretion, multiple new vessels form at the junction between the vascularized central portion of the retina and the outer portions that are not yet vascularized (Eldweik & Mantagos, 2016). High concentrations of VEGF in the vitreous encourage the proliferation of retinal blood vessels beyond the retina and into the vitreous humor (Dogra et al., 2017).

ROP may regress if circulation to the peripheral avascular retina can be reestablished and excess vessels are reabsorbed. Residual scarring at the neovascular ridge may persist and, with shrinking of this scar tissue, place traction on the retina, which can lead to detachment.

RISK FACTORS

Despite many years of research, we do not have a full understanding of why some premature infants are affected by ROP, whereas others of a similar gestational age, weight, and degree of illness may not develop the disease. Birth weight and gestational age remain the single most significant risk factors (Dogra et al., 2017; Lin & Binenbaum 2019); very few infants who are closer to term or of larger birth weight develop ROP. Low serum IGF-1 levels, hyperoxic exposure, and fluctuations in arterial oxygen concentrations are additional known risks, and are discussed here.

Low serum IGF-1 levels are also present in premature neonates with comorbidities, including intraventricular hemorrhage (IVH), bronchopulmonary dysplasia (BPD), and necrotizing enterocolitis (NEC; Hellström et al., 2003). This may explain the elevated risk of ROP in neonates with these conditions. The rate of postnatal weight gain has been postulated to be a surrogate marker for serum levels of IGF-1 with slower weight gain suggesting continued low levels of IGF-1 (Lin & Binenbaum, 2019). The recommendations from the American Academy of Pediatrics (AAP) to screen infants with a birth weight between 1,500 and 2,000 grams who have an unstable clinical course will capture infants with conditions that lead to low IGF-1 levels. Monitoring the rate of postnatal growth as a surrogate marker for low IGF-1 levels may also aid in predicting infants at increased risk of ROP (Lin & Binenbaum, 2019).

Exposure of the premature infant to an oxygen-enriched environment has long been held as an important risk factor for the development of ROP. Despite the physiologic link between hyperoxia and suppression of VEGF, the exact role of oxygen in the development of ROP has been elusive. An early study by Kinsey and colleagues (1977) failed to find a correlation between arterial oxygen levels and the development of ROP. Other studies did find a link between the duration of high oxygen exposure and subsequent development of ROP (Flynn et al., 1992; Gallo et al., 1993).

Some research found a link between fluctuating levels of arterial oxygen and the development of ROP (Hartnett, 2010; York et al., 2004). It is postulated that the period of recovery following each hypoxic event results in the formation of reactive oxygen species, which cause injury to mitochondria and may lead to modifications in gene expression (Beharry et al., 2018). This relationship was studied in the Supplemental Therapeutic Oxygen for Prethreshold Retinopathy of Prematurity (STOP-ROP) study. The large, multicentered trial evaluated the safety and efficacy of avoiding fluctuations in arterial oxygen levels by maintaining oxygen saturations (SpO_2) in specific ranges. Study protocol called for the maintenance of SpO_2 between 96% and 99%, as compared to standard practice of 89% and 94% in infants with prethreshold ROP. Researchers found that the higher SpO_2 target did not reduce the severity of ROP and resulted in more adverse pulmonary complications. A small reduction in progression to threshold disease was noted in the supplemental oxygen group compared to the group of infants with saturations maintained at 89% to 94% (32% vs. 46%), a finding that was not seen in infants with plus disease (ROP accompanied by enlarged posterior veins and tortuous arterioles; 57% vs. 52%; STOP-ROP Multicenter Study Group, 2000).

In the late 2000s, several large trials were conducted to examine targeted SpO_2 levels (85%–89% vs. 91%–95%) and outcomes, including death, neurodevelopmental outcome, and ROP. A meta-analysis of these trials found a higher risk of death in the group of infants in the lower SpO_2 target group compared to the higher target group (19.9% vs. 17.1%, $p = 0.01$; Askie et al., 2018). Treatment for ROP was required in 10.9% (220 of 2,020 subjects) of infants in the lower saturation group compared to 14.9% (308 of 2,065 infants) in the higher target group ($p < .001$).

More recent work has implicated oxidative stress, or pro-oxidant antioxidant balance (PAB), as a key factor in predicting the risk of ROP (Deliyanti et al., 2016); Boskabadi and associates (2021) enrolled 154 neonates with a birth weight of less than 1,500 grams and measured PAB on day 1 of life. These authors found that infants who went on to develop ROP had a significantly higher PAB ($p < .0001$) compared to those infants without ROP. This work is congruent with a number of other studies that have identified the connection between oxidative stress and inflammation. Several studies have demonstrated elevated levels of proinflammatory factors, including interleukin-6 (IL-6), interleukin-18 (IL-18), interleukin-1B (IL-1B), and cyclooxygenase-2, in the retina of infants with ROP (Rivera et al., 2013; Sennlaub et al., 2003; Sood et al., 2010; Zhou et al., 2016).

Numerous other risk factors have been identified, including low birth weight (Binenbaum et al., 2012; Good et al., 2005), PDA (Tsui et al., 2013), history of an IVH (Mohamed et al., 2013; Tsui et al., 2013), history of bacteremia (Mohamed et al., 2013; Tsui et al., 2013), White race (Husain et al., 2013), hyperglycemia (Mohamed et al., 2013), male sex, small for gestational age, lack of antenatal exposure to steroids, ventilator support on day 28 of life, and NEC (Gonski et al., 2019). Intrauterine and postnatal inflammation as well as maternal smoking have also been linked to an increased risk of ROP (Higgins, 2019; Wickramasinghe et al., 2021; Box 29.1).

PREVENTATIVE STRATEGIES

A number of strategies have been employed in an attempt to reduce the incidence of ROP, the need for pharmacologic therapy, and deleterious progression of the disease. Most obvious is a reduction in the rate of preterm birth. Antenatal care and immediate care of the preterm infant influence the risk of ROP. Appropriate use of antenatal corticosteroids has been shown to reduce both the incidence and severity of ROP (Travers et al., 2017).

Postnatal care practices that are associated with a reduced incidence of ROP include delayed cord clamping, maintenance of euthermia, and maintaining strict infection-control practices. Delayed cord clamping has been shown to reduce the incidence of anemia and decrease the need for blood transfusions, both of which impact the development of ROP (Lundgren et al., 2019; Lust et al., 2019). Specific to thermoregulation, a retrospective study of 9,833 neonates born at fewer than 33 weeks found that the lowest rates of adverse outcomes, including ROP, occurred when admission temperatures remained between 97.7°F/36.5°C and 99°F/37.2°C ($\alpha > 0$ [$p < .05$]; Lyu et al., 2015). In addition to maintaining a euthermic state, recall that most low-birth-weight infants require respiratory support and supplemental oxygen because of lung immaturity. In addition, care practices in the NICU that reduce the risk of infection, including those related to central lines, should be addressed through an ongoing process of quality improvement (Darlow & Husain, 2019).

Minimizing Hyperoxia

Prolonged oxygen exposure is associated with an increased risk of ROP (Klinger et al., 2010; J. Lee & Dammann, 2012; Lundgren et al., 2017). However, the precise role of oxygen in the development of ROP is not yet fully understood. There is evidence that oxygen exposure in preterm infants increases the risk of ROP (Higgins, 2019). There is also some evidence to suggest that both fluctuating blood oxygen levels and the duration of oxygen exposure may influence the severity of ROP (Das et al., 2018; Gantz et al., 2020; Kaufman et al., 2014). Despite large studies examining the

BOX 29.1 Risk Factors for Retinopathy of Prematurity

Prematurity (<32 weeks' gestation)
Low birth weight
Small for gestational age
Lack of prenatal steroids
Exposure to exogenous oxygen
Fluctuations in arterial oxygen levels
Presence of IVH, BPD, NEC, and PDA
Reduced postnatal weight gain
Bacteremia
Hyperglycemia
Prolonged mechanical ventilation
White race
Male sex
Maternal smoking

BPD, bronchopulmonary dysplasia; IVH, intraventricular hemorrhage; NEC, necrotizing enterocolitis; PDA, patent ductus areteriosus.

optimal range of inspired oxygen, gaps in our understanding remain. There is current consensus that oxygen saturations of 91% to 95% result in a lower mortality than more restrictive saturation targets (Askie et al., 2018; Darlow et al., 2018). Providers should ensure that infants receiving supplemental oxygen have continuous saturation monitoring with equipment that is calibrated to ensure accurate measurements.

Lability in the cardiorespiratory status in preterm infants makes it challenging to maintain targeted saturation levels. Early case-control studies examine the importance of quality-improvement approaches to carefully regulating oxygen saturation levels to reduce the risk of ROP (Chow et al., 2003; Vanderveen et al., 2006). A systematic review of 16 studies involving 574 infants and 2,935 nurses found that there was low compliance in oxygen saturation targeting, inappropriate upper alarm limits, and difficulty maintaining the oxygen saturation below the prescribed upper limits (van Zanten et al., 2015).

Strategies to improve compliance include having policies in place outlining the saturation targets and to ensure compliance with alarm limits. Education should be provided regarding the need to be cautious in administering supplemental oxygen during handling or with procedures. Quality-improvement practices, such as audits to ensure compliance with alarm limits, may also reduce the amount of time infants spend outside of the targeted saturation range (van Zanten et al., 2015; van Zanten, Pauws, et al., 2017).

New technologies may also play a role in reducing the incidence of ROP. Automated response systems that adjust the levels of inspired oxygen in response to changes in oxygen saturation may provide better control of hyperoxia (van Zanten et al., 2015; van Zanten, Kuypers, et al., 2017). The use of near-infrared spectroscopy (NIRS) to measure regional cerebral tissue oxygenation may provide an estimate of retinal oxygen levels, thereby providing more precise data than the current methods of measuring systemic oxygen saturation (Richter et al., 2019; Vesoulis et al., 2016).

Nutrition

Both intrapartum and postnatal growth failure have been shown to increase the low-birth-weight infant's risk of developing ROP (Lin & Binenbaum, 2019). Prenatal strategies aimed at identifying growth-restricted infants, and correcting deficits when possible, should be addressed.

Adequate nutrition during the neonatal period supports brain development and improves neurodevelopmental outcomes as well as reduces the risk of ROP (Harding et al., 2017). In particular, there is some evidence to support the use of mother's breast milk to reduce ROP. A meta-analysis of nine case-control and cohort studies found that, compared to a diet of formula, infants receiving human milk were less likely to develop severe or any ROP (Bharwani et al., 2016). However, not all studies have shown a similar benefit. Miller and colleagues (2018) performed a systematic review and meta-analysis examining the benefits of human milk and found that, if present, the benefits of human milk in relationship to ROP are likely to be small (relative risk [RR]: 0.65 for exclusive human milk compared to exclusive formula feeding, 95% confidence interval [CI]: 0.31–1.34, four studies including 1,256 infants).

Caffeine

Caffeine is frequently used in treating apnea of prematurity in low-birth-weight infants. Follow-up data from the Caffeine for Apnea of Prematurity (CAP) trial demonstrated a significant reduction in severe ROP in infants receiving caffeine compared to a placebo (odds ratio [OR]: 0.61, 95% CI: 0.42–0.89, $p = .01$; Schmidt et al., 2007).

Benchmarking

Neonatal organizations, such as the Eunice Kennedy Shriver National Institutes of Health Child Health and Development (NICHD)'s Neonatal Research Network, Vermont Oxford Network (VON), and the Canadian Neonatal Network (CNN), provide standardization across the specialty of neonatal health. This standardization includes data collection and measurement of key quality indicators, which lead to better collaboration with other care providers in research, education, and quality improvement (Edwards & Horbar, 2019). Participating in the research and quality-improvement activities offered by a neonatal network is an important step in improving approaches to problems such as ROP.

RETINOPATHY OF PREMATURITY SCREENING

ROP affects a select group of infants, primarily those born at less than 28 weeks' gestation. ROP progresses in a relatively predictable pattern that provides the opportunity for timely screening and intervention (Fierson et al., 2018). An effective screening program is critical to ensure that infants who would benefit from treatment are identified in a timely manner to avoid untoward outcomes. Because of the potentially life-altering nature of untreated or delayed treatment of ROP, screening programs will result in some lower risk infants being screened.

Screening should be performed by an experienced ophthalmologist who is familiar with preterm infant examinations. The schedule of examinations should be based on the infant's gestational age at birth with ongoing exams based on the presence and severity of disease. Because some infants will be transferred or discharged from the NICU prior to complete retinal vascularization, an effective screening program will also include a program to ensure that discharged infants continue to receive timely and appropriate follow-up (Fierson et al., 2018).

The AAP screening guideline includes the following recommendations (Fierson et al., 2018):

- Screen all infants with a gestational age of less than 30 weeks' or a birth weight of less than 1,500 grams and infants with a birth weight between 1,500 and 2,000 grams who are determined to be at risk for ROP. This may include infants who required inotropic support and infants receiving supplemental oxygen for a prolonged period of time (more than a few days).
- Examinations should be done by an experienced ophthalmologist using binocular indirect ophthalmoscopy after pupillary dilation.
- The International Classification of Retinopathy of Prematurity Revisited (ICROP) should be used to classify the retinal findings (International Committee for the Classification of Retinopathy of Prematurity, 2005).
- Screening should be initiated according to the infant's postmenstrual age. Note that the recommendations for infants born at 22 and 23 weeks' gestation are extrapolated. Controversy exists as to whether or not screening should begin earlier for infants born at this gestation.
- The timing of follow-up examinations is determined by the examining ophthalmologist and is based on the finding of the exam. Specific recommendations can be found in the AAP Clinical Practice Guideline (Fierson et al., 2018).
- The decision to discharge an infant from the routine screening examination should be based on the retinal findings in combination with the infant's age. Specific guidance can be found in the AAP Clinical Practice Guideline (Fierson et al., 2018).
- The use of digital retinal images captured as part of a remote screening program should be adopted cautiously and follow the AAP guidelines (Fierson et al., 2018). An indirect ophthalmologic exam performed by a qualified ophthalmologist should be undertaken at least once before treatment or discharge from the screening program occurs.

Screening should be done following dilation of the pupils with a mydriatic agent. Cycloplegic mydriatic agents (e.g., cyclopentolate, tropicamide) have rapid onset of action, with peak dilation occurring between 20 and 60 minutes. Phenylephrine may also be used, usually in combination with either cyclopentolate or tropicamide. Some studies have shown that the combination of a cycloplegic agent with phenylephrine was both safe and effective in optimizing pupil dilation (Alpay et al., 2019; Neffendorf et al., 2015). Others have noted that these drugs have been associated with reduced milk intake, abdominal distension, and reduced pulse rates on the day following instillation and that infants should be closely monitored following screening (Obata et al., 2021). Other symptoms of systemic absorption include tachycardia and agitation. Ophthalmic proparacaine 0.5% and oral sucrose should be provided prior to examination to mitigate pain. Excess medication should be wiped away quickly to avoid absorption. Application of gentle pressure over the nasolacrimal duct for 1 minute following instillation of the eye drops will also reduce systemic absorption.

CLASSIFICATION OF RETINOPATHY OF PREMATURITY

Once identified during the ophthalmic screening exam, ROP is classified according to standards established by the ICROP. These standards were first developed in 1984 by ophthalmologists from six countries and subsequently updated in 1987 and 2005 (International Committee for the Classification of Retinopathy of Prematurity, 2005). Both the AAP and the Canadian Paediatric Society (CPS) recommend the use of this classification system to describe and record retinal findings during screening examinations (Fierson et al., 2018; Jeffries & Canadian Paediatric Society, Fetus and Newborn Committee, 2016).

Using the ICROP system, the location of disease in the eye is determined by dividing the retina into three concentric areas centered on the optic disc (Figure 29.1). Zone I extends twice the distance from the optic nerve (the center of zone I) to the macula. Zone II circles around zone I with the nasal ora serrata as a border. Zone III is the crescent area on the temporal side not encompassed by zone II. The extent of the disease is expressed as the number of clock hours of the retina involved. ROP is divided into five stages (Table 29.1).

When any stage of ROP is accompanied by enlarged posterior veins and tortuous arterioles, the term *plus disease* is used (for example, stage 3+). Other findings of plus disease include poor pupillary dilation and vitreous haze (International Committee for the Classification of Retinopathy of Prematurity, 2005). The presence of plus disease increases the likelihood that the disease will progress rapidly and significantly increases the chances of an unfavorable visual outcome.

The term *pre-plus disease* is used when abnormal dilation and tortuosity of the vessels is present but not yet severe enough to be classed as plus disease. Pre-plus disease may progress to plus disease as dilation increases (International Committee for the Classification of Retinopathy of Prematurity, 2005).

In some infants larger than 1,000 grams, an unusually aggressive pattern of ROP, formerly termed *Rush disease*, may occur. The newer term for this finding is *aggressive posterior ROP* (*AP-ROP;* International Committee for the Classification of Retinopathy of Prematurity, 2005). AP-ROP, most commonly seen in zone I, is characterized by ill-defined, dilated, and tortuous vessels in the posterior portion of the eye. Shunts are present between the vessels and hemorrhages may occur. AP-ROP does not progress through the usual stages; rather, if left untreated, it rapidly moves to severe ROP with retinal detachment (Dogra et al., 2017; Hartnett, 2017).

FIGURE 29.1 Zones of retinopathy of prematurity.

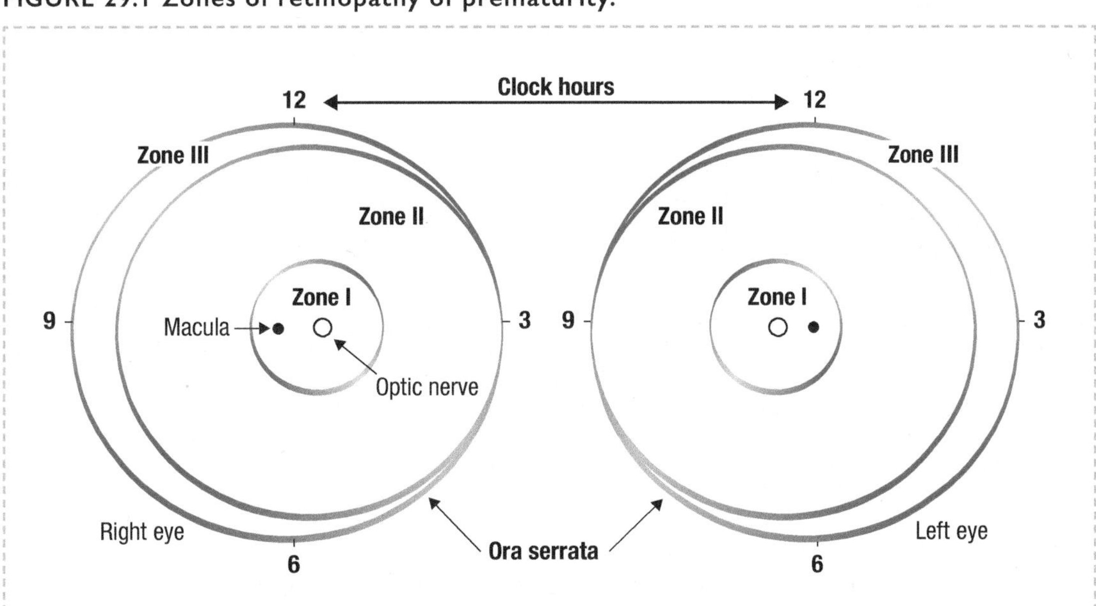

Design credit: Drawing courtesy of Amanda Smith, MSN, NNP-BC.
Source: From Jnah, A. J., & Trembath, A. N. (2018). *Fetal and neonatal physiology for the advanced practice nurse*. Springer Publishing Company.

TABLE 29.1 Stages of Retinopathy of Prematurity

STAGE	DESCRIPTION
1	A sharp demarcation line separating the avascular from the vascularized portion of the retina
2	The presence of an elevated ridge of tissue, often with small tufts of new blood vessels seen posterior to the ridge
3	The ridge of new blood vessels extends beyond the retina into the vitreous
4	Partial retinal detachment
5	Total retinal detachment

Source: Eldweik, L., & Mantagos, I. S. (2016). Role of VEGF inhibition in the treatment of retinopathy of prematurity. *Seminars in Ophthalmology, 31*(1–2), 163–168. https://doi.org/10.3109/08820538.2015.1114847

Previously, ROP was divided into threshold and prethreshold disease to define the need for treatment. Following the Early Treatment for Retinopathy of Prematurity Randomized Trial (ETROP; 2003), which confirmed the efficacy of treating high-risk prethreshold disease, the terms *threshold* and *prethreshold* disease were replaced with *type 1 ROP* and *type 2 ROP* (Fierson et al., 2018). The development of type 1 ROP is noted to peak at 35 weeks' gestation (ETROP, 2003).

Type 1 ROP (aggressive requiring treatment) is characterized by (ETROP, 2003):

- any-stage ROP with plus disease in zone I,
- stage 3 ROP with no plus disease in zone I, and,
- stage 2 or 3 ROP with plus disease in zone II.

Type 2 ROP (more indolent, less aggressive disease) is characterized by:

- stage 1 or 2 ROP without plus disease in zone I, and
- stage 3 ROP without plus disease in zone II.

HISTORICAL PERSPECTIVE: SEMINAL AND OTHER NOTEWORTHY STUDIES

The earliest treatment for ROP, introduced in the 1960s, was cryotherapy, which used a liquid nitrogen probe to freeze the avascular retina and stop vessel proliferation. The most well-known study of cryotherapy, the CRYO-ROP study, enrolled 9,751 infants born at less than 1,251 grams in 23 U.S. health centers; enrollment was halted early because of the demonstrated benefit of cryotherapy. Researchers had a robust follow-up regimen and reported results after 3 months, 1 year, 3½ years, 5½ years, and 10 years. In the study, 291 infants (6%) developed threshold ROP and were randomized to either the control group or treated with cryotherapy within 72 hours of diagnosis. Cryotherapy significantly reduced unfavorable visual outcomes (posterior retinal detachment, a retinal fold involving the macula, or retrolental tissue). Poor visual outcomes occurred in 31.1% of treated eyes compared to 51.4% of control eyes at 3 months (Cryotherapy for Retinopathy of Prematurity Cooperative Group, 1990b). Visual outcomes measured 1 year after treatment suggested that 35% of treated eyes had an unfavorable functional outcome compared to 56.3% in untreated eyes (Cryotherapy for Retinopathy of Prematurity Cooperative Group, 1990a). At 10 years, 247 children remained in follow-up. Benefit persisted at the 10-year follow-up for unfavorable distance visual acuity (44.4% in treated eyes vs. 62.1% in control eyes) and for fundus status (27.2% vs. 47.9%). Of interest, 41.4% of the control infants had a retinal detachment, whereas this complication occurred in only 22% of the treated eyes (Cryotherapy for Retinopathy of Prematurity Cooperative Group, 2001).

Laser Photocoagulation

Following the 2012 recommendation from the American Academy of Ophthalmology (Simpson et al., 2012), laser ablation therapy has replaced cryotherapy in the treatment of most cases of ROP. Compared to cryotherapy, laser treatment can be delivered to a more precise target area, is less traumatic to surrounding tissues, and causes less discomfort (Chan-Ling et al., 2018).

The most well-known study examining the efficacy of laser treatment of ROP, the ETROP trial, screened 7,000 infants with a birth weight of less than 1,251 grams and identified a cohort of 401 infants requiring treatment for ROP. These infants were randomized to earlier treatment (prethreshold) or conventionally timed treatment (threshold disease) with laser therapy. Results of this study suggested that laser treatment prior to threshold disease reduced unfavorable structural outcomes from 15.4% to 9.1% (Good et al., 2005). This study resulted in the adoption of laser treatment as the preferred therapy for ROP and also resulted in the adoption of type 1 ROP to describe eye findings requiring treatment (ETROP, 2003).

CURRENT PHARMACOLOGIC TREATMENT STRATEGIES

The AAP clinical practice guidelines (Fierson et al., 2018) recommend treatment when an infant is diagnosed with type 1 ROP. These recommendations come from results of the ETROP Study (Early Treatment for Retinopathy of Prematurity Cooperative Group, 2010), which found that visual outcomes are improved if treatment is initiated early. Fierson and colleagues (2018) note that the presence of plus disease is more important in determining the need for treatment than the number of clock hours in which disease is present.

Once determined that it is required, treatment should be initiated within 72 hours to decrease the risk of irreversible retinal detachment. Following treatment, the infant should have a follow-up examination within 3 to 7 days to determine the need for additional therapy (Fierson et al., 2018). The type of treatment selected depends on a number of factors, including local expertise and availability of treatment modalities. The treatment also depends on the location and severity of the disease. Currently, two types of treatment are available: laser photocoagulation and VEGF inhibitor injections. Although a number of VEGF inhibitors have been studied in neonates, only two, bevacizumab and ranibizumab, are widely used in North America and will be reviewed here.

Vascular Endothelial Growth Factor Inhibitors

The recognition of the role of VEGF in the vasoproliferative phase of ROP has led to the use of VEGF inhibitors to prevent progression of type 1 ROP. In adults, VEGF inhibitors have been used to treat conditions such as diabetic retinopathy (Bressler et al., 2017) and macular degeneration (Holekamp, 2019).

Several VEGF inhibitors have been studied in neonates, including the recombinant monoclonal antibodies bevacizumab (Avastin); ranibizumab (Lucentis); pegaptanib (Macugen), which is a pegylated oligonucleotide; and aflibercept (VEGF Trap-Eye), a fusion protein (Eldweik & Mantagos, 2016; VanderVeen & Cataltepe, 2019; Wallace & Wu, 2013). Of these, bevacizumab has been most extensively studied; however, none of the VEGF drugs on the market have received Food and Drug Administration (FDA) approval for treatment of ROP (A. Bancalari & Schade, 2020). Bevacizumab has been approved by the FDA for the treatment of solid tumors, including colon, breast, and ovarian cancers (Jordan, 2014), but has been used off label for a number of ocular conditions in which aberrant blood vessel growth occurs. The other agents have been approved for ocular diagnoses in adults (VanderVeen & Cataltepe, 2019).

The use of VEGF inhibitors in treating ROP is based on evidence suggesting that moderating the activity of VEGF can reduce the accelerated growth of retinal vessels, which occurs when the peripheral avascular retina becomes hypoxic (Hartnett et al., 2008; Zeng et al., 2007), and also reduces the disordered blood vessel growth characteristic of the second phase of ROP (Jiang et al., 2014). Unlike lasers, VEGF inhibitors do not destroy the tissue of the peripheral retina; theoretically, these drugs cause fewer changes to the structure of the eye and therefore result in better visual outcomes (Eldweik & Mantagos, 2016).

BEVACIZUMAB/RANIBIZUMAB

Mechanism of Action/Core Pharmacokinetic Principles

Bevacizumab (Avastin) and ranibizumab (Lucentis) are recombinant, monoclonal antibodies that prevent VEGF from binding to endothelial receptors (Eldweik & Mantagos, 2016). Bevacizumab is a full-length monoclonal antibody, whereas ranibizumab is an engineered antibody fragment

(Fab; Eldweik & Mantagos, 2016). Ranibizumab has a shorter half-life than bevacizumab, which may be advantageous in reducing the risks of systemic suppression of VEGF (Menke et al., 2015; Mota et al., 2012).

The first reports of use of bevacizumab for the treatment of ROP were published in 2007 (Chung et al., 2007; Travassos et al., 2007). Early research examined this drug as a single therapy or as an adjuvant to laser treatment (Law et al., 2010; Mintz-Hittner et al., 2011). In some centers, bevacizumab has also been used as a rescue treatment if laser was not successful (M. A. Bancalari et al., 2014). Despite being used for almost 15 years in the neonatal population, there are few well-controlled prospective studies investigating its use (VanderVeen et al., 2017).

The first multicentered randomized controlled study of bevacizumab, the BEAT-ROP study, was published in 2011 (Mintz-Hittner et al., 2011). These researchers randomized 150 neonates to either laser therapy or bevacizumab and found that ROP recurred in six of 140 eyes (4%) in the bevacizumab-treated group compared to 32 of 146 eyes (22%) in the laser group. For posterior zone II ROP, the rate of recurrence did not differ. Researchers concluded that, compared to laser, bevacizumab was of benefit in halting the progression of ROP in zone I but not in posterior zone II. This is in contrast to other studies that have found that anti-VEGF therapy results in a better outcome for posterior disease than with laser therapy (Hwang et al., 2015; Lepore et al., 2014; A. L. Wu & Wu, 2018; W. C. Wu et al., 2011).

The 2-year follow-up of children in the BEAT-ROP study found that those treated with bevacizumab had a significantly lower rate of severe myopia (1.7%) compared to those treated with laser therapy (36.4%; $p < .001$; Geloneck et al., 2014). These findings suggest that bevacizumab may result in less structural alteration of the eye than laser therapy. This theory has been supported by findings from a group of Turkish studies that demonstrated a lower rate of refractive errors in eyes treated with bevacizumab and ranibizumab compared to laser therapy (Gunay et al., 2015, 2017; Kabataş et al., 2017).

A 5-year retrospective analysis of 28 patients (54 eyes) published by Hwang and associates (2015) found a higher rate of recurrence but a lower rate of myopia in infants treated with bevacizumab compared to those treated with laser. These findings are similar to a meta-analysis of 10 studies published in 2018 (Li et al., 2018). Authors of this analysis concluded that, compared to laser therapy, the need for retreatment was significantly increased with anti-VEGF treatment (OR: 2.52, 95% CI: 1.37–4.66; $p = 0.003$) but there was a lower incidence of myopia and eye complications (OR: 0.29; 95% CI: 0.10–0.82; $p = .02$).

There have been a small number of studies that examined the use of ranibizumab for treatment of ROP. Zhang and colleagues (2017) randomized 50 neonates with type 1 ROP in zone II to receive bilateral treatment with ranibizumab (0.3 mg) or laser treatment. All of the eyes treated with ranibizumab show regression of ROP but 52% required retreatment compared to only one patient in the laser group. These findings were in contrast with another smaller study (19 infants) of infants with aggressive posterior ROP who were treated with either 0.12 mg or 0.2 mg of ranibizumab. Sixteen infants survived and, of those, 88.9% (8/9) who received the lower dose and 85.6% of infants (6/7) receiving the higher dose did not require retreatment (Stahl et al., 2018).

In 2018, an updated Cochrane review (Sankar et al., 2018) was published that reported on the results of six trials of 383 infants. Four trials compared laser therapy with bevacizumab (Karkhaneh et al., 2016; Lepore et al., 2014; Mintz-Hittner et al., 2011; O'Keeffe et al., 2016), one trial compared ranibizumab with laser treatment (Zhang et al., 2017), and the sixth trial compared pegaptanib plus laser with combined cryo- and laser therapy (Autrata et al., 2012). Reviewers concluded that when used as monotherapy, bevacizumab or ranibizumab compared to laser therapy reduced the risk of refractive errors in childhood but did not reduce the risk of retinal detachment or recurrence of ROP. Further, these drugs might result in a higher risk of recurrence requiring retreatment in infants with disease in zone II. Pegaptanib used in conjunction with laser therapy resulted in a lower risk of recurrence of ROP and retinal detachment. These findings are tempered by low-quality evidence and the lack of information about long-term systemic effects of these drugs. The authors suggest further research before routine use of these drugs can be recommended (Sankar et al., 2018).

Administration

Bevacizumab and ranibizumab are administered via intravitreal injection after topical anesthesia. This can be done at the bedside; comfort strategies, such as bundling, use of a pacifier, or oral sucrose, can be used as adjuvant measures; and a normal feeding schedule can be maintained

(Vanderveen & Cataltepe, 2019). The treatment time for these drugs is short and this, combined with bedside administration, is advantageous for infants who are clinically unstable. An additional benefit of VEGF inhibitors is that they can be administered in the presence of media opacity, tunica vasculosa lentis, and poor pupillary dilation. These conditions make laser therapy difficult (A. L. Wu & Wu, 2018).

Dosing Recommendations

Optimal dosing of bevacizumab is still under investigation with recommended dosages ranging between 0.25 and 1.25 mg in research protocols (Han et al., 2018; Wallace et al., 2018). The BEAT-ROP study used a dosing regimen of 0.625 mg, which is half of the normal adult dose (Mintz-Hittner et al., 2011), but others have suggested that, to avoid systemic side effects, a lower dose be used (Harder et al., 2014; Spandau, 2013). Han and colleagues (2018) compared doses of 0.25 mg and 0.625 mg in eight infants with stage 3+ in zone I or posterior zone II ROP and found no difference in the short-term outcomes between the two groups. In this study, one eye was injected with the lower dose and the other eye received the higher dose. This protocol limited the ability to control for the systemic effects of the drug or the possibility that the higher dose may have resulted in a treatment effect in the eye receiving a lower dose. A dose-finding study (Wallace et al., 2017) used a strategy of dose deescalation in 61 infants with type 1 ROP beginning with doses of 0.25 mg for the first group of infants; then, if treatment was successful, the dose was reduced to 0.125 mg, 0.063 mg, and 0.031 mg with each subsequent group. These researchers concluded that the lowest dose studied (0.031 mg) was successful in treating ROP in nine of nine eyes.

Clinical-Monitoring Pearls

Following treatment, a regimen of antibiotics and dexamethasone eye drops is usually used to reduce inflammation and prevent infection (A. Bancalari & Schade, 2020). Treatment effects are usually seen within 24 to 48 hours postinjection. Infants should be monitored for signs of infection (rare), including erythema, eye discharge, fever, and systemic signs of illness.

Follow-up ophthalmologic examinations should begin 3 to 7 days after the injection to determine the effectiveness of the treatment. Follow-up should continue until retinal vascularization is complete or until it can be determined that reactivation of the ROP has not occurred (Fierson et al., 2018). Unlike laser therapy, reactivation of proliferative ROP tends to occur later; therefore, a longer period of follow-up should be pursued (Fierson et al., 2018). Some studies reported ROP recurrences as late as 65 to 70 weeks' postmenstrual age (Geloneck et al., 2014; Honda et al., 2008; Hu et al., 2012; Quinn et al., 2014).

The ocular complications of bevacizumab include hyphema, endophthalmitis, vitreous hemorrhage, retinal detachment, glaucoma, and cataracts (Hu et al., 2012; Jamrozy-Witkowska et al., 2011; Pertl et al., 2015; VanderVeen & Cataltepe, 2019). The most common early problem occurring with VEGF inhibitors is treatment failure requiring retreatment (Vanderveen & Cataltepe, 2019). Results of some studies have suggested that the rate of complications with VEGF therapy is no greater than that of laser therapy (Morrison et al., 2018; Pertl et al., 2015). The Postnatal Growth and Retinopathy of Prematurity (G-ROP) study group published an analysis of 512 infants (1,004 eyes) in which 970 eyes received laser treatment and 34 received bevacizumab. In the laser group, the rate of ocular complications was 2.6%, vitreous hemorrhage occurred in 5.4%, and disease progression occurred in 9.2%. None of the infants in the bevacizumab group experienced complications, hemorrhage, or disease progression (Morrison et al., 2018).

W. C. Wu and colleagues' study of 27 patients (49 eyes) receiving bevacizumab for stage 3 or 4a ROP found vitreous or preretinal hemorrhages in four eyes (8%), and in four eyes additional treatment with laser therapy was required for ongoing ROP. Some studies of bevacizumab have reported cases of fibrotic traction, some resulting in retinal detachment (Honda et al., 2008; B. J. Lee et al., 2012; W. C. Wu et al., 2011; Zepeda-Romero et al., 2010). A systematic review of eight prospective and 15 retrospective studies involving 385 eyes treated with bevacizumab found that accelerated fibrovascular involution causing traction and progression to retinal detachment was the most common adverse effect reported, occurring in eight eyes (Hapsari & Sitorus, 2014).

Recurrence of ROP is seen with both laser treatment and anti-VEGF injections. In the case of bevacizumab, the risk of recurrence is reported to persist over a longer period. In the retrospective review of nine patients (17 eyes) with recurrent ROP following bevacizumab injections, the range of time for recurrence was 4 weeks to 35 weeks following treatment. Five eyes in this study progressed to retinal detachment with the age at detachment ranging from 49 to 69 weeks' postmenstrual age (Hu et al., 2012). Moran and colleagues (2014) conducted a study of 14 infants with either posterior zone II or bilateral stage 3 ROP who received bevacizumab in one eye and laser therapy for the other eye. ROP requiring treatment recurred in three eyes treated with bevacizumab and one eye from the laser group. Time to recurrence was 37 weeks' postmenstrual age in the laser group and 50 to 52 weeks' postmenstrual age in the eyes treated with bevacizumab. Developmental examinations and brain MRIs in the Moran study showed no adverse outcomes attributed to bevacizumab.

A follow-up study, using digital retinal imaging and fluorescein angiography of 20 infants with zone I ROP in which one eye was treated with bevacizumab and the other eye treated with laser therapy, found that at 4 years of age, the eyes treated with bevacizumab all showed abnormalities in the posterior pole or periphery of the retina. Peripheral abnormalities included avascular areas, vessel leakage, abnormal vessel growth or tangles, and, at the pole, hyperfluorescent lesions or absence of the foveal avascular zone (Lepore et al., 2018). Of note, no data on visual outcomes were presented in this study. A similar study by Tahija and colleagues (2014) found that abnormal retinal vascularization persisted in 11 of 20 eyes treated with bevacizumab.

Concerns remain regarding the long-term effects of VEGF inhibitors. It is currently not feasible to localize the delivery of these drugs to only one area of a treated eye. Inhibiting vascular growth in the diseased portion of the retina may impact normal blood vessel growth and development. Premature infants have an impaired retinal-blood barrier, which allows bevacizumab to enter the circulation and reduce systemic levels of VEGF (Eldweik & Mantagos, 2016; Sato et al., 2012). Decreased levels of VEGF may persist for up to 8 weeks after ROP treatment with bevacizumab (W. C. Wu et al., 2015). This finding raises concerns about the potential impact of bevacizumab on organs, such as the brain, heart, lung, and kidney, which are dependent on VEGF for vascularization.

Several studies have examined the neurodevelopmental outcomes of infants receiving bevacizumab with mixed results. A Canadian retrospective study comparing 27 infants receiving bevacizumab with 97 infants receiving laser therapy found that significant neurodevelopmental disabilities (bilateral blindness, bilateral deafness, severe cerebral palsy, or Bayley scores <70) were 3.1 times higher in the bevacizumab group compared to the group receiving laser therapy (Morin et al., 2016). The nonrandomized nature of this study results in more infants with zone I disease being treated with bevacizumab compared to the laser group. Zone I disease is a marker for more serious illness, which may account for the neurodevelopmental findings. One of the centers from the BEAT-ROP study published 18- to 28-month follow-up data and found no differences in neurodevelopmental outcomes in seven infants receiving bevacizumab compared to nine receiving laser therapy (Kennedy & Mintz-Hittner, 2018). A retrospective case series of 61 children at 2 years of age who had received either laser only, bevacizumab, or a combination of bevacizumab and laser found no difference in Bayley scores in the bevacizumab or laser-only groups, but did find significant mental and psychomotor impairments in the group receiving combination therapy (Lien et al., 2016). A 5-year follow-up study of 13 patients (18 eyes) treated with bevacizumab found that median vision was 20/25 with 12 eyes developing low myopia. One patient had a delay in growth and neurodevelopment; the remaining patients were within the normal range (Martínez-Castellanos et al., 2013).

Laser Photocoagulation

Laser photocoagulation continues to be used in the treatment of ROP, either as an initial treatment or following ROP recurrence in eyes treated with anti-VEGF therapy (Kim et al., 2014; Yoon et al., 2017). Combining laser therapy with bevacizumab or ranibizumab offers the potential benefit of lower dosing of the anti-VEGF medication along with a requirement for a smaller area of laser application (Kim et al., 2014).

Infants with more aggressive posterior ROP and flat neovascularization have been shown to benefit from two sessions of laser therapy rather than one. A study of 29 infants randomized each eye to either a single laser session or two sessions 7 days apart. Infants receiving two sessions of laser had fewer and smaller vitreous hemorrhages compared to infants treated with one session of laser therapy (Vinekar et al., 2015).

Laser therapy is usually carried out under general anesthesia although some studies have supported the use of opioids, such as morphine, fentanyl, or remifentanil, to avoid the need for intubation and general anesthesia (Kirwan et al., 2007; Örge et al., 2013; Piersigilli et al., 2019). Safety precautions recommended for laser therapy should be in place wherever the procedure takes place.

Complications of laser treatment include localized edema, hyphema, retinal hemorrhage, cataracts, variations in ocular pressure, and an increase in refractive errors. In some cases, laser therapy causes destruction of the peripheral avascular retina, which limits the child's field of vision (A. Bancalari & Schade, 2020; Laser ROP Study Group, 1994).

Retinal Detachment Treatment

Two treatments are used to manage stage 4 and 5 ROP. A lens-sparing vitrectomy (LSV), usually performed when progressive stage 4 ROP is diagnosed, involves removal of the vitreous and scar tissue, allowing the retina to contact the posterior wall of the eye. Once retinal detachment has occurred, scleral buckling (SB) can be performed. SB involves the placement of a silicone band around the eye, which alters the shape of the eye and pushes the retina back toward the rear wall of the eye, where it can reattach.

LSV is more commonly used but SB may be indicated if there is peripheral traction or folding (Hansen & Hartnett, 2019). LSV is recommended for stage 4 ROP in posterior zone II or zone I or in stage 5 disease in which the retina is not in close proximity to the lens, whereas a scleral buckle is more commonly used with peripheral detachment of the retina or rhegmatogenous detachments caused by breaks or holes in the retina (Hansen & Hartnett, 2019). SB done concurrently with bevacizumab injections has also been studied and shown to be successful. A study of the concurrent use of SB and bevacizumab was undertaken in nine infants (13 eyes) in which nine eyes were stage 4a, two were stage 4b, and two were stage 5. All four eyes with stage 4b and stage 5 ROP required vitrectomy, whereas macular attachment was achieved in all eyes with stage 4a ROP (Shah et al., 2016).

In a follow-up study of 66 infants in the ETROP study who underwent vitrectomy with or without SB, successful attachment was achieved in 16/48 eyes. At 9 months, 30% of the 56 eyes had macular attachment after vitrectomy with or without SB, whereas macular attachment occurred in 60% of the 10 eyes after SB alone. Favorable visual acuity was achieved in 13 of 78 eyes, all with stage 4a disease. Surgery was undertaken in 11 eyes with stage 5 ROP; six of the 11 eyes had no light perception, three had light perception only, and two had some vision (Repka et al., 2006). It is speculated that infants in the ETROP study had a more aggressive form of ROP, which may account for the difference in success rates compared to those seen in other studies (Hubbard, 2008).

LSV for infants with stage 4a, 4b, or 5 was studied by Nudleman and colleagues (2015). In their retrospective review of 496 eyes from 351 patients treated between 1992 and 2013, successful reattachment occurred in 82.1% of eyes with stage 4a, 69.5% for stage 4b, and 42.6% for eyes with stage 5. Follow-up of these infants demonstrated lens opacities in 26.6% of treated eyes. Macor and colleagues (2021) found that in 10 eyes (7 infants) treated with LSV for stage 4a ROP, vitreous hemorrhage occurred in two eyes and in the remaining eight eyes mean visual acuity at 36 months was 20/80 and all eyes required correction for myopic refraction.

Reported complications of SB and LSV include myopia, retinal tears, cataracts, and glaucoma (Clark & Mandal, 2008; Macor et al., 2021; Nudleman et al., 2015). SB is reported to result in higher rates of myopia which improve after the buckle is removed (Choi & Yu, 2000). Poor outcomes for all surgical interventions are predicted by the presence of plus disease, vitreous haze, and continued neovascularization (Hartnett, 2003).

PROGNOSIS

Infants born prematurely are at risk of ocular dysfunction regardless of whether or not they have ROP. Early work by Fledelius (1996) demonstrated changes in the growth and shape of the premature infant's cornea and lens, leading to a greater incidence of myopia and astigmatism. Mild ROP does not appear to worsen these refractive errors; however, more severe cases increase the severity of these vision changes (Fielder et al., 2015; Larsson & Holmstrom, 2003; Norman et al., 2019). Progressive myopia, which stabilizes around 3 years of age, has been linked to severe ROP (Fielder et al., 2015). Rates of glaucoma and cataracts are higher in infants with ROP (Bremer et al., 2012; Davitt et al., 2013; Fierson et al., 2018) as are other visual problems, including amblyopia (Fierson et al., 2018), anisometropia (Wang et al., 2013), strabismus (Fierson et al., 2018; VanderVeen et al., 2011), astigmatism (Wang et al., 2013), and nystagmus (Siatkowski et al., 2013).

The visual prognosis for ROP is also dependent on the location of the disease. ROP in zone I responds less favorably to laser therapy and is linked to poorer visual and anatomic outcomes (Good, 2004; Spandau et al., 2013).

Treatment of severe ROP with laser therapy has been shown to increase the risk of both cataracts and glaucoma (Chang & Rao, 2021). Laser therapy is also linked to a higher incidence of corneal damage and dry eye syndrome. To date, these findings have not been seen in neonates treated with anti-VEGF pharmacotherapy.

Late reactivation of the neovascular ridge in ex-preterm adults has been reported and can occur both in treated and untreated eyes. Retinal tears and detachments can also occur in adult patients with a history of ROP (Chang & Rao, 2021).

CONCLUSIONS

ROP is a multifactorial disease that affects infants who are premature and of low birth weight. Globally, it remains one of the leading causes of childhood blindness. Although multiple risk factors, including increased or fluctuating levels of oxygen, have been identified, the precise relationship between these risk factors and the development of severe disease remains to be determined.

A comprehensive screening program with a well-developed plan for following at-risk infants is an important part of preventing progressive ROP. The two mainstays of treatment, laser therapy and VEGF inhibitors, have limited efficacy and the potential for concerning adverse effects. Anti-VEGF drugs, although widely used to treat ROP, have not been approved for this purpose by the FDA and raise the concern for yet-unknown long-term systemic side effects. Continued research efforts are needed, both to better understand the pathophysiology of ROP and to determine optimal treatments that reduce the risk of visual impairment without causing untoward side effects.

LEARNING TOOLS AND RESOURCES

Advice From the Authors

Debbie Fraser, MN, NNP, CNeoN(C), FCAN

Every NICU should have a process in place to ensure timely screening, ongoing monitoring, and postdischarge follow-up. An organized approach is critical to avoid missing neonates who meet the criteria for treatment. Current strategies for treatment include intraocular bevacizumab or laser therapy. Each of these treatments has risks and benefits as well as potential adverse effects that clinicians must be aware of and monitor for.

William Diehl-Jones, PhD, RN, MSc, BScN

The risk of retinopathy of prematurity is inversely related to gestational age. Although the exact etiology of this disease is unknown, risk factors include prematurity, low birth weight, and postnatal exposure to oxygen therapy. All NICUs should have strategies in place to reduce exposure of premature infants to conditions of hyperoxia. Approaches can include putting posters or crib cards at each bedside identifying the desired oxygen saturation limits, alarm limit audits, and regular education for care providers.

Discussion Prompts

1. What factors increase the risk of ROP?
2. What are the stages of ROP?
3. At what stage of disease should treatment be considered?
4. How is the choice of treatment for ROP made? For what type of ROP is laser therapy preferred?

Mind Map

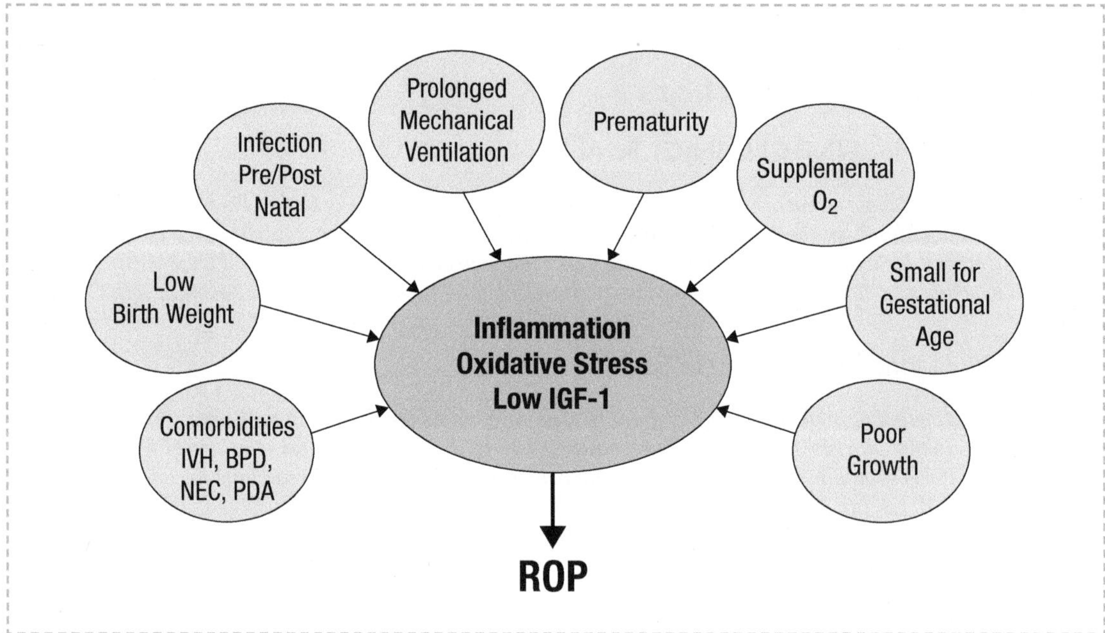

Note: This mind map reflects the design team's interpretation of a portion of one or more concepts addressed in this chapter. Readers should regard the mind maps woven throughout this textbook as examples of multisensory study tools that can be developed to encourage conceptual understanding. Readers are encouraged to develop their own unique mind maps in consultation with academic faculty or clinical preceptors. BPD, bronchopulmonary dysplasia; IGF, insulin-like growth factor; IVH, intraventricular hemorrhage; NEC, necrotizing enterocolitis; PDA, patent ductus arteriosus; ROP, retinopathy of prematurity.
Design credit: Dr. W. Diehl-Jones.

REFERENCES

References for this chapter are online and available at https://connect.springerpub.com/content/book/978-0-8261-5884-0/part/partVIII/toc-part/ch29.

PART IX

Special Circumstances

chapter 30

Central Venous Catheter Care and Occlusion

Elizabeth Sharpe

LEARNING OBJECTIVES

After completing this chapter, the reader should be able to:

- Describe at least two considerations in vascular access device selection.
- Describe at least two benefits of peripherally inserted central catheters in neonates.
- Identify appropriate catheter tip location for a peripherally inserted central catheter.
- Discuss preventive strategies for catheter occlusion.
- Describe instillation of clearing agents for management of catheter occlusion.

INTRODUCTION

As more small and fragile neonates survive, there is increasing need to provide them with nourishing and therapeutic fluids. These fluids constitute lifesaving intravenous therapy. The central vascular access device (CVAD), or central venous catheter, is the requisite lifeline for the infusion of these fluids. Central venous catheters commonly used in the NICU include peripherally inserted central venous catheters (PICCs), umbilical venous catheters, and tunneled (Broviac) catheters.

The establishment and maintenance of reliable central venous access is a mainstay in care of critical and extremely low-birth-weight neonates. Therefore, we explore the different types of central venous catheters and their definitions and care in this chapter. A special focus on PICCs highlights the prevention and management of catheter occlusion, including the use of clearing agents. This content is particularly important for APRNs, as PICC insertion and maintenance is often the responsibility of the APRN team.

DEFINITION, BENEFITS, AND RISKS

PICCs are defined as central by the location of the catheter tip in the superior vena cava (SVC) or the inferior vena cava (IVC; Food and Drug Administration [FDA], 1989; Gorski et al., 2021; Sharpe et al., 2022). The central-tip location enables direct release of infusate into the vena cava. Here, solutions are immediately subject to powerful hemodynamic flow, which dilutes the infusate and minimizes risk of damage to the vascular endothelium (Kluckow & Evans, 2000). The use of PICCs (vs. peripheral intravenous [PIV] catheters) makes it possible to deliver highly concentrated parenteral nutrition and highly osmolar medications with minimal risks. When properly maintained, PICCs offer reliable long-term vascular access compared with PIVs, which when used as the primary modality for the infusion of parenteral nutrition and medications require interval replacement. This leads to interruptions in care (and nutrition), pain, and discomfort.

Neonatal APRNs must be able to identify the recommended locations for the insertion of a PICC. These anatomic locations include the basilic, cephalic, greater and lesser saphenous, posterior auricular, temporal, or external jugular veins. PICCs inserted into the upper extremities (basilic, cephalic, posterior auricular, or temporal veins) should be advanced such that the catheter tip resides in the SVC. In comparison, PICCs placed into the lower extremities (greater or lesser saphenous veins) should be advanced such that the catheter tip resides both above the diaphragm and within the IVC (FDA, 1989; Gorski et al., 2021; Sharpe et al., 2022). Placement of PICC catheter tips within the SVC or IVC is associated with the lowest incidence of complications, which are discussed later in this chapter (Colacchio et al., 2012; Dhillon et al., 2020; Goldwasser et al., 2017; Jain et al., 2013; Racadio et al., 2001; Sertic et al., 2018).

A central venous catheter inserted into an upper or lower vein and with tip placement outside the SVC or IVC is considered a "midline" catheter. Midline catheters placed into an upper extremity peripheral vein should have the terminal tip located at the axilla. Midline catheters placed in veins in the scalp should have the terminal tip located in the jugular vein and above the clavicle. Midline catheters placed in peripheral veins in the lower extremity should have the terminal tip located below the inguinal crease (Gorski et al., 2021).

INDICATIONS FOR USE

Vascular access device selection is multifactorial and should encompass patient needs; consideration of the intended duration of therapy; and the chemical, osmolar, and irritant properties of potential infusates (Sharpe et al., 2022). Patients who are PICC candidates include very-low-birth-weight premature infants, infants transitioning from umbilical catheters or requiring more than 6 days of intravenous therapy, infants with gastrointestinal or congenital cardiac disorders, infants who have reached venous exhaustion, or infants unable to receive therapy using another device (Gordon et al., 2017; Levit et al., 2020).

Although there is no single specific criteria for a PICC, interprofessional NICU teams should take the following factors into consideration:

- Use umbilical venous catheters for medications and parenteral nutrition and blood products, particularly within the first 48 to 72 hours after birth to initiate therapies (Gorski et al., 2021).
- Use PICC or CVAD (or midline catheter) when the duration of intravenous therapy is likely to exceed 6 days (O'Grady et al., 2011).
- Use PICC or CVAD for infusion of parenteral nutrition solutions/emulsions with an osmolarity higher than 900 mOsm/L (Ayers et al., 2020; Gorski et al., 2021).
- Do not use midline catheters for continuous vesicant therapy, parenteral nutrition, or infusates with extremes of pH or osmolarity greater than 900 mOsm/L (Gorski et al., 2021).

MONITORING OF VASCULAR ACCESS DEVICES

Expert panels recommend that vascular access devices, particularly those used in neonates, are assessed hourly or more frequently (Sharpe et al., 2022). Bedside clinicians should document the following as part of this interval assessment:

- condition of the insertion site (color, temperature, leakage, bleeding)
- visualization of the length of exposed catheter (exposed length should be compared with the procedure note, which documents the length of the catheter at the time of insertion)
- dressing integrity
- condition of infusion tubing (e.g., condition of catheter tubing connections, presence of precipitate or blood in tubing)
- infusion pump settings

Complications

Complications associated with PICCs and other CVADs include catheter occlusion, leaking, dislodgment, central line-associated bloodstream infection (CLABSI), catheter migration resulting in loss of suboptimal tip location and function as a centrally positioned device, and phlebitis. The most common of the aforementioned complications include occlusion, leaking, dislodgment, and infection (Isemann et al., 2012). Catheter occlusion is a common complication that is significantly associated with interrupted or delayed therapy. Less common complications include thrombosis, pneumothorax, nerve injury, and pericardial or pleural effusions (Sharpe et al., 2022). As occlusion of PICCs or CVADs can critically interrupt care, further discussion focuses on this most frequently occurring complication.

CATHETER OCCLUSION

Hallmark signs of occlusion include infusion pump alarms and the inability to flush the catheter or aspirate blood. The most common cause is the development of thrombus in or surrounding the catheter. Other causes of catheter occlusion include mechanical and chemical causes, as well as vascular calcifications. Mechanical causes include kinking or compression of the catheter, known as *pinch-off syndrome*. Chemical causes occur when infusates, such as parenteral nutrition components and certain medications, interact and produce crystals or precipitates, which can occlude PICCs and CVADs. These most often result due to a calcium and phosphorus imbalance within the parenteral nutrition solution (Doellman, 2011).

Although the most common etiology for an occlusion is thrombotic, a thorough assessment must be performed and should guide clinical management. Begin by visually inspecting the insertion site, tubing, and infusion device. Next, assess the patency of the device by attempting to aspirate fluid or blood through the catheter (Gorski et al., 2021; Sharpe et al., 2022). The result obtained after the aspiration attempt allows clinicians to characterize the degree of occlusion as a partial occlusion, withdrawal occlusion, or complete occlusion. Partial occlusions manifest with sluggish flow, resistance to flushing and aspiration, and a high pressure reading on infusion devices. Withdrawal occlusion is suspected when the infusions can be administered without resistance, but clinicians are unable to aspirate blood through the catheter. In contrast, a complete inability to infuse or withdraw fluid or blood denotes a complete occlusion (Figure 30.1; Broadhurst et al., 2019).

PREVENTION OF CATHETER OCCLUSION

Neonates are especially at risk of occlusion due to the small internal lumen size of PICC catheters (e.g., 1.9 French [Fr], 1.4 Fr, and 1.1 Fr) and CVADs used in this population. Use of evidence-based protocols for maintaining these devices and preventing occlusion is critical to each infant's successful completion of therapy. Hospital-based protocols should include the following:

- specialized training for bedside clinicians, specific to PICC and CVAD assessment and maintenance of catheter integrity
- hourly monitoring of the insertion site
- prompt response to equipment alarms
- pharmacy collaboration to screen for potential precipitate-forming coinfusions
- nursing collaboration to screen medications and infusing solutions for potential precipitate-forming coinfusions before beginning an infusion, to avoid obstructions
- flushing before and after medication administration
- heparinization of continuous infusion fluids (Shah & Shah, 2008)
- maintenance of a minimum hourly infusion rate to ensure patency, based on institutional outcome data

The following strategies support catheter patency and successful management:

- **Continuous infusion:** Maintaining a minimum continuous infusion rate with heparin through PICCs is associated with increased duration of therapy. The most commonly reported minimum infusion rates range from 0.5 to 2 mL/hr, with the majority reporting a rate of 1 mL/hr (Sharpe et al., 2013).

FIGURE 30.1 Classes of thrombotic occlusion.

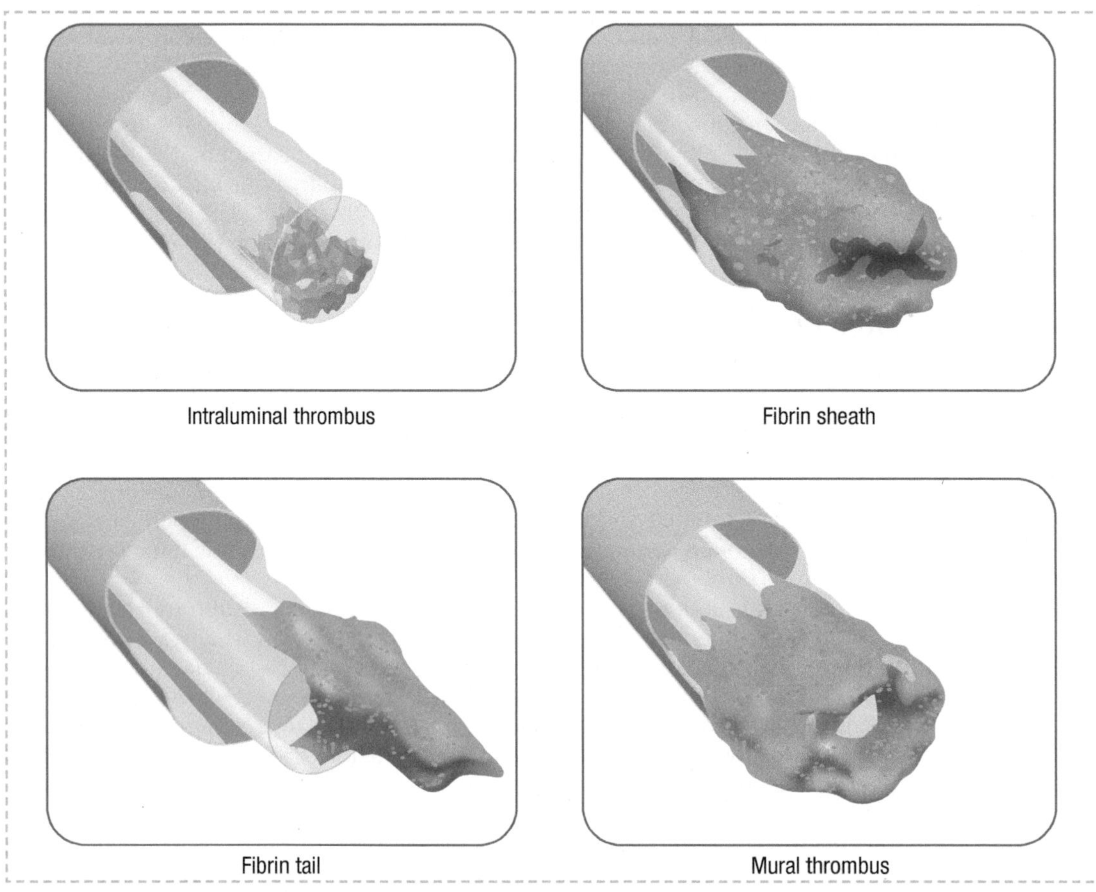

Note: Fibrin deposits, as well as fully formed thrombi, can produce a plug residing within the lumen of a catheter (an intraluminal thrombus) or can form a sock-like sheath that covers the exterior of the catheter tip. The insoluble material can also form a "tail" at the catheter tip, interfering with blood withdrawal. Thrombi forming along the wall of the vein but exterior to the catheter (mural thrombi) can also interfere with fluid flow through the central venous access device.
Source: From Genentech "Types of Occlusions" (https://www.cathflo.com/catheter-management/types-catheter-occlusions.html).

- **Flushing:** There should be a protocol in place for consistent flushing and heparin locking of PICCs that are used intermittently. There is inadequate evidence to recommend a specific volume of flush. However, flushing with at least twice the priming volume of the catheter, any extension tubing, and add-on devices should clear the catheter. The most commonly reported flush volumes range from 0.5 to 2 mL, with the majority reporting 1 mL (Sharpe et al., 2013). For intermittent locking, flush every 6 hours with 1 mL of 10 units/mL heparin (Doellman, 2011). Catheters should be flushed before and after administration of medications, although it remains unclear whether 0.9% saline is adequate or heparin is superior (Boord, 2019; Bradford et al., 2016; Gorski et al., 2021).

HISTORICAL PERSPECTIVE: SEMINAL AND OTHER NOTEWORTHY STUDIES

The spectrum of parenteral nutrition intravenous therapy has expanded and become more complex since its humble beginnings. In 1968, Stanley Dudrick published his case of a 2,300-gram (5 lb., 1 oz) infant with small bowel atresia who received a nutrient solution of 25% glucose, minerals, and vitamins for 44 days. He described the novel method of inserting a no. 24 polyvinyl catheter into the external jugular vein, positioning the catheter tip in the SVC for optimal dilution (Wilmore & Dudrick, 1968). This pioneering intervention sustained the patient, even achieving weight gain until the infant could begin enteral feeds on the 45th postoperative day. This has now evolved into modern total parenteral nutrition (Dudrick & Palesty, 2011). In 1973, Jonathan Shaw described delivering parenteral nutrition through medical-grade silastic tubing in peripheral veins in the upper and lower extremities and scalp (Shaw, 1973). This extraordinary accomplishment became a seminal step toward current utilization of PICCs in neonates today.

As the need arose, with the use of PICCs and CVADs becoming commonplace in NICUs and the duration of therapy increased, neonatal clinicians adopted pharmacologic clearing agents effectively used in other populations (e.g., pediatric cancer wards) to mitigate catheter obstructions. Next, increased attention was paid to fluid compatibilities and other causes of occlusion to encourage patency and reduce the need for clearing agents. These events led to the development of formalized training programs for PICC insertion and maintenance, as well as hospital-based training programs for bedside nurses who care for infants with central venous catheters.

CURRENT PHARMACOLOGIC MANAGEMENT OF CATHETER OCCLUSION

Management of catheter occlusion calls for a comprehensive assessment of the patient's active diseases, infused therapies, duration of the intended course of therapies, and any newly anticipated intravenous therapy needs. Clinicians may attempt to clear the catheter, discontinue the catheter, or place an alternate less invasive vascular access device. To avoid subsequent procedures and discomfort to the patient, initial attempts to clear the catheter are generally prudent. Interventions to restore patency are guided by the suspected cause, which includes mechanical, chemical, or thrombotic processes (Table 30.1). Chemical occlusion can occur with phenytoin, mannitol, and parenteral nutrition. Thorough review of infusates and solutions should inform the selection of the most appropriate clearing agents according to the suspected medication or solutions (Table 30.2; Broadhurst et al., 2019; Gorski et al., 2021).

Physical instillation of catheter clearing agents is aimed at diluting and dissolving the occlusive matter at the chemical level to enable removal of the degraded material and regain catheter patency. Although clinicians may be more familiar with heparin, heparin is an anticoagulant. Although heparin decreases coagulability, it is not effective as a clearing agent after thrombus formation (Shah & Shah, 2008). Rather, alteplase is the drug of choice for treating a thrombotic occlusion.

Recombinant Tissue Plasminogen Activator: Alteplase

Tissue plasminogen activator (tPA) is a thrombolytic substance that occurs naturally in the body. Alteplase is a recombinant DNA-manufactured tissue plasminogen activator (rtPA) approved in

TABLE 30.1 Types of Occlusions

TYPE OF OCCLUSION	CAUSE	ASSESSMENT	MANAGEMENT
Mechanical	• Improper securement or kinking • Compression of catheter as in pinch-off syndrome • Catheter tip malpositioned	• Change in length of external catheter, loose or constricting dressing • Pain or arrhythmias during infusion	• Change of dressing and add-on devices • Repositioning of the patient • Radiographic evaluation, possible removal
Chemical	• Crystallized medication • Precipitates	• Visible precipitate in tubing	• Instillation of clearing agents
Thrombotic	• Blood forms a thrombus	• Visible blood or streaking in tubing or needleless connector	• Instillation of alteplase

Sources: From Broadhurst, D., Cernusca, C., Cook, C., Hill, J., Naayer, K., Paquet, F., & Raynak, A. (2019). *CVAA occlusion management guideline for central venous access devices (CVADs)* (2nd ed.). Canadian Vascular Access Association; Gorski, L.A., Hadaway, L., Hagle, M. E., Broadhurst, D., Clare, S., Kleidon, T., Meyer, B. M., Nickel, B., Rowley, S., Sharpe, E., & Alexander, M. (2021). Infusion therapy standards of practice (8th ed.). *Journal of Infusion Nursing, 44*(1S Suppl. 1), S1–S224. https://doi.org/10.1097/NAN.0000000000000396.

TABLE 30.2 Clearing Agents Based on Etiology of Occlusion

ETIOLOGY OF OCCLUSION	CLEARING AGENT	DOSE/GUIDELINES
Thrombus	Alteplase	For patients <30 kg: 110% of the internal lumen volume of CVAD, not to exceed 2 mg/2 mL. Dwell time = 30 minutes. Attempt to aspirate. If not successful, reassess after 120 minutes. If still occluded, a second dose may be instilled (Blaney et al., 2006; Genentech).
Drug with a low pH Calcium phosphate	HCl L-cysteine	Instill 0.5 mL of 0.1-N HCl from 1-mL syringe, irrigating gently for 1–2 minutes. If patency is not immediately restored, allow to instill for an hour, then reassess, and may repeat hourly (Werlin et al., 1995). Instill L-cysteine at a dose appropriate to the catheter volume per hospital protocol for clearing catheter occlusion (Pai & Plogsted, 2014). Instill 0.2–1 mL of 0.1-N HCl for 1–2 hours. If patency is not immediately restored, allow to instill for an hour, then reassess, and may repeat hourly. If patency is restored, flush with 5 mL of normal saline (Baskin et al., 2009).
Drug with a high pH	Sodium bicarbonate	Instill 1 mL of 1 mEq/mL sodium bicarbonate (Kerner et al., 2006).
Lipid emulsion	70% ethanol	Instill 0.55 mL/kg 70% ethanol to a max of 3 mL. Allow to instill for 1–2 hours, then assess, and may repeat once (Werlin et al., 1995).

CVAD, central venous access device; HCl, hydrochloric acid.

2001 by the FDA for restoration of central venous catheter function (FDA, 2001). In fact, alteplase is the *only* drug approved for restoration of central venous catheter patency for use in neonates (Taketomo, 2023).

In a prospective study of 310 patients aged 2 weeks through 18 years old, with 55 patients younger than 2 years old, alteplase achieved 82.9% restoration of catheter patency, with only two serious adverse events attributed to the study drug (one case of sepsis and one case of catheter rupture), demonstrating safety and efficacy in pediatric patients (Blaney et al., 2006). In a literature review of 10 studies composed of pediatric patients, overall efficacy for restoration of CVAD function ranged from 50% to 90% (Anderson et al., 2013). Case reports have described successful outcomes in treating thrombosis with alteplase in neonate (Erdinç et al., 2013; Khan et al., 2008).

MECHANISM OF ACTION/PHARMACOKINETIC PRINCIPLES

Alteplase is chemically identical to endogenously synthesized tPA and exhibits a strong affinity for fibrin. The mechanism of action of alteplase is two fold. Alteplase binds to fibrin (on the thrombus) and activates the conversion of inactive plasminogen to active plasmin. The release of plasmin leads to fibrinolysis and the formation of fibrin degradation products (e.g., d-dimer; Burcham & Rosenthal, 2018; Taketomo, 2023).

Pharmacokinetic data are limited to studies of intravenous infusions of alteplase for deep vein thrombosis in adults, which is not the indication for use in neonates and infants when clearing a PICC occlusion. The large molecular size of alteplase limits its use to parenteral administration only.

DOSING RECOMMENDATIONS

Alteplase should be reconstituted with sterile water for injection, not bacteriostatic water, and is compatible with sodium chloride 0.9% (Genentech). The reported administered concentration is 0.25 to 1 mg/mL (Taketomo, 2023; Soylu, 2010). The injected volume should equal 110% of the capacity of the catheter (completely fill the catheter). The solution should remain in the catheter for 120 minutes and then be completely aspirated from the catheter. This procedure may be repeated a second time, if the first attempt is unsuccessful (Genentech).

It is important that the APRN who is instilling alteplase has specialized knowledge of PICC and CVAD management (Broadhurst et al., 2019; Sharpe et al., 2022). In addition, if attempting to clear a dual-lumen catheter, if occlusion is suspected in one lumen, both lumens should be attempted to be cleared (Broadhurst et al., 2019; Gorski et al., 2021). It is recommended that lumens are cleared one at a time and not concurrently.

FIGURE 30.2 Clearing catheter occlusion.

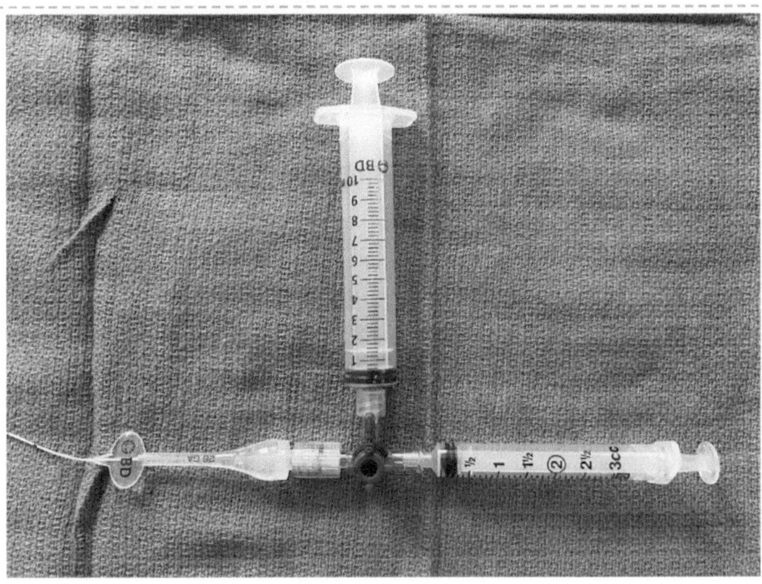

Procedure for Clearing Catheter Occlusion

1. Stop current infusion before and during instillation.
2. Clamp catheter with gauze, protecting the catheter to prevent air entry. Do not place hemostats directly on the catheter.
3. Attach the three-way stopcock in OFF position to the catheter.
4. Attach an empty, sterile 10-mL syringe to the middle port of the three-way stopcock (Figure 30.2).
5. Attach the clearing agent in a 3-mL or 10-mL syringe to the straight pathway of the three-way stopcock.
6. Turn the stopcock to the OFF position to the clearing agent.
7. Use the 10-mL syringe to gently aspirate the catheter until the plunger is pulled back to the 3-mL mark. This creates negative pressure, drawing the clearing agent into the catheter lumen.
8. Allow dwell time specific to the clearing agent.
9. Reassess patency, attempting to withdraw and discard degraded contents.
10. If patency is achieved, flush the catheter per hospital protocol. If occlusion persists, repeat dose specific to clearing agent guidelines.
11. If instillation of the clearing agent is unsuccessful in achieving catheter patency, reevaluate patient needs and consider alternate management or device (Broadhurst et al., 2019; Cummings-Winfield & Mushani-Kanji, 2009; Doellman et al., 2015).

CLINICAL-MONITORING PEARLS

Infants treated with alteplase should be monitored carefully for signs of sepsis, bleeding, and thrombosis in the days following drug administration.

CONCLUSIONS

Preservation of CVADs is paramount. Concerted care should incorporate evidence-based best practices. Many of the strategies described in this chapter are based on evidence gained from experiences with the pediatric and adult populations. Although new knowledge continues to emerge, a need remains for more high-level evidence surrounding catheter occlusion management in our tiny patients.

LEARNING TOOLS AND RESOURCES

Advice From the Author

Elizabeth Sharpe, DNP, APRN, NNP-BC, VA-BC, FAANP, FAAN

Early detection of complications like catheter occlusion enables your greatest breadth of options for management. Circle back to the original decision for placing the device and reconsider the patient's status, needs, benefits, risks, and options. Consider all aspects of the patient's therapy needs and how they have changed. There may be more options than you think!

Discussion Prompts

1. Discuss current preventive strategies for catheter occlusion that you see incorporated into your hospital's protocol. How do those strategies compare with the recommendations reviewed in this chapter?
2. Compare partial and complete occlusion and the associated presenting signs.
3. Analyze the interval monitoring policy and criteria for discontinuation of CVADs and PICCs in your unit. Do these protocols align with best practices for infection control?

Mind Map

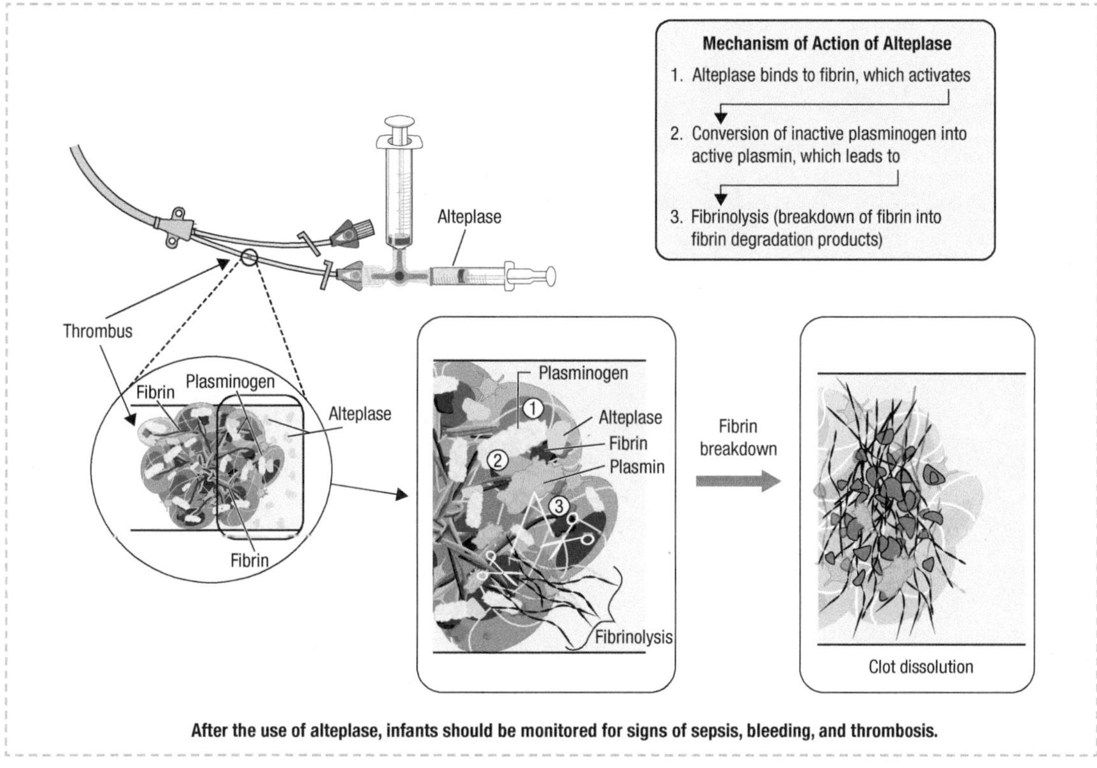

Note: This mind map reflects the design team's interpretation of a portion of one or more concepts addressed in this chapter. Readers should regard the mind maps woven throughout this textbook as examples of multisensory study tools that can be developed to encourage conceptual understanding. Readers are encouraged to develop their own unique mind maps in consultation with academic faculty or clinical preceptors. Design credit: Erin McDowell, MSN, RNC-NIC, c-ELBW. Created with Biorender.com.

REFERENCES

References for this chapter are online and available at https://connect.springerpub.com/content/book/978-0-8261-5884-0/part/partIX/toc-part/ch30.

PART X

Appendix

chapter 31

Formulary

Amy J. Jnah and Amy L. Brown

COMMON CENTRAL NERVOUS SYSTEM MEDICATIONS

DRUG CLASS: Central Nervous System Stimulant

MEDICATION NAME	FDA APPROVED FOR USE IN NICU?	MECHANISM OF ACTION	HALF-LIFE (BIRTH–AGE 2)	COMMON INDICATIONS FOR USE IN THE NICU	CLINICAL MONITORING CONSIDERATIONS
Caffeine citrate	Yes, limited to the treatment of apnea of prematurity in preterm infants.[2]	Inhibits adenosine A_1 and A_2 receptors and phosphodiesterase. The effect is stimulation of the medullary respiratory center and an increase in sensitivity to carbon dioxide levels. Neonates exhibit increased respiratory drive and diaphragmatic contractility.	Neonates: 72 to 96 hours[1] Infants (>9 months): 5 hours[1]	• Apnea of prematurity • Pre-extubation respiratory stimulant	• HR • Feeding tolerance **NOTE**: Serum drug concentration may be obtained in infants with prior exposure to theophylline, or with hepatic or renal disease.

Note: Content included in this table is intended for educational purposes only. The status of the FDA approvals and PK data may change over time. Readers are encouraged to consult package inserts for the most current information. Medications selected are considered to be among the top 100 most commonly prescribed medications in the NICU, per Stark, A., Smith, P. B., Hornik, C. P., Zimmerman, K. O., Hornik, C. D., Pradeep, S., Clark, R. H., Benjamin, D. K., Jr., Laughon, M., Greenberg, R. G. (2022). Medication use in the neonatal intensive care unit and changes from 2010 to 2018. *The Journal of Pediatrics, 240,* 66–71.e4. https://doi.org/10.1016/j.jpeds.2021.08.075.

FDA, U.S. Food and Drug Administration; HR, heart rate; PK, pharmacokinetic.

Sources: [1]Taketomo, C. K. (Ed.). (2023). *Pediatric & neonatal dosage handbook: An extensive resource for clinicians treating pediatric and neonatal patients* (29th ed.). Lexicomp/Wolters Kluwer; [2]Roxane Laboratories. (2020 April). *Cafcit.* https://www.accessdata.fda.gov/drugsatfda_docs/label/2000/20793s11lbl.pdf

DRUG CLASS: Barbiturate Anticonvulsant

MEDICATION NAME	FDA APPROVED FOR USE IN NICU?	MECHANISM OF ACTION	HALF-LIFE (BIRTH–AGE 2)	COMMON INDICATIONS FOR USE IN THE NICU	CLINICAL MONITORING CONSIDERATIONS
Phenobarbital • *Abortive therapy for neonatal seizures* • *Use with caution in preterm infants: May accelerate neuronal apoptosis*[3]	Yes	Long-acting anticonvulsant. GABA agonist that inhibits synaptic activity in the central nervous system and therefore inhibits seizure activity; blocks the release of excitatory neurotransmitters, including glutamate receptor AMPA (the primary excitatory neurotransmitter in the brain) and others dependent upon calcium channels, which also inhibits seizure activity; inhibits polysynaptic midbrain reticular formation, which elicits a sedative-hypnotic effect.	60–160 hours[1]	• Neonatal seizures (including prophylaxis) • Paroxysmal activity • Neonatal abstinence syndrome (polysubstance) • Hyperbilirubinemia	• Blood pressure • Comorbid conditions (e.g., neonatal encephalopathy and receiving therapeutic hypothermia) and higher cumulative dose may exacerbate risk for adverse effects[2] • Drug–drug interactions (barbiturates induce the synthesis of many CYP450 enzymes, which can enhance the metabolism and clearance of other drugs) • Gastrointestinal function (poor feeding) • HR • Hepatic function • Level of sedation • Respiratory rate • Renal function **NOTE:** Monitor serum drug concentration (therapeutic range is typically 15–40 mcg/mL).

Note: Content included in this table is intended for educational purposes only. The status of the FDA approvals and PK data may change over time. Readers are encouraged to consult package inserts for the most current information. Medications selected are considered to be among the top 100 most commonly prescribed medications in the NICU, per Stark, A., Smith, P. B., Hornik, C. P., Zimmerman, K. O., Hornik, C. D., Pradeep, S., Clark, R. H., Benjamin, D. K., Jr., Laughon, M., Greenberg, R. G. (2022). Medication use in the neonatal intensive care unit and changes from 2010 to 2018. *The Journal of Pediatrics, 240*, 66–71.e4. https://doi.org/10.1016/j.jpeds.2021.08.075.

CYP450, cytochrome P450; FDA, U.S. Food and Drug Administration; GABA, gamma aminobutyric acid; HR, heart rate.

Sources: [1]Taketomo, C. K. (Ed.). (2023). *Pediatric & neonatal dosage handbook: An extensive resource for clinicians treating pediatric and neonatal patients* (29th ed.). Lexicomp/Wolters Kluwer; [2]Sharpe, C., Reiner, G. E., Davis, S. L., Nespeca, M., Gold, J. J., Rasmussen, M., Kuperman, R., Harbert, M. J., Michelson, D., Joe, P., Wang, S., Rismanchi, N., Le, N. M., Mower, A., Kim, J., Battin, M. R., Lane, B., Honold, J., Knodel, E., . . . Haas, R. H. (2020). Levetiracetam versus phenobarbital for neonatal seizures: A randomized controlled trial. *Pediatrics, 145*(6), Article e20193182. https://doi.org/10.1542/peds.2019-3182; [3]Bittigau, P., Sifringer, M., Genz, K., Reith, E., Pospischil, D., Govindarajalu, S., Dzietko, M., Pesditschek, S., Mai, I., Dikranian, K., & Olney, J. W. (2002) Antiepileptic drugs and apoptotic neurodegeneration in the developing brain. *Proceedings of the National Academy of Sciences of the United States of America, 99*(23), 15089–15094. https://doi.org/10.1073/pnas.222550499

DRUG CLASS: Benzodiazepine Anticonvulsants

MEDICATION NAME	FDA APPROVED FOR USE IN NICU?	MECHANISM OF ACTION	HALF-LIFE (BIRTH–AGE 2)	COMMON INDICATIONS FOR USE IN THE NICU	CLINICAL MONITORING CONSIDERATIONS
Lorazepam • *Use with caution in preterm infants: may accelerate neuronal apoptosis.*[3]	No	GABA agonist; the benzodiazepine binds to the neuron at the GABAa receptor (separate location from where GABA binds to the receptor), which encourages increased GABA binding (allosteric effect) at a different locus on the neuron. As a result, chloride channels open, then chloride enters the neuron and hyperpolarizes it, making it less likely to fire an action potential. This creates a sedative (antianxiety) effect and encourages muscle relaxation.	Term neonates (intravenous dosing): 40.2 ± 16.5 hours[1] Infants (5 months–3 years): 15.8 hours[1]	• Neonatal seizures • Status epilepticus • Sedation/anxiolytic	• Blood pressure • HR • Neurologic function (seizure secondary to drug withdrawal; neurotoxicity; myoclonus; hyper- or hypotonia; chorea; dyskinesia) • Renal function • Hepatic function • Respiratory status
Midazolam • *Use with caution in preterm infants: may accelerate neuronal apoptosis*[3]	IV: Yes Oral: ≥6 months of age	GABA agonist; the benzodiazepine binds to the neuron at the GABAa receptor (separate location from where GABA binds to the receptor), which encourages increased GABA binding (allosteric effect) at a different locus on the neuron. As a result, chloride channels open, then chloride enters the neuron and hyperpolarizes it, making it less likely to fire an action potential. This creates a sedative (antianxiety) effect and encourages muscle relaxation.	Preterm infants (26–34 weeks): 2.6–17.7 hours[1] Late preterm and term neonates: 4–12 hours[1] Critically ill neonates: 6.5–12 hours[1]	• Refractory seizures • Sedation/anxiolytic[2] • Status epilepticus	• Blood pressure (hypotension) • HR • Respiratory status • Neurologic function (epileptiform activity, myoclonus, hyper- or hypotonia)[3]

Note: Content included in this table is intended for educational purposes only. The status of the FDA approvals and PK data may change over time. Readers are encouraged to consult package inserts for the most current information. Medications selected are considered to be among the top 100 most commonly prescribed medications in the NICU, per Stark, A., Smith, P. B., Hornik, C. P., Zimmerman, K. O., Hornik, C. D., Pradeep, S., Clark, R. H., Benjamin, D. K., Jr., Laughon, M., Greenberg, R. G. (2022). Medication use in the neonatal intensive care unit and changes from 2010 to 2018. *The Journal of Pediatrics, 240,* 66–71.e4. https://doi.org/10.1016/j.jpeds.2021.08.075.

FDA, U.S. Food and Drug Administration; GABA, gamma aminobutyric acid; HR, heart rate; PMA, postmenstrual age.

Sources: [1]Taketomo, C. K. (Ed.). (2023). *Pediatric & neonatal dosage handbook: An extensive resource for clinicians treating pediatric and neonatal patients* (29th ed.). Lexicomp/Wolters Kluwer; [2]Ng, E., Taddio, A., & Ohlsson, A. (2012). Intravenous midazolam infusion for sedation of infants in the neonatal intensive care unit. *Cochrane Database of Systematic Reviews,* (6), Article CD002052. https://doi.org/10.1002/14651858.CD002052.pub2; [3]Bittigau, P., Sifringer, M., Genz, K., Reith, E., Pospischil, D., Govindarajalu, S., Dzietko, M., Pesditschek, S., Mai, I., Dikranian, K., & Olney, J. W. (2002). Antiepileptic drugs and apoptotic neurodegeneration in the developing brain. *Proceedings of the National Academy of Sciences of the United States of America, 99*(23), 15089–15094. https://doi.org/10.1073/pnas.222550499

DRUG CLASS: Hydantoin Anticonvulsant

MEDICATION NAME	FDA APPROVED FOR USE IN NICU?	MECHANISM OF ACTION	HALF-LIFE (BIRTH–AGE 2)	COMMON INDICATIONS FOR USE IN THE NICU	CLINICAL MONITORING CONSIDERATIONS
Fosphenytoin • *Use with caution in preterm infants: may accelerate neuronal apoptosis*[3]	Yes	Prodrug of phenytoin. Blocks voltage-gated sodium channels, which inhibit the transmission of repetitive action potentials at the focal point of the seizure.[2]	Neonates, infants, and children: 2.5–18.5 minutes (for conversion from fosphenytoin to phenytoin; see below)	• Neonatal seizures • Status epilepticus	• Blood glucose • Blood pressure • Heart rhythm • Hepatic function • Level of sedation • Renal function • Respiratory rate **NOTE:** Monitor serum drug concentration (therapeutic range of total phenytoin is 8 to 15 mcg/mL in neonates and 10–20 mcg/mL in infants, free phenytoin is 1–2.5 mcg/mL).
Phenytoin • *Use with caution in preterm infants: may accelerate neuronal apoptosis*[3]	Yes	Blocks voltage-gated sodium channels, which inhibit the transmission of repetitive action potentials at the focal point of the seizure.[2]	Neonates: Significantly prolonged due to decreased clearance (range 7–194 hours)[1]	• Neonatal seizures • Status epilepticus	• Blood glucose • Blood pressure (hypotension) • Heart rhythm (arrythmias) • Hepatic function • Level of sedation • Renal function • Respiratory function (respiratory depression) • Purple glove syndrome if given intravenously **NOTE:** Serum concentrations may be decreased when coadministered with enteral feedings. Monitor serum drug concentration (therapeutic range total phenytoin is 8–15 mcg/mL in neonates and 10–20 mcg/mL in infants, free phenytoin is 1–2.5 mcg/mL).

Note: The term *prodrug* refers to a drug that is inactive when administered, and, once metabolized, is enzymatically or chemically converted to an active form. Content included in this table is intended for educational purposes only. The status of the FDA approvals and PK data may change over time. Readers are encouraged to consult package inserts for the most current information. Medications selected are considered to be among the top 100 most commonly prescribed medications in the NICU, per Stark, A., Smith, P. B., Hornik, C. P., Zimmerman, K. O., Hornik, C. D., Pradeep, S., Clark, R. H., Benjamin, D. K., Jr., Laughon, M., Greenberg, R. G. (2022). Medication use in the neonatal intensive care unit and changes from 2010 to 2018. *The Journal of Pediatrics, 240*, 66–71.e4. https://doi.org/10.1016/j.jpeds.2021.08.075.
FDA, U.S. Food and Drug Administration.

Sources: [1]Taketomo, C. K. (Ed.). (2023). *Pediatric & neonatal dosage handbook: An extensive resource for clinicians treating pediatric and neonatal patients* (29th ed.). Lexicomp/Wolters Kluwer; [2]Gupta, M., & Tripp, J. (2022, July 11). Phenytoin. In *StatPearls* [Internet]. StatPearls Publishing. https://www.ncbi.nlm.nih.gov/books/NBK551520; [3]Bittigau, P., Sifringer, M., Genz, K., Reith, E., Pospischil, D., Govindarajalu, S., Dzietko, M., Pesditschek, S., Mai, I., Dikranian, K., Olney, J. W., & Ikonomidou, C. (2002). Antiepileptic drugs and apoptotic neurodegeneration in the developing brain. *Proceedings of the National Academy of Sciences of the United States of America, 99*(23), 15089–15094. https://doi.org/10.1073/pnas.222550499

DRUG CLASS: Racetam Anticonvulsant

MEDICATION NAME	FDA APPROVED FOR USE IN NICU?	MECHANISM OF ACTION	HALF-LIFE (BIRTH–AGE 2)	COMMON INDICATIONS FOR USE IN THE NICU	CLINICAL MONITORING CONSIDERATIONS
Levetiracetam	Yes, ≥1 month of age	Mechanism of action is not fully understood. Among infants with hypoxic-ischemic injury at-risk for seizures, the drug appears to inhibit voltage-dependent N-type calcium channels, reducing the incidence of cellular apoptosis at the level of the hippocampus and cerebral cortex.[2]	Term neonates: 5.3–32.7 hours Infants and children (<4 years of age): 5.3 ± 1.3 hours[1]	• Neonatal seizures	• Blood pressure • Complete blood count • Gastrointestinal function (poor feeding) • Hepatic function • Level of sedation • Renal function

Note: Content included in this table is intended for educational purposes only. The status of the FDA approvals and PK data may change over time. Readers are encouraged to consult package inserts for the most current information. Medications selected are considered to be among the top 100 most commonly prescribed medications in the NICU, per Stark, A., Smith, P. B., Hornik, C. P., Zimmerman, K. O., Hornik, C. D., Pradeep, S., Clark, R. H., Benjamin, D. K., Jr., Laughon, M., Greenberg, R. G. (2022). Medication use in the neonatal intensive care unit and changes from 2010 to 2018. *The Journal of Pediatrics, 240,* 66–71.e4. https://doi.org/10.1016/j.jpeds.2021.08.075.

FDA, U.S. Food and Drug Administration.

Sources: [1]Taketomo, C. K. (Ed.). (2023). *Pediatric & neonatal dosage handbook: An extensive resource for clinicians treating pediatric and neonatal patients* (29th ed.). Lexicomp/Wolters Kluwer; [2]Falsaperla, R., Vitaliti, G., Mauceri, L., Romano, C., Pavone, P., Motamed-Gorji, N., Matin, N., Lubrano, R., & Corsello, G. (2017). Levetiracetam in neonatal seizures as first-line treatment: A prospective study. *Journal of Pediatric Neurosciences, 12*(1), 24–28. https://doi.org/10.4103/jpn.JPN_172_16

DRUG CLASS: Analgesics/Opioids

MEDICATION NAME	FDA APPROVED FOR USE IN NICU?	MECHANISM OF ACTION	HALF-LIFE (BIRTH–AGE 2)	COMMON INDICATIONS FOR USE IN THE NICU	CLINICAL MONITORING CONSIDERATIONS
Fentanyl • **Use with caution: Drug is *50–100 times more potent than morphine.***	No	Synthetic opioid analgesic that binds selectively to mu-opioid receptors on neurons in the brain, suppressing action potentials. The downstream signaling that follows inhibits the ascending pain response and raises the pain threshold (yielding its analgesic effect). In addition, calcium conductance is blocked, which decreases excitatory neurotransmitter release while permitting the release of dopamine. The effect is relaxation, euphoria, and, with prolonged use, drug dependence.[2]	Neonates: 5.3–21 hours[5] Infants and children (5 months–5 years of age) receiving intravenous infusion: 2.4 hours[1] ***Infants with increased intraabdominal pressure may exhibit a prolonged half-life.***	• Sedation/ anesthesia • Analgesia	• HR (bradycardia) • Blood pressure (hypotension) • Hepatic function • Neurologic function (opioid tolerance) • Level of sedation • Renal function • Respiratory effort • Pain scores **NOTE:** The onset of action is approximately 2–3 minutes[5] *and* duration of action is 60 minutes.[5] Rapid administration is associated with risk for chest wall rigidity.
Methadone	No	Synthetic opioid analgesic that binds selectively to opioid receptors on neurons in the brain and gastrointestinal smooth muscle. The effect is analgesia, euphoria, and sedation. In addition, nociceptive afferent neurons within the peripheral nervous system are inhibited, further decreasing the transmission of pain sensation. Last, methadone antagonizes (blocks) NMDA glutamate receptors, which raises the pain threshold, especially as it relates to neuropathic pain.[3]	Neonates: 16–63 hours Children: 3.8–62 hours[1]	• Opioid withdrawal (neonatal abstinence syndrome)	• HR and rhythm (bradycardia, QTc prolongation) • Hepatic function • Level of sedation • Neurologic function (opioid tolerance) • Renal function • Respiratory effort

Morphine	IV: Yes Oral: ≥2 years of age	Opioid analgesic that binds primarily to mu-opioid receptors on neurons in the brain, suppressing action potentials. The downstream signaling that follows inhibits the ascending pain response and raises the pain threshold. In addition, nociceptive afferent neurons within the peripheral nervous system are inhibited, further decreasing the transmission of pain sensation.[4]	Preterm neonates: 10.6 hours[1] Term neonates: 7.6 hours[1] Infants (1–3 months of life): 6.2 hours[1] Infants (3–6 months of life): 4.5 hours[1]	• Sedation/ anesthesia • Analgesia • Opioid withdrawal (neonatal abstinence syndrome)	• HR (bradycardia) • Blood pressure (hypotension) • Hepatic function • Level of sedation • Neurologic function (opioid tolerance) • Renal function • Pain scores

Note: Content included in this table is intended for educational purposes only. The status of the FDA approvals and PK data may change over time. Readers are encouraged to consult package inserts for the most current information. Medications selected are considered to be among the top 100 most commonly prescribed medications in the NICU, per Stark, A., Smith, P. B., Hornik, C. P., Zimmerman, K. O., Hornik, C. D., Pradeep, S., Clark, R. H., Benjamin, D. K., Jr., Laughon, M., Greenberg, R. G. (2022). Medication use in the neonatal intensive care unit and changes from 2010 to 2018. *The Journal of Pediatrics, 240*, 66–71.e4. https://doi.org/10.1016/j.jpeds.2021.08.075.

FDA, U.S. Food and Drug Administration; HR, heart rate; NMDA, N-methyl-D-aspartate.

Sources: [1]Taketomo, C. K. (Ed.). (2023). *Pediatric & neonatal dosage handbook: An extensive resource for clinicians treating pediatric and neonatal patients* (29th ed.). Lexicomp/Wolters Kluwer; [2]Ramos-Matos, C. F., Bistas, K. G., & Lopez-Ojeda, W. (2022, May 30). Fentanyl. In *StatPearls* [Internet]. StatPearls Publishing. https://www.ncbi.nlm.nih.gov/books/NBK459275; [3]Durrani, M., & Bansal, K. (2022, August 1). Methadone. In *StatPearls* [Internet]. StatPearls Publishing. https://www.ncbi.nlm.nih.gov/books/NBK562216; [4]Murphy, P. B., Bechmann, S., & Barrett, M. J. (2022, June 20). Morphine. In *StatPearls* [Internet]. StatPearls Publishing. https://www.ncbi.nlm.nih.gov/books/NBK526115; [5]Pacifici, G. M. (2015). Clinical pharmacology of fentanyl in preterm infants. A review. *Pediatrics and Neonatology, 56*(3), 143–148. https://doi.org/10.1016/j.pedneo.2014.06.002

DRUG CLASS: Alpha-2-Agonist Sedative

MEDICATION NAME	FDA APPROVED FOR USE IN NICU?	MECHANISM OF ACTION	HALF-LIFE (BIRTH–AGE 2)	COMMON INDICATIONS FOR USE IN THE NICU	CLINICAL MONITORING CONSIDERATIONS
Dexmedetomidine	No	Alpha-agonist that inhibits the release of norepinephrine by blocking alpha receptors (primarily A2 receptors) at the brainstem. This sympatholytic activity yields the effects of sedation, hypnosis, and analgesia.	Preterm neonates (28–<36 weeks): 3–9.1 hours[1] Term neonates (36–44 weeks): 1–9.4 hours[1] Infants & children (<2 years of age): 1.5–3.3 hours[1]	• Sedation/anesthesia • Analgesia	• Blood pressure (hypotension) • HR (bradycardia) • Level of sedation • Renal function • Pain scores
Clonidine	No	Activates inhibitory neurons in the medulla, which reduces excitatory input to the sympathetic nervous system, and, in doing so, lowers the HR and blood pressure. Among neonates with neonatal abstinence syndrome, clonidine reduces activity at hyperactive noradrenergic receptors and aids in the reduction of opioid withdrawal.	Neonates: 14–17 hours Children: 8–12 hours	• Neonatal abstinence syndrome (adjunctive therapy) • SSRI/SNRI withdrawal • Autonomic symptoms	• Blood pressure • HR • Hepatic function • Renal function • NAS withdrawal symptoms

Note: Content included in this table is intended for educational purposes only. The status of the FDA approvals and PK data may change over time. Readers are encouraged to consult package inserts for the most current information. Medications selected are considered to be among the top 100 most commonly prescribed medications in the NICU, per Stark, A., Smith, P. B., Hornik, C. P., Zimmerman, K. O., Hornik, C. D., Pradeep, S., Clark, R. H., Benjamin, D. K., Jr., Laughon, M., Greenberg, R. G. (2022). Medication use in the neonatal intensive care unit and changes from 2010 to 2018. *The Journal of Pediatrics, 240,* 66–71.e4. https://doi.org/10.1016/j.jpeds.2021.08.075.

FDA, U.S. Food and Drug Administration; HR, heart rate; NAS, neonatal abstinence syndrome; PO, by mouth; SNRI, serotonin and norepinephrine reuptake inhibitors; SSRI, selective serotonin reuptake inhibitors.

Source: [1]Taketomo, C. K. (Ed.). (2023). *Pediatric & neonatal dosage handbook: An extensive resource for clinicians treating pediatric and neonatal patients* (29th ed.). Lexicomp/Wolters Kluwer.

DRUG CLASS: Neuromuscular Blocker/Paralytic

MEDICATION NAME	FDA APPROVED FOR USE IN NICU?	MECHANISM OF ACTION	HALF-LIFE (BIRTH–AGE 2)	COMMON INDICATIONS FOR USE IN THE NICU	CLINICAL MONITORING CONSIDERATIONS
Vecuronium	Neonates and infants <7 weeks of age: No Infants >7 weeks of age: Yes	Nondepolarizing neuromuscular blocker that elicits skeletal muscle relaxation (paralysis) by binding to nicotinic cholinergic receptors at motor end plates. Binding inhibits the action of acetylcholine and prevents depolarization. The effect is muscle fasciculations that progress in a caudal direction (starting with the eyes), followed by paralysis. Recovery of muscle movement occurs in the opposite (cephalad) direction.	Neonates: No data Infants (>1 month): 65 minutes[1]	• Rapid sequence intubation (when used with atropine and opioid) • Neuromuscular blockade	• Blood pressure • HR • Hepatic function • Level of paralysis • Renal function **NOTE:** The approximate onset of action is 2–3 minutes and duration of action is 50–70 minutes.[1]

Note: Content included in this table is intended for educational purposes only. The status of the FDA approvals and PK data may change over time. Readers are encouraged to consult package inserts for the most current information. Medications selected are considered to be among the top 100 most commonly prescribed medications in the NICU, per Stark, A., Smith, P. B., Hornik, C. P., Zimmerman, K. O., Hornik, C. D., Pradeep, S., Clark, R. H., Benjamin, D. K., Jr., Laughon, M., Greenberg, R. G. (2022). Medication use in the neonatal intensive care unit and changes from 2010 to 2018. *The Journal of Pediatrics, 240*, 66–71.e4. https://doi.org/10.1016/j.jpeds.2021.08.075.

FDA, U.S. Food and Drug Administration; HR, heart rate.

Source: [1]Taketomo, C. K. (Ed.). (2023). *Pediatric & neonatal dosage handbook: An extensive resource for clinicians treating pediatric and neonatal patients* (29th ed.). Lexicomp/Wolters Kluwer.

DRUG CLASS: Neuropathic Pain

MEDICATION NAME	FDA APPROVED FOR USE IN NICU?	MECHANISM OF ACTION	HALF-LIFE (BIRTH–AGE 2)	COMMON INDICATIONS FOR USE IN THE NICU	CLINICAL MONITORING CONSIDERATIONS
Gabapentin	No	Inhibits calcium ion channels in the central nervous system, which inhibits heightened sensitivity to normal gastrointestinal activity (visceral hyperalgesia)	Neonates: No data Infants (>1 month): 4.7 hours[1]	• Visceral hyperalgesia	• Abrupt discontinuation of treatment increases the risk for irritability, tachycardia, and emesis[2] • Growth velocity • Level of sedation • Renal function

Note: Content included in this table is intended for educational purposes only. The status of the FDA approvals and PK data may change over time. Readers are encouraged to consult package inserts for the most current information. Medications selected are considered to be among the top 100 most commonly prescribed medications in the NICU, per Stark, A., Smith, P. B., Hornik, C. P., Zimmerman, K. O., Hornik, C. D., Pradeep, S., Clark, R. H., Benjamin, D. K., Jr., Laughon, M., Greenberg, R. G. (2022). Medication use in the neonatal intensive care unit and changes from 2010 to 2018. *The Journal of Pediatrics, 240*, 66–71.e4. https://doi.org/10.1016/j.jpeds.2021.08.075.

FDA, U.S. Food and Drug Administration.

Sources: [1]Taketomo, C. K. (Ed.). (2023). *Pediatric & neonatal dosage handbook: An extensive resource for clinicians treating pediatric and neonatal patients* (29th ed.). Lexicomp/Wolters Kluwer; [2]Edwards, L., DeMeo, S., Hornik, C. D., Cotten, C. M., Smith, P. B., Pizoli, C., Hauer, J. M., & Bidegain, M. (2016). Gabapentin use in the neonatal intensive care unit. *Journal of Pediatrics, 169*, 310–312. https://doi.org/10.1016/j.jpeds.2015.10.013

COMMON RESPIRATORY SYSTEM MEDICATIONS

DRUG CLASS: Bronchodilators

MEDICATION NAME	FDA APPROVED FOR USE IN NICU?	MECHANISM OF ACTION	HALF-LIFE (BIRTH–AGE 2)	COMMON INDICATIONS FOR USE IN THE NICU	CLINICAL MONITORING CONSIDERATIONS
Albuterol	No	Relaxes bronchial smooth muscle by action on beta-2 receptors with little effect on HR	Not reported	• Bronchopulmonary dysplasia • Bronchospasm • Hyperkalemia	• HR (tachycardia) • Serum electrolytes (hypokalemia, hypoglycemia)
Aminophylline	No	Inhibits adenosine A_1 and A_2 receptors and phosphodiesterase. The effect is stimulation of the medullary respiratory center and an increase in sensitivity to carbon dioxide levels. Neonates exhibit increased respiratory drive and diaphragmatic contractility.	Preterm neonates: 30 hours[1] Term neonates: 25 hours[1] Children 1–4 years: 3.4 hours[1]	• Bronchopulmonary dysplasia • Bronchospasm	• HR (tachycardia) • Hepatic function • Respiratory rate (tachypnea) • Renal function Kinetic Monitoring: Serum drug concentration should be obtained approximately 72 hours into therapy (and weekly thereafter), and in infants with signs of toxicity (tachycardia, emesis, agitation). Therapeutic concentration is <10 mcg/mL in neonates and <20 mcg/mL in older infants.
Ipratropium	No	Ipratropium is an acetylcholine antagonist that blocks muscarinic cholinergic receptors. This decreases the production of cyclic guanosine monophosphate at parasympathetic sites in the bronchial smooth muscle, which encourages bronchodilation.	Not reported	• Bronchopulmonary dysplasia	• Respiratory function (paroxysmal bronchospasm)

(continued)

DRUG CLASS: Bronchodilators *(continued)*

MEDICATION NAME	FDA APPROVED FOR USE IN NICU?	MECHANISM OF ACTION	HALF-LIFE (BIRTH–AGE 2)	COMMON INDICATIONS FOR USE IN THE NICU	CLINICAL MONITORING CONSIDERATIONS
Epinephrine (Racemic)	No	Sympathomimetic catecholamine and non-selective alpha adrenergic receptor agonist. Activity at alpha receptors increases vascular smooth muscle contraction (vasoconstriction). In theory, this vasoconstrictive state decreases inflammation associated with airway constriction. Among infants with croup, the leakage of fluid from the interstitial space and into the capillary arterioles that occurs during the disease process is reversed. Racemic epinephrine induces a state of fluid resorption, which decreases laryngeal edema.	Not reported	• Acute laryngeal edema or stridor • Acute bronchospasm • Bronchial asthma • Viral croup	• Blood pressure (hypertension) • HR and rhythm (tachycardia or arrythmia)
Epinephrine (Nebulized)	No	Agonist at alpha-, beta-1, and beta-2 adrenergic receptors resulting in relaxation of smooth muscle of the bronchial tree, cardiac stimulation increasing contractility and HR and dilation of the skeletal muscle vasculature. Alpha-agonist activity causes vasoconstriction of vascular smooth muscle, most notably in the skin and splanchnic circulation (gastrointestinal organs). Beta-adrenergic stimulation increases myocardial contractility and HR. In addition, beta-adrenergic stimulation relaxes skeletal and pulmonary smooth muscle, leading to bronchodilation.	Less than 5 minutes[1]	• Bronchospasm • Upper airway obstruction • Airway edema • Croup • Respiratory Syncytial virus (RSV) bronchiolitis	• Blood pressure • HR and heart rhythm • Serum electrolytes (hypokalemia, hypomagnesemia)

Note: Content included in this table is intended for educational purposes only. The status of the FDA approvals and PK data may change over time. Readers are encouraged to consult package inserts for the most current information. Medications selected are considered to be among the top 100 most commonly prescribed medications in the NICU, per Stark, A., Smith, P. B., Hornik, C. P., Zimmerman, K. O., Hornik, C. D., Pradeep, S., Clark, R. H., Benjamin, D. K., Jr., Laughon, M., Greenberg, R. G. (2022). Medication use in the neonatal intensive care unit and changes from 2010 to 2018. *The Journal of Pediatrics, 240,* 66–71.e4. https://doi.org/10.1016/j.jpeds.2021.08.075.

FDA, U.S. Food and Drug Administration; HR, heart rate.

Source: [1]Taketomo, C. K. (Ed.). (2023). *Pediatric & neonatal dosage handbook: An extensive resource for clinicians treating pediatric and neonatal patients* (29th ed.). Lexicomp/Wolters Kluwer.

DRUG CLASS: Exogenous Lung Surfactants

MEDICATION NAME	FDA APPROVED FOR USE IN NICU?	MECHANISM OF ACTION	HALF-LIFE (BIRTH–AGE 2)	COMMON INDICATIONS FOR USE IN THE NICU	CLINICAL MONITORING CONSIDERATIONS
Beractant	Yes: prevention of RDS in premature infants <1,250 grams; newborns with surfactant deficiency; treatment of RDS in newborns with confirmatory features requiring mechanical ventilation.	A natural bovine lung extract containing phospholipids, neutral lipids, fatty acids, and surfactant-associated proteins that augments endogenous lung surfactant and prevents alveolar collapse during expiration by lowering surface tension between air and alveolar surfaces.	Not reported	• MAS • RDS	• Blood pressure (hypotension secondary to pulmonary hemorrhage) • HR (bradycardia) • Respiratory function (tidal volume and oxygenation) • Respiratory secretions (pulmonary hemorrhage)
Calfactant	Yes: prevention of RDS in premature infants <29 weeks' gestation; treatment of RDS in newborns <72 hours of age with confirmatory features requiring mechanical ventilation.	An extract of natural surfactant from calf lungs that includes phospholipids, neutral lipids, and hydrophobic surfactant-associated proteins B and C (SP-B and SP-C). Augments endogenous lung surfactant and prevents alveolar collapse during expiration by lowering surface tension between air and alveolar surfaces.	Not reported	• MAS • RDS	• Blood pressure (hypotension secondary to pulmonary hemorrhage) • HR (bradycardia) • Respiratory function (tidal volume and oxygenation) • Respiratory secretions (pulmonary hemorrhage)

(*continued*)

DRUG CLASS: Exogenous Lung Surfactants (*continued*)

MEDICATION NAME	FDA APPROVED FOR USE IN NICU?	MECHANISM OF ACTION	HALF-LIFE (BIRTH–AGE 2)	COMMON INDICATIONS FOR USE IN THE NICU	CLINICAL MONITORING CONSIDERATIONS
Poractant alfa	Yes; for the treatment of RDS in premature infants	An extract of natural porcine lung surfactant consisting of 99% polar lipids (mainly phospholipids) and 1% hydrophobic low-molecular-weight proteins (surfactant-associated proteins SP-B and SP-C). Augments endogenous lung surfactant and prevents alveolar collapse during expiration by lowering surface tension between air and alveolar surfaces.	Not reported	• MAS • RDS	• Blood pressure (hypotension secondary to pulmonary hemorrhage) • HR (bradycardia) • Respiratory function (tidal volume and oxygenation) • Respiratory secretions (pulmonary hemorrhage)

Note: Content included in this table is intended for educational purposes only. The status of the FDA approvals and PK data may change over time. Readers are encouraged to consult package inserts for the most current information. Medications selected are considered to be among the top 100 most commonly prescribed medications in the NICU, per Stark, A., Smith, P. B., Hornik, C. P., Zimmerman, K. O., Hornik, C. D., Pradeep, S., Clark, R. H., Benjamin, D. K., Jr., Laughon, M., Greenberg, R. G. (2022). Medication use in the neonatal intensive care unit and changes from 2010 to 2018. *The Journal of Pediatrics, 240*, 66–71.e4. https://doi.org/10.1016/j.jpeds.2021.08.075.

FDA, U.S. Food and Drug Administration; HR, heart rate; MAS, meconium aspiration syndrome; RDS, respiratory distress syndrome.

DRUG CLASS: Pulmonary Vasodilator

MEDICATION NAME	FDA APPROVED FOR USE IN NICU?	MECHANISM OF ACTION	HALF-LIFE (BIRTH–AGE 2)	COMMON INDICATIONS FOR USE IN THE NICU	CLINICAL MONITORING CONSIDERATIONS
Nitric oxide	Yes; for term and preterm neonates >34 weeks' gestation	Selective pulmonary vascular smooth muscle relaxant. Drug molecules bind to cytosolic guanylate cyclase, which initiates a cascade of events leading to increased synthesis of cyclic GMP, a messenger molecule that pulls calcium from vascular smooth muscle cells and induces a state of vasodilation.	*Duration of action*: 2–5 seconds[1]	• Hypoxic respiratory failure with evidence of pulmonary hypertension	• Oxygenation • Blood pressure • Serum methemoglobin

Note: Content included in this table is intended for educational purposes only. The status of the FDA approvals and PK data may change over time. Readers are encouraged to consult package inserts for the most current information. Medications selected are considered to be among the top 100 most commonly prescribed medications in the NICU, per Stark, A., Smith, P. B., Hornik, C. P., Zimmerman, K. O., Hornik, C. D., Pradeep, S., Clark, R. H., Benjamin, D. K., Jr., Laughon, M., Greenberg, R. G. (2022). Medication use in the neonatal intensive care unit and changes from 2010 to 2018. *The Journal of Pediatrics, 240*, 66–71.e4. https://doi.org/10.1016/j.jpeds.2021.08.075.

FDA, U.S. Food and Drug Administration; GMP, guanosine 3',5'-monophosphate.

Source: [1]Ignarro, L. J. (1989). Biological actions and properties of endothelium-derived nitric oxide formed and released from artery and vein. *Circulation Research, 65*(1), 1–21. https://doi.org/10.1161/01.res.65.1.1

DRUG CLASS: Mucolytic Agent

MEDICATION NAME	FDA APPROVED FOR USE IN NICU?	MECHANISM OF ACTION	HALF-LIFE (BIRTH–AGE 2)	COMMON INDICATIONS FOR USE IN THE NICU	CLINICAL MONITORING CONSIDERATIONS
Dornase alpha • *Commonly prescribed in infants with cystic fibrosis (CTFR gene mutation)*	No	Mucolytic agent that lyses the DNA material that accumulates in the lining of the respiratory tract of infants with repetitive bacterial infections (i.e., pseudomonas). The removal of accumulated DNA material reduces airway congestion and the viscosity of respiratory mucus. This aids its normal movement up the respiratory tract and expulsion (by way of coughing).	Not reported in neonates and infants	• Cystic fibrosis • Rhinosinusitis	• Respiratory function (cough) • Skin integrity (rash)

Note: Content included in this table is intended for educational purposes only. The status of the FDA approvals and PK data may change over time. Readers are encouraged to consult package inserts for the most current information. Medications selected are considered to be among the top 100 most commonly prescribed medications in the NICU, per Stark, A., Smith, P. B., Hornik, C. P., Zimmerman, K. O., Hornik, C. D., Pradeep, S., Clark, R. H., Benjamin, D. K., Jr., Laughon, M., Greenberg, R. G. (2022). Medication use in the neonatal intensive care unit and changes from 2010 to 2018. *The Journal of Pediatrics, 240*, 66–71.e4. https://doi.org/10.1016/j.jpeds.2021.08.075.
FDA, U.S. Food and Drug Administration.

DRUG CLASS: Nebulized Steroids

MEDICATION NAME	FDA APPROVED FOR USE IN NICU?	MECHANISM OF ACTION	HALF-LIFE (BIRTH–AGE 2)	COMMON INDICATIONS FOR USE IN THE NICU	CLINICAL MONITORING CONSIDERATIONS
Budesonide	Neonates: No Infants (>1 year of age): Yes[1]	Inhaled corticosteroid that modulates protein synthesis and depresses migration of inflammatory cells (i.e., PMN leukocytes, mast cells, eosinophils, macrophages, and fibroblasts) and inflammatory mediators (i.e., cytokines). Reverses capillary permeability. The effect is reduced inflammation at the site of injury.	4 hours[3]	• Bronchopulmonary dysplasia	• Blood pressure (hypertension) • Respiratory rate (tachypnea) • Growth velocity
Fluticasone	No	Inhaled corticosteroid that modulates protein synthesis and depresses migration of inflammatory cells including PMN leukocytes, eosinophils, monocytes, macrophages, mast cells, and dendritic cells. Agonist at beta-2 adrenergic receptors, which encourages smooth muscle relaxation and decreases mucus production. The effect is reduced inflammation at the site of injury.[2]	Not reported in neonates and infants	• Bronchopulmonary dysplasia	• Blood pressure (hypertension) • Respiratory rate (tachypnea) • Growth velocity

Note: Content included in this table is intended for educational purposes only. The status of the FDA approvals and PK data may change over time. Readers are encouraged to consult package inserts for the most current information. Medications selected are considered to be among the top 100 most commonly prescribed medications in the NICU, per Stark, A., Smith, P. B., Hornik, C. P., Zimmerman, K. O., Hornik, C. D., Pradeep, S., Clark, R. H., Benjamin, D. K., Jr., Laughon, M., Greenberg, R. G. (2022). Medication use in the neonatal intensive care unit and changes from 2010 to 2018. *The Journal of Pediatrics, 240*, 66–71.e4. https://doi.org/10.1016/j.jpeds.2021.08.075.

FDA, U.S. Food and Drug Administration; PMN, polymorphonuclear.

Sources: [1]Taketomo, C. K. (Ed.). (2023). *Pediatric & neonatal dosage handbook: An extensive resource for clinicians treating pediatric and neonatal pctients* (29th ed.). Lexicomp/Wolters Kluwer; [2]Remien, K., & Bowman, A. (2022, November 14). Fluticasone. In *StatPearls* [Internet]. StatPearls Publishing. https://www.ncbi.nlm.nih.gov/books/NBK542161; [3]Yeh, T. F., Lin, H. C. Chang, C. H., Wu, T. S., Su, B. H., Li, T. C., Pyati, S., & Tsai, C. H. (2008). Early intratracheal instillation of budesonide using surfactant as a vehicle to prevent chronic lung disease in preterm infants: A pilot study. *Pediatrics, 121*(5), e1310–e1318. https://doi.org/10.1542/peds.2007-1973

COMMON CARDIOVASCULAR MEDICATIONS

DRUG CLASS: ACE Inhibitors

MEDICATION NAME	FDA APPROVED FOR USE IN NICU?	MECHANISM OF ACTION	HALF-LIFE (BIRTH–AGE 2)	COMMON INDICATIONS FOR USE IN THE NICU	CLINICAL MONITORING CONSIDERATIONS
Captopril	No	Inhibits the normal physiologic function of ACE by blocking the conversion of angiotensin I to angiotensin II. Prevents the breakdown of bradykinin. Collectively, this results in vasodilation (reducing preload) and decreased aldosterone secretion.	1.2–12.4 hours[1] (infants with CHF) 0.98–2.3 hours[1] in children	• CHF • Hypertension	• Blood glucose • Blood pressure • Hydration/fluid balance • Renal function • Serum electrolytes **NOTE:** Use with caution in preterm infants, as drug may impair final stages of renal development.[2]
Enalapril Enalaprilat	Liquid formulation approved for infants >1 month	Inhibits the normal physiologic function of ACE, blocking the conversion of angiotensin I to angiotensin II. Prevents the breakdown of bradykinin. Collectively, this results in vasodilation (reducing preload) and decreased aldosterone secretion.	PO: 4.2–13.4 hours[1] (neonates) PO: 1.3–6.3 hours[1] (infants and children) IV: 5.9–15.6 hours[1] (neonates) IV: 5.1–20.8 hours (infants and children)	• CHF • Hypertension	• Blood pressure • Hydration/fluid balance • Renal function • Serum electrolytes **NOTE:** Use with caution in preterm infants, as drug may impair final stages of renal development.[2]

Note: Content included in this table is intended for educational purposes only. The status of the FDA approvals and PK data may change over time. Readers are encouraged to consult package inserts for the most current information. Medications selected are considered to be among the top 100 most commonly prescribed medications in the NICU, per Stark, A., Smith, P. B., Hornik, C. P., Zimmerman, K. O., Hornik, C. D., Pradeep, S., Clark, R. H., Benjamin, D. K., Jr., Laughon, M., Greenberg, R. G. (2022). Medication use in the neonatal intensive care unit and changes from 2010 to 2018. *The Journal of Pediatrics, 240,* 66–71.e4. https://doi.org/10.1016/j.jpeds.2021.08.075.

ACE, angiotensin-converting enzyme; CHF, congestive heart failure; FDA, U.S. Food and Drug Administration.

Sources: [1]Taketomo, C. K. (Ed.). (2023). *Pediatric & neonatal dosage handbook: An extensive resource for clinicians treating pediatric and neonatal patients* (29th ed.). Lexicomp/Wolters Kluwer; [2]Ravisankar, S., Kuehn, D., Clark, R. H., Greenberg, R. G., Smith, P. B., & Hornik, C. P. (2017). Antihypertensive drug exposure in premature infants from 1997 to 2013. *Cardiology in the Young,* 27(5), 905–911. https://doi.org/10.1017/S1047951116001591

DRUG CLASS: Adrenergic Agonists, Sympathomimetic

MEDICATION NAME	FDA APPROVED FOR USE IN NICU?	MECHANISM OF ACTION	HALF-LIFE (BIRTH–AGE 2)	COMMON INDICATIONS FOR USE IN THE NICU	CLINICAL MONITORING CONSIDERATIONS
Dobutamine	Yes	Stimulates myocardial alpha-1, beta-1, & beta-2 adrenergic receptors. *Alpha-1 receptors* exert an effect on vascular smooth muscle and cardiomyocytes, increasing smooth muscle contraction, myocardial contractility, and gluconeogenesis, as well as decreasing insulin release. *Beta-1 receptors* exert an effect on the sinoatrial node, atrial and ventricular muscles, and conduction system, thereby increasing HR, conduction velocity, myocardial contractility, and renin synthesis. *Beta-2 receptors* are located in the bronchial, atrial, and ventricular smooth muscles; activation increases HR, myocardial contractility, smooth muscle relaxation, bronchial relaxation, glycogenolysis, and insulin secretion, and decreases intestinal motility. Collectively, this results in positive inotropic and chronotropic actions on the myocardium, lowering central venous pressure.[1]	No data in neonates and infants 2 minutes (adults)[1,2]	• Hypoperfusion • Hypotension • Septic shock	• Blood pressure • HR and rhythm • Hydration/fluid balance • Serum electrolytes
Dopamine	Yes	Effects are dose-dependent. At *low doses*, dopaminergic receptors are primarily stimulated, which results in focused vasodilation of the renal and intestinal systems, and coronary system. The effect is increased renal blood flow, urine output, and sodium losses in the urine, and sometimes hypotension. *Moderate doses* stimulate both dopaminergic and beta-1 adrenergic receptors. Beta-1 receptor activation elicits the release of norepinephrine from sympathetic nerve endings. This results in positive chronotropic and inotropic effects on the myocardium (not the periphery), which increases HR and cardiac contractility. *At high doses*, alpha-1 adrenergic receptors are stimulated, eliciting vasoconstriction. Effects include smooth muscle contraction, increased myocardial contractility, gluconeogenesis, and decreased insulin release. Dopaminergic effects are suppressed at high doses.[1]	2 minutes (term infants)[2] 4–5 minutes (preterm infants)[2]	• Hypoperfusion • Hypotension • Increase in urine output • Septic shock	• Blood glucose • Blood pressure • HR and rhythm • Hydration/fluid balance • Renal function

(*continued*)

DRUG CLASS: Adrenergic Agonists, Sympathomimetic *(continued)*

MEDICATION NAME	FDA APPROVED FOR USE IN NICU?	MECHANISM OF ACTION	HALF-LIFE (BIRTH–AGE 2)	COMMON INDICATIONS FOR USE IN THE NICU	CLINICAL MONITORING CONSIDERATIONS
Epinephrine (systemic)	No	Agonist at alpha-, beta-1, and beta-2 adrenergic receptors. Alpha-agonist activity causes vasoconstriction of vascular smooth muscle, most notably in the skin and splanchnic circulation (gastrointestinal organs). Beta-adrenergic stimulation increases myocardial contractility and HR. In addition, beta-adrenergic stimulation relaxes skeletal and pulmonary smooth muscle, leading to bronchodilation.[1]	Less than 5 minutes[1]	• Newborn resuscitation • Hypoperfusion • Hypotension • Septic shock	• Blood pressure • Blood glucose • HR and rhythm • Lactate
Norepinephrine	No	Agonist at alpha-adrenergic receptors. Alpha-agonist activity causes vasoconstriction of vascular smooth muscle, most notably in the skin and splanchnic circulation (gastrointestinal organs). Alpha-2 agonist activity may induce preferential systemic more than pulmonary vasoconstriction. Minimal beta-1 agonist activity is observed.	No data in neonates and infants 2 minutes (adults)[1]	• Hypotension in the setting of persistent pulmonary hypertension of the newborn • Septic shock	• Blood pressure • HR • Integrity of infusion site (central venous catheter preferred) • Peripheral perfusion

Note: Content included in this table is intended for educational purposes only. The status of the FDA approvals and PK data may change over time. Readers are encouraged to consult package inserts for the most current information. Medications selected are considered to be among the top 100 most commonly prescribed medications in the NICU, per Stark, A., Smith, P. B., Hornik, C. P., Zimmerman, K. O., Hornik, C. D., Pradeep, S., Clark, R. H., Benjamin, D. K., Jr., Laughon, M., Greenberg, R. G. (2022). Medication use in the neonatal intensive care unit and changes from 2010 to 2018. *The Journal of Pediatrics, 240,* 66–71.e4. https://doi.org/10.1016/j.jpeds.2021.08.075.

FDA, U.S. Food and Drug Administration; HR, heart rate.

Sources: [1]Taketomo, C. K. (Ed.). (2023). *Pediatric & neonatal dosage handbook: An extensive resource for clinicians treating pediatric and neonatal patients* (29th ed.). Lexicomp/Wolters Kluwer; [2]Bhatt-Mehta, V., & Nahata, M. C. (1989). Dopamine and dobutamine in pediatric therapy. *Pharmacotherapy, 9*(5), 303–314. https://doi.org/10.1002/j.1875-9114.1989.tb04142.x

DRUG CLASS: Antihypertensive Agent/Vasodilator

MEDICATION NAME	FDA APPROVED FOR USE IN NICU?	MECHANISM OF ACTION	HALF-LIFE (BIRTH–AGE 2)	COMMON INDICATIONS FOR USE IN THE NICU	CLINICAL MONITORING CONSIDERATIONS
Hydralazine	No	Selectively relaxes arteriolar smooth muscle (not venous smooth muscle), likely by blocking calcium from entering the smooth muscle (calcium induces vasoconstriction). The result is a reduction in blood pressure with increased cardiac output.	No data in neonates and infants 3–7 hours (adults)[1]	• Heart failure • Hypertension • Hypertensive emergency	• Blood pressure • HR

Note: Content included in this table is intended for educational purposes only. The status of the FDA approvals and PK data may change over time. Readers are encouraged to consult package inserts for the most current information. Medications selected are considered to be among the top 100 most commonly prescribed medications in the NICU, per Stark, A., Smith, P. B., Hornik, C. P., Zimmerman, K. O., Hornik, C. D., Pradeep, S., Clark, R. H., Benjamin, D. K., Jr., Laughon, M., Greenberg, R. G. (2022). Medication use in the neonatal intensive care unit and changes from 2010 to 2018. *The Journal of Pediatrics, 240*, 66–71.e4. https://doi.org/10.1016/j.jpeds.2021.08.075.

FDA, U.S. Food and Drug Administration; HR, heart rate.

Source: [1]Taketomo, C. K. (Ed.). (2023). *Pediatric & neonatal dosage handbook: An extensive resource for clinicians treating pediatric and neonatal patients* (29th ed.). Lexicomp/Wolters Kluwer.

DRUG CLASS: Antiarrhythmic Agents

MEDICATION NAME	FDA APPROVED FOR USE IN NICU?	MECHANISM OF ACTION	HALF-LIFE (BIRTH–AGE 2)	COMMON INDICATIONS FOR USE IN THE NICU	CLINICAL MONITORING CONSIDERATIONS
Adenosine	Yes	Acts on adenosine receptors located within the AV node. Adenosine draws potassium out of cardiomyocytes and inhibits the influx of calcium. This prolongs the time necessary for depolarization, slowing cardiac conduction (action potential).[1]	No data in neonates and infants <10 seconds (adults)[1]	• Supraventricular tachycardia	• Blood pressure • HR and rhythm **NOTE:** Competition from concurrent caffeine dosing for apnea of prematurity is possible (higher adenosine dose may be required to achieve a therapeutic effect).
Digoxin • *Additional therapeutic category: Cardiac glycoside*	Yes	Cardiac glycoside with positive inotropic and negative chronotropic activity. Heart failure: Inhibits Na/K ATPase pump in myocardial cells, resulting in a transient increase of intracellular Na, which promotes Ca influx leading to increased contractility. SVT: Stimulates the parasympathetic nervous system, slowing electrical conduction in the AV node, thereby decreasing HR.	Preterm neonates: 61–170 hours[1] Term neonates: 35–45 hours[1] Infants: 18–25 hours[1]	• Congestive heart failure • Supraventricular tachycardia	• Blood pressure • HR and heart rhythm (arrythmias are associated with toxicity) • Serum electrolytes • Renal function **NOTE:** Periodic monitoring of plasma drug concentration is recommended in infants with renal or hepatic insufficiency, or with signs of toxicity.

Note: Content included in this table is intended for educational purposes only. The status of the FDA approvals and PK data may change over time. Readers are encouraged to consult package inserts for the most current information. Medications selected are considered to be among the top 100 most commonly prescribed medications in the NICU, per Stark, A., Smith, P. B., Hornik, C. P., Zimmerman, K. O., Hornik, C. D., Pradeep, S., Clark, R. H., Benjamin, D. K., Jr., Laughon, M., Greenberg, R. G. (2022). Medication use in the neonatal intensive care unit and changes from 2010 to 2018. *The Journal of Pediatrics, 240,* 66–71.e4. https://doi.org/10.1016/j.jpeds.2021.08.075.

ATP, adenosine triphosphate; AV, atrioventricular; FDA, U.S. Food and Drug Administration; HR, heart rate; SVT, supraventricular tachycardia.

Source: [1]Taketomo, C. K. (Ed.). (2023). *Pediatric & neonatal dosage handbook: An extensive resource for clinicians treating pediatric and neonatal patients* (29th ed.). Lexicomp/Wolters Kluwer.

DRUG CLASS: Anticholinergic

MEDICATION NAME	FDA APPROVED FOR USE IN NICU?	MECHANISM OF ACTION	HALF-LIFE (BIRTH–AGE 2)	COMMON INDICATIONS FOR USE IN THE NICU	CLINICAL MONITORING CONSIDERATIONS
Atropine	No	Acetylcholine antagonist that acts at muscarinic receptors and, in doing so, inhibits vagal activation of the sinoatrial node. This vagolytic mechanism of action prevents reflex bradycardia.	6.9 ± 3 hours[1]	• Intubation	• Blood pressure • HR (sinus tachycardia) • Oxygenation

Note: Content included in this table is intended for educational purposes only. The status of the FDA approvals and PK data may change over time. Readers are encouraged to consult package inserts for the most current information. Medications selected are considered to be among the top 100 most commonly prescribed medications in the NICU, per Stark, A., Smith, P. B., Hornik, C. P., Zimmerman, K. O., Hornik, C. D., Pradeep, S., Clark, R. H., Benjamin, D. K., Jr., Laughon, M., Greenberg, R. G. (2022). Medication use in the neonatal intensive care unit and changes from 2010 to 2018. *The Journal of Pediatrics, 240,* 66–71.e4. https://doi.org/10.1016/j.jpeds.2021.08.075.

FDA, U.S. Food and Drug Administration; HR, heart rate.

Source: [1]Taketomo, C. K. (Ed.). (2023). *Pediatric & neonatal dosage handbook: An extensive resource for clinicians treating pediatric and neonatal patients* (29th ed.). Lexicomp/Wolters Kluwer.

DRUG CLASS: Beta-Adrenergic Blockers

MEDICATION NAME	FDA APPROVED FOR USE IN NICU?	MECHANISM OF ACTION	HALF-LIFE (BIRTH–AGE 2)	COMMON INDICATIONS FOR USE IN THE NICU	CLINICAL MONITORING CONSIDERATIONS
Propranolol	Hemangeol® has limited FDA approval for infants ≥5 weeks of age and weighing ≥2 kg.	Nonselective beta-adrenoreceptor antagonist and class II antiarrhythmic agent that blocks beta-1 and beta-2 adrenergic receptor stimulation in the myocardium. The net effect is decreased cardiac conduction, contractility, and cardiac output (beta-1 block), as well as mild vasoconstriction (beta-2 block). Among patients with infantile hemangioma, propranolol inhibits angiogenesis by downregulating growth factors in the vascular endothelium, which stops growth and hastens the natural involution of the hemangioma.	Neonates: Possible increased half-life compared to infants, children, and adults[1] Infants (35–150 days old): 3.5 hrs[1]	• Hypertension • Infantile hemangioma • Supraventricular tachycardia / tachyarrythmias • TET spells • Thyrotoxicosis	• Blood glucose • Blood pressure • HR and heart rhythm (arrythmias are associated with toxicity) • Renal function
Labetalol	No	Selective antagonist at alpha-1 receptor sites, eliciting vasodilation and reduced vascular resistance (decreasing the blood pressure). Nonselective antagonist at beta receptors, eliciting decreased cardiac contractility, HR, and myocardial oxygen demand.	No data in neonates and infants Adults: 5–8 hours[1]	• Hypertension • Hypertensive emergency	• Blood pressure • HR • Heart function (heart failure is a risk) • Renal function

Note: Content included in this table is intended for educational purposes only. The status of the FDA approvals and PK data may change over time. Readers are encouraged to consult package inserts for the most current information. Medications selected are considered to be among the top 100 most commonly prescribed medications in the NICU, per Stark, A., Smith, P. B., Hornik, C. P., Zimmerman, K. O., Hornik, C. D., Pradeep, S., Clark, R. H., Benjamin, D. K., Jr., Laughon, M., Greenberg, R. G. (2022). Medication use in the neonatal intensive care unit and changes from 2010 to 2018. *The Journal of Pediatrics, 240*, 66–71.e4. https://doi.org/10.1016/j.jpeds.2021.08.075.

FDA, U.S. Food and Drug Administration; HR, heart rate; TET, tetralogy of Fallot.

Source: [1]Taketomo, C. K. (Ed.). (2023). *Pediatric & neonatal dosage handbook: An extensive resource for clinicians treating pediatric and neonatal patients* (29th ed.). Lexicomp/Wolters Kluwer.

DRUG CLASS: Calcium Channel Blocker

MEDICATION NAME	FDA APPROVED FOR USE IN NICU?	MECHANISM OF ACTION	HALF-LIFE (BIRTH–AGE 2)	COMMON INDICATIONS FOR USE IN THE NICU	CLINICAL MONITORING CONSIDERATIONS
Amlodipine	No	Gradually interacts with calcium channel receptor sites, which inhibit the influx of calcium into the cardiomyocyte. Selective action at the vascular smooth muscle during phase 2 of the cardiac action potential. The effect is relaxation of the vascular smooth muscle (reducing the blood pressure) without a negative inotropic effect.[1]	No data in neonates Infants (>1 year of age): 21.8 hours[3]	• Hypertension	• Blood pressure • HR • General appearance (flushing) • Renal function
Nicardipine	No	Blocks the influx of calcium into the cardiomyocyte, selectively, at the vascular smooth muscle during phase 2 of the cardiac action potential. The effect is relaxation of the vascular smooth muscle (reducing the blood pressure) without a negative inotropic effect.[1,2]	No data in neonates and infants Adults: 40 minutes[2]	• Hypertension	• Blood pressure • General appearance (flushing) • HR (tachycardia) • Hepatic function • Renal function

Note: Content included in this table is intended for educational purposes only. The status of the FDA approvals and PK data may change over time. Readers are encouraged to consult package inserts for the most current information. Medications selected are considered to be among the top 100 most commonly prescribed medications in the NICU, per Stark, A., Smith, P. B., Hornik, C. P., Zimmerman, K. O., Hornik, C. D., Pradeep, S., Clark, R. H., Benjamin, D. K., Jr., Laughon, M., Greenberg, R. G. (2022). Medication use in the neonatal intensive care unit and changes from 2010 to 2018. *The Journal of Pediatrics, 240*, 66–71.e4. https://doi.org/10.1016/j.jpeds.2021.08.075.

FDA, U.S. Food and Drug Administration; HR, heart rate.

Sources: [1]Taketomo, C. K. (Ed.). (2023). *Pediatric & neonatal dosage handbook: An extensive resource for clinicians treating pediatric and neonatal patients* (29th ed.). Lexicomp/Wolters Kluwer; [2]Graham, D. J., Dow, R. J., Freedman, D., Mroszczak, E., & Ling, T. (1984). Pharmacokinetics of nicardipine following oral and intravenous administration in man. *Postgraduate Medical Journal, 60*(Suppl. 4), 7–10; [3]van der Vossen, A. C., Cransberg, K., de Winter, B. C. M., Schreuder, M. F., van Rooij-Kouwenhoven, R. W. G., Vulto, A. G., & Hanff, L. M. (2020). Use of amlodipine oral solution for the treatment of hypertension in children. *International Journal of Clinical Pharmacy, 42*(3), 848–852. https://doi.org/10.1007/s11096-020-01000-9

DRUG CLASS: Carbonic Anhydrase Inhibitor/Diuretic

MEDICATION NAME	FDA APPROVED FOR USE IN NICU?	MECHANISM OF ACTION	HALF-LIFE (BIRTH–AGE 2)	COMMON INDICATIONS FOR USE IN THE NICU	CLINICAL MONITORING CONSIDERATIONS
Acetazolamide	No	Inhibits carbonic anhydrase enzymes in the proximal tubule of the nephron, enzymes which normally encourage bicarbonate reabsorption. The inhibition of carbonic anhydrase enzymes encourages the secretion of bicarbonate, potassium, sodium, and water into the tubule while preserving the serum chloride concentration.[2]	No data in neonates and infants Adults: 2.4–5.8 hours[1]	• Metabolic alkalosis[2] • Edema	• Complete blood count • Growth velocity • Hepatic function • Renal function • Serum electrolytes

Note: Content included in this table is intended for educational purposes only. The status of the FDA approvals and PK data may change over time. Readers are encouraged to consult package inserts for the most current information. Medications selected are considered to be among the top 100 most commonly prescribed medications in the NICU, per Stark, A., Smith, P. B., Hornik, C. P., Zimmerman, K. O., Hornik, C. D., Pradeep, S., Clark, R. H., Benjamin, D. K., Jr., Laughon, M., Greenberg, R. G. (2022). Medication use in the neonatal intensive care unit and changes from 2010 to 2018. *The Journal of Pediatrics, 240,* 66–71.e4. https://doi.org/10.1016/j.jpeds.2021.08.075.
FDA, U.S. Food and Drug Administration.
Sources: [1]Taketomo, C. K. (Ed.). (2023). *Pediatric & neonatal dosage handbook: An extensive resource for clinicians treating pediatric and neonatal patients* (29th ed.). Lexicomp/Wolters Kluwer; [2]Tam, B., Chhay, A., Yen, L., Tesoriero, L., Ramanathan, R., Seri, I., & Friedlich, P. S. (2014). Acetazolamide for the management of chronic metabolic alkalosis in neonates and infants. *American Journal of Therapeutics, 21*(6), 477–481. https://doi.org/10.1097/MJT.0b013e31825e792c

DRUG CLASS: Endothelin Receptor Antagonist

MEDICATION NAME	FDA APPROVED FOR USE IN NICU?	MECHANISM OF ACTION	HALF-LIFE (BIRTH–AGE 2)	COMMON INDICATIONS FOR USE IN THE NICU	CLINICAL MONITORING CONSIDERATIONS
Bosentan	No	Inhibits endothelin-1, a potent vasoconstrictor, by way of antagonism at endothelin-1 A and B receptors.[1]	No data in neonates and infants	• Persistent pulmonary hypertension of the newborn	• Blood pressure • Complete blood count (leukopenia, anemia) • Hepatic function • Oxygen demand

Note: Content included in this table is intended for educational purposes only. The status of the FDA approvals and PK data may change over time. Readers are encouraged to consult package inserts for the most current information. Medications selected are considered to be among the top 100 most commonly prescribed medications in the NICU, per Stark, A., Smith, P. B., Hornik, C. P., Zimmerman, K. O., Hornik, C. D., Pradeep, S., Clark, R. H., Benjamin, D. K., Jr., Laughon, M., Greenberg, R. G. (2022). Medication use in the neonatal intensive care unit and changes from 2010 to 2018. *The Journal of Pediatrics, 240,* 66–71.e4. https://doi.org/10.1016/j.jpeds.2021.08.075.
FDA, U.S. Food and Drug Administration.
Sources: [1]Mandell, E., Kinsella, J. P., & Abman, S. H. (2021). Persistent pulmonary hypertension of the newborn. *Pediatric Pulmonology, 56*(3), 661–669. https://doi.org/10.1002/ppul.25073

DRUG CLASS: Loop Diuretics/Antihypertensive Agents

MEDICATION NAME	FDA APPROVED FOR USE IN NICU?	MECHANISM OF ACTION	HALF-LIFE (BIRTH–AGE 2)	COMMON INDICATIONS FOR USE IN THE NICU	CLINICAL MONITORING CONSIDERATIONS
Furosemide	No	Inhibits the sodium-potassium-chloride ($Na^+/K^+/2Cl^-$) cotransport system, which blocks the reabsorption of sodium, chloride, and potassium at the proximal and distal tubules as well as ascending loop of Henle. This facilitates losses of water, sodium, chloride, magnesium, and calcium to the urine.[2]	No data in neonates and infants Adults: 30 minutes–2 hours[1]	• Edema (peripheral or pulmonary) • Postblood transfusion therapy to prevent fluid overload • Tachypnea	• Audiology screening test results • Fluid status • Heart sounds • Hepatic function • Metabolic bone disease • Renal function • Serum electrolytes
Bumetanide	No	Inhibits the reabsorption of sodium and chloride at the ascending loop of Henle. This facilitates losses of water, sodium, chloride, magnesium, and calcium to the urine.[2]	Neonates (preterm/term): 6 hours[1] Infants (<2 months): 2.5 hours[1] Infants (>2–6 months): 1.5 hours[1]	• Edema	• Audiology screening test results • Blood pressure • Heart sounds • Hepatic function • Hydration/Fluid status • Metabolic bone disease • Renal function • Serum electrolytes

Note: Content included in this table is intended for educational purposes only. The status of the FDA approvals and PK data may change over time. Readers are encouraged to consult package inserts for the most current information. Medications selected are considered to be among the top 100 most commonly prescribed medications in the NICU, per Stark, A., Smith, P. B., Hornik, C. P., Zimmerman, K. O., Hornik, C. D., Pradeep, S., Clark, R. H., Benjamin, D. K., Jr., Laughon, M., Greenberg, R. G. (2022). Medication use in the neonatal intensive care unit and changes from 2010 to 2018. *The Journal of Pediatrics, 240,* 66–71.e4. https://doi.org/10.1016/j.jpeds.2021.08.075.

FDA, U.S. Food and Drug Administration.

Sources: [1]Taketomo, C. K. (Ed.). (2023). *Pediatric & neonatal dosage handbook: An extensive resource for clinicians treating pediatric and neonatal patients* (29th ed.). Lexicomp/Wolters Kluwer; [2]Thompson, E. J., Benjamin, D. K., Greenberg, R. G., Kumar, K. R., Zimmerman, K. O., Laughon, M., Clark, R. H., Smith, P. B., & Hornik, C. P. (2020). Pharmacoepidemiology of furosemide in the neonatal intensive care unit. *Neonatology, 117*(6), 780–784. https://doi.org/10.1159/000510657

DRUG CLASS: Potassium-Sparing Diuretics

MEDICATION NAME	FDA APPROVED FOR USE IN NICU?	MECHANISM OF ACTION	HALF-LIFE (BIRTH–AGE 2)	COMMON INDICATIONS FOR USE IN THE NICU	CLINICAL MONITORING CONSIDERATIONS
Spironolactone	No	Competes with aldosterone at mineralocorticoid receptors located within the distal collecting tubule. This inhibits potassium excretion at the distal collecting tubule. Sodium reabsorption decreases, whereas serum concentrations of potassium and hydrogen increase.[1,2]	No data in neonates and infants Adults: 1–2 hours[1]	• Bronchopulmonary dysplasia • Congenital adrenal hyperplasia • Edema • Hypertension	• Blood pressure • Hydration/Fluid status • Renal function • Serum electrolytes

Note: Content included in this table is intended for educational purposes only. The status of the FDA approvals and PK data may change over time. Readers are encouraged to consult package inserts for the most current information. Medications selected are considered to be among the top 100 most commonly prescribed medications in the NICU, per Stark, A., Smith, P. B., Hornik, C. P., Zimmerman, K. O., Hornik, C. D., Pradeep, S., Clark, R. H., Benjamin, D. K., Jr., Laughon, M., Greenberg, R. G. (2022). Medication use in the neonatal intensive care unit and changes from 2010 to 2018. *The Journal of Pediatrics, 240,* 66–71.e4. https://doi.org/10.1016/j.jpeds.2021.08.075.

FDA, U.S. Food and Drug Administration.

Sources: [1]Taketomo, C. K. (Ed.). (2023). *Pediatric & neonatal dosage handbook: An extensive resource for clinicians treating pediatric and neonatal patients* (29th ed.). Lexicomp/Wolters Kluwer; [2]Bestic, M. L., & Reed, M. D. (2012). Common diuretics used in the preterm and term infant: What's changed? *NeoReviews, 13*(7), e410–e419. https://doi.org/10.1542/neo.13-7-e410

DRUG CLASS: Thiazide Diuretics

MEDICATION NAME	FDA APPROVED FOR USE IN NICU?	MECHANISM OF ACTION	HALF-LIFE (BIRTH–AGE 2)	COMMON INDICATIONS FOR USE IN THE NICU	CLINICAL MONITORING CONSIDERATIONS
Chlorothiazide	Yes (oral only)	Inhibits the sodium-chloride transporter, which reduces membrane permeability to chloride and sodium at the distal collecting tubule. The result is diuresis (increased excretion of sodium, chloride, and water in the urine). Losses of potassium and hydrogen ions, phosphate, and bicarbonate also occur.[1,2]	No data in neonates and infants Adults: 45–120 minutes[1]	• Bronchopulmonary dysplasia • Congenital diabetes insipidus • Edema • Heart failure • Hyperinsulinemia/hypoglycemia • Hypertension	• Audiology screening results • Blood glucose • Blood pressure • Fluid status • Renal function • Serum electrolytes (hyponatremia, hypokalemia)
Hydrochlorothiazide	Yes	Inhibits the sodium-chloride transporter, which reduces membrane permeability to chloride and sodium at the distal collecting tubule. The result is increased excretion of sodium, chloride, and water in the urine.[1,2]	No data in neonates and infants Adults: 6–15 hours[1]	• Bronchopulmonary dysplasia • Congenital diabetes insipidus • Edema • Hypercalciuria • Hypertension	• Audiology screening results • Blood glucose • Blood pressure • Fluid status • Renal function • Serum electrolytes (hyponatremia, hypokalemia)

Note: Content included in this table is intended for educational purposes only. The status of the FDA approvals and PK data may change over time. Readers are encouraged to consult package inserts for the most current information. Medications selected are considered to be among the top 100 most commonly prescribed medications in the NICU, per Stark, A., Smith, P. B., Hornik, C. P., Zimmerman, K. O., Hornik, C. D., Pradeep, S., Clark, R. H., Benjamin, D. K., Jr., Laughon, M., Greenberg, R. G. (2022). Medication use in the neonatal intensive care unit and changes from 2010 to 2018. *The Journal of Pediatrics, 240*, 66–71.e4. https://doi.org/10.1016/j.jpeds.2021.08.075.

FDA, U.S. Food and Drug Administration.

Sources: [1]Taketomo, C. K. (Ed.). (2023). *Pediatric & neonatal dosage handbook: An extensive resource for clinicians treating pediatric and neonatal patients* (29th ed.). Lexicomp/Wolters Kluwer; [2]Bestic, M. L., & Reed, M. D. (2012). Common diuretics used in the preterm and term infant: What's changed? *NeoReviews, 13*(7), e410–e419. https://doi.org/10.1542/neo.13-7-e410

DRUG CLASS: Nonsteroidal Anti-Inflammatory Drugs

MEDICATION NAME	FDA APPROVED FOR USE IN NEONATES?	MECHANISM OF ACTION	HALF-LIFE (BIRTH–AGE 2)	COMMON INDICATIONS FOR USE IN THE NICU	CLINICAL MONITORING CONSIDERATIONS
Acetaminophen	No	Inhibits peroxidase, which prevents the conversion of arachidonic acid into prostaglandins. This leads to constriction of the smooth muscle wall of the ductus arteriosus and anatomical ductal closure. In addition, inhibition of prostaglandin synthesis in the central nervous system is thought to elicit analgesia and antipyresis.	Neonates: 4–25 hours[1] Infants: 1–5 hours[1]	• Analgesia • Closure of PDA	For analgesia: • Pain scores and indices For PDA closure: • Hepatic function • Renal function
Ibuprofen	Yes, limited approvals Oral analgesia: ≥6 months of age IV ibuprofen lysine: ≤32 weeks' gestation and weighing 500–1,500 grams	Inhibits cyclooxygenase (COX-1 and COX-2), which prevents the conversion of arachidonic acid into prostaglandins. This leads to constriction of the smooth muscle wall of the ductus arteriosus and anatomical ductal closure. In addition, inhibition of prostaglandin synthesis in the central nervous system is thought to elicit analgesia and antipyresis.	Data in neonates is highly variable Oral dosing in infants >3 months: 1.6±0.7 hours[1] IV dosing in infants (6 months–2 years): 1.8 hours[1]	• Analgesia • Closure of PDA	• Blood glucose • Cardiovascular function (pulmonary hypertension) • Complete blood count • Gastrointestinal integrity • Hepatic function • Renal function • Serum electrolytes • Signs of bleeding • Signs and symptoms of infection

Indomethacin	Yes, limited approval IV: Limited to PDA closure among neonates weighing, 500–1,750 grams	Inhibits cyclooxygenase (COX-1 and COX-2), which prevents the conversion of arachidonic acid into prostaglandins. This leads to constriction of the smooth muscle wall of the ductus arteriosus and anatomical ductal closure.	Neonates (<2 weeks): 20 hours Neonates and infants (>2 weeks): 11 hours[1]	• Closure of PDA • IVH prevention	• Blood glucose • Cardiovascular function • Complete blood count • Gastrointestinal integrity • Hepatic function • Renal function • Serum electrolytes • Signs of bleeding • Signs and symptoms of infection

Note: Content included in this table is intended for educational purposes only. The status of the FDA approvals and PK data may change over time. Readers are encouraged to consult package inserts for the most current information. Medications selected are considered to be among the top 100 most commonly prescribed medications in the NICU, per Stark, A., Smith, P. B., Hornik, C. P., Zimmerman, K. O., Hornik, C. D., Pradeep, S., Clark, R. H., Benjamin, D. K., Jr., Laughon, M., Greenberg, R. G. (2022). Medication use in the neonatal intensive care unit and changes from 2010 to 2018. *The Journal of Pediatrics, 240*, 66–71.e4. https://doi.org/10.1016/j.jpeds.2021.08.075.

COX, cyclooxygenase; FDA, U.S. Food and Drug Administration; IV, intravenous; IVH, intraventricular hemorrhage; PDA, patent ductus arteriosus.

Source: [1]Taketomo, C. K. (Ed.). (2023). *Pediatric & neonatal dosage handbook: An extensive resource for clinicians treating pediatric and neonatal patients* (29th ed.). Lexicomp/Wolters Kluwer.

DRUG CLASS: Phosphodiesterase Inhibitors

MEDICATION NAME	FDA APPROVED FOR USE IN NICU?	MECHANISM OF ACTION	HALF-LIFE (BIRTH–AGE 2)	COMMON INDICATIONS FOR USE IN THE NICU	CLINICAL MONITORING CONSIDERATIONS
Milrinone	No	Selective phosphodiesterase inhibitor in cardiac and vascular tissue. Increases cardiac output by decreasing afterload and causes pulmonary artery vasodilatation and subsequently leads to a reduction in pulmonary artery pressure by increasing cAMP.	No data in neonates Infants: 3.15 ± 2 hours[1]	• Heart failure • Persistent pulmonary hypertension of the newborn • Postoperative low cardiac output syndrome • Shock	• Blood pressure • HR • Renal function • Serum electrolytes
Sildenafil	No	Inhibits the ability of phosphodiesterase type 5 to degrade cGMP, a nucleotide that decreases vascular tone. The accumulation of cGMP reduces smooth muscle tone within the pulmonary vasculature, which decreases pulmonary vascular resistance.	Neonates (day 1 of life): 55.9 hours[1] Neonates (day 7 of life): 47.7 hours[1]	• Persistent pulmonary hypertension of the newborn	• Blood pressure • HR • Hepatic function • Oxygenation

Note: Content included in this table is intended for educational purposes only. The status of the FDA approvals and PK data may change over time. Readers are encouraged to consult package inserts for the most current information. Medications selected are considered to be among the top 100 most commonly prescribed medications in the NICU, per Stark, A., Smith, P. B., Hornik, C. P., Zimmerman, K. O., Hornik, C. D., Pradeep, S., Clark, R. H., Benjamin, D. K., Jr., Laughon, M., Greenberg, R. G. (2022). Medication use in the neonatal intensive care unit and changes from 2010 to 2018. *The Journal of Pediatrics, 240,* 66–71.e4. https://doi.org/10.1016/j.jpeds.2021.08.075.

cAMP, cyclic adenosine monophosphate; cGMP, cyclic guanosine monophosphate; FDA, U.S. Food and Drug Administration; HR, heart rate.

Source: [1]Taketomo, C. K. (Ed.). (2023). *Pediatric & neonatal dosage handbook: An extensive resource for clinicians treating pediatric and neonatal patients* (29th ed.). Lexicomp/Wolters Kluwer.

DRUG CLASS: Prostaglandin Vasodilator

MEDICATION NAME	FDA APPROVED FOR USE IN NICU?	MECHANISM OF ACTION	HALF-LIFE (BIRTH–AGE 2)	COMMON INDICATIONS FOR USE IN THE NICU	CLINICAL MONITORING CONSIDERATIONS
Alprostadil	Yes, limited to temporarily maintain patency of ductus arteriosus pending corrective or palliative cardiovascular surgery.[1]	Selective relaxation of vascular and ductus arteriosus smooth muscle	5–10 minutes	• Congenital diaphragmatic hernia with severe pulmonary hypertension • Ductus arteriosus patency (congenital cyanotic heart defects)	• Blood pressure • Gastrointestinal function • Oxygenation • Respiratory rate • Skin color • Serum pH • Temperature

Note: Content included in this table is intended for educational purposes only. The status of the FDA approvals and PK data may change over time. Readers are encouraged to consult package inserts for the most current information. Medications selected are considered to be among the top 100 most commonly prescribed medications in the NICU, per Stark, A., Smith, P. B., Hornik, C. P., Zimmerman, K. O., Hornik, C. D., Pradeep, S., Clark, R. H., Benjamin, D. K., Jr., Laughon, M., Greenberg, R. G. (2022). Medication use in the neonatal intensive care unit and changes from 2010 to 2018. *The Journal of Pediatrics, 240*, 66–71.e4. https://doi.org/10.1016/j.jpeds.2021.08.075.

FDA, U.S. Food and Drug Administration.

Source: [1]Center for Drug Evaluation and Research. (1998, January 20). *Approval package for Alprostadil injection.* https://www.accessdata.fda.gov/drugsatfda_docs/anda/98/074815ap.pdf

COMMON GASTROINTESTINAL SYSTEM MEDICATIONS

DRUG CLASS: Antacid

MEDICATION NAME	FDA APPROVED FOR USE IN NICU?	MECHANISM OF ACTION	HALF-LIFE (BIRTH–AGE 2)	COMMON INDICATIONS FOR USE IN THE NICU	CLINICAL MONITORING CONSIDERATIONS
Aluminum and magnesium hydroxide	No	Neutralizes gastric acidity and increases gastric pH by acting as a buffer. Inhibits pepsin's ability to break down proteins in the stomach.	Not reported	• Esophagitis • Gastritis • GERD • Hiatal hernia	• Gastrointestinal function (constipation) • Renal function • Serum electrolytes (hyperalbuminemia, hypophosphatemia, hypermagnesemia)

Note: Content included in this table is intended for educational purposes only. The status of the FDA approvals and PK data may change over time. Readers are encouraged to consult package inserts for the most current information. Medications selected are considered to be among the top 100 most commonly prescribed medications in the NICU, per Stark, A., Smith, P. B., Hornik, C. P., Zimmerman, K. O., Hornik, C. D., Pradeep, S., Clark, R. H., Benjamin, D. K., Jr., Laughon, M., Greenberg, R. G. (2022). Medication use in the neonatal intensive care unit and changes from 2010 to 2018. *The Journal of Pediatrics, 240,* 66–71.e4. https://doi.org/10.1016/j.jpeds.2021.08.075. FDA, U.S. Food and Drug Administration; GERD, gastroesophageal reflux disease.

DRUG CLASS: Histamine H2 Antagonist

MEDICATION NAME	FDA APPROVED FOR USE IN NICU?	MECHANISM OF ACTION	HALF-LIFE (BIRTH–AGE 2)	COMMON INDICATIONS FOR USE IN THE NICU	CLINICAL MONITORING CONSIDERATIONS
Famotidine	Yes	Inhibits histamine binding at H2 receptors of the gastric parietal cells, which inhibits gastric acid secretion.	Neonates and infants (<3 months of age): 8.1 ± 3.5 hours to 10.5 ± 5.4 hours[1] Infants (3–12 months of age): 4.5 ± 1.1 hours[1] Infants and children (>12 months –12 years of age): 2.3 ± 0.4 hours[1]	• Gastrointestinal ulcerations • GERD • Hypersecretory conditions	• Feeding tolerance • Renal function

Note: Content included in this table is intended for educational purposes only. The status of the FDA approvals and PK data may change over time. Readers are encouraged to consult package inserts for the most current information. Medications selected are considered to be among the top 100 most commonly prescribed medications in the NICU, per Stark, A., Smith, P. B., Hornik, C. P., Zimmerman, K. O., Hornik, C. D., Pradeep, S., Clark, R. H., Benjamin, D. K., Jr., Laughon, M., Greenberg, R. G. (2022). Medication use in the neonatal intensive care unit and changes from 2010 to 2018. *The Journal of Pediatrics, 240,* 66–71.e4. https://doi.org/10.1016/j.jpeds.2021.08.075. FDA, U.S. Food and Drug Administration; GERD, gastroesophageal reflux disease.

Sources: [1]Taketomo, C. K. (Ed.). (2023). *Pediatric & neonatal dosage handbook: An extensive resource for clinicians treating pediatric and neonatal patients* (29th ed.). Lexicomp/Wolters Kluwer.

DRUG CLASS: Proton-Pump Inhibitor

MEDICATION NAME	FDA APPROVED FOR USE IN NICU?	MECHANISM OF ACTION	HALF-LIFE (BIRTH–AGE 2)	COMMON INDICATIONS FOR USE IN THE NICU	CLINICAL MONITORING CONSIDERATIONS
Lansoprazole	No	Inhibits hydrogen-potassium-ATPase, which is the enzyme that causes the secretion of hydrochloric acid by the gastric parietal cell.	Less than 2 hours[1,3] *Acid inhibitory effect lasts >24 hours.*[2]	• Esophagitis (secondary to GERD) • Gastrointestinal ulcerations	• Feeding tolerance • Hepatic function
Omeprazole	Yes, >1 month of age	Inhibits hydrogen-potassium-ATPase, which is the enzyme that causes the secretion of hydrochloric acid by the gastric parietal cell.	30 minutes–2 hours	• Esophagitis (secondary to GERD) • Gastrointestinal ulcerations	• Feeding tolerance • Hepatic function (alkaline phosphatase level)

Note: Content included in this table is intended for educational purposes only. The status of the FDA approvals and PK data may change over time. Readers are encouraged to consult package inserts for the most current information. Medications selected are considered to be among the top 100 most commonly prescribed medications in the NICU, per Stark, A., Smith, P. B., Hornik, C. P., Zimmerman, K. O., Hornik, C. D., Pradeep, S., Clark, R. H., Benjamin, D. K., Jr., Laughon, M., Greenberg, R. G. (2022). Medication use in the neonatal intensive care unit and changes from 2010 to 2018. *The Journal of Pediatrics, 240,* 66–71.e4. https://doi.org/10.1016/j.jpeds.2021.08.075. FDA, U.S. Food and Drug Administration; GERD, gastroesophageal reflux disease.

Sources: [1]Taketomo, C. K. (Ed.). (2023). *Pediatric & neonatal dosage handbook: An extensive resource for clinicians treating pediatric and neonatal patients* (29th ed.). Lexicomp/Wolters Kluwer; [2]Zhang, W., Kukulka, M., Witt, G., Sutkowski-Markmann, D., North, J., & Atkinson, S. (2008). Age-dependent pharmacokinetics of lansoprazole in neonates and infants. *Pediatric Drugs, 10*(4), 265–274. https://doi.org/10.2165/00148581-200810040-00005; [3]IBM Watson Health. (2021). *IBM Micromedex NEOFAX* [electronic version]. https://www.ibm.com/products/micromedex-neofax-pediatrics

DRUG CLASS: Anti-Flatulence

MEDICATION NAME	FDA APPROVED FOR USE IN NICU?	MECHANISM OF ACTION	HALF-LIFE (BIRTH–AGE 2)	COMMON INDICATIONS FOR USE IN THE NICU	CLINICAL MONITORING CONSIDERATIONS
Simethicone	Yes	Nonsystemic surfactant that reduces surface tension among gastrointestinal gas bubbles. This action causes the bubbles to disperse, which facilitates elimination and relief of gas pains.[1]	Not reported	• Gas pain	• Gastrointestinal function (loose stools)[2]

Note: Content included in this table is intended for educational purposes only. The status of the FDA approvals and PK data may change over time. Readers are encouraged to consult package inserts for the most current information. Medications selected are considered to be among the top 100 most commonly prescribed medications in the NICU, per Stark, A., Smith, P. B., Hornik, C. P., Zimmerman, K. O., Hornik, C. D., Pradeep, S., Clark, R. H., Benjamin, D. K., Jr., Laughon, M., Greenberg, R. G. (2022). Medication use in the neonatal intensive care unit and changes from 2010 to 2018. *The Journal of Pediatrics, 240,* 66–71.e4. https://doi.org/10.1016/j.jpeds.2021.08.075. FDA, U.S. Food and Drug Administration.

Sources: [1]Taketomo, C. K. (Ed.). (2023). *Pediatric & neonatal dosage handbook: An extensive resource for clinicians treating pediatric and neonatal patients* (29th ed.). Lexicomp/Wolters Kluwer; [2]IBM Watson Health. (2021). *IBM Micromedex NEOFAX* [electronic version]. https://www.ibm.com/products/micromedex-neofax-pediatrics

DRUG CLASS: Nutritional Supplements

MEDICATION NAME	FDA APPROVED FOR USE IN NICU?	MECHANISM OF ACTION	HALF-LIFE (BIRTH–AGE 2)	COMMON INDICATIONS FOR USE IN THE NICU	CLINICAL MONITORING CONSIDERATIONS
Vitamin A	Yes, specific to IM dosing for vitamin A deficiency	Vitamin supplement used in preterm infants for the prevention of BPD. Four mechanisms of action are proposed: (a) promotes normal lung development by facilitating epithelial cell growth, differentiation, development, and maturation; (b) decreases oxygen-induced lung damage; (c) exerts an anti-infective effect by modulating the immune response; and (d) facilitates lung tissue repair.	12 days[2]	• Prevention of BPD • Vitamin A deficiency (in preterm infants)	• Hepatic assessment (hepatomegaly) • Neurologic assessment (Bulging fontanel in the absence of IVH, irritability, lethargy)[3] • Skin changes[3]
Cholecalciferol (Vitamin D_3)	Yes	Stimulates calcium and phosphate absorption from the small intestine, promotes secretion of calcium from bone to blood; promotes renal tubule phosphate resorption[1]	19–25 hours (adults)	• Vitamin D deficiency, prevention or treatment	• Hepatic function (alkaline phosphatase) • Renal function • Serum 25(OH)D monitoring (interval measurements, as needed) • Serum electrolytes (calcium, phosphorus)
Ferrous sulfate (oral)	Yes	Augments or replaces endogenous iron stores, which facilitate oxygen transport[1]	Not reported	• Iron deficiency, prevention or treatment • Adjunctive therapy with epoetin dosing	• Ferritin • Hemoglobin, hematocrit • Reticulocyte count

Note: Content included in this table is intended for educational purposes only. The status of the FDA approvals and PK data may change over time. Readers are encouraged to consult package inserts for the most current information. Medications selected are considered to be among the top 100 most commonly prescribed medications in the NICU, per Stark, A., Smith, P. B., Hornik, C. P., Zimmerman, K. O., Hornik, C. D., Pradeep, S., Clark, R. H., Benjamin, D. K., Jr., Laughon, M., Greenberg, R. G. (2022). Medication use in the neonatal intensive care unit and changes from 2010 to 2018. *The Journal of Pediatrics, 240*, 66–71.e4. https://doi.org/10.1016/j.jpeds.2021.08.075.

BPD, bronchopulmonary dysplasia; FDA, U.S. Food and Drug Administration; IM, intramuscular; IVH, intraventricular hemorrhage.

Sources: [1]Taketomo, C. K. (Ed.). (2023). *Pediatric & neonatal dosage handbook: An extensive resource for clinicians treating pediatric and neonatal patients* (29th ed.). Lexicomp/Wolters Kluwer; [2]IBM Watson Health. (2021). *IBM Micromedex NEOFAX* [electronic version]. https://www.ibm.com/products/micromedex-neofax-pediatrics; [3]Rakshasbhuvankar, A. A., Simmer, K., Patole, S. K., Stoecklin, B., Nathan, E. A., Clarke, M. W., & Pillow, J. J. (2021). Enteral vitamin A for reducing severity of bronchopulmonary dysplasia: A randomized trial. *Pediatrics, 147*(1), Article e2020009985. https://doi.org/10.1542/peds.2020-009985

COMMON HEMATOLOGIC SYSTEM MEDICATIONS

DRUG CLASS: Erythropoietin-Stimulating Agent

MEDICATION NAME	FDA APPROVED FOR USE IN NICU?	MECHANISM OF ACTION	HALF-LIFE (BIRTH–AGE 2)	COMMON INDICATIONS FOR USE IN THE NICU	CLINICAL MONITORING CONSIDERATIONS
Epoetin alfa	Yes, >1 month of age for anemia associated with chronic kidney disease	Stimulates terminal erythropoiesis within the bone marrow by binding to erythropoietin receptors on progenitor cells. This elicits a hierarchical and stepwise signaling process, which ultimately leads to increased proliferation of mature red blood cells. Stimulates increased neurogenesis, oligodendrocyte differentiation and maturation, and white matter integrity. A decrease in neuronal apoptosis and inflammation is also reported.	Neonates (<32 weeks' PMA) IV dosing: 8.1 ± 2.7 hours[1] Neonates (<32 weeks' PMA) SubQ dosing: 71 ± 4.1 hours[1] Neonates (≥32 weeks' PMA): SubQ dosing: 7.9 hours[1]	• Anemia of prematurity	• Ferritin level • Hemoglobin • Reticulocyte count

Note: Content included in this table is intended for educational purposes only. The status of the FDA approvals and PK data may change over time. Readers are encouraged to consult package inserts for the most current information. Medications selected are considered to be among the top 100 most commonly prescribed medications in the NICU, per Stark, A., Smith, P. B., Hornik, C. P., Zimmerman, K. O., Hornik, C. D., Pradeep, S., Clark, R. H., Benjamin, D. K., Jr., Laughon, M., Greenberg, R. G. (2022). Medication use in the neonatal intensive care unit and changes from 2010 to 2018. *The Journal of Pediatrics, 240*, 66–71.e4. https://doi.org/10.1016/j.jpeds.2021.08.075.

FDA, U.S. Food and Drug Administration; PMA, postmenstrual age; SubQ, subcutaneous.

Source: [1]Taketomo, C. K. (Ed.). (2023). *Pediatric & neonatal dosage handbook: An extensive resource for clinicians treating pediatric and neonatal patients* (29th ed.). Lexicomp/Wolters Kluwer.

DRUG CLASS: Enzyme

MEDICATION NAME	FDA APPROVED FOR USE IN NICU?	MECHANISM OF ACTION	HALF-LIFE (BIRTH–AGE 2)	COMMON INDICATIONS FOR USE IN THE NICU	CLINICAL MONITORING CONSIDERATIONS
Hyaluronidase	Yes	Hydrolyzes hyaluronic acid, which increases the permeability of connective tissue. This facilitates the diffusion (egress) of vesicant fluids from a site of extravasation.	Not reported	• Extravasation	• Skin integrity • Pulses and perfusion (increased risk for altered perfusion and compartment syndrome distal to extravasation) • Vital signs (pain related)

Note: Content included in this table is intended for educational purposes only. The status of the FDA approvals and PK data may change over time. Readers are encouraged to consult package inserts for the most current information. Medications selected are considered to be among the top 100 most commonly prescribed medications in the NICU, per Stark, A., Smith, P. B., Hornik, C. P., Zimmerman, K. O., Hornik, C. D., Pradeep, S., Clark, R. H., Benjamin, D. K., Jr., Laughon, M., Greenberg, R. G. (2022). Medication use in the neonatal intensive care unit and changes from 2010 to 2018. *The Journal of Pediatrics, 240,* 66–71.e4. https://doi.org/10.1016/j.jpeds.2021.08.075.
FDA, U.S. Food and Drug Administration.

DRUG CLASS: Colony-Stimulating Factor

MEDICATION NAME	FDA APPROVED FOR USE IN NICU?	MECHANISM OF ACTION	HALF-LIFE (BIRTH–AGE 2)	COMMON INDICATIONS FOR USE IN THE NICU	CLINICAL MONITORING CONSIDERATIONS
Filgrastim	Yes	Stimulates the synthesis of neutrophils	Neonates: ~4 hours[1]	• Neutropenia	• Neutrophil count • Platelet count • Renal function • Hepatic function • Temperature

Note: Content included in this table is intended for educational purposes only. The status of the FDA approvals and PK data may change over time. Readers are encouraged to consult package inserts for the most current information. Medications selected are considered to be among the top 100 most commonly prescribed medications in the NICU, per Stark, A., Smith, P. B., Hornik, C. P., Zimmerman, K. O., Hornik, C. D., Pradeep, S., Clark, R. H., Benjamin, D. K., Jr., Laughon, M., Greenberg, R. G. (2022). Medication use in the neonatal intensive care unit and changes from 2010 to 2018. *The Journal of Pediatrics, 240,* 66–71.e4. https://doi.org/10.1016/j.jpeds.2021.08.075.
FDA, U.S. Food and Drug Administration.
Source: [1]Taketomo, C. K. (Ed.). (2023). *Pediatric & neonatal dosage handbook: An extensive resource for clinicians treating pediatric and neonatal patients* (29th ed.). Lexicomp/Wolters Kluwer.

COMMON ENDOCRINE SYSTEM MEDICATIONS

DRUG CLASS: Adrenal Corticosteroids

MEDICATION NAME	FDA APPROVED FOR USE IN NEONATES?	MECHANISM OF ACTION	HALF-LIFE (BIRTH–AGE 2)	COMMON INDICATIONS FOR USE IN THE NICU	CLINICAL MONITORING CONSIDERATIONS
Dexamethasone	No	Long-acting corticosteroid that elicits anti-inflammatory and immunosuppressive activity	Extremely-low-birth-weight infants (with BPD): 9.26 ± 3.34 hours[1] Infants (>4 months) and children: 4.34 ± 4.14 hours[1]	• Airway edema • BPD (to facilitate extubation)	• Blood pressure • Blood glucose • Growth velocity • Hemoglobin concentration • Infection • Renal function • Serum electrolytes • Echocardiogram (hypertrophic cardiomy-opathy)
Hydrocortisone	No	Short-acting corticosteroid that elicits anti-inflammatory and immunosuppressive activity	~3 hours	• BPD • Congenital adrenal hyperplasia • Hypoglycemia (refractory) • Hypotension	• Cortisol • Blood pressure • Blood glucose • Growth velocity • Hemoglobin concentration • Infection • Renal function • Serum electrolytes

Note: Content included in this table is intended for educational purposes only. The status of the FDA approvals and PK data may change over time. Readers are encouraged to consult package inserts for the most current information. Medications selected are considered to be among the top 100 most commonly prescribed medications in the NICU, per Stark, A., Smith, P. B., Hornik, C. P., Zimmerman, K. O., Hornik, C. D., Pradeep, S., Clark, R. H., Benjamin, D. K., Jr., Laughon, M., Greenberg, R. G. (2022). Medication use in the neonatal intensive care unit and changes from 2010 to 2018. *The Journal of Pediatrics, 240*, 66–71.e4. https://doi.org/10.1016/j.jpeds.2021.08.075.

BPD, bronchopulmonary dysplasia; FDA, U.S. Food and Drug Administration.

Source: [1]Taketomo, C. K. (Ed.). (2023). *Pediatric & neonatal dosage handbook: An extensive resource for clinicians treating pediatric and neonatal patients* (29th ed.). Lexicomp/Wolters Kluwer.

DRUG CLASS: Insulin

MEDICATION NAME	FDA APPROVED FOR USE IN NEONATES?	MECHANISM OF ACTION	HALF-LIFE (BIRTH–AGE 2)	COMMON INDICATIONS FOR USE IN THE NICU	CLINICAL MONITORING CONSIDERATIONS
Regular insulin	No	Regulates the metabolism of macronutrients (carbohydrates, protein, fat) by stimulating hepatic glycogen synthesis.[1]	Onset of action: ~30–60 minutes	• Refractory hyperglycemia	• Glucose (hypoglycemia) • Renal function • Serum electrolytes (hypokalemia)

Note: Content included in this table is intended for educational purposes only. The status of the FDA approvals and PK data may change over time. Readers are encouraged to consult package inserts for the most current information. Medications selected are considered to be among the top 100 most commonly prescribed medications in the NICU, per Stark, A., Smith, P. B., Hornik, C. P., Zimmerman, K. O., Hornik, C. D., Pradeep, S., Clark, R. H., Benjamin, D. K., Jr., Laughon, M., Greenberg, R. G. (2022). Medication use in the neonatal intensive care unit and changes from 2010 to 2018. *The Journal of Pediatrics, 240*, 66–71.e4. https://doi.org/10.1016/j.jpeds.2021.08.075.

FDA, U.S. Food and Drug Administration.

Source: [1]Taketomo, C. K. (Ed.). (2023). *Pediatric & neonatal dosage handbook: An extensive resource for clinicians treating pediatric and neonatal patients* (29th ed.). Lexicomp/Wolters Kluwer.

DRUG CLASS: Thyroid Product

MEDICATION NAME	FDA APPROVED FOR USE IN NEONATES?	MECHANISM OF ACTION	HALF-LIFE (BIRTH–AGE 2)	COMMON INDICATIONS FOR USE IN THE NICU	CLINICAL MONITORING CONSIDERATIONS
Levothyroxine	Yes, for the treatment of congenital hypothyroidism	Regulates metabolism, growth, and development in the thyroid gland, including promotion of gluconeogenesis, mobilization of glycogen stores, and stimulation of protein synthesis.[1]	9–10 days (adults)[1]	• Congenital hypothyroidism	• Blood pressure • Growth velocity • HR • Renal function • Thyroid function (TSH, free T4)

Note: Content included in this table is intended for educational purposes only. The status of the FDA approvals and PK data may change over time. Readers are encouraged to consult package inserts for the most current information. Medications selected are considered to be among the top 100 most commonly prescribed medications in the NICU, per Stark, A., Smith, P. B., Hornik, C. P., Zimmerman, K. O., Hornik, C. D., Pradeep, S., Clark, R. H., Benjamin, D. K., Jr., Laughon, M., Greenberg, R. G. (2022). Medication use in the neonatal intensive care unit and changes from 2010 to 2018. *The Journal of Pediatrics, 240*, 66–71.e4. https://doi.org/10.1016/j.jpeds.2021.08.075.

FDA, U.S. Food and Drug Administration; HR, heart rate.

Source: [1]Taketomo, C. K. (Ed.). (2023). *Pediatric & neonatal dosage handbook: An extensive resource for clinicians treating pediatric and neonatal patients* (29th ed.). Lexicomp/Wolters Kluwer.

DRUG CLASS: Bile Acid Sequestrants

MEDICATION NAME	FDA APPROVED FOR USE IN NEONATES?	MECHANISM OF ACTION	HALF-LIFE (BIRTH–AGE 2)	COMMON INDICATIONS FOR USE IN THE NICU	CLINICAL MONITORING CONSIDERATIONS
Cholestyramine	No	Binds to bile acids at the intestinal lumen, preventing the normal reabsorption of bile acids and reducing the quantity of stools. Consequently, this action may interfere with fat digestion and the absorption of fat-soluble vitamins.[1]	Not reported	• Cholestasis • Congenital chloride diarrhea	• Growth velocity • Serum electrolytes (delayed/reduced absorption of thiazide diuretics with concomitant use) • Stooling frequency • Thyroid function

Note: Content included in this table is intended for educational purposes only. The status of the FDA approvals and PK data may change over time. Readers are encouraged to consult package inserts for the most current information. Medications selected are considered to be among the top 100 most commonly prescribed medications in the NICU, per Stark, A., Smith, P. B., Hornik, C. P., Zimmerman, K. O., Hornik, C. D., Pradeep, S., Clark, R. H., Benjamin, D. K., Jr., Laughon, M., Greenberg, R. G. (2022). Medication use in the neonatal intensive care unit and changes from 2010 to 2018. *The Journal of Pediatrics, 240,* 66–71.e4. https://doi.org/10.1016/j.jpeds.2021.08.075.
FDA, U.S. Food and Drug Administration.
Source: [1]Taketomo, C. K. (Ed.). (2023). *Pediatric & neonatal dosage handbook: An extensive resource for clinicians treating pediatric and neonatal patients* (29th ed.). Lexicomp/Wolters Kluwer.

DRUG CLASS: Gallstone Dissolution Agent

MEDICATION NAME	FDA APPROVED FOR USE IN NICU?	MECHANISM OF ACTION	HALF-LIFE (BIRTH–AGE 2)	COMMON INDICATIONS FOR USE IN THE NICU	CLINICAL MONITORING CONSIDERATIONS
Ursodeoxycholic acid	No	Decreases the cholesterol content of bile and bile stones by reducing the secretion of cholesterol from the liver and the fractional reabsorption of cholesterol by the intestines.[1]	3–6 days[2]	• Biliary atresia • Cholestasis	• Hepatic function • Feeding tolerance

Note: Content included in this table is intended for educational purposes only. The status of the FDA approvals and PK data may change over time. Readers are encouraged to consult package inserts for the most current information. Medications selected are considered to be among the top 100 most commonly prescribed medications in the NICU, per Stark, A., Smith, P. B., Hornik, C. P., Zimmerman, K. O., Hornik, C. D., Pradeep, S., Clark, R. H., Benjamin, D. K., Jr., Laughon, M., Greenberg, R. G. (2022). Medication use in the neonatal intensive care unit and changes from 2010 to 2018. *The Journal of Pediatrics, 240,* 66–71.e4. https://doi.org/10.1016/j.jpeds.2021.08.075.
FDA, U.S. Food and Drug Administration.
Sources: [1]Taketomo, C. K. (Ed.). (2023). *Pediatric & neonatal dosage handbook: An extensive resource for clinicians treating pediatric and neonatal patients* (29th ed.). Lexicomp/Wolters Kluwer; [2]IBM Watson Health. (2021). *IBM Micromedex NEOFAX* [electronic version]. https://www.ibm.com/products/micromedex-neofax-pediatrics

COMMON INFECTIOUS DISEASE MEDICATIONS

DRUG CLASS: Antiviral Agents

MEDICATION NAME	FDA APPROVED FOR USE IN NICU?	MECHANISM OF ACTION	HALF-LIFE (BIRTH–AGE 2)	COMMON INDICATIONS FOR USE IN THE NICU	CLINICAL MONITORING CONSIDERATIONS
Acyclovir • *Most commonly prescribed antiviral agent*	Parenteral: Yes, for the treatment and prophylaxis of HSV-1 and HSV-2. Oral: Yes, after parenteral treatment for HSV infections	Inhibits viral DNA polymerase synthesis and terminates viral replication[2]	Neonates and infants (<3 months): 3.8 ± 1.2 hours[1] Infants (>3 months–<12 years): 2.36 ± 0.97 hours[1]	• HSV • VZV	• Complete blood count (neutropenia, anemia, thrombocytopenia) • Liver function (hyperbilirubinemia) • Renal function (hematuria, interstitial nephritis, and obstruction from formation of acyclovir crystals)

Note: Content included in this table is intended for educational purposes only. The status of the FDA approvals and PK data may change over time. Readers are encouraged to consult package inserts for the most current information. Medications selected are considered to be among the top 100 most commonly prescribed medications in the NICU, per Stark, A., Smith, P. B., Hornik, C. P., Zimmerman, K. O., Hornik, C. D., Pradeep, S., Clark, R. H., Benjamin, D. K., Jr., Laughon, M., Greenberg, R. G. (2022). Medication use in the neonatal intensive care unit and changes from 2010 to 2018. *The Journal of Pediatrics, 240,* 66–71.e4. https://doi.org/10.1016/j.jpeds.2021.08.075.

FDA, U.S. Food and Drug Administration; HSV, herpes simplex virus; VZV, varicella zoster virus.

Sources: [1]Taketomo, C. K. (Ed.). (2023). *Pediatric & neonatal dosage handbook: An extensive resource for clinicians treating pediatric and neonatal patients* (29th ed.). Lexicomp/Wolters Kluwer; [2]Whitley, R. J. (2012). The use of antiviral drugs during the neonatal period. *Clinics in Perinatology, 39*(1), 69–81. https://doi.org/10.1016/j.clp.2011.12.004

DRUG CLASS: Antiretroviral Agents

MEDICATION NAME	FDA APPROVED FOR USE IN NICU?	MECHANISM OF ACTION	HALF-LIFE (BIRTH–AGE 2)	COMMON INDICATIONS FOR USE IN THE NICU	CLINICAL MONITORING CONSIDERATIONS
Zidovudine	Yes	Thymidine analog that inhibits HIV-specific reverse transcriptase enzyme, preventing viral synthesis and replication	Preterm neonates: 6.3 hours[1] Term infants: 3.1 hours[1] Infants (14 days–3 months): 1.9 hours[1] Infants/children (3 months–12 years): 1.5 hours[1]	• Congenital HIV • Prevention of perinatal HIV transmission	• Complete blood count (anemia, neutropenia)

Note: Content included in this table is intended for educational purposes only. The status of the FDA approvals and PK data may change over time. Readers are encouraged to consult package inserts for the most current information. Medications selected are considered to be among the top 100 most commonly prescribed medications in the NICU, pe- Stark, A., Smith, P. B., Hornik, C. P., Zimmerman, K. O., Hornik, C. D., Pradeep, S., Clark, R. H., Benjamin, D. K., Jr., Laughon, M., Greenberg, R. G. (2022). Medication use in the neonatal intensive care unit and changes from 2010 to 2018. *The Journal of Pediatrics, 240*, 66–71.e4. https://doi.org/10.1016/j.jpeds.2021.08.075.

FDA, U.S. Food and Drug Administration.

Source: [1]Taketomo, C. K. (Ed.). (2023). *Pediatric & neonatal dosage handbook: An extensive resource for clinicians treating pediatric and neonatal patients* (29th ed.). Lexicomp/Wolters Kluwer.

DRUG CLASS: Aminoglycoside Antibiotics

MEDICATION NAME	FDA APPROVED FOR USE IN NICU?	MECHANISM OF ACTION	HALF-LIFE (BIRTH–AGE 2)	COMMON INDICATIONS FOR USE IN THE NICU	CLINICAL MONITORING CONSIDERATIONS
Amikacin	Yes	Inhibits protein synthesis in aerobic gram-negative bacteria. The aminoglycoside reaches a bacterial ribosome by way of oxygen-dependent active transport. Next, the drug molecule binds irreversibly at the 30S subunit, explores the surface of the ribosome, and induces ribosomal dysfunction.	Neonates (day of life 1–3 with birth weight <2,500 g): 7–9 hours Term infants (>7 days of life): 4–5 hours	• Gram-negative sepsis (e.g., *Pseudomonas, Klebsiella sp., Enterobacter, Serratia, Proteus,* and *Escherichia coli*) • Synergy for gram-positive sepsis (e.g., *group B Streptococcus*)	• Newborn hearing screen test result (ototoxicity) • Renal function (nephrotoxicity) • Serum drug concentration monitoring may be indicated
Gentamicin	Yes	Inhibits protein synthesis in aerobic gram-negative bacteria. The aminoglycoside reaches a bacterial ribosome by way of oxygen-dependent active transport. Next, the drug molecule binds irreversibly at the 30S subunit, explores the surface of the ribosome, and induces ribosomal dysfunction.	Neonates (<1 week of life): 3–11.5 hours[1] Neonates (7–30 days of life): 3–6 hours[1] Infants: 4 ± 1 hour[1]	• Gram-negative sepsis (e.g., *Pseudomonas, Klebsiella sp., Enterobacter, Serratia, Proteus,* and *E. coli*) • Synergy for gram-positive sepsis (e.g., *group B Streptococcus*)	• Newborn hearing screen test result (ototoxicity) • Renal function (nephrotoxicity) • Serum concentrations
Tobramycin	Yes	Inhibits protein synthesis in aerobic gram-negative bacteria. The aminoglycoside reaches a bacterial ribosome by way of oxygen-dependent active transport. Next, the drug molecule binds irreversibly at the 30S subunit, explores the surface of the ribosome, and induces ribosomal dysfunction.	Neonates ≤1,200 g: 11 hours[1] Neonates >1,200 g; 2–9 hours[1] Infants: 4 ± 1 hour[1]	• Gram-negative sepsis (e.g., *Pseudomonas, Klebsiella sp., Enterobacter, Serratia, Proteus,* and *Escherichia coli*) • Synergy for gram-positive sepsis (e.g., *group B Streptococcus*)	• Newborn hearing screen test result (ototoxicity) • Renal function (nephrotoxicity) • Serum concentrations

Note: A typical bacterial cell is comprised of thousands of ribosomes. Numerous antibiotics, including aminoglycosides, bind to a portion of the ribosome and interfere with translation. This leads to faulty protein synthesis and over time, cell death.

Content included in this table is intended for educational purposes only. The status of the FDA approvals and PK data may change over time. Readers are encouraged to consult package inserts for the most current information. Medications selected are considered to be among the top 100 most commonly prescribed medications in the NICU, per Stark, A., Smith, P. B., Hornik, C. P., Zimmerman, K. O., Hornik, C. D., Pradeep, S., Clark, R. H., Benjamin, D. K., Jr., Laughon, M., Greenberg, R. G. (2022). Medication use in the neonatal intensive care unit and changes from 2010 to 2018. *The Journal of Pediatrics, 240,* 66–71.e4. https://doi.org/10.1016/j.jpeds.2021.08.075.

FDA, U.S. Food and Drug Administration.

Source: [1]Taketomo, C. K. (Ed.). (2023). *Pediatric & neonatal dosage handbook: An extensive resource for clinicians treating pediatric and neonatal patients* (29th ed.). Lexicomp/Wolters Kluwer.

DRUG CLASS: Penicillin Antibiotics

MEDICATION NAME	FDA APPROVED FOR USE IN NICU?	MECHANISM OF ACTION	HALF-LIFE (BIRTH–AGE 2)	COMMON INDICATIONS FOR USE IN THE NICU	CLINICAL MONITORING CONSIDERATIONS
Amoxicillin	Yes	Inhibits bacterial cell wall biosynthesis of susceptible gram-positive and gram-negative pathogens, which leads to bacterial cell death.[2]	Neonates: 5.2 ± 1.9 hours[1]	• Prophylaxis for urinary tract infections • Pyelectasis	• Hepatic function (with prolonged therapy) • Maculopapular rash (increased risk with concurrent congenital CMV infection) • Renal function
Ampicillin *Combination therapy with gentamicin accelerates killing of group B Streptococcus*	Yes	Inhibits bacterial cell wall biosynthesis of susceptible gram-positive and gram-negative pathogens, which leads to bacterial cell death.[3]	Neonates (0–7 days of life) 3–6 hours[4] Neonates (>7 days of life) and infants: 2–3.5 hours[4]	• Gram-positive sepsis (e.g., Group B *Streptococci, Listeria monocytogenes, Enterococcus)*	• Hematologic function • Hepatic function (elevated liver enzymes, with prolonged therapy) • Renal function • Serum electrolytes (hypokalemia)
Nafcillin	Yes	Inhibits bacterial cell wall biosynthesis of susceptible gram-positive pathogens, which leads to bacterial cell death.	Neonates (0–21 days of life): 2.2–5.5 hours[1] Infants (4–9 weeks): 1.2–2.3 hours[1] Infants (>1 month and children through age 2): 0.75–1.9 hours[1]	• Penicillinase-producing *Staphylococcus* (e.g., osteomyelitis, bacteremia, septicemia, meningitis)[1]	• Hematologic function (neutropenia) • Renal function • Hepatic function (total bilirubin) • Injection site reactions
Oxacillin	Yes	Inhibits bacterial cell wall biosynthesis of susceptible gram-positive pathogens, which leads to bacterial cell death.	Preterm infants: 3 hours[4] Neonates (day of life 8–15): 1.6 hours[1] Infants and children through age 2: 0.9–1.8 hours[1]	• Penicillinase-producing *Staphylococcus* (e.g., osteomyelitis, bacteremia, septicemia, meningitis)[1]	• Hematologic function (neutropenia) • Hepatic function (elevated liver enzymes) • Renal function • Urinalysis (hematuria)

(*continued*)

DRUG CLASS: Penicillin Antibiotics (*continued*)

MEDICATION NAME	FDA APPROVED FOR USE IN NICU?	MECHANISM OF ACTION	HALF-LIFE (BIRTH–AGE 2)	COMMON INDICATIONS FOR USE IN THE NICU	CLINICAL MONITORING CONSIDERATIONS
Penicillin G aqueous	Yes	Inhibits bacterial cell wall biosynthesis of penicillin-susceptible gram-positive pathogens, which leads to bacterial cell death.	Neonates (0–6 days of life): 3.1 hours[1] Neonates (≥14 days of life): 1.4 hours *Half-life decreases as renal clearance improves.*	• Bacteremia (e.g., group B *Streptococcus, Listeria monocytogenes)* • Congenital syphilis *(Treponema pallidum*)	• Renal function • Hepatic function (biliary function) • Serum electrolytes • Complete blood count (neutropenia)
Piperacillin-tazobactam	Neonates and infants <2 months of age: No Infants ≥2 months of age: for intra-abdominal infections and nosocomial pneumonia	Inhibits bacterial cell wall biosynthesis of susceptible gram-positive and gram-negative pathogens, which leads to bacterial cell death.	Premature neonates: 2.5–4.5 hours[1] Term neonates: 2–3.6 hours[1] Infants (<6 months): 1.4 hours[1] Infants (>6 months): 0.7–0.9 hours[1] *Septic shock and renal insufficiency prolong the half-life (up–14 hours)*.[4]	• Gram-negative sepsis or meningitis (e.g., *Escherichia coli, Klebsiella, Haemophilus influenza, Neisseria gonorrhoeae, N. meningitidis*) • Gram-positive sepsis (e.g., group B *Streptococci, Listeria monocytogenes, Enterococcus)* • Anaerobic infections (e.g., necrotizing enterocolitis)	• Hematologic function • Hepatic function (elevated liver enzymes, with prolonged therapy) • Renal function • Serum electrolytes (hypokalemia)

Note: Content included in this table is intended for educational purposes only. The status of the FDA approvals and PK data may change over time. Readers are encouraged to consult package inserts for the most current information. Medications selected are considered to be among the top 100 most commonly prescribed medications in the NICU, per Stark, A., Smith, P. B., Hornik, C. P., Zimmerman, K. O., Hornik, C. D., Pradeep, S., Clark, R. H., Benjamin, D. K., Jr., Laughon, M., Greenberg, R. G. (2022). Medication use in the neonatal intensive care unit and changes from 2010 to 2018. *The Journal of Pediatrics, 240*, 66–71.e4. https://doi.org/10.1016/j.jpeds.2021.08.075.

CMV, cytomegalovirus; FDA, U.S. Food and Drug Administration.

Sources: [1]Taketomo, C. K. (Ed.). (2023). *Pediatric & neonatal dosage handbook: An extensive resource for clinicians treating pediatric and neonatal patients* (29th ed.). Lexicomp/Wolters Kluwer; [2]Preferred Pharmaceuticals. (2022, March). *Amoxicillin, for suspension* (Package insert). https://dailymed.nlm.nih.gov/dailymed/lookup.cfm?setid=b23637eb-16ff-4e92-96e5-d6efd5cc4ee8; [3]G.C. Hanford Manufacturing Co. (2017, October). *Ampicillin for injection, USP* (Package insert). https://www.fda.gov/media/127633/download; [4]Wilson, C. B., Nizet, V., Maldonado, Y. A., Remington, J. S., & Klein, J. O. (Eds.). (2016). *Remington and Klein's infectious diseases of the fetus and newborn infant* (8th ed.). Elsevier/Saunders.

DRUG CLASS: Cephalosporins

MEDICATION NAME (GENERATION)	FDA APPROVED FOR USE IN NICU?	MECHANISM OF ACTION	HALF-LIFE (BIRTH–AGE 2)	COMMON INDICATIONS FOR USE IN THE NICU	CLINICAL MONITORING CONSIDERATIONS
Cefazolin (first)	Neonates: No Infants (≥1 month): Yes	Beta-lactam antibiotic that exhibits bactericidal activity by binding to penicillin-binding proteins on the membrane of the bacterial cell wall. PBPs are necessary to maintain cell wall integrity (rigidity). This weakens the bacterial cell wall, induces lysis, and inhibits further bacterial cell wall synthesis. **Effective against most gram-positive bacteria and some gram-negative bacteria (e.g., *Escherichia coli*).**	Neonates (day of life 0–7): 4.5–5 hours[3] Neonates (>3 weeks of age) and infants: 3 hours[3]	• Perioperative prophylaxis	• Bone marrow suppression • Hematologic function (eosinophilia) • Renal function • Hepatic function • Gastrointestinal abnormalities (diarrhea) • Seizure activity (indicates toxicity)
Cephalexin (first)	Neonates: No Infants (>1 year): Yes	Beta-lactam antibiotic that exhibits bactericidal activity by binding to penicillin-binding proteins on the membrane of the bacterial cell wall. PBPs are necessary to maintain cell wall integrity (rigidity). This weakens the bacterial cell wall, induces lysis, and inhibits further bacterial cell wall synthesis. **Effective against most gram-positive bacteria and some gram-negative bacteria (e.g., *E. coli*).**[2]	Neonates: 5 hours[1]	• Perioperative prophylaxis	• Bone marrow suppression • Hematologic function (eosinophilia) • Renal function • Hepatic function • Gastrointestinal abnormalities (diarrhea) • Seizure activity (indicates toxicity)

(*continued*)

DRUG CLASS: Cephalosporins *(continued)*

MEDICATION NAME (GENERATION)	FDA APPROVED FOR USE IN NICU?	MECHANISM OF ACTION	HALF-LIFE (BIRTH–AGE 2)	COMMON INDICATIONS FOR USE IN THE NICU	CLINICAL MONITORING CONSIDERATIONS
Ceftazidime (third)	Yes	Beta-lactam antibiotic that exhibits bactericidal activity by binding to penicillin-binding proteins on the membrane of the bacterial cell wall. PBPs are necessary to maintain cell wall integrity (rigidity). This weakens the bacterial cell wall, induces lysis, and inhibits further bacterial cell wall synthesis. **Variable efficacy against gram-positive bacteria with increased bactericidal activity against gram-negative bacteria compared to second-generation cephalosporins.**	<23 days: 2.2–4.7 hours[3]	• Bacteremia • Bacterial meningitis • Lower respiratory tract infections • *Pseudomonas aeruginosa* infection	• Bone marrow suppression • Hematologic function (eosinophilia) • Renal function • Hepatic function • Gastrointestinal abnormalities (diarrhea) • Signs of fungal infection (increased risk with preterm infants) • Seizure activity (indicates toxicity)
Cefotaxime (third)	Yes	Beta-lactam antibiotic that exhibits bactericidal activity by binding to penicillin-binding proteins on the membrane of the bacterial cell wall. PBPs are necessary to maintain cell wall integrity (rigidity). This weakens the bacterial cell wall, induces lysis, and inhibits further bacterial cell wall synthesis. **Variable efficacy against gram-positive bacteria with increased bactericidal activity against gram-negative bacteria compared to second-generation cephalosporins.**	Low-birth-weight neonates and infants (<1,500 grams): 4.6 hours[3] Neonates and infants >1,500 grams: 3.4 hours[3]	• Bacteremia • Bacterial meningitis • Lower respiratory tract infections	• Hematologic function (eosinophilia, leukopenia) • Renal function • Hepatic function • Gastrointestinal abnormalities including loose stool and colonization with resistant organisms (e.g., *Pseudomonas, Enterobacter, Enterococcus*) • Signs of fungal infection (increased risk with preterm infants)

Ceftriaxone (third)	Yes	Beta-lactam antibiotic that exhibits bactericidal activity by binding to penicillin-binding proteins on the membrane of the bacterial cell wall. PBPs are necessary to maintain cell wall integrity (rigidity). This weakens the bacterial cell wall, induces lysis, and inhibits further bacterial cell wall synthesis. **Variable efficacy against gram-positive bacteria with increased bactericidal activity against gram-negative bacteria compared to second-generation cephalosporins.**	Neonates (0–4 days): 16 hours[1] Neonates (9–30 days): 9 hours[1] Infants: 4–6.6 hours[1]	• Bacteremia • Bacterial meningitis • Lower respiratory tract infections	• Hematologic function (eosinophilia, leukopenia) • Renal function • Hepatic function • Gastrointestinal abnormalities including loose stool and colonization with resistant organisms (e.g., *Pseudomonas, Enterobacter, Enterococcus*) • Signs of fungal infection (increased risk with preterm infants)
Cefepime (fourth)	Neonates: No Infants (≥2 months): Yes	Beta-lactam antibiotic that exhibits bactericidal activity by binding to penicillin-binding proteins on the membrane of the bacterial cell wall. PBPs are necessary to maintain cell wall integrity (rigidity). This weakens the bacterial cell wall, induces lysis, and inhibits further bacterial cell wall synthesis. **Effective against gram-positive and gram-negative bacteria.**	Neonates (0–14 days of life): 4.5 hours[3] Neonates and infants (>14 days of life): 1.8 hours[3]	• Gram-negative sepsis and meningitis **NOTE:** Poor bactericidal activity against *P. aeruginosa*, enterococci, and *Listeria monocytogenes*[3]	• Bone marrow suppression • Hematologic function (eosinophilia) • Renal function • Hepatic function • Gastrointestinal abnormalities (diarrhea) • Signs of fungal infection (increased risk with preterm infants) • Seizure activity (indicates toxicity)

Note: Both first- and second-generation cephalosporins are most effective at lysing gram-positive bacteria. As the drug generation increases to the second and third generations, gram-positive bactericidal activity varies; bactericidal activity against gram-negative bacteria increases. Therefore, third-generation cephalosporins have a mixed capacity to treat both gram-positive and gram-negative bacteria (higher efficacy toward gram-negative species). Fourth-generation cephalosporins are active against gram-positive and gram-negative bacteria. Content included in this table is intended for educational purposes only. The status of the FDA approvals and PK data may change over time. Readers are encouraged to consult package inserts for the most current information. Medications selected are considered to be among the top 100 most commonly prescribed medications in the NICU, per Stark, A., Smith, P. B., Hornik, C. P., Zimmerman, K. O., Hornik, C. D., Pradeep, S., Clark, R. H., Benjamin, D. K., Jr., Laughon, M., Greenberg, R. G. (2022). Medication use in the neonatal intensive care unit and changes from 2010 to 2018. *The Journal of Pediatrics, 240*, 66–71.e4. https://doi.org/10.1016/j.jpeds.2021.08.075.

FDA, U.S. Food and Drug Administration; PBP, penicillin-binding protein.

Sources: [1]Taketomo, C. K. (Ed.). (2023). *Pediatric & neonatal dosage handbook: An extensive resource for clinicians treating pediatric and neonatal patients* (29th ed.). Lexicomp/Wolters Kluwer; [2]Pragma Pharmaceuticals. (2018, December). *Keflex®* (Package insert). https://www.accessdata.fda.gov/drugsatfda_docs/label/2018/050405s107lbl.pdf; [3]Wilson, C. B., Nizet, V., Maldonado, Y. A., Remington, J. S., & Klein, J. O. (Eds.). (2016). *Remington and Klein's infectious diseases of the fetus and newborn infant* (8th ed.). Elsevier/Saunders.

DRUG CLASS: Glycopeptide Antibiotic

MEDICATION NAME	FDA APPROVED FOR USE IN NICU?	MECHANISM OF ACTION	HALF-LIFE (BIRTH–AGE 2)	COMMON INDICATIONS FOR USE IN THE NICU	CLINICAL MONITORING CONSIDERATIONS
Vancomycin	Yes[1]	This glycopeptide antibiotic prevents the linking (polymerization) of peptidoglycans in the bacterial cell wall, which weakens the wall, permits leakage of cellular contents, and results in cell death. Bactericidal activity is only effective against gram-positive bacteria.	Neonates (day of life 0–7; <2 kg): 6.7 hours[2] Neonates (day of life 0–7; >2 kg): 5.9[2] Infants and children through age 2: 4 hours[2]	• Resistant gram-positive bacteria (e.g., methicillin-resistant *Staphylococcus aureus*, ampicillin-resistant *Enterococcus*, coagulase-negative *Staphylococcus*)	• Renal function • Trough level should be monitored. • Penetrates meninges only with concomitant inflammation; monitoring for therapeutic response is important

Note: Content included in this table is intended for educational purposes only. The status of the FDA approvals and PK data may change over time. Readers are encouraged to consult package inserts for the most current information. Medications selected are considered to be among the top 100 most commonly prescribed medications in the NICU, per Stark, A., Smith, P. B., Hornik, C. P., Zimmerman, K. O., Hornik, C. D., Pradeep, S., Clark, R. H., Benjamin, D. K., Jr., Laughon, M., Greenberg, R. G. (2022). Medication use in the neonatal intensive care unit and changes from 2010 to 2018. *The Journal of Pediatrics, 240*, 66–71.e4. https://doi.org/10.1016/j.jpeds.2021.08.075.

FDA, U.S. Food and Drug Administration.

Sources: [1]Taketomo, C. K. (Ed.). (2023). *Pediatric & neonatal dosage handbook: An extensive resource for clinicians treating pediatric and neonatal patients* (29th ed.). Lexicomp/Wolters Kluwer; [2]Wilson, C. B., Nizet, V., Maldonado, Y. A., Remington, J. S., & Klein, J. O. (Eds.). (2016). *Remington and Klein's infectious diseases of the fetus and newborn infant* (8th ed.). Elsevier/Saunders.

DRUG CLASS: Anaerobic Antibiotics

MEDICATION NAME	FDA APPROVED FOR USE IN NICU?	MECHANISM OF ACTION	HALF-LIFE (BIRTH–AGE 2)	COMMON INDICATIONS FOR USE IN THE NICU	CLINICAL MONITORING CONSIDERATIONS
Clindamycin	Yes[1]	Bacteriostatic antibiotic that inhibits bacterial protein synthesis by binding to 23S RNA of the 50S subunit of ribosomes.	Preterm infants: 8.7 hours[2] Term infants: 3.6 hours[2]	• Anaerobic infections (e.g., necrotizing enterocolitis) • Bacterial infections (e.g., *Staphylococcus, Streptococcus,* methicillin resistance)	• Hepatic function
Metronidazole	Yes	This nitromidazole antibiotic enters the bacterial cell by way of passive diffusion. Once in the cell, the drug molecule is chemically reduced, a process that produces toxic free radicals. The presence of these free radicals leads to apoptosis and cell death.	Neonates (<14 days of life): 24 hours[2] Neonates (>14 days of life) and infants: 15 hours[2]	• Anaerobic infections (e.g., necrotizing enterocolitis, meningitis, bacteremia) • Protozoal infections	• Renal function • Complete blood count with differential

Note: Content included in this table is intended for educational purposes only. The status of the FDA approvals and PK data may change over time. Readers are encouraged to consult package inserts for the most current information. Medications selected are considered to be among the top 100 most commonly prescribed medications in the NICU, per Stark, A., Smith, P. B., Hornik, C. P., Zimmerman, K. O., Hornik, C. D., Pradeep, S., Clark, R. H., Benjamin, D. K., Jr., Laughon, M., Greenberg, R. G. (2022). Medication use in the neonatal intensive care unit and changes from 2010 to 2018. *The Journal of Pediatrics, 240,* 66–71.e4. https://doi.org/10.1016/j.jpeds.2021.08.075.

FDA, U.S. Food and Drug Administration.

Sources: [1]Taketomo, C. K. (Ed.). (2023). *Pediatric & neonatal dosage handbook: An extensive resource for clinicians treating pediatric and neonatal patients* (29th ed.). Lexicomp/Wolters Kluwer; [2]Wilson, C. B., Nizet, V., Maldonado, Y. A., Remington, J. S., & Klein, J. O. (Eds.). (2016). *Remington and Klein's infectious diseases of the fetus and newborn infant* (8th ed.). Elsevier/Saunders.

DRUG CLASS: Macrolide Antibiotics

MEDICATION NAME	FDA APPROVED FOR USE IN NICU?	MECHANISM OF ACTION	HALF-LIFE (BIRTH–AGE 2)	COMMON INDICATIONS FOR USE IN THE NICU	CLINICAL MONITORING CONSIDERATIONS
Azithromycin	Neonates: No Infants (≥6 months): Yes	Binds irreversibly at the large 50S subunit, inhibiting translation (elongation) of the bacterial ribosome and inhibition of bacterial growth.	Neonates: 26–83 hours Infants(>4 months): 54.5 hours[1]	• Chlamydia conjunctivitis • Chlamydia pneumonia • Pertussis • Acute otitis media in infants with confirmed *Haemophilus influenzae, Streptococcus pneumoniae, or Moraxella catarrhalis*	• Hepatic function • Gastrointestinal function (nonbilious vomiting, irritability) **NOTE:** Treatment >42 days linked to increased risk for hypertrophic pyloric stenosis.
Erythromycin	Yes	Inhibits ribosomal function by binding to the bacterial ribosome Prokinetic/gastrointestinal motility agent	Neonates (≤15 days of life): 1.9–2.1 hours[1] Neonates (>15 days of life) and infants: 2.4 ± 0.3 hours[1]	• Pertussis in infants >1 month of life	• Hepatic function • Gastrointestinal function (increased risk for pyloric stenosis in newborns exposed to therapy) • Respiratory function (gasping syndrome observed in some infants subject to doses containing benzyl alcohol)

Note: Content included in this table is intended for educational purposes only. The status of the FDA approvals and PK data may change over time. Readers are encouraged to consult package inserts for the most current information. Medications selected are considered to be among the top 100 most commonly prescribed medications in the NICU, per Stark, A., Smith, P. B., Hornik, C. P., Zimmerman, K. O., Hornik, C. D., Pradeep, S., Clark, R. H., Benjamin, D. K., Jr., Laughon, M., Greenberg, R. G. (2022). Medication use in the neonatal intensive care unit and changes from 2010 to 2018. *The Journal of Pediatrics, 240*, 66–71.e4. https://doi.org/10.1016/j.jpeds.2021.08.075.
FDA, U.S. Food and Drug Administration.
Source: [1]Taketomo, C. K. (Ed.). (2023). *Pediatric & neonatal dosage handbook: An extensive resource for clinicians treating pediatric and neonatal patients* (29th ed.). Lexicomp/Wolters Kluwer.

DRUG CLASS: Carbapenem Antibiotics

MEDICATION NAME	FDA APPROVED FOR USE IN NICU?	MECHANISM OF ACTION	HALF-LIFE (BIRTH–AGE 2)	COMMON INDICATIONS FOR USE IN THE NICU	CLINICAL MONITORING CONSIDERATIONS
Meropenem	Yes	Inhibits bacterial peptidoglycan synthesis within the bacterial cell wall, which weakens the wall, permits leakage of cellular contents, and produces cell death.[2]	Neonates and infants ≤3 months of age: 2.7 hours[1] Infants and children 3 months–2 years of age: 1.5 hours[1]	• Gram-positive and gram-negative pathogens (aerobic and anaerobic) • Extended spectrum and chromosomal beta-lactamase producers (e.g., *Enterobacteriaceae, Pseudomonas*)	• Renal function • Hepatic function • Neurologic status

Note: Content included in this table is intended for educational purposes only. The status of the FDA approvals and PK data may change over time. Readers are encouraged to consult package inserts for the most current information. Medications selected are considered to be among the top 100 most commonly prescribed medications in the NICU, per Stark, A., Smith, P. B., Hornik, C. P., Zimmerman, K. O., Hornik, C. D., Pradeep, S., Clark, R. H., Benjamin, D. K., Jr., Laughon, M., Greenberg, R. G. (2022). Medication use in the neonatal intensive care unit and changes from 2010 to 2018. *The Journal of Pediatrics, 240,* 66–71.e4. https://doi.org/10.1016/j.jpeds.2021.08.075.

FDA, U.S. Food and Drug Administration.

Sources: [1]Taketomo, C. K. (Ed.). (2023). *Pediatric & neonatal dosage handbook: An extensive resource for clinicians treating pediatric and neonatal patients* (29th ed.). Lexicomp/Wolters Kluwer; [2]Wilson, C. B., Nizet, V., Maldonado, Y. A., Remington, J. S., & Klein, J. O. (Eds.). (2016). *Remington and Klein's infectious diseases of the fetus and newborn infant* (8th ed.). Elsevier/Saunders.

DRUG CLASS: Oxazolidinone Antibiotic

MEDICATION NAME	FDA APPROVED FOR USE IN NICU?	MECHANISM OF ACTION	HALF-LIFE (BIRTH–AGE 2)	COMMON INDICATIONS FOR USE IN THE NICU	CLINICAL MONITORING CONSIDERATIONS
Linezolid	Yes	Inhibits bacterial protein synthesis and multiplication by binding to the bacterial ribosome cell wall at the 50S subunit.	Neonates (day of life 0–7; <34 weeks' gestation): 5.6 hours[1,2] Infants (7–89 days of life; 25–40 weeks' gestation): 5.9 hours[2]	• Vancomycin-resistant *Enterococcus faecium* infections • Pneumonia secondary to MRSA *or Streptococcus pneumoniae*	• Renal function • Hepatic function • Complete blood count (thrombocytopenia, anemia)

Note: Content included in this table is intended for educational purposes only. The status of the FDA approvals and PK data may change over time. Readers are encouraged to consult package inserts for the most current information. Medications selected are considered to be among the top 100 most commonly prescribed medications in the NICU, per Stark, A., Smith, P. B., Hornik, C. P., Zimmerman, K. O., Hornik, C. D., Pradeep, S., Clark, R. H., Benjamin, D. K., Jr., Laughon, M., Greenberg, R. G. (2022). Medication use in the neonatal intensive care unit and changes from 2010 to 2018. *The Journal of Pediatrics, 240*, 66–71.e4. https://doi.org/10.1016/j.jpeds.2021.08.075.

FDA, U.S. Food and Drug Administration; MRSA, methicillin-resistant *Staphylococcus aureus*.

Sources: [1]Taketomo, C. K. (Ed.). (2023). *Pediatric & neonatal dosage handbook: An extensive resource for clinicians treating pediatric and neonatal patients* (29th ed.). Lexicomp/Wolters Kluwer; [2]Wilson, C. B., Nizet, V., Maldonado, Y. A., Remington, J. S., & Klein, J. O. (Eds.). (2016). *Remington and Klein's infectious diseases of the fetus and newborn infant* (8th ed.). Elsevier/Saunders.

DRUG CLASS: Systemic Antifungals

MEDICATION NAME	FDA APPROVED FOR USE IN NICU?	MECHANISM OF ACTION	HALF-LIFE (BIRTH–AGE 2)	COMMON INDICATIONS FOR USE IN THE NICU	CLINICAL MONITORING CONSIDERATIONS
Amphotericin B	Amphotericin B deoxycholate: No Liposomal amphotericin B: Yes (≥1 month of age)	Antifungal agent that selectively binds to ergosterol, a sterol located within the fungal cell membrane. The result is oxidative damage and the formation of ion channels, which increase membrane permeability. Leakage of cellular contents (protons and cations) occurs, which leads to cell death.	Preterm neonates and infants (after first dose): 24–48 hours[3] Preterm neonates and infants (subsequent dosing): 14.8 hours[3]	• Invasive candidiasis (e.g., *Candida albicans, C. parapsilosis, C. tropicalis*)	• Renal function • Serum electrolytes • Complete blood count with differential
Fluconazole	Yes	Antifungal agent that inhibits the synthesis of ergosterol, a sterol located in the fungal cell membrane, by inhibiting the normal activity of the cytochrome P450 enzyme 14-demethylase. (Normally, 14-demethylase facilitates the conversion of lanosterol to ergosterol.) This increases cell wall permeability and leakage of cellular contents, and leads to cell death.	Preterm neonates (26–29 weeks): 73.6–46.6 hours (decreasing with advancing postnatal age)[1]	• Invasive candidiasis (e.g., *C. albicans, C. parapsilosis, C. tropicalis*)	• Hepatic function • Renal function (creatinine >1.3 mg/dL yields >70% reduction in drug clearance)[2]

Note: Content included in this table is intended for educational purposes only. The status of the FDA approvals and PK data may change over time. Readers are encouraged to consult package inserts for the most current information. Medications selected are considered to be among the top 100 most commonly prescribed medications in the NICU, per Stark, A., Smith, P. B., Hornik, C. P., Zimmerman, K. O., Hornik, C. D., Pradeep, S., Clark, R. H., Benjamin, D. K., Jr., Laughon, M., Greenberg, R. G. (2022). Medication use in the neonatal intensive care unit and changes from 2010 to 2018. *The Journal of Pediatrics, 240,* 66–71.e4. https://doi.org/10.1016/j.jpeds.2021.08.075.

FDA, U.S. Food and Drug Administration

Sources: [1]Taketomo, C. K. (Ed.). (2023). *Pediatric & neonatal dosage handbook: An extensive resource for clinicians treating pediatric and neonatal patients* (29th ed.). Lexicomp/Wolters Kluwer; [2]Turner, K., Manzoni, P., Benjamin, D. K., Cohen-Wolkowiez, M., Smith, P. B., & Laughon, M. M. (2012). Fluconazole pharmacokinetics and safety in premature infants. *Current Medicinal Chemistry, 19*(27), 4617–4620. https://doi.org/10.2174/092986712803306367; [3]Testoni, D., Smith, P. B., & Benjamin, D. K., Jr. (2012). The use of antifungal therapy in neonatal intensive care. *Clinics in Perinatology, 39*(1), 83–98. https://doi.org/10.1016/j.clp.2011.12.008

DRUG CLASS: Oral and Topical Antifungals

MEDICATION NAME	FDA APPROVED FOR USE IN NICU?	MECHANISM OF ACTION	HALF-LIFE (BIRTH–AGE 2)	COMMON INDICATIONS FOR USE IN THE NICU	CLINICAL MONITORING CONSIDERATIONS
Nystatin (oral/paste)	Yes	Binds to ergosterol, a sterol that maintains fungal cell integrity, and increases fungal cell membrane permeability. This causes a leakage of intracellular components from the fungal cell, acidification, and cell death.	Not reported (poorly absorbed)	• Oral candidiasis • Diaper dermatitis	• Gastrointestinal function (consistency of stools; osmolarity of suspension exceeds 3,000 mOsm/L) • Therapeutic response (given poor oral absorption and negligible topical absorption through intact skin, clinicians usually maintain therapy for 48–72 hours after symptoms have resolved)
Clotrimazole	No	Inhibits ergosterol synthesis by interacting with CYP450 enzyme 14-alpha demethylase. This interaction restricts 14-alpha demethylase activity, which is necessary for the conversion of lanosterol to ergosterol, the sterol that maintains fungal cell wall integrity. In doing so, the fungal cell wall is weakened. This causes a leakage of intracellular components from the fungal cell, acidification, and cell death.	Not reported	• Diaper dermatitis	• Therapeutic response (given negligible topical absorption through intact skin, clinicians usually maintain therapy for 48–72 hours after symptoms have resolved)

Note: Content included in this table is intended for educational purposes only. The status of the FDA approvals and PK data may change over time. Readers are encouraged to consult package inserts for the most current information. Medications selected are considered to be among the top 100 most commonly prescribed medications in the NICU, per Stark, A., Smith, P. B., Hornik, C. P., Zimmerman, K. O., Hornik, C. D., Pradeep, S., Clark, R. H., Benjamin, D. K., Jr., Laughon, M., Greenberg, R. G. (2022). Medication use in the neonatal intensive care unit and changes from 2010 to 2018. *The Journal of Pediatrics, 240,* 66–71.e4. https://doi.org/10.1016/j.jpeds.2021.08.075.
FDA, U.S. Food and Drug Administration

DRUG CLASS: Immune Globulin

MEDICATION NAME	FDA APPROVED FOR USE IN NICU?	MECHANISM OF ACTION	HALF-LIFE (BIRTH–AGE 2)	COMMON INDICATIONS FOR USE IN THE NICU	CLINICAL MONITORING CONSIDERATIONS
IVIG	No	Immune replacement therapy. Among infants with HDN, IVIG blocks binding at Fc receptors, which protects antibody-coated red blood cells from phagocytosis by maternal IgG antibodies.[1]	Neonates/Infants: no data Adults: 14–40 days (variable)	• Immune thrombocytopenia • HDN, immune mediated	• Gastrointestinal function (increased risk for necrotizing enterocolitis) • IVIG volume overload (changes in respiratory rate, HR, blood pressure, skin coloration, abdominal distention) • Renal function

Note: Content included in this table is intended for educational purposes only. The status of the FDA approvals and PK data may change over time. Readers are encouraged to consult package inserts for the most current information. Medications selected are considered to be among the top 100 most commonly prescribed medications in the NICU, per Stark, A., Smith, P. B., Hornik, C. P., Zimmerman, K. O., Hornik, C. D., Pradeep, S., Clark, R. H., Benjamin, D. K., Jr., Laughon, M., Greenberg, R. G. (2022). Medication use in the neonatal intensive care unit and changes from 2010 to 2018. *The Journal of Pediatrics, 240,* 66–71.e4. https://doi.org/10.1016/j.jpeds.2021.08.075.

FDA, U.S. Food and Drug Administration; HDN, hemolytic disease of the newborn; HR, heart rate; IgG, immunoglobulin G; IVIG, intravenous immune globulin.

Source: [1]Pan, J., Zhan, C., Yuan, T., Chen, X., Ni, Y., Shen, Y., Chen, W., Wu, T., & Yu, H. (2021). Intravenous immunoglobulin G in the treatment of ABO hemolytic disease of the newborn during the early neonatal period at a tertiary academic hospital: A retrospective study. *Journal of Perinatology, 41*(6), 1397–1402. https://doi.org/10.1038/s41372-021-00963-5

DRUG CLASS: Monoclonal Antibody

MEDICATION NAME	FDA APPROVED FOR USE IN NICU?	MECHANISM OF ACTION	HALF-LIFE (BIRTH–AGE 2)	COMMON INDICATIONS FOR USE IN THE NICU	CLINICAL MONITORING CONSIDERATIONS
Palivizumab	Yes	Monoclonal antibody that exhibits anti-RSV activity by neutralizing RSV particles and inhibiting RSV replication[2]	Infants <24 months without preexisting CHD: 20–24.5 days[1]	• RSV prophylaxis	• Injection site (rash) • Temperature (fever)

Note: Content included in this table is intended for educational purposes only. The status of the FDA approvals and PK data may change over time. Readers are encouraged to consult package inserts for the most current information. Medications selected are considered to be among the top 100 most commonly prescribed medications in the NICU, per Stark, A., Smith, P. B., Hornik, C. P., Zimmerman, K. O., Hornik, C. D., Pradeep, S., Clark, R. H., Benjamin, D. K., Jr., Laughon, M., Greenberg, R. G. (2022). Medication use in the neonatal intensive care unit and changes from 2010 to 2018. *The Journal of Pediatrics, 240,* 66–71.e4. https://doi.org/10.1016/j.jpeds.2021.08.075.

CHD, congenital heart defect; FDA, U.S. Food and Drug Administration; RSV, respiratory syncytial virus.

Sources: [1]Taketomo, C. K. (Ed.). (2023). *Pediatric & neonatal dosage handbook: An extensive resource for clinicians treating pediatric and neonatal patients* (29th ed.). Lexicomp/Wolters Kluwer; [2]MedImmune. (2014, March). *Synagis: Highlights of prescribing information* (Package insert). https://www.accessdata.fda.gov/drugsatfda_docs/label/2014/103770s5185lbl.pdf

Index

Note: Page numbers in *italics* denote figures and tables.